CLINICAL MANUAL AND REVIEW OF TRANSESOPHAGEAL ECHOCARDIOGRAPHY

Second Edition

Edited by

Joseph P. Mathew, MD, MHSc.
Professor of Anesthesiology
Chief, Division of Cardiothoracic Anesthesiology
Duke University Medical Center
Durham, North Carolina

Madhav Swaminathan, MD, FASE, FAHA
Associate Professor of Anesthesiology
Director, Perioperative Echocardiography
Duke University Medical Center
Durham, North Carolina

Chakib M. Ayoub, MD
Associate Professor
Department of Anesthesiology
American University of Beirut Medical Center
Beirut, Lebanon
Clinical Assistant Professor
Department of Anesthesiology
Yale University School of Medicine
New Haven, Connecticut

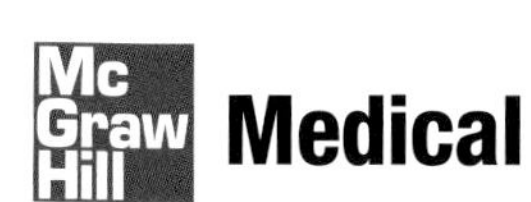

New York / Chicago / San Francisco / Lisbon / London / Madrid / Mexico City
Milan / New Delhi / San Juan / Seoul / Singapore / Sydney / Toronto

The McGraw-Hill Companies

Clinical Manual and Review of Transesophageal Echocardiography, Second Edition

3 4 5 6 7 8 9 0 CTPS/CTPS 14 13 12

Set ISBN 978-0-07163807-4; MHID 0-07-163807-5
Book ISBN 978-0-07-163476-2; MHID 0-07-163476-2
CD ISBN 978-0-07-163477-9; MHID 0-07-163477-0

Notice

Medicine is an ever-changing science. As new research and clinical experience broaden our knowledge, changes in treatment and drug therapy are required. The editors and the publisher of this work have checked with sources believed to be reliable in their efforts to provide information that is complete and generally in accord with the standards accepted at the time of publication. However, in view of the possibility of human error or changes in medical sciences, neither the editors nor the publisher nor any other party who has been involved in the preparation or publication of this work warrants that the information contained herein is in every respect accurate or complete, and they disclaim all responsibility for any errors or omissions or for the results obtained from use of the information contained in this work. Readers are encouraged to confirm the information contained herein with other sources. For example and in particular, readers are advised to check the product information sheet included in the package of each drug they plan to administer to be certain that the information contained in this work is accurate and that changes have not been made in the recommended dose or in the contraindications for administration. This recommendation is of particular importance in connection with new or infrequently used drugs.

This book was set in Adobe Garamond by Glyph International.
The editors were Brian Belval and Regina Y. Brown.
The production supervisor was Sherri Souffrance.
Project management was provided by Gita Raman, Glyph International.
The cover designer was Thomas DePierro.
China Translation & Printing Services, Ltd., was printer and binder.

Cataloging in Publication data is on file with the Library of Congress.

Contents

To my children, Jonathan, Eliza, and Susanna–dearly loved and precious gifts from God. May you always walk in truth and grace knowing that the One who calls you is faithful and He also will bring it to pass.

Joseph P. Mathew

To my wife, my closest friend, for her unconditional support.
To our children, for making it all worthwhile.
And to my mentors, for their remarkable vision.

Madhav Swaminathan

To all four that are the most precious to me:
My wife Aline
It is her unconditional, never-ending love and support which make all things possible;
My children
Maurice the intellectual, for his compassionate and ambitious nature,
Marc the charismatic, for his native wit, integrity, and determination,
Paul, the rising star …

Chakib M. Ayoub

Contributors

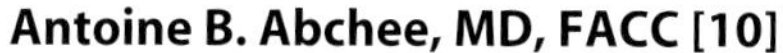
Antoine B. Abchee, MD, FACC [10]
Associate Professor of Clinical Medicine
Department of Internal Medicine
American University of Beirut
Beirut, Lebanon

David B. Adams, RCS, RDCS [2]
Cardiac Diagnostic Unit
Duke University Medical Center
Durham, North Carolina

Brian P. Barrick, MD [1]
Assistant Professor
Department of Anesthesiology
University of North Carolina
Chapel Hill, North Carolina

Shahar Bar-Yosef, MD [13, 25]
Assistant Professor
Anesthesiology and Critical Care Medicine
Duke University Medical Center
Durham, North Carolina

Angus Christie, MD [21]
Associate Residency Director
Department of Anesthesiology and Pain Management
Maine Medical Center
Portland, Maine

Jose Coddens, MD [16, 19]
Staff Anesthesiologist
Anesthesia and Intensive Care Medicine
Onze Lieve Vrouw Clinic
Aalst, Belgium

Issam El-Rassi, MD [8]
Senior Lecturer
Cardiac Surgery
Hotel-Dieu de France Hospital
Beirut, Lebanon

Stephanie S.F. Fischer, MD [18]
Cardiothoracic Anesthesiologist
Private Practice
Sea Point, South Africa

Manuel L. Fontes, MD [15]
Associate Professor of Anesthesiology and Critical Care
Department of Anesthesiology
Weill Cornell Medical College
New York, New York

Laura Ford-Mukkamala, DO, FACC [6]
Clinical Cardiologist
Southeastern Cardiology Associates
Columbus, Georgia

Emily Forsberg, RDCS, PA-C [2]
Park Nicollet Heart and Vascular Center
St. Louis Park, Minnesota

Linda D. Gillam, MD, MPH [6]
Professor of Clinical Medicine
Department of Medicine
Columbia University
New York, New York

Kathryn E. Glas, MD, MBA, FASE [20]
Associate Professor
Department of Anesthesiology
Emory University
Atlanta, Georgia

Katherine Grichnik, MD, FASE [3, 27]
Professor
Department of Anesthesiology
Duke University Medical Center
Durham, North Carolina

Hillary B. Hrabak, BS, RDCS [2]
Cardiac Sonographer
Cardiac Diagnostic Unit
Duke University Medical Center
Durham, North Carolina

Christopher C. C. Hudson, MD, FRCPC [16]
Assistant Professor
Department of Anesthesiology
University of Ottawa
Ottawa, Ontario, Canada

Jordan K. C. Hudson, MD, FRCPC [22]
Assistant Professor
Department of Anesthesiology
University of Ottawa
Ottawa, Ontario, Canada

Victor Jebara, MD [8]
Professor and Chief
Thoracic and Cardiovascular Surgery
Hotel-Dieu de France Hospital
Beirut, Lebanon

Bettina Jungwirth, MD [24]
Assistant Professor
Department of Anesthesiology
Klinik fuer Anaesthesiologie
Muenchen, Germany

Blaine A. Kent, MD, FRCPC [11]
Chief, Division of Cardiac Anesthesia
Department of Anesthesiology
Capital District Health Authority / Dalhousie University
Halifax, Nova Scotia
Canada

Ryan E. Lauer, MD [5]
Assistant Professor
Department of Anesthesiology
Loma Linda University
Loma Linda, California

Frederick W. Lombard, MD [21]
Assistant Professor
Department of Anesthesiology
Duke University Medical Center
Durham, North Carolina

G. Burkhard Mackensen, MD, PhD [24]
Associate Professor
Department of Anesthesiology
Duke University Medical Center
Durham, North Carolina

Aman Mahajan, MD, PhD [24]
Professor and Chief
Cardiothoracic Anesthesiology
Ronald Reagan UCLA Medical Center
Los Angeles, California

Feroze Mahmood, MD [4]
Assistant Professor
Anesthesia and Critical Care
Beth Israel Deaconess Medical Center
Harvard Medical School
Boston, Massachusetts

Carlo E. Marcucci, MD [24]
Director of Cardiothoracic Anesthesiology
Department of Anesthesiology
University Hospital Lausanne (CHUV)
Lausanne, Vaud
Switzerland

Jonathan B. Mark, MD [13, 25]
Professor
Department of Anesthesiology
Veterans Affairs Medical Center
Durham, North Carolina

Susan M. Martinelli, MD [17]
Assistant Professor
Department of Anesthesiology
University of North Carolina
Chapel Hill, North Carolina

Andrew Maslow, MD [14]
Clinical Associate Professor
Department of Anesthesiology
Brown University Medical Center
Providence, Rhode Island

Robina Matyal, MD [4]
Instructor in Anesthesia
Anesthesia and Critical Care
Beth Israel Deaconess Medical Center
Harvard Medical School
Boston, Massachusetts

Carmelo A. Milano, MD [17]
Associate Professor
Department of Surgery
Duke University Medical Center
Durham, North Carolina

George V. Moukarbel, MD, FASE [10]
Advanced Echocardiography Fellow
Cardiovascular Diseases
Brigham and Women's Hospital
Harvard Medical School
Boston, Massachusetts

Alina Nicoara, MD [12]
Assistant Professor
Department of Anesthesiology
Duke University Medical Center
Durham, North Carolina

Wendy L. Pabich [3]
Assistant Professor
Department of Anesthesiology
Duke University Medical Center
Durham, North Carolina

Mathew V. Patteril, MD [18]
Consultant Anaesthetist and Deputy Clinical Director
Department of Anaesthesia and Pain Management
University Hospitals of Coventry and Warwickshire
Coventry, United Kingdom

Mihai V. Podgoreanu, MD, FASE [1]
Assistant Professor
Department of Anesthesiology
Duke University Medical Center
Durham, North Carolina

Wanda M. Popescu, MD [12]
Assistant Professor
Department of Anesthesiology
Yale University School of Medicine
New Haven, Connecticut

Edward K. Prokop, MD [1]
Director, Cardiac Diagnostic Unit
Department of Radiology
Hospital of St. Raphael
New Haven, Connecticut

Joseph G. Rogers, MD [17]
Associate Professor
Department of Medicine
Duke University Medical Center
Durham, North Carolina

Rebecca A. Schroeder, MD [13, 25]
Associate Professor
Department of Anesthesiology
Duke University Medical Center
Durham, North Carolina

Svati H. Shah, MD, MHS, FACC [23]
Assistant Professor
Department of Medicine
Duke University Medical Center
Durham, North Carolina

Jack S. Shanewise, MD, FASE [26]
Professor of Clinical Anesthesiology
Department of Anesthesiology
Columbia University Medical Center
New York, New York

Andrew Shaw, MB, FRCA, FCCM [22]
Associate Professor
Department of Anesthesiology
Duke University Medical Center
Durham, North Carolina

Stanton K. Shernan, MD, FAHA, FASE [14, 20]
Associate Professor
Anesthesiology, Perioperative and Pain Medicine
Brigham and Women's Hospital
Harvard Medical School
Boston, Massachusetts

Nikolaos I. Skubas, MD, FASE, DSc [15]
Associate Professor
Department of Anesthesiology
Weill Cornell Medical College
New York, New York

Ghassan Sleilaty, MD [8]
Fellow
Division of Cardiovascular and Thoracic Surgery
Hotel-Dieu de France Hospital
Beirut, Lebanon

Justiaan Swanevelder MB, ChB, MMed, FCA(SA), FRCA [7]
Consultant Anaesthetist
University Hospitals of Leicester NHS Trust
Glenfield Hospital
Leicester, United Kingdom

Mark A. Taylor, MD, FASE [9]
Assistant Professor
Department of Anesthesiology
The Western Pennsylvania Hospital-Forbes Regional Campus
Monroeville, Pennsylvania

Christopher A. Troianos, MD [9]
Professor and Chair
Department of Anesthesiology
Western Pennsylvania Hospital
Pittsburgh, Pennsylvania

Johannes van der Westhuizen, MBChB, MMed (Anes) [7]
Consultant Anesthesiologist
Anesthesiology
Haumann and Partners
Bloemfontein, South Africa

Matthew Wood, MD [27]
Staff Anesthesiologist
West End Anesthesia Group
Bon Secours St. Mary's Hospital
Richmond, Virginia

Foreword

Echocardiography, termed one of cardiology's ten greatest discoveries of the twentieth century, has been singled out as the most important noninvasive application for cardiac diagnosis since the invention of the electrocardiogram.[1] As with any seminal contribution, the story of the echocardiogram is composed of many scenes.[2] The story begins in the 18th century with Lazzaro Spallanzani's observation that bats navigate by use of inaudible echoes. The saga continues with Pierre and Marie Curie whose important work on piezoelectricity led to the ability to create ultrasonic waves. World War II brought the application of SONAR (Sound Navigation and Ranging system) to maturity. Gradually, scientists initiated investigations to determine if ultrasound could be applied to medical diagnosis. Despite the failure of many researchers to discover a suitable method for use of ultrasound in the medical arena, cardiologist Dr. Inge Edler and his co-investigator, physicist Dr. Carl Hertz, were able to see the promise of this imaging tool and make it practical for clinical care. It is noteworthy that the unit of frequency, the hertz (Hz) was named after his uncle, Heinrich Hertz. Parenthetically, Carl Hertz also invented the inkjet printer! On October 29, 1953, Edler and Hertz recorded the first real-time echocardiographic images of the heart. Since that discovery, the application of echocardiography has gone in a number of different directions to enhance (1) its utility in a variety of different clinical settings, (2) image acquisition, and (3) augmentation of data retrieval for a given examination.

Transesophageal echocardiography (TEE) is a core component of perioperative cardiovascular monitoring and diagnosis. Just as electrocardiography and arterial and cardiac catheterization originated in cardiac operating rooms, TEE has followed a similar path and is now employed in a large number of noncardiac surgeries and intensive care units. Similar to Edler and Hertz's pioneering the clinical application of ultrasound, the contemporary anesthesiologist must adapt new technologies to sophisticated surgical procedures. It is said that the major achievements of modern surgery would not have taken place without the accompanying vision of pioneers in anesthesiology. The adaptation of echocardiography to the monitoring of anesthetized patients is just *the* case in point.

With this rich tradition as a background, Drs. Joseph Mathew, Madhav Swamninathan, and Chakib Ayoub, internationally respected echocardiographers and educators, have significantly revised their popular textbook *Clinical Manual and Review of Transesophageal Echocardiography* in a second edition. This represents a herculean editorial challenge as to the educational framework required by the various audiences who use this book to guide clinical care as well as study for Board examinations: resident, fellow, and attending physician. The challenge is to make this text useful to the novice and serve as a resource for the experienced clinician. With so many "echo textbooks" available, why choose this one? First the editors' aggregate experience in the use of echocardiography represents more than 50 years of teaching and clinical care. Consequently, they understand the didactic and clinical pitfalls in image acquisition, interpretation, and clinical application. Their lavish use of graphics, both echocardiograms and associated drawings, are striking in their clarity and the simplicity of the message for each figure. As improvements in the field have occurred, they are also mirrored in this edition. Chief among these is the novel use of three-dimensional imaging, particularly as it applies to valvular heart surgery. As TEE moves beyond cardiac surgery, new training paradigms are required, and the text meets these needs in three chapters devoted to noncardiac surgical settings. Finally, for those studying for Board certification or re-certification, two chapters, nearly 1000 review questions, and a practice TEE examination are devoted to this important educational component.

In conclusion, Clinical Manual and Review of Transesophageal Echocardiography (Second Edition) represents a narrative and graphic standard that will enhance the knowledge of the reader and facilitate application of exemplary clinical care to high-risk patients in the perioperative period.

REFERENCES

1. Mehta NJ, Khan IA. Cardiology's 10 greatest discoveries of the 20th century. *Texas Heart Inst J.* 2002;29:164-171.
2. Singh S, Goyal A. The origin of echocardiography. *Texas Heart Inst J.* 2007;34:431-438.

Paul Barash, MD

Professor of Anesthesiology
Yale University School of Medicine
New Haven, Connecticut

Preface

Since the publication of the first edition of the *Clinical Manual and Review of Transesophageal Echocardiography* in 2005, the field has continued to grow at a rapid pace. In order to maintain its place as a standard reference manual, this edition has been completely reorganized and expanded to offer concise yet comprehensive coverage of the key principles, concepts, and developing practices of transesophageal echocardiography (TEE). This second edition was written with pride and gratitude by numerous contributing authors and is offered to anesthesiologists, cardiologists, cardiothoracic surgeons, emergency room physicians, intensivists, and sonographers. Each chapter has been thoroughly revised and updated to provide a summary of the physiology, pathophysiology, tomographic views, and the required two-dimensional, M-mode, color-flow, and Doppler echocardiography data for both normal and common disease states. New chapters on ultrasound artifacts, quantitative echocardiography, tricuspid and pulmonic valves, right heart function, heart failure surgery, epicardial and epiaortic ultrasonography, TEE in nonoperative settings, three-dimensional echocardiography, and the board certification process have also been added. Whenever possible, important clinical information has been integrated with the principles of cardiovascular physiology. In addition, narrative and bulleted text, charts, and graphs were effectively blended in order to speed access to key clinical information for the purpose of improving clinical management. Finally, an increased number of chapter-ending standardized review questions along with a new companion CD, which includes a practice test, offer readers an opportunity to test their knowledge and to prepare for the certification exams.

In this edition we welcome our new co-editor, Dr. Madhav Swaminathan, and several new authors. We gratefully acknowledge the contributions of all our authors, who are prominent experts in their fields, and we are thankful for their hard work, dedication, and selfless commitment to this second edition. It is their excellence, attention to detail, passion for echocardiography, and vast knowledge that allowed this project to proceed smoothly. We are also thankful to the many readers of the first edition who offered words of encouragement and even advice on how the book could be improved—many of those suggestions have been incorporated into this edition. Despite the changes, however, we hope that we have retained the elements that made the first edition so useful to the novice echocardiographer. Finally, we once again recognize and are indebted to those who instilled in us the passion for echocardiography and for discovery: Drs. Paul Barash, Fiona Clements, Ed Prokop, and Terry Rafferty, as well as Elizabeth Davis, LPN, RDCS.

Our sincere appreciation also goes to our assistants, Melinda Macalino, Jaime Cooke, and Rabih Mukalled, for their dedication, enthusiasm, and patience. In addition, we would like to thank Marsha Gelber, Regina Brown, Brian Belval, and the staff at McGraw-Hill for their continued support with this project.

Joseph P. Mathew

Madhav Swaminathan

Chakib M. Ayoub

Physics of Ultrasound Imaging

1

Brian P. Barrick, Mihai V. Podgoreanu, and Edward K. Prokop

BASICS OF ULTRASOUND[1-3]

Nature and Properties of Ultrasound Waves

Humans can hear sound waves with frequencies between 20 Hz and 20 KHz. Frequencies higher than this range are termed as ultrasound. A *sound* wave can be described as a mechanical, longitudinal wave comprised of cyclic compressions and rarefactions of molecules in a medium. This is in contrast to electromagnetic waves, which do not require a medium for propagation. The amplitude of these cyclic changes can be measured in any of three **acoustic variables**.

- **Pressure:** Routinely measured in pascals
- **Density:** Units of mass per unit volume (eg, kg/cm^3)
- **Distance:** Units of length (eg, millimeters, centimeters)

Three parameters can be used to describe the absolute and relative strength ("loudness") of a sound wave.

- **Amplitude:** The amount of change in one of the above acoustic variables. Amplitude is equal to the difference between average and the maximum (or minimum) values of an acoustic variable (or half the "peak-to-peak" amplitude).
- **Power:** The rate of energy transfer, expressed in watts (joules/second). Power is proportional to the *square* of the amplitude.
- **Intensity:** The energy per unit cross-sectional area in a sound beam, expressed in watts per square centimeter (W/cm^2). This is the parameter used most frequently when describing the biological safety of ultrasound (US).

The operator can modify all of the above parameters. Note that this is *not* the same as adjusting receiver gain, which is a postprocessing function.

Changes (usually in intensity) can also be expressed in a *relative, logarithmic* scale known as **decibels (dB)**. In common practice, the lowest-intensity audible sound (10^{-12} W/cm^2) is assigned the value of 0 dB. An increase of 3 dB represents a two-fold increase in intensity while an increase of 10 dB represents a ten-fold increase in intensity. This means that a sound with an intensity of 120 dB is one trillion times as intense as a sound of 0 dB.

Four additional parameters that are inherent to the sound generator (transducer) and/or the medium through which the sound propagates are also used. When referring to a single transducer (piezoelectric) element in a pulsed ultrasound system, these parameters *cannot* be manipulated by the operator.

- **Period:** The duration of a single cycle. Typical values for clinical ultrasound are 0.1 to 0.5 microseconds (μs).
- **Frequency (f):** The number of cycles per unit time. One cycle per second is 1 hertz (Hz). Ultrasound (US) is defined as a sound wave with a frequency greater than 20,000 Hz. Values that are relevant in clinical imaging modalities such as echocardiography and vascular ultrasound range from 2 to 15 megahertz (MHz).

Period and frequency are *reciprocals*. Period = $1/f$.

- **Wavelength (λ):** The distance traveled by sound in 1 cycle (0.1 to 0.8 mm)

Wavelength and frequency are *inversely proportional*, and are related by propagation speed through the formula $\lambda = c/f$.

- **Propagation speed (c):** The speed of sound in a medium, determined by characteristics of the medium through which it propagates. Propagation speed does *not* depend on the amplitude or frequency of the sound wave. It is directly proportional to the stiffness and inversely proportional to the density of the medium.

Sound propagates at 1540 m/s for average human soft tissue, including heart muscle, blood, and valve tissue. Other useful values are 330 m/s for air and 4080 m/s for skull bone. Because the propagation speed in the heart is constant at 1540 m/s, the wavelength of any transducer frequency can be calculated as:

$$\lambda\ (\text{mm}) = 1.54/f\ (\text{MHz})$$

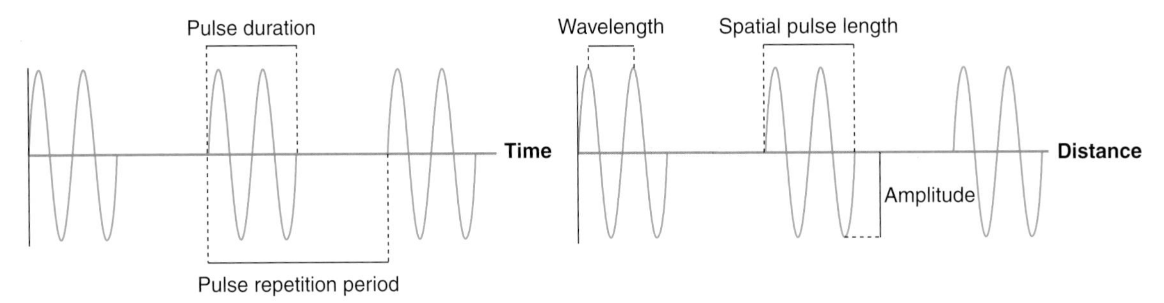

FIGURE 1–1. Physical parameters describing continuous and pulsed ultrasound waves.

Properties of Pulsed Ultrasound

Continuous waves are not useful for structural imaging. Instead, US systems use brief pulses of acoustic signal. These are emitted from the transducer during the "on" time and received during the "off" time. One pulse typically consists of 3 to 5 cycles.

Pulsed US can be described by 5 parameters (Figure 1–1):

- **Pulse duration:** The time a pulse is "on", which is *very short* (0.5 to 3 μs).
- **Pulse repetition period:** The time from the *start* of a pulse to the *start* of the next pulse, and *includes the listening time.* Typical values are 0.1 to 1 ms.
- **Spatial pulse length:** The distance from the start to the end of a pulse (0.1 to 1 mm).
- **Duty factor:** The percentage of time the transducer is actively transmitting US, usually 0.1% to 1%.

This means that the transducer element acts as a receiver over 99% of the time.

- **Pulse repetition frequency (PRF):** The number of pulses that occur in 1 second, expressed in hertz (Hz). PRF is reciprocal to pulse repetition period. Typical values are 1000 to 10,000 Hz (not to be confused with the frequency of the US within a pulse, which is many times greater).

PRF is inversely proportional to imaging depth. Because sound takes time to propagate, a deeper image requires more listening time. Therefore, with a deeper image, the transducer can emit fewer pulses per second. This concept will also be important for the discussion of Doppler ultrasound.

The relation between the depth of a reflector and the time it takes for a US pulse to travel from the transducer to the reflector and back to the transducer (time-of-flight) is called the *range equation*:

$$\text{Distance to Reflector (mm)} = \text{Propagation Speed (mm/}\mu\text{s)} \times \text{Time-of-Flight (}\mu\text{s)}/2$$

This allows the US systems to calculate the distance to a certain structure by measuring only the time-of-flight. Assuming that soft tissue has a uniform propagation speed of 1540 m/s, or 1.54 mm/μs, *time-of-flight increases by 13 μs means for every 1 cm of depth of the reflector.* This value is important for imaging and for Doppler US.

Propagation of Ultrasound Through Tissues

The most important effect of a medium on the US wave is *attenuation*, the gradual decrease in intensity (measured in dB) of a US wave. Attenuation results from three processes.

- **Absorption:** Conversion of sound energy to heat energy.
- **Scattering:** Diffuse spread of sound from a border with small irregularities.
- **Reflection:** Return of sound to the transducer from a relatively smooth border between two media. *It is reflection that is important for imaging.*

Different tissues attenuate by different processes and at different rates.

- Air bubbles reflect much of the US that engages them, and appear very echo dense (bright). Since sound attenuates the most in air, information distal to an air bubble is often lost as a result.
- Lung, being mostly air filled, causes much scatter and results in the most attenuation of US by tissue.
- Bone absorbs and reflects US, resulting in somewhat less attenuation than lung.
- Soft tissue and blood attenuate even less than bone.
- Water attenuates sound very little, mostly by absorption with very little reflection. It is therefore very echo lucent (appears black on image).

Within soft tissue, attenuation is proportional to both the US frequency and path length, and can be expressed by the following equation:

$$\text{Attenuation (in dB)} = 0.5\ \text{dB/(cm} \bullet \text{MHz)} \times \text{Path Length (in cm)} \times \text{Frequency (in MHz)}$$

Therefore, one may conclude that, high-frequency US has greater attenuation and poor penetration, and is less effective at imaging deeper structures.

Less than 1% of the incident US is usually reflected at the boundary between different soft tissues. The interfaces between air and tissue, and between bone and tissue are strong reflectors and can result in several types of artifacts (see Chapter 3).

As the US beam strikes a boundary between two media, three phenomena may occur:

- Reflection can be further broken down into *specular reflection* and *diffuse reflection* or *backscatter*.
- Transmission.
- Refraction.

Reflection of the transmitted US signal from internal structures is the basis of US imaging. It can occur only if there is a difference in the *acoustic impedance* (*measured in MRayls*) between the 2 media, and is dependent on the angle of incidence of the US beam at the interface. Acoustic impedance is a property of the media, *not* of the US beam. It is directly proportional to both density and propagation speed of the material.

Specular reflectors have large, smooth surfaces, or have irregularities that are larger than the wavelength of the US beam. They are angle dependent, reflecting US best at normal incidence (90°, or perpendicular to the boundary).

Scatter reflectors (the "signal" used in US imaging) have irregularities that are about the same size or smaller than the wavelength of US that strikes the boundary. Scatter reflectors are also not angle dependent. A special type of scattering is termed *Rayleigh scattering*, and this occurs when US strikes an object much smaller than the beam's wavelength (such as a red blood cell). Sound is scattered uniformly in all directions.

Refraction is a process associated with transmission and refers to the change of wave direction upon crossing the interface between two media. Refraction can occur only when the propagation speeds in the 2 media are different and the incident angle is oblique (Figure 1–2). Refraction is described by *Snell's law*:

Sine (Refracted Angle)/Sine (Incident Angle) = Speed of Sound in Medium 2/Speed of Sound in Medium 1

Thus, if the speed of sound in medium 2 is *less* than the speed of sound in medium 1, then the transmission (refracted) angle is *less* than the incident angle. Similarly, if the speed of sound in medium 2 is *greater* than the speed of sound in medium 1, then the transmission angle is *greater* than the incident angle.

Because it violates the assumption that US travels in a straight line, refraction may result in image artifacts (eg, second copy of a true reflector).

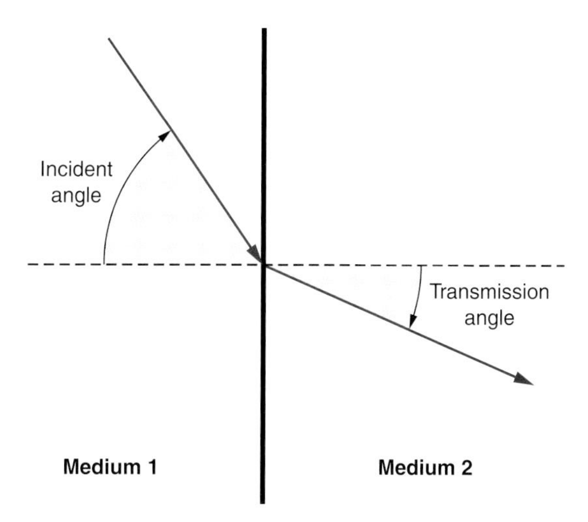

FIGURE 1–2. An illustration demonstrating refraction. In this example, the propagation speed of medium 1 is greater than medium 2, resulting in a lower transmission angle.

ULTRASOUND TRANSDUCERS

Simply put, an ultrasound transducer is a device that converts electrical energy into high-frequency acoustic energy, and vice versa. US transducers contain crystals that change shape when an electrical potential is applied (*reverse piezoelectric effect*), as during sound transmission, and also create voltage when mechanically deformed (*piezoelectric effect*), as during sound reception. The most common crystals in US systems are composed of lead, zirconate, and titanate (PZT). The frequency of the US generated by each piezoelectric element is related to the thickness and the propagation speed of the crystal by the formula:

Frequency (MHz) = the *Material's* Propagation Speed (mm/μs)/Twice the Thickness (mm)

In addition to the crystal, there is a backing material that is designed to limit the ringing of the crystal. This leads to a shorter pulse length, and improves resolution of the picture. The backing layer also increases the range of frequencies (or bandwidth) around the resonant frequency of the crystal. A wide bandwidth in an imaging transducer is useful because it gives the operator a limited ability to adjust the frequency of the US beam, optimizing imaging. Frequencies used in transesophageal echocardiography (TEE) typically range from 2.0 to 7.0 MHz.

There is also a matching layer in front of the crystal. This layer is designed to have an acoustic impedance

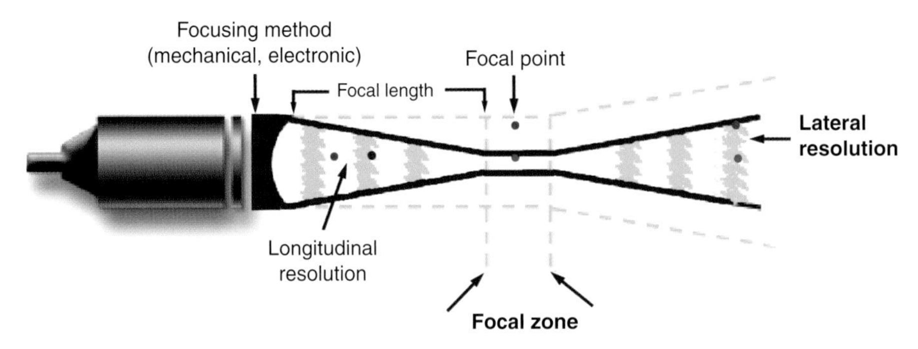

FIGURE 1–3. Anatomy of an ultrasound beam.

between that of the transducer material and the soft tissue it contacts, increasing transmission of US. The ideal matching layer has a thickness of one-quarter of the wavelength.

The sound beam produced by a single crystal whose thickness is one-half the wavelength of emitted sound spreads in a hemispherical pattern. The beam emitted by a US transducer composed of several crystals, however, has a characteristic hourglass shape due to constructive and destructive interference of the wavelets from each crystal. This is referred to as *Huygens principle*. The *focal point* or *focus* is the location where the beam reaches its minimum diameter and maximal intensity (Figure 1–3). Here the beam is about half the width of the transducer. The near area, or area between the transducer and focus, is also called the Fresnel zone. The far area after the focus is called the Fraunhofer zone.

The simplest transducer can be comprised of a single piezoelectric crystal that produces a two-dimensional (2D) image via *mechanical scanning*. More commonly, multiple elements are arranged in arrays. In *linear switched arrays*, the simplest type of array, the elements are arranged in a line and fire simultaneously. In *phased arrays* (linear, annular, or convex), the elements fire with very small time delays, in the order of 10 nanoseconds. Phased arrays allow for electronic focusing and steering of the US beam.

If all of the elements fired simultaneously, as in a linear switched array, the image would be rectangular and the focus would be fixed. Changing the pattern of time delays in element firing, as in phased arrays, allows for steering of the beam, resulting in a wider scan area (sector shaped). It also allows for adjustment of the focal point.

Modern US systems (including TEE) are equipped with phased arrays that are located at the tip of the TEE probe. Biplane probes had two orthogonal arrays, and only allowed imaging at 0° and 90°. However, the 2D multiplane probes in common use now have a single array that can be electronically rotated by adjusting a switch located in the handle of the TEE probe.

Major advances have allowed three-dimensional (3D) TEE to become a reality in the operating room. Older systems utilized 256 elements, arranged in different planes to generate a 3D data set (but could not produce a real-time image). Matrix array transducers, first used in transthoracic echocardiography (TTE), are essentially phased arrays that utilize over 3000 fully sampled elements, yielding a pyramidal 3D dataset in real time (Table 1–1). The only currently available real-time 3D TEE transducer utilizes 2400 elements and piezoelectric crystals that are purer and more uniform to allow multiplane 2D and Doppler imaging, simultaneous display of 2 orthogonal planes, and real-time 3D imaging.[4]

INSTRUMENTATION

Components of an Ultrasound System

Any US system has six components:

Transducer: Converts electrical energy into acoustic energy and vice versa.

Pulser: Controls the electrical signals sent to the transducer. Controls PRF, pulse amplitude, and pulse repetition period. It is also responsible for electronic steering and focusing in phased arrays.

Receiver: Processes returning signals to produce an image on a display. Processing occurs in the following order:

1. *Amplification*: Overall gain, 50 to 100 dB.
2. *Compensation*: More specifically, time gain compensation. Adjusts for increased attenuation with depth.
3. *Compression*: Reduces the dynamic range of the signals to match the dynamic range of the system's electrical components. Does *not* change the relative value of the returning signals.
4. *Demodulation*: Makes the image more suitable for viewing.

Table 1–1. Summary of Transducer Properties.

Transducer Type	Image Shape	Steering Technique	Focusing Technique	Crystal Defect
Mechanical	Sector	Mechanical	Fixed	Image loss
Linear switched array	Rectangular	None	Fixed	Vertical line dropout
Linear phased array	Sector	Electronic	Electronic	Poor steering and focusing
Annular phased array	Sector	Mechanical	Electronic	Horizontal line dropout
Convex sequential array	Blunted sector	None	Fixed	Vertical line dropout
Convex phased array	Blunted sector	Electronic	Electronic	Poor steering and focusing
Vector array	Flat top sector	Electronic	Electronic	Poor steering and focusing
Matrix array	Sector	Electronic	Electronic	Poor steering and focusing

Reproduced with permission from Edelman SK. *Understanding Ultrasound Physics*. 3rd edition. Woodlands, TX: Education for the Sonographic Professional, Inc; 2004.

a. Rectification converts all returning signals to positive amplitude.
b. Smoothing converts signal bursts into a single deflection for each reflector.

5. *Rejection*: Elimination of low level signals.

Display: Consists of a cathode ray tube or computer monitor screen.

Storage media: Archiving of data (video tape, optical disk, DVD).

Master synchronizer: Integrates all the individual components of the system.

Ultrasound Imaging

The modes of displaying returning echoes are as follows:

A (amplitude) mode: No longer used in clinical echocardiography. Displays upward deflections with height proportional to the amplitude of the returning echo and location proportional to the depth of the reflector (x-axis: reflector depth; y-axis: amplitude of echo). This mode only displays 1 scan line.

B (brightness) mode: Displays spots with brightness proportional to the amplitude of the echo and location proportional to the depth of the reflector (x-axis: reflector depth; z-axis: amplitude of echoes; there is no y-axis). B-mode echocardiography can be further classified as:

- **M (motion) mode:** A continuous B-mode display. Displays 1 scan line versus time. Allows for a high frame rate, accuracy of linear measurements, and tracking of motion of reflectors (x-axis: time; y-axis: reflector depth).
- **Two-dimensional imaging** is a line of B-mode echo data moved in an arc through a section of tissue in a back-and-forth fashion. This can be achieved with mechanical or electronic steering of the B-mode echo beam. Images are generated as series of *frames* displayed in rapid fashion to produce the impression of constant motion.

Determinants of Two-Dimensional Resolution

The ability of a US system to image accurately is termed *resolution. Spatial resolution* is defined as the minimum separation between two reflectors where they can still be identified as different structures. Spatial resolution has been described in terms of distinguishing structures parallel to the US beam (***longitudinal*** *or* ***axial*** *resolution*) or perpendicular to the US beam (***lateral*** *resolution*).

Synonyms for *longitudinal* resolution include *axial, radial, range,* and *depth* (LARRD). Synonyms for *lateral* resolution include *angular, transverse,* and *azimuth* (LATA).

Longitudinal Resolution = Spatial Pulse Length/2

Therefore, longitudinal resolution can be improved by shortening the spatial pulse length. Given the same number of cycles per pulse, higher frequency US will result in a shorter pulse length. Longitudinal resolution is typically better than lateral resolution.

Lateral resolution is approximately equal to the US beam diameter. It can be improved by electronic focusing, making the beam width narrowest in the area of interest. Increasing US frequency will result in a deeper area of focus, less divergence in the far field, and decreased beam width.

Note that *both* longitudinal and lateral resolutions are improved with high-frequency US. **In choosing the settings of a US system, there is a trade-off between the ability to obtain high-resolution images and the ability to image deeper structures (Figure 1–4).**

The ability to accurately locate moving structures at a given time is termed *temporal resolution.* Temporal resolution is proportional to the number of frames per second (*frame rate*). Factors that improve temporal resolution (by increasing the frame rate) are:

1. Minimizing imaging depth
2. Using single focus imaging (1 pulse/line)
3. Using a narrow sector
4. Minimizing line density

Because using multi-focus imaging and high line density results in better lateral resolution, improving temporal resolution is achieved at the expense of spatial resolution (Figure 1–5).

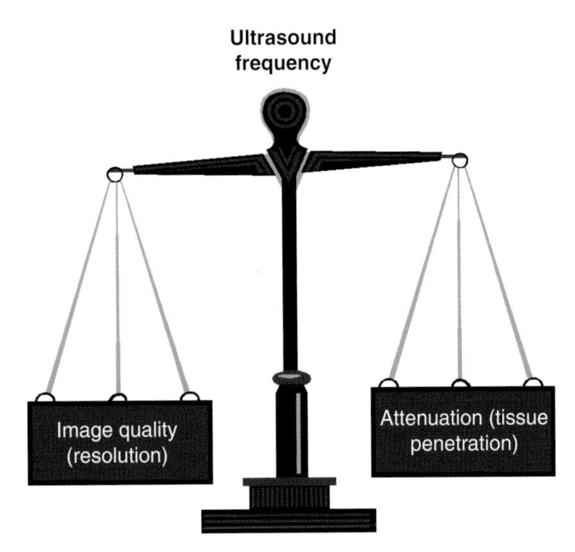

FIGURE 1–4. Relation between ultrasound frequency, image resolution, and tissue penetration. Image resolution improves at higher frequencies but at the expense of tissue penetration.

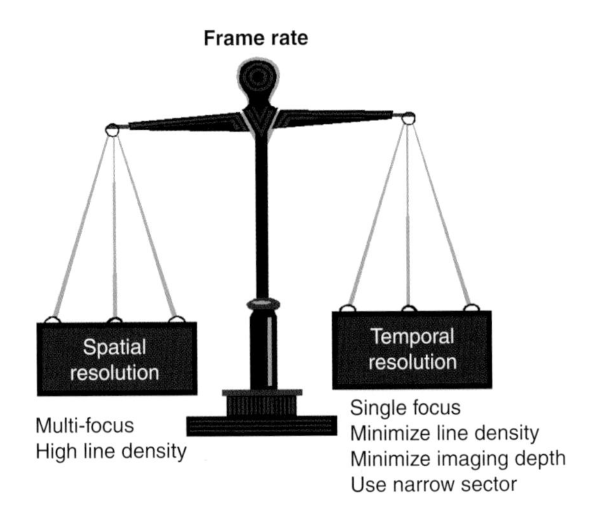

FIGURE 1–5. Relation between frame rate, spatial resolution, and temporal resolution. Improving temporal resolution is achieved at the expense of spatial resolution.

PRINCIPLES OF DOPPLER ULTRASOUND

The *Doppler effect* is defined as the *change* in the frequency of sound emitted or reflected by a moving object. The amount of change is termed the *Doppler shift.* It is important to note that though both the transmitted and reflected frequencies are ultrasonic (MHz range), the actual Doppler shift is in the audible range (20 to 20,000 Hz).

The most common applications of Doppler US are to measure velocity (magnitude and direction) of blood flow and, more recently, tissue. The *Doppler equation* is as follows:

$$\text{Doppler Shift (expressed in Hz)} = (2 \times v \times Fi \times \text{Cosine } \theta)/c$$

v = Velocity of the moving object
Fi = Incident frequency, or frequency emitted by the transducer
θ = Angle between the incident US beam and the direction of movement
c = Propagation speed of US in the medium (a constant 1540 m/s in soft tissue)

If the object is moving directly toward ($\theta = 0°$) or away from ($\theta = 180°$) the transducer, and v is expressed in units of m/s, then cosine θ is 1 and the equation simplifies to the following:

$$\text{Doppler Shift} = (v \times Fi)/770$$

Because the Doppler shift varies with the cosine of the angle of beam incidence (θ), the maximum measurable velocity decreases as θ increases. When movement is perpendicular (90°) to the beam, no Doppler shift is detected. Therefore, only measurements obtained with θ smaller than 20° are considered accurate.

In practice, the machine *measures* a Doppler shift and *calculates* a velocity. It also assumes θ is 0° or 180°. Rearranging the simplified Doppler equation gives us the following:

$$v = 770 \times (\text{Doppler Shift}/Fi)$$

When reflected (backscattered) signals are received at the transducer, the difference between the transmitted and reflected frequency is determined, analyzed by fast Fourier transform, and then displayed on the screen as Doppler envelope. This process is known as spectral analysis and results in a display of the following:

- Direction of blood flow: Flow toward the transducer results in an increased frequency (positive Doppler shift displayed above the baseline), whereas flow away from the transducer results in a decreased frequency (negative Doppler shift displayed below the baseline).
- Velocity or frequency shift.
- Signal amplitude.

Spectral Doppler (in contrast to color Doppler) can be further divided into pulsed wave and continuous wave.

Pulsed-Wave Doppler

Pulsed-wave Doppler uses one crystal that alternates between sending and receiving a US beam. A timed pulse allows sampling from a discrete area of about 1 to 3 mm, selected by the operator, known as the *sample volume.* This allows for *range discrimination* (Figure 1–6). Since the same element acts as both sender and receiver, the transducer must wait for the pulse to complete a round trip before emitting another pulse. As an example, if the sampling volume is 5 cm from the probe, the transducer must wait 65 μs until sending the next pulse.

Because sampling is intermittent, the pulse repetition frequency limits the maximum Doppler shift (and

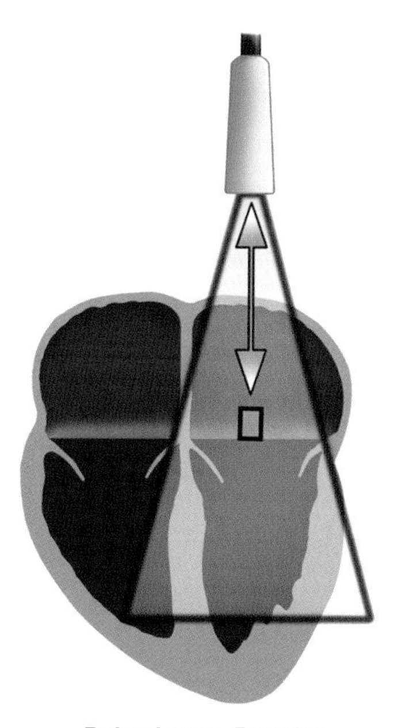

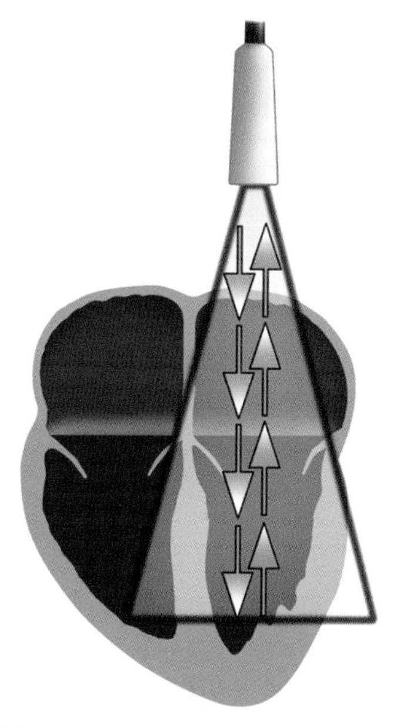

FIGURE 1–6. Characteristics of pulsed-wave and continuous-wave Doppler.

thus maximum velocity) that can be measured accurately. Velocities higher than this maximum velocity will appear to wrap around on the display, a phenomenon known as *aliasing* (see Chapter 3). The *Doppler frequency **shift** at which aliasing occurs,* equal to PRF divided by 2, is termed the *Nyquist limit.*

For example, if a 5 MHz transducer can only send out about 15,000 pulses per second, the Nyquist limit is 7500 Hz (15,000/2). Using the velocity equation above, the maximum velocity that can be measured without aliasing is about 1.15 m/s [770 × (7500/ 5,000,000)].

Methods to avoid aliasing include the following:

1. Use of continuous-wave Doppler
2. Changing view to bring area of interest closer to the probe (shallower depth)
3. Use of a transducer with a lower incident frequency (results in lower Doppler shift for given flow velocity; see the equation above)
4. Adjusting the scale to its maximum
5. Moving baseline up or down (makes picture "prettier" but does not eliminate aliasing)

From a practical standpoint, pulsed-wave Doppler should be used when measuring relatively low flow velocities (less than ~1.2 m/s) in specific areas of interest (eg, pulmonary vein flow, mitral valve inflow).

Compared to imaging ultrasound, pulsed-wave Doppler requires greater output power, longer pulse lengths, and a higher pulse repetition frequency.

When the velocity of the tissue becomes the object of measurement (Doppler tissue imaging), the system is set as a low-pass filter. This means that low velocity, high amplitude signals are preferentially displayed.

Continuous-Wave Doppler

Continuous-wave Doppler uses two crystals simultaneously in the transducer: one to constantly send US waves and the other to continuously receive. The PRF can thus be extremely high. This continuous sampling allows determination of high-velocity flow. However, because echoes come from anywhere along the length of the beam, continuous sampling prevents determination of the location of maximum measured velocity, termed *range ambiguity* (see Figure 1–6).

Continuous-wave Doppler should be used when measuring velocities greater than ~1.2 m/s (eg, regurgitant jets, stenotic valves).

Color-Flow Doppler

Color-flow Doppler is a *pulsed* US technique that color codes Doppler information and superimposes it on a 2D image, providing information on the direction of flow and semiquantitative information on the *mean* velocities of flow. It has the characteristics of pulsed-wave Doppler (range discrimination and aliasing). Color-flow Doppler uses packets of multiple pulses (3 to 20 per scan line), and therefore has a low temporal resolution (Figure 1–7). It then employs spectral analysis methods to estimate the mean velocity at each depth. The information on the direction of flow and the magnitude of the Doppler shift are displayed as *color maps,* which can be *velocity maps* or *variance maps* (Figure 1–8). A variance map contains information on the quality of flow (ie, laminar vs turbulent); however, turbulent flow and signal aliasing will result in an apparent wide range of velocities. Also, in the case of color-flow Doppler, aliasing may introduce confusion as to the direction of flow. Color-flow and spectral Doppler imaging use a high-pass filter to eliminate tissue motion artifacts.

A typical (but not uniform) convention for color Doppler velocity maps is for red to indicate flow toward the probe and for blue to indicate flow away from the probe (BART = Blue Away Red Toward). A region that is black on color-flow Doppler imaging represents an area where there is no measured Doppler shift.

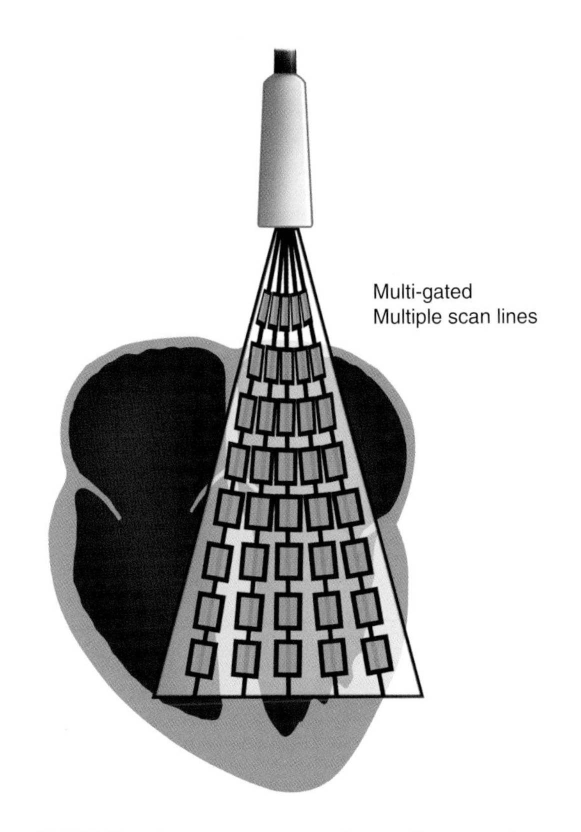

FIGURE 1–7. Characteristics of color-flow Doppler.

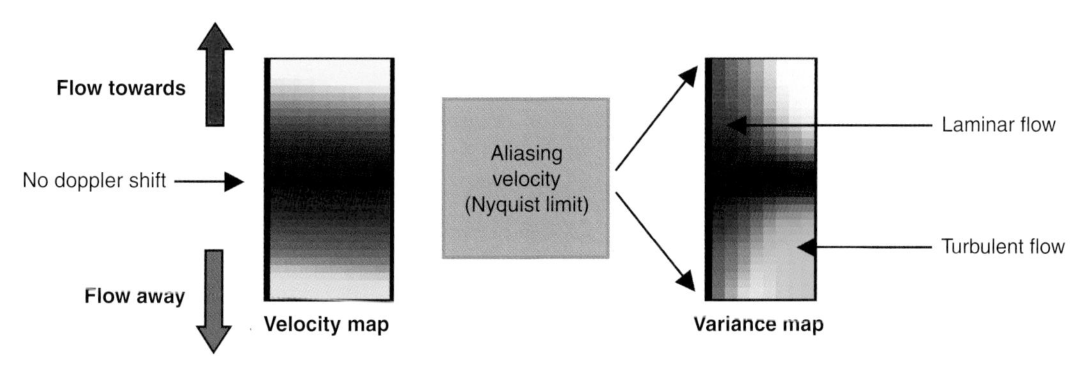

FIGURE 1–8. Characteristics of color-flow maps.

BIOEFFECTS

US bioeffects include *thermal effects* and *cavitation*. In addition, mechanical effects (vibration) may be of concern. *Thermal bioeffects* consist of a temperature elevation resulting from the absorption and scattering of US by biologic tissue and is related to beam intensity (the spatial peak and temporal average intensity; SPTA). The SPTA limits are 100 mW/cm^2 for unfocused beams and 1 W/cm^2 for focused beams. *Cavitation* results from the interaction of US with microscopic gas bubbles. Stable cavitation refers to forces that cause the bubbles to contract and expand. Transient cavitation results in breaking the bubbles and releasing energy, producing perhaps more pronounced effects on tissues at the microscopic level. The *mechanical index (MI)*, a calculated and unitless number, is used to convey the likelihood of bioeffects from cavitation. Cavitation bioeffects are more likely with a higher MI.

The U.S. Food and Drug Administration (FDA) limits the maximum intensity output of cardiac ultrasound systems to less than 720 W/cm^2 due to concerns of possible tissue and neurological damage from mechanical injury.

REFERENCES

1. Edelman SK. *Understanding Ultrasound Physics.* 3rd ed. Woodlands, TX: Education for the Sonographic Professional, Inc; 2004.
2. Edelman SK. *Ultrasound Physics and Instrumentation.* Woodlands, TX: Education for the Sonographic Professional, Inc; 2007.
3. Weyman AE. *Principles and Practice of Echocardiography.* Philadelphia: Lea & Febiger; 1993.
4. Jungwirth B, Mackensen GB. Real-time 3-dimensional echocardiography in the operating room. *Semin Cardiothorac Vasc Anesth.* 2008;12(4):248-264.
5. Reynolds T. *The Echocardiographer's Pocket Reference.* Phoenix: Arizona Heart Institute; 2000.

REVIEW QUESTIONS[1-3,5]

Basics of Ultrasound

Select the *one best* answer for each item.

1. Which of the following is *not* an acoustic variable?
   a. Pressure
   b. Density
   c. Distance
   d. Intensity

2. Which of the following sound wave frequencies is ultrasonic?
   a. 10 Hz
   b. 10 MHz
   c. 10 kHz
   d. 10,000 Hz

3. An increase in the strength of the US pulse will increase:
   a. Frequency
   b. Intensity
   c. Pulse duration
   d. Pulse repetition frequency

4. If imaging depth decreases, pulse repetition frequency:
   a. Decreases
   b. Does not change
   c. Increases
   d. Varies

5. An example of a Rayleigh scatterer is the:
   a. Red blood cell
   b. Kidney
   c. Mitral valve
   d. Pericardium

6. If the frequency is doubled, period:
   a. Increases two-fold
   b. Decreases
   c. Does not change
   d. Increases ten-fold

7. The wavelength in soft tissue of sound with a frequency of 2 MHz is:
   a. 6.16 mm
   b. 3.08 mm
   c. 1.54 mm
   d. 0.77 mm

8. The speed of sound is slowest in:
   a. Air
   b. Fat
   c. Soft tissue
   d. Bone

9. Which of the following parameters of sound are determined by the sound source *and* the medium?
   a. Frequency
   b. Wavelength
   c. Amplitude
   d. Propagation speed

10. Reflection occurs when the two media at the boundary have:
    a. Identical acoustic impedances
    b. Different acoustic impedances
    c. Identical densities and propagation speeds
    d. Different temperatures

11. All of the following are true of refraction *except*:
    a. It is a change in direction of wave propagation when traveling from one medium to another.
    b. It occurs when there are different propagation speeds and oblique incidence.
    c. It is described by Snell's law.
    d. It occurs with different propagation speeds and normal incidence.

12. A sound beam strikes the boundary between two media at an incident angle of 45° and is partly reflected and transmitted. If medium A has an impedance of 1.25 MRayls and a propagation speed of 1540 m/s, and medium B has an impedance of 1.85 MRayls and a propagation speed of 2.54 km/s, what is the angle of *reflection*?
    a. 45°
    b. 30°
    c. 60°
    d. 15°

13. A sound beam strikes the boundary between two media at an incident angle of 45° and is partly reflected and transmitted. If the propagation speed of the second medium is slower than the propagation speed of the first medium, then the transmission angle is:
    a. Equal to the incident angle
    b. Greater than the incident angle
    c. Less than the incident angle
    d. Cannot be determined

14. A sound wave leaves its source and travels through a liquid. If the speed of sound through that liquid is 600 m/s and the echo returns to the source 1 s later, at what distance is the source from the reflector?
    a. 1540 m
    b. 770 m
    c. 600 m
    d. 300 m

15. The amplitude of a wave is:
    a. The difference between the average and maximum (or minimum) values of an acoustic variable
    b. Determined initially by the medium
    c. Cannot be changed by the sonographer
    d. Twice the average amplitude

16. Intensity is inversely proportional to:
    a. Beam area
    b. Power
    c. Amplitude
    d. Amplitude squared

17. The speed of sound in a medium increases when:
    a. Elasticity of the medium increases
    b. Density of the medium increases
    c. Stiffness of the medium decreases
    d. Stiffness of the medium increases

18. Increasing the frequency of a transducer:
    a. Increases wavelength
    b. Improves axial resolution
    c. Increases depth of penetration
    d. Increases pulse duration

19. Propagation speed:
    a. Can be changed by the sonographer
    b. Is an average of 1540 km/s in soft tissue
    c. Is slower in a liquid than a solid
    d. Is determined by the sound source

20. Attenuation of an ultrasound beam results from:
    a. Absorption
    b. Reflection

c. Scattering
d. All of the above

21. Compared with backscatter, specular reflections are:
    a. Diffuse
    b. Random
    c. Well seen when sound strikes the reflector at 90°
    d. Occur when the wavelength is larger than the irregularities in the boundary

22. Pulsed ultrasound is described by:
    a. Duty factor
    b. Repetition frequency
    c. Spatial length
    d. All of the above

23. Pulse repetition frequency:
    a. Is determined by the sound source and the medium
    b. Can be changed by the sonographer
    c. Increases as imaging depth increases
    d. Is directly proportional to pulse repetition period

24. When a sound beam strikes a reflector at 90° incidence, it is considered as:
    a. Obtuse
    b. Oblique
    c. Normal
    d. Acute

25. Sound waves can be characterized as:
    a. Electrical
    b. Transverse
    c. Longitudinal
    d. Spectral

Transducers

Select the *one best* answer for each item.

1. Which piezoelectric effect does a US transducer use during the transmission phase?
   a. Doppler effect
   b. Reverse piezoelectric effect
   c. Direct piezoelectric effect
   d. Indirect piezoelectric effect

2. The most common piezoelectric material currently used includes all of the following *except*:
   a. Lead
   b. Zirconate
   c. Titanate
   d. Tourmaline

3. The optimal thickness for the matching layer as a fraction of the wavelength is:
   a. One-eighth
   b. One-fourth
   c. One-half
   d. Three-fourths

4. All of the following are true of linear switched or sequential arrays except:
   a. They produce a rectangular image display.
   b. Defective crystal creates a line of dropout from top to bottom.
   c. They have a fixed transmit focus.
   d. Elements are fired in a sequence to create an image.

5. In a phased array transducer, beam steering and focusing are produced by:
   a. Manually rotating the transducer
   b. Mechanically rotating the transducer
   c. Changing the timing of pulses to the piezoelectric elements
   d. Changing the resonant frequency of the piezoelectric elements

6. In an M-mode tracing, the x-axis represents:
   a. Depth
   b. Time
   c. Amplitude
   d. Frequency

7. The damping material in an ultrasound transducer increases the following:
   a. Pulse duration
   b. Spatial pulse length
   c. Duty factor
   d. Bandwidth

8. The region or zone between the transducer and the focal point is known as the:
   a. Far zone
   b. Fresnel zone
   c. Fraunhofer zone
   d. Focal zone

9. At the focus, the beam diameter is:
   a. One-fourth the transducer diameter
   b. Half the transducer diameter
   c. Double the transducer diameter
   d. Equal to the transducer diameter

10. In a linear phased array transducer:
    a. Image shape is a blunted sector.
    b. Steering is mechanical.
    c. Focusing is electronic.
    d. Crystal defect produces a vertical line dropout.

Instrumentation

Select the *one best* answer for each item.

1. The US modality providing the best temporal resolution is:
   a. A mode
   b. B mode
   c. Three dimensional
   d. M mode

2. Increasing transducer output:
   a. Creates identical changes in the image as an increase in overall gain
   b. Cannot be controlled by the sonographer
   c. Causes no change in the brightness of the image
   d. Decreases the energy output of the transducer

3. Which of the following is used to create an image of uniform brightness from top to bottom?
   a. Compression
   b. Time gain compensation
   c. Demodulation
   d. Overall gain

4. The ability to distinguish two objects that are parallel to the US beam's main axis is called:
   a. Axial resolution
   b. Lateral resolution
   c. Transverse resolution
   d. Azimuth resolution

5. If the US image shows no weak reflectors on the image, the best corrective action is to:
   a. Increase overall gain.
   b. Increase the transducer output power.
   c. Decrease the reject level.
   d. Use a high-frequency transducer.

6. The principal display modes for ultrasound include:
   a. M mode
   b. A mode
   c. B mode
   d. All of the above

7. Temporal resolution can be improved by:
   a. Using multi-focus
   b. Using a wide sector
   c. Minimizing line density
   d. Maximizing depth of view

8. Components of a US system include:
   a. Pulser
   b. Receiver
   c. Master synchronizer
   d. All of the above

9. Lateral resolution can be increased by:
   a. Increasing beam diameter
   b. Decreasing transducer frequency
   c. Focusing
   d. Increasing gain

Doppler

Select the *one best* answer for each item.

1. The difference between the transmitted and reflected frequencies is known as the:
   a. Bernoulli equation
   b. Doppler principle
   c. Doppler shift
   d. Gorlin equation

2. Velocity is defined by:
   a. Magnitude
   b. Direction
   c. Neither a nor b
   d. Both a and b

3. When the angle between the sound beam and the direction of motion is 90°, the measured velocity is equal to:
   a. True velocity
   b. Zero
   c. 20% of true velocity
   d. 50% of true velocity

4. Current spectral analysis is achieved by:
   a. Fast Fourier transform
   b. Multi-filter analysis
   c. Zero-crossing detector
   d. Time interval histogram

5. Modal velocity represents:
   a. Average Doppler velocity
   b. Greatest amplitude returned Doppler shift
   c. Maximum Doppler velocity
   d. None of the above

6. Wall motion–induced frequency shifts are:
   a. High amplitude, low velocity, low frequency
   b. Low amplitude, low velocity, low frequency
   c. High amplitude, high velocity, high frequency
   d. High amplitude, low velocity, high frequency

7. Doppler wall motion filters are:
   a. Low pass
   b. High pass

c. Zero pass
d. One pass

8. The maximal detectable frequency shift or one-half of the PRF is known as:
a. Doppler effect
b. Propagation speed
c. Nyquist limit
d. Peak Doppler shift

9. The following pulsed Doppler spectral display demonstrates:

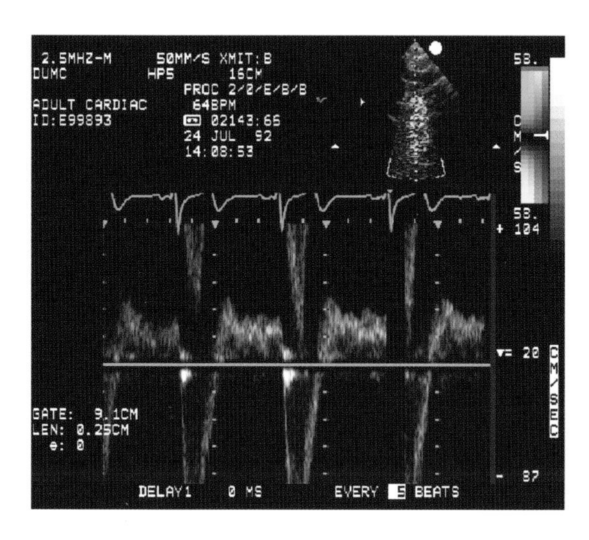

a. Reverberation
b. Aliasing
c. Mirroring
d. Side lobe

10. Color-flow Doppler measures the:
a. Peak velocity
b. Mean velocity
c. Modal velocity
d. Instantaneous velocity

11. When color-flow Doppler is used, the number of US pulses per scan line is called:
a. Line density
b. Frame rate
c. Nyquist limit
d. Packet size

12. The color map below is a:

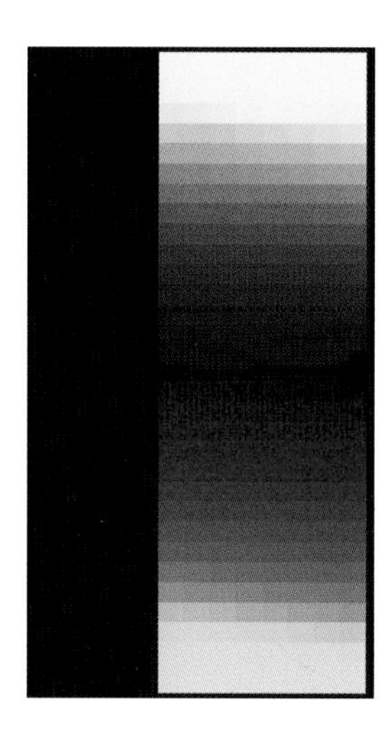

a. Normal map
b. Velocity map
c. Variance map
d. Aliased map

13. The color map below is a:

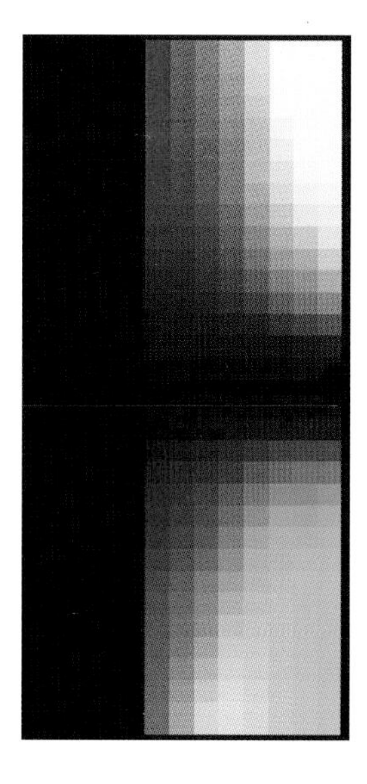

a. Normal map
b. Velocity map
c. Variance map
d. Aliased map

14. In the figure below, the arrow points to a region (black) where:

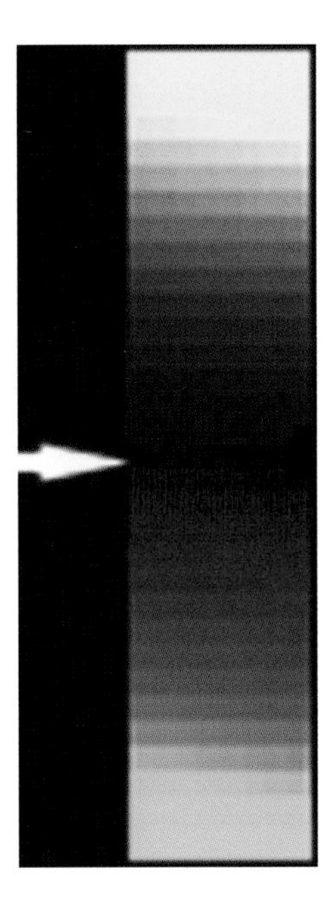

a. There is no flow.
b. There is no Doppler shift.
c. There is turbulent flow.
d. There is laminar flow.

15. A color Doppler examination is performed with the color map shown. If a red blood cell is traveling perpendicular to the direction of the sound beam, the color that will appear on the image for this red blood cell is:

a. Red
b. Orange
c. Black
d. Yellow

16. If the aliasing velocity of the color scale below is 40 cm/s, laminar flow toward the probe at 50 cm/s would appear:

a. Red
b. Blue
c. Yellow
d. Green

17. When a Doppler shift is displayed above the zero baselines:
a. Reflected frequency is less than the transmitted frequency.
b. Red blood cells are moving away from the transducer.
c. Sound source and reflector are approaching each other.
d. It is called a negative Doppler shift.

18. Continuous-wave Doppler:
a. Cannot measure very high velocities
b. Transmits and receives ultrasound constantly
c. Is prone to aliasing artifact
d. Is characterized as a wide bandwidth transducer

19. The Doppler spectral display graphically demonstrates:
a. Direction of blood flow
b. Velocity of blood flow

c. Duration of blood flow
d. All of the above

20. A 5-MHz transducer with a pulse repetition frequency of 5600 Hz is imaging to a depth of 5.6 cm. The Nyquist frequency is:
a. 2.8 MHz
b. 2.8 dB
c. 2.8 kHz
d. 2500 Hz

21. Compared with pulsed *imaging* (2D), pulsed-wave Doppler:
a. Causes less acoustic exposure
b. Has lower output power
c. Uses shorter pulse repetition periods
d. Uses shorter pulse lengths

22. Color Doppler:
a. Reports average velocities
b. Uses continuous-wave US
c. Does not provide range resolution
d. Is not subject to aliasing

23. The following principle is true of color Doppler imaging:
a. Red always represents flow toward the transducer.
b. Turbulent flow is indicated as black.
c. Blue always indicates flow away from the transducer.
d. Color Doppler examinations tend to have lower temporal resolution.

24. Blood flow in the imaged vessel is moving from:

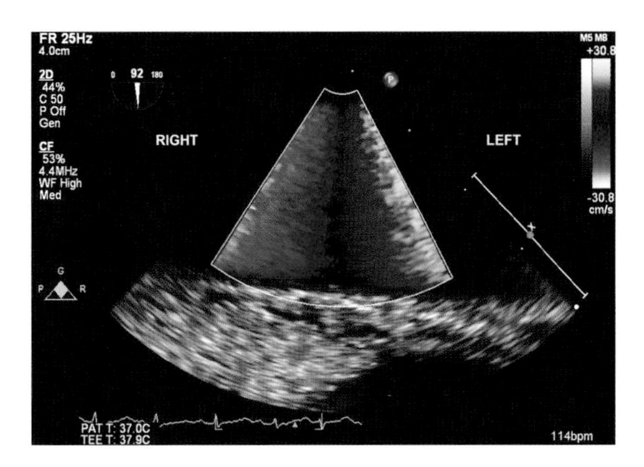

a. Right to left (as labeled on the image)
b. Right to left and then left to right
c. Left to right (as labeled on the image)
d. Left to right and then right to left

Bioeffects

Select the *one best* answer for each item.

1. The most relevant intensity with respect to tissue heating is:
a. SPTA
b. SPTP
c. SATP
d. SATA

2. Which of the following modalities has the lowest intensity value?
a. Pulsed-wave Doppler
b. Continuous-wave Doppler
c. M mode/B mode
d. All of the above have the same intensity

3. Contraction and expansion of gas bubbles is known as:
a. Transient cavitation
b. Stable cavitation
c. Attenuation
d. Particle motion

4. US bioeffects can be caused by all of the following *except*:
a. Thermal effects
b. Mechanical effects
c. Scan conversion
d. Cavitation

5. A number developed to predict the likelihood of cavitation-induced bioeffects is called:
a. Duty factor
b. Mechanical index
c. Pulsatility index
d. Resistivity index

6. Acoustic exposure to the patient is increased by:
a. Increase in receiver gain
b. Decrease in pulse repetition frequency
c. Application of reject
d. Increase in examination time

Understanding Ultrasound System Controls

2

Hillary Hrabak, Emily Forsberg, and David Adams

It is crucial for clinicians performing transesophageal (TEE) examinations to understand how the controls on an ultrasound machine alter the display. Without this knowledge, it is impossible to consistently optimize images, and unskilled manipulations may misrepresent diagnostic information and result in missed diagnoses. This chapter describes the controls found on most ultrasound machines, how they affect the image, and how they are used to optimize the ultrasound image. Table 2–1 presents the most commonly used controls for two-dimensional (2D) imaging.

PREPARING THE MACHINE

After providing power to the machine itself, a TEE *probe* must be connected to the machine, register as compatible with the machine, and be selected from other possible transducer options. The basic parameters for the ultrasound examination may be defined by choosing an appropriate TEE *preset.* The preset provides a starting point for basic machine settings such as depth, gain, and image processing settings. The operator can adjust all the machine's variables from the initially fixed settings, as needed. Adjustments to the preset can be saved permanently under a different preset name when desired. *Patient identification* (name and medical record number) and any other relevant information should be entered into the machine before beginning an exam. This includes date of birth, sex, videotape number, name of person performing the examination, location, and a number of other qualifiers.

The five most common modes used during TEE examinations are 2D gray-scale imaging, color Doppler, pulsed-wave (PW) Doppler, continuous-wave (CW) Doppler, and three-dimensional (3D) imaging. The usual buttons to enable these modes are *2D, Color, PW, CW,* and *3D.* Other scanning modes, such as *M-mode* and *angio,* are often available but are minimally important in comparison. Figure 2–1 is an example of four common ultrasound control panels. While the number and layout of buttons and controls are different, there are many similarities. This chapter focuses on controls that affect 2D imaging, color Doppler, pulsed-wave Doppler, and continuous-wave Doppler. Three-dimensional imaging is a new and exciting addition to TEE, especially for the evaluation of the mitral valve, and will be briefly discussed at the end of this chapter.

TWO-DIMENSIONAL IMAGING AND BASIC IMAGE MANIPULATION

Two-dimensional gray-scale imaging is a type of B-mode imaging (*B* is for brightness) in which the various amplitudes of returning ultrasound signals are displayed in multiple shades of gray. Higher amplitude signals are closer to white, whereas lower amplitude signals are displayed as closer to black. The many different shades of gray form an image or representative picture of the patient's cardiac anatomy. TEE probes generate a sector or pie-shaped display of gray-scale images, with the top portion of the sector showing the tissue closest to the transducer. Of the five modes, the 2D display mode is most commonly used and manipulated during a TEE examination. Two-dimensional imaging also provides a reference point from which to activate all three forms of Doppler (color, PW, and CW).

GAIN

Overall gain or amplification is the first postprocessing function performed by the receiver and is the most important variable to adjust during a study. Overall gain controls the degree of amplification that returning signals undergo before display. By increasing gain, small voltages are changed into larger voltages by an operator-specified level of amplification. Gain is also the one control that is misused most often, with the most common mistake being the addition of too much gain to an image. Although additional gain can make the picture brighter and structures more obvious, using too much gain, or over gaining, will destroy image resolution. The appropriate amount of gain for any given image becomes apparent when reflectors and tissue interfaces

Table 2–1. Commonly Used Controls for 2D Imaging.

2D Variable	Knob(s)	Function
Gain	Gain	Amplifies returning signals before display
TGC/DGC	TGC/DGC toggles	Selectively amplifies returning signals before display (horizontally)
LGC	LGC toggles	Selectively amplifies returning signals before display (vertically)
Compression	Compression	Changes the difference between the highest and lowest received amplitudes (shades of gray)
Power	Power (dB)	Controls rate at which energy is propagated into an imaged medium
Frequency	Dependent on probe	Determines number of times/second a sound wave completes a cycle
Focal zone	Focal zone	Alters the placement of the narrowed region that designates an area of improved resolution
Depth	Depth	Selects how shallow or deep an area is imaged
Sector size	Size, trackball	Narrows or widens the image sector
Zoom	Zoom	Magnifies a particular area of interest within the sector
Freeze	Freeze	Stops or starts live imaging
Measurement	Freeze, caliper, trace, enter, erase	Quantifies features of a 2D image
Harmonics	Harmonics	Uses frequencies created by the tissues, rather than the fundamental frequency, to create an image
Annotation	Annotation	Adds text or picture to image

2D, two-dimensional; dB, decibel; DGC, depth gain compensation; LGC, lateral gain compensation; TGC, time gain compensation.

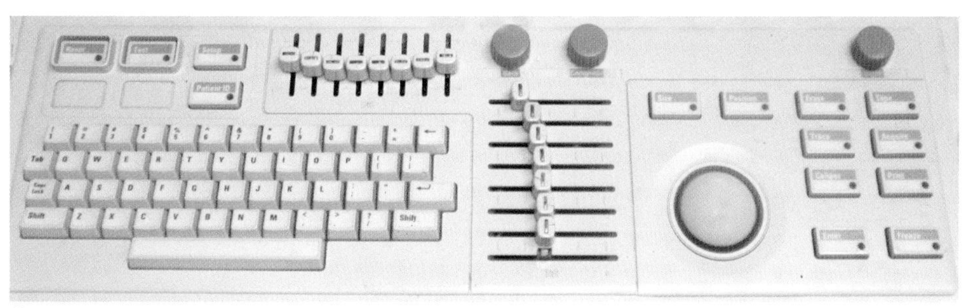

A

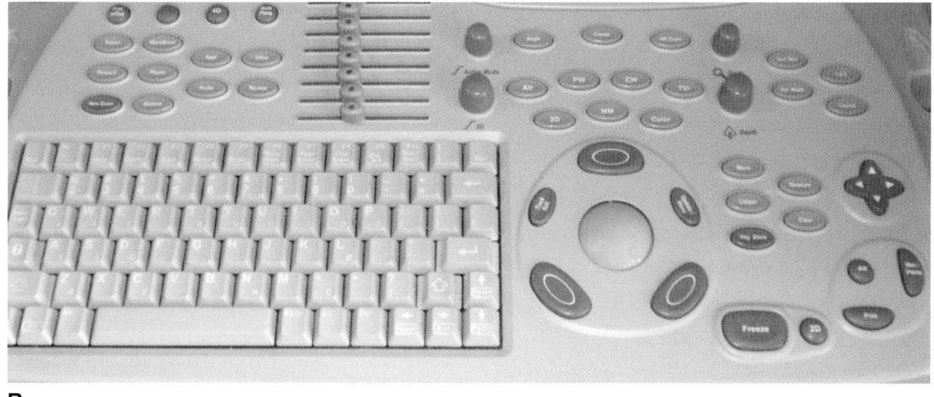

B

FIGURE 2–1. Typical control panels on cardiac ultrasound machines. While they look different there are shared controls such as TGCs on all systems.

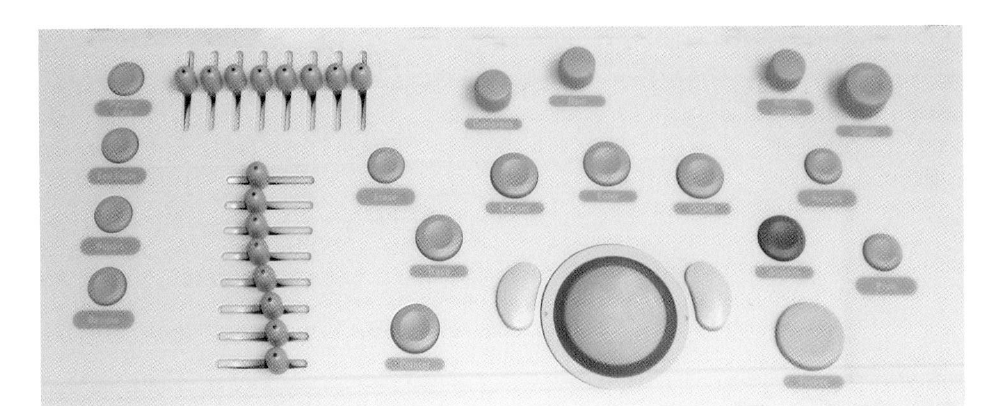

C

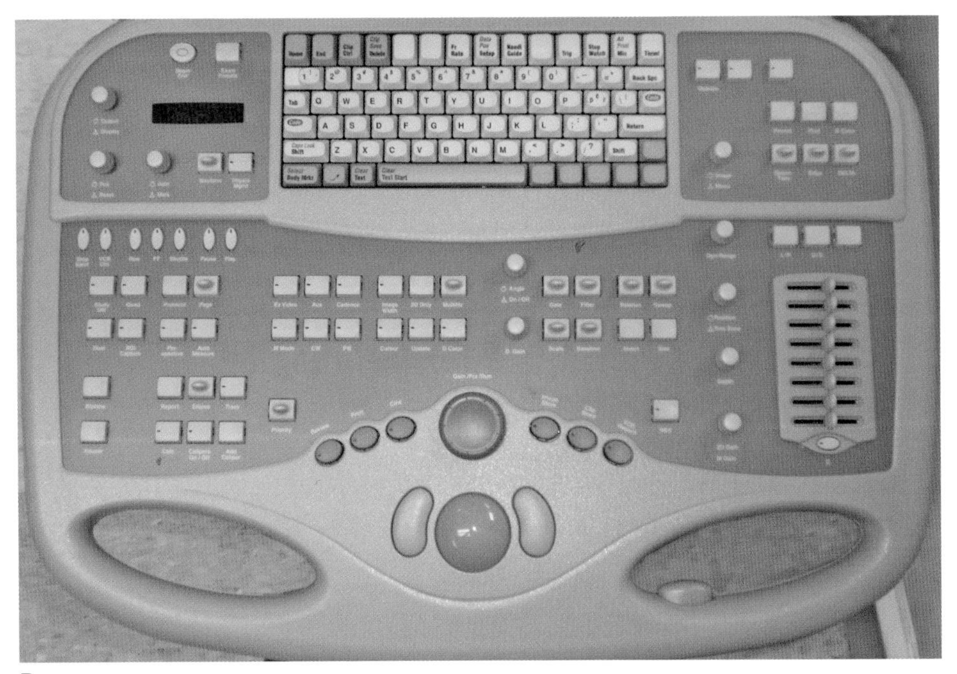

D

FIGURE 2–1. *(Continued)*

can be seen, but fluid and blood appear as totally black and echo-free. Myocardium should be adequately dispersed with reflectors by setting it at a medium shade of gray, but the muscle should not approach the look of a solid white band. Only the pericardium, certain states of abnormal thickening, calcification, tissue infiltration, and surgically altered valves should be hyperechoic (very bright). Gain should be added incrementally if the picture is entirely black or if the only structures seen with clarity are normally hyperechoic. Figure 2–2 shows a TEE image with varying gain settings. Figure 2–2A is an example of overall gain setting being too low, while Figure 2–2B is proper gain setting. Figure 2–2C shows the same image with a gain setting that is too high.

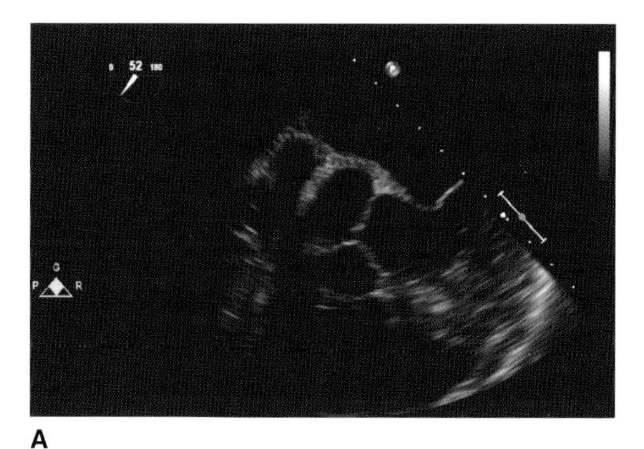

A

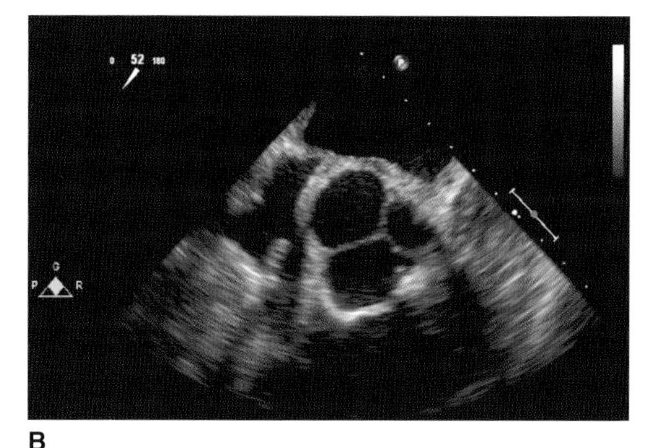

B

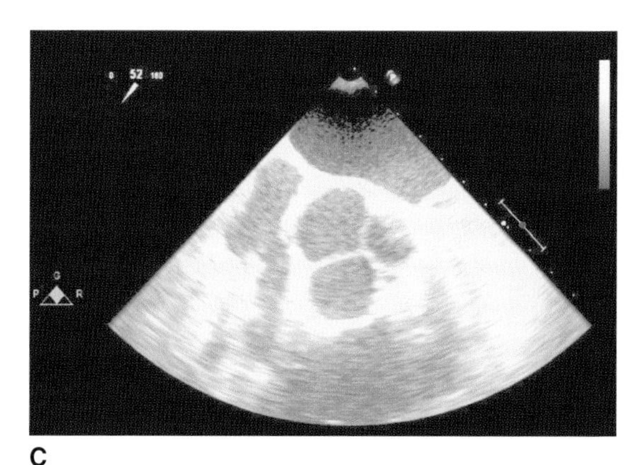

C

FIGURE 2–2. The effect of overall gain on an ultrasound image. **(A)** shows an image that is under gained, while in **(B)** there is optimal gain. Compare this to **(C)** where there is obviously too much overall gain.

TIME OR DEPTH GAIN COMPENSATION

The second postprocessing function of the receiver is compensation, commonly known as time gain compensation (TGC) or depth gain compensation (DGC). Compensation makes up for energy loss from the sound beam due to attenuation. Attenuation is the loss of intensity and amplitude of the ultrasound beam as it travels deeper into the body. Strong returning signals from the near field (close to the transducer) need to be suppressed, whereas signals from the far field (deeper depths) require higher amplification.

TGC/DGC is seen on the machine as a column of toggles that can be manipulated along a horizontal plane. By sliding a toggle to the right, the operator increases the gain at that given depth. The TGC/DGC is normally placed at a diagonal slope of variable steepness in which the upper, or near field, toggles are often set at a lower degree of compensation, whereas the lower, or far field, toggles are often set at a higher degree of compensation. A pattern of gradual change from one toggle to the next avoids a "striped" appearance to the ultrasound picture.

LATERAL GAIN COMPENSATION

Lateral gain compensation (LGC) is present on only some ultrasound machines. LGC toggles are similar to TGC/DGC toggles but act selectively on the y-axis of the picture to change the gain in vertical portions. LGCs help to bring out myocardial walls that may be hypoechoic (lacking in brightness) due to technique or positioning. However, the operator must be selective in using compensation of the gray scale because some sections of the image may not require any compensation.

COMPRESSION

Compression is another postprocessing function that is just as important as gain. Compression alters the difference between the highest and lowest echo amplitudes received by taking the received amplitudes and fitting them into a gray-scale range that the machine can display. Dynamic range (how many shades of gray appear within the image) is determined by the degree of compression applied to returning signals. Compression changes the dynamic range of the ultrasound signal with an inverse relationship. Increasing the compression produces an image with more shades of gray, whereas decreasing the compression provides a highly contrasted image with strong white and black components. Sharply decreasing the compression may be a tempting method to improve structure delineation, but it will sacrifice low-amplitude targets. Most presets will start the operator with midlevel value of compression and gain. Figure 2–3 shows the effect of compression on an image of a mitral valve. Figure 2–3A shows a high compression

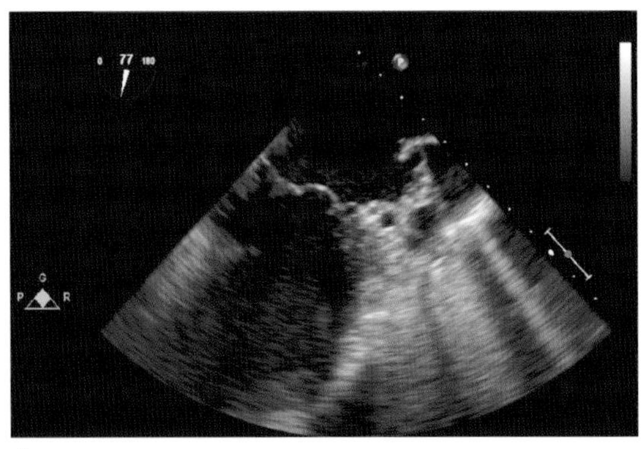
A

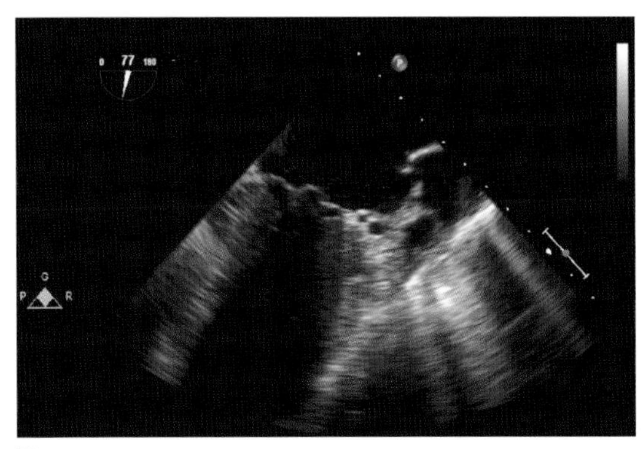
B

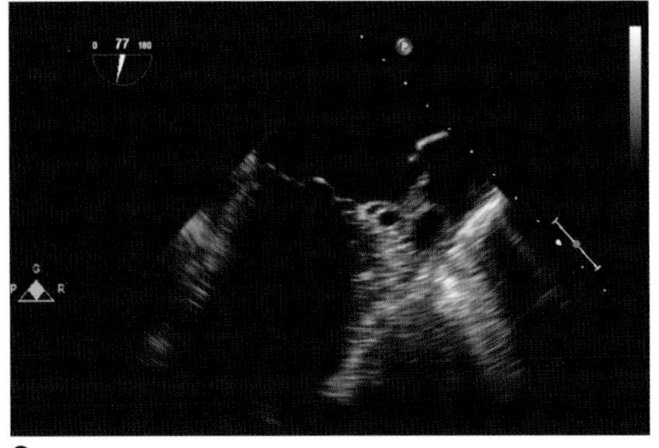
C

FIGURE 2–3. The effect of different compression settings on an ultrasound image. **(A)** shows an image that has a high compression setting, while in **(B)** there is an optimal compression setting. Compare this to **(C)** where there is a low compression setting.

setting so the image has too many low amplitude targets. Figure 2–3B presents a medium compression setting. The image has the optimal gray-scale information. Figure 2–3C depicts a low compression setting, so the image has little gray-scale information.

POWER

Power can be indirectly assessed by *decibel* (dB) settings, *mechanical index (MI)*, and *thermal index (TI)*. Power, expressed in watts (W) or milliwatts (mW), describes the rate at which energy is propagated into the imaged medium. Intensity, power per unit area (mW/cm^2 or some unit variation), is a concept that closely relates to power. Intensity may not be entirely uniform throughout tissues, so intensity levels predict more accurately the risk of bioeffects than do power levels. When looking at an image, changing the output power from the transducer appears to have an effect similar to that of changing the overall gain; however, alteration of power is less preferable than increasing the overall gain. Any increase in output power can raise the amount of energy that transfers into the biologic tissue, increasing risk of bioeffects. Adjustment of gain settings do not change the amount of energy transferred into the tissue. Changes in overall gain setting adjust signals that have already traveled through tissues. **Thus, gain variables should always be adjusted before ever attempting to change the power.**

Most machines do not describe the power level in watts or milliwatts. Instead, they *indirectly* describe power in terms of decibels. The *3-dB rule*, intended to help clinicians understand alterations in power, states that an increase of 3 dB doubles the power or intensity from an original value, whereas a decrease of 3 dB halves the power or intensity from an original value. The exact power or intensity levels are not presented on the display, so manufacturers have placed two more variables on the display screen to help clinicians estimate power and intensity levels. The two variables shown on the display are the *mechanical index* and the *thermal index*. The MI conveys the likelihood of *cavitation* resulting from the ultrasonic energy during the examination. Cavitation refers to activity (oscillation or bursting) of microscopic gas bubbles within the tissues due to exposure to ultrasound energy. The TI is the ratio of output power emitted by the transducer to the power needed to raise tissue temperature by 1° Celsius.

FREQUENCY

Frequency is defined as the number of cycles per second. The frequency of most TEE probes is between 5 and 7 MHz (5,000,000 to 7,000,000 cycles/s). The frequency of the ultrasound probe can have a dramatic effect on image quality of the TEE. Lower transmitted frequencies will create very different images than higher transmitted frequencies. *Resolution* is the ability to detect two targets positioned closely to one another. When the wavelength is shorter (higher frequencies), the axial resolution is better. Improved resolution generates a more accurate anatomic rendering of structures displayed by ultrasound. However, the lower the sound source frequency, the more effective it is in penetrating tissue and not falling subject to attenuation. Unfortunately, low frequencies yield poorer resolution in their resulting images when compared with high-frequency images. A TEE can be performed at a higher frequency than a chest wall echocardiogram. This is largely due to the fact that the heart is closer to the probe and there is less interference from bone, lung, and other tissue.

The imaging frequency is dependent on the transducer used; however, each probe has a *frequency bandwidth*. Frequency bandwidth is the range of frequencies any selected probe is able to transmit. Broadband transducers are commonly used because of their ability to transmit over a wide range of frequencies. Some ultrasound systems offer a wide bandwidth and allow an operator to select a part of the bandwidth spectrum that is most appropriate to make the images. During a TEE, the highest possible frequency should be used to distinguish targets on the display. Such a strategy takes advantage of the close proximity of the heart to the TEE probe and will produce more highly resolved images.

HARMONICS

Standard transducers transmit and receive frequencies that are the same or within a very close range. The frequency from such a transducer is known as the *fundamental frequency*. As the beam propagates through tissues, it distorts and creates additional frequencies that are multiples of the fundamental frequency. These additional frequencies are the *harmonic frequencies* and are created by the tissues themselves. Whereas the fundamental frequency may undergo a large amount of distortion, the harmonic frequencies do not. In patients with poor sound transmission due to obesity or dense muscle tissue, the harmonic frequencies may produce a better image than the fundamental frequency. In general, it should be unnecessary to use the harmonics during a TEE because of the proximity of the transducer to the heart. In fact, when using harmonics, the image likely will have poorer resolution than the image created with the fundamental frequency. During contrast studies, harmonics will improve image quality whether using agitated saline solution or one of the transpulmonary contrast agents. Figure 2–4 demonstrates the differences between a fundamental low frequency (Figure 2–4A), a fundamental high frequency (Figure 2–4B), and a

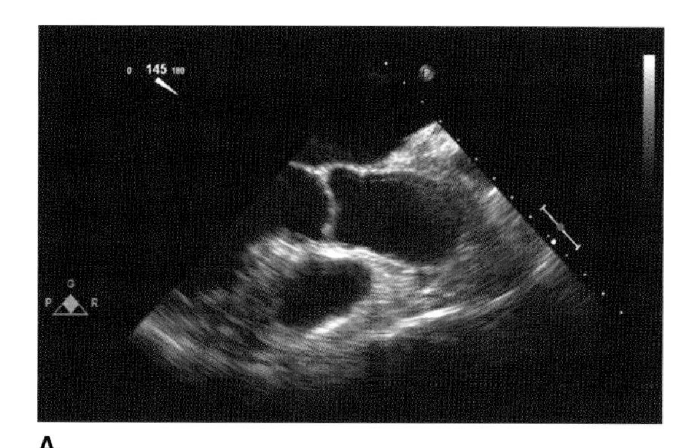

A

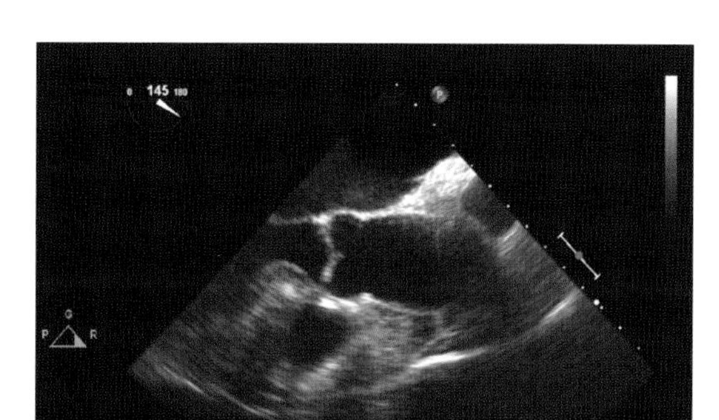

B

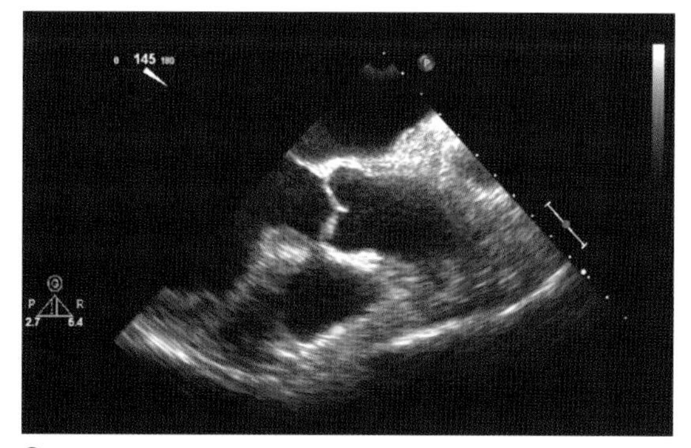

C

FIGURE 2–4. The effect of changes in frequency and harmonics on TEE images of the aorta and aortic valve. **(A)** shows an image obtained in fundamental imaging at a lower frequency, while in **(B)** the fundamental frequency has been shifted higher. Compare this to **(C)** where harmonic imaging has been used.

harmonic image (Figure 2–4C). Notice how harmonic imaging makes the aortic valve appear thicker in the harmonic image compared to the fundamental images.

FOCAL ZONE

Because the ultrasound beam does not necessarily maintain the same width as it travels into the depths of tissue, many systems use a technique known as *focusing* to better evaluate a specific depth. Focusing the ultrasound beam is a process accomplished by mechanical or electronic means and is available as a system control. As the beam proceeds deeper into the tissue, the beam gradually tapers to a narrow region known as the *focal zone*. The central point of the focal zone is the *focal point*, an area that will have the highest intensity (mW/cm^2) of the transmitted ultrasound energy from the transducer. Of interest to the echocardiographer is the fact that manipulation of focal zones produces a higher quality image because it produces better returning signals for the machine to process and display.

DEPTH

All machines have a control that increases or decreases the overall image depth. Decreasing the depth increases the frame rate by reducing the amount of information that the machine has to process and shortening the time required for the beam to travel to and return from a target of interest. Regardless of frame rate, some cardiac views require a deeper field of view for adequate display. Each machine has a limit as to how deep it is able to image. Although this can become a limitation in transthoracic echocardiograms of extremely obese patients, depth is seldom a limiting factor in acquiring a TEE picture. Figure 2–5 shows an example of the use of deep (Figure 2–5A) and shallow (Figure 2–5B) depth settings.

SECTOR SIZE

Reducing the width of the sector is another excellent way to increase frame rate and isolate an area of interest. Just as depth will reduce the amount of information that needs to be processed, so will narrowing the sector. See Figure 2–6 for a display of wide (Figure 2–6A) and narrow (Figure 2–6B) sector images.

COLOR DOPPLER

All forms of Doppler analysis on the ultrasound machine, including color Doppler, are based on the *Doppler effect*, the perceived change in frequency that occurs between a sound source and a sound receiver. When a reflector is stationary and the transducer is stationary, no Doppler shift occurs. In the human body,

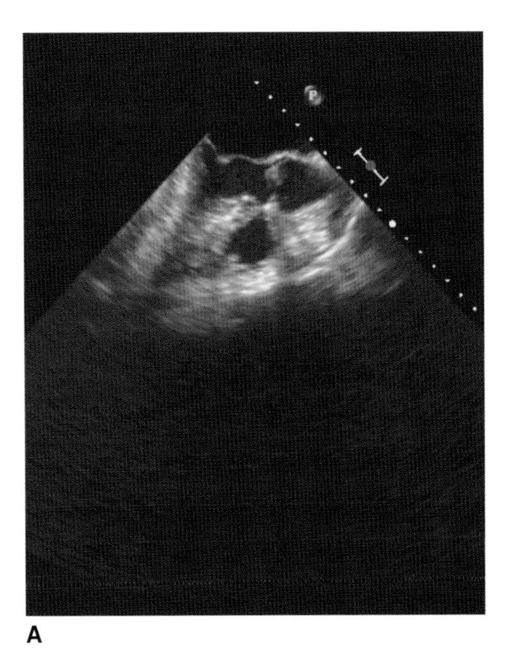

A

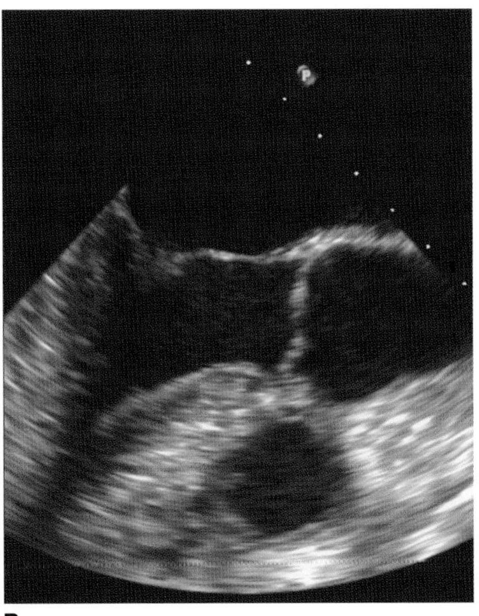

B

FIGURE 2–5. An echocardiographic image obtained at a very deep depth setting **(A)** compared to an image obtained with the depth decreased **(B)**.

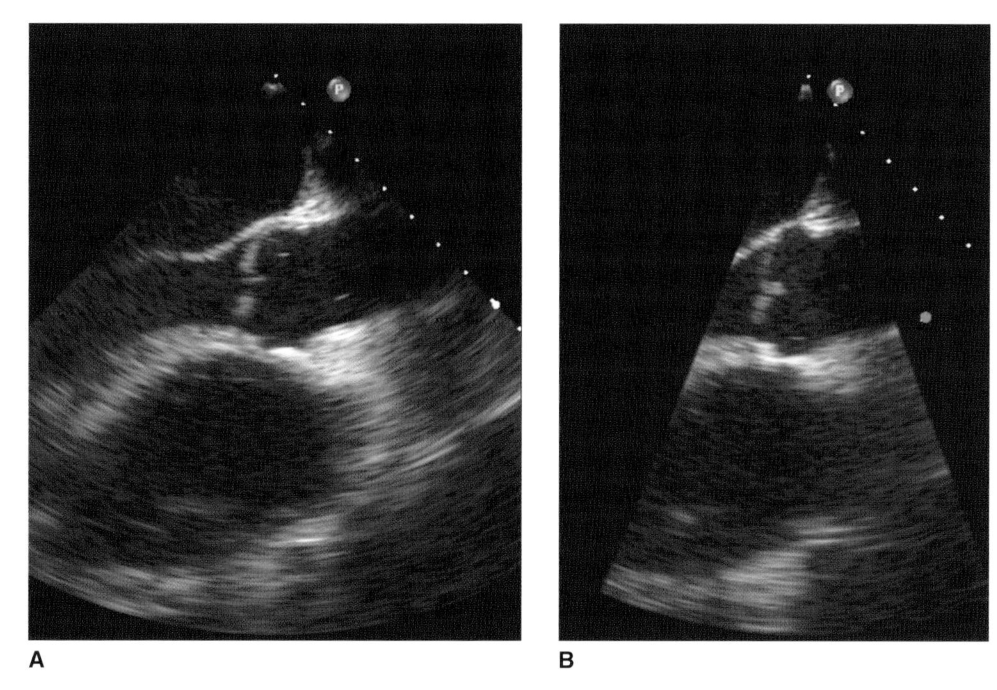

FIGURE 2–6. Alterations in the sector width. In **(A)** the sector size is set at a wide angle (90°) compared to **(B)** where the sector size has been narrowed significantly.

the constantly moving red blood cells serve as the reflector creating the Doppler shift. It should be remembered that color Doppler provides data only on moving reflectors and that stationary reflectors detected within each color packet are eliminated from processing. Color Doppler is commonly layered over a 2D image to provide information on blood flow within the context needed to adequately interpret the color data.

The direction of flow, relative to the transducer, is always shown on the machine's display with a color map. Manufacturers frequently provide a red-and-blue color map, with red designating flow toward the probe and blue representing flow away from the probe. The machine operator can change many color display properties. A *color invert* option will flip the color map; this would present blue as flow toward the probe, and red as flow away from the probe. Figure 2–7 depicts this color-invert option. The *color map* can also be changed to display flows in an entirely new set of hues or intensities. One set of color maps are *velocity maps*, these display Doppler velocities with two preselected colors (typically red and blue). Some color maps add an element of green or yellow to differentiate between laminar and turbulent flows; these are *variance maps*. While using a variance map, color Doppler analyzes velocities, direction of flow, and areas of turbulent versus laminar flow. Figure 2–8 shows examples of mitral regurgitation by TEE using two different color maps. Figure 2–8A shows a velocity map, a map of direction and velocity. Figure 2–8B is an example of a variance map, showing direction, velocity, and turbulence.

The color mode also has an adjustable *scale*. The numbers above and below the color map indicate the range of mean velocities that can be displayed, typically in centimeters per second, without aliasing. Usually, the machine calculates an optimal scale based largely on depth. Lowering the scale number lowers the pulse repetition frequency and therefore the Nyquist limit (pulse repetition frequency/2 = Nyquist limit). Although the lower scale is more sensitive to flow, it is more susceptible to aliasing. Raising the scale will reduce sensitivity to flow, raise the pulse repetition frequency and Nyquist limit, and make the color display less likely to alias. Figure 2–9A shows normal diastolic flow through the mitral valve in diastole. In Figure 2–9B, the Doppler scale has been lowered to 15.4 cm/s resulting in distortion of the normal diastolic flow. Altering the scale may be beneficial in select instances, but the scale should be left alone most of the time, and particularly when grading valvular regurgitation.

Quality of color imaging depends on the number of pulses per *color packet*, or packet size, and on the *frame rate* of the overall picture with color. Each tiny color packet represents the *mean* velocity within that particular

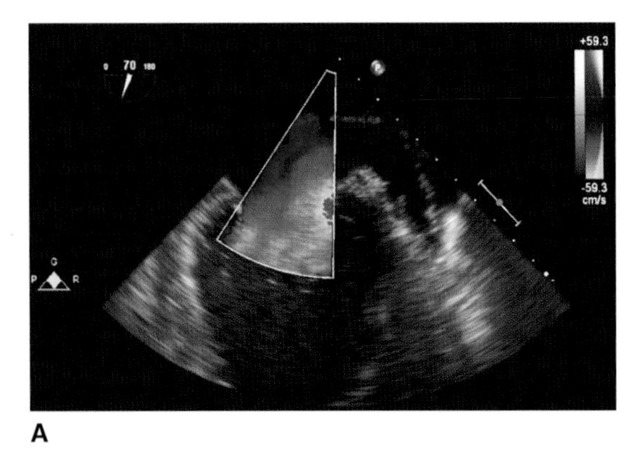

A

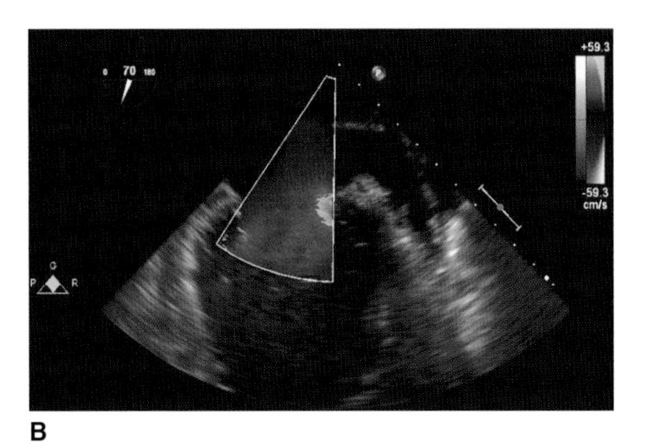

B

FIGURE 2–7. An example of how the color-flow Doppler map direction can be changed. In **(A)** the map is directed in the typical position where flow towards the probe is red and flow away is blue. Flow through the mitral valve in diastole is seen as blue. In **(B)** the color Doppler map has been inverted so that flow towards the probe is blue and flow away is red. Thus, the flow through the mitral valve in diastole is now red.

color packet. The more pulses in the color packet, the more accurate the received data and the color representation, but these variables must be balanced carefully because a larger number of pulses in the color packets also decreases frame rates. The frame rate of the image with color Doppler can be highly dependent on the machine operator. For optimal imaging, the depth should be kept as shallow as possible to have the highest frame rate. The color box also should be as narrow as possible and fully cover the area of interest. Wider color boxes will lower frame rates because more time is required to interrogate a flow in a larger area. In contrast, the length of the color box has a minimal effect on the frame rate. Keyboard controls, such as trackball, size, and position controls, can be used to change the length, width, and placement, respectively, of the color box.

Smoothing determines the degree to which the color packets progressively transition into adjacent color packets. A low smoothing setting will make the individual color packets highly independent of one another and create a speckled impression of color flow. A high

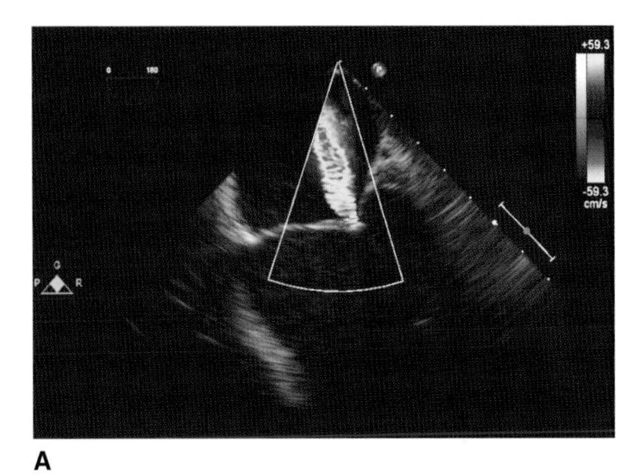

A

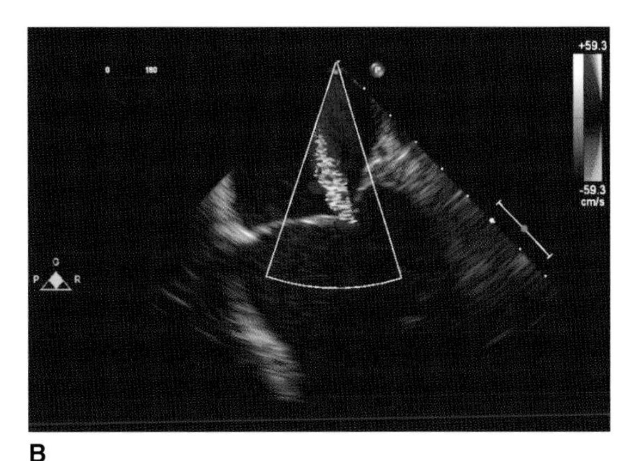

B

FIGURE 2–8. Color-flow Doppler imaging using an enhanced or velocity map **(A)** versus a turbulent map **(B)**. In **(A)** there is direction and velocity information, while in **(B)** there is the added information for the detection of turbulence in this mitral regurgitation jet.

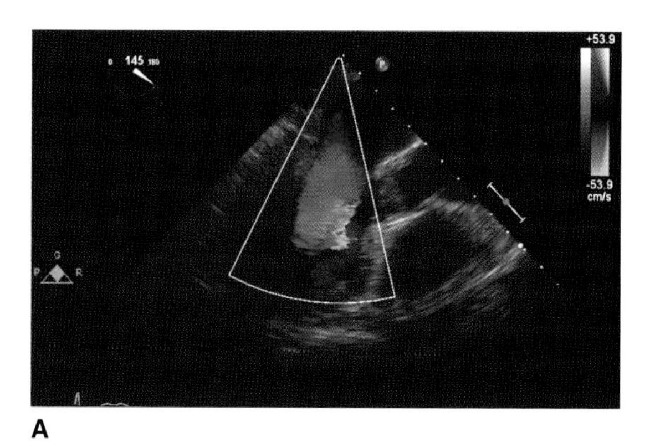

A

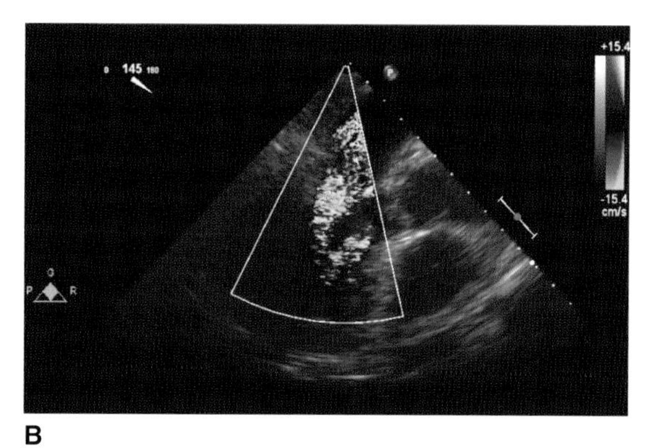

B

FIGURE 2–9. Shifting the scale of the color-flow Doppler. In **(A)** the scale is set at the normal default setting and flow through the mitral valve in diastole is optimally seen. In **(B)** the Nyquist limit has been set to a much lower value and the flow through the mitral valve in diastole now appears as a mosaic, which may be mistaken for turbulent blood flow. Lowering the scale for color Doppler helps in optimizing low-velocity flow, but should not be used for normal-velocity flow.

degree of smoothing will make the color packets appear as though they were blended together. The appearance of color filling improves with higher levels of smoothing. If the color appears bright and flashy within the color box, it may help to decrease the *color gain*. Table 2–2 lists the most commonly used controls for adjusting the color Doppler display.

PULSED-WAVE AND CONTINUOUS-WAVE DOPPLER

PW Doppler samples velocities at a specific point along the beam axis. A gate designates the sampling point and its position within a 2D image, and the trackball moves the pulse sample gate within the ultrasound image. The disadvantage of PW lies in its susceptibility to aliasing. This type of Doppler is best for low-velocity flows or selecting a specific area to interrogate blood flow.

CW Doppler possesses a clear advantage over PW Doppler in its lack of a Nyquist limit. This means that the high-velocity flows will not alias. However, if the scale on the Doppler waveform display is set too low, it may appear to wrap around in the same manner as PW Doppler. If this occurs, the scale (cm/s) can be increased to the desired velocity range. CW Doppler is not depth specific. While using CW, the ultrasound machine samples all along the beam axis, constantly sending and receiving Doppler signals. Figure 2–10 compares the Doppler spectral traces of a high-velocity jet in a patient with mitral regurgitation. Figure 2–10A shows a PW Doppler trace with the sample site in the mitral valve orifice. The flow is aliased and an accurate peak velocity cannot be measured. In Figure 2–10B, the CW Doppler spectral trace shows no aliasing and the peak velocity of the mitral regurgitation is easy to accurately measure.

Table 2–2. Commonly Used Controls for Adjusting Color Doppler Display.

Color Variable	Knob(s)	Function
Map	Map	Provides key to convert velocities into colors
Scale	Scale	Specifies range of velocities that can be expressed by color and the Nyquist limit
Invert	Invert	Inverts assignment of specified color to direction of flow
Sector placement	Position, trackball	Determines placement of color box
Sector size	Size, trackball	Determines size of color box
Gain	Gain	Amplifies color Doppler signal before display
Baseline	Baseline	Shifts the zero baseline of the color-scale velocities
Smoothing	Smoothing	Determines degree of separation of color packets

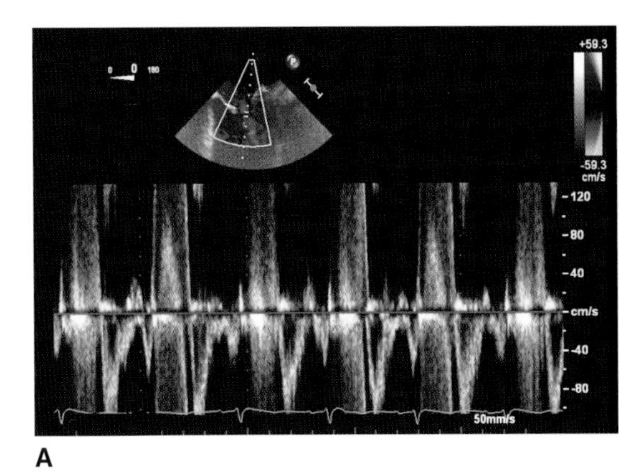

A

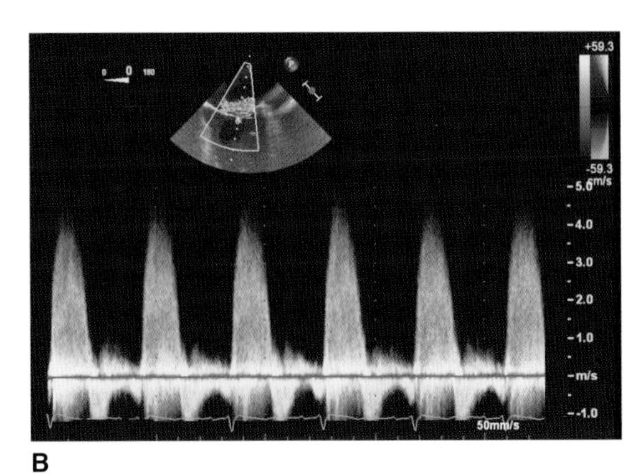

B

FIGURE 2–10. Mitral regurgitation obtained with PW versus CW Doppler. In **(A)** with PW there is aliasing of the systolic flow so that an accurate velocity cannot be obtained. **(B)** shows the full Doppler velocity when using CW.

PW and CW Doppler placements are straightforward and take very little time to learn. It is of primary importance to have the beam axis at an angle as close as possible to 0° (parallel) with blood flow. On the sector display, the dotted line designating Doppler beam placement is positioned within the area of interest using the position button and the trackball. When using PW Doppler mode, the sample gate can move freely vertically along the beam path. Only flow at the point designated by the sample gate will be displayed. Very small, incremental changes in beam axis or sample gate placement can produce significant changes in pressures, velocities, and patterns of flow. Hypertrophic obstructive cardiomyopathy (HOCM) investigation consistently proves the importance of good sample gate and beam axis position. In CW Doppler mode, an operator can adjust only the focal point of the beam, without eliminating any specific depths from the overall Doppler display.

PW and CW Doppler displays may need to be "cleaned up" before they are acceptable for acquisition. Relevant information should be extracted and refined from the Doppler display. Once Doppler sampling placement is optimal, the resulting Doppler signal can be easily manipulated. Common controls to manipulate the signal include Doppler *sweep speed, gain, scale, baseline, compression,* and *reject.* In case Doppler uniformity is preferred, a *Doppler invert* button is also available. The Doppler invert feature will flip the image vertically along the baseline to display flows toward the transducer below the baseline and flows away from the transducer above the baseline. Even though Doppler invert provides no additional Doppler information, it can make a more aesthetically pleasing comparison of Doppler frames during interpretation.

Sweep speed changes the number and width of Doppler waveforms that can be displayed in a single picture. Increasing the sweep speed effectively zooms in on one or a few Doppler waveforms at a time. High sweep speed is optimal for patients in normal sinus rhythm with multiple uniform Doppler readings over time. Conversely, sweep speed should be reduced for a patient with significant Doppler variations between cardiac cycles or for arrhythmic patients. Other common indications for very slow sweep speed include assessment of tamponade or constriction, for which the presence or absence of respiratory variation needs to be demonstrated. Figure 2–11 is an example of three spectral traces with various sweep speeds.

Gain amplifies or de-amplifies the returning signal from the moving red blood cells. The gain is often preset, but changing gain can compensate for low- or high-density red blood cell movement. The Doppler spectral signal itself should be a midlevel gray, and the Doppler background should be black. If the signal is bright white, Doppler gain should be reduced. If it is very faint or totally black but present, Doppler gain should be increased. Increasing the audio volume to hear the Doppler shift may be helpful in optimizing the spectral trace. Audio volume provides critical information when using Pedoff-style probes, which produce Doppler signals with no 2D image for guidance. Figure 2–12 compares a Doppler spectral trace with too low a gain setting (see Figure 2–12A) with optimal gain setting (see Figure 2–12B). Figure 2–12C is an example of a very high Doppler gain setting.

The *scale setting* controls the highest and lowest velocity (cm/s) levels that can be presented on the Doppler display. If the baseline is in the center of the Doppler display y-axis, then the highest velocities that can be detected above and below the baseline (toward and away from the probe) should be the same. If a flow velocity is very high or very low, it may be necessary to alter the Doppler scale.

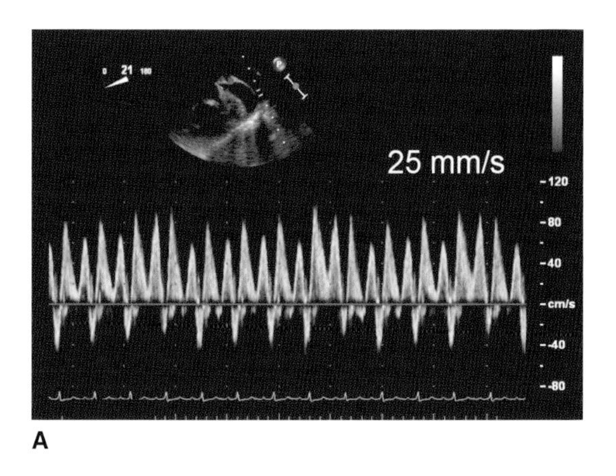

A

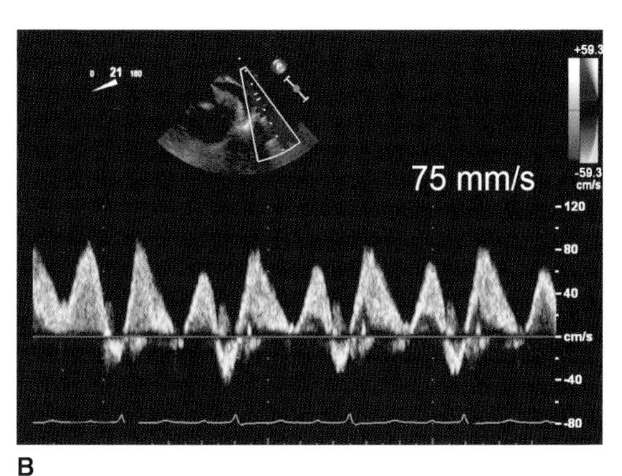

B

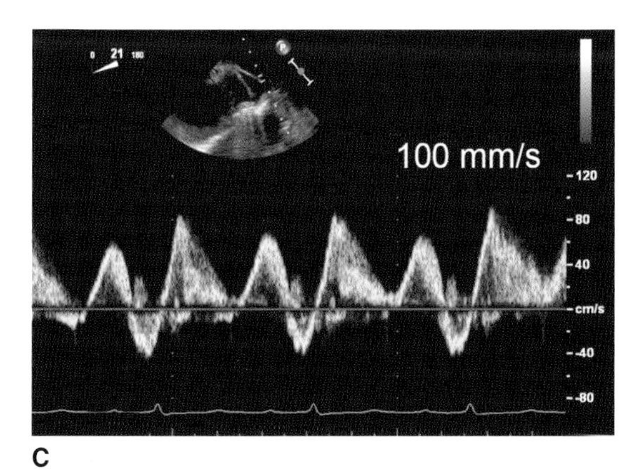

C

FIGURE 2–11. Flow from a pulmonary vein into the left atrium by pulsed Doppler. The spectral trace is seen at a very low sweep speed in **(A)** (25 mm/s). The medium setting for sweep speed is shown in **(B)** (75 mm/s), and a very fast sweep speed (100 mm/s) is shown in **(C)**.

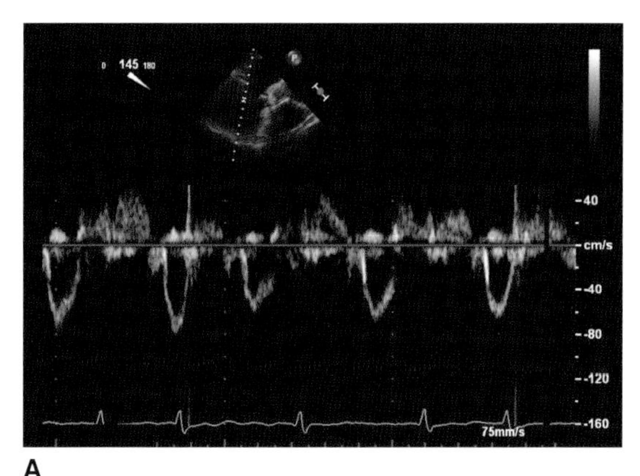

A

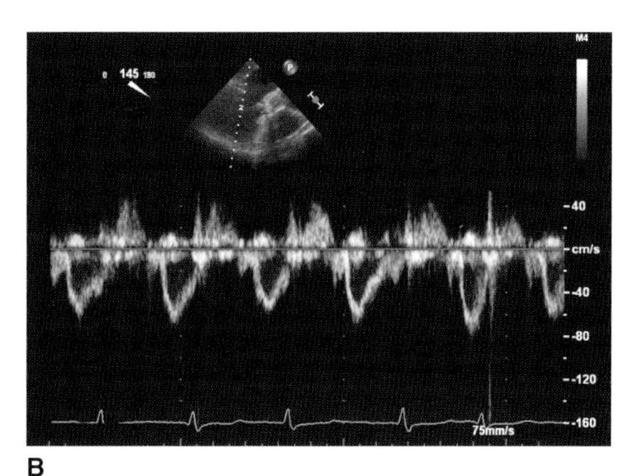

B

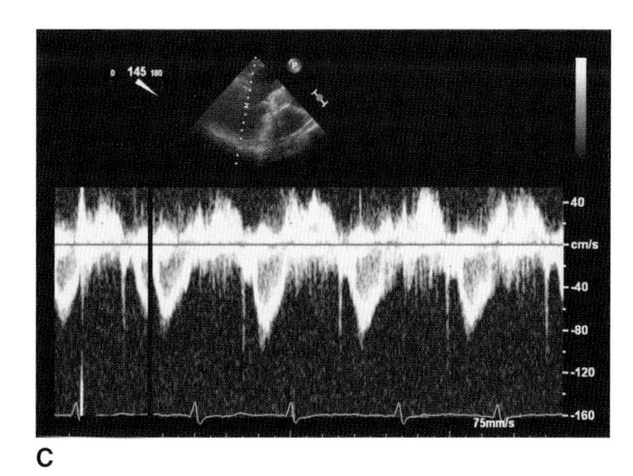

C

FIGURE 2–12. The effect of gain on the Doppler spectral trace. In **(A)** there is a very low gain setting so that the complete spectral trace is not seen. In **(B)** there is an optimal setting for gain, and in **(C)** there is a high gain setting.

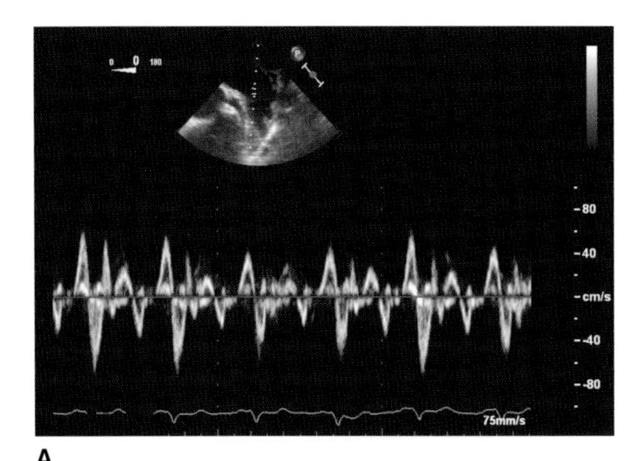

A

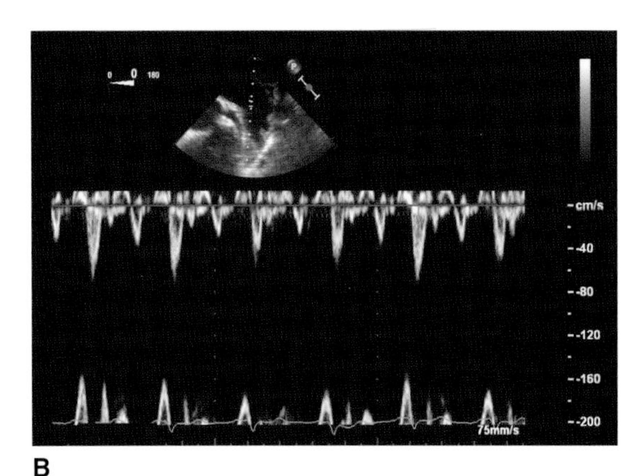

B

FIGURE 2–13. The effect of baseline shift on a Doppler spectral trace. In **(A)**, the baseline is positioned in the middle of the trace, while in **(B)** the baseline has been shifted to the top of the spectral trace.

The *baseline* is a horizontal line showing the zero velocity point over time. Velocities can be shown symmetrically above and below the baseline. The alternative is to eliminate unwanted information by raising or lowering the zero velocity point along the y-axis of the Doppler display to focus attention on flow above or below the baseline. Figure 2–13 depicts the effect of shifting the Doppler spectral trace baseline.

Doppler *compression* changes the number of gray shades assigned to the spectral display. Increasing the numerical level of Doppler compression creates a softer, smoother, gray Doppler display. A lower numerical level of Doppler compression creates a harsh display with more black-and-white contrast and fewer shades of gray. Figure 2–14 shows an example of changing the compression on the Doppler spectral trace. Figure 2–14A is an example of high Doppler compression setting showing

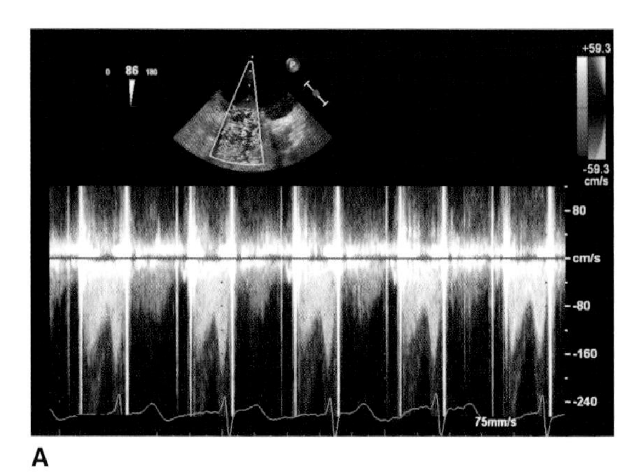

A

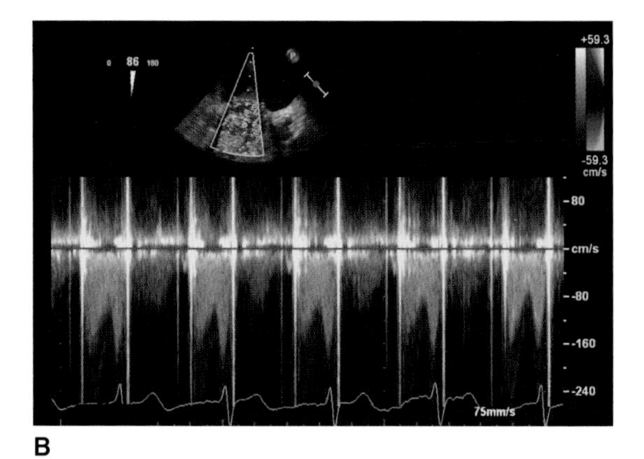

B

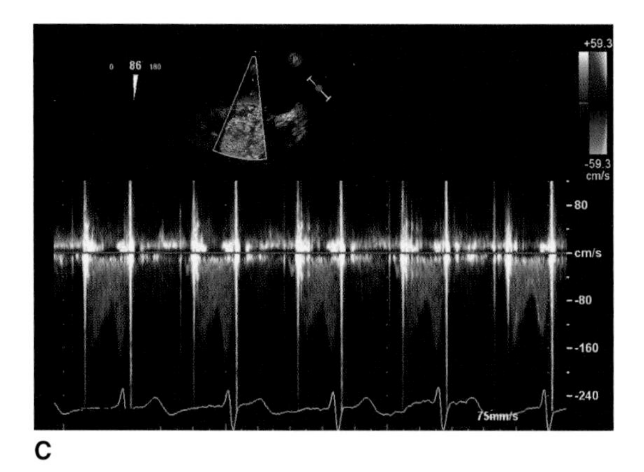

C

FIGURE 2–14. The effect of compression on the Doppler spectral trace. **(A)** is a very high compression setting so that the low amplitude noise is displayed. In **(B)** there is an optimal setting for compression, and in **(C)** there is a low compression setting so that some of the information is missing from the spectral trace.

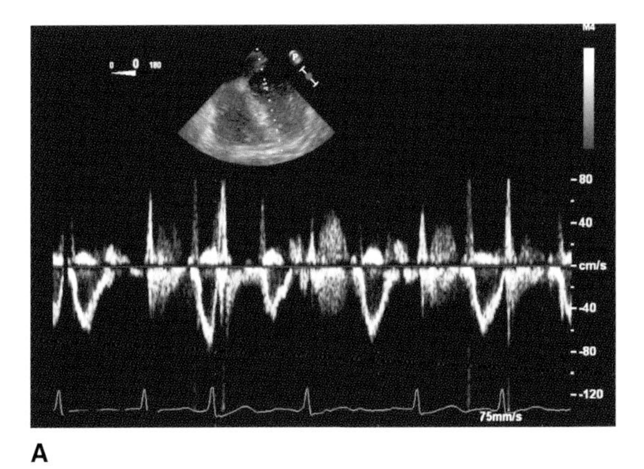

A

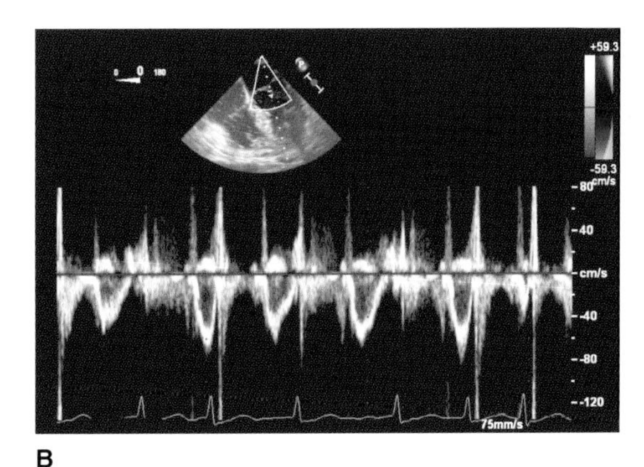

B

FIGURE 2–15. Application of Doppler reject. In **(A)** the reject control is at a high setting so that a lot of the background noise is not displayed. In **(B)** the reject is set lower and more of the background noise is seen.

too many low amplitude signals. In Figure 2–14B, the trace displays optimal shades of gray. In Figure 2–14C, the spectral trace is at a lower compression setting.

Reject is a function that can eliminate low-velocity signals, which usually are seen near the baseline. Reject brings the Doppler background to black or close to it. Reject also helps to define the borders of the Doppler signal. When tracing or measuring, the reject should be set at an acceptable level to eliminate baseline noise. Figure 2–15 shows the use of reject on the Doppler spectral trace. Figure 2–15A shows a spectral trace with reject set higher, thus eliminating the background noise. Figure 2–15B shows an example of low reject with more background noise seen on the display.

Doppler measurements are often necessary for a complete cardiac assessment. Relevant controls to accomplish this task include freeze, caliper, trace, enter, erase, and the trackball. Caliper measurements of PW and CW Doppler can be made with the caliper, trackball, and enter controls, and typically are used for machine calculations of instantaneous velocity and pressure. Traced Doppler measurements, made by using the trace, trackball, and enter buttons, provide information on peak velocity, and peak and mean pressure gradients. The erase button may be pressed one or more times to remove one or all Doppler measurements from the image waveforms. Figure 2–16 shows examples of typical Doppler measurements. Figure 2–16A displays a simple caliper measurement of an aortic stenosis Doppler velocity and peak gradient. Figure 2–16B shows the same Doppler spectral trace with more advanced measurements performed under the system's analysis package.

Doppler measurements can be recorded inside or outside the machine analysis package. The analysis package on any machine is intended to label, identify, and present measurements in an organized manner. Calculations can be simplified: once certain Doppler measurements are accumulated, the machine may be able to compute additional helpful values by using previously programmed ultrasound equations. Table 2–3 lists the most commonly used controls for PW and CW Doppler variables.

ZOOM

Zooming an area of interest is another good way to isolate a part of cardiac anatomy or to remove unwanted information from the display sector. Zooming trims from the x- and y-axes of the sector, increases frame rate, and increases spatial resolution. *Zoom* can be selected on the machine and an initial zoom box will appear. Zoom parameters for the box can be changed by using the size and position buttons, and the trackball until the area of interest is adequately covered. Figure 2–17A shows a normal, full-sector-size image. Figure 2–17B shows a zoomed view of the same image, focusing on the left atrial appendage.

FREEZE

Although the freeze button is fairly simple and straightforward, it should not be underestimated. When measuring 2D, PW, or CW images, an operator must first freeze the image and sometimes scroll backward or forward in time to obtain the correct frame. Individual frames can be compared and scrolled as needed. In TEE, the freeze button should be used whenever the probe is not actively needed (eg, when introducing the probe into the esophagus, after completion of the examination, or during cardiopulmonary bypass). Freezing

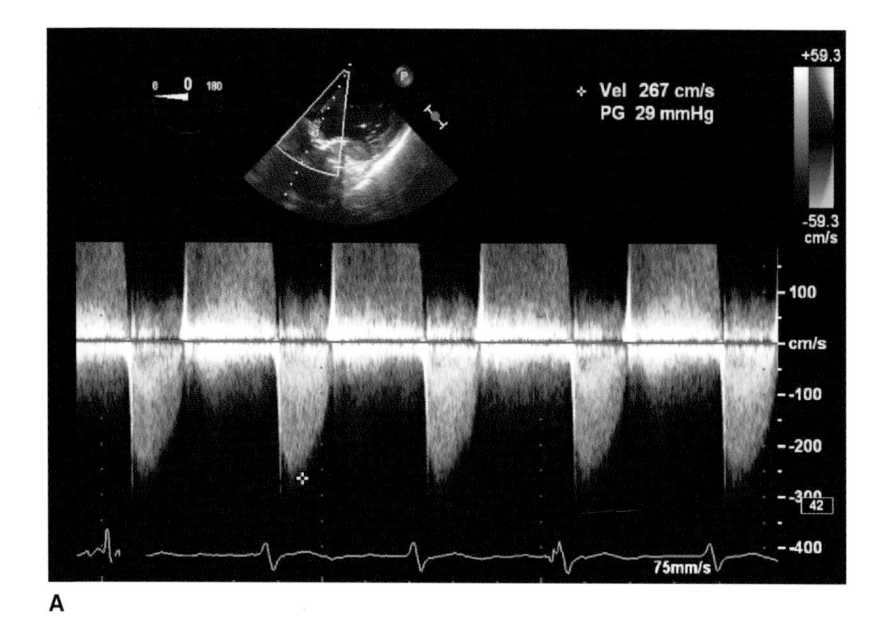

A

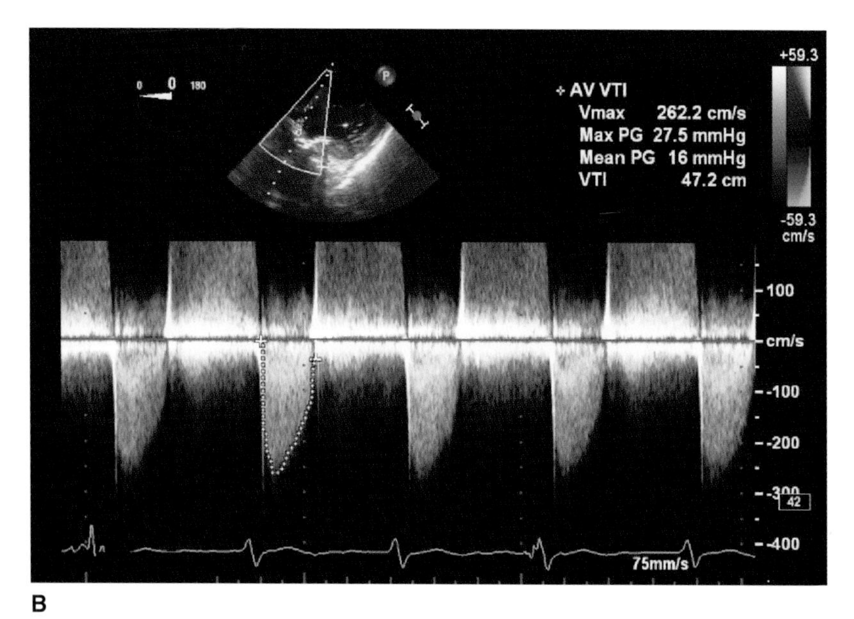

B

FIGURE 2–16. Measurement of aortic stenosis **(A)** shows a simple measurement of the peak velocity and peak gradient in a patient with aortic stenosis. **(B)** shows the same spectral trace that now has more advanced measurements performed.

the image stops probe sound transmission, thus decreasing the chance of the probe overheating.

MEASUREMENTS

All echocardiographic images can be measured and quantified. Buttons used for gray-scale assessments may include *freeze*, *caliper*, *trace*, *enter*, and *erase*. Measurements of 2D images can be made outside or inside the analysis package. If measurements are made within the analysis package, the operator will need to select the *analysis* or *measurement package* button and then the proper name for the subsequent measurement. A pair of calipers is provided for exact linear measurements of

Table 2–3. Commonly Used Controls for PW and CW Doppler.

PW/CW Variable	Knob(s)	Function
Sample placement	Position, trackball	Specifies location of Doppler beam
Scale	Scale	Specifies range of velocities that can be displayed and the Nyquist limit (PW)
Sweep speed	Sweep speed	Changes number of cycles that can be shown on the x-axis of the Doppler display
Gain	Gain	Amplifies PW and CW Doppler signals before display
Baseline	Baseline	Positions the zero baseline of the Doppler display
Compression	Compression	Changes the difference between the highest and lowest received amplitudes (shades of gray)
Reject	Reject	Eliminates low-velocity signals near zero baseline
Invert	Invert	Determines the presentation of signals as above or below zero baseline regardless of direction of flow
Measurements	Freeze, caliper, trace, enter, erase	Quantifies features of a PW or CW Doppler spectral display

CW, continuous wave; PW, pulsed wave.

gray-scale images. The first caliper has to be entered onto a point to have the second caliper appear. Once the second caliper is set, then the machine calculates the linear distance between the two points. Multiple linear caliper measurements can be made. Calipers are removed by using the erase button. To obtain the area or circumference of an object, the *trace*, *trackball*, and *enter* buttons are commonly used. On some ultrasound machines, once the trace function is selected, the first given caliper is set to a starting point and the trackball is used to follow the borders of the desired region. When the border is outlined and the dotted tracing line

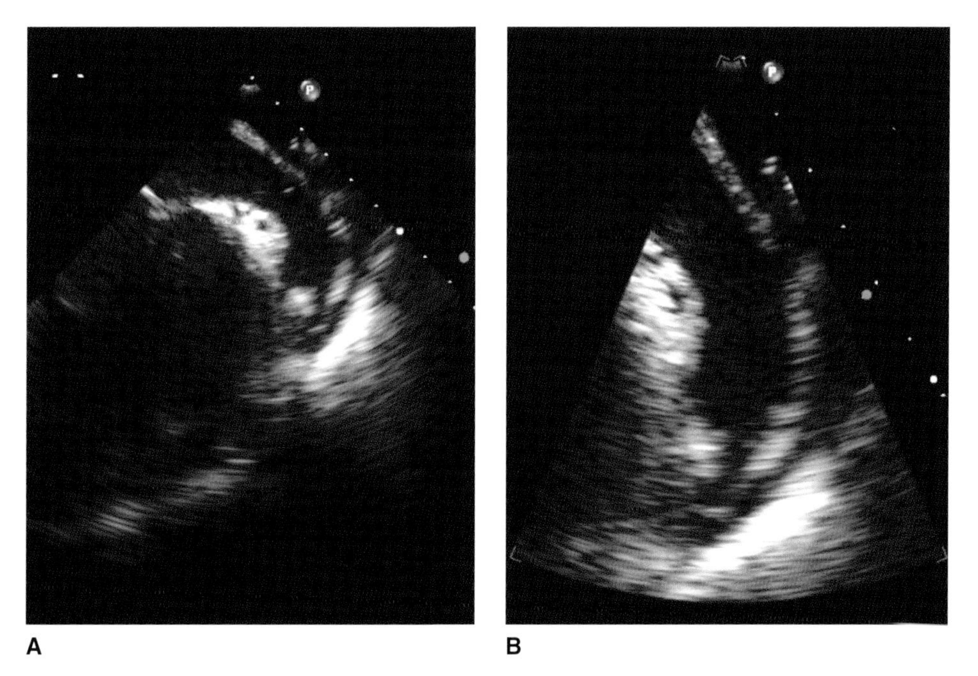

FIGURE 2–17. Using the zoom control. In **(A)** the left atrial appendage is viewed with zoom turned off. In **(B)** the system zoom has been turned on and the left atrial appendage appears much larger.

is returned to the starting point, the outline must be entered before the machine will calculate any area. The operator has the ability to backtrack a traced line or completely remove any given trace by using the erase function.

ANNOTATION

Annotations are labels that are in the form of text or pictures; they can be used to accompany an image for communication. Nonstandard views, unusual anatomic variations, or highly edited standard views may need some further explanation. It is also helpful to annotate when a standard view is not available or is of very poor quality. Naming anatomic landmarks, body positioning of the patient, relationships to other anatomic points of reference, or timing of events is often helpful for the interpreting physician. For example, it may be useful to label an image as a pre- or postsurgical event. Applied comments should be removed after the image is recorded so that later pictures are not confusing as a result of incorrect labeling.

THREE-DIMENSIONAL IMAGING

Three-dimensional TEE is a new diagnostic tool that has already proven to be helpful in the preoperative assessment of mitral valve disease. This is especially true for mitral valve prolapse patients being considered for repair rather than replacement. Once a 3D TEE image is obtained, it can be rotated and cropped in order to display specific anatomy, and then these images can be saved as still pictures or moving loops. Figure 2–18 is an example of a flail mitral valve imaged with a 3D TEE probe pre- and post-repair. The 3D has been cropped and rotated into the "surgeon's" view so that the mitral valve is viewed from the left atrium down towards the ventricle.

The 3D TEE image can also be saved as a dataset from which additional images can be derived after the study is completed. Emerging software is available for on-line or off-line analysis of these 3D datasets, and can provide additional information on valve size and structure. Figure 2–19 is an example of this type of

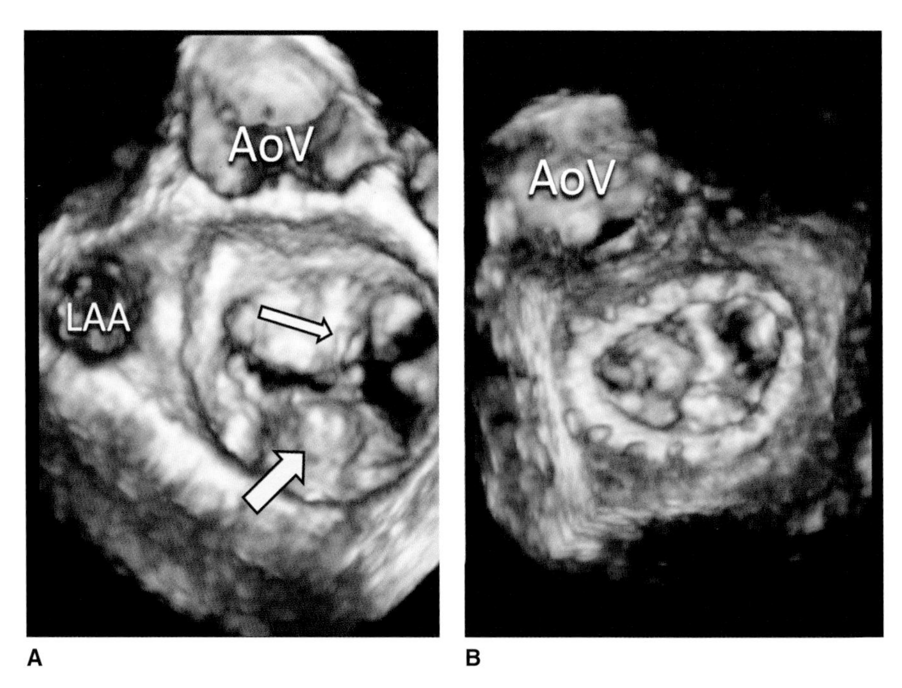

FIGURE 2–18. Three-dimensional TEE examples of the mitral valve from the left atrial side. **A:** Mitral valve prolapse *(large arrow)* of the posterior leaflet (P2 segment) with a torn chordae *(small arrow)*. **B:** Annuloplasty ring after mitral valve repair. AoV = aortic valve; LAA = left atrial appendage.

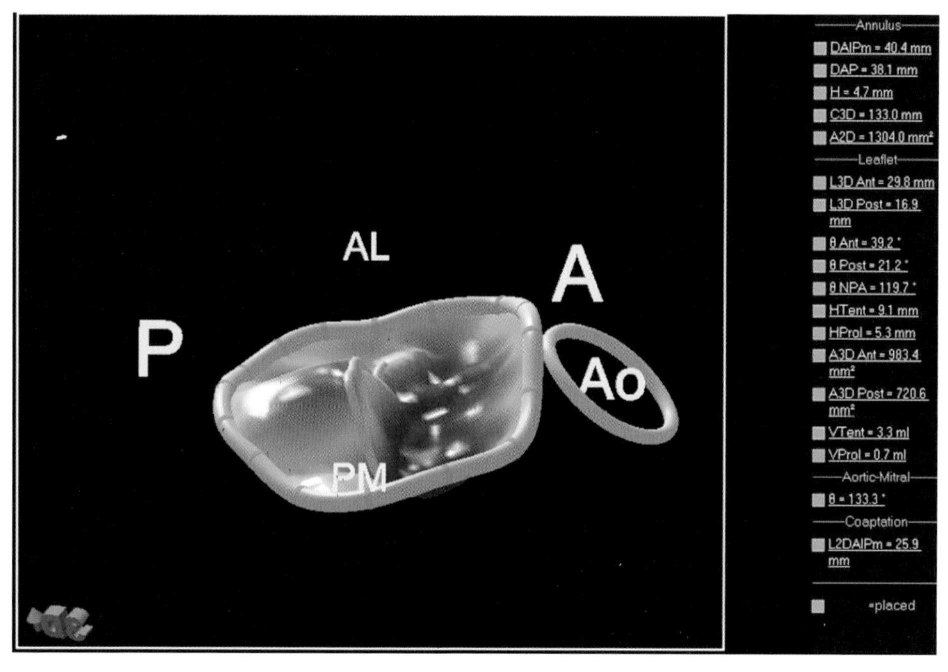

FIGURE 2–19. An example of mitral valve quantification using software to model the mitral annulus and leaflet geometry.

derived information obtained from a 3D TEE dataset. Further research is required to verify the clinical utility of these data.

CONCLUSION

Image quality and diagnostic accuracy depend heavily on the knowledge and skill of the clinician operating the ultrasound machine. Awareness of the basic knobs associated with 2D, color Doppler, PW Doppler, and CW Doppler is absolutely essential for performing a good TEE examination. In addition to the controls for adjusting a 2D TEE image, 3D TEE adds a variety of tools for manipulating 3D data sets. Although simple display manipulation may seem difficult at first, image optimization becomes second nature with time and experience.

REVIEW QUESTIONS

1. Which of the following is *NOT* a common mode used during TEE examinations?
   a. Color Doppler
   b. Speckle tracking
   c. Continuous-wave Doppler
   d. Two-dimensional gray-scale imaging

2. Two-dimensional gray scale is considered what type of imaging?
   a. Ionizing
   b. Darkness
   c. Quantitative
   d. Brightness

3. The most important control for two-dimensional gray-scale imaging is:
   a. TGC
   b. Gain
   c. Color Doppler
   d. Compression

4. Time gain compensation (TGC) is a control that allows the operator to:
   a. Help with color Doppler.
   b. Make a pretty picture.
   c. Compensate for ultrasound attenuation.
   d. Decrease the power into the patient's tissue.

5. The two-dimensional compression control changes:
   a. The peak velocity in CW Doppler
   b. The 2D sector to get rid of extra targets outside of the image

c. The difference between highest and lowest shade of gray
d. The amount of artifacts seen in the picture

6. The zoom control is used for which of the following?
a. It enhances color-flow Doppler.
b. It magnifies an area of interest within the image.
c. It makes the entire image appear bigger on the display.
d. It helps position a pulse Doppler sample volume.

7. Annotation is used for which of the following purposes?
a. Adding text to the image
b. Helping to determine which view you're looking at
c. Constructing an ultrasound report within the image
d. Controlling the overall system gain

8. Ultrasound harmonic frequencies are the result of:
a. Side lobe artifacts
b. A strong reflector in the near field
c. Propagation of the ultrasound through tissue
d. A strong ultrasound reflector in the far field

9. The Doppler effect is best described as:
a. What happens when ultrasound travels over a short distance
b. What happens when ultrasound travels over a large distance
c. The result of artifacts created by the ultrasound machine
d. A change in frequency that occurs between a sound source and receiver

10. By convention, which of the following is the direction of color-flow Doppler maps in cardiac ultrasound?
a. Red towards, blue away
b. Blue towards, red away
c. Red towards, green away
d. Green towards, red away

11. Which of the following colors is added to denote turbulent flow in color Doppler systems?
a. Red
b. Gray
c. Blue
d. Green

12. An ultrasound machine that transmits and receives using the same frequency is operating in which of the following ways?
a. Tissue Doppler
b. Harmonic imaging
c. Fundamental imaging
d. Spectral tracking

13. In pulsed-wave Doppler echocardiography, which of the following statements is true?
a. Aliasing is rarely a problem.
b. The size of the sample gate cannot be changed.
c. High-velocity flows can be accurately measured.
d. Combined with 2D imaging, you can localize where flow is occurring.

14. Which of the following is typically *NOT* a hyperechoic structure?
a. Pericardium
b. Pacer lead
c. Myocardial hypertrophy
d. Bioprosthetic MV annular ring

15. Lowering the Nyquist limit is useful in:
a. Evaluating MR
b. Interrogating a PFO
c. Increasing frame rate
d. Imaging at a shallow depth

16. CW Doppler is often used in evaluating:
a. PV flow
b. Stenotic valves
c. LAA velocities
d. Annular velocities

17. In the setting of probe overheating, which machine control can assist in decreasing probe temperature?
a. Gain
b. Output power
c. Freeze
d. Depth

18. Which spectral Doppler trace can be mistaken for the other?
a. TR and PS
b. PV and hepatic vein flow
c. Aliased MR and TS
d. MR and LVOT obstruction

19. A normal MV may appear thickened due to the improper use of which machine control?
a. Gain
b. Reject
c. Increased depth
d. Lateral gain compensation (LGC)

20. Improper use of which machine control could appear as an effusion on the display?
a. Time gain compensation (TGC)
b. Output power
c. Compression
d. Color Doppler

21. Which function will not increase frame rate?
    a. Zoom
    b. Sector size
    c. Depth
    d. CW Doppler

22. Which of the following color maps only show direction and velocity?
    a. Variance
    b. Velocity

23. On a patient's TEE, MR is shown with color Doppler using the color map invert function. The jets' primary color would be:
    a. Blue
    b. Red

24. Output power is the same as overall gain.
    a. True
    b. False

25. The highest frame rate will occur using a ________ color sector.
    a. Large
    b. Small

Anatomic Variants and Ultrasound Artifacts

3

Wendy L. Pabich and Katherine Grichnik

Anatomic variants are variations in normal anatomy that can be misinterpreted as pathological conditions. Many anatomic variants are remnant structures from embryological development and fetal circulation, particularly in the atria. Anatomic variants are seen in multiple image planes and persist despite changes in transducer frequency, gain, compression, and depth. *Ultrasound artifacts* are errors in imaging most commonly due to a violation of the assumptions that are inherent in any ultrasound system. All imaging systems assume that sound travels in a straight line, travels directly back from a reflector, and travels at exactly 1540 m/s through soft tissue. Additionally, it is assumed that the ultrasound beam is very thin, reflections are entirely from structures within the main axis of the beam, and the intensity of reflections is related only to the tissue characteristics of the reflector.[1] Artifacts cross known anatomic planes and boundaries and typically disappear with alternate imaging planes and when remedial actions are taken. It is vital to be familiar with the common anatomic variations and ultrasound imaging artifacts to ensure accurate echocardiographic interpretation and to avoid unnecessary interventions.[2]

DEVELOPMENT OF ANATOMIC VARIANTS[3]

The atria and the sinus venosus evolve in the 4th week of embryonic development. Initially, the sinus venosus receives venous blood from left and right sinus horns (Figure 3–1A and B). In time, the veins to the left sinus horn are obliterated and the remnants become the coronary sinus. The right sinus horn, on the other hand, enlarges and forms the smooth-walled part of the right atrium (RA), known as the sinus venarum. As the RA expands, the sinus venarum displaces the trabeculated tissue of the primitive RA into the periphery and into the right atrial appendage (which may have prominent pectinate muscles). Right and left venous valves mark the junction of the original sinus venarum and the primitive RA. The left venous valve disappears as it fuses with the developing atrial septum. The right venous valve of the right sinus venosus horn develops inferiorly into (1) the valve of the inferior vena cava (IVC) or the eustachian valve, which directs fetal blood flow from the IVC across the foramen ovale, and (2) the valve to the coronary sinus or the thebesian valve (Figure 3–2). Superiorly, the convergence of the smooth sinus venarum and the trabeculated RA is the crista terminalis. Concurrently, the atrial septum forms with migration of the septum primum to obliterate the ostium primum, followed by the migration of the septum secundum to cover the ostium secundum. This migration leads to the characteristic thin-walled appearance of the foramen ovale, with incomplete septation leading to the possibility of a patent foramen ovale.

In the left atrium (LA), the smooth tissue of the pulmonary veins is incorporated into the wall of the left atrium and it displaces the primitive atrial trabeculated tissue almost entirely into the left atrial appendage. The ridge of tissue at the junction of the smooth left superior pulmonary vein and the trabeculated left atrial appendage is called the ligament of Marshall or, more colloquially, the coumadin ridge (since this structure was initially misinterpreted as a thrombus requiring anticoagulation). During the 8th week of embryonic development, the distal end of the left common cardinal vein degenerates, and the proximal portion connects via the left brachiocephalic vein to the right brachiocephalic vein, forming the superior vena cava (SVC). The left posterior cardinal vein also degenerates and the remnants of the left sinus horn, receiving venous drainage from the heart, become the coronary sinus. Failure of the left posterior cardinal vein to resorb results in a persistent left superior vena cava (PLSVC) that drains into and dilates the coronary sinus.

ANATOMIC VARIANTS BY LOCATION

The anatomic variants are best classified by location, although some variant structures can appear in more than one cardiac chamber.

Right Atrium

CRISTA TERMINALIS

The crista terminalis is seen at the junction of the SVC and the RA, forming a structure that may appear to

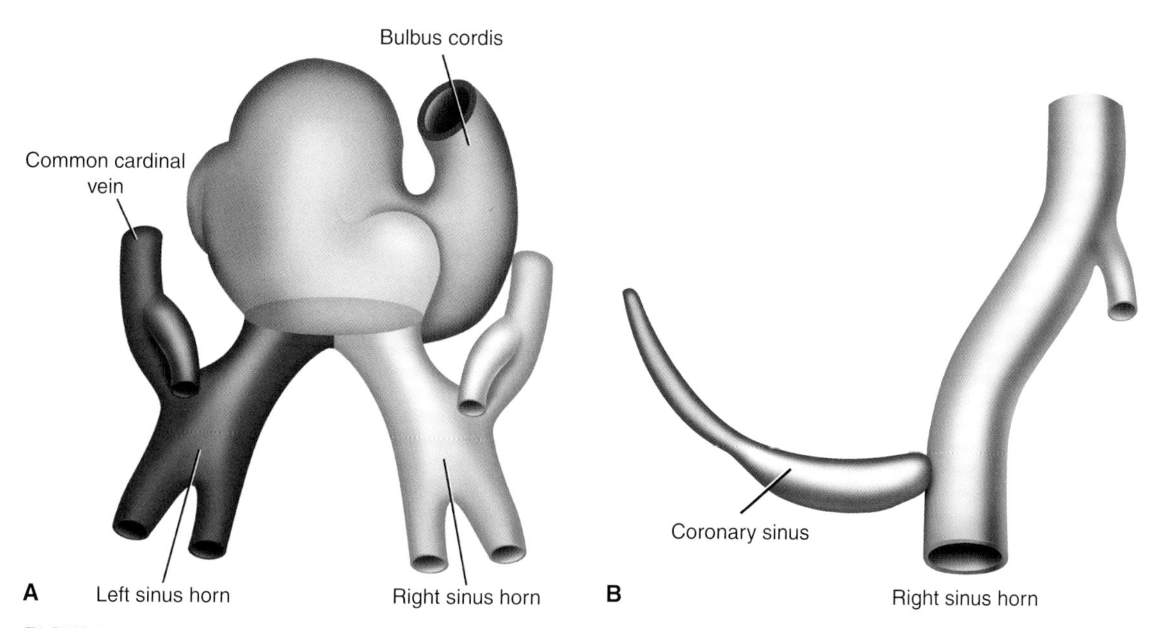

FIGURE 3–1. **A:** Illustration of the right and left sinus venosus horns as they join the developing heart.[3] **B:** The remnant of the left sinus venosus horn becomes the coronary sinus, which joins the right sinus venosus horn on the posterior aspect of the developing heart.[3]

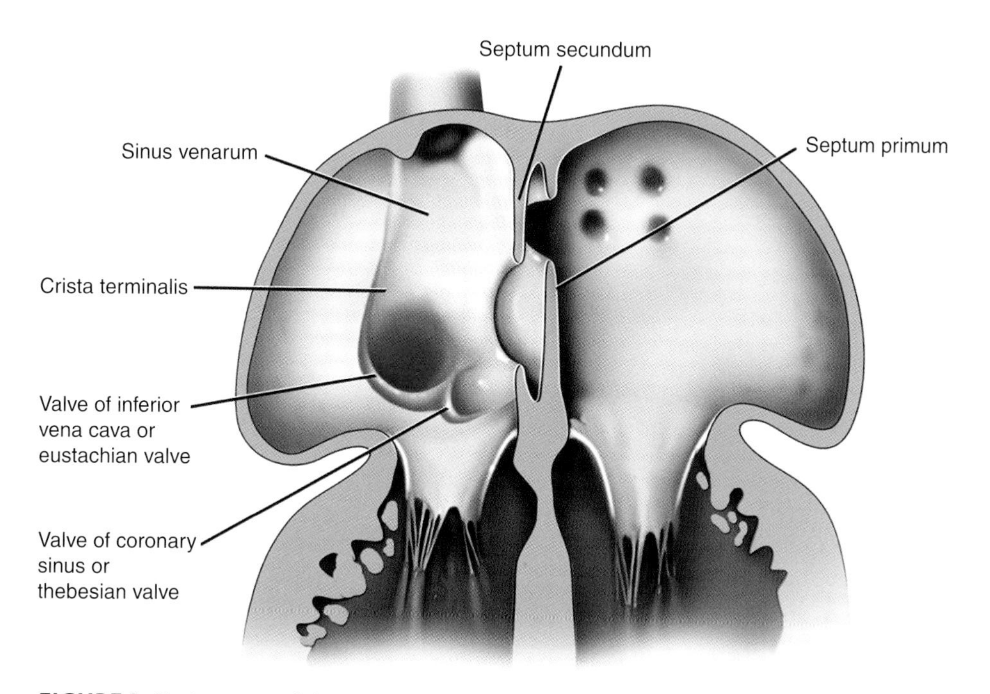

FIGURE 3–2. Anatomy of the right atrium demonstrating the crista terminalis, atrial septum, and the eustachian and thebesian valves.

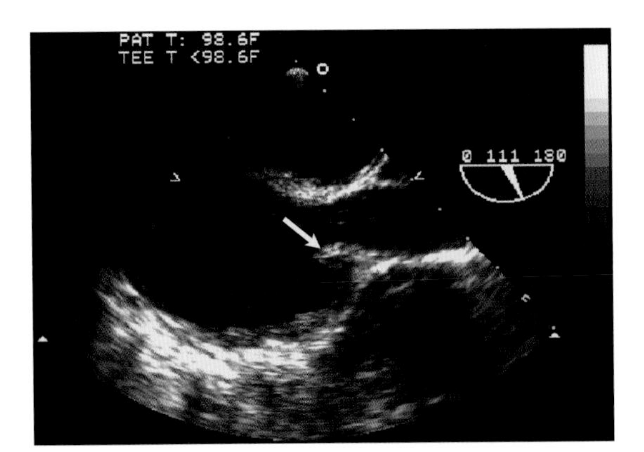

FIGURE 3–3. The crista terminalis is shown at the arrow.

protrude longitudinally into the RA towards the IVC. This structure is often visualized in the midesophageal (ME) bicaval view and should not be mistaken for thrombus or tumor (Figure 3–3). Of note, the crista terminalis is thought to be a location where atrial tachydysrhythmias originate due to the high density of adrenergic nerve fibers, and thus may be a site for ablation therapy.[4]

EUSTACHIAN VALVE

The eustachian valve can be found in multiple views including the ME bicaval view and right ventricular (RV) inflow-outflow views (Figure 3–4). It is seen at the junction of the IVC and RA in approximately 25% of individuals and appears as an elongated, membranous, sometimes undulating structure that can extend from the IVC to the border of the fossa ovalis. Usually it is of no physiological consequence, but it can be confused with an intracardiac thrombus, cause turbulent atrial blood flow, complicate IVC cannulation, or serve as a site for endocarditis or thrombus formation.[5] Occasionally it may also appear to bisect the right atrium, simulating cor triatriatum dexter, but a eustachian valve is distinguished by a lack of flow disturbance on colorflow Doppler examination.[6]

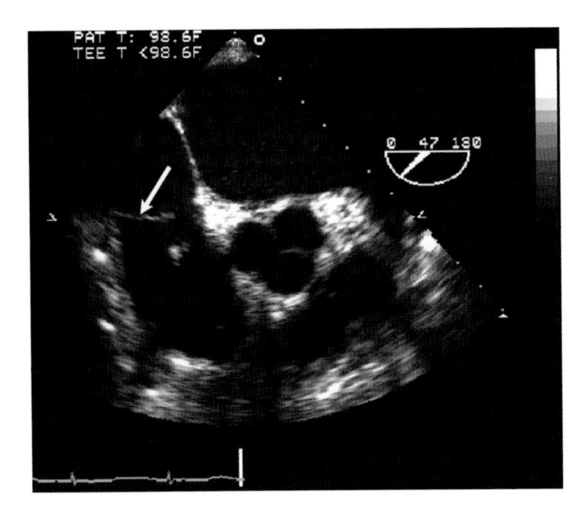

FIGURE 3–4. The eustachian valve is shown at the arrow. A pulmonary artery catheter is also seen inferior to the eustachian valve as a round structure in the right atrium creating an acoustic shadow.

THEBESIAN VALVE

The thebesian valve is a structure that can be seen as a thin piece of tissue guarding the entrance to the coronary sinus in the ME four-chamber view with the probe slightly advanced towards the tricuspid valve. It can also be seen in a modified bicaval view inferior to the left atrium in the atrioventricular groove (Figure 3–5). This valve serves to prevent retrograde flow into the coronary sinus during atrial contraction and is inconsequential unless it inhibits cannulation of the coronary sinus for retrograde cardioplegia catheter placement or biventricular pacing wire advancement.[7]

CHIARI NETWORK

The Chiari network is a thin, mobile, membranous structure seen within the RA in multiple imaging views (Figure 3–6) that is thought to be a remnant of sinus venosus–derived structures. It is similar to but usually more extensively attached to intracardiac structures than the eustachian valve. The Chiari network is typically perforated and associated with the IVC orifice; however, the primary site of origin can vary to include the RA wall, interatrial septum, or the coronary sinus. The Chiari network moves toward the tricuspid valve during atrial contraction followed by a rapid posterior

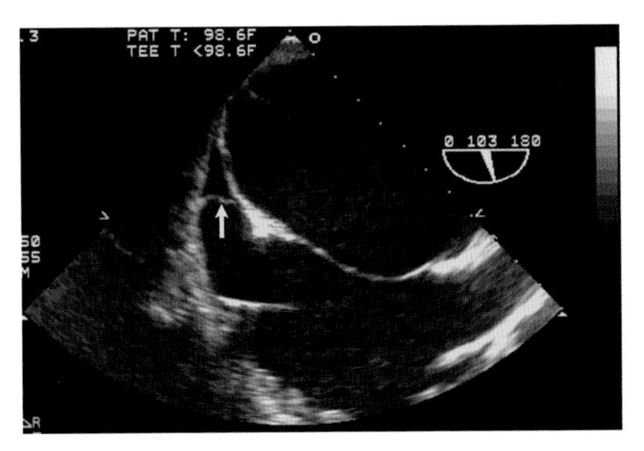

FIGURE 3–5. The thebesian valve *(arrow)* is shown at the mouth of the coronary sinus.

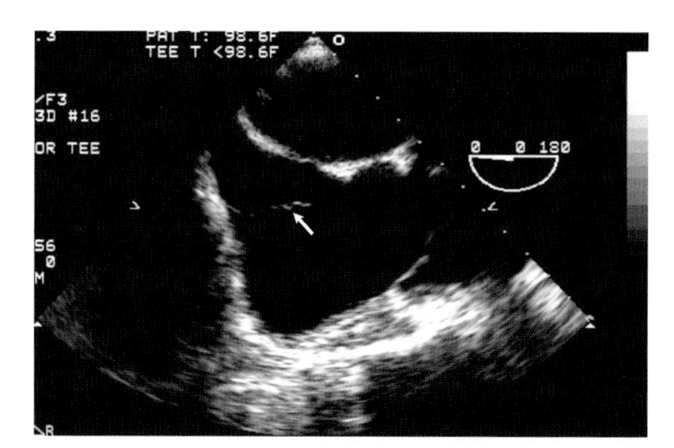

FIGURE 3–6. The Chiari network is shown at the arrow.

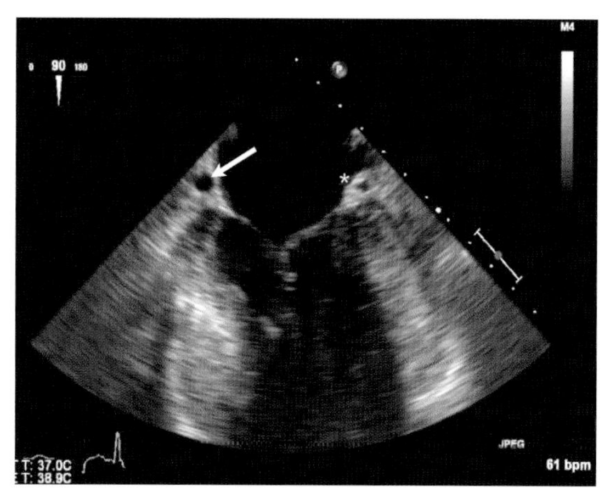

FIGURE 3–8. A normal coronary sinus is shown at the arrow. The circular echolucency on the right side of the image *(near the asterisk)* may be the coronary sinus or the circumflex artery.

motion at the onset of ventricular systole. It has little clinical significance except that it has been associated with a patent foramen ovale, interatrial septal aneurysm, and paradoxical embolization. It is seen in 2% to 3% of all patients at autopsy and by TEE.[8]

PERSISTENT LEFT SUPERIOR VENA CAVA (PLSVC)

The coronary sinus is best seen with slight probe advancement in the ME four-chamber view as an echolucency in the RA, just superior to the tricuspid valve (Figure 3–7). Since it courses in the atrioventricular groove superior to the mitral valve annulus,[9] it can also be seen in a modified ME bicaval view as it curves around the atrium in the atrioventricular groove (see Figure 3–5), or in cross-section in the ME two-chamber view (Figure 3–8). It is a useful structure to identify in order to assist with the placement of coronary sinus catheters for retrograde cardioplegia delivery and pacing wires for biventricular pacing. Despite echocardiographic guidance, injury to the coronary sinus during these procedures is not uncommon.[10] Understanding the normal anatomy of the coronary sinus is also important for identification of an inferior sinus venosus defect. The coronary sinus is normally less than 1 cm wide and approximately 3 cm long, but can dilate as a consequence of right heart volume or pressure overload.[11] Coronary sinus dilation can result from atrial hypertension, tricuspid regurgitation, or a PLSVC that drains into the coronary sinus (Figure 3–9).[12] A PLSVC can also be seen between the left upper pulmonary vein and the left atrial appendage in the ME four-chamber view (Figure 3–10). Diagnosis of a PLSVC is suggested by a dilated coronary sinus (> 1.1 cm) and confirmed by injection of agitated saline into a left upper extremity vein resulting in opacification of the coronary sinus as the PLSVC flow enters the coronary sinus (see Figure 3–10) and then into the RA.

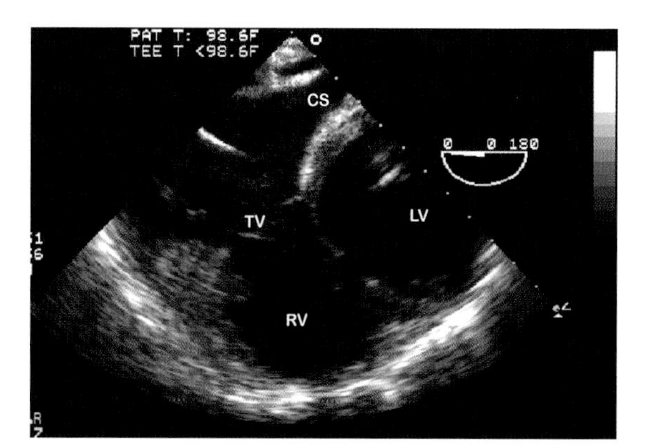

FIGURE 3–7. Dilated coronary sinus (CS) is shown just superior to the tricuspid valve (TV). A pulmonary artery catheter is visible in the right atrium. (RV, right ventricle; LV, left ventricle.)

PATENT FORAMEN OVALE

The normal foramen ovale is seen best in a ME bicaval view; it appears as a thin slice of tissue bound by thicker ridges of tissue, one of which appears as a "flap." Up to 30% of the population may have a probe patent foramen ovale (PFO), with the possibility of right to left intracardiac shunting (Figure 3–11) when right atrial pressure exceeds that of the left atrium.[13] TEE evaluation of the foramen ovale should include 2D assessment for flap movement and color-flow Doppler assessment, optimized for measurement of lower velocity flow.

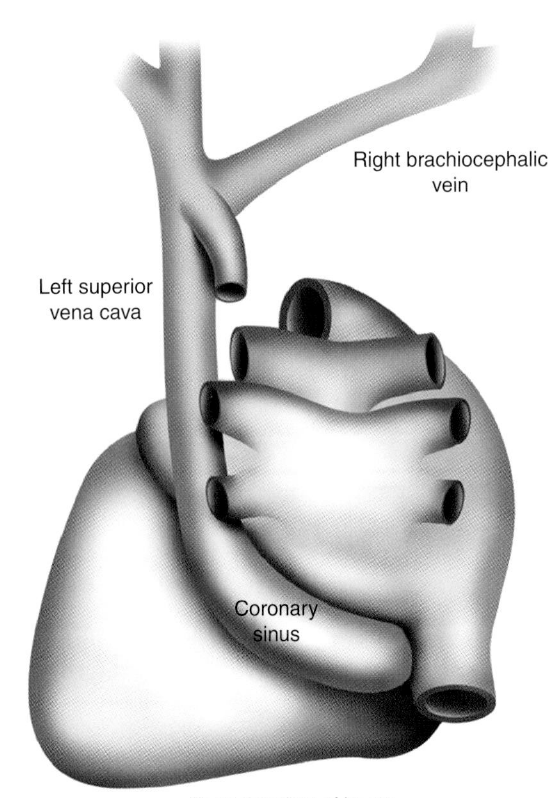

FIGURE 3–9. A drawing of a persistent left superior vena cava.

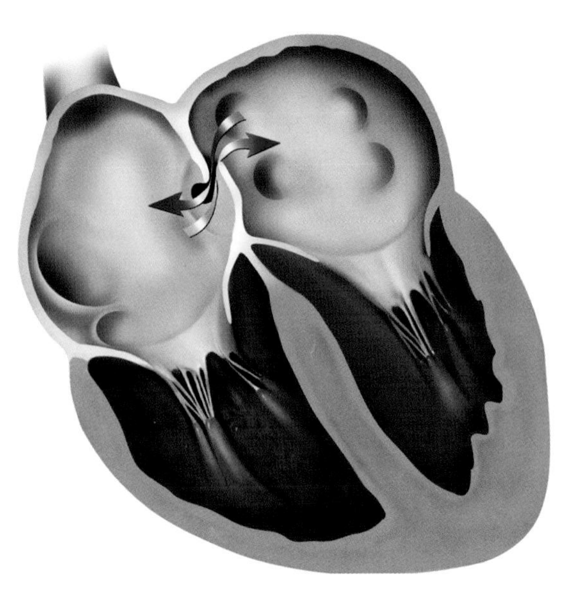

FIGURE 3–11. A drawing of persistent foramen ovale.

Injection of agitated saline (a "bubble study") along with a Valsalva maneuver is typically used to provoke right to left shunting. In such a study, the bubbles should be injected after the Valsalva maneuver produces a decrease in RA volume, and the Valsalva should be released (so as to transiently increase RA pressure over LA pressure) when the microbubbles are first seen to enter the RA. Admixture of agitated saline with small quantities of blood has been reported to improve the acoustic signal of the microbubbles. The bubble study is positive if bubbles appear in the left atrium within five cardiac cycles (Figure 3–12).

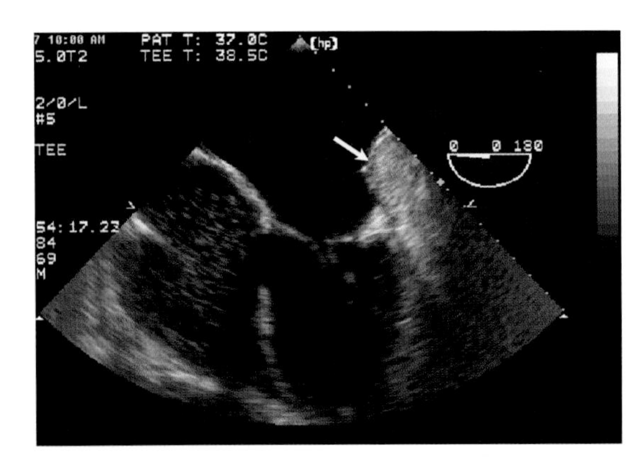

FIGURE 3–10. Opacification of the coronary sinus *(arrow)* after injection of agitated saline into a left arm vein. The bubbles have coursed into the right atrium and ventricle as well.

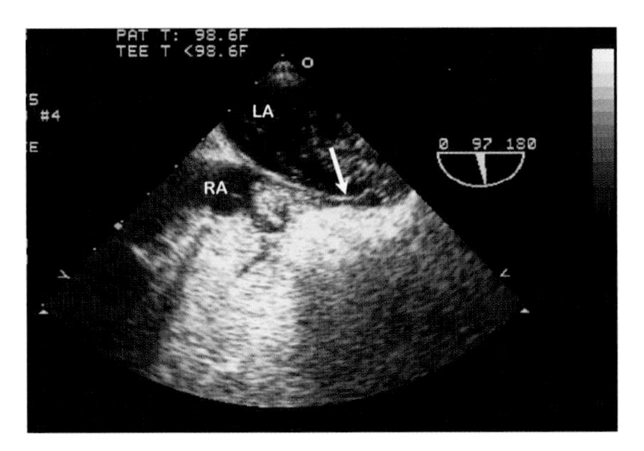

FIGURE 3–12. Positive bubble study in a patient with a patent foramen ovale (PFO). The arrow points to the PFO through which bubbles *(left of arrow)* have entered the left atrium (LA). (RA, right atrium.)

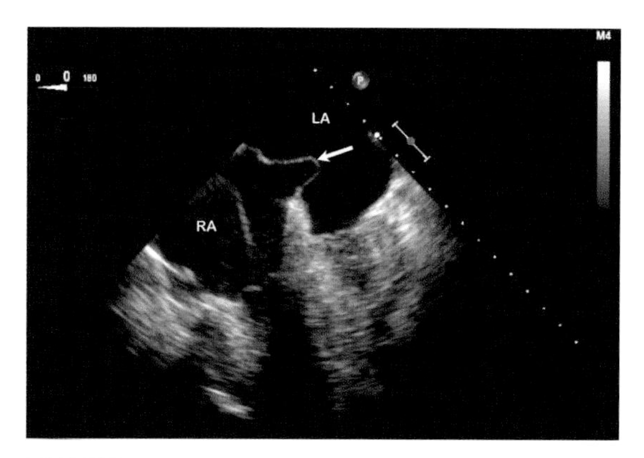

FIGURE 3–13. An interatrial septal aneurysm is demonstrated at the arrow. (LA, left atrium; RA, right atrium.)

ATRIAL SEPTAL ANEURYSM

This condition may be idiopathic or may develop as the result of right heart dysfunction and elevated right-sided pressures.[13] The interatrial septum is enlarged and seen to be undulating between each atrium during the cardiac cycle (Figure 3–13). An interatrial septal aneurysm is defined as constituting more than 1.5 cm of the atrial septum and extending 1.5 cm into either atrial chamber (Figure 3–14). The grading system for these aneurysms is largely based on the extent of excursion into the left and right atrium (see Appendix H). Atrial septal aneurysms have been associated with PFO and Chiari network and may predispose to thrombus formation, resulting in potential paradoxical embolism and stroke.[14] Percutaneously inserted closure devices for PFOs may be efficacious in patients with paradoxical emboli.[15]

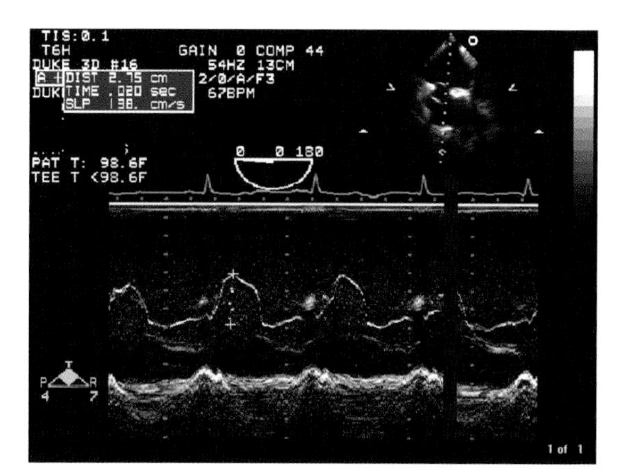

FIGURE 3–14. The image demonstrates the use of M-mode to measure the excursion of an interatrial septal aneurysm.

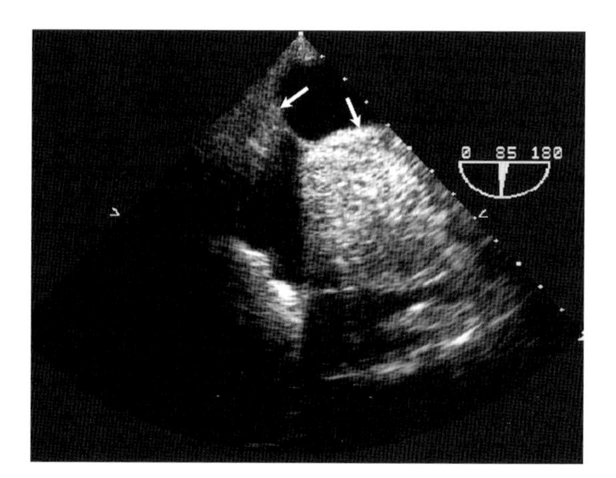

FIGURE 3–15. Lipomatous hypertrophy of the interatrial septum *(arrows)*. The thin flap of the fossa ovalis is seen in between the hypertrophied sections of the atrial septum.

LIPOMATOUS HYPERTROPHY OF THE ATRIAL SEPTUM

Lipomatous thickening of the interatrial septum is often quite striking, and may mimic an infiltrative process. This benign process creates a dumbbell-like appearance of the superior and inferior atrial septum, and is characterized by the lack of involvement of the fossa ovalis (Figure 3–15). The echogenic fat may also involve the right atrial wall, a finding that is associated with coronary artery disease and obesity.[16]

TRABECULATIONS

Trabeculations seen on echocardiographic examinations represent the muscle bundles on the endocardial surface of the heart and are more characteristic of the RA, right atrial appendage, and right ventricle than the left atrium and ventricle. Right ventricular hypertrophy may accentuate these trabeculations.

PECTINATE MUSCLES

A series of parallel ridges known as pectinate muscles course across the anterior endocardial surfaces of the left and right atria, including both appendages. Pectinate muscles are more apparent in the RA than in the left atrium (Figure 3–16). Prominent pectinate muscles can be distinguished from a mass or thrombus by their movement in synchrony with cardiac tissue, whereas a thrombus is often asynchronous with cardiac motion and is associated with arrhythmias such as atrial fibrillation or low flow states such as mitral stenosis.[17]

RIGHT ATRIAL APPENDAGE (RAA)

The RAA is most commonly seen in a ME bicaval view where the crista terminalis separates the SVC and RAA. Occasionally, the prominent trabeculations or pectinate

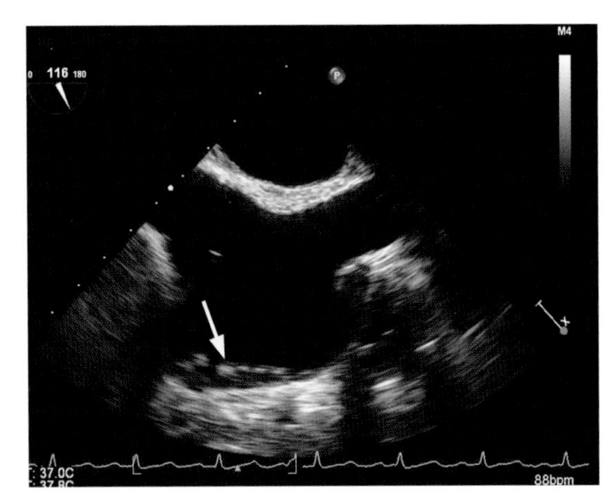

FIGURE 3–16. Pectinate muscles are demonstrated in the periphery of the right atrium as small round echo densities—like "pearls on a string."

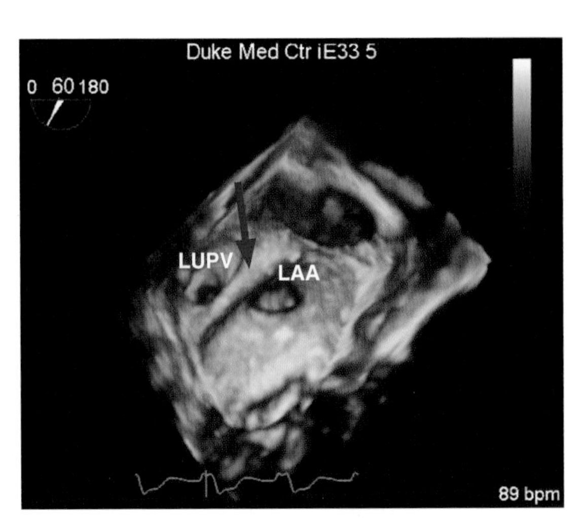

FIGURE 3–18. Three-dimensional image of the ligament of Marshall *(arrow)*. (LAA, left atrial appendage; LUPV, left upper pulmonary vein.)

muscles can also be seen. The RAA can also appear as an echo-free space anterior to the ascending aorta and near the right ventricular outflow tract in the ME aortic valve long-axis view.

Left Atrium

Ligament of Marshall

The atrial tissue separating the entrance of the left upper pulmonary vein (LUPV) from the left atrial appendage (LAA) commonly has multiple appearances, including a globular fatty appearance, often resembling a "Q-tip" (Figures 3–17 and 3–18). It is commonly referred to as the "warfarin" or "coumadin ridge" because it has historically been misinterpreted as a thrombus leading to treatment with anticoagulants. The ligament of Marshall is an important landmark for electrophysiological ablation procedures as it is thought to contribute to the maintenance of atrial fibrillation.[18]

Left Atrial Appendage (LAA)

The LAA is best seen in an ME two-chamber view where it is separated from the left superior pulmonary vein by the ligament of Marshall (Figure 3–19). Trabeculations and pectinate muscles in the LAA can be distinguished from thrombus by their synchronous movement and similar density to other cardiac tissue.

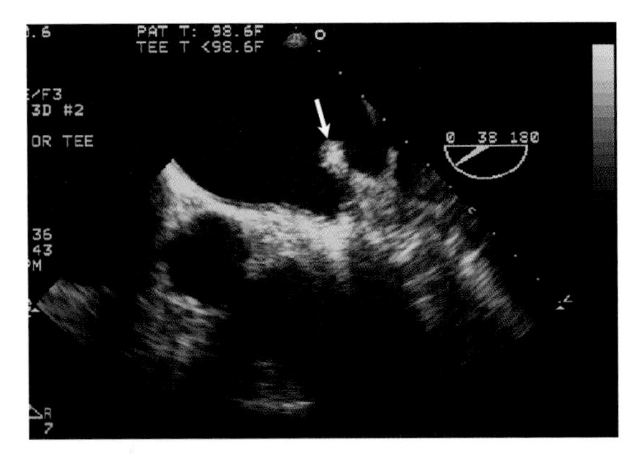

FIGURE 3–17. Ligament of Marshall or "coumadin ridge" is shown at the arrow. It often looks like a Q-tip and separates the left upper pulmonary vein and the left atrial appendage.

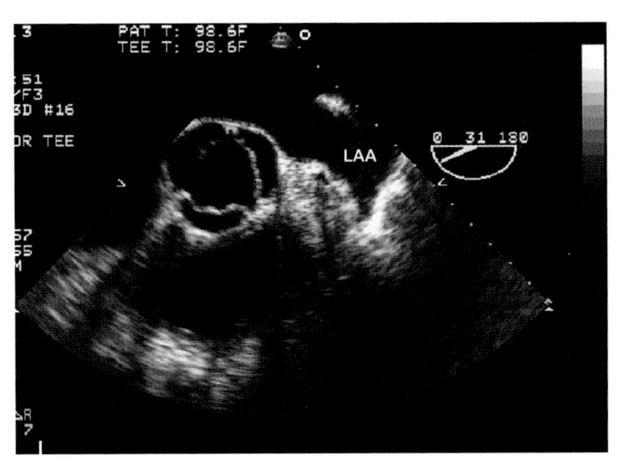

FIGURE 3–19. A normal left atrial appendage is shown. (LAA, left atrial appendage.)

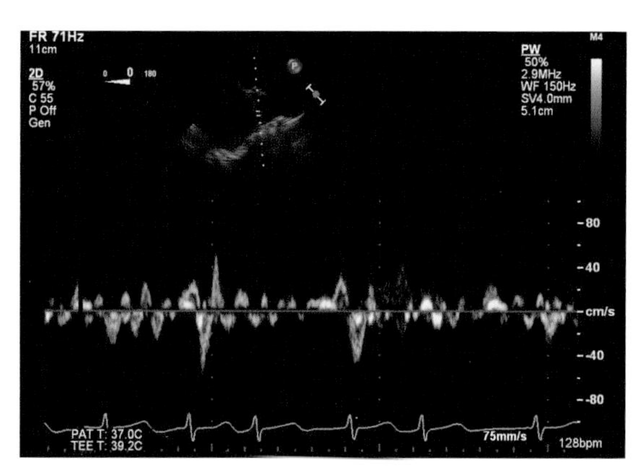

FIGURE 3–20. Pulsed Doppler flow in the left atrial appendage from a patient with atrial fibrillation demonstrating flow greater than 40 cm/s.

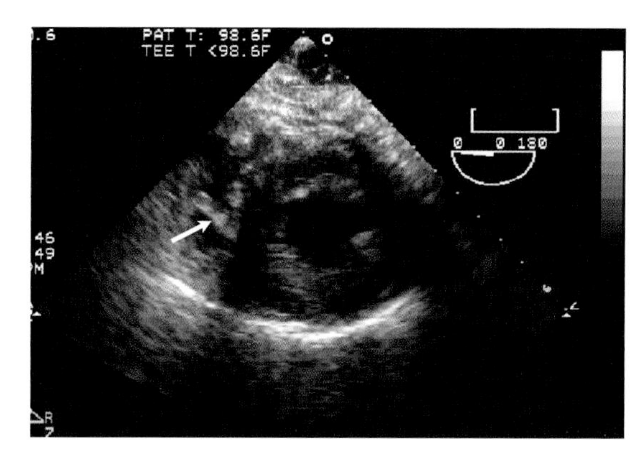

FIGURE 3–22. A moderator band in the right ventricle is demonstrated in short-axis at the arrow.

Transesophageal echocardiography (TEE) is superior to transthoracic echocardiography (TTE) for identification of a cardiac embolic source in patients with a history of transient ischemic attack (TIA) or stroke.[19] In addition to 2D imaging, color-flow Doppler, pulsed-wave Doppler, tissue Doppler, power Doppler, contrast echo, and 3D imaging can enhance the diagnostic process for thrombi.[20,21] Pulsed Doppler is the most commonly applied technique and is performed by placing the pulsed-wave Doppler sample at the mouth of the LAA. A velocity greater than 40 cm/s in the LAA decreases the likelihood of a thrombus (Figure 3–20). Thirty to fifty percent of people also have a bilobed or multilobed left atrial appendage (Figure 3–21).[22] These are often characterized by a round circle of normal-appearing tissue within the LAA which represents one lobe of the LAA that is angulated relative to the other lobe.

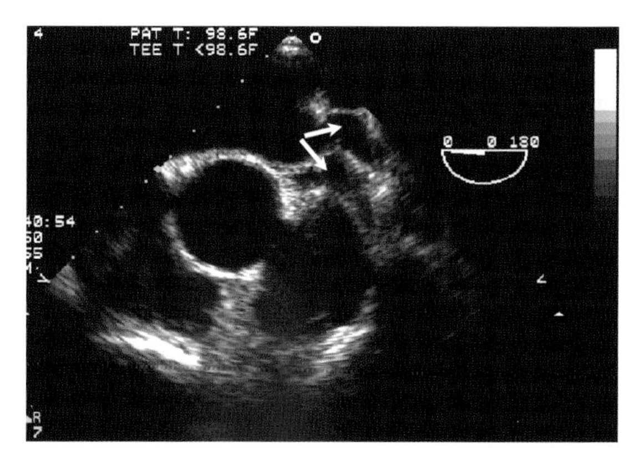

FIGURE 3–21. A bilobed left atrial appendage is demonstrated at the arrows. Note the ligament of Marshall is located posteriorly, appearing as a "Q tip."

Right Ventricle

MODERATOR BAND

The moderator band is the most prominent muscle band that lies in the apical third of the right ventricle (RV) and is associated with the anterior papillary muscle of the RV.[23] It can be seen in long- (LAX) or short-axis (SAX) views (Figure 3–22) and can be confused with a tumor or thrombus. The moderator band is involved with the conduction system as Purkinje fibers may course through it. The left ventricle (LV) does not usually have a moderator band.

Left Ventricle

FALSE TENDONS AND LV BANDS

"False tendons" are finer, usually filamentous structures compared to the RV moderator band and have also been called false chordae tendineae (Figure 3–23). They usually occur between the ventricular septum and the free wall, and have an association with murmurs and arrhythmias, but they are usually of little clinical significance, other than the potential for misinterpretation as a thrombus.[24] Occasionally, larger bands can occur in the LV, but unlike the RV moderator band, they are not usually associated with the conduction system (Figure 3–24).

LAMBL'S EXCRESCENCES

Lambl's excrescences are small filamentous structures arising from the aortic valve leaflets, usually on the aortic side of the leaflets (Figure 3–25). They occur along the line of leaflet coaptation and are usually multiple.

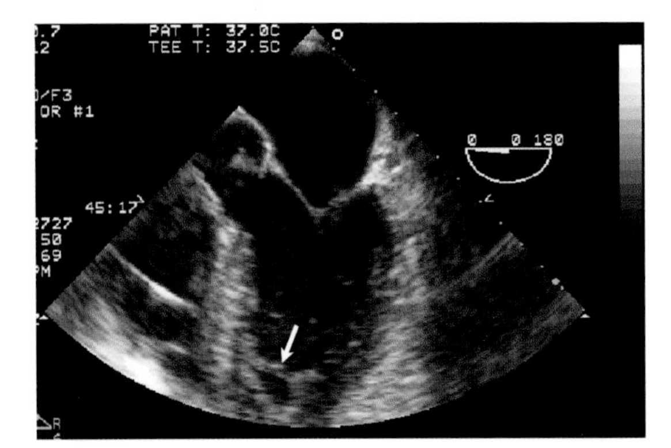

FIGURE 3–23. A false tendon in the left ventricle is shown at the arrow. The linear echo density in the right ventricle is a side lobe artifact from the pulmonary artery catheter.

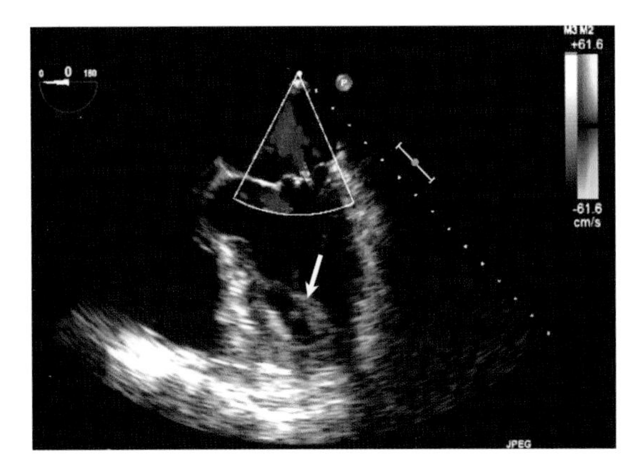

FIGURE 3–24. A large left ventricular band is shown at the arrow.

A clinical history is usually required to distinguish these from thrombi, vegetations, and cardiac neoplasms. Distinguishing Lambl's excrescences from papillary fibroelastomas is a common clinical challenge. Papillary fibroelastomas are less likely to be filamentous and more likely to have multiple fronds. On pathological examination, they are also rich in an acid mucopolysaccharide matrix and smooth muscle cells. Lambl's excrescences do not have a clearly defined clinical significance, but have been thought to be associated with stroke. The decision to excise these when noted as an incidental finding is variable and largely dictated by a history of embolic events.[25]

NODULE OF ARANTIUS

This nodule-like appearance at the coaptation point of the three aortic cusps results from thickening in the middle of the free edge of the aortic valve cusps from the wear and tear of valvular opening and closing.[26] The nodule can become calcified and appear as a mass on the aortic valve leaflets, or can hypertrophy and lead to aortic regurgitation.

Extracardiac Spaces

PERICARDIAL EFFUSION

The normal pericardial sac contains about 15 to 30 mL of pericardial fluid that is not typically seen with TEE. However, a larger effusion separates the myocardium from the pericardium and creates an echo-free space that is easily visualized (Figure 3–26). The clinical significance of an effusion depends upon the degree of ventricular and atrial compression and the rate of fluid accumulation, and can be identified by signs such as diastolic right ventricular collapse (see Chapter 15).[27]

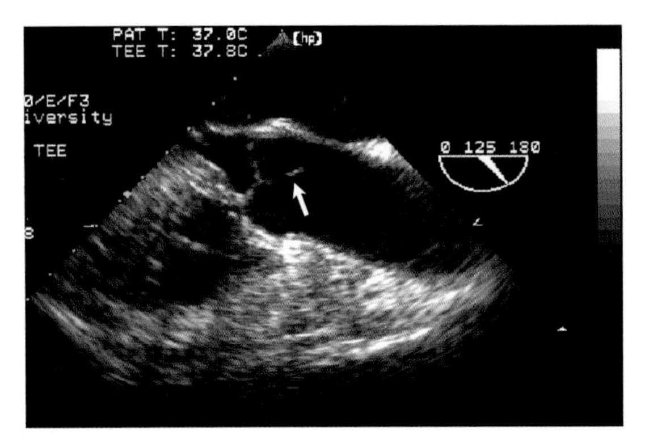

FIGURE 3–25. Lambl's excrescence is shown at the arrow.

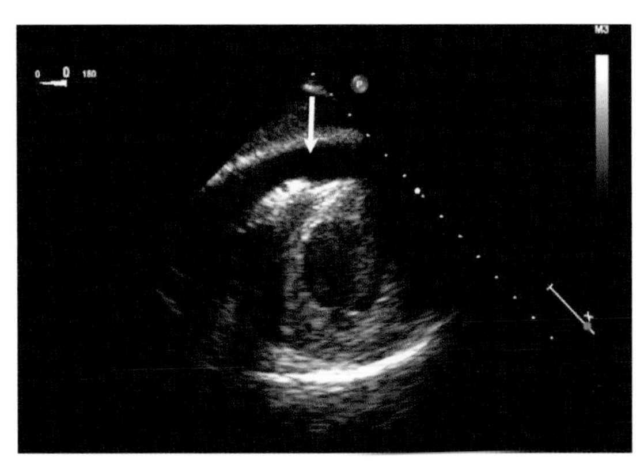

FIGURE 3–26. A pericardial effusion is demonstrated at the arrow.

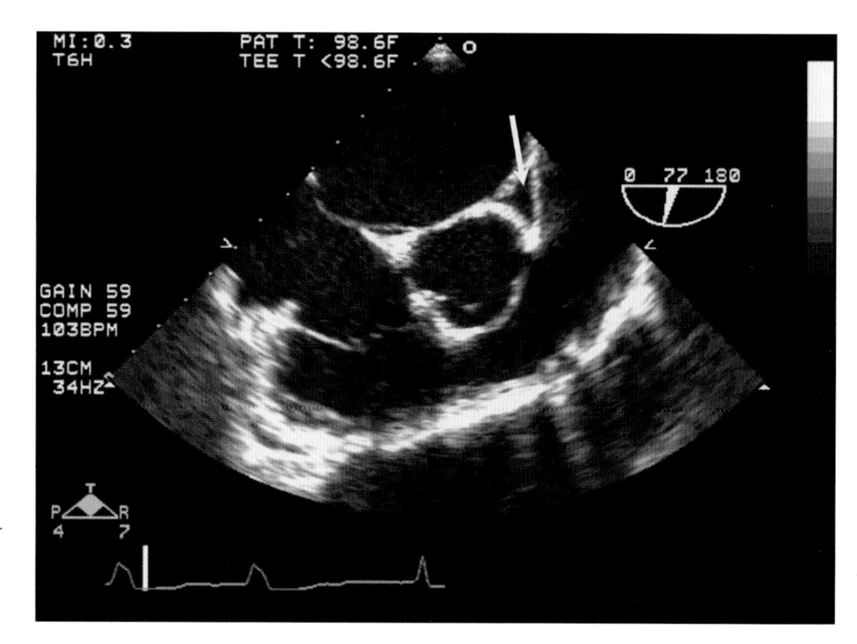

FIGURE 3–27. The transverse sinus is shown at the arrow. It is a pericardial reflection noted between the left atrium, the pulmonary artery, and the aorta.

The pericardial sac may also be calcified or thickened, leading to constrictive pericarditis. Of note, pericardial fat is often confused with a pericardial effusion.[28]

Transverse and Oblique Sinuses

The transverse sinus is formed by a reflection of pericardium between the posterior wall of the ascending aorta, the anterior left atrium, and the posterior pulmonary artery (Figure 3–27). It may be misinterpreted as a cyst or abscess cavity, and has even been reported to contain a hemagioma.[29] The transverse sinus should not have color flow in it, but can contain fibrinous material, fat, or fluid. The oblique sinus is another, more inferior pericardial reflection located posteriorly between the entry of the four pulmonary veins into the left atrium (Figure 3–28). The oblique sinus is not well visualized with TEE, but may be seen on transthoracic echo posterior to the left atrium in the parasternal long-axis view.

Pleural Effusion

Pleural effusions, lateral to the heart, can easily be identified by TEE. Left pleural effusions can be seen lateral and posterior, near the descending thoracic aorta (Figure 3–29). Right pleural effusions can be seen lateral to the heart, superior to the liver. TEE has been shown to be accurate in the identification of pleural fluid in the cardiac surgical patient, with the ability to detect a median of 125 mL of fluid on the left and 225 mL on the right.[1]

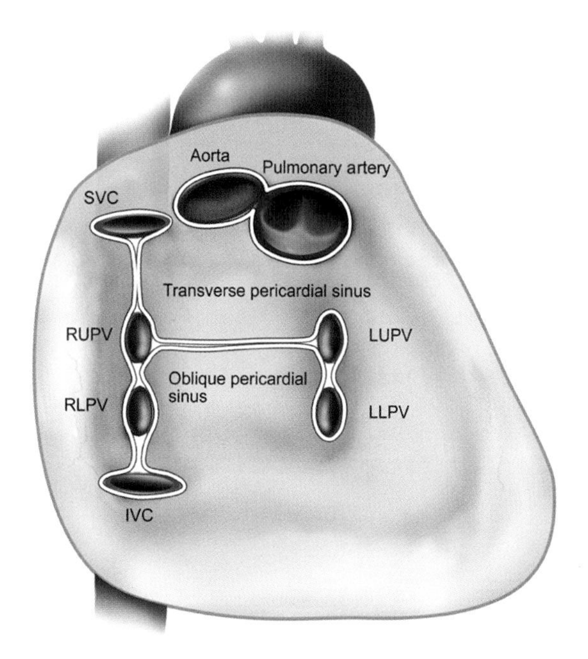

FIGURE 3–28. A drawing of the oblique pericardial sinus, located posterior to the left atrium (LA), between the entry of the four pulmonary veins into the LA. (SVC, superior vena cava; IVC, inferior vena cava; LUPV, left upper pulmonary vein; LLPV, left lower pulmonary vein; RUPV, right upper pulmonary vein; RLPV, right lower pulmonary vein.)

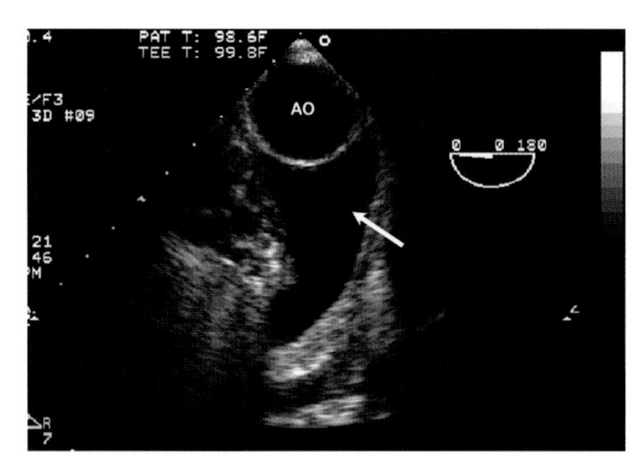

FIGURE 3–29. A pleural effusion adjacent to the descending thoracic aorta (AO) is seen at the arrow.

ULTRASOUND ARTIFACTS

An artifact is any structure in an ultrasound image that does not have a corresponding anatomic tissue structure. Although artifacts are largely related to the physics of ultrasound, they can also result from operator fault or equipment failure. Artifacts can be broadly categorized as (1) missing structures, (2) degraded images, (3) falsely perceived objects, and (4) misregistered locations.[30]

Missing Structures

Missing structures are related to the resolution of the ultrasound beam or to shadowing from a structure that reflects ultrasound so strongly that distal structures are not imaged or are "shadowed."

Resolution

Resolution is a property of ultrasound that allows one to differentiate two separate structures that are closely approximated.[1] Lateral resolution allows one to distinguish objects in a horizontal plane and is determined by the bandwidth of the ultrasound probe. With *lateral resolution* artifact, two structures that are closer together than the width of the ultrasound beam will appear as a single merged structure. Thus, a small reflector such as an air bubble may also be displayed as a wide line rather than a round point. Longitudinal resolution allows one to distinguish objects in a longitudinal plane and is related to spatial pulse length. *Longitudinal resolution* artifact occurs when one reflection is created from two structures that are closer than one-half the spatial pulse length. Higher frequency transducers have better longitudinal resolution while lateral resolution is optimal in the focal zone where the ultrasound beam width is narrowest (Figure 3–30). Therefore, resolution (lateral and longitudinal) can be improved by increasing frequency, placing the area of interest in the focal zone, and decreasing the overall gain to better visualize distinct objects.

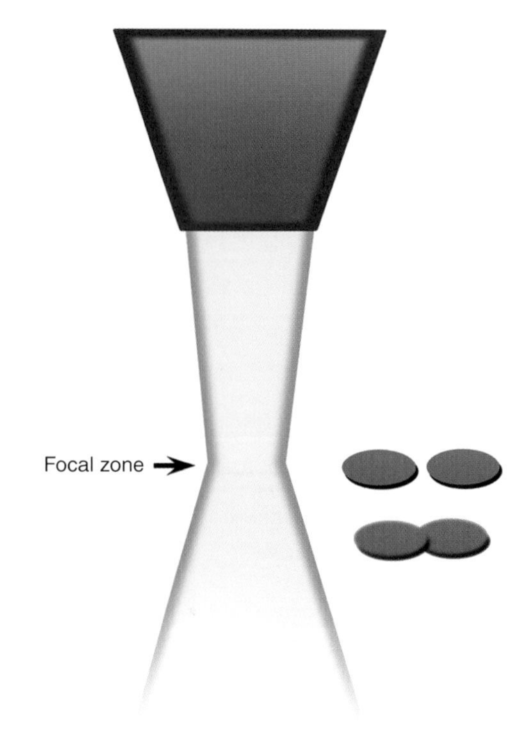

FIGURE 3–30. The ability to resolve two objects that are close together is optimal at the focal zone of the ultrasound beam, as illustrated.

Acoustic Shadowing

High-density structures with high acoustic impedance can prevent the ultrasound beam from penetrating beyond them, causing an echolucent shadow deep to the dense object. Prosthetic valves, patches, or implants are common examples of such structures (Figure 3–31).[31] Similarly, heavily calcified structures such as valves, mitral valve annuli, or chordae tendineae can also cause *shadowing*. Large shadows can be problematic as they can obstruct the evaluation of important cardiac structures (Figure 3–32),[32] and alternate views may be required (Figure 3–33). For example, a prosthetic valve in the aortic position is best evaluated in the transgastric long-axis or deep transgastic views so that acoustic shadowing from the prosthesis does not obscure perivalvular leaks or other valve dysfunction. An *edge shadow* is a special type of shadowing that results from the refraction and divergence of sound along the edge of a curved structure.

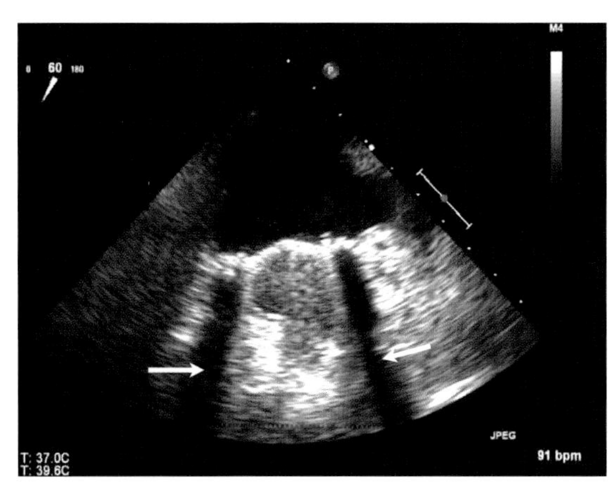

FIGURE 3–31. The image demonstrates acoustic shadows from a St. Jude prosthetic valve (in the closed position in this image).

Degraded Images

REVERBERATIONS

Reverberations typically occur when the sound wave bounces back and forth between two strong reflectors (eg, calcified structures, metallic objects, catheters, and air/fluid interfaces). Successive reflections returning to the transducer result in repeated, equally spaced images extending from the object, away from the transducer—the first two reflections closest to the transducer being real. Less commonly, reverberations can occur when a strong ultrasound signal returns to the transducer from a single reflector and is reflected back to the tissues. Once again, repeated images of the structure appear on the screen, but this time at distances that are multiples of the actual object's distance from the transducer (Figure 3–34). Reverberations are commonly seen in the descending thoracic aorta (Figure 3–35). Diagnostic criteria for reverberant images in the descending aorta include displacement parallel to aortic walls (as opposed to free movement of a flap, for example), blood flow superimposed on the artifact during color-flow Doppler imaging, and similar blood velocities on both sides of the image.[33] When

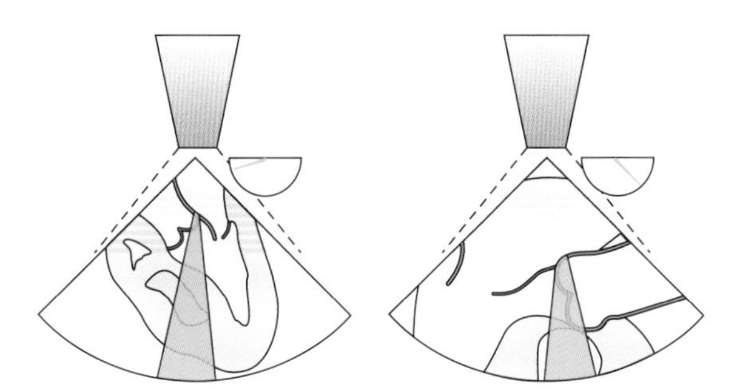

FIGURE 3–32. An illustration of how acoustic shadowing impairs prosthetic valvular assessment in the midesophageal four-chamber and midesophageal aortic valve long-axis views.

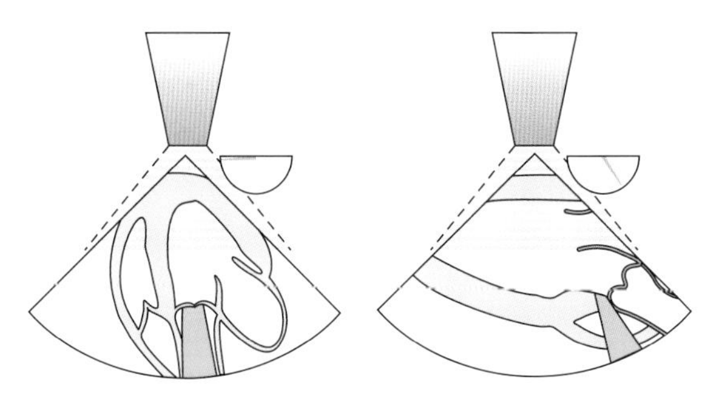

FIGURE 3–33. Acoustic shadows appear away from the prosthetic valve in the deep transgastric and transgastric long-axis views, allowing valve assessment.

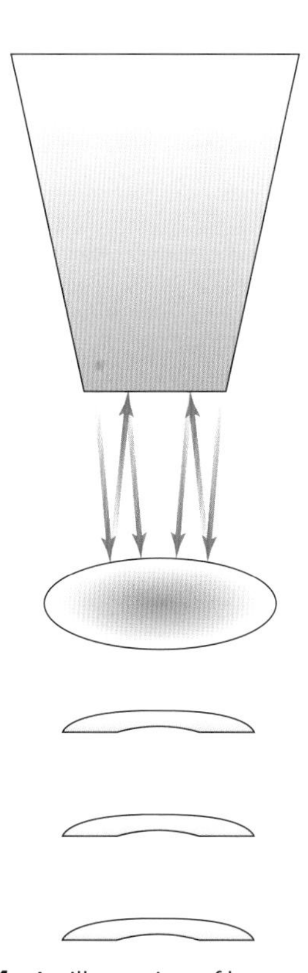

FIGURE 3–34. An illustration of how reverberations are formed when the surface of the ultrasound probe itself serves as a reflector.

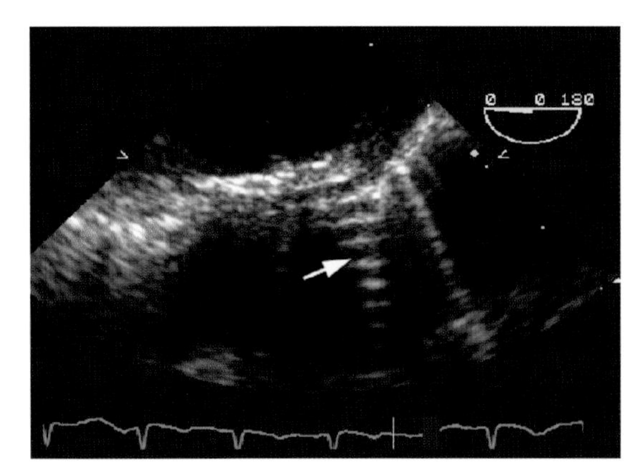

FIGURE 3–35. Reverberation artifact *(arrow)* in a long-axis view of the aortic arch.

closely spaced reverberations merge to form a single line deep to the echo-dense object, they are known as a *comet tail* or *ring down* artifact.

Acoustic Noise/Near Field Clutter

Structures too close to the transducer can be obscured by high-amplitude oscillations of its piezoelectric elements in a phased array system.[1] This is often observed in the LA and the descending aorta when imaging with a TEE probe, and can be improved by adjusting the gain settings. It is very noticeable with epiaortic and epicardial scanning, and can be minimized by physically separating the transducer from the tissue of interest with fluid or gel.

Electrical Noise

This artifact often occurs in the operating room from electrical interference and appears as "snow" on an image display. Newer transducer and ultrasound systems have incorporated electrocautery suppression software to limit this artifact.

Enhancement

Enhancement occurs when a deeper object appears more reflective (brighter) than it should because the ultrasound beam has traveled through a region with abnormally low attenuation. It is commonly seen with the anterior pericardium in a transgastric view. Adjusting the ultrasound time-gain compensation can minimize enhancement.

Falsely Perceived Objects

Refraction Artifact

When sound waves travel through relatively homogeneous media, they are propagated in essentially straight lines. However, when an ultrasound beam crosses an interface of tissues or fluid with different propagation speeds, the ultrasound beam changes direction.[1] The ultrasound system,

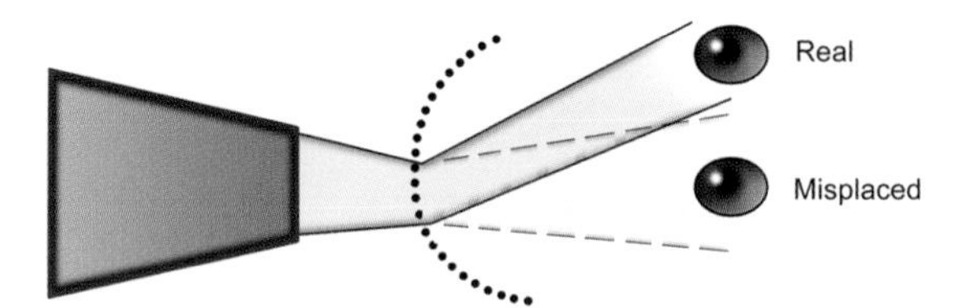

FIGURE 3–36. An illustration of how refraction results in a misplaced ultrasound image.

however, assumes that sound travels in a straight line from the transducer and will therefore place a second copy of an object seen in the path of the refracted wave, side by side with (at the same depth as) the true image of the object (Figure 3–36).

Mirror Images

Mirror image artifacts are produced when a strong reflector redirects the ultrasound beam, resulting in a second copy being placed deeper to the real structure. The structure that acts as a mirror lies on a direct line between the transducer and the artifact, and the true reflector and artifact are equal distances from the mirror (Figure 3–37). Mirror images that occur commonly in the descending aorta and in the aortic arch are sometimes referred to as a reverberation, but if there is only one copy, it is more aptly described as a mirror. Mirror artifacts can appear in any image plane, often causing confusion about the identity, nature, and pathology of the mirror image.[34]

Misregistered Locations

Side Lobes

The lateral edges of the ultrasound transducer can generate extraneous but weaker beams of ultrasound that diverge from the direction of the main ultrasound beam. Reflected signals from such extraneous beams are, however, interpreted as if they resulted from the direction of

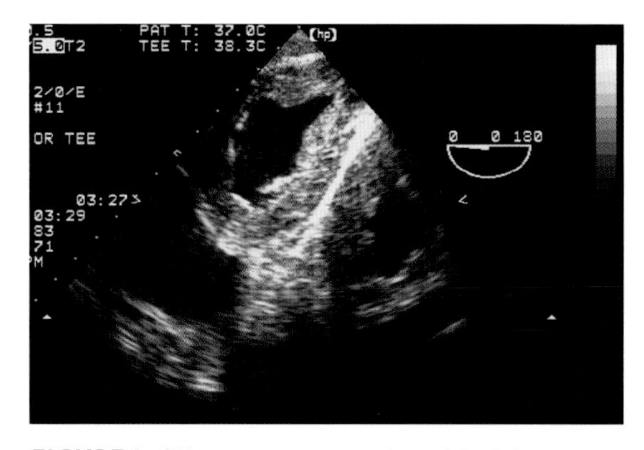

FIGURE 3–37. Mirror image artifact of the left ventricle.

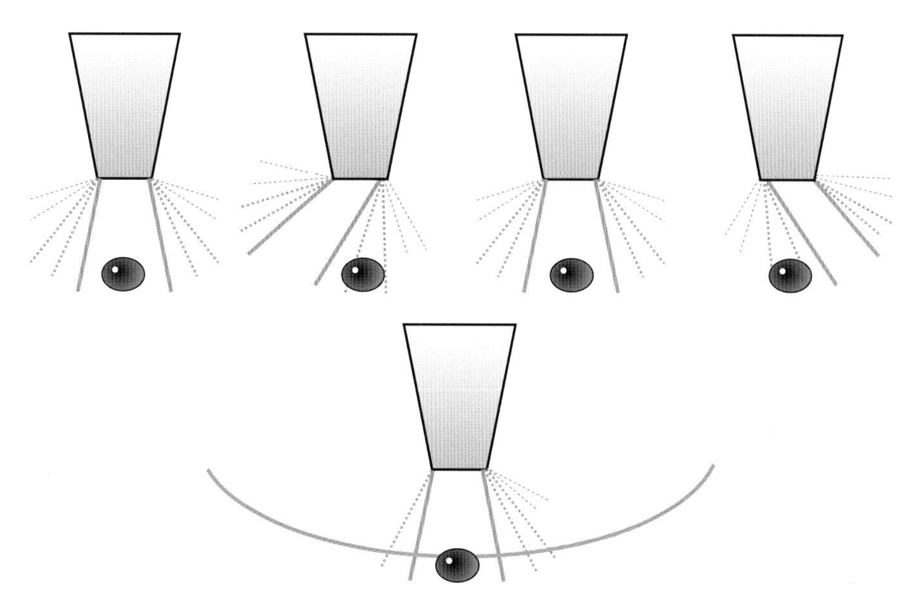

FIGURE 3–38. An illustration of how side lobes are formed.

the main beam. The energy in these extraneous beams is typically much less than the main beam and often no erroneous image is created. However, when the extraneous ultrasound beams contact very reflective structures, a *side lobe* artifact appears as a curvilinear object at a uniform distance from the transducer (Figure 3–38).[1] Side lobe artifacts create uncertainty when they appear as an unexpected object or linear structure in a cardiac chamber[35] (Figure 3–39) or when imaging for the presence of aortic dissection.[33] Unlike true dissections (Figure 3–40),

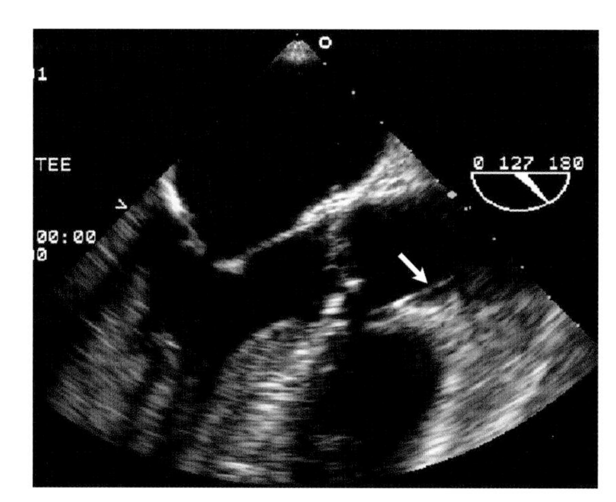

FIGURE 3–39. A side lobe artifact in the ascending aorta in a midesophageal aortic valve long-axis view from a calcified plaque at the sinotubular junction. This artifact is not to be confused with an aortic dissection.

side lobe artifacts tend to be displaced parallel to aortic walls and have similar blood flow velocities on both sides of the artifact. Imaging with multiple planes can also aid in distinguishing the true reflector from the artifact.

SPEED ERRORS

A *speed error* artifact occurs when the sound wave travels through an object that has a propagation speed different from that of soft tissue. If the propagation speed is slower than that in soft tissue, reflectors are placed deeper on the image than they really are because sound is traveling slower than the ultrasound system assumes. Similarly, if the propagation speed is faster, the reflector will be shallower.

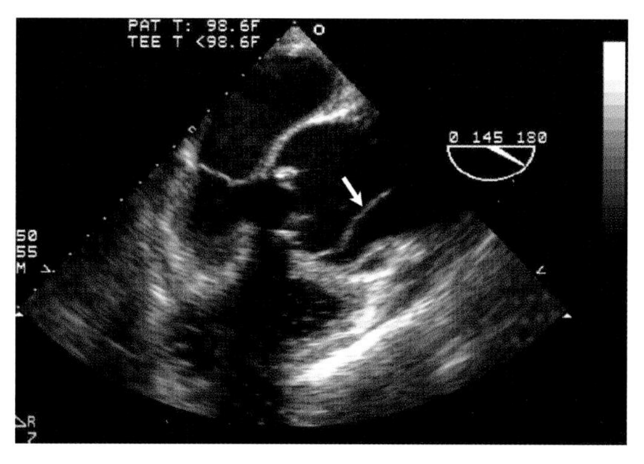

FIGURE 3–40. A true aortic dissection in a midesophageal aortic valve long-axis view. The dissection flap is seen at the arrow.

ALIASING

Aliasing of Doppler flow can introduce confusion regarding the direction of blood flow and can prevent measurement of a peak velocity. Aliasing is produced when the Doppler frequency shift exceeds one-half the pulse repetition frequency (PRF), also known as the Nyquist limit. The PRF determines the maximal Doppler shift, or maximum velocity, that is reliably measured by the transducer. When the velocity of the sound wave in question is greater than the Nyquist limit, the system cannot sample frequently enough to accurately detect the velocity. As a result, the signal is displayed as starting correctly, but once it reaches the Nyquist limit it "wraps around" the scale, appearing to come from the opposite side of the baseline (Figure 3–41). Aliasing does not occur with continuous-wave Doppler, as with this modality the system is continuously sending and receiving ultrasound; thus, it can accurately measure all velocities. The aliasing artifact can be overcome by increasing the velocity scale to the maximum, using a lower-frequency transducer (lower Doppler shifts), selecting a shallower depth (increased PRF), using continuous-wave Doppler, or shifting the baseline. As color-flow Doppler is a pulsed ultrasound technique, it can alias as well (Figure 3–42). In this situation, when the blood flow velocity exceeds the Nyquist limit, the flow is assigned the color on the opposite end of the color bar—giving the impression (if one was only to look at the color) that the blood flow had turned around to flow in the opposite direction (Figure 3–43). However, this is just the color Doppler version of "wrap around."

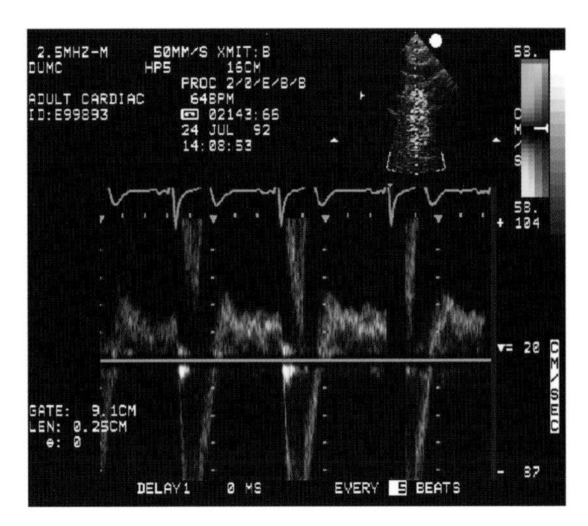

FIGURE 3–41. This image demonstrates pulsed-wave Doppler aliasing artifact, with "wraparound" of the Doppler signal.

GHOSTING AND CLUTTER

Movement of heart muscle or vessel walls produces very low-frequency Doppler shifts that can be detected by ultrasound systems. In spectral Doppler, these low-frequency shifts are known as *clutter*, while in color-flow Doppler, they are known as a *ghosting artifact.*

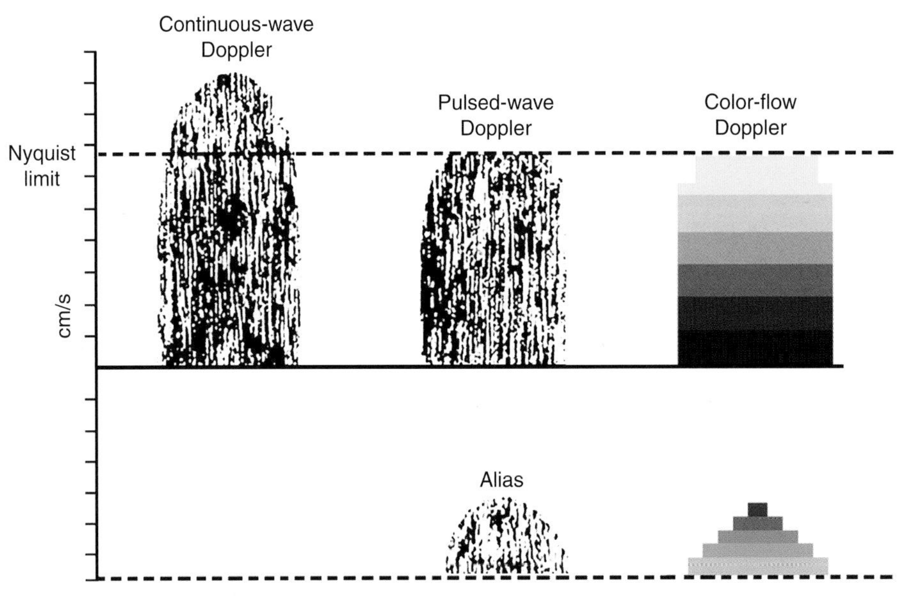

FIGURE 3–42. Pulsed-wave Doppler and color-flow Doppler are subject to aliasing artifact, but continuous-wave Doppler is not.

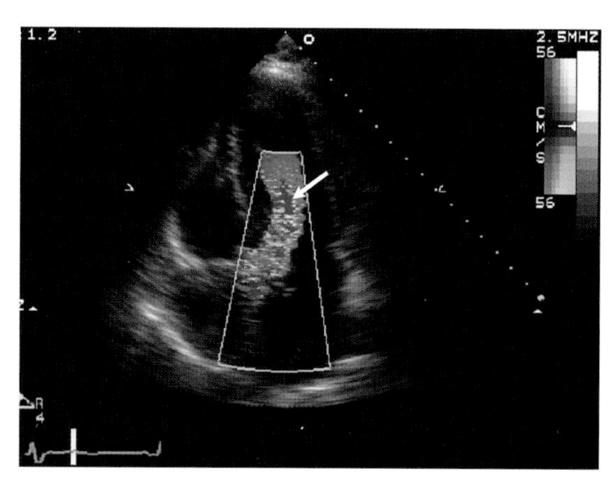

FIGURE 3–43. Color-flow Doppler aliases in the left ventricular outflow tract in a deep transgastric view; the blood flow going from the left ventricle towards the aorta changes from blue to red as the velocity of flow in the outflow tract exceeds the set Nyquist limit.

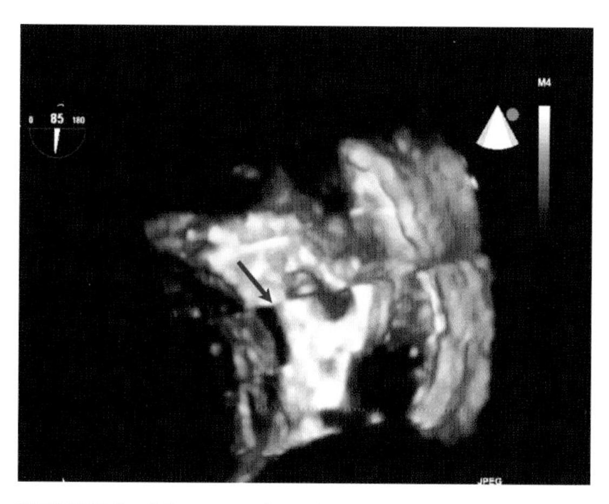

FIGURE 3–44. A "stitch artifact" is demonstrated. This may occur with the acquisition of a full-volume image during a disturbance of cardiac rhythm or with patient or operator movement.

THREE-DIMENSIONAL ECHOCARDIOGRAPHY

Just as 2D echocardiography reveals normal anatomic variants and is subject to artifacts, so is 3D echocardiography. The anatomic variants are the same as seen in 2D imaging, but must be identified as such with 3D imaging. Similarly, many of the artifacts seen with 2D echocardiography are also seen with 3D echocardiography, including side lobe generation and attenuation of beam intensity, leading to blurry images in the far field.[36,37] Two other artifacts are particularly relevant to 3D imaging. First, a "stitch" artifact may occur with the acquisition of a full-volume image during a disturbance of cardiac rhythm, patient movement, or operator movement. This is because a full-volume image is acquired from several sub-volume images, which are "stitched" together to create a full-volume image. If any one of the sub-volume images does not match the other sub-volumes with respect to cardiac cycle or position, then a jagged or blurred interface occurs in the image (Figure 3–44). This 3D imaging artifact does not occur with real-time 3D imaging where sub-volumes are not melded together; real-time *full-volume* imaging would, however, still be subject to a "stitch" artifact.[38] A dropout artifact can also occur when the z-axis is not monitored properly, the gain setting is too low (no image acquired), or the gain setting is too high (leading to masking).[36,37]

ARTIFACTS OF DISPLAY

The interpretation of a 2D or 3D image can be confused by inappropriate use of spectral gain, color-flow sector size, image depth, and/or changes in the color-flow velocity scale or color-flow gain.

SUMMARY

Appropriate interpretation of ultrasound images is necessary to diagnose both pathological and normal conditions, thereby leading to suitable interventions. Thus, it is important to be familiar with the common variants and artifacts as well as the common pathological conditions that variants and artifacts may be confused with.

A few key questions or observations may assist in determining if a structure is pathologic or is simply a normal anatomic variant or ultrasound artifact:

1. Is the density and texture of the structure the same as the rest of the heart? If yes, then the structure is likely to be a variant.
2. Does the structure move synchronously with the rest of the heart? If yes, then the structure is likely to be a variant.
3. Does the structure appear in multiple planes and views? If yes, then the structure is not likely to be an artifact.
4. Does the structure cross anatomic boundaries? If yes, then it is likely to be an artifact.
5. Look for secondary signs and clues. For example, if the patient has poor left ventricular function and/or is in atrial fibrillation, then a thrombus in either atrial appendage or the LV is likely.
6. Use various views to reduce the impact of artifacts; for example, use a deep transgastric view to assess prosthetic aortic valves to avoid acoustic shadow interference.

7. Use agitated saline injections to identify shunts, persistent left superior vena cavae, or distinguish intracardiac spaces from extracardiac spaces.

REFERENCES

1. Edelman S. Artifacts. In: Edelman S, ed. *Understanding Ultrasound Physics.* 3rd ed. Woodlands: Education for the Sonographic Professional, Inc; 2007:329-351.
2. Feigenbaum H, Armstrong WF, Ryan T. Masses, tumors and source of embolus. In: Feigenbaum H, Armstrong WF, Ryan T, eds. *Feigenbaum's Echocardiography.* 6th ed. Philadelphia: Lippincott Williams & Wilkins; 2005:701-702.
3. Sadler TW. Cardiovascular system. In: Sadler TW, ed. *Langman's Medical Embryology.* 8th ed. Philadelphia: Lippincott Williams & Wilkins; 2006:208-259.
4. Zhao QY, Huang H, Tang YH, et al. Relationship between autonomic innervation in crista terminalis and atrial arrhythmia. *J Cardiovasc Electrophysiol.* 2009;20(5):551-557.
5. Escota-Villanueva J, Lacambra-Blasco I, Gonzalvo C. Images in cardiovascular medicine. Eustachian valve thrombosis. *Circulation.* 2008;118(13):e504.
6. Yavuz T, Nazli C, Kinay O, Kutsal A. Giant eustachian valve with echocardiographic appearance of divided right atrium. *Tex Heart Inst J.* 2002;29(4):336-338.
7. Hill AJ, Ahlberg SE, Wilkoff BL, Iaizzo PA. Dynamic obstruction to coronary sinus access: the thebesian valve. *Heart Rhythm.* 2006;3(10):1240-1241.
8. Pellett AA. The Chiari network in an echocardiography student. *Echocardiography.* 2004;21(1):91-93.
9. Tops LF, Van de Veire NR, Schuijf JD, et al. Noninvasive evaluation of coronary sinus anatomy and its relation to the mitral valve annulus: implications for percutaneous mitral annuloplasty. *Circulation.* 2007;115(11):1426-1432.
10. Agrifoglio M, Barili F, Kassem S, et al. Sutureless patch-and-glue technique for the repair of coronary sinus injuries. *J Thorac Cardiovasc Surg.* 2007;134(2):522-523.
11. Lee MS, Shah AP, Dang N, et al. Coronary sinus is dilated and outwardly displaced in patients with mitral regurgitation: quantitative angiographic analysis. *Catheter Cardiovasc Interv.* 2006;67(3):490-494.
12. Ratliff HL, Yousufuddin M, Lieving WR, et al. Persistent left superior vena cava: case reports and clinical implications. *Int J Cardiol.* 2006;113(2):242-246.
13. Augoustides JG, Weiss SJ, Ochroch AE, et al. Analysis of the interatrial septum by transesophageal echocardiography in adult cardiac surgical patients: anatomic variants and correlation with patent foramen ovale. *J Cardiothorac Vasc Anesth.* 2005;19(2):146-149.
14. Burger AJ, Sherman HB, Charlamb MJ. Low incidence of embolic strokes with atrial septal aneurysms: a prospective, long-term study. *Am Heart J.* 2000;139(1 Pt 1):149-152.
15. Wahl A, Krumsdorf U, Meier B, et al. Transcatheter treatment of atrial septal aneurysm associated with patent foramen ovale for prevention of recurrent paradoxical embolism in high-risk patients. *J Am Coll Cardiol.* 2005;45(3):377-380.
16. O'Connor S, Recavarren R, Nichols LC, Parwani AV. Lipomatous hypertrophy of the interatrial septum: an overview. *Arch Pathol Lab Med.* 2006;130(3):397-399.
17. Bilen E, Yasar AS, Bilge M, Kurt M. A prominent pectinate muscle mimicking a pathological cardiac mass. *Echocardiography.* 2008;25(6):662.
18. Tan AY, Chou CC, Zhou S, et al. Electrical connections between left superior pulmonary vein, left atrium, and ligament of Marshall: implications for mechanisms of atrial fibrillation. *Am J Physiol Heart Circ Physiol.* 2006;290(1):H312-H322.
19. de Bruijn SF, Agema WR, Lammers GJ, et al. Transesophageal echocardiography is superior to transthoracic echocardiography in management of patients of any age with transient ischemic attack or stroke. *Stroke.* 2006;37(10):2531-2534.
20. Ruiz-Arango A, Landolfo C. A novel approach to the diagnosis of left atrial appendage thrombus using contrast echocardiography and power Doppler imaging. *Eur J Echocardiogr.* 2008;9(2):329-333.
21. Parvathaneni L, Mahenthiran J, Jacob S, et al. Comparison of tissue Doppler dynamics to Doppler flow in evaluating left atrial appendage function by transesophageal echocardiography. *Am J Cardiol.* 2005;95(8):1011-1014.
22. Thomas L. Assessment of atrial function. *Heart Lung Circ.* 2007;16(3):234-242.
23. Ho SY, Nihoyannopoulos P. Anatomy, echocardiography, and normal right ventricular dimensions. *Heart.* 2006 2006;92(suppl 1):i2-i13.
24. Loukas M, Louis RG Jr, Black B, Pham D, Fudalej M, Sharkees M. False tendons: an endoscopic cadaveric approach. *Clin Anat.* 2007;20(2):163-169.
25. Jaffe W, Figueredo VM. An example of Lambl's excrescences by transesophageal echocardiogram: a commonly misinterpreted lesion. *Echocardiography.* 2007;24(10):1086-1089.
26. Ho SY. Structure and anatomy of the aortic root. *Eur J Echocardiogr.* 2009;10(1):i3-i10.
27. Hoit BD. Pericardial disease and pericardial tamponade. *Crit Care Med.* 2007;35(8 suppl):S355-S364.
28. Kanna B, Osorio F, Dharmarajan L. Pericardial fat mimicking pericardial effusion on two-dimensional echocardiography. *Echocardiography.* 2006;23(5):400-402.
29. Fitzsimons B, Koch CG. Transverse sinus hemangioma. *Anesth Analg.* 2008;106(1):63-64.
30. Heller LB, Aronson S. Imaging artifacts and pitfalls. In: Savage RM SA, Thomas JD, Shanewise JS, Shernan SK, eds. *Comprehensive Textbook of Intraoperative Transesophageal Echocardiography.* Philadelphia: Lippincott Williams & Wilkins, Wolters Kluwer Health; 2004:39-48.
31. Tempe DK, Ramamurthy P, Datt V, Goyal G, Banerjee A, Narang P. An unusual transesophageal echocardiographic finding after Gore-Tex patch closure of an atrial septal defect. *J Cardiothorac Vasc Anesth.* 2006;20(5):751-752.
32. Barbetseas J, Brili S, Stamatopoulos I, et al. Pitfalls leading to misdiagnosis of a normally functioning prosthetic aortic valve as stenotic. *Echocardiography.* 2007;24(7):773-779.
33. Vignon P, Spencer KT, Rambaud G, et al. Differential transesophageal echocardiographic diagnosis between linear artifacts and intraluminal flap of aortic dissection or disruption. *Chest.* 2001;119(6):1778-1790.
34. Adams MS, Alston TA. Echocardiographic reflections on a pericardium. *Anesth Analg.* 2007;104(3):506.

35. Skubas N, Brown NI, Mishra R. Diagnostic dilemma: a pacemaker lead inside the left atrium or an echocardiographic beam width artifact? *Anesth Analg.* 2006;102(4):1043-1044.
36. Yang HS, Bansal RC, Mookadam F, Khandheria BK, Tajik AJ, Chandrasekaran K. Practical guide for three-dimensional transthoracic echocardiography using a fully sampled matrix array transducer. *J Am Soc Echocardiogr.* 2008;21(9):979-989.
37. Hung J, Lang R, Flachskampf F, et al. 3D echocardiography: a review of the current status and future directions. *J Am Soc Echocardiogr.* 2007;20(3):213-233.
38. Brekke S, Rabben SI, Stoylen A, et al. Volume stitching in three-dimensional echocardiography: distortion analysis and extension to real time. *Ultrasound Med Biol.* 2007;33(5):782-796.

REVIEW QUESTIONS

Select the *one best* answer for each question.

1. Identify the structure:

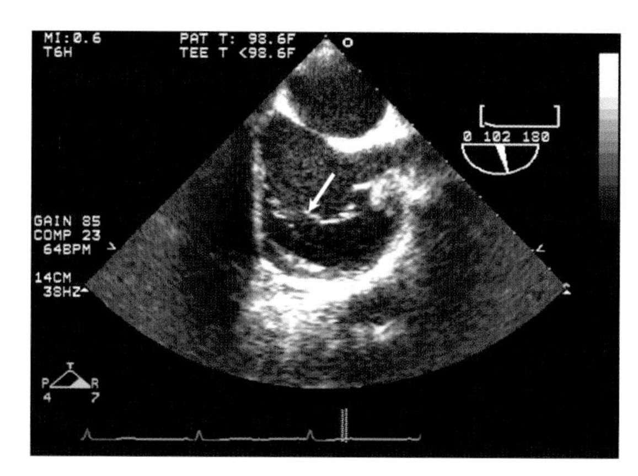

a. Chiari network
b. Eustachian valve
c. Pacing wire
d. Venous cannula

2. Identify the artifact:

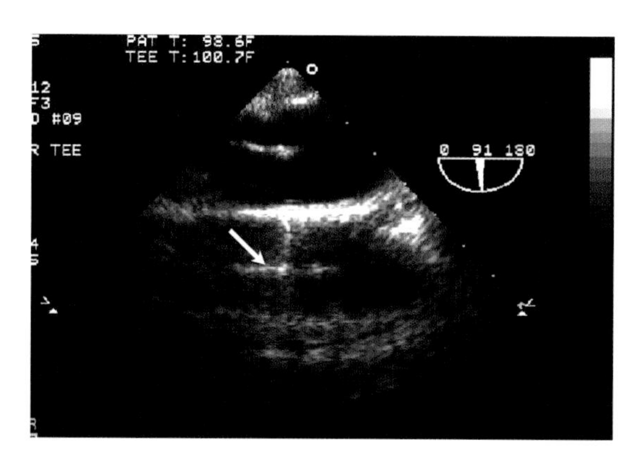

a. Reverberation
b. Mirror image
c. Side lobe
d. Near field clutter

3. Identify the structure at the arrow:

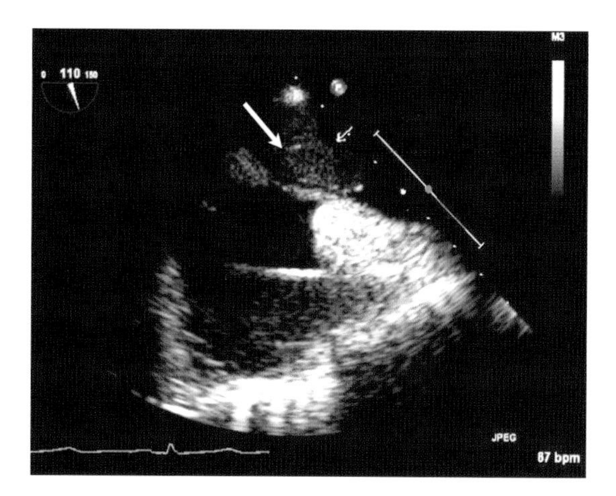

a. Cor triatriatum
b. Myxoma
c. Mitral annular calcification
d. Lipomatous hypertrophy of the interatrial septum

4. Identify the variant or pathology:

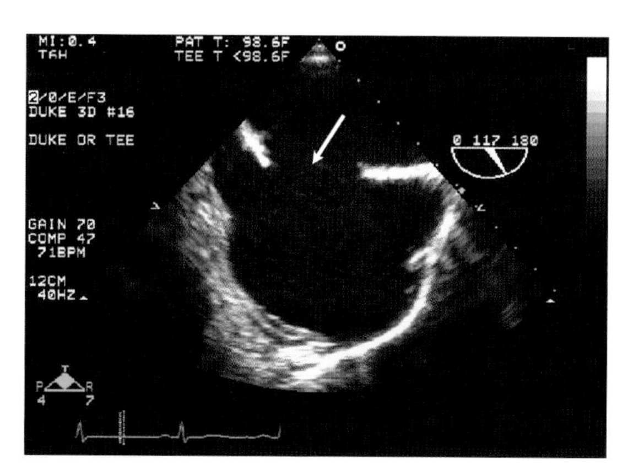

a. Atrial septal defect
b. Crista terminalis
c. Lipomatous hypertrophy of the interatrial septum
d. Eustachian valve

5. What is the artifact seen?

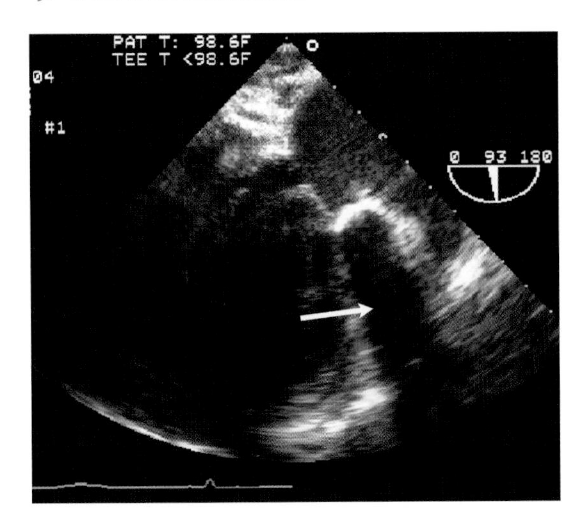

a. Near field clutter
b. Mirror image
c. Acoustic shadow
d. Reverberation

6. Identify the structure at the arrow:

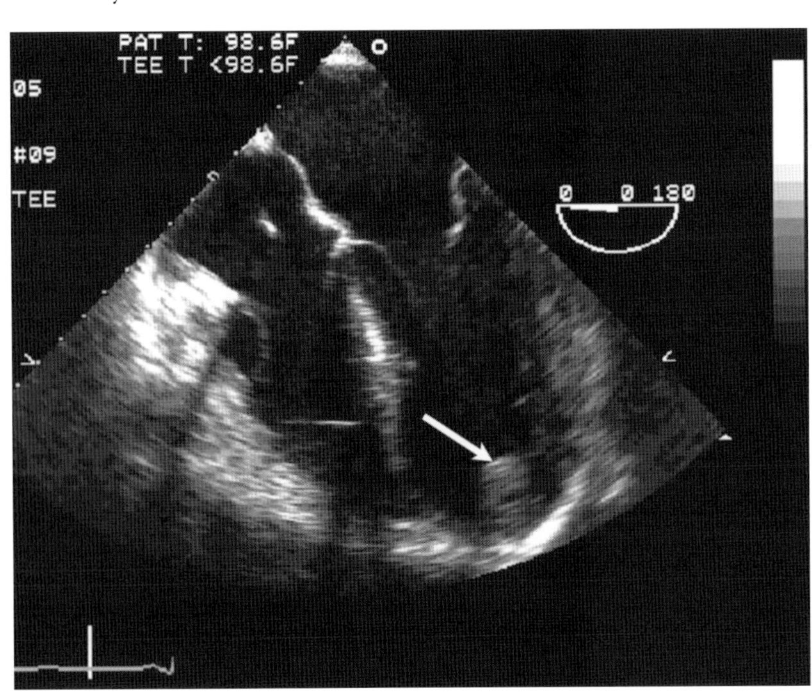

a. Moderator band
b. Papillary muscle
c. Left ventricular band
d. Left ventricular thrombus

7. Identify the source of the flow:

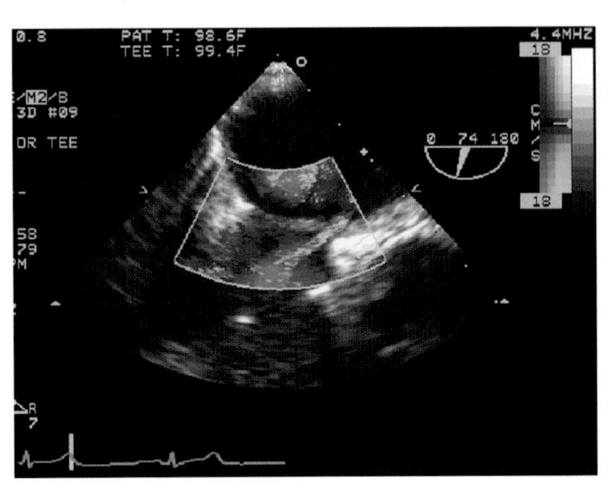

a. Right atrium to left atrium via patent foramen ovale
b. Right atrium to left atrium via atrial septal defect
c. Left atrium to right atrium via patent foramen ovale
d. Left atrium to right atrium via atrial septal defect

8. Identify the structure at the arrow:

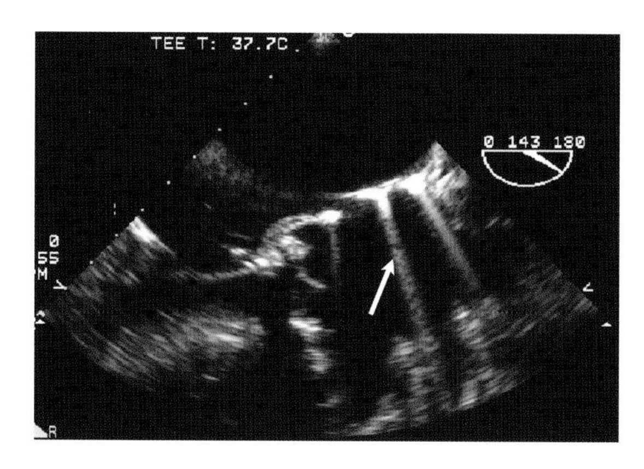

a. Side lobe
b. Mirror image
c. Reverberation
d. Range ambiguity

9. Identify the structure at the arrow:

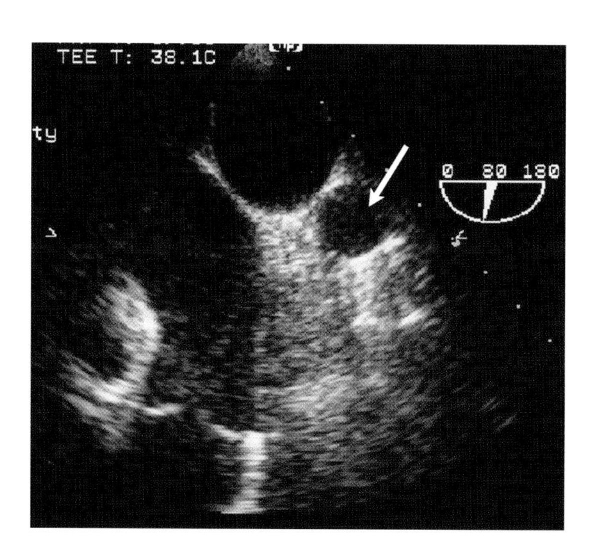

a. Transverse sinus
b. Oblique sinus
c. Ascending pulmonary artery
d. Brachiocephalic vein

10. Identify the structure at the arrow:

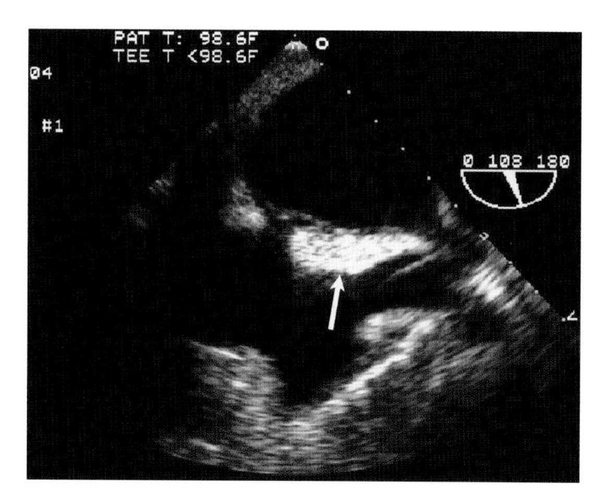

a. Myxoma of the atrial septum
b. Nodulus Aranti
c. Interatrial septal hypertrophy
d. Superior vena caval thrombus

11. What does the following image illustrate?

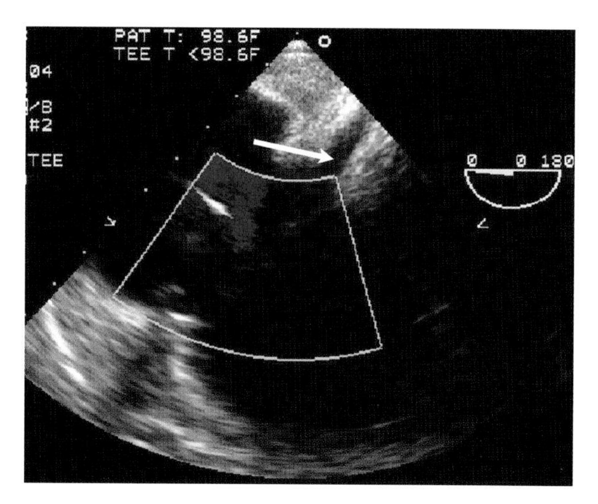

a. Persistent left superior vena cava
b. Normal coronary sinus
c. Dextrocardia
d. Persistent right superior vena cava

12. What is the structure at the arrow?

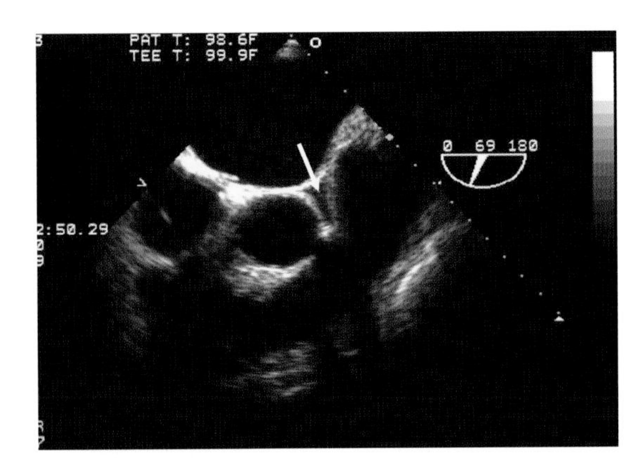

a. Persistent left superior vena cava
b. Left atrial appendage
c. Transverse sinus
d. Ascending pulmonary artery

13. What is the structure at the arrow?

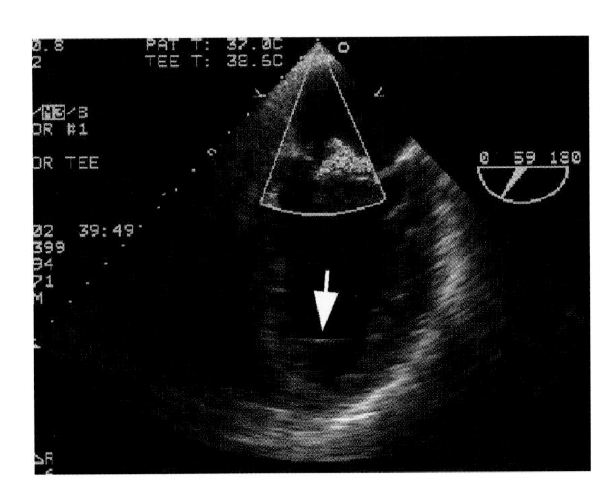

a. Side lobe
b. Aortic dissection
c. Reverberation
d. Comet tail

14. What is seen in the periphery of the right atrium?

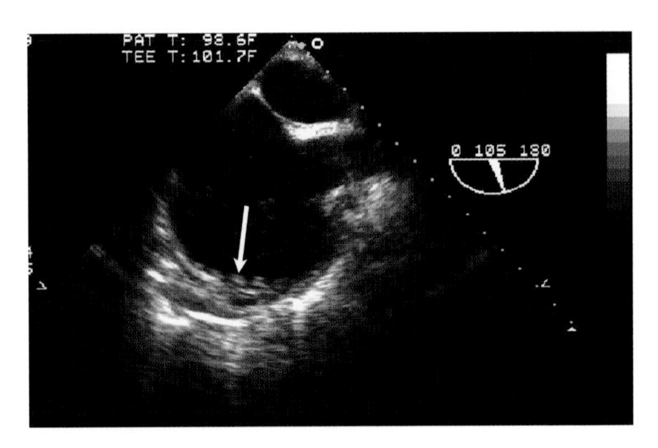

a. Right atrial myxoma
b. Pectinate muscle
c. Lambl's excrescence
d. Nodulus Aranti

15. Identify the structure at the arrow:

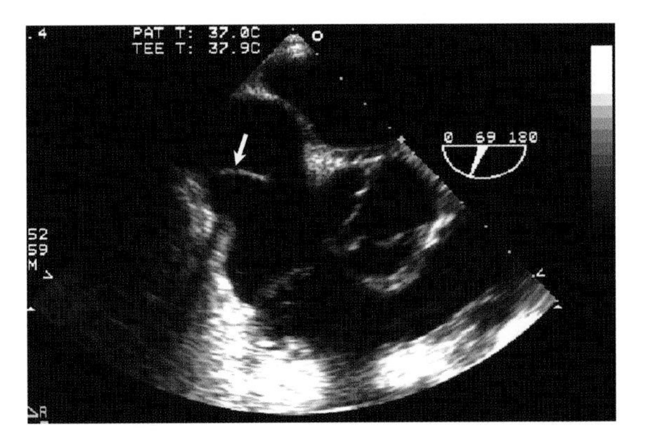

a. Chiari network
b. Eustachian valve
c. Pacing wire
d. Venous cannula

16. What does the following image demonstrate?

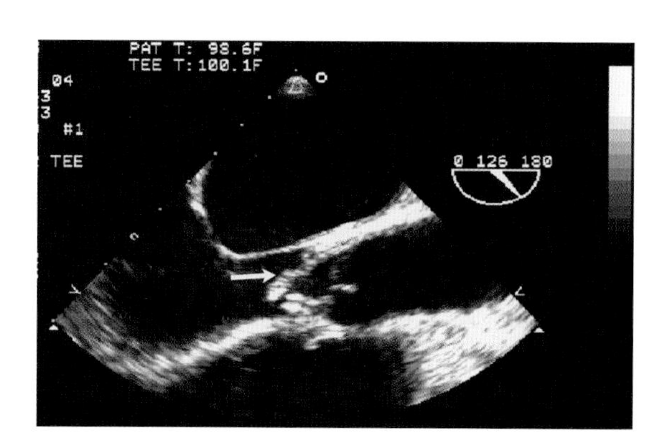

a. Fibroelastoma
b. Lambl's excrescence
c. Flail aortic valve
d. Endocarditis

17. What is the structure at the arrow?

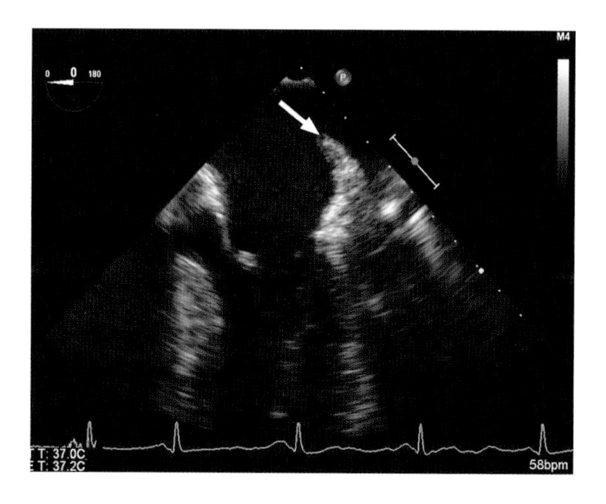

a. Crista terminalis
b. Eustachian valve
c. Thebesian valve
d. Ligament of Marshall

18. The arrow demonstrates:

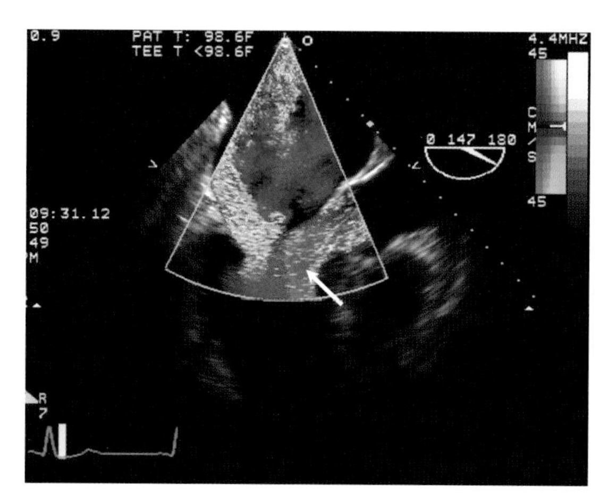

a. Continuous-wave Doppler aliasing
b. Over-gain of the color-flow Doppler
c. Baseline shift of the color-flow Doppler
d. Color-flow Doppler aliasing

19. The structure at the arrow is:

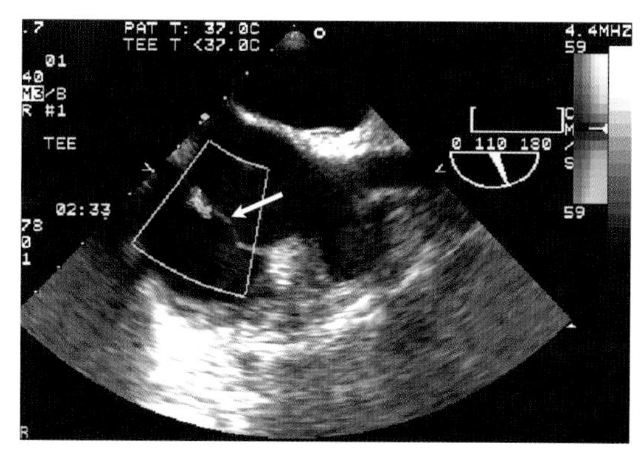

a. Ebstein anomaly
b. Eustachian valve
c. Normal tricuspid valve
d. Patent foramen ovale

20. Based on this image, what is the likely additional anatomic variant?

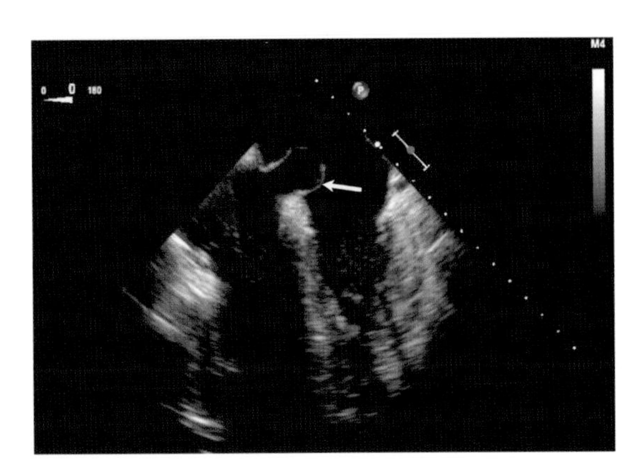

a. Atrial septal defect
b. Ventricular septal defect
c. Chiari network
d. Eustachian valve

21. The echolucency at the arrow is:

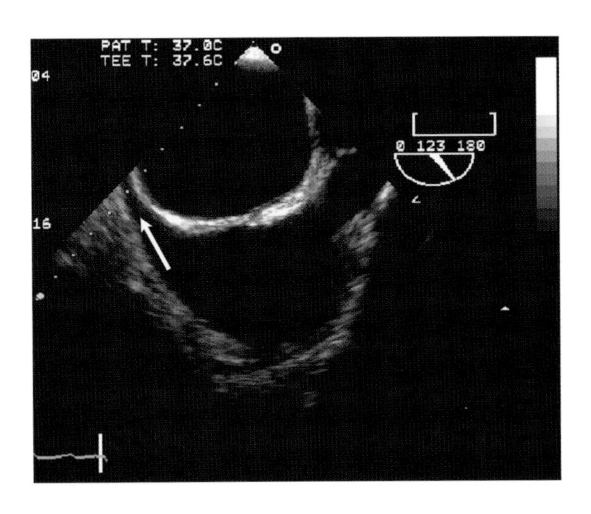

a. Transverse sinus
b. Oblique sinus
c. Inferior vena cava
d. Coronary sinus

22. Identify the structure at the arrow:

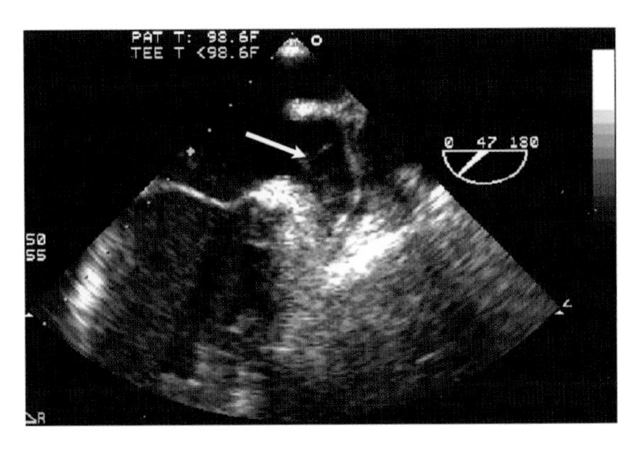

a. Right atrial appendage thrombus
b. Left atrial appendage thrombus
c. Left atrial appendage pectinate muscle
d. Left upper pulmonary vein clot

23. The arrow demonstrates:

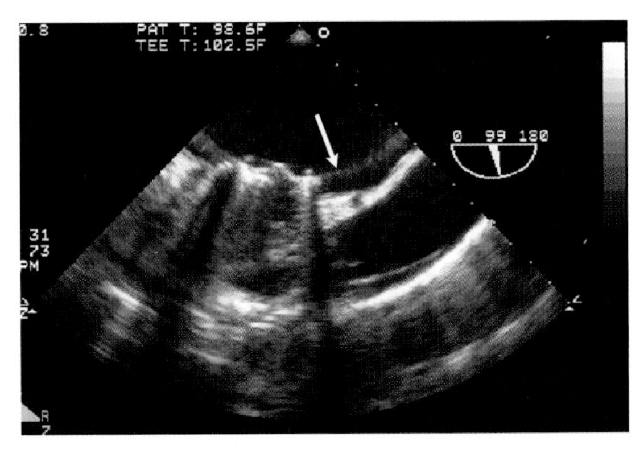

a. Acoustic shadowing
b. Side lobe
c. Reverberation
d. Mirror image

24. The structure at the arrow is:

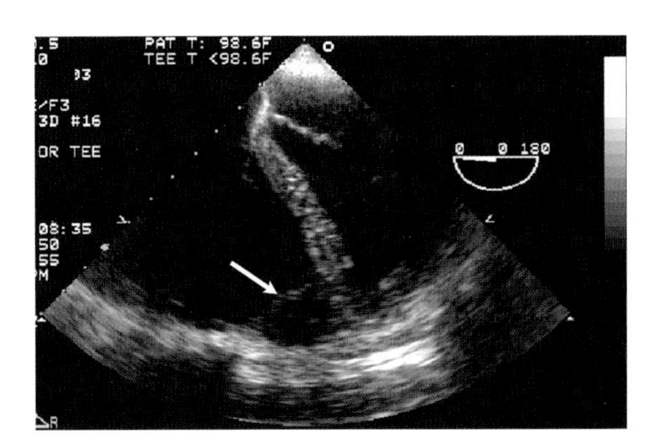

a. Side lobe
b. Papillary muscle
c. Moderator band
d. False tendon

25. The arrow points to an artifact called:

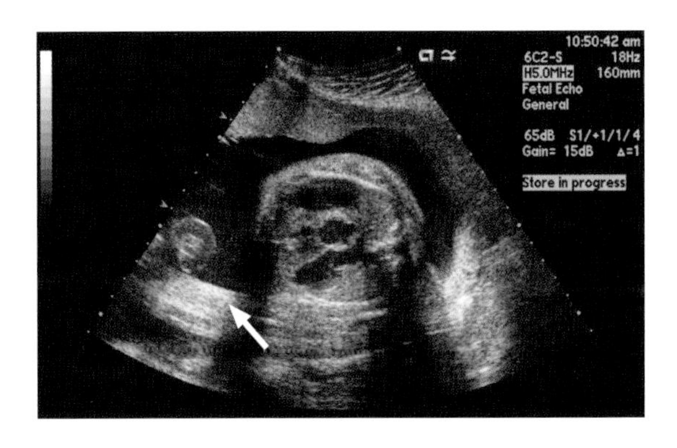

a. Near field clutter
b. Enhancement
c. Acoustic shadow
d. Side lobe

26. The structure at the arrow is:

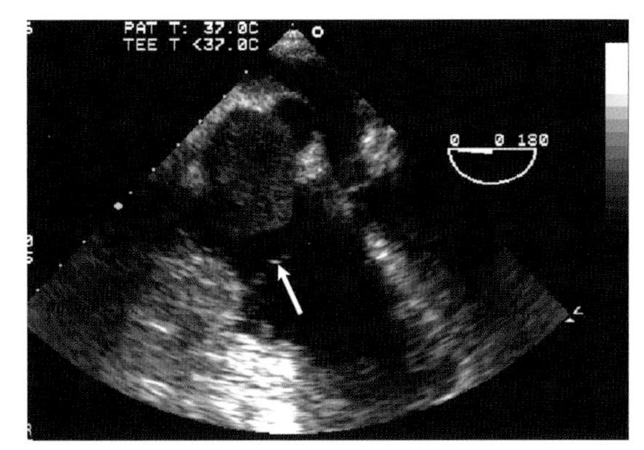

a. Eustachian valve
b. Mitral valve
c. Tricuspid valve
d. Thebesian valve

27. The structure at the arrow is:

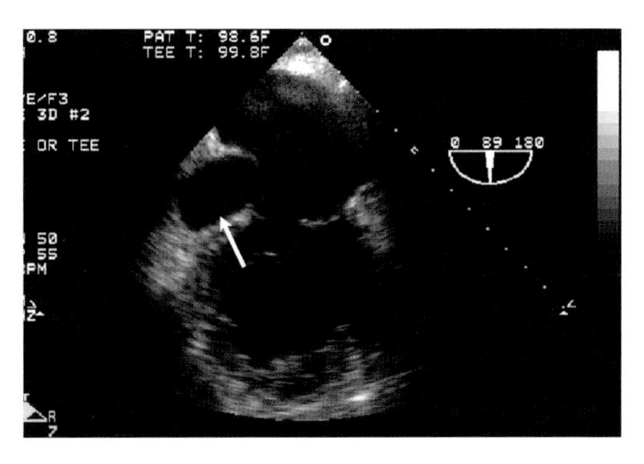

a. Right ventricular cyst
b. Inferior vena cava
c. Aortic outflow tract
d. Dilated coronary sinus

28. The structure at the arrow is:

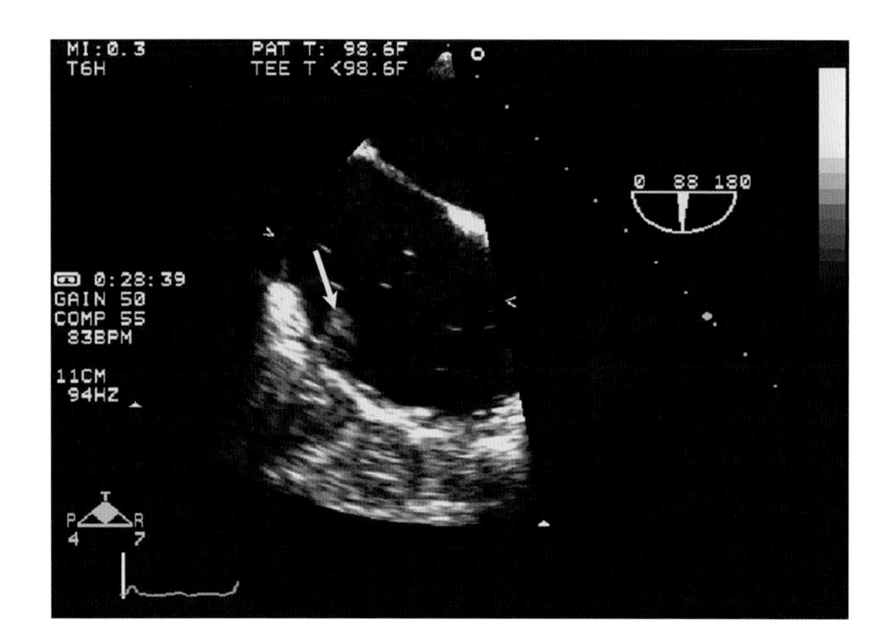

a. Thrombus
b. Tricuspid valve
c. Pectinate muscles
d. Crista terminalis

29. The structure at the arrow is:

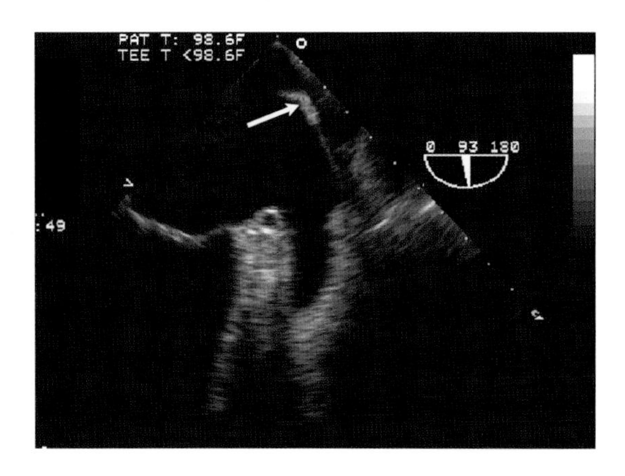

a. Crista terminalis
b. Ligament of Marshall
c. Interatrial septum
d. Eustachian valve

30. The structure at the arrow is:

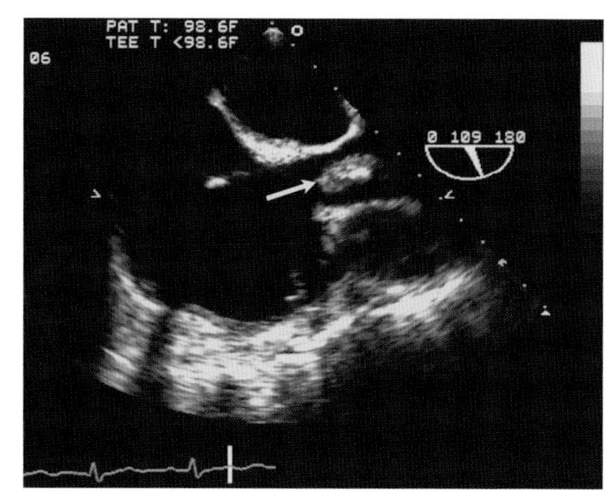

a. Crista terminalis
b. Eustachian valve
c. Thrombus
d. Pulmonary artery catheter

31. The space at the arrow is:

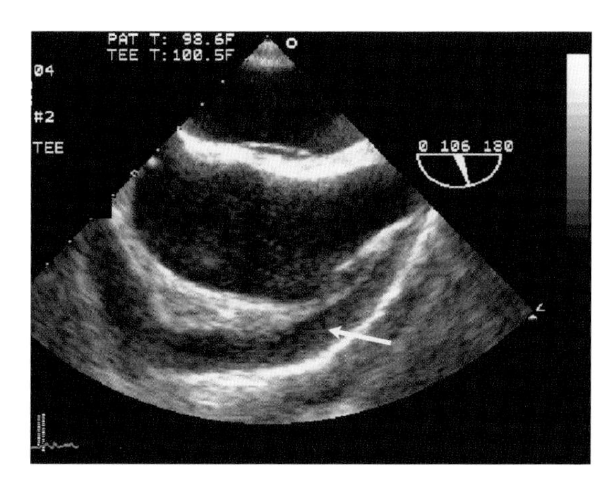

a. Pericardial effusion
b. Right atrium
c. Mirror image
d. Right ventricle

32. The space at the arrow is:

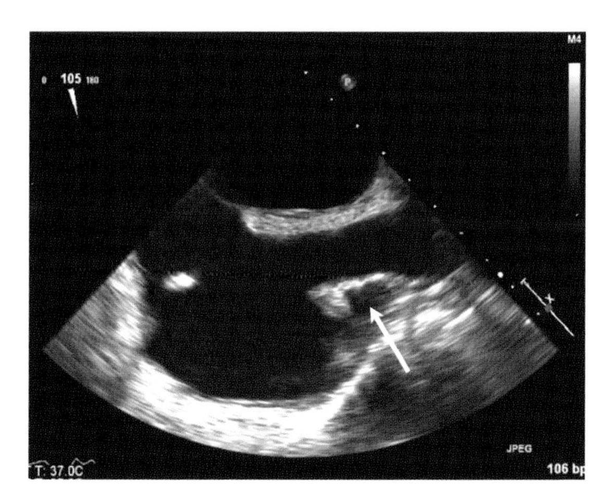

a. Right upper pulmonary vein
b. Left upper pulmonary vein
c. Right atrial appendage
d. Tricuspid valve annulus

33. The sinus venosus leads to the formation of:
a. Eustachian valve, crista terminalis, and moderator band
b. Crista terminalis, eustachian valve, and thebesian valve
c. Eustachian valve, moderator band, and transverse sinus
d. Crista terminalis, transverse sinus, and thebesian valve

34. The purpose of the thebesian valve is to:
a. Direct superior vena cava blood flow in utero
b. Direct inferior vena cava blood flow in utero
c. Direct blood flow into the coronary sinus
d. Prevent retrograde blood flow into the coronary sinus

35. An atrial septal aneurysm is associated with:
a. Thebesian valve and patent foramen ovale
b. Chiari network and moderator band
c. Chiari network and patent foramen ovale
d. Thebesian valve and Chiari network

36. Lipomatous hypertrophy of the interatrial septum is associated with:
a. Coronary artery disease
b. Patent foramen ovale
c Chiari network
e. Persistent left superior vena cava

37. The transverse sinus is seen between the:
a. Left atrium, left upper pulmonary vein, aorta
b. Right atrium, right upper pulmonary vein, aorta
c. Left atrium, pulmonary artery, aorta
a. Right atrium, pulmonary artery, aorta

38. The crista terminalis separates the:
a. Superior vena cava from the eustachian valve
b. Superior vena cava from the right atrial appendage
c. Left atrium from the ascending pulmonary artery
d. Right atrium from the transverse sinus

39. Discrimination of two objects can be improved by:
a. Imaging at the focal zone and decreasing frequency
b. Decreasing the depth and increasing frequency
c. Increasing the depth and increasing frequency
d. Imaging at the focal zone and increasing depth

40. Acoustic shadowing is caused by:
a. A change in the ultrasound medium
b. Dense structures with high acoustic impedance
c. High-amplitude oscillations of piezoelectric crystals
d. The ultrasound beam bouncing between reflective surfaces

41. A patent foramen ovale is best diagnosed using:
a. Agitated saline injection into a peripheral left arm vein
b. Agitated saline injection with a Valsalva maneuver

c. Appearance of bubbles in the left atrium in six cardiac cycles
d. Appearance of bubbles in the right atrium in two cardiac cycles

42. Pectinate muscles may be distinguished from thrombus by:
a. Being associated with atrial fibrillation
b. Being similar in density to the right atrial appendage tissue
c. Undulating throughout the cardiac cycle
d. Appearing in different areas in various TEE views

43. Anatomic variants associated with the conduction system of the heart include:
a. Moderator band, persistent left superior vena cava, eustachian valve
b. Persistent left superior vena cava, eustachian valve, ligament of Marshall
c. Ligament of Marshall, left upper pulmonary vein, moderator band
d. Left upper pulmonary vein, moderator band, persistent left superior vena cava

44. Nodules of Arantius are:
a. Associated with ventricular dysrhythmias
b. Located on the ventricular side of the mitral valve leaflet
c. An important landmark for aortic dissections
d. Located in the free edge of the aortic valve cusps

45. Pericardial fat may be confused with:
a. Pericardial effusion
b. Moderator band
c. Left ventricular thrombus
d. Atrial septal defect

46. Side lobes occur due to:
a. A change in acoustic medium and density
b. Reflection from an object with high density
c. Extraneous divergent beams from the transducer
d. High-amplitude oscillations of piezoelectric crystals

47. Mirror images always appear:
a. On a straight line with and deeper to the real structure
b. On a straight line with and more shallow than the real structure
c. Lateral from and deeper to the real structure
d. Lateral from and more shallow than the real structure

48. The oblique sinus is seen:
a. Anterior to the left atrium, right atrium, and ascending aorta
b. Posterior to the left atrium between the inlet of the pulmonary veins
c. Superior to the superior vena cava and crista terminalis
a. Inferior to the right atrial appendage and coronary sinus

49. The coronary sinus:
a. Is guarded by the eustachian valve
b. Is a pericardial reflection
c. Is in the atrioventricular groove
d. Is normally 1.5 cm wide and 5 cm long

50. The eustachian valve:
a. Directs blood flow in utero toward the foramen ovale
b. Is associated with the superior vena cava
c. Oscillates randomly within the right heart
d. Is associated with right heart volume overload

Quantitative Echocardiography

4

Feroze Mahmood and Robina Matyal

PRINCIPLES OF DOPPLER ECHOCARDIOGRAPHY

Christian Doppler, in his 1842 paper titled, "On the Coloured Light of the Binary Stars and Some Other Stars of the Heavens," was the first to note that stars moving towards the earth emitted blue light while stars moving away from earth radiated red light. Thus, he postulated that the observed frequency of a wave depends on the relative speed of the source and the observer. Although Doppler himself never extended the principle to other natural phenomena, the common observation that the pitch of sound is different for a locomotive approaching the listener than one moving away led to a more widespread application of Doppler's initial observation.

In clinical echocardiography, the Doppler technique depends upon an analysis of the frequency and wavelength of an emitted ultrasound beam. Frequency is defined as the number of waves passing though a certain point in 1 second, and is a fundamental property of the sound waves. It is expressed in units of hertz (Hz) and determines the resolution and the depth of penetration of the medium. However, the Doppler assessment of ultrasound waves depends upon not just the absolute emitted frequency, but the relative change in frequency as the sound waves are reflected back (by red blood cells) towards the transducer. The frequency of the reflected sound waves increases when the red blood cells are moving towards the transducer and decreases when red blood cells are moving away from the transducer (Figure 4–1). This relative change in the frequency, known as the Doppler shift, enables the echocardiographer to assess the direction, speed, and turbulence of blood flow, which in turn helps to objectively quantify intracardiac pressures and the severity of valvular stenosis and regurgitation.

DOPPLER SHIFT

The Doppler shift is defined as the change in frequency of the reflected ultrasound waves and is described by the following mathematical relationship[1]:

$$\Delta f = 2f_t \times (v \times \text{Cos}\theta)/c$$

Δf = Difference between the transmitted frequency (f_t) and received frequency
v = Velocity of red blood cells
θ = Angle between the Doppler beam and the direction of blood flow
c = Speed of ultrasound in blood (1540 m/s)

When the Doppler beam is parallel to the direction of blood flow, the cosine of θ is 1 and the Doppler shift is most accurately calculated, but with increases in θ there is a progressive decrease in the measured Doppler shift. This underestimation of Doppler shift remains clinically insignificant until θ exceeds 20° and the associated percentage error exceeds 7% (Figure 4–2).[2] When the Doppler beam is perpendicular to the direction of flow, the Doppler shift is recorded as zero since the cosine of 90 is zero. It is therefore essential to align the Doppler beam as parallel to the direction of blood flow as possible for an accurate measurement of speed and direction of flow.

Doppler Display

All ultrasound systems are equipped to create both a spectral display and an audio component of the beat-to-beat Doppler data during acquisition. The loudness and pitch of this audio signal varies with the strength and quality of the Doppler data, and experienced echocardiographers have been known to use the audio component alone to acquire and record the maximal velocity. The loudness/pitch of the audio signal can also be used to qualitatively diagnose the presence of stenosis; however, the information obtained from audio analysis is qualitative and subjective and should not be used as the sole means of quantification.[1]

On the other hand, quantitative Doppler data on a spectral display provides a high degree of spatial and temporal resolution. Before the Doppler information can be displayed as distinct envelopes (velocity profiles over time) on the spectral display, the raw Doppler data undergo significant post-acquisition manipulation (demodulation, fast Fourier transformation, and chirp-Z transformation) to isolate the required frequencies.[1] If the returning frequency is higher than the transmitted frequency, it is referred

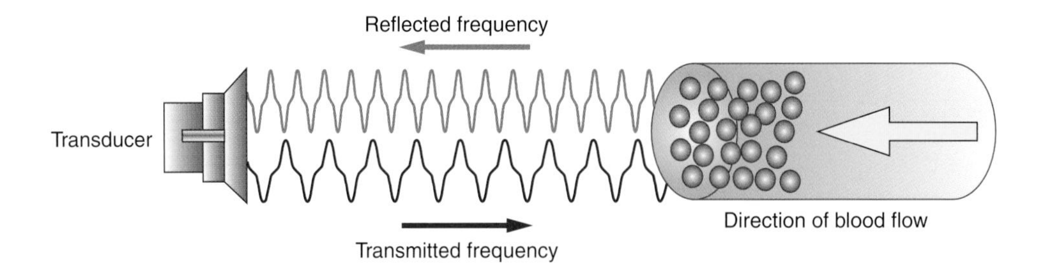

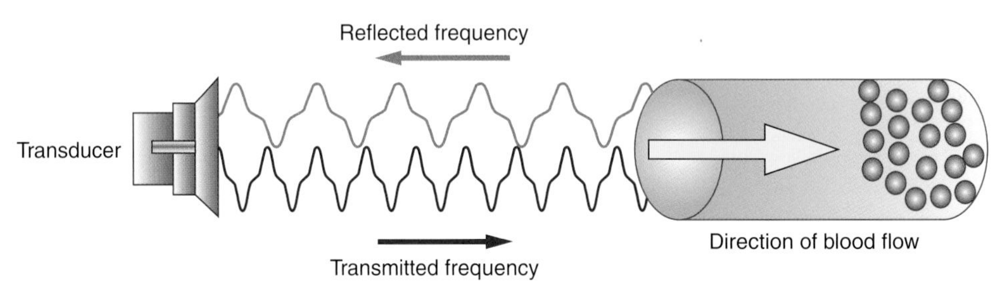

FIGURE 4–1. Principle of Doppler shift. The frequency (cycles/second) of the reflected sound waves increases when the red blood cells are moving towards the transducer and decreases when red blood cells are moving away from the transducer.

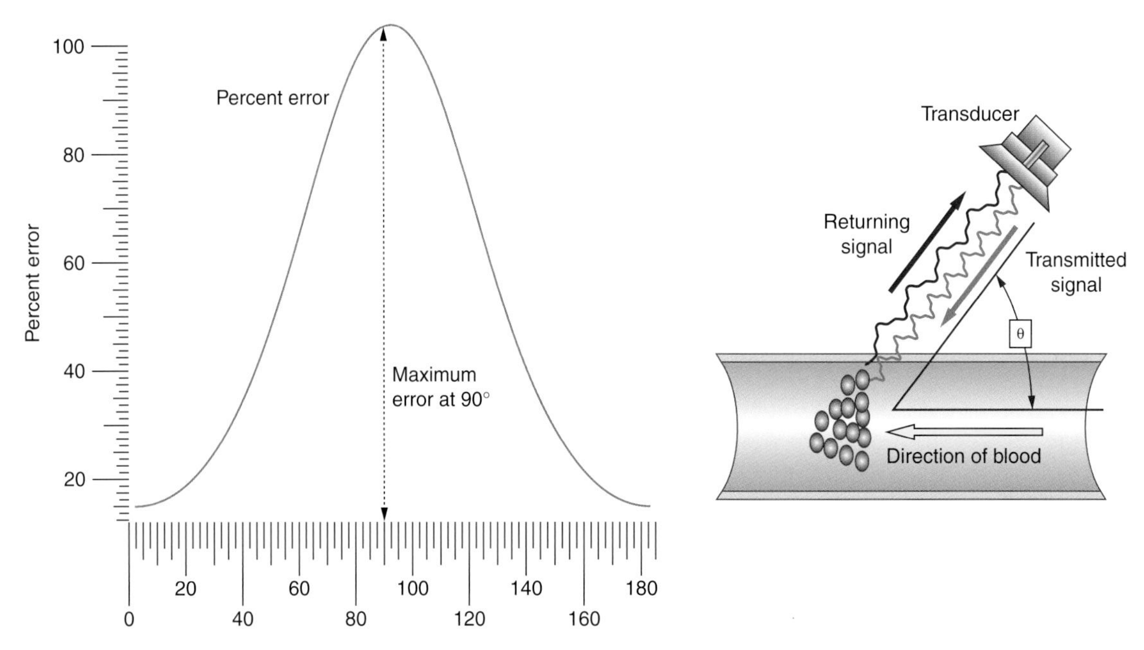

FIGURE 4–2. When the Doppler beam is parallel to the direction of blood flow, the Doppler shift is most accurately calculated, but with increases in θ there is a progressive decrease in the measured Doppler shift. This error is clinically insignificant when θ is less than 20°.

to as a "positive Doppler shift" (blood moving towards the transducer) and is displayed above the baseline. If the returning frequency is less than the transmitted frequency, it is called a "negative Doppler shift" (blood moving away from transducer) and is displayed below the baseline.

It is important to remember that a simultaneous display of the two-dimensional (2D) image and Doppler information requires a time-share arrangement between two independent functions of the transducer. In the case of a continuous spectral display, the 2D image display is rapidly switched on and off, giving the impression of a continuous image alongside the spectral display. Thus, there is always some reduction in the quality of 2D and Doppler data when a simultaneous imaging mode is used.[1]

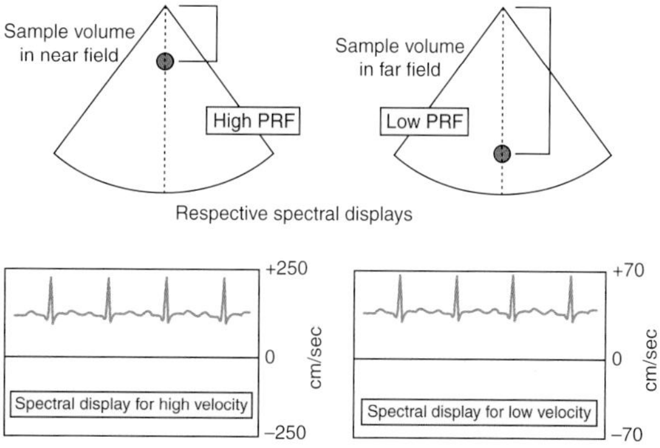

FIGURE 4–3. Imaging depth and pulse repetition frequency. At a greater imaging depth, the pulse repetition frequency is lower.

DOPPLER MODALITIES

Doppler can be used either in "pulse" or "continuous" mode to interrogate intracardiac flow patterns. Both these modalities have strengths and weaknesses that are suited for specific situations.

Pulsed-Wave Doppler (PWD)

PWD utilizes a single ultrasound crystal that alternates between transmission and reception. As a consequence, the maximal frequency shift (and thus maximum velocity) that can be measured is limited to one-half the pulse repetition frequency (also known as the Nyquist limit). When this maximal frequency shift is exceeded, aliasing or a wrapping around of the velocities is seen on the spectral Doppler display. In general, the maximum measurable velocity without aliasing with PWD is less than 2 m/s. The pulse repetition frequency (PRF) is directly related to the depth of placement of the sample volume, ie, the longer the time it takes for the sound to travel back to the transducer, the lower the PRF (Figure 4–3). An advantage of PWD is that the operator can select the specific site of measurement by manually positioning the sample volume during conventional 2D echocardiography, thus providing "range resolution" or the ability to identify the exact location of the recorded velocity (Figure 4–4). Simultaneous display of the location of the sample volume and

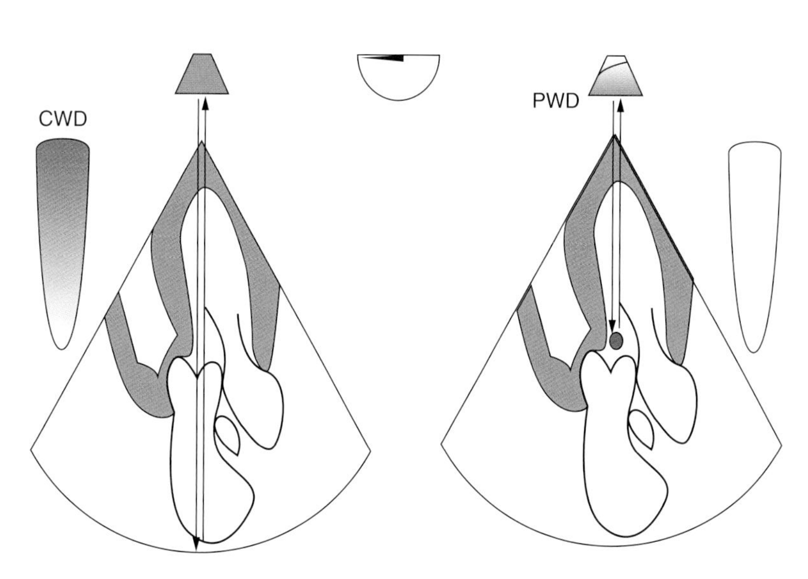

FIGURE 4–4. PWD allows the operator to measure a specific site by manually positioning the sample volume. CWD measures the highest velocity in the path of the ultrasound beam, thus suffering from "range ambiguity" or the inability to discriminate the precise location of the highest recorded velocity. The velocity envelopes obtained with CWD are typically shaded, representing the multiple velocities measured in the course of the ultrasound beam.

the spectral Doppler data is also possible with some sacrifice of the quality of the 2D image as well as the Doppler signal. The distance from the transducer determines the size and three-dimensional shape of the sample volume. The farther the sample volume is placed from the transducer, the larger it becomes due to progressive divergence of the ultrasound beam from the transducer.

During transmission of a PWD beam, the signals returning to the transducer are interpreted on the basis of the time it takes for them to return to the transducer, a process referred to as "time-gating." During time-gating, signals returning after a specific time from a preselected depth are chosen for interpretation, and all other returning signals are selectively ignored by the ultrasound system. Time-gating is described by the following mathematical relationship:

$$\text{Time Delay} = 2d/C$$

d = Depth
C = Speed of sound in blood

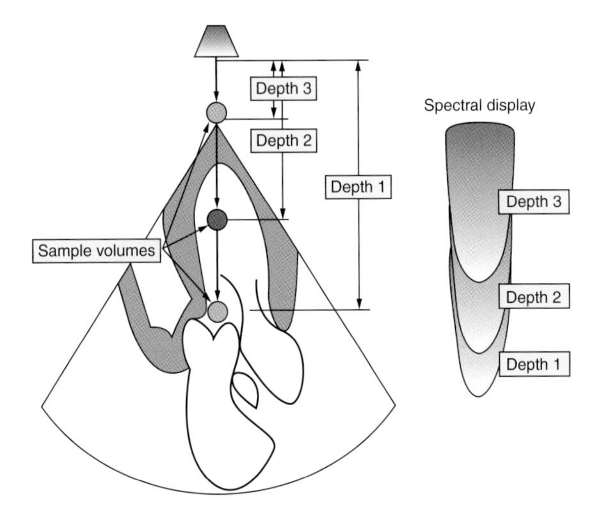

FIGURE 4–5. High pulse repetition frequency pulsed-wave Doppler is used to resolve the velocity of multiple high-velocity lesions that are in series.

High Pulse Repetition Frequency (HPRF) Doppler

A technique to measure high velocities with PWD employs special transducers with the ability to emit multiple pulses. Since any emitted pulse does continue beyond the primary sampling depth (albeit weaker), the net effect is increased sampling at locations beyond the primary depth. Depending on the number of pulses, the Nyquist limit can be increased by a factor of 2 or more. The increase in sampling frequency is, however, at the expense of range ambiguity. The primary application of HPRF Doppler is in resolving the velocity of multiple high-velocity lesions that are in series (Figure 4–5).

Continuous-Wave Doppler (CWD)

In the continuous-wave mode, the ultrasound transducer utilizes two crystals—one to continuously send an ultrasound beam and another to constantly receive the reflected wave (see Figure 4–4). Since there is one crystal dedicated to receiving the reflection, the maximal frequency shift that can be detected is not limited by the pulse repetition frequency, and very high velocities can be recorded without aliasing. However, the CWD signal is not time-gated and measures the highest velocity in the path of the ultrasound beam, thus suffering from "range ambiguity" or the inability to discriminate the precise location of the highest recorded velocity. The velocity envelopes obtained with CWD are typically shaded, representing the multiple velocities measured in the course of the ultrasound beam.

Color-Flow Doppler

Color-flow Doppler is a pulsed ultrasound technique that color codes Doppler information and superimposes it on a 2D image, displaying information on the direction and the mean velocities of flow as color maps. Blood flow directed towards the transducer is commonly (but not exclusively) color-coded in shades of red, while blood flowing away from the transducer is color-coded in shades of blue. Lighter shades within each of these colors typically represent higher velocities. Color-flow Doppler uses packets of multiple pulses (3 to 20 per scan line), and therefore has a low temporal resolution. It has the characteristics of pulsed-wave Doppler (range discrimination and aliasing), but color-flow Doppler aliases at a lower velocity than traditional PWD because of the reduction in PRF associated with the simultaneous generation of a gray-scale and a color image.

Doppler Tissue Imaging

Conventional Doppler modalities are designed to calculate the intracardiac or intravascular blood flow velocities (ie, high-velocity and low-amplitude signals). Doppler tissue imaging (DTI) is geared to detect velocities of the actual myocardial tissue (ie, low-velocity, high-amplitude signals).[3-5] Current echocardiography systems come equipped with presets for measuring DTI signals, and are generally set to measure myocardial velocities in the range of 0.2 to 0.4 cm/s and detect amplitudes greater than 20 dB. In contrast, the amplitude of the movement of red blood cells is generally less than 15 dB.[6] The DTI signals can be displayed as a spectral tracing, in association with color-flow Doppler signals, or as color-encoded 2D signals.

UTILIZATION OF DOPPLER FOR HEMODYNAMIC ASSESSMENT

Two-dimensional and Doppler imaging can be used to obtain comprehensive hemodynamic data, but it should be remembered that these data, while providing a more objective measure of cardiac performance, should always be interpreted within the context of the patient's clinical condition.

Measurement of Flow

In circulation, the blood flow and velocity are phasic, ie, change throughout the cardiac cycle. A Doppler spectrum of the velocity of blood flowing through a conduit will yield a curve during systole that has velocity (cm/s) on the y-axis and time (s) on the x-axis. When this curve is integrated, it yields a velocity-time integral (VTI) in units of centimeters (velocity [cm/s] time [s] = VTI [cm]). The VTI is a manifestation of the stroke distance (ie, the distance the stroke volume travels over time during a single systolic ejection period). The product of VTI (cm) and cross-sectional area (CSA; cm^2) will yield stroke volume (SV; cm^3):

$$\text{Stroke Volume (SV)} = \text{Stroke Distance (VTI)} \times \text{Cross Sectional Area (CSA)}$$

Cardiac output can then be calculated as:

$$\text{Cardiac Output} = \text{Stroke Volume} \times \text{Heart Rate}$$

Cardiac index can be calculated as:

$$\text{Cardiac Index} = \text{Cardiac Output/Body Surface Area}$$

The calculation of SV through a conduit assumes laminar flow, a flat flow profile in which velocities are

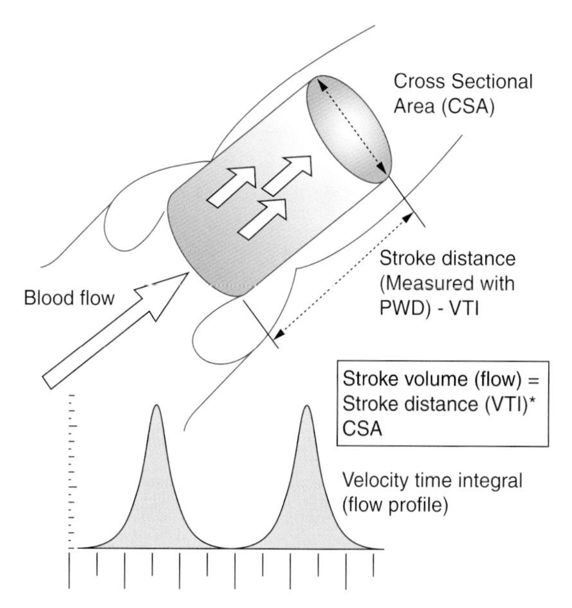

FIGURE 4–6. Calculation of cardiac output from the left ventricular outflow tract (LVOT). (PWD, pulsed-wave Doppler.)

uniform, constant diameter of the conduit, velocity measured at the same point as the diameter, velocity measured represents the mean velocity during the entire ejection period, and accurate measurement of the conduit diameter (a common source of error). Stroke volume can be measured at any conduit in the heart; however, the preferred site for such calculation is the left ventricular outflow tract (LVOT) (Figure 4–6). Other intracardiac sites such as the pulmonic and mitral valves have a dynamic conduit diameter during the cardiac cycle, and at times the velocity profile is parabolic, where velocities vary across the parabola.

In echocardiography, it is assumed that a conduit or orifice, such as the LVOT, is circular. The CSA is calculated from the diameter measurements by using the equation for area of a circle:

$$
\begin{aligned}
\text{CSA} &= \pi \times r^2, \text{ where r is the radius} \\
&= \pi \times (D/2)^2, \text{ where D is the diameter and D/2 is the radius (r)} \\
&= \pi \times D^2/4 \\
&= \pi/4 \times D^2, \text{ where } \pi = 3.14 \\
&= 0.785 \times D^2
\end{aligned}
$$

The diameter of the LVOT is calculated from the midesophageal long-axis window, and LVOT VTI is calculated from the deep transgastric window (Figure 4–7).

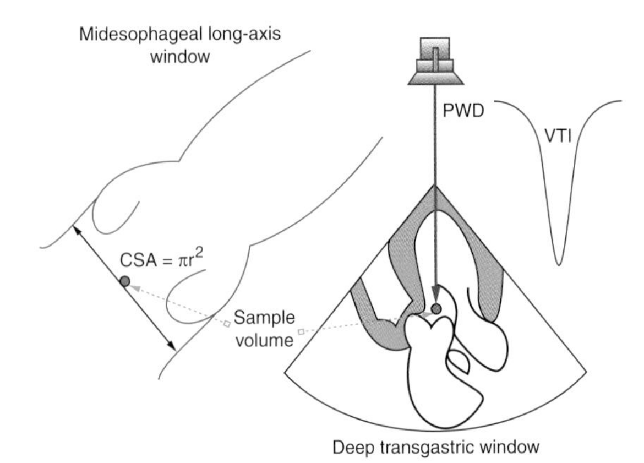

FIGURE 4–7. Imaging windows used to calculate stroke volume. The midesophageal long-axis view is used to measure left ventricular outflow tract (LVOT) diameter, and the deep transgastric long-axis view is used to measure the LVOT velocity-time integral (VTI). (CSA, cross-sectional area; PWD, pulsed-wave Doppler.)

Measurement of Intracardiac Shunts

The ratio of pulmonary (Q_p) to systemic (Q_s) flow is a useful parameter to assess the magnitude of shunting, with a ratio greater than 1.5 generally considered significant. Q_p/Q_s calculation requires calculation of the stroke volume at the right ventricular outflow tract (RVOT) and the left ventricular outflow tract (LVOT). Thus, for atrial or ventricular shunts:

$$Q_p/Q_s = (CSA_{RVOT} \times TVI_{RVOT})/(CSA_{LVOT} \times TVI_{LVOT})$$

For shunts occurring through a patent ductus arteriosus:

$$Q_p/Q_s = (CSA_{LVOT} \times TVI_{LVOT})/(CSA_{RVOT} \times TVI_{RVOT})$$

Conservation of Flow

Assuming a constant flow of fluid through a conduit at a certain velocity, if there is a stenosis in the conduit, the velocity of fluid will increase at the site of stenosis to conserve flow. This concept is known as the *continuity of flow* and sometimes as the *conservation of flow*:

$$Flow_{Larger\ Conduit} = Flow_{Stenosis}$$

As described above, constant flow (cm^3/s) in a conduit is the product of cross-sectional area (CSA) of the conduit (cm^2) and the average velocity of the fluid (cm/s). Thus,

$$CSA_{Larger\ Conduit} \times Velocity_{Larger\ Conduit} = CSA_{Stenosis} \times Velocity_{Stenosis}$$

When three variables are known, the fourth is easily determined with this equation, commonly known as the *continuity equation*.

In aortic stenosis, flow across the aortic valve is equal to the flow across the LVOT (Figure 4–8) and in order to determine the stenotic area, the continuity equation can be reordered as:

$$CSA_{Stenosis} = \frac{CSA_{Larger\ Conduit} \times Velocity_{Larger\ Conduit}}{Velocity_{Stenosis}}$$

Thus:

$$\text{Aortic Valve Area} = \frac{CSA_{LVOT} \times VTI_{LVOT}}{VTI_{Aortic\ Valve}}$$

Mitral valve area can also be similarly calculated, but it must be remembered that the transmitral flow must be the same as left ventricular SV, a condition that is met only in the absence of ventricular shunts and mitral and aortic regurgitation.

$$\text{Mitral Valve Area} = \frac{CSA_{LVOT} \times VTI_{LVOT}}{VTI_{Mitral\ Valve}}$$

The principles of flow conservation can also be applied to assess regurgitant volumes and fractions. For this calculation, one valve is considered the "reference valve," but it should be remembered that the assumption that the mitral valve orifice is circular may not always be valid. In the absence of aortic stenosis or regurgitation (see Chapters 7 and 9), SV_{LVOT} can be substituted for $SV_{Aortic\ Valve}$

$$\text{Regurgitant Volume}_{Mitral\ Valve} = SV_{Mitral\ Valve} - SV_{LVOT}$$
$$= (CSA_{Mitral} \times VTI_{Mitral}) - (CSA_{LVOT} \times VTI_{LVOT})$$

$$\text{Regurgitant Volume}_{Aortic\ Valve} = SV_{LVOT} - SV_{Mitral\ Valve}$$
$$= (CSA_{LVOT} \times VTI_{LVOT}) - (CSA_{Mitral} \times VTI_{Mitral})$$

$$\text{Regurgitant Fraction}_{Valve}\ (\%) = \frac{\text{Regurgitant Volume}_{Valve}}{\text{Stroke Volume}_{Valve}} \times 100$$

$$\text{Effective Regurgitant Orifice Area (EROA)} = \frac{\text{Regurgitant Volume}_{Mitral\ Valve}}{VTI_{Mitral\ Regurgitant\ Jet}}$$

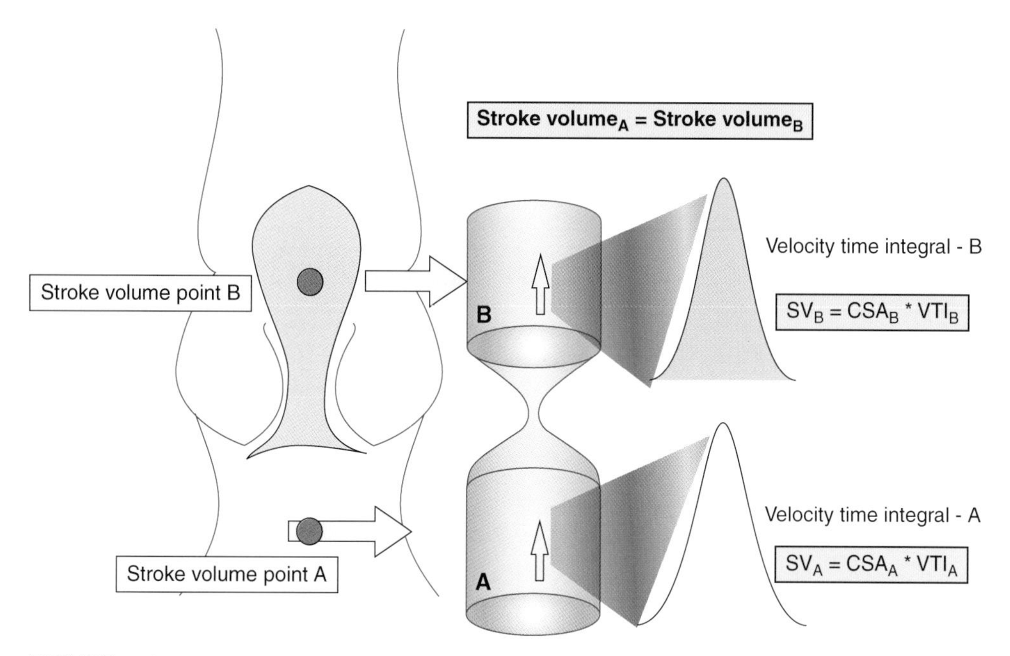

FIGURE 4–8. Principles of the continuity equation. (SV, stroke volume; CSA, cross-sectional area; PWD, pulsed-wave Doppler; CWD, continuous-wave Doppler; VTI, velocity-time integral.)

Velocity Acceleration

When molecules move within a large cavity toward a small orifice, as in stenotic and regurgitant lesions, the velocity increases over a large area and the velocity profile is hemispherical, with the cavity of the hemisphere facing the orifice. The velocity over the surface of the hemisphere is the same (isovelocity), and because it is proximal to the orifice, the surface area is known as *proximal isovelocity surface area* (PISA). The product of the (iso)velocity (cm/s) and the surface area of the hemispherical velocity profile (cm^2) yields the flow (cm^3).

$$\text{Flow} = \text{PISA} \times \text{Velocity}_{\text{Hemisphere Surface}}$$

If the flow approaching the orifice is examined with color-flow Doppler, with the color scale set so that the accelerated velocity exceeds the Nyquist limit, aliasing will take place and a semicircular shell of a contrasting color will appear to cap the orifice (Figure 4–9). To obtain this shell, the baseline for the color scale should be shifted in the direction of the jet of interest (eg, towards the transesophageal echocardiography [TEE] transducer for mitral regurgitation). The semicircular shell is in fact a hemisphere in three dimensions, and its surface area can be calculated as that of a sphere:

$$\text{Surface Area of a Sphere} = 4\pi \times r^2,$$
where r is the radius of the hemisphere
$$\text{Surface Area of a Hemisphere (PISA)} = (4\pi \times r^2)/2 = 2\pi \times r^2$$

The velocity at the surface of the hemispherical velocity profile is the Nyquist limit (aliasing velocity) on the color-flow Doppler scale. Thus,

$$\text{Flow} = \text{PISA} \times \text{Velocity}_{\text{Aliasing}}$$

By the principle of conservation of flow, the flow through an orifice is the same as the flow where the PISA is located:

$$\text{PISA} \times \text{Velocity}_{\text{Aliasing}} = \text{CSA}_{\text{Orifice}} \times \text{Peak Velocity}_{\text{Orifice}}$$

In the setting of stenosis, the valve area can be calculated by reordering the equation as:

$$\text{CSA}_{\text{Stenotic Orifice}} = \frac{\text{PISA} \times \text{Velocity}_{\text{Aliasing}}}{\text{Peak Velocity}_{\text{Stenotic Orifice}}}$$

For a regurgitant lesion, the calculation of the effective regurgitant orifice area (EROA) employs the peak velocity of the regurgitant jet so that:

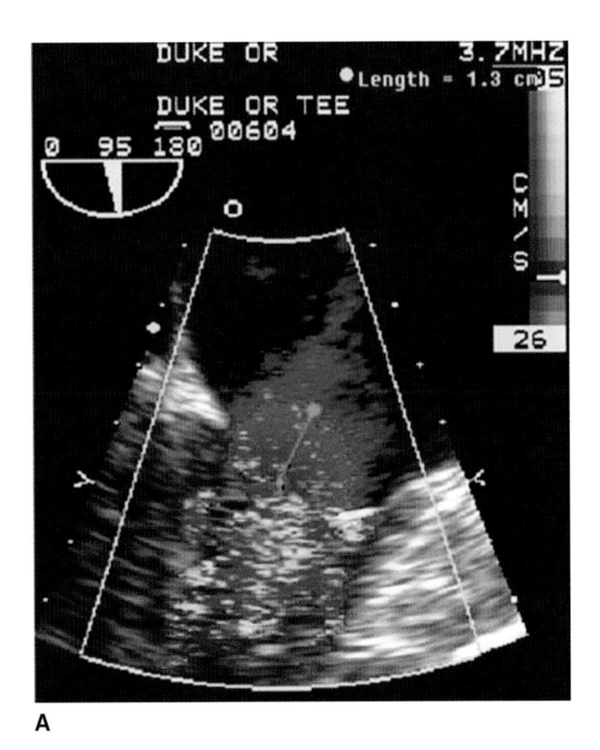

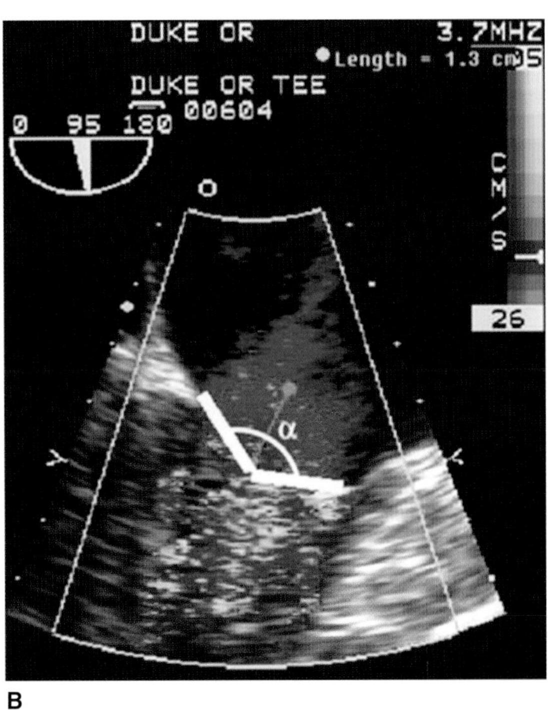

FIGURE 4–9. Color-flow Doppler examination of transmitral flow in mitral stenosis. **A:** Velocity acceleration as flow approaches the stenotic orifice is demonstrated by aliasing of color flow, which shows a shell of proximal isovelocity surface area. The edge of the proximal isovelocity surface area is defined by the transition from blue to red color. In this case, the aliasing velocity is 26 cm/s and the radius of the hemisphere is 1.3 cm. **B:** The angle (α) subtended by the mitral leaflets is shown.

$$CSA_{\text{Regurgitant Orifice}} = \frac{PISA \times Velocity_{\text{Aliasing}}}{\text{Peak Velocity}_{\text{Regurgitant Jet}}}$$

The PISA radius should be measured at the same time as the peak velocity of the jet, and this can be more readily accomplished using color M-mode imaging. PISA has been validated for mitral valve assessment, but is not commonly applied to TEE assessment of the aortic valve. PISA is performed in diastole and on the left atrial side for assessment of mitral stenosis severity, and during systole and on the left ventricular side for calculation of the EROA (Figure 4–10). Summarizing, the assessment of the mitral valve:

$$\text{Mitral Valve Area} = \frac{2\pi r^2 \times Velocity_{\text{Aliasing}}}{\text{Peak Velocity}_{\text{Transmitral}}} \quad \text{(Figure 4-11)}$$

$$EROA = \frac{2\pi r^2 \times Velocity_{\text{Aliasing}}}{\text{Peak Velocity}_{\text{Mitral Regurgitant Jet}}} \quad \text{(Figure 4-12)}$$

True hemispheric shells require a flat valve surface area, and because the mitral valve surface area is not flat, an angle correction term is sometimes used to increase the accuracy of volumetric flow assessment:

$$PISA = 2\pi \times r^2 \times \alpha/180$$

where α is the angle subtended by the mitral leaflets (see Figure 4–9). However, this technique of angle correction is limited by the inability to readily measure α with existing ultrasound system software.

Measurement of Pressure

BERNOULLI EQUATION[1]

A Dutch-Swiss mathematician, Daniel Bernoulli, in 1798 proposed the principle that the total energy in a steady flowing fluid column remains constant, such that when the velocity (kinetic energy) increases, it is accompanied by a simultaneous decrease in pressure (potential energy). This principle helped to explain the development of a pressure gradient across a narrowing,

PISA for Mitral Stenosis

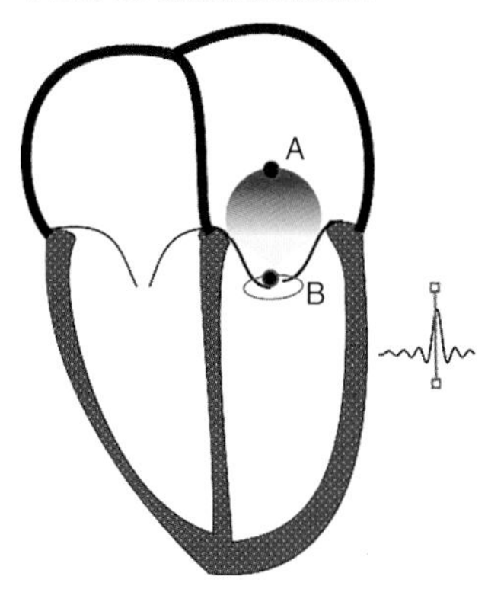

1. Measured during diastole
2. Left atrial side of the mitral valve
3. Stroke volume at point A
4. Stroke volume at point B
5. Equation solved for mitral valve area

PISA for Mitral Regurgitation

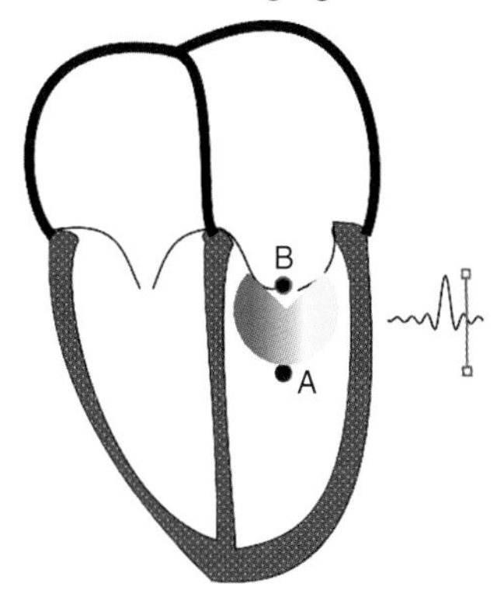

1. Measured during systole
2. Left ventricular side of the mitral valve
3. Stroke volume at point A
4. Stroke volume at point B
5. Equation solved for EROA

FIGURE 4–10. Application of the PISA principle for assessment of mitral stenosis and mitral regurgitation. (PISA, proximal isovelocity surface area.)

ie, there is an increase in distal velocity with a simultaneous drop in pressure (Figure 4–13). The Bernoulli equation can be applied to compressible and noncompressible fluids or even gases, and is expressed as:

Pressure Difference = Convective Acceleration + Flow Acceleration + Viscous Friction

or

$$P_1 - P_2 = \Delta P = \frac{1}{2}\rho(V_2^2 - V_1^2) + \rho \int_1^2 \frac{dv}{dt}\, ds + R(\mu, v)$$

$P_1 - P_2$ = Pressure difference between the two locations
ρ = Mass density of blood (gm/cm^3)
V_1 = Velocity proximal to stenosis (m/s)
V_2 = Velocity at vena contracta (m/s)
dv/dt = Acceleration
s = Distance over which flow accelerates
R = Viscous resistance
μ = Viscosity
v = Velocity of blood flow (m/s)

During routine clinical echocardiography, acceleration at peak velocities (dv/dt) is zero and viscous

Aliasing velocity
Isovelocity shell
PISA radius
35 cm/sec
A wave
E wave

Mitral valve area = $2\pi r^2$ (PISA) *Velocity$_{Aliasing}$/Velocity$_{Peak\ transmitral}$

FIGURE 4–11. PISA for mitral stenosis. (PISA, proximal isovelocity surface area.)

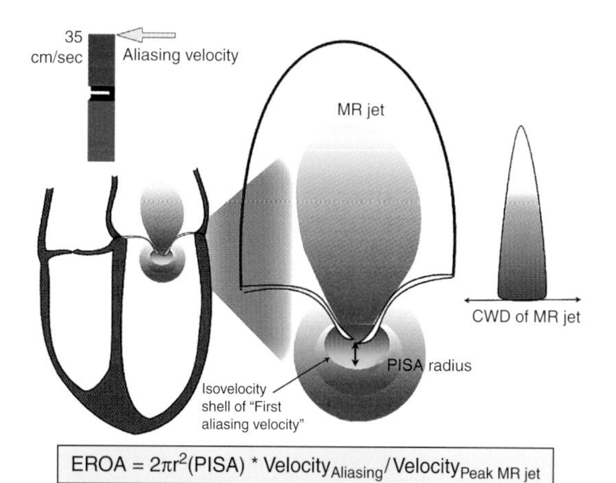

FIGURE 4–12. PISA for mitral regurgitation. (MR, mitral regurgitation; CWD, continuous-wave Doppler; PISA, proximal isovelocity surface area.)

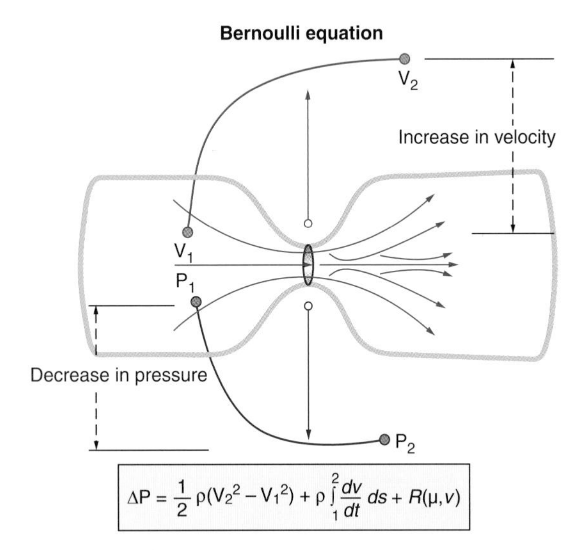

FIGURE 4–13. Principles of the Bernoulli equation.

acceleration is negligible, and hence both terms can be ignored. One-half of the mass density of blood ($1/2\rho$) is equal to 4 (after correction for units of measure), hence the Bernoulli equation can be *modified* as:

$$\Delta P = 4(V_2^2 - V_1^2)$$

The proximal velocity (V_1) is also generally very low and can often (but not always) be ignored, thus further *simplifying* the equation:

$$\Delta P = 4V_2^2$$

Limitations of the Bernoulli Equation

Significant error can be introduced into the calculation in specific situations when the assumptions inherent in simplifying the equation are violated. For example, flow acceleration (inertial force) can become significant with some prosthetic valves, where a greater than normal force is required to open the valve. Similarly, the presence of viscous friction is negligible with laminar flow, but should be accounted for in lesions with tubular obstructions greater than 4 cm in length and orifices less than 0.1 cm^2. The simplified Bernoulli equation also ignores the proximal velocity (V_1), but in conditions such as high cardiac output states, sub-aortic obstruction, significant aortic regurgitation, and intracardiac shunts, the proximal velocity (V_1) can be significant (>1.5 m/s), leading to an overestimation of the pressure gradient if the modified (rather than the simplified) Bernoulli equation is not applied. Finally, alterations in the blood viscosity, such as an increase in hematocrit to 60%, may lead to an underestimation of gradients, as $1/2\ \rho$ may be higher from an increase in the mass density of blood.

Applications of the Bernoulli Equation

Peak and Mean Gradients The Bernoulli equation is most commonly used to determine the peak instantaneous gradients across stenotic valves. The peak instantaneous gradient is measured with continuous-wave Doppler, and most echocardiography machines can automatically calculate the peak gradient by simply positioning the cursor at the highest point of the velocity envelope (Figure 4–14).

$$\text{Peak Instantaneous Gradient} = 4 \times (V_{Peak})^2$$

Mean pressure gradients are calculated as the average of multiple successive peak instantaneous peak gradients measured over time during the particular ejection phase (see Figure 4–14).

Intracardiac Pressure Measurements Estimation of intracardiac chambers is one of the most common forms of application of the modified Bernoulli equation. This

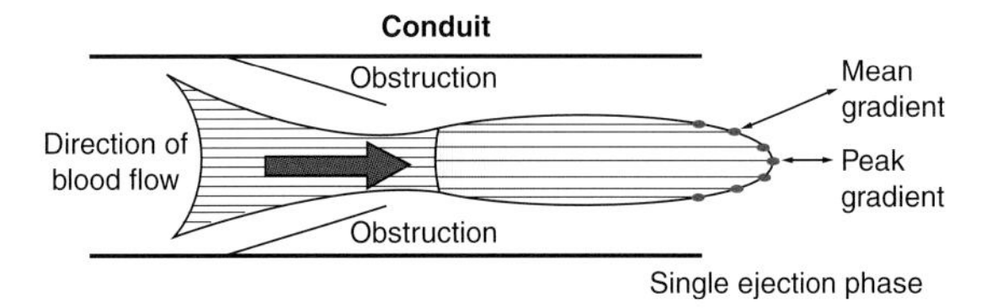

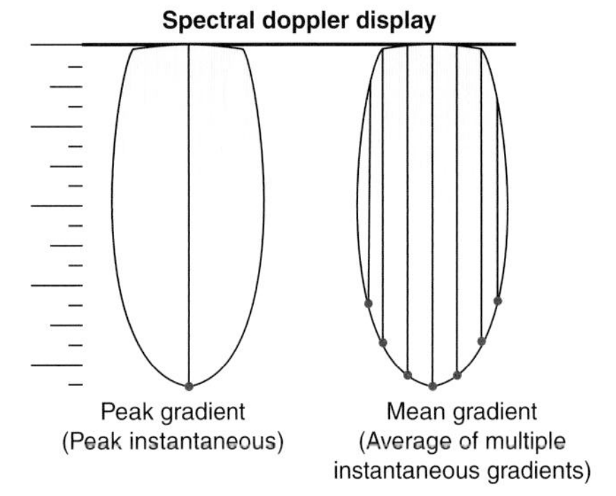

FIGURE 4–14. Measurement of peak and mean gradients. Mean pressure gradients are calculated as the average of multiple successive peak instantaneous peak gradients measured over time.

method requires the presence of a regurgitant jet or the presence of a shunt jet. The estimation of intracardiac pressures is performed in the following steps (Figure 4–15)[2]:

1. Utilization of continuous-wave Doppler to measure the peak velocity of the jet
2. Conversion of peak velocity into pressure gradient with the Bernoulli equation
3. Estimation of pressure in the origination chamber (P_{OC})
4. Estimation of pressure in the receiving chamber (P_{RC})
5. Calculation of pressures (Figure 4–15):
   a. $P_{OC} = 4v^2 + P_{RC}$
   b. $P_{RC} = P_{OC} - 4v^2$

Using this methodology, numerous intracardiac pressures can be measured depending upon the presence or absence of regurgitation jets:

Right Heart Pressures

1. Right ventricular systolic pressure (RVSP) using tricuspid regurgitant (TR) jet

$$RVSP = 4\,(V_{Peak\ TR})^2 + \text{Right Atrial Pressure (CVP)}$$

In the absence of pulmonic stenosis or right ventricular outflow tract obstruction, RVSP is equal to pulmonary artery systolic pressure.

2. Right ventricular systolic pressure in the presence of a ventricular septal defect (VSD)

$$RVSP = \text{Left Ventricular Systolic Pressure} - 4\,(V_{Peak\ VSD})^2$$

3. Pulmonary artery mean pressures (PAMP) using pulmonary regurgitant (PR) jet

$$PAMP = 4\,(V_{Peak\ PR})^2 + \text{Right Atrial Pressure (CVP)}$$

4. Pulmonary artery diastolic pressures (PADP) using pulmonary regurgitant (PR) jet

$$PADP = 4\,(V_{End\text{-}Diastolic\ PR})^2 + \text{Right Atrial Pressure (CVP)}$$

5. Pulmonary artery systolic pressure (PASP) in the presence of a patent ductus arteriosus (PDA)

$$PASP = \text{Systolic Blood Pressure} - 4\,(V_{Peak\ PDA})^2$$

Left Heart Pressures

1. Left atrial pressure (LAP) from a mitral regurgitant (MR) jet

$$LAP = \text{Left Ventricular Systolic Pressure} - 4\,(V_{Peak\ MR})^2$$

In the absence of aortic stenosis or left ventricular outflow tract obstruction, systolic blood pressure can be substituted for left ventricular systolic pressure.

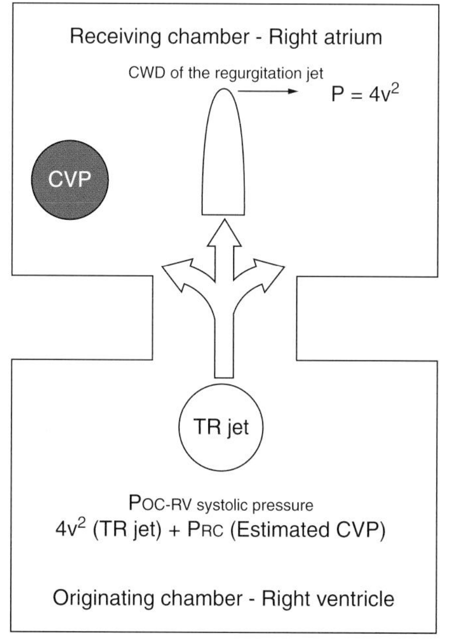

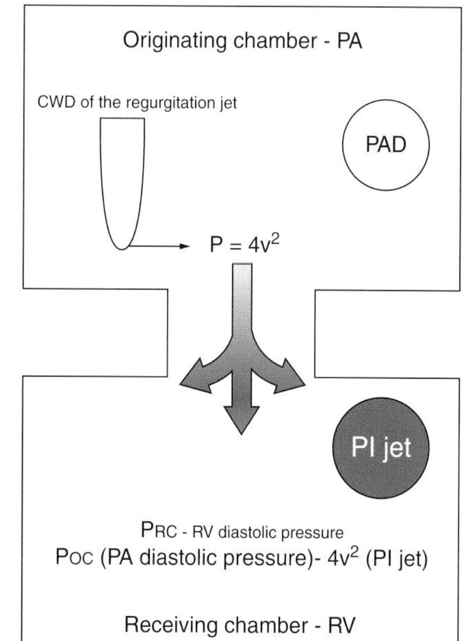

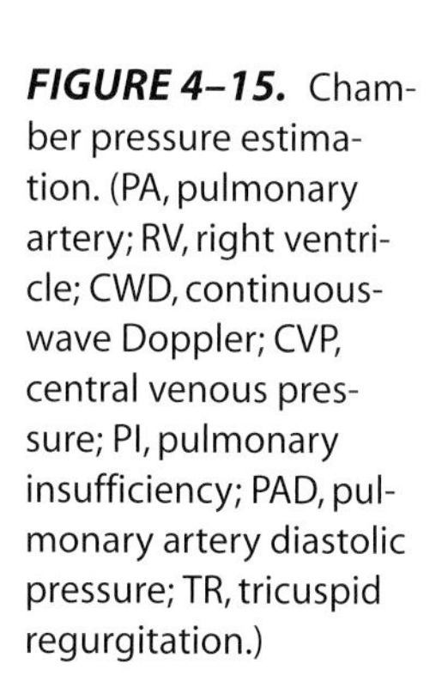

FIGURE 4–15. Chamber pressure estimation. (PA, pulmonary artery; RV, right ventricle; CWD, continuous-wave Doppler; CVP, central venous pressure; PI, pulmonary insufficiency; PAD, pulmonary artery diastolic pressure; TR, tricuspid regurgitation.)

2. Left atrial pressure in the presence of a patent foramen ovale (PFO)

$$LAP = 4\,(V_{Peak\ PFO})^2 + \text{Right Atrial Pressure (CVP)}$$

3. Left ventricular end-diastolic pressure (LVEDP) from an aortic regurgitant (AR) jet

$$LVEDP = \text{Diastolic Blood Pressure} - 4\,(V_{End\text{-}Diastolic\ AR})^2$$

Measurement of Resistance

Systemic vascular resistance (SVR) and pulmonary vascular resistance (PVR) are typically calculated from invasive hemodynamic measurements; however, Doppler echocardiography can provide a noninvasive assessment of vascular resistance. Units for measuring vascular resistance are dyne·s·cm^{-5}, pascal seconds per cubic meter (Pa·s/m^3), or mm Hg/L/min, which is referred to as a Wood unit (WU). The WU value is multiplied by 8 to convert to Pa·s/m^3 or by 80 to obtain the value in dyn·s·cm^{-5}. Normal SVR values range from 10 to 14 WU, while a normal PVR is 1 WU.

The ratio of peak mitral regurgitant velocity to the time-velocity integral of the LVOT flow (V_{MR}/TVI_{LVOT}) measured by Doppler echocardiography has been shown by Abbas et al[7] to correlate positively with SVR measurements (WU) obtained invasively (r = 0.84, 95% CI = 0.7 to 0.92). Furthermore, a calculated ratio greater than 0.27 identified patients with elevated SVR (>14 WU) with 70% sensitivity and 77% specificity, whereas a ratio less than 0.2 had a 92% sensitivity and 88% specificity to identify SVR less than 10 WU.

Similarly, Doppler echocardiography has been shown to provide a clinically reliable noninvasive method to determine PVR[8]:

$$PVR\ (WU) = \frac{V_{TR}}{TVI_{RVOT}} \times 10$$

where V_{TR} = peak tricuspid regurgitant velocity and TVI_{RVOT} = right ventricular outflow tract time-velocity integral. Furthermore, the ratio of V_{TR}/TVI_{RVOT} compared favorably to invasive PVR measurements (r = 0.93, 95% CI = 0.87 to 0.96), and a ratio greater than 0.175 had a sensitivity of 77% and a specificity of 81% to determine PVR greater than 2 WU.[8] Scapellato et al[9] have also described a method of estimating PVR using the preejection period (PEP), acceleration time (AcT), and total systolic time (TT) derived from pulmonary systolic flow:

$$PVR = -0.156 + \{1.154 \times [(PEP/AcT)/TT)]\}$$

Although these methods have the advantage of being simple and easily applicable, they may not be as reliable in patients with pulmonary arterial hypertension (PAH). More recently, Haddad et al[10] reported that the ratio of systolic pulmonary artery pressure/(HR × TVI_{RVOT}) correlated very well with invasive measurements of PVR indexed to body surface area (PVRI; r = 0.86; 95% CI = 0.76 to 0.92). A cutoff value of 0.076 provided a sensitivity of 86% and specificity of 82% to determine PVRI greater than 15 WU/m^2. A cutoff value of 0.057 increased sensitivity to 97% but decreased specificity to 65%. Similarly, Kouzu et al[11] showed that the ratio of the peak tricuspid regurgitant pressure gradient over the time–velocity integral of right ventricular outflow (PG_{TR}/TVI_{RVOT}) provided a reliable estimation of PVR over a wide range of PAH values and from various causes, including intracardiac shunts. In addition, a PG_{TR}/TVI_{RVOT} ratio greater than 7.6 was suggestive of poor prognosis for patients with PAH without an intracardiac shunt.

Measurement of Contractility

A relatively load-independent index of left ventricular systolic performance is peak dP/dt, or the maximum rate of rise of left ventricular pressure during systole. The echocardiographic method for deriving this parameter is based on the continuous-wave Doppler recording of the mitral regurgitant spectrum, wherein the time for velocity to rise from 1 m/s to 3 m/s is measured, and the pressure change from 1 m/s to 3 m/s is calculated by the Bernoulli equation as 32 mm Hg ($4 \times 3^2 - 4 \times 1^2$). dP/dt is then calculated with the following equation:

$$\text{Left Ventricular } dP/dt = 32 \times 1000/dt \text{ in Milliseconds}$$

Normal values for this parameter are 1610 ± 290 mm Hg/s. Although relatively afterload dependent, dP/dt is preload dependent.

Right ventricular dP/dt may be calculated by using the continuous-wave tricuspid regurgitant spectrum in a manner analogous to the approach used for left ventricular dP/dt. Because even hypertensive right ventricular pressures are typically lower than those of the left ventricle, the convention is to make the calculation based on the rise in velocity between 1 and 2 m/s. The pressure change from 1 m/s to 2 m/s is calculated by the Bernoulli equation as 12 mm Hg ($4 \times 2^2 - 4 \times 1^2$). dP/dt is then calculated as:

$$\text{Right Ventricular } dP/dt = 12 \times 1000/dt \text{ in Milliseconds}$$

A value greater than 1000 mm Hg/s is generally associated with normal right ventricular function.

CHAMBER QUANTIFICATION[12]

There has been a lack of standardization of values for cardiac chamber quantification with echocardiography, particularly TEE. Comparison of TEE measurements with transthoracic echocardiography (TTE) standards has also added to the confusion and led to the impression that the measurements made during echocardiography are somehow less accurate than with other imaging modalities such as magnetic resonance imaging (MRI). However, despite differences in imaging planes, in general, the same range of normal values are recommended for both TEE and TTE.

To make reliable measurements with echocardiography, it is essential that all conditions be optimized for image acquisition, display, and archiving. The echocardiographer should make an effort to minimize translational movements of the heart, make adjustments to maximize image resolution, avoid apical foreshortening of the left ventricle, and optimize endocardial definition. Furthermore, it is important to identify systole and diastole with simultaneous display of the electrocardiogram (ECG) and to make measurements at the appropriate point in the cardiac cycle. For patients with arrhythmias, it is critical that measurements be averaged over multiple cardiac cycles.[12]

Cardiac Cycle

End-diastole is identified temporally along the ECG tracing as the onset of the QRS complex. However, end-diastole can also be defined as the frame after mitral valve closure or as the frame with the largest cardiac dimension. End-systole is defined as the frame preceding mitral valve opening or the frame with the smallest cardiac dimension.[12]

Quantification of Left Ventricle (LV)

A variety of echocardiographic techniques have been proposed to quantify LV dimensions and volumes (Table 4–1). Of the many potential LV measurements, septal wall thickness (SWT), inferolateral (posterior)

Table 4–1. Advantages and limitations of left ventricular quantification methods.

Dimension/Volumes	Use/Advantages	Limitations
Linear		
M-mode	- Reproducible - High frame rates - Wealth of accumulated data - Most representative in normally shaped ventricles	- Beam orientation frequently off axis - Single dimension may not be representative in distorted ventricles - Most representative in normally shaped ventricles
2D-guided	- Assures orientation perpendicular to ventricular long axis	- Lower frame rates than in M-Mode - Single dimension only
Volumetric		
Biplane Simpson	- Corrects for shape distortions - Minimizes mathematic assumptions	- Apex frequently foreshortened - Endocardial dropout - Relies on only two planes - Few accumulated data on normal population
Area length	- Partial correction for shape distortion	- Based on mathematic assumptions - Few accumulated data
Mass		
M-mode or 2D-guided	- Wealth of accumulated data	- Inaccurate in ventricles with regional abnormalities - Beam orientation (M-mode) - Small errors magnified - Overestimates LV mass
Area length	- Allows for contribution of papillary muscles	- Insensitive to distortion in ventricular shape
Truncated ellipsoid	- More sensitive to distortions in ventricular shape	- Based on a number of mathematic assumptions - Minimal normal data

ABBREVIATIONS: 2D, two-dimensional; LV, left ventricle.

Reproduced with permission from Lang RM, Bierig M, Devereux RB, et al. Recommendations for chamber quantification: a report from the American Society of Echocardiography's Guidelines and Standards Committee and the Chamber Quantification Writing Group, developed in conjunction with the European Association of Echocardiography, a branch of the European Society of Cardiology. *J Am Soc Echocardiogr.* 2005;18(12):1440-1463.

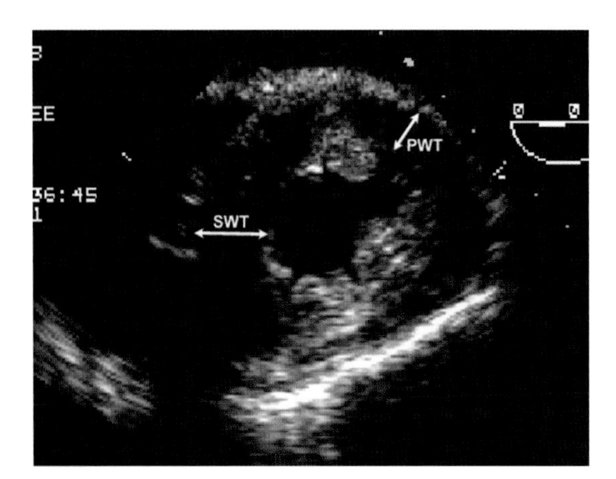

FIGURE 4–16. Measurement of left ventricular posterior (inferolateral) and septal (anteroseptal) wall thickness. (PWT, posterior wall thickness; SWT, septal wall thickness.)

wall thickness (PWT), and internal dimensions during systole (LVIDs) and diastole (LVIDd) are the most clinically relevant. PWT and SWT are best assessed in the transgastric mid–short axis view (Figure 4–16) in diastole. LV diameters are ideally measured from the midesophageal two-chamber and the transgastric two chamber views (Figure 4–17), but care should be taken to avoid apical foreshortening. LVID is measured at the minor axis of the LV (ie, at the tips of the mitral valve leaflets), and the range for normal systolic and diastolic measures at this level are 3.3 ± 0.5 cm and 4.7 ± 0.4 cm, respectively (Tables 4–2, 4–3).[12] While 2D or M-mode can be used to make these measurements, temporal resolution is better with M-mode leading to more accurate measurements. When M-mode is applied, the distance between leading edge echoes is measured.

The current method of choice for LV volume measurement is the biplane method of disks (modified

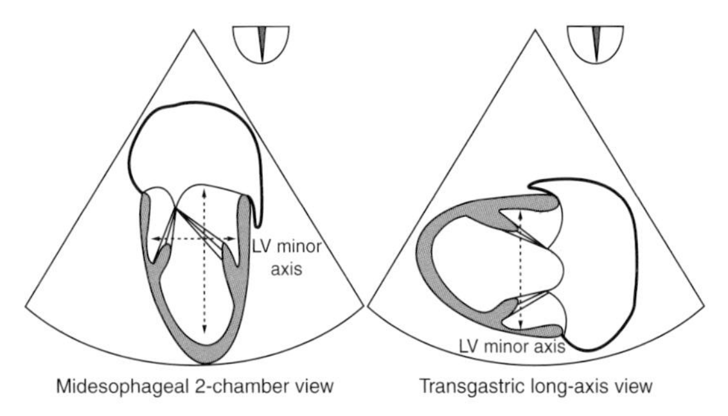

FIGURE 4–17. Measurement of left ventricular (LV) internal dimensions.

Simpson rule). It is based on modeling the left ventricle as a series of stacked cylindrical disks capped by an elliptical disk apex. The volume for each cylindrical disk is quantified by using the equation:

$$V = (\pi \times D_1/2 \times D_2/2) \times H$$

where D_1 and D_2 are orthogonal diameters of the cylinder, and H is the height of the cylinder. Fortunately, the operator can rely on ultrasound system software to make these calculations, but measurements averaged from two orthogonal views (midesophageal four-chamber and two-chamber) are recommended, particularly when extensive wall-motion abnormalities are present. Reference values for LV systolic and diastolic volumes are provided in Table 4–3.

LV mass is the total weight of the myocardium and is equal to the product of the volume of the myocardium and the specific density of cardiac muscle. LV mass can be derived from the transgastric mid-papillary short-axis view using a simple geometric cube formula:

$$\text{LV Mass} = 0.8 \times \{1.04 \times [(\text{LVIDd} + \text{PWTd} + \text{SWTd})^3 - (\text{LVIDd})^3]\} + 0.6\ \text{g}$$

The formula is based on the assumption that the LV is a prolate ellipse and is accurate only when there are no major distortions in LV geometry. Since LV dimensions are cubed, even a small error in diameter measurements is significantly amplified. Calculation of LV mass by TEE is comparable with TTE; however, TEE measurements are higher by an average of 6 gm/m^2 (see Table 4–2).[12]

Indexing LV dimensions to body surface area remains controversial, because such indexing has been shown to underestimate the incidence of LV hypertrophy in overweight and obese individuals. Furthermore, the total LV mass differs between men and women even when indexed for body surface area, and it is unclear whether indexing improves the predictive value of these measures for the occurrence of cardiovascular events.

Recently, three-dimensional (3D) echocardiography has been utilized to calculate LV dimensions and shapes. Since 3D echocardiography does not make assumptions about the shape of the ventricle, volumetric measurements have been shown to be more accurate and comparable to gold standards such as MRI. The 3D calculations of LV volumes and dimensions have been primarily obtained with the matrix 3D TTE transducer. It remains to be seen whether images acquired with the recently introduced 3D matrix TEE probe will demonstrate similar degrees of accuracy and reproducibility.

Table 4–2. Reference values for left ventricle mass and geometry.

	Women				Men			
	Reference Range	Mildly Abnormal	Moderately Abnormal	Severely Abnormal	Reference Range	Mildly Abnormal	Moderately Abnormal	Severely Abnormal
Linear method								
LV mass, g	67-162	163-186	187-210	≥211	88-224	225-258	259-292	≥293
LV mass/BSA, g/m²	43-95	96-108	109-121	≥122	49-115	116-131	132-148	≥149
LV mass/height, g/m	41-99	100-115	116-128	≥129	52-126	127-144	145-162	≥163
LV mass/height, g/m	18-44	45-51	52-58	≥59	20-48	49-55	56-63	≥64
Relative wall thickness, cm	0.22-0.42	0.43-0.47	0.48-0.52	≥0.53	0.24-0.42	0.43-0.46	0.47-0.51	≥0.52
Septal thickness, cm	0.6-0.9	1.0-1.2	1.3-1.5	≥1.6	0.6-1.0	1.1-1.3	1.4-1.6	≥1.7
Posterior wall thickness, cm	0.6-0.9	1.0-1.2	1.3-1.5	≥1.6	0.6-1.0	1.1-1.3	1.4-1.6	≥1.7
2D method								
LV mass, g	66-150	151-171	172-182	>193	96-200	201-227	228-254	>255
LV mass/BSA, g/m²	44-88	89-100	101-112	≥113	50-102	103-116	117-130	≥131

ABBREVIATIONS: LV, left ventricle; BSA, body surface area; 2D, two-dimensional.

Reproduced with permission from Lang RM, Bierig M, Devereux RB, et al. Recommendations for chamber quantification: a report from the American Society of Echocardiography's Guidelines and Standards Committee and the Chamber Quantification Writing Group, developed in conjunction with the European Association of Echocardiography, a branch of the European Society of Cardiology. *J Am Soc Echocardiogr.* 2005;18(12):1440-1463.

Table 4–3. Reference values for left ventricular dimensions and volumes.

	Women				Men			
	Reference Range	Mildly Abnormal	Moderately Abnormal	Severely Abnormal	Reference Range	Mildly Abnormal	Moderately Abnormal	Severely Abnormal
LV dimension								
LV diastolic diameter	3.9-5.3	5.4-5.7	5.8-6.1	≥6.2	4.2-5.9	6.0-6.3	6.4-6.8	≥6.9
LV diastolic diameter/BSA, cm/m²	2.4-3.2	3.3-3.4	3.5-3.7	≥3.8	2.2-3.1	3.2-3.4	3.5-3.6	≥3.7
LV diastolic diameter height, cm/m	2.5-3.2	3.3-3.4	3.5-3.6	≥3.7	2.4-3.3	3.4-3.5	3.6-3.7	≥3.8
LV volume								
LV diastolic volume, mL	56-104	105-117	118-130	≥131	67-155	156-178	179-201	≥201
LV diastolic volume/BSA, mL/m²	*35-75*	*76-86*	*87-96*	*≥97*	*35-75*	*76-86*	*87-96*	*≥97*
LV systolic volume, mL	19-49	50-59	60-69	≥70	22-58	59-70	71-82	≥83
LV systolic volume/BSA, mL/m²	*12-30*	*31-36*	*37-42*	*≥43*	*12-30*	*31-36*	*37-42*	*≥43*

ABBREVIATIONS: LV, left ventricle; BSA, body surface area.

Reproduced with permission from Lang RM, Bierig M, Devereux RB, et al. Recommendations for chamber quantification: a report from the American Society of Echocardiography's Guidelines and Standards Committee and the Chamber Quantification Writing Group, developed in conjunction with the European Association of Echocardiography, a branch of the European Society of Cardiology. *J Am Soc Echocardiogr.* 2005;18(12):1440-1463.

Quantification of Right Ventricle (RV)

The normal RV is a low-pressure and highly compliant cardiac chamber. While it typically appears smaller than the LV, in fact it has almost the same volume as the LV. Since it is crescent shaped, has greater trabeculations, and is structurally more complex, it is incompletely visualized from a single 2D echocardiographic view.[13,14] When using TEE for RV assessment, the midesophageal four-chamber view, with the multiplane angle adjusted to 10° to 20° to maximize tricuspid annulus diameter, should be used for measurement of RV size, wall thickness, and fractional area change (Figure 4–18 and Table 4–4). Normal RV free wall thickness as measured in the midesophageal four-chamber view at end-diastole is generally less than 0.5 cm.[12] The right ventricular outflow tract (RVOT) extends from the anterosuperior aspect of the RV to the pulmonary artery and includes the pulmonic valve (Figure 4–19). The diameter of the RVOT is best measured from the midesophageal RV inflow-outflow view (Figure 4–19).

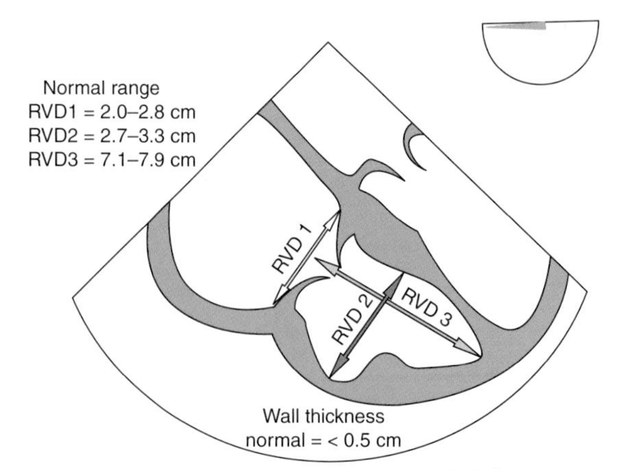

FIGURE 4–18. Measurement of right ventricular diameters. (RVD, right ventricular diameter.)

Quantification of Left Atrium (LA) and Right Atrium (RA)

LA size should be measured at end-systole, because the LA achieves its greatest dimension at that point in the cardiac cycle.[12] The LA gradually enlarges with worsening diastolic dysfunction, and therefore LA dimensions can be followed over time to assess response to therapy and to assess prognosis. TEE measurement of LA dimensions is problematic and unreliable. This is because in most cases the LA size exceeds the maximal span of the ultrasound beam, and hence cannot be measured accurately. It is recommended that the LA be estimated from multiple imaging planes. Also, for purposes of risk stratification, LA volumes assessed with transthoracic echo have shown a greater prognostic value than LA size. The reference ranges for LA diameter in men and women are 3.0 to 4.0 cm and 2.7 to 3.8 cm, respectively.[12]

There are limited data available on the best transthoracic or TEE view to assess the RA size or volume.

Table 4–4. Reference values for right ventricular (RV), right ventricular outflow tract (RVOT), and pulmonary artery (PA) dimensions.

	Reference Range	Mildly Abnormal	Moderately Abnormal	Severely Abnormal
RV dimension (Figure 4–18)				
Basal RV diameter (RVD1), cm	2.0-2.8	2.9-3.3	3.4-3.8	≥3.9
Mid-RV diameter (RVD2), cm	2.7-3.3	3.4-3.7	3.8-4.1	≥4.2
Base-to-apex length (RVD3), cm	7.1-7.9	8.0-8.5	8.6-9.1	≥9.2
RVOT diameters (Figure 4–19)				
Subpulmonary region (RVOT1), cm	2.5-2.9	3.0-3.2	3.3-3.5	≥3.6
Pulmonic annulus (RVOT2), cm	1.7-2.3	2.4-2.7	2.8-3.1	≥3.2
PA diameter (Figure 4–19)				
Above pulmonic valve (MPA), cm	1.5-2.1	2.2-2.5	2.6-2.9	≥3.0

RVD, right ventricular diameter.

Reproduced with permission from Lang RM, Bierig M, Devereux RB, et al. Recommendations for chamber quantification: a report from the American Society of Echocardiography's Guidelines and Standards Committee and the Chamber Quantification Writing Group, developed in conjunction with the European Association of Echocardiography, a branch of the European Society of Cardiology. *J Am Soc Echocardiogr.* 2005;18(12):1440-1463.

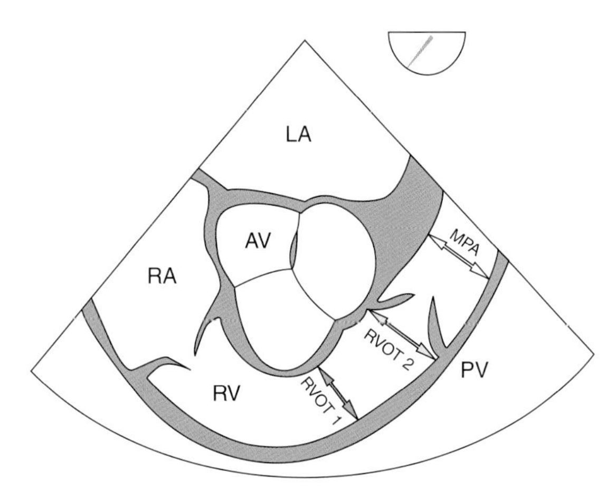

FIGURE 4–19. Measurement of right ventricular outflow tract diameter. (LA, left atrium; RA, right atrium; RV, right ventricle; RVOT, right ventricular outflow tract; MPA, main pulmonary artery; AV, aortic valve; PV, pulmonic valve.)

As with the LA, the RA size should be estimated from multiple echocardiographic windows. It is also believed that RA volume may be a more accurate and reproducible estimate of size than a linear measure.

REFERENCES

1. Weyman AE. *Principles and Practice of Echocardiography.* 2nd ed. Philadelphia: Lea & Febiger; 1994.
2. Anderson B. *Echocardiography: The Normal Examination and Echocardiographic Measurements.* 2nd ed. Hoboken: John Wiley & Sons; 2007.
3. Alam M, Wardell J, Andersson E, Samad BA, Nordlander R. Characteristics of mitral and tricuspid annular velocities determined by pulsed wave Doppler tissue imaging in healthy subjects. *J Am Soc Echocardiogr.* 1999;12(8):618-628.
4. Nishimura RA, Miller FA Jr, Callahan MJ, Benassi RC, Seward JB, Tajik AJ. Doppler echocardiography: theory, instrumentation, technique, and application. *Mayo Clin Proc.* 1985;60(5):321-343.
5. Quinones MA, Otto CM, Stoddard M, Waggoner A, Zoghbi WA. Recommendations for quantification of Doppler echocardiography: a report from the Doppler Quantification Task Force of the Nomenclature and Standards Committee of the American Society of Echocardiography. *J Am Soc Echocardiogr.* 2002;15(2):167-184.
6. Miyatake K, Yamagishi M, Tanaka N, et al. New method for evaluating left ventricular wall motion by color-coded tissue Doppler imaging: in vitro and in vivo studies. *J Am Coll Cardiol.* 1995;25(3):717-724.
7. Abbas AE, Fortuin FD, Patel B, Moreno CA, Schiller NB, Lester SJ. Noninvasive measurement of systemic vascular resistance using Doppler echocardiography. *J Am Soc Echocardiogr.* 2004;17(8):834-838.
8. Abbas AE, Fortuin FD, Schiller NB, Appleton CP, Moreno CA, Lester SJ. A simple method for noninvasive estimation of pulmonary vascular resistance. *J Am Coll Cardiol.* 2003;41(6): 1021-1027.
9. Scapellato F, Temporelli PL, Eleuteri E, Corra U, Imparato A, Giannuzzi P. Accurate noninvasive estimation of pulmonary vascular resistance by Doppler echocardiography in patients with chronic failure heart failure. *J Am Coll Cardiol.* 2001;37(7): 1813-1819.
10. Haddad F, Zamanian R, Beraud AS, et al. A novel non-invasive method of estimating pulmonary vascular resistance in patients with pulmonary arterial hypertension. *J Am Soc Echocardiogr.* 2009;22(5):523-529.
11. Kouzu H, Nakatani S, Kyotani S, Kanzaki H, Nakanishi N, Kitakaze M. Noninvasive estimation of pulmonary vascular resistance by Doppler echocardiography in patients with pulmonary arterial hypertension. *Am J Cardiol.* 2009;103(6):872-876.
12. Lang RM, Bierig M, Devereux RB, et al. Recommendations for chamber quantification: a report from the American Society of Echocardiography's Guidelines and Standards Committee and the Chamber Quantification Writing Group, developed in conjunction with the European Association of Echocardiography, a branch of the European Society of Cardiology. *J Am Soc Echocardiogr.* 2005;18(12):1440-1463.
13. Haddad F, Couture P, Tousignant C, Denault AY. The right ventricle in cardiac surgery, a perioperative perspective: II. Pathophysiology, clinical importance, and management. *Anesth Analg.* 2009;108(2):422-433.
14. Haddad F, Couture P, Tousignant C, Denault AY. The right ventricle in cardiac surgery, a perioperative perspective: I. Anatomy, physiology, and assessment. *Anesth Analg.* 2009;108(2): 407-421

REVIEW QUESTIONS

Select the *one best* answer for each question.

1. Frequency is defined as:
   a. Number of wavelengths passing through a certain point
   b. Number of pulses passing through a certain point
   c. Number of positive deflections of a wave passing through a certain point
   d. Number of negative deflections of a wave passing through a certain point
   e. Number of pulses divided by the number of wavelengths

2. The units of frequency are:
   a. Meters/second
   b. Pulses/second
   c. Centimeters
   d. Seconds
   e. Hertz

3. Frequency determines:
   a. Resolution
   b. Brightness
   c. Contrast
   d. Compensation
   e. Attenuation

4. The Doppler principle is based on the:
   a. Change in speed of the returning sound waves
   b. Change in speed of emitted sound waves
   c. Change in frequency of the returning sound waves
   d. Change in angle of the returning sound waves
   e. Change in resolution

5. The Doppler shift is most accurately calculated when the angle between the emitted and reflected sounds is:
   a. 90°
   b. 30°
   c. 0°
   d. 45°
   a. 120°

6. The underestimation of Doppler shift is significantly increased when the angle of reflection increases more than:
   a. 15°
   b. 30°
   c. 10°
   d. 20°
   e. 25°

7. Misalignment of the Doppler beam with the blood flow:
   a. Can cause underestimation of the gradient
   b. Can cause overestimation of the gradient
   c. Does not affect the calculation of gradient
   d. Affects the gradient calculation but the correction factor is built into the calculation
   e. Occurs only during transthoracic echocardiography

8. During continuous-wave Doppler interrogation:
   a. Sound waves are emitted continuously but received intermittently.
   b. Sound waves are emitted intermittently but received continuously.
   c. Sound waves are emitted and received continuously.
   d. Sound waves are only emitted and not received by the transducer.
   e. Sound waves are not emitted and only received.

9. Continuous-wave Doppler:
   a. Is time-gated
   b. Measures the lowest velocity in the pathway of the beam
   c. Is not affected by the angle between the emitted and reflected signals
   d. Can be used to avoid aliasing
   e. Can only be used in conjunction with color-flow Doppler

10. Pulsed-wave Doppler:
    a. Should be used to detect high velocities to avoid aliasing
    b. Utilizes the time delay to analyze the reflected signals reaching the transducer
    c. Analyzes all the returning signals in the pathway of the ultrasound beam
    d. Is not affected by the angle between the emitted and the returning signals
    e. Generates "shaded" envelopes because it samples all the velocities in its pathway.

11. Pulse repetition frequency:
    a. Is inversely related to the depth of placement of the sample volume
    b. Is determined by the source, ie, the transducer *and* the medium
    c. Is the number of cycles per second generated by the transducer
    d. Is directly related to pulse repetition period
    e. Is exactly half of the Nyquist limit

12. High pulse repetition frequency Doppler:
    a. Utilizes continuous-wave Doppler to analyze multiple high velocities
    b. Is only used to analyze tissue motion
    c. Is based on analysis of successive pulsed-wave Doppler sample volumes to analyze velocities at multiple locations in series
    d. Considerably increases the spatial accuracy of the pulsed-wave Doppler
    e. Is a combination of pulsed-wave and continuous-wave Doppler

13. Color-flow Doppler:
    a. Is a continuous-wave Doppler signal
    b. Is a combination of continuous- and pulsed-wave Doppler signals
    c. Does not alias
    d. Is a pulsed-wave Doppler signal
    e. Use leads to an increase in the pulse repetition frequency

14. Doppler tissue imaging:
    a. Is used to assess high-velocity and low-amplitude signals
    b. Can be used to grade aortic valve stenosis
    c. Is designed to detect low-velocity myocardial tissue velocities
    d. Cannot be used to analyze diastolic function
    e. Is not angle dependent

15. Which one of the following is *NOT* an assumption of the continuity equation:
    a. Non-laminar flow
    b. Constant diameter of the outflow tract
    c. Measurement of Doppler velocity-time integral exactly at the measurement of the outflow tract diameter
    d. Parallel alignment of the Doppler beam with blood flow
    e. Flat profile of the blood flow

16. The greatest source of error in the continuity equation is:
    a. Calculation of the velocity-time integral
    b. Misalignment of Doppler beam
    c. Calculation of the left ventricular outflow tract diameter
    d. High velocity of blood
    e. The presence of severe stenosis

17. The proximal isovelocity surface area method for the diagnosis of mitral stenosis:
    a. Is based on calculation of mean gradient across the mitral valve
    b. Is based on identification of isovelocity shells of flow acceleration on the left ventricular aspect of the mitral valve
    c. Is based on the continuity equation
    d. Requires an accurate calculation of the mitral annular diameter
    e. Utilizes the peak transmitral E velocity obtained by the pulsed-wave Doppler

18. Which one of the following is *NOT* a component of the Bernoulli equation:
    a. Proximal velocity (V_1)
    b. Distal velocity (V_2)
    c. Density of the liquid (ρ)
    d. Diameter of the blood vessel (D)
    e. Viscous resistance (R)

19. In the *simplified* Bernoulli equation, which of the following components of the original equation is not ignored?
    a. Distal velocity (V_2)
    b. Proximal velocity (V_1)
    c. Distance over which the pressure decreases (ds)
    d. Resistance (R)
    e. Density of blood (ρ)

20. Which of the following *cannot* be estimated with the modified Bernoulli equation?
    a. Peak gradient
    b. Mean gradient
    c. Peak right ventricular systolic pressure estimation even in the absence of tricuspid regurgitation
    d. Pulmonary artery end-diastolic pressure in the presence of pulmonary regurgitation
    e. Left atrial pressure in the presence of mitral regurgitation

21. Which of the following statements about identification of cardiac cycle stages by echocardiography is *NOT* correct?
    a. End-diastole can be defined as the onset of the QRS complex on ECG.
    b. End-diastole can be defined as the frame after mitral valve closure.
    c. End-diastole can be defined as the frame with the largest left ventricular dimension.
    d. End-systole can be defined as the frame with the smallest left ventricular dimension.
    e. End-systole can be defined as the frame preceding aortic valve closure.

22. Left ventricular dimensions should be measured at:
    a. Left ventricular major axis at the base of the papillary muscles
    b. Left ventricular minor axis at the tips of mitral leaflets
    c. Base of the left ventricle at the level of the mitral annulus
    d. In the deep transgastric window at 110°
    e. Midesophageal position at 0°

23. M-mode:
    a. Cannot be used for chamber quantification
    b. Can only be used to assess wall thickness
    c. Measures slightly higher left ventricular dimensions as compared to two-dimensional echo for the same left ventricle
    d. Can only be used to calculate left atrial diameter
    e. Can only be used to measure end-diastolic diameter of left ventricle

24. Left ventricular diameters are best measured:
    a. At right angles to the axis of the ultrasound beam
    b. At 0° (parallel) to the long axis of the left ventricle
    c. At 45° to the long axis of the left ventricle
    d. At 120° to the long axis of the left ventricle
    e. At the minor axis of the left ventricle regardless of the rotation

25. The normal right ventricle has:
    a. More volume than the left ventricle
    b. Less volume than the left ventricle
    c. The same volume as the left ventricle
    d. A volume that changes with every beat due to excessive compliance
    e. A fixed volume despite changes in preload and afterload

26. The recommended view for right ventricular chamber quantification by TEE is:
    a. Midesophageal four-chamber view
    b. Midesophageal long-axis view
    c. Deep transgastric view at 120°
    d. Midesophageal short-axis view of the right ventricular inflow and outflow at 50°
    e. Transgastric view at 90°

27. The recommended view for measurement of the right ventricular outflow tract is the:
    a. Midesophageal right ventricular inflow-outflow view between 50° and 60°
    b. Midesophageal four-chamber view
    c. Midesophageal long-axis view at 120°
    d. Upper esophageal view at 90°
    e. Transgastric view at 120°

28. Speed of propagation of ultrasound waves:
    a. Is *not* determined by the tissue in which it travels
    b. Can be changed on the ultrasound system
    c. Is a multiple of frequency (Hz) and amplitude
    d. Does not change with changing frequency for a specific medium
    e. Is 1540 m/sec in lung tissue

29. Duty factor of an ultrasound system is:
    a. The percentage of time the system is emitting the pulse
    b. Measured as cycles/second
    c. Determined by the source of the sound wave and the medium
    d. Fixed and cannot be changed
    e. Directly related to the amplitude of the wave

30. Which of the following is not a component of the Doppler equation?
    a. Transmitted frequency
    b. Change in frequency
    c. Cosine theta
    d. Speed of sound
    e. Frame rate

31. The phenomena of the returning frequency being higher than the transmitted frequency is called:
    a. Phase shift
    b. Positive Doppler shift
    c. Negative Doppler shift
    d. Fourier transformation
    e. Wave analysis

32. Range ambiguity can be defined as:
    a. Inability to utilize the focus control
    b. Poor two-dimensional image leading to inaccurate measurements
    c. Inability of the pulsed-wave Doppler to measure high intracardiac velocities
    d. Inability of the continuous-wave Doppler to locate the site of the high velocity
    e. Aliasing observed during Doppler tissue imaging

33. During pulsed-wave Doppler interrogation, the depth of the "sample volume":
    a. Is automatically calculated by the ultrasound system
    b. Is fixed and cannot be changed
    c. Can be changed by the sonographer
    d. Keeps changing automatically with the increase/decrease in velocity
    e. In irrelevant, because all the velocities in the Doppler path are measured

34. During pulsed-wave Doppler echocardiography, the size of the "sample volume":
    a. Is fixed and cannot change
    b. Keeps increasing as the depth increases
    c. Is not determined by the depth of the sample volume
    d. Is determined by the speed of the blood
    e. Is determined by the frequency change

35. The Nyquist limit is:
    a. One-half of the pulse repetition frequency
    b. Twice the pulse repetition frequency
    c. Equal to the pulse repetition frequency
    d. One-fourth of the pulse repetition frequency
    e. Four times as much as the pulse repetition frequency

36. A low frequency transducer will enable the transducer to record:
    a. Higher velocities at an given depth without aliasing
    b. Lower velocities at any given depth without aliasing
    c. The same velocities without aliasing
    d. Lower velocities with aliasing
    e. Higher velocities at greater depths

37. Aliasing during color-flow Doppler examination:
    a. Occurs at a higher velocity than during pulsed-wave Doppler examination of the same flow
    b. Occurs at a lower velocity than during pulsed-wave Doppler examination of the same flow
    c. Occurs at the same velocity as during pulsed-wave Doppler examination of the same flow
    d. Does not occur because it is based on continuous-wave Doppler
    e. Is only determined by the depth of the color-flow Doppler interrogation

38. The pulmonary valve is not used for cardiac output calculation with continuity equation because:
    a. It has a dynamic diameter during the cardiac cycle.
    b. The flow is non-laminar
    c. There is a low velocity of ejection.
    d. There is always regurgitation.
    e. There is always poor alignment of the Doppler beam.

39. Regurgitant volume through the mitral valve can be calculated by:
    a. Comparing the stroke volume at the aortic and mitral valves
    b. Comparing the stroke volume at the mitral and tricuspid valves
    c. Comparing the stroke volume at the aortic and tricuspid valves
    d. Comparing the stroke volume at the aortic and pulmonary valves
    e. Comparing the stroke volume at the mitral and pulmonary valves

40. Calculation of left ventricular (LV) mass is performed by:
    a. Subtraction of the LV volume enclosed in the endocardium from the LV volume enclosed in the epicardium
    b. Measuring the LV mass from images obtained from the CT scan
    c. Assuming the LV to be of a perfect circle
    d. Transthoracic echo only
    e. Cardiac magnetic resonance imaging only

41. Indexing of normal left ventricular (LV) dimensions to body surface area leads to:
    a. Overestimation of LV diameters in females
    b. Underestimation of LV hypertrophy in obese individuals
    c. Underestimation of LV hypertrophy in normal-sized individuals
    d. Overestimation of LV diameters in obese individuals
    e. Underestimation of LV hypertrophy in females

42. The right ventricle:
    a. Can be comprehensively visualized in the midesophageal windows
    b. Wall thickness should be measured in the deep transgastric position
    c. Diameter should be measured in the midesophageal long-axis view at 135°
    d. Is crescentic in shape
    e. Is more noncompliant than the left ventricle

43. Left atrial size should be measured at:
    a. End-diastole when it achieves its greatest dimension
    b. End-systole when it achieves its greatest dimension
    c. Mid-diastole when all its walls can be visualized
    d. Mid-systole when it achieves its greatest dimension
    e. Early systole when it achieves its smallest dimension

44. Left atrial dimensions:
    a. Are of not much clinical significance
    b. Are useful only for planning mitral valve surgery
    c. Are useful to quantify and follow the response to therapy in diastolic dysfunction
    d. Cannot be accurately calculated with transthoracic echocardiography
    e. Can be reliably performed with transesophageal echo

45. M-mode echocardiography:
    a. Has a better temporal resolution due to a higher frame rate
    b. Has a better spatial resolution due to a higher frame rate
    c. Is used to visualize slow-moving intracardiac structures due to a lower frame rate
    d. Cannot be used in conjunction with color-flow Doppler
    e. Is ideal to measure higher gradients due to a high frame rate

46. During left ventricular volume measurement with TEE:
    a. Measurements are doubled during calculation hence there is less error.
    b. Measurements are cubed hence there is more error.
    c. Unlike transthoracic echocardiography, there is no error.
    d. Three-dimensional echocardiography has been definitely established to be superior to two-dimensional echocardiography.
    e. Left ventricular distortions in shape have no effect on the accuracy of calculations.

47. Left ventricular mass calculation with TEE:
    a. Does not show any correlation with LV mass measured with TTE
    b. Generally measures more LV mass, greater than 6 gm/m^2 as measured with TTE
    c. Generally measures less LV mass, less than 6 gm/m^2 as measured with TTE
    d. Cannot be performed
    e. Requires only the calculation of left ventricular internal diameter during systole

48. A patient is found to have a peak velocity of 6.3 m/sec on continuous-wave Doppler interrogation of the aortic valve in the deep transgastric window. Based on the Bernoulli equation, the peak gradient across the aortic valve is:
    a. 100 mm Hg
    b. 120 mm Hg
    c. 164.5 mm Hg
    d. 158.8 mm Hg
    e. 132.9 mm Hg

49. The peak gradient across the aortic valve is found to be 39.6 mm Hg. Based on the Bernoulli equation the corresponding peak velocity across the valve would be:
    a. 4 m/sec
    b. 3.15 m/sec
    c. 2 m/sec
    d. 5.15 m/sec
    e. 1.5 m/sec

For questions 50-53: A 60-year-old female suffers a cardiac arrest during a total hip replacement. An emergent TEE is performed and the following TEE data are obtained:

Pulmonary artery diameter = 2.5 cm
Pulmonary artery velocity-time integral = 11 cm
LVOT diameter = 2.0 cm
LVOT velocity = 1 m/sec
Aortic valve peak velocity = 4.5 m/sec
Tricuspid regurgitant jet peak velocity = 4 m/sec
Heart rate = 100 beats/min
CVP = 15 mm Hg
Systemic blood pressure = 90/40 mm Hg

50. Based on the above data, the stroke volume of the patient is:
    a. 25.5 mL
    b. 35.8 mL
    c. 60.4 mL
    d. 53.9 mL
    e. 58.2 mL

51. Based on the above data, the cardiac output of the patient is:
    a. 2.5 L/min
    b. 3.8 L/min
    c. 5.4 L/min
    d. 6.5 L/min
    e. 4.5 L/min

52. Based on the above data, the aortic valve area by continuity equation is:
    a. 1.5 cm^2
    b. 1.1 cm^2
    c. 0.9 cm^2
    d. 0.69 cm^2
    e. 0.81 cm^2

53. The estimated peak right ventricular systolic pressure in this patient would be:
    a. 35 mm Hg
    b. 66.4 mm Hg
    c. 57 mm Hg
    d. 79 mm Hg
    e. 45.9 mm Hg

For questions 54-57: During a routine intraoperative TEE examination, the following data are obtained:

LVOT peak velocity = 0.5 m/sec
LVOT VTI = 12 cm
LVOT diameter = 2.15 cm
Heart rate = 64 beats/min
Aortic valve peak velocity = 4.4 m/s
Aortic valve VTI = 22 cm

54. The peak gradient across the aortic valve would be:
    a. 44 mm Hg
    b. 33 mm Hg
    c. 77 mm Hg
    d. 85 mm Hg
    e. 66 mm Hg

55. The stroke volume in this patient would be:
    a. 23.5 mL
    b. 22.3 mL
    c. 43.5 mL
    d. 37.8 mL
    e. 51.9 mL

56. The cardiac output in this patient would be:
    a. 3.5 L/min
    b. 2.8 L/min
    c. 4.2 L/min
    d. 5.1 L/min
    e. 1.9 L/min

57. The aortic valve area in this patient is:
    a. 1.9 cm^2
    b. 1.1 cm^2
    c. 1.0 cm^2
    d. 0.7 cm^2
    e. 0.9 cm^2

For questions 58-59: During an intraoperative TEE examination for mitral regurgitation (MR), a proximal flow convergence is noted at a Nyquist limit of 50 cm/s, with a proximal isovelocity surface area (PISA) radius of 1.0 cm, and a peak MR jet velocity of 5 m/s. The patient's blood pressure was 110/60 mm Hg.

58. Based on the PISA equation, the effective regurgitant orifice area (EROA) in this patient is:
    a. 0.62 cm^2
    b. 0.71 cm^2
    c. 0.55 cm^2
    d. 0.43 cm^2
    e. 0.21 cm^2

59. Calculate this patient's LAP.
    a. 5 mm Hg
    b. 8 mm Hg
    c. 10 mm Hg
    d. 14 mm Hg
    e. 19 mm Hg

For questions 60-64: A 48-year-old male is undergoing coronary artery bypass graft surgery. During the intraoperative TEE examination, it is noticed that he has moderate left ventricular dilatation, with at least 2+ mitral regurgitation. The following data are obtained:

LVOT diameter = 2.5 cm
LVOT VTI = 15 cm
Mitral annulus diameter = 3.7 cm
Mitral annulus VTI = 12 cm
PISA radius = 0.7 cm
PISA aliasing velocity = 45 cm/s
Peak mitral regurgitation jet velocity = 445 cm/s
Mitral regurgitation VTI = 180 cm

60. The stroke volume through the LVOT in this patient would be:
    a. 73.6 cm^3
    b. 82 cm^3
    c. 55 cm^3
    d. 45 cm^3
    e. 66 cm^3

61. The stroke volume through the mitral valve would be:
    a. 100 cm^3
    b. 118 cm^3
    c. 147 cm^3
    d. 129 cm^3
    e. 133 cm^3

62. Regurgitant volume in this patient would be:
    a. 66.8 cm^3
    b. 55.4 cm^3
    c. 44.9 cm^3
    d. 76.8 cm^3
    e. 59.3 cm^3

63. The regurgitant fraction in this patient would be:
    a. 55.3%
    b. 66.8%
    c. 42.9%
    d. 55.2 %
    e. 33.9%

64. Based on the PISA equation, the mitral regurgitant orifice area is:
    a. 0.51 cm^2
    b. 0.31 cm^2
    c. 0.39 cm^2
    d. 0.48 cm^2
    e. 0.42 cm^2

65. The maximum velocity through a persistent patent ductus arteriousus is 4 m/s and the blood pressure is 90/60 mm Hg. The pulmonary artery systolic pressure is:
    a. 4 mm Hg
    b. 26 mm Hg
    c. 74 mm Hg
    d. 90 mm Hg
    e. 116 mm Hg

For questions 66-68: During the intraoperative TEE examination of a 58-year-old male undergoing coronary artery bypass graft surgery, it is noticed that he has tricuspid and aortic regurgitation. His blood pressure is 110/60 and his CVP is 10 mm Hg. Continuous-wave Doppler examination of the pulmonic and aortic valves revealed the following profile:

Peak pulmonary regurgitant velocity = 1.69 m/s
End-diastolic pulmonary regurgitant velocity = 1.43 m/s
End-diastolic aortic regurgitant velocity = 2.2 m/s

66. Calculate the pulmonary artery mean pressure.
    a. 12.2 mm Hg
    b. 14.8 mm Hg
    c. 16.3 mm Hg
    d. 18.1 mm Hg
    e. 21.4 mm Hg

67. Calculate the pulmonary artery diastolic pressure.
    a. 12.2 mm Hg
    b. 14.8 mm Hg
    c. 16.3 mm Hg
    d. 18.2 mm Hg
    e. 21.4 mm Hg

68. Calculate the left ventricular end-diastolic pressure.
    a. 18.2 mm Hg
    b. 24.8 mm Hg
    c. 40.6 mm Hg
    d. 46.1 mm Hg
    e. 50.4 mm Hg

69. The continuous-wave spectral Doppler interrogation of an MR jet showed a 42 millisecond period between 1 m/s and 3 m/s of the MR velocity. The LV dP/dt is:
    a. 402 mm Hg/s
    b. 505 mm Hg/s
    c. 761 mm Hg/s
    d. 978 mm Hg/s
    e. 1006 mm Hg/s

Transesophageal Tomographic Views

5

Ryan Lauer and Joseph P. Mathew

GUIDELINES AND CLINICAL INDICATIONS FOR A COMPREHENSIVE TRANSESOPHAGEAL EXAMINATION

Transesophageal echocardiography (TEE) training and certification have become standardized with the use of recognized nomenclature and tomographic views. A consistent nomenclature has the advantage of not only facilitating communication between physicians but also promoting the performance of comprehensive examinations. Familiarity with standard views enables the echocardiographer to spot abnormalities more easily and compare sequential images. However, in some patients, it will not be possible to obtain a complete set of perfect two-dimensional views because of time constraints, or because the patient's body habitus or anatomy impedes the ability to develop the appropriate imaging planes. With practice, a complete TEE examination generally can be performed in 10 minutes or less, with images recorded on videotape or, preferably, in a digital format. A written report should then be generated as part of the patient's medical record (see Chapter 25). Recommendations presented in this chapter primarily pertain to the widely available TEE equipment, which permits multiplane two-dimensional imaging. As experience with the newly available real-time three-dimensional (3D) TEE grows, standardized recommendations are sure to follow.

Guidelines for a comprehensive TEE examination have been established jointly by the American Society of Echocardiography and the Society of Cardiovascular Anesthesiologists.[1] The indications for performing a TEE examination continue to evolve on the basis of evidence attesting to its value and the weight of expert opinion and are listed in Table 5–1.[2]

In fact, the decision to perform a TEE examination is influenced not only by the patient's clinical condition but also by the setting in which the examination is to be done and the procedure or operation that is being done on the patient. Often, a combination of factors, each one a doubtful indication for TEE by itself, add up to a strong indication for a TEE examination. Further, a single TEE examination can answer, in a matter of minutes, a number of questions that would otherwise require several different tests. For example, a patient on a balloon pump who is unstable after coronary surgery can be examined with TEE specifically to evaluate the location of the intraaortic balloon pump, global left ventricular function, regional function that might reflect specific bypass graft patency, mitral valve competence, right ventricular function, and the presence of pericardial fluid collections. Important contraindications to performing a TEE examination are discussed in Chapter 25.

PRINCIPLES OF PROBE MANIPULATION AND IMAGE DISPLAY

Probe Insertion

The TEE probe can usually be inserted into an anesthetized patient by displacing the mandible anteriorly and inserting the probe gently in the midline. Recent evidence, however, suggests that insertion of the probe under direct laryngoscopic visualization reduces the number of insertion attempts as well as the incidence of oropharyngeal mucosal injury and postoperative odynophagia (pain with swallowing).[3] The transducer should never be forced through resistance upon entry into or passage through the esophagus. The tip of the transducer also should be maintained in the neutral position, and the control wheels (see following paragraph) must always be unlocked whenever advancing or withdrawing the probe. Flexion of the probe tip while in the esophagus should be performed with great caution and never with excessive force. Suctioning of gastric fluid and air with an "in-and-out" placement of an orogastric tube prior to probe insertion significantly improves the quality of transgastric images. Probe insertion in an awake patient presents additional challenges that are discussed in Chapter 25.

Probe Manipulation

To view a particular image, the probe can be manipulated in four ways. First, it can be positioned in the esophagus to a certain depth; this technique is referred to as *advancing* and *withdrawing* the probe. Four esophageal

Table 5–1. Recommendations for the use of TEE in the perioperative period.

I. Cardiac and Thoracic Aortic Procedures

- *Cardiac and Thoracic Aortic Surgery*
  - For adult patients without contraindications, TEE should be used in all open heart (eg, valvular procedures) and thoracic aortic surgical procedures, and should be considered in CABG surgeries as well to
    - Confirm and refine the preoperative diagnosis
    - Detect new or unsuspected pathology
    - Adjust the anesthetic and surgical plan accordingly
    - Assess results of the surgical intervention
  - In small children, the use of TEE should be considered on a case-by-case basis because of risks unique to these patients (eg, bronchial obstruction)
- *Catheter-Based Intracardiac Procedures*
  - For patients undergoing transcatheter intracardiac procedures, TEE may be used

II. Noncardiac Surgery

- TEE may be used when the nature of the planned surgery or the patient's known or suspected cardiovascular pathology might result in severe hemodynamic, pulmonary, or neurologic compromise
- If equipment and expertise are available, TEE should be used when unexplained life-threatening circulatory instability persists despite corrective therapy

III. Critical Care

- For critical care patients, TEE should be used when diagnostic information that is expected to alter management cannot be obtained by TTE or other modalities in a timely manner

Abbreviations: TEE, transesophageal echocardiography; TTE, transthoracic echocardiography; CABG, coronary artery bypass graft.
Source: Practice Guidelines for Perioperative Transesophageal Echocardiography. An Updated Report by the American Society of Anesthesiologists and the Society of Cardiovascular Anesthesiologists Task Force on Transesophageal Echocardiography. Anesthesiology 2010;112:1084-1096.

"windows" are used to obtain TEE views corresponding to different positions within the esophagus (Figure 5–1). For example, many views will be obtained at a depth of about 35 cm from the teeth when the probe head (transducer) is generally posterior to the left atrium. This depth corresponds to a midesophageal position. Upper esophageal views would be obtained with the probe closer to a depth of 25 cm; transgastric views at about 40 cm and deep transgastric views might be obtained with the probe advanced to a depth of 50 cm. The second aspect of probe manipulation consists of flexion of the probe tip in four different directions by using the two control wheels located on the probe handle. The large wheel controls forward and backward movements of the probe tip. Forward motion of the probe tip is called *anteflexion*, in which the probe is flexed toward the sternum (Figure 5–2A). Backward motion of the tip is called *retroflexion*, when the probe is flexed back toward the spine (see Figure 5–2B). The smaller control wheel flexes the probe tip to the patient's left and right and those motions are so described (Figure 5–3A and B). *Lateral flexion* to the left and right is much less useful than anteflexion and retroflexion.

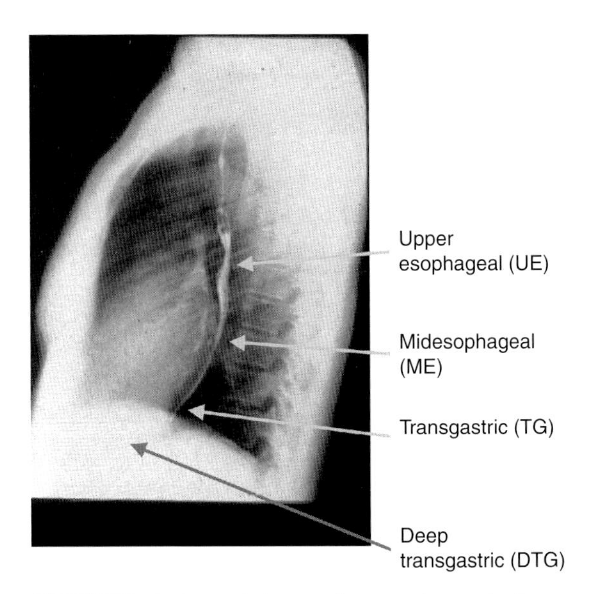

FIGURE 5–1. Lateral chest radiogram shows the location of the windows used for transesophageal tomographic views.

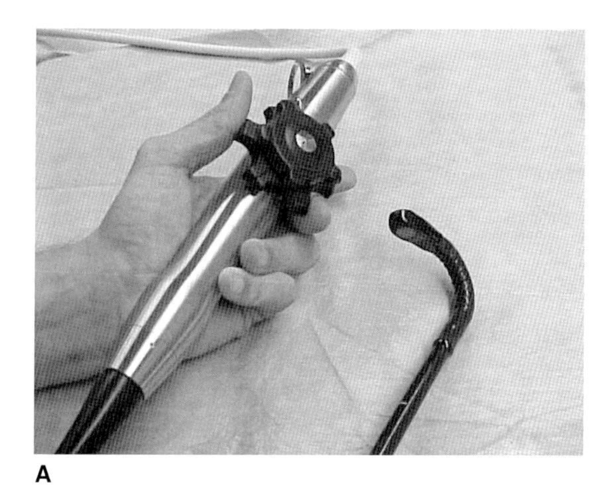

A

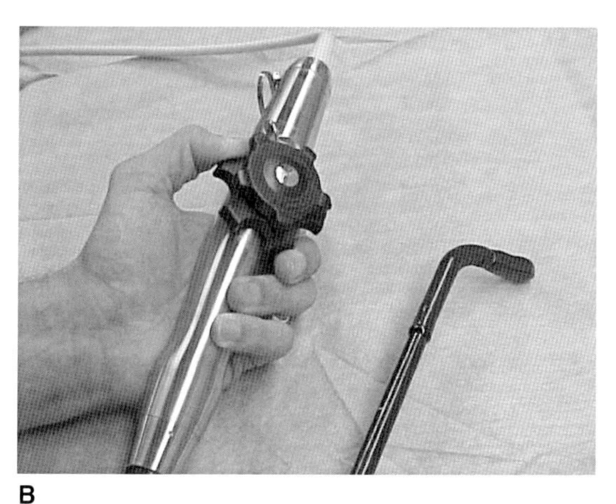

B

FIGURE 5–2. Probe manipulation. **A:** Anteflexion. **B:** Retroflexion.

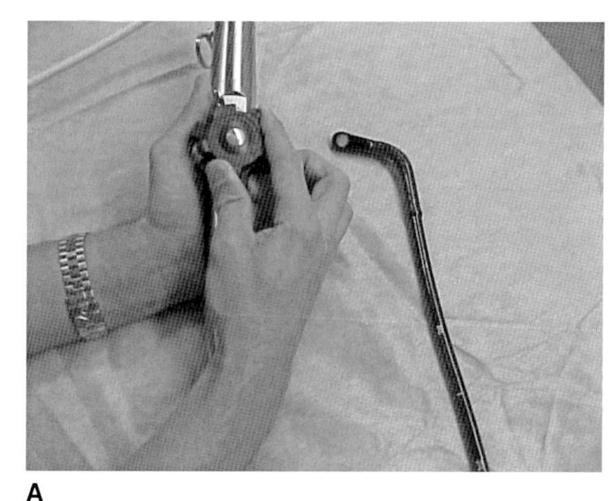

A

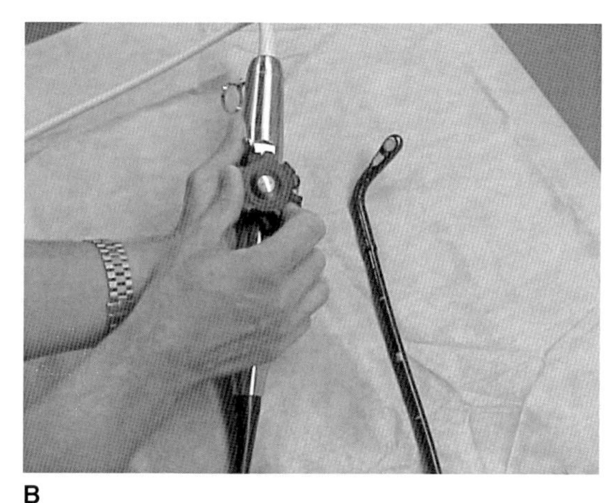

B

FIGURE 5–3. Probe manipulation. **A:** Lateral flexion to the left. **B:** Lateral flexion to the right.

Third, the imaging plane provided by the transducer can be *rotated* axially through 180° by means of the lever or buttons located on the probe handle (Figure 5–4A and B). Multiplane probes permit this plane to be *rotated forward* from the 0° horizontal to a 90° plane, thus providing a vertical or longitudinal plane, and over to the horizontal plane again at 180° (a mirror image of that present at 0°). The imaging plane then can be *rotated back* from 180° toward 0° by electronically rotating the scanning plane backward (see Figure 5–4B). Fourth, the probe can be turned manually to the right and left sides of the patient, and this is referred to as *turning* to avoid confusion with the term *rotation*, which is applied to the electronic rotation of the scanning plane from 0° to 180°.

Image Display

By convention, the transducer location (within the esophagus) appears at the top of the images, with the near field close to the transducer at the top and the far field below. The depth of the tissue being imaged is indicated by the centimeter markers at the sides of the image and on most machines by a numeric notation for the depth of field. At 0° the imaging plane is directed anteriorly from the esophagus through the heart, and the patient's right side is presented on the left of the image display (when facing the display; Figure 5–5). Rotation to 90° progresses counterclockwise (the TEE probe tip is the clock face) from the 0° plane and presents the inferior portion of the heart

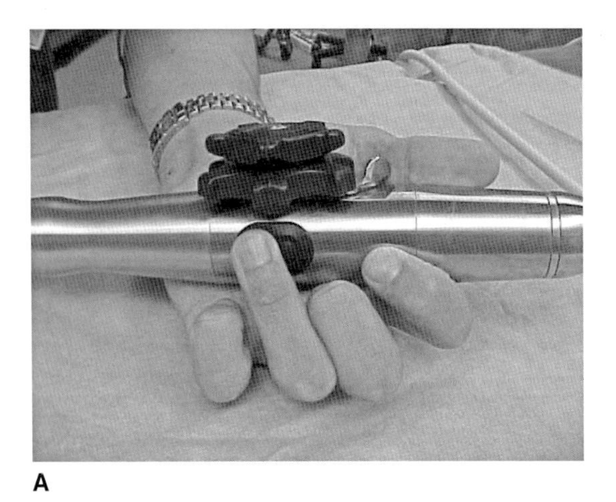

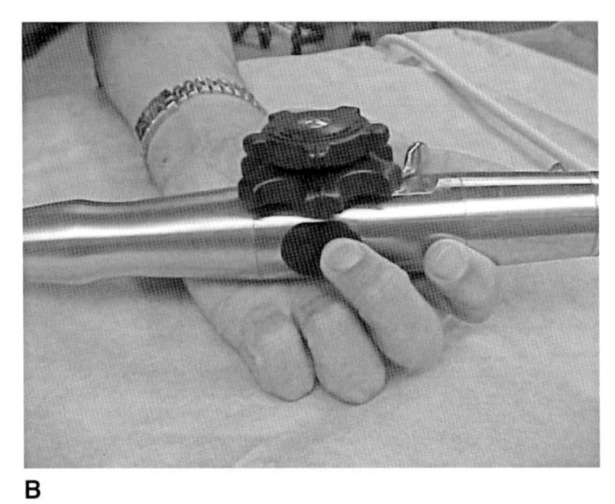

A B

FIGURE 5–4. Rotation of the multiplane angle. **A:** Forward. **B:** Backward.

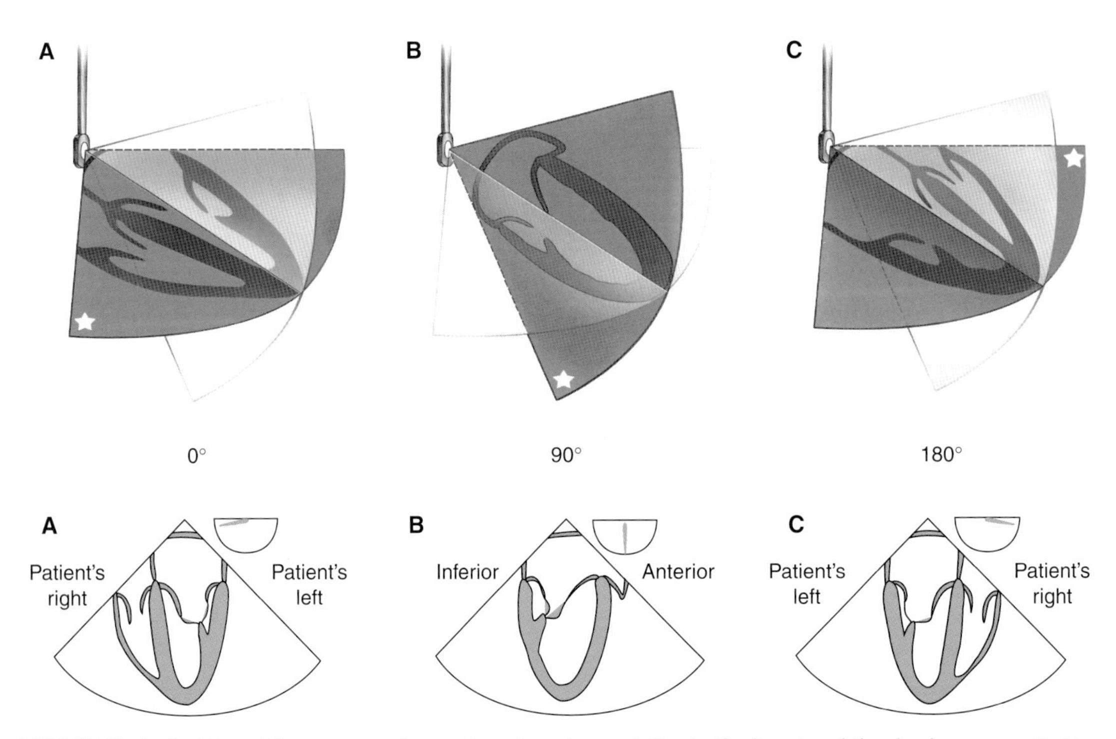

FIGURE 5–5. Position of the transesophageal imaging plane relative to the heart and the display screen. **A:** At 0°, the imaging plane is directed anteriorly from the esophagus through the heart, and the patient's right side is presented on the left of the image display. **B:** Forward rotation to 90° progresses in a counterclockwise direction (probe as the clock face) from the 0° plane and presents the inferior portion of the heart on the left side of the display and the anterior portion on the right side. Note the change in the position of the white star on the imaging plane when the multiplane angle is rotated. **C:** Rotation to 180° places the patient's left side on the left side of the display, thus creating a mirror image of the 0° imaging plane. Backward rotation results in a clockwise rotation of the imaging plane.

on the left side of the display and the anterior portion on the right side. Rotation to 180° places the patient's left side on the left side of the display, thus creating a mirror image of the 0° imaging plane.

THE COMPLETE TEE EXAMINATION

A complete examination currently includes three ultrasound modes:

1. Two-dimensional imaging to examine cardiac anatomy
2. Color-flow Doppler imaging to visualize blood flow velocities
3. Spectral Doppler
   a. Pulsed wave, to measure blood flow velocities at specific locations
   b. Continuous wave, to measure high velocities that exceed the limits of pulsed Doppler and are commonly associated with abnormal flow jets

Although not a part of current recommendations, 3D TEE is expected to rapidly become more standard because of the added insights it provides into cardiac anatomy and function. The reader is therefore strongly encouraged to become facile with 3D imaging (see Chapter 24).

RECOMMENDED TOMOGRAPHIC VIEWS

The complete examination should include the 20 views shown in Figure 5–6. The sequence in which these should be obtained is not rigidly fixed, but a specific order will permit the consistent performance of a comprehensive examination. One such sequence may start with midesophageal views, proceed to transgastric views, and end with the upper esophageal views. At times the echocardiographer may wish to go straight to an imaging plane that will answer a specific question such as the severity of regurgitation; however, a complete examination should always follow. Although 20 views are suggested for the complete examination, it may well be necessary to examine some nonstandard views. As every patient's anatomy is different, one must not too rigidly follow suggested imaging depths or multiplane angles. A solid understanding of the anatomy provides the echocardiographer insight when a view is not ideal from a "standard" location. Three-dimensional imaging may be a useful guide in defining precise angulation necessary for "standard" views.

The complete examination, as presented in the remainder of this chapter, will focus in turn on the following structures:

- Left ventricle (LV)
- Mitral valve
- Aortic valve, aortic root, and LV outflow tract (LVOT)
- Left atrium and pulmonary veins, right atrium, and atrial septum
- Right ventricle (RV), tricuspid valve, and pulmonary valve
- Thoracic aorta

LEFT VENTRICLE

- Views

  Midesophageal four chamber, two chamber, and long axis

  Transgastric two chamber and basal, mid-papillary, and apical short axis

- Assessment

  Contractility (fractional area change and ejection fraction)

  Segmental wall motion

  Chamber dimensions (dilation and hypertrophy)

  Masses (thrombus and tumor)

Assessment of the LV begins with the midesophageal four-chamber view to examine the size and overall contractility of the LV (Figure 5–7). This view is obtained at a depth of approximately 35 cm when the transducer is posterior to the left atrium. A 16-cm depth of field is usually appropriate to ensure that the entire apex is visualized. Forward rotation to 10° to 20° aligns the imaging plane with the true longitudinal plane of the LV, maximizes the tricuspid annular dimension, and excludes the aortic valve. A greater forward rotation may be required in patients with dilated ventricles or in patients undergoing redo procedures in whom adhesions can alter the normal lay of the heart within the pericardial sac. Gentle retroflexion is often also necessary to avoid foreshortening the ventricle and to visualize the left ventricular apex. The American Heart Association has recommended standardization of myocardial segmentation and nomenclature for tomographic imaging of the heart by any imaging modality (coronary angiography, nuclear cardiology, echocardiography, cardiovascular magnetic resonance, cardiac computed tomography, and positron emission

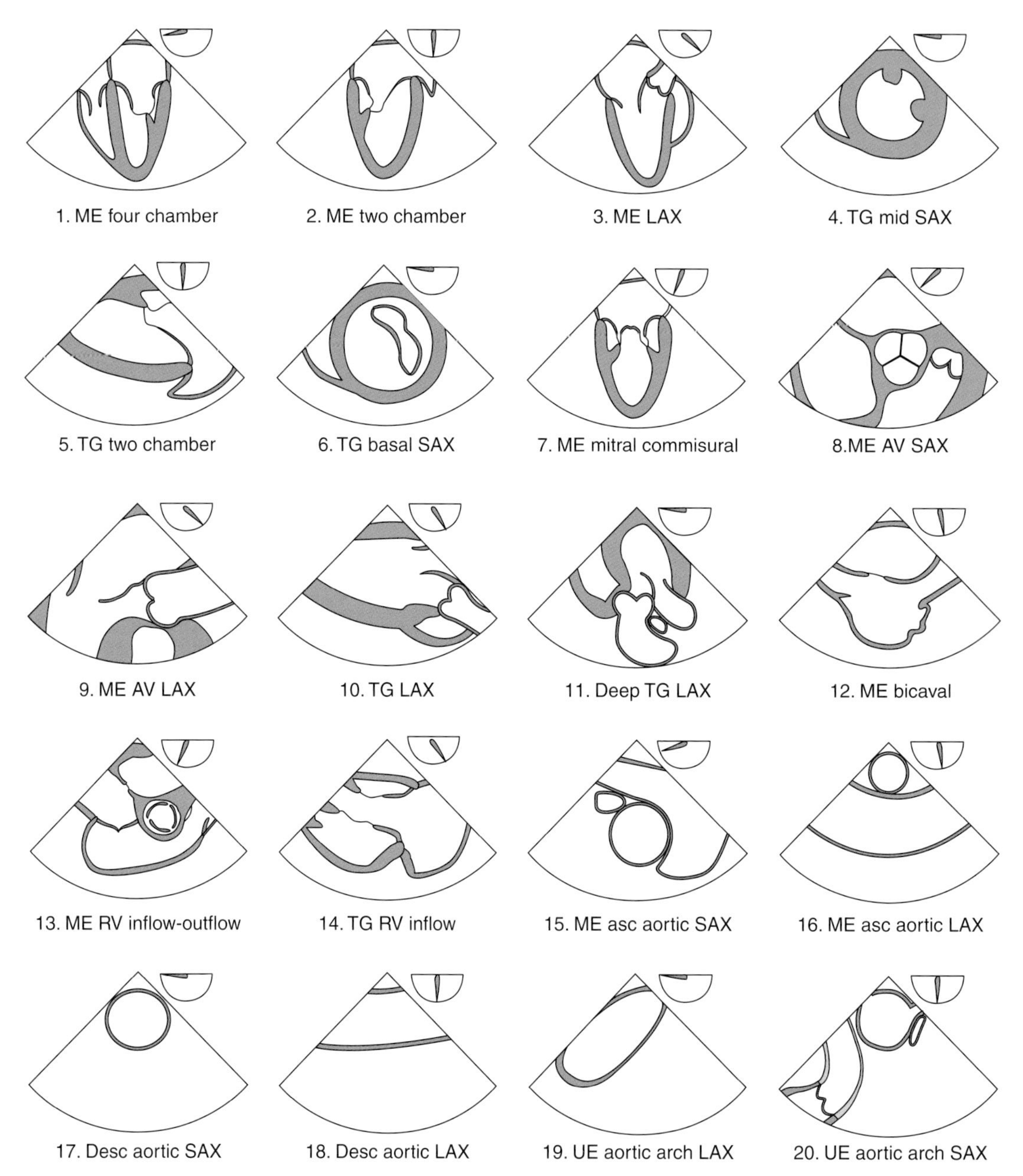

FIGURE 5–6. The 20 two-dimensional tomographic views recommended for a complete transesophageal examination. Approximate multiplane angles are indicated by the icons adjacent to each view. (asc, ascending; AV, aortic valve; desc, descending; LAX, long axis; ME, midesophageal; RV, right ventricle; SAX, short axis; TG, transgastric; UE, upper esophageal.) *(Reproduced with permission from Shanewise JS, Cheung AT, Aronson S, et al. ASE/SCA guidelines for performing a comprehensive intraoperative multiplane transesophageal echocardiography examination: recommendations of the American Society of Echocardiography Council for Intraoperative Echocardiography and the Society of Cardiovascular Anesthesiologists Task Force for Certification in Perioperative Transesophageal Echocardiography. Anesth Analg. 1999;89:870.)*

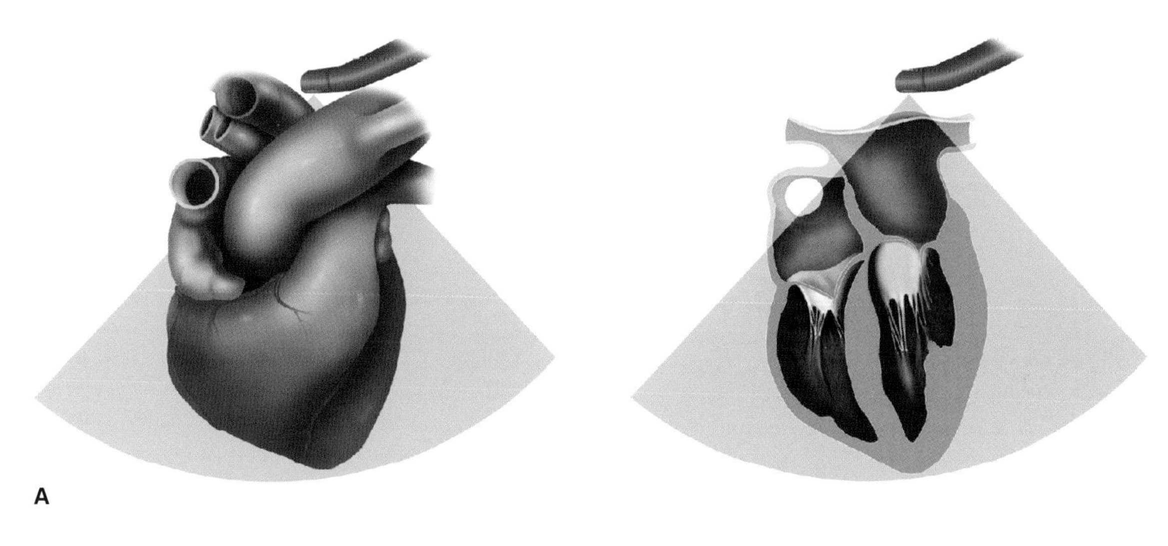

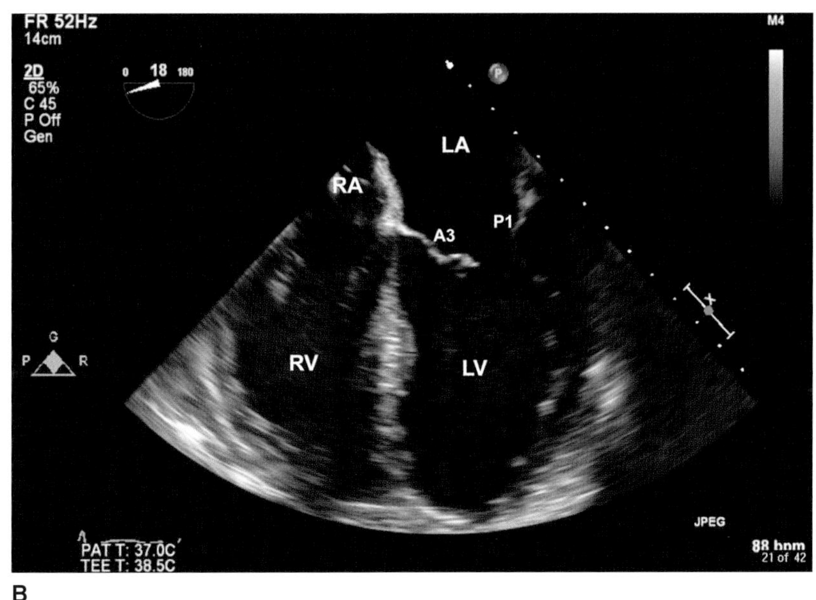

FIGURE 5–7. Anatomic **(A)** and ultrasound **(B)** illustration of the imaging plane as it cuts through the heart for the midesophageal four-chamber view. The basal, mid, and apical septal and lateral myocardial segments as well as the A3 segment of the anterior leaflet and the P1 scallop of the posterior leaflet are seen in this view. (RA, right atrium; RV, right ventricle; LA, left atrium; LV, left ventricle.)

computed tomography) and this recommendation will be followed in this chapter.[4] Thus, in the midesophageal four-chamber view, the basal and mid-inferoseptal and -anterolateral myocardial segments, the apical septal and lateral segments, and the apical cap are visible.

Further forward rotation to 80° to 100° depicts the midesophageal two-chamber view (Figure 5–8) and rotation to 120° to 160° shows the long-axis view (Figure 5–9). While all three views are forms of long-axis views of the LV, only the imaging plane shown in Figure 5–9 is actually called the long-axis view. As with the four-chamber view, these imaging planes are used primarily to assess overall contractility and regional wall motion. In the two-chamber view, the basal, mid, and apical anterior and inferior myocardial segments are seen, and the long-axis view permits assessment of the

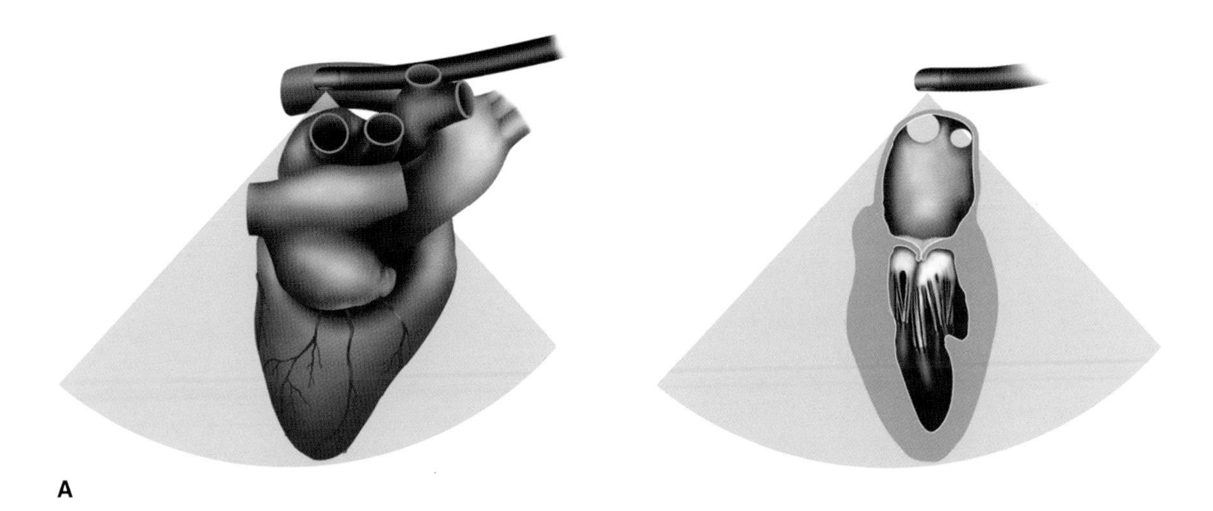

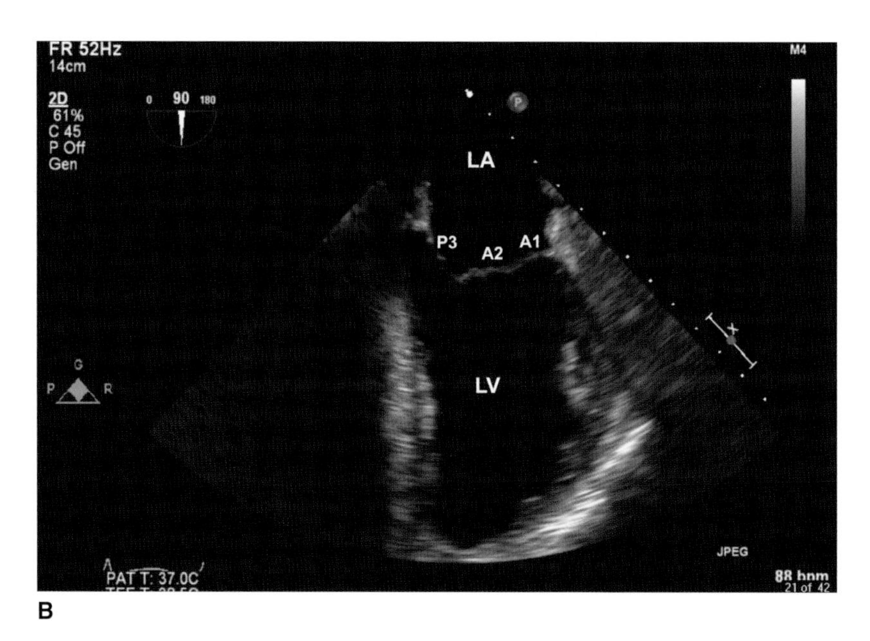

FIGURE 5–8. Anatomic **(A)** and ultrasound **(B)** illustration of the imaging plane as it cuts through the heart for the midesophageal two-chamber view. The basal, mid, and apical anterior and inferior myocardial segments as well as the P3 scallop of the posterior leaflet and the A1 and A2 segments of the anterior leaflet are seen in this view. (LA, left atrium; LV, left ventricle.)

basal and mid-anteroseptal and -inferolateral segments and the apical septal and lateral segments. The apical cap also is visualized in these two views.

Once the midesophageal views have been acquired, the TEE probe should be advanced to the transgastric position. Anteflexion of the tip of the probe is necessary to produce the basal (Figure 5–10), midpapillary (Figure 5–11), and apical (Figure 5–12) short-axis views. Care should be taken to ensure that the entire LV is seen on the image, which usually requires a depth of field of 12 cm and some probe turning. The LV also should appear circular, particularly with the basal short-axis view, where excessive anteflexion commonly results in imaging of the membranous portion of the interventricular septum and/or portions of the LVOT, making it difficult to accurately categorize myocardial segments

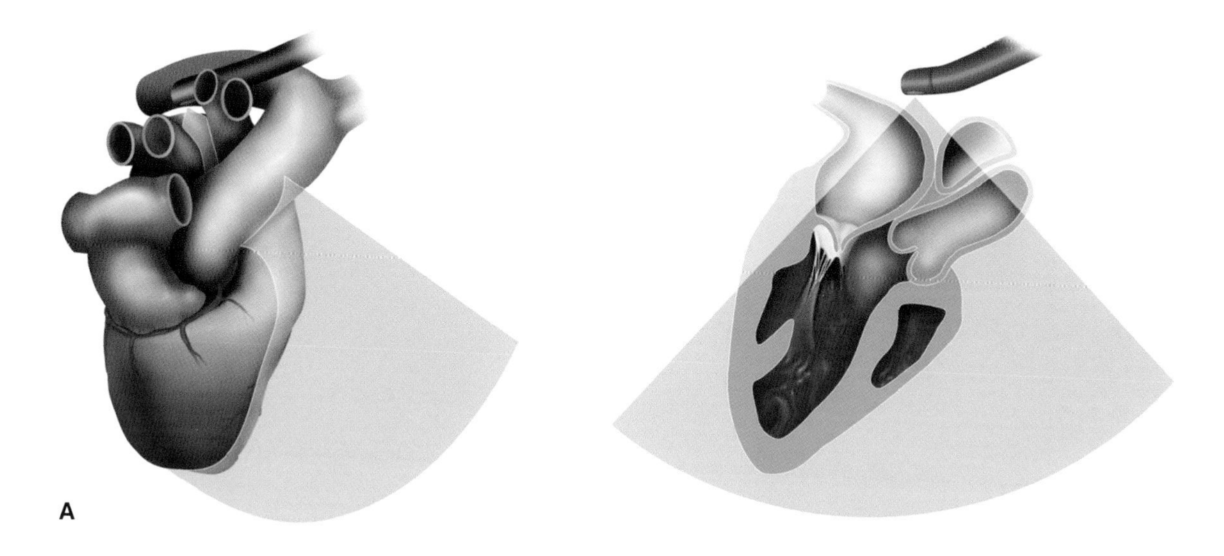

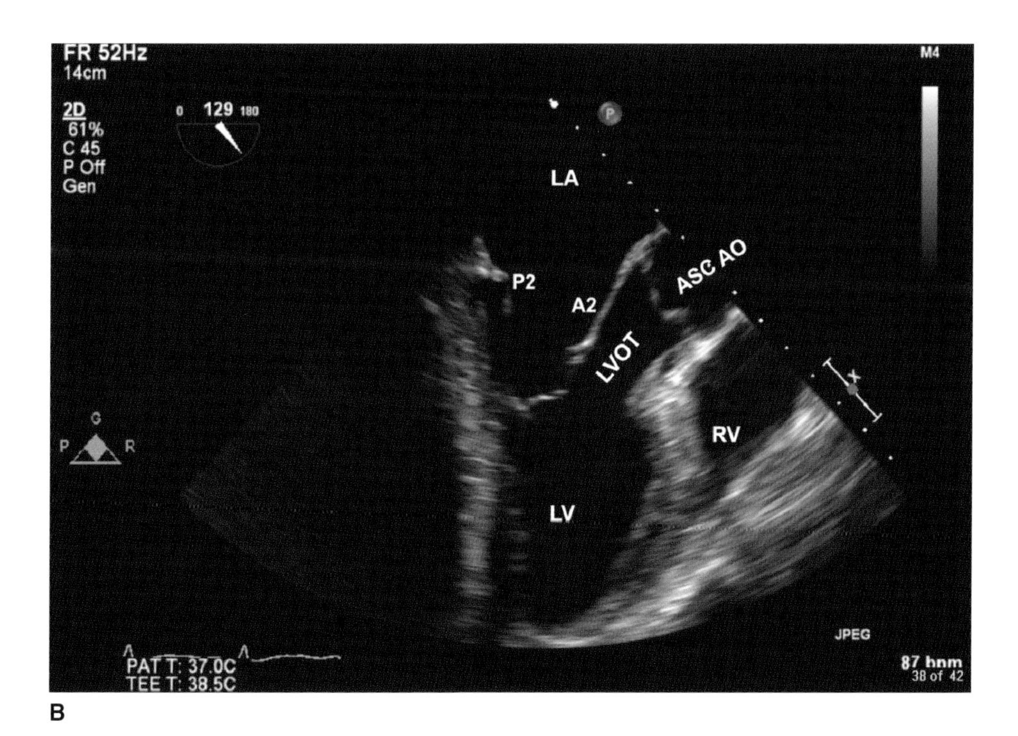

FIGURE 5–9. Anatomic **(A)** and ultrasound **(B)** illustration of the imaging plane as it cuts through the heart for the midesophageal long-axis view. The basal and mid anteroseptal and inferolateral myocardial segments as well as the A2 segment of the anterior leaflet and the P2 scallop of the posterior leaflet are seen in this view. (RV, right ventricle; LA, left atrium; LV, left ventricle; LVOT, left ventricular outflow tract; ASC AO, ascending aorta.)

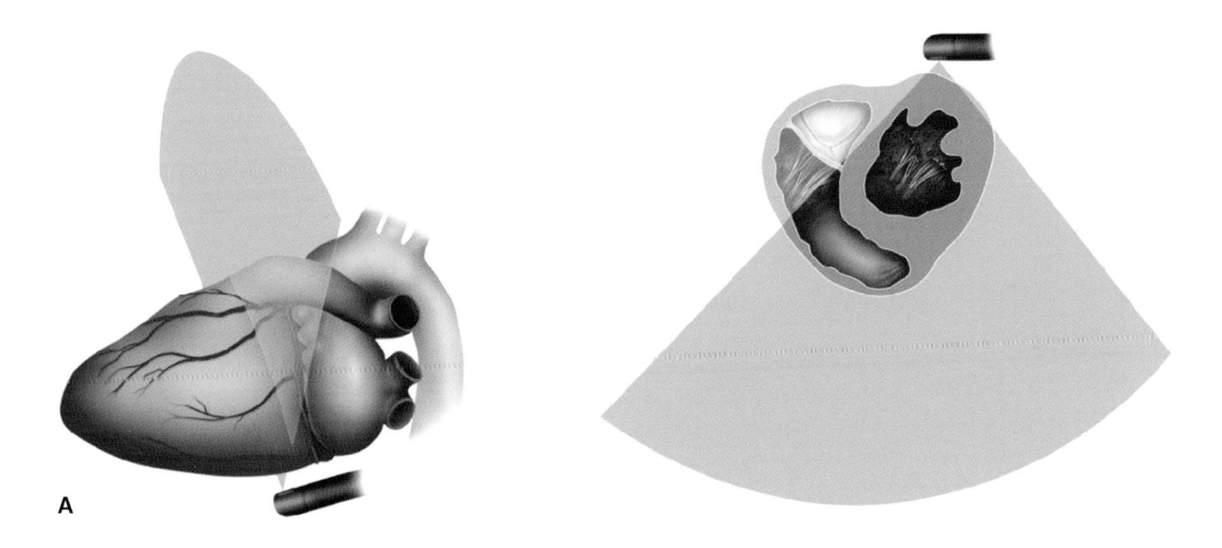

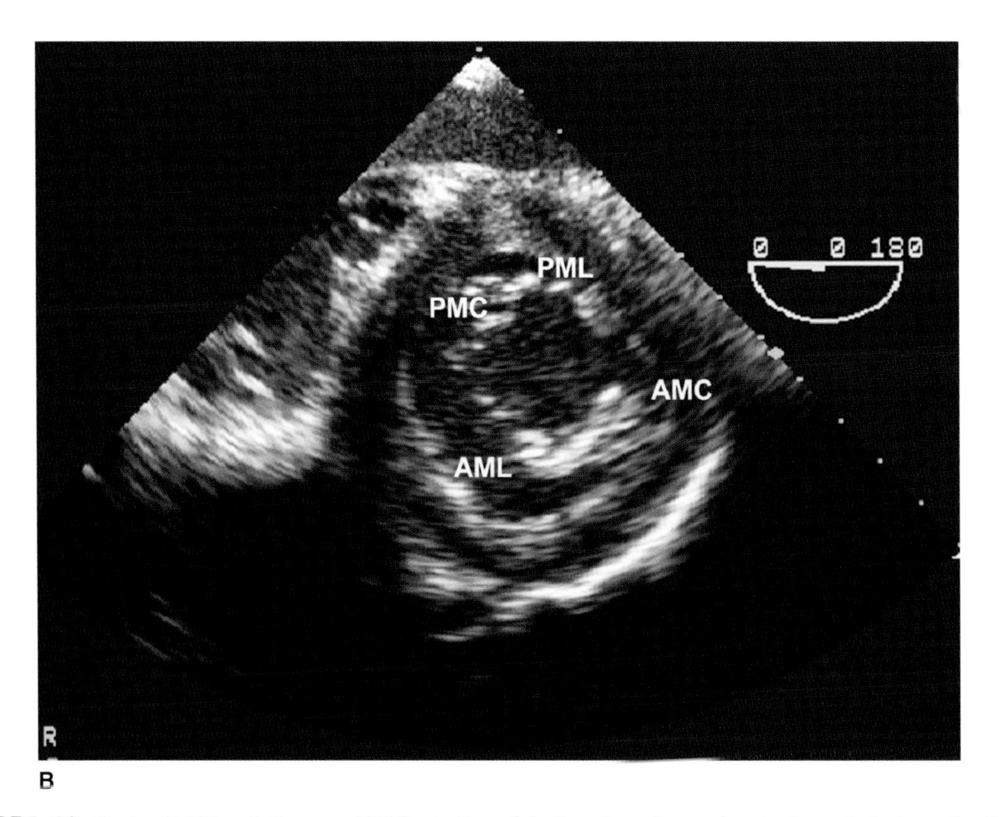

FIGURE 5–10. Anatomic **(A)** and ultrasound **(B)** illustration of the imaging plane as it cuts through the heart for the transgastric basal short-axis view. (AML, anterior mitral leaflet; PML, posterior mitral leaflet; AMC, anterolateral mitral commissure; PMC, posteromedial mitral commissure.)

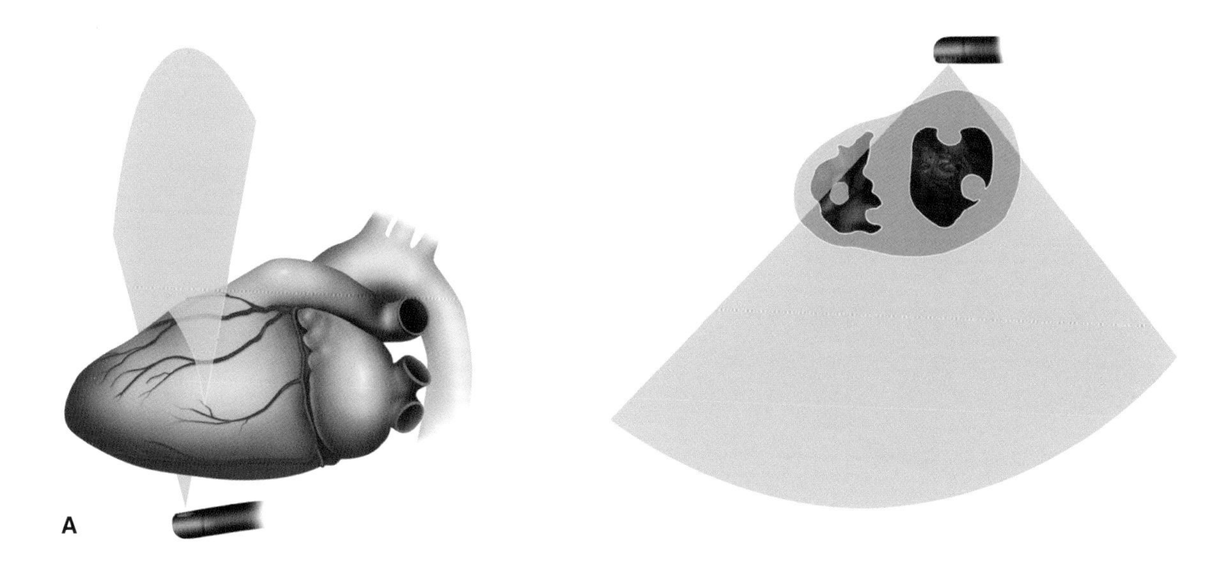

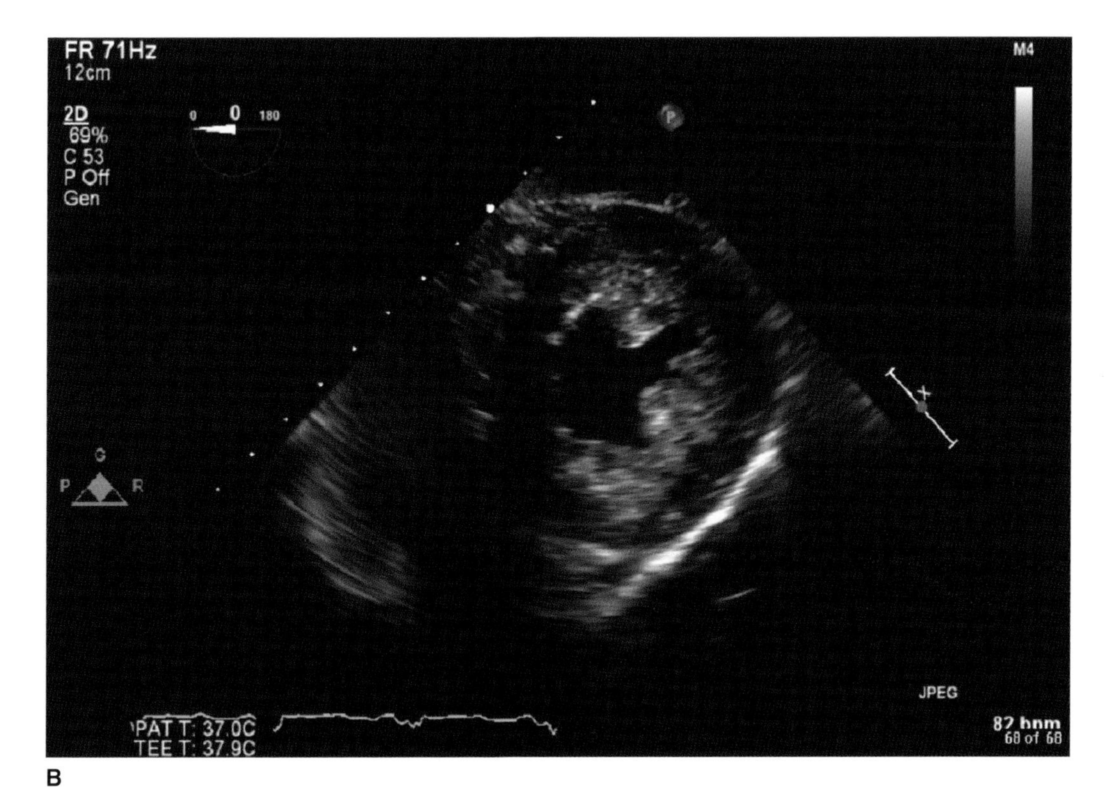

FIGURE 5–11. Anatomic **(A)** and ultrasound **(B)** illustration of the imaging plane as it cuts through the heart for the transgastric mid short-axis view.

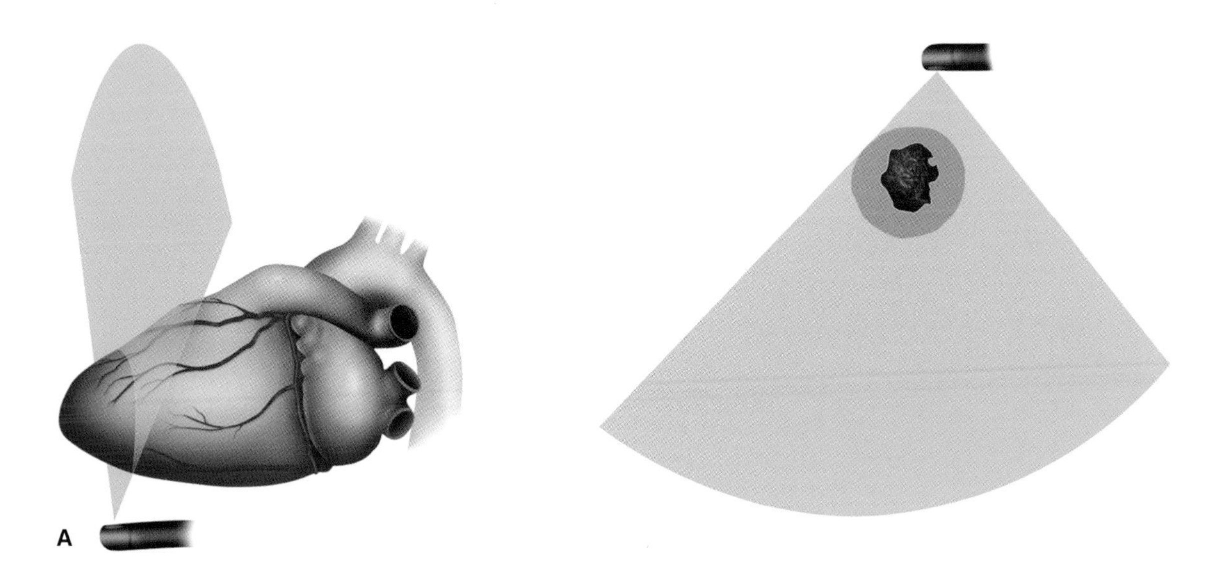

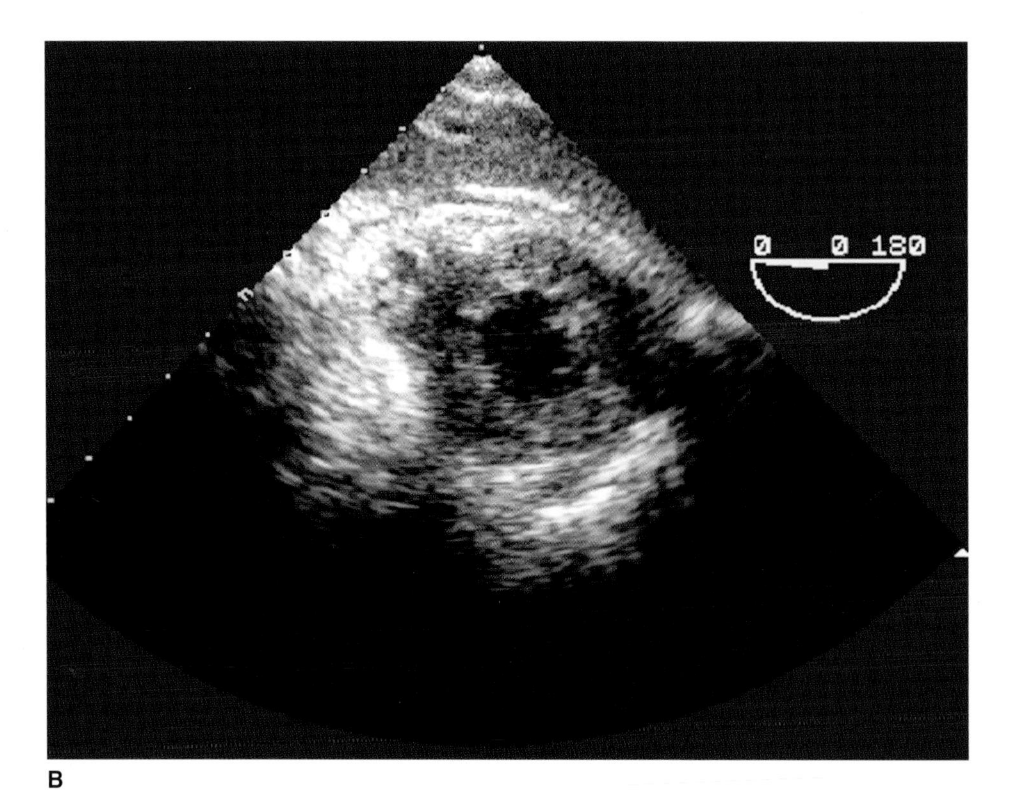

FIGURE 5–12. Anatomic **(A)** and ultrasound **(B)** illustration of the imaging plane as it cuts through the heart for the transgastric apical short-axis view.

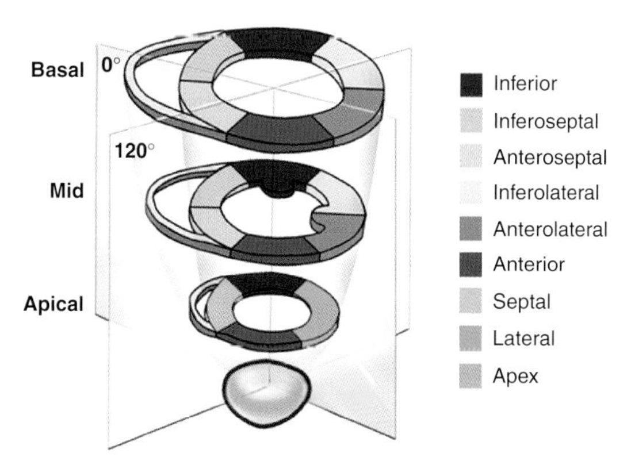

FIGURE 5–13. Left ventricular segmentation and nomenclature using the scheme for standardization between all imaging modalities as proposed by the American Heart Association Writing Group on Myocardial Segmentation and Registration for Cardiac Imaging. *(From Cerqueira MD, Weissman NJ, Dilsizian V, et al. Standardized myocardial segmentation and nomenclature for tomographic imaging of the heart: a statement for healthcare professionals from the Cardiac Imaging Committee of the Council on Clinical Cardiology of the American Heart Association. Circulation. 2002;105:539.)*

and thus assess regional wall motion abnormalities. Tangential imaging planes may be corrected by reducing the anteflexion, advancing the probe, or lateral flexion of the tip of the probe.

The transgastric short-axis views are useful for evaluating wall thickness and chamber size. LV hypertrophy is defined as an *end-diastolic* wall thickness greater than 1.1 cm in the midpapillary short-axis view. LV enlargement is considered to be present when the *end-diastolic* diameter measured from endocardium to endocardium in the midpapillary short-axis view is larger than 5.4 cm. Measurement errors are commonly produced by including a portion of the papillary muscles within the measurement or by using images that lack a clear definition of the endocardial or epicardial border. End-diastole may be confirmed by using the image coinciding with the onset of the QRS complex on the electrocardiogram.

Wall motion analysis is best performed with the transgastric short-axis views. The LV is divided into equal thirds, perpendicular to the long axis of the heart (Figure 5–13). The basal third extends from the mitral annulus to the tips of the papillary muscles, the mid-cavity view includes the entire length of the papillary muscles, and the apical region extends from the papillary muscles to just before the end of the cavity. The apical cap (17th segment) is the area beyond the end of the LV cavity.[4] Myocardial segments are named with reference to the long axis of the ventricle and the circumferential location on the short-axis view. The attachment of the RV to the LV is used to identify and separate the septum from the LV anterior and inferior walls. The basal and mid-cavity imaging planes are divided into six segments of approximately 60° each; however, because the LV tapers as it approaches the apex, the apical imaging plane consists of only four segments. In general, regional wall motion is appreciated most easily from short-axis views, but it is worth remembering that the same segments can be visualized with midesophageal views of the LV. In particular, the apex is likely to be overlooked in short-axis imaging of the LV. Each myocardial segment should be examined for inward endocardial motion and for percentage of thickening during systole. Normally, the myocardium thickens by greater than 30%. Mild hypokinesia is represented by 10% to 30% wall thickening; severe hypokinesia by less than 10% wall thickening; akinesia by failure to thicken at all; and dyskinesia by outward bulging of the myocardium during systole. Thus, an old, transmural myocardial infarct will appear as a region of thinner myocardium that may be akinetic or even dyskinetic.

From the midpapillary short-axis view, forward rotation to 90° produces the transgastric two-chamber view (Figure 5–14). This imaging plane is particularly useful for imaging the apex, which is now on the left side of the screen, with the mitral valve and subvalvular apparatus on the right side. The inferior wall is seen at the top and the anterior wall at the bottom of the display.

Coronary Blood Supply to the Left Ventricular Segments

In general, segmental coronary supply is derived as indicated by Figures 5–15 and 5–16. However, considerable variation may be present, particularly in the apical segments. For example, the apical inferior segment is supplied by the posterior descending coronary branch, which may arise from the right coronary (right dominant circulation) or the left anterior descending coronary (left dominant circulation). Likewise, the apical lateral segment may be supplied by the circumflex or the left anterior descending coronary. If the motions of the apical lateral segment and the midlevel inferolateral and anterolateral segments are abnormal at the same time, the apical lateral segment likely was served by the circumflex coronary and not by the left anterior descending coronary. Therefore, apical wall motion abnormalities should be examined with other segmental wall motion abnormalities in mind.

MITRAL VALVE

- Views

  Midesophageal four chamber, two chamber, mitral commissural, and long axis

  Transgastric long axis and basal short axis

  Three dimensional

- Assessment

  Valve and annular morphology

  Stenosis

  Regurgitation

  Mitral inflow

A thorough understanding of mitral valve anatomy is essential for the echocardiographer. The valve can roughly be divided into supporting structures (annulus, papillary muscles, and chordae tendineae) and leaflets (anterior and posterior). The mitral annulus is a saddle-shaped structure with two axes. The longer axis parallels the line of coaptation in the lower portion of the "saddle" and runs in a mostly medial to lateral orientation. The shorter axis, perpendicular to the line of coaptation, runs between the high points of the "saddle" in a mostly anterior to posterior orientation. As seen in Figure 5–17C, the anterior portion of the mitral annulus is continuous with the aortic valve annulus. The annulus is strongest here, where it has structural support from the fibrous skeleton of the heart, and is weakest posteriorly, where the fibrous tissue is less dense. The papillary muscles and chordae tendineae form the rest of the supporting structure of the mitral valve. The papillary muscles originate from the anterolateral and posteromedial portions of the ventricular walls and are named as such. The anterolateral papillary muscle is supplied by branches from the left anterior descending coronary artery and from the marginal branches of the left circumflex artery. In 71% of patients presenting for coronary surgery, the anterolateral papillary muscle had a dual-vessel supply while 29% had a single-vessel supply.[5] The posteromedial papillary muscle receives a variable supply from the left circumflex artery and branches of the right coronary artery, but in 63% of patients, it was perfused by a single vessel, commonly the right coronary artery.[5]

The anatomy of the mitral leaflets has been described most commonly using terminology developed by Carpentier, thus allowing standardized communication between physicians on leaflet pathology. The crescent-shaped posterior mitral leaflet has three scallops, which, in Carpentier's terminology, are known as P1, P2, and P3, with P1 being the most anterior, P2 in the middle, and P3 the most posterior. The anterior leaflet attaches to the same fibrous skeleton of the heart as the left and noncoronary cusps of the aortic valve. It is not scalloped, but the portions coapting with the posterior leaflet are termed A1, A2, and A3, from anterior to posterior. The anterolateral and posteromedial commissures are associated with their respective papillary muscles, and each is attached to portions of both mitral leaflets. Thus, the chordae originating from the anterolateral papillary muscle support the anterolateral commissure and the adjoining halves of the anterior and posterior leaflets (A1, P1, and part of A2 and P2) while the posteromedial papillary muscle's chordae support the posteromedial commissure and the adjoining halves of the anterior and posterior leaflets (A3 and P3 and part of A2 and P2).[6] The orientation of the mitral valve as seen in the basal short-axis image and in Figure 5–17A and B does not correspond to the orientation of the valve as seen by the operating surgeon who sees the anterior leaflet sitting on top of the posterior leaflet (see Figure 5–17C). Three-dimensional TEE now makes it possible to view the mitral valve leaflets from the same perspective as the surgeon (see Figure 5–17 C).

A systematic examination of the mitral valve begins with optimization of the ultrasound image. The depth of view should be decreased so as to only view the mitral valve leaflets and subvalvular apparatus. This enlarges the areas of interest and increases the frame rate (temporal resolution). The overall gain should be adjusted down until the blood pool just turns black, thereby decreasing the likelihood that the leaflets will artifactually appear thickened. Increasing the transducer frequency will also improve leaflet resolution. In each of following views the valve should first be examined in two dimensions (2D) and then with a color-flow Doppler sector that includes the left atrial portion to assess the regurgitant jet and the LV aspect of the valve to assess flow convergence.

Examination of the mitral valve frequently includes four midesophageal views, two transgastric views, and 3D views. The midesophageal four-chamber view is a frequent starting place as it provides an overall sense of the valve function or pathology. The imaging plane (20° to 30°) transects the mitral valve in an oblique plane relative to the valve commissures, thus showing the A3 segment of the anterior leaflet to the left of the display and the P1 scallop of the posterior leaflet to the right of the display (Figure 5–7). By slightly withdrawing or anteflexing the probe, the tomographic plane will transect the valve closer to the anterolateral commissure, bringing the left ventricular outflow tract into view, while slightly

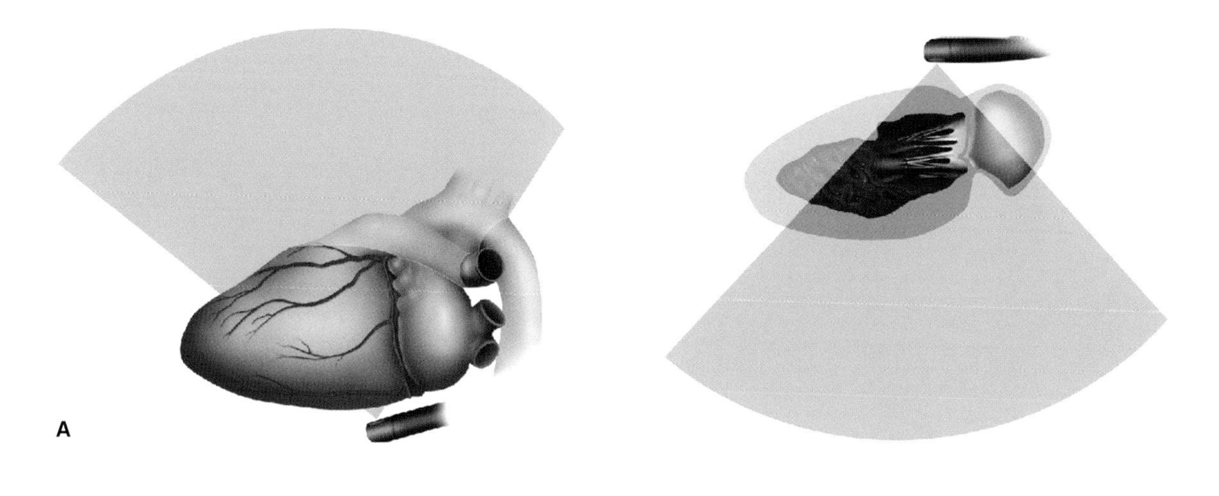

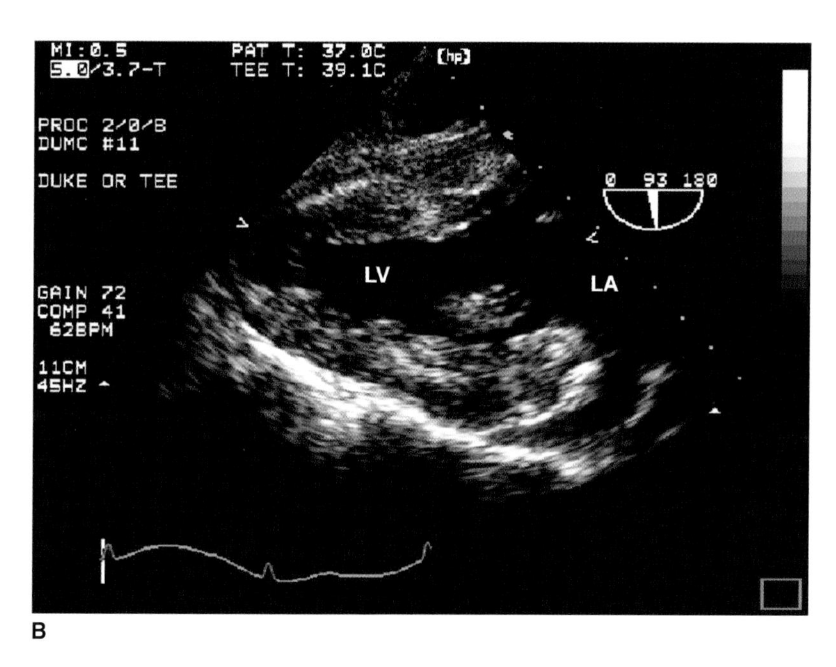

FIGURE 5–14. Anatomic **(A)** and ultrasound **(B)** illustration of the imaging plane as it cuts through the heart for the transgastric two-chamber view. (LA, left atrium; LV, left ventricle.)

advancing or retroflexing the probe transects the valve more toward the posteromedial commissure. Next, the midesophageal mitral valve commissural view is obtained by rotating the multiplane angle forward to about 60° (Figure 5–18). In this view, three parts to the mitral leaflets are visible, as the posterior leaflet is captured at the posteromedial (P3 to the left of the display) and anterolateral (P1 to the right of the display) portions, with the anterior leaflet (A2) appearing in between. Imaging with color-flow Doppler in this view can help to determine the origin of a regurgitant jet and localize it to either commissure. The long axis of the mitral annulus can be measured in this view as well.

Rotating the multiplane angle forward to approximately 90° creates the midesophageal two-chamber view. P3 is always seen on the left of the image, while A1 and A2 are typically seen on the right of the image (Figure 5–8). By turning the probe to the left more of the posterior

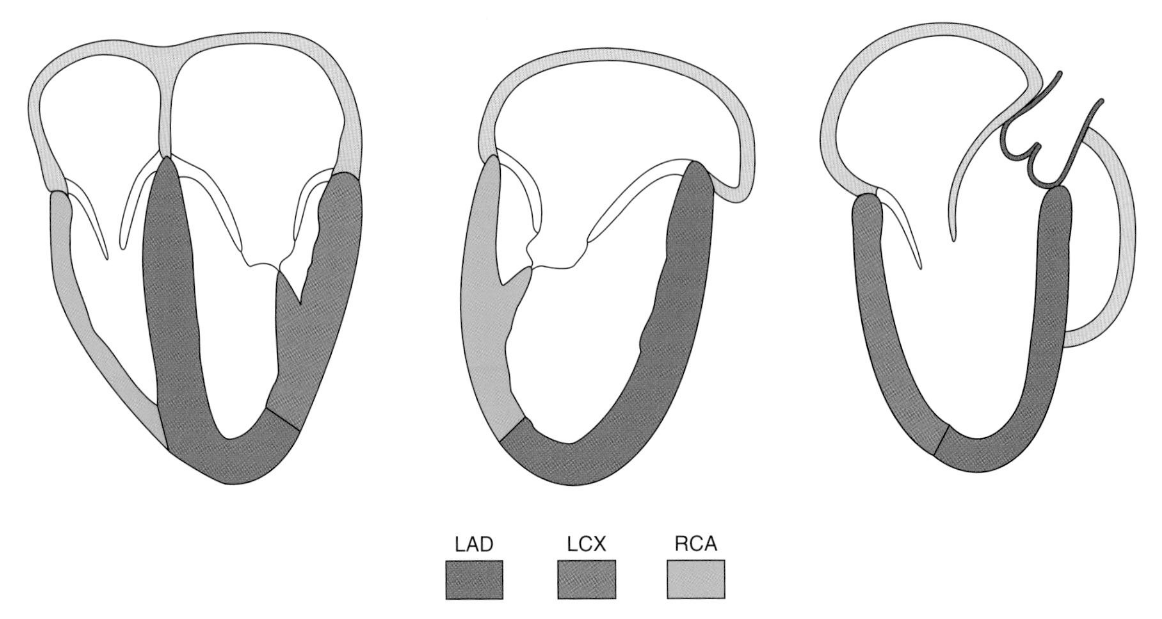

FIGURE 5–15. Regions of myocardium perfused by each of the major coronary arteries as seen in the three standard midesophageal views. (LAD, left anterior descending; LCX, left circumflex artery; RCA, right coronary artery.)

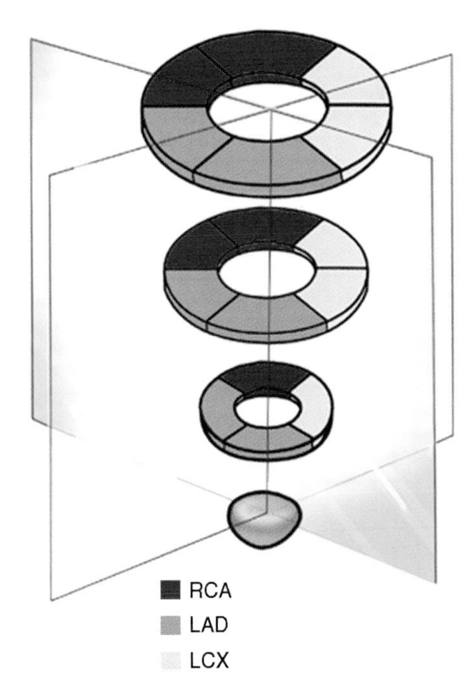

FIGURE 5–16. Assignment of the myocardial segments to the territories of the major coronary arteries as seen in transgastric short-axis views. (LAD, left anterior descending; LCX, left circumflex artery; RCA, right coronary artery.)

leaflet (P2, P1) is visualized on the right, while turning the probe to the right visualizes more of the anterior leaflet (A2, A3) on the right. Finally, the multiplane angle is rotated forward (between 120° and 150°) until both the mitral valve and aortic valve are seen but neither papillary muscle is in view (midesophageal long-axis view). In this view, A2 is typically seen on the right with P2 on the left (Figure 5–9). As the image plane cuts perpendicularly through the line of coaptation, all segments of both leaflets can be assessed by simply turning the probe (left for A1/P1 and right for A3/P3). The short axis of the mitral annulus can be measured here, and it is the best imaging plane for measurement of vena contracta.

Before leaving the midesophageal views, two pulsed Doppler flow profiles should be examined: (a) a mitral inflow flow profile that provides information about the diastolic function of the LV (see Chapter 12) and is used for evaluating mitral stenosis by the pressure half-time method (see Chapter 7) and (b) pulmonary vein flow, used in the evaluation of LV diastolic function and severity of mitral insufficiency (see Chapter 7).

For the transgastric views, the probe is withdrawn and anteflexed from the mid-papillary short-axis view, as necessary, to bring the mitral valve clearly into view (see Figure 5–10). The image then corresponds to the anatomic orientation shown in Figure 5–17A, with the posteromedial commissure in the upper left of the display and the anterolateral commissure to the lower right.

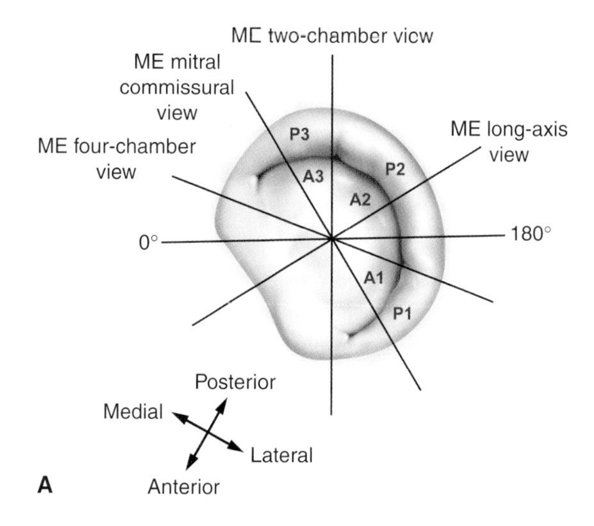

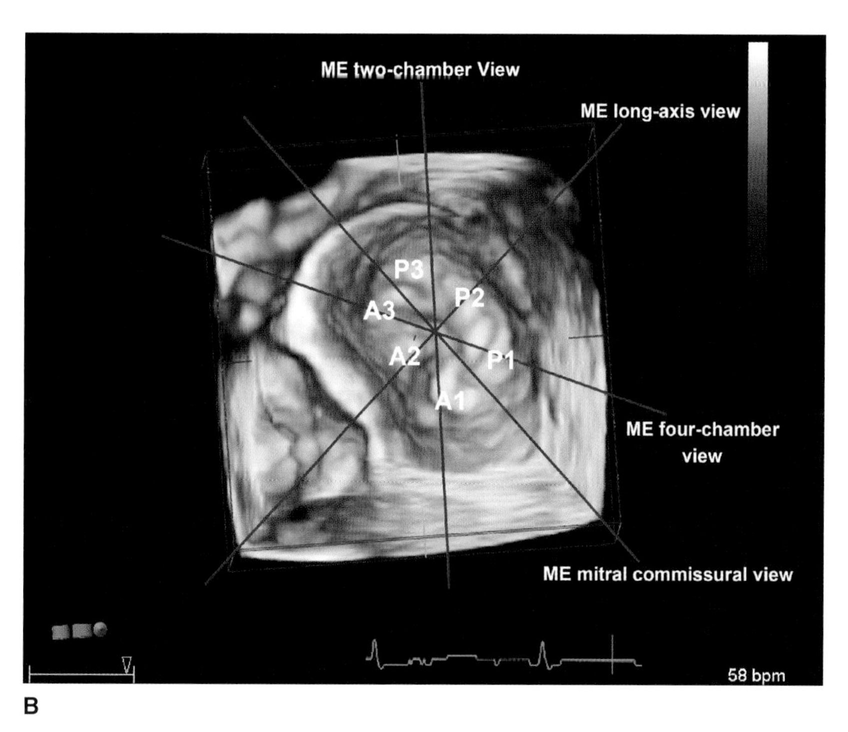

FIGURE 5–17. **A:** Anatomy of the mitral valve. The three scallops of the posterior mitral leaflet (P1, P2, and P3) and their corresponding anterior segments (A1, A2, and A3) are shown schematically **(A)** and in a 3D image **(B)**, illustrating how the valve is transected by the midesophageal (ME) views. **C:** Three-dimensional view of the mitral valve from the atrial perspective with the image rotated to match the surgeon's orientation to the mitral valve while standing on the patient's right side. The relationship of the mitral and aortic valves (AOV) is also seen in this image, with the anterior portion of the mitral annulus in continuity with the aortic annulus. *(**A** modified with permission from Shanewise JS, Cheung AT, Aronson S, et al. ASE/SCA guidelines for performing a comprehensive intraoperative multiplane transesophageal echocardiography examination: recommendations of the American Society of Echocardiography Council for Intraoperative Echocardiography and the Society of Cardiovascular Anesthesiologists Task Force for Certification in Perioperative Transesophageal Echocardiography. Anesth Analg. 1999;89:870.)*

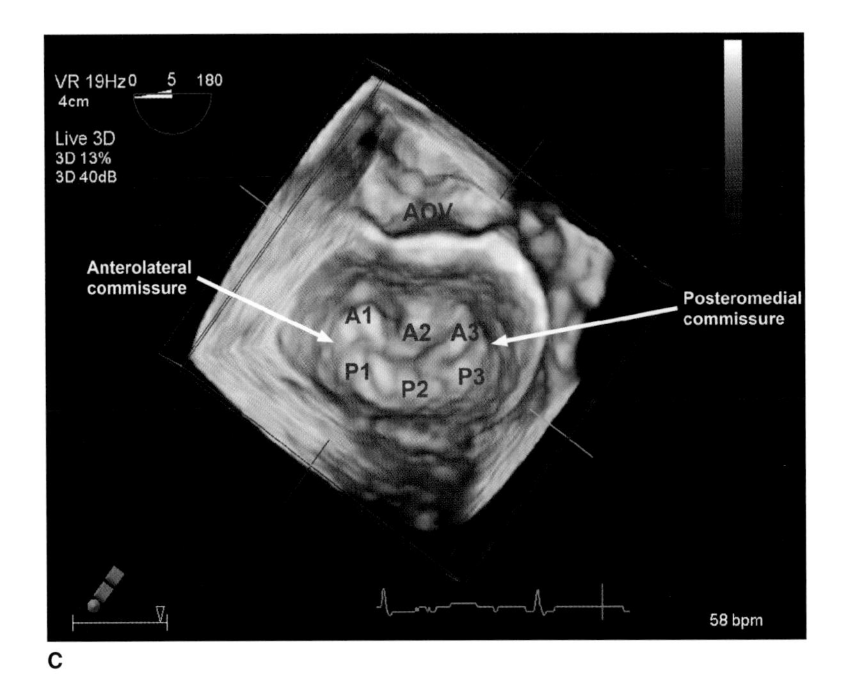

C

FIGURE 5–17. *(Continued)*

This imaging plane (Figure 5–10) sometimes can be helpful with color-flow Doppler to find the origin of a regurgitant jet. The transgastric two-chamber view is often very good for displaying the papillary muscles and chordae tendineae (subvalvular apparatus). The chordae to the posteromedial papillary muscle are seen at the top of the display, and those to the anteromedial papillary muscle are at the bottom.

Real-time 3D TEE is increasingly being adopted for the routine evaluation of the mitral valve. Several methods exist for acquiring 3D image sets with the current technology—live 3D, 3D zoom, 2D full volume, and 3D color full volume (see Chapter 24). The 3D zoom function is most commonly used to rapidly acquire the so-called *en face* or "surgeon's" view that displays the anterior mitral leaflet above with posterior leaflet below and the aortic valve at about 12 o'clock (see Figure 5–17C). Once acquired, the mitral valve can be viewed from the left atrium or be easily manipulated to view the ventricular surface. Although it requires greater processing time, information from a full-volume acquisition is valuable since it provides greater resolution and a larger field of view, providing a more detailed image of the subvalvular apparatus. It should be noted that routine 3D imaging will render obsolete the 2D categorization of mitral leaflets as defined in the preceding paragraphs.

AORTIC VALVE, AORTIC ROOT, AND LEFT VENTRICULAR OUTFLOW TRACT

- Views
  - Midesophageal aortic short and long axis
  - Transgastric long axis and deep transgastric long axis
- Assessment
  - Valve and annular morphology
  - LVOT, annular, sinotubular junction, and aortic root dimensions
  - Stenosis: valvular, subvalvular, supravalvular
  - Regurgitation
  - LVOT and transvalvular flow

The four views listed above allow examination of the aortic annulus, the aortic cusps, the sinuses of Valsalva, the sinotubular junction, the origins of the right and left main coronaries, the proximal ascending aorta, and

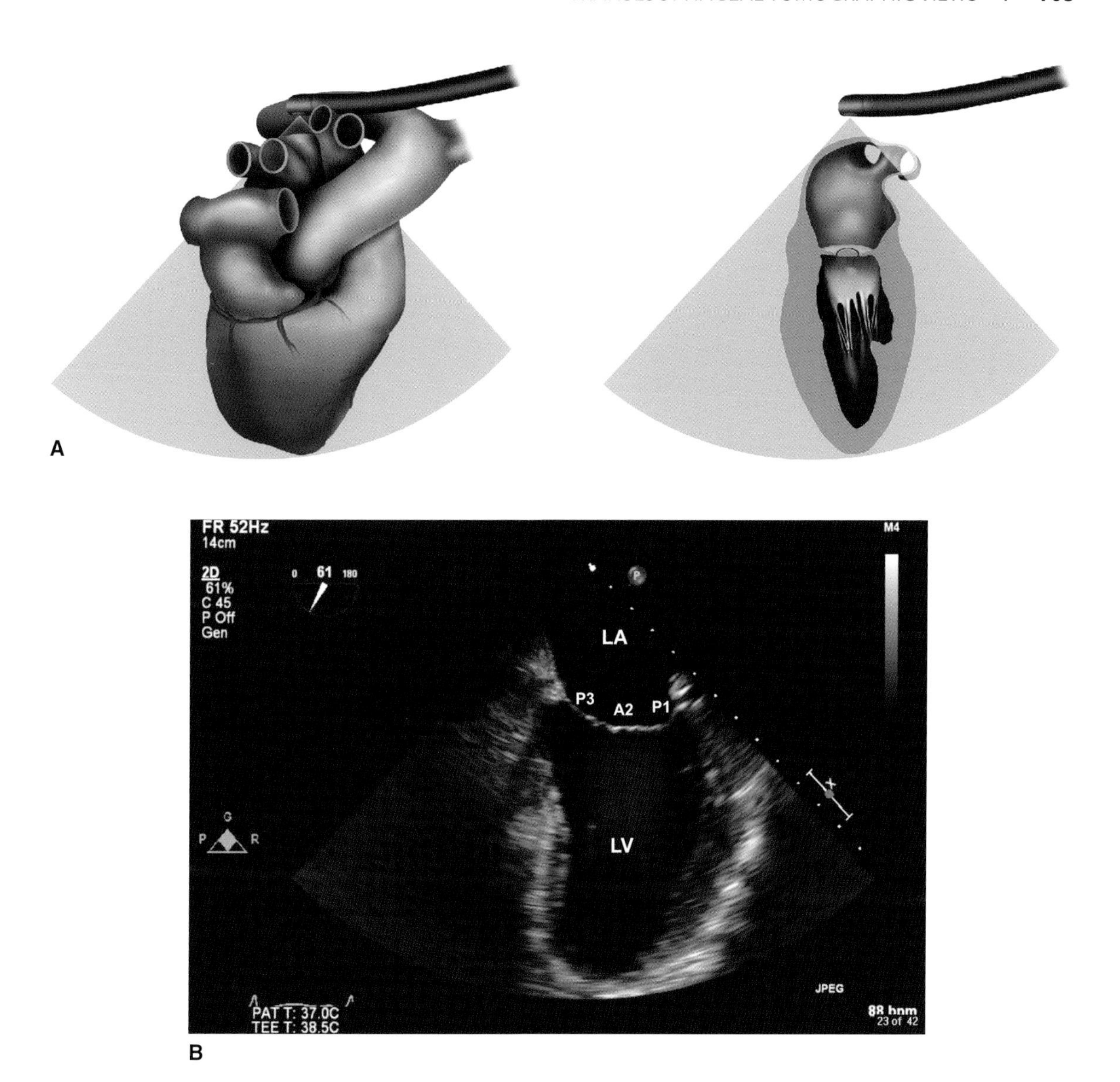

FIGURE 5–18. Anatomic **(A)** and ultrasound **(B)** illustration of the imaging plane as it cuts through the heart for the midesophageal mitral commissural view. In this view, P3 is seen to the left of the display, P1 to the right of the display, and A2 appears in between. (LA, left atrium; LV, left ventricle.)

the LVOT. The LVOT is of particular interest for the occasional subvalvular membrane mimicking true aortic valve stenosis, for ventricular septal defects, and for the detection of outflow tract obstruction that may occur with LV septal hypertrophy (e.g. hypertrophic obstructive cardiomyopathy; see Chapter 14) or after mitral valve repair (systolic anterior motion).

The midesophageal aortic valve short-axis view is obtained by placing the aortic valve in the center of the screen, usually with a depth of field of 10 to 12 cm, and then rotating the angle forward to 30° to 60° to display the three cusps of the aortic valve as the "Mercedes-Benz" sign (Figure 5–19). Minimal anteflexion also may be necessary to optimize the view. The noncoronary, right and left cusps should be specifically identified (see Figure 5–19); the thickness and mobility of the leaflets should be noted, and the addition of color will reveal the origin of regurgitant jets. This view is also used to measure the

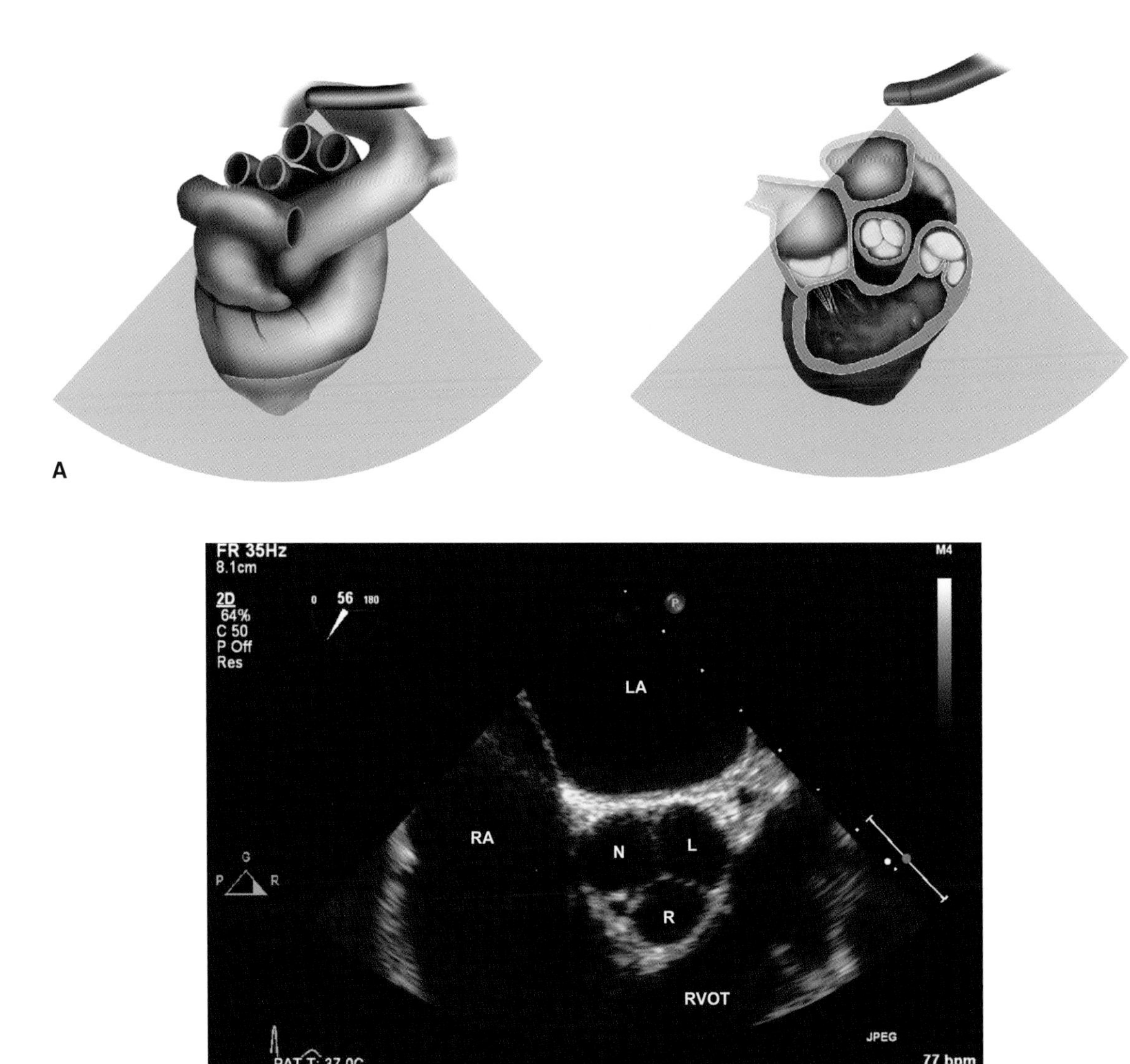

FIGURE 5–19. Anatomic **(A)** and ultrasound **(B)** illustration of the imaging plane as it cuts through the heart for the aortic valve short-axis view. (RA, right atrium; LA, left atrium; RVOT, right ventricular outflow tract; L, left coronary cusp; N, noncoronary cusp; R, right coronary cusp.)

valve orifice by planimetry. Forward rotation of the angle from this point to about 120° brings the midesophageal aortic valve long-axis plane into view. However, to carefully examine the aortic valve in the long axis, the depth of field should be adjusted to 10 to 12 cm, and the angle may need to be rotated forward to 120° to 160° to visualize as much of the LVOT, aortic valve, and ascending aorta as possible (Figure 5–20). This imaging plane permits further assessment of leaflet mobility and morphology as well as measurement of the sinotubular junction, proximal ascending aorta, LVOT, and aortic valve annulus, identified as the points of attachment of the valve cusps to the aortic wall. The aortic valve cusp at the bottom of the display is the right coronary cusp, but the other cusp can be the left or noncoronary cusp, depending on the imaging plane. Aortic regurgitation is best assessed with color-flow Doppler from this view. The transgastric long-axis view is developed from the

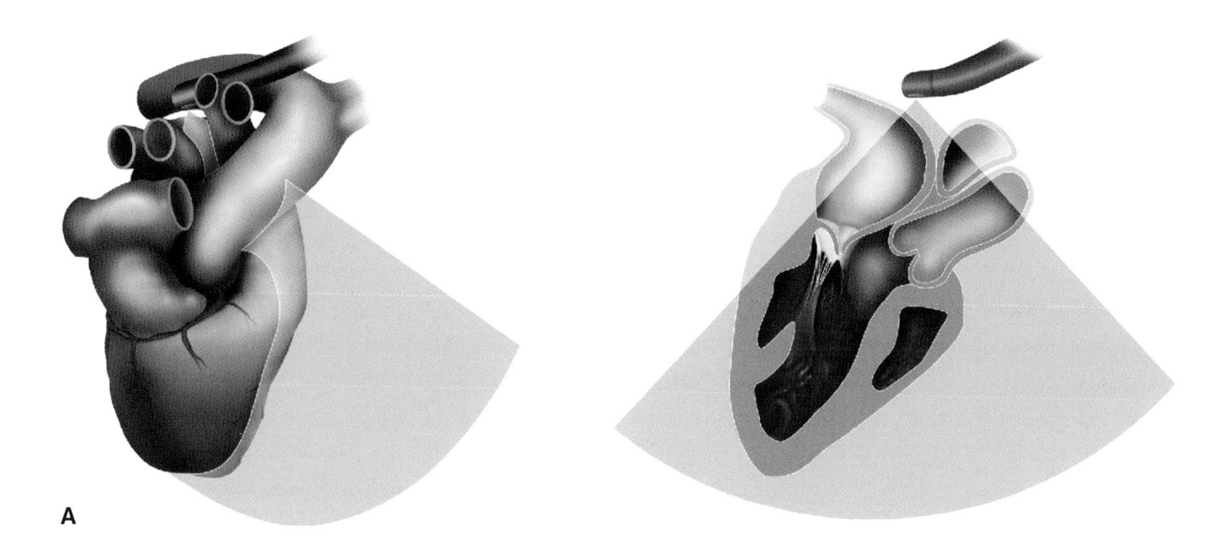

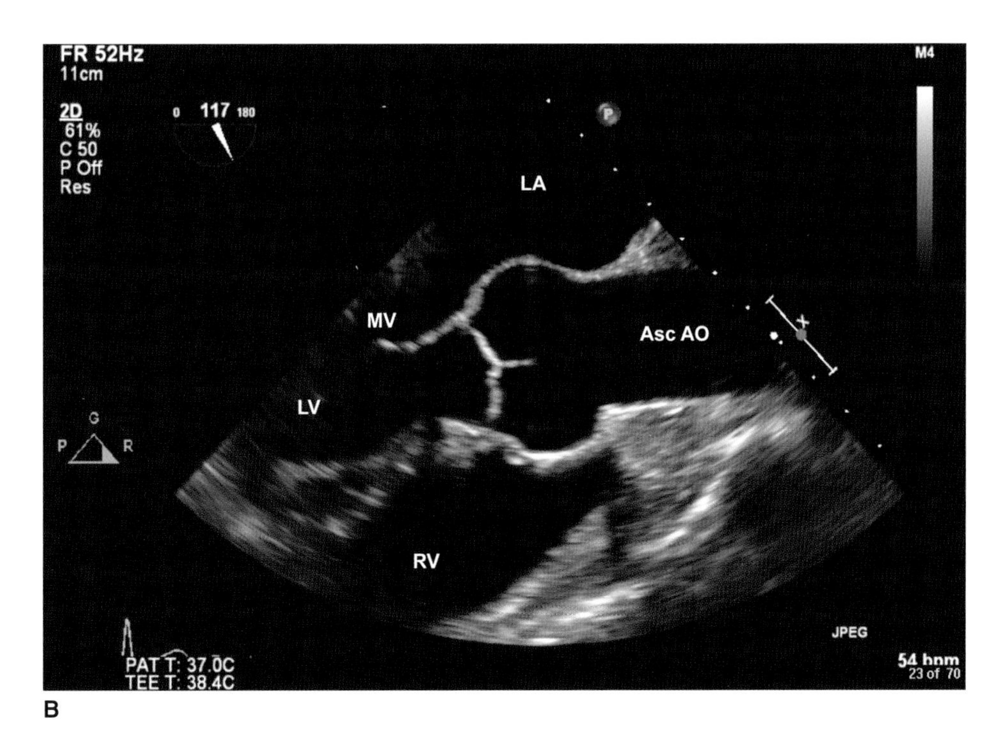

FIGURE 5–20. Anatomic **(A)** and ultrasound **(B)** illustration of the imaging plane as it cuts through the heart for the aortic valve long-axis view. The aortic valve cusp at the bottom of the display is the right coronary cusp, but the other cusp may be the left or noncoronary cusp, depending on the imaging plane. (LA, left atrium; LV, = left ventricle; RV, right ventricle; MV, mitral valve; Asc Ao, ascending aorta.)

transgastric short-axis view by rotating the angle forward to 90° to 120° and often turning the probe slightly to the right (Figure 5–21). To obtain the deep transgastric view, the tip of the TEE probe first must be advanced deep into the stomach and positioned adjacent to the LV apex. At this point, the probe is anteflexed and slowly withdrawn until contact with the stomach is again achieved, thus creating an imaging plane originating at the apex (Figure 5–22). Occasionally, lateral flexion of the probe tip to the left can be helpful. The transgastric long-axis and deep transgastric long-axis views put the aortic valve in the far field, so these views are not helpful for closely assessing valve anatomy. However, if a prosthetic mitral valve casts an acoustic shadow on the aortic valve in the midesophageal window, then these views will minimize the effect of shadowing and permit at least a cursory color-flow Doppler examination of the aortic valve. However, the real value of these views is for measuring the blood flow velocity through the LVOT and the aortic valve with pulsed- or continuous-wave Doppler, because the blood flow stream is better aligned (more parallel) with the Doppler beam (Figure 5–23).

LEFT ATRIUM, LEFT ATRIAL APPENDAGE, PULMONARY VEINS, ATRIAL SEPTUM, RIGHT ATRIUM, RIGHT ATRIAL APPENDAGE, CORONARY SINUS, AND VENA CAVAE

- Views
  - Midesophageal four and two chamber
  - Bicaval
- Assessment
  - Atrial dimensions
  - Atrial masses (appendage thrombus and tumors)
  - Pulmonary venous flow
  - Atrial septal defects
  - Coronary sinus dimensions and catheter placement
  - Vena caval dimensions and catheter placement

To evaluate the left atrium, the depth of field first should be reduced to 10 cm in the midesophageal four-chamber view to enlarge the left atrium on the display screen. Advancing and withdrawing the probe allows for the complete examination of the left atrium from its superior to its inferior margins. However, because the probe is situated immediately posterior to the left atrium, the exact superior margin is often difficult to quantify.

The left atrial appendage is best examined in the midesophageal two-chamber view. It arises from the superior part of the left atrium, appearing on the right side of the display screen as a triangular structure. Imaging the appendage through additional planes and with 3D is often useful in identifying pathology (see Chapter 24). It is separated from the left superior pulmonary vein by a normal ridge of tissue that frequently has been mistaken for a mass or thrombus and is therefore popularly called the *coumadin ridge* (see Chapter 3). The left atrial appendage should be evaluated for the presence of thrombus in all patients with enlarged atria or atrial fibrillation.

The left upper pulmonary vein enters the atrium just lateral to the appendage and is identified by withdrawing slightly from the midesophageal four-chamber view and turning the probe to the left (Figure 5–24). Depending on the orientation of the heart within the mediastinum, forward rotation to 20° to 30° often will optimize the alignment of the Doppler beam with the pulmonary vein flow. To find the left lower pulmonary vein, the probe is further turned minimally to the left and advanced 1 to 2 cm. Color-flow Doppler imaging is often useful to identify the pulmonary vein flow. Returning to the superior part of the left atrium and turning the probe to the right locates the right pulmonary veins. The right upper vein will appear on the left side of the screen, entering the left atrium in an anterior-to-posterior direction. Advancing the probe 1 to 2 cm and turning slightly to the right identifies the right lower vein. Doppler examination of the pulmonary vein flow is conducted with a pulsed-wave Doppler cursor placed 1 to 2 cm into the vein (see Chapter 12). Interrogation of the left upper pulmonary vein results in an angle most parallel to vein flow and is therefore more accurate than the right upper pulmonary vein; both lower pulmonary veins enter the atrium nearly perpendicular to the Doppler beam, and are therefore least useful.

The interatrial septum should be examined in the four-chamber view by advancing and withdrawing the probe and turning it, as necessary, to see the thicker limbus regions anteriorly and posteriorly that surround the thin, central fossa ovalis. Normally, the septum bulges slightly into the right atrium because left atrial pressure is 2 to 3 mm Hg higher than the right atrial pressure. However, in volume-depleted patients on a ventilator, the septum may wave back and forth between the atria. The atrial septum should be examined for

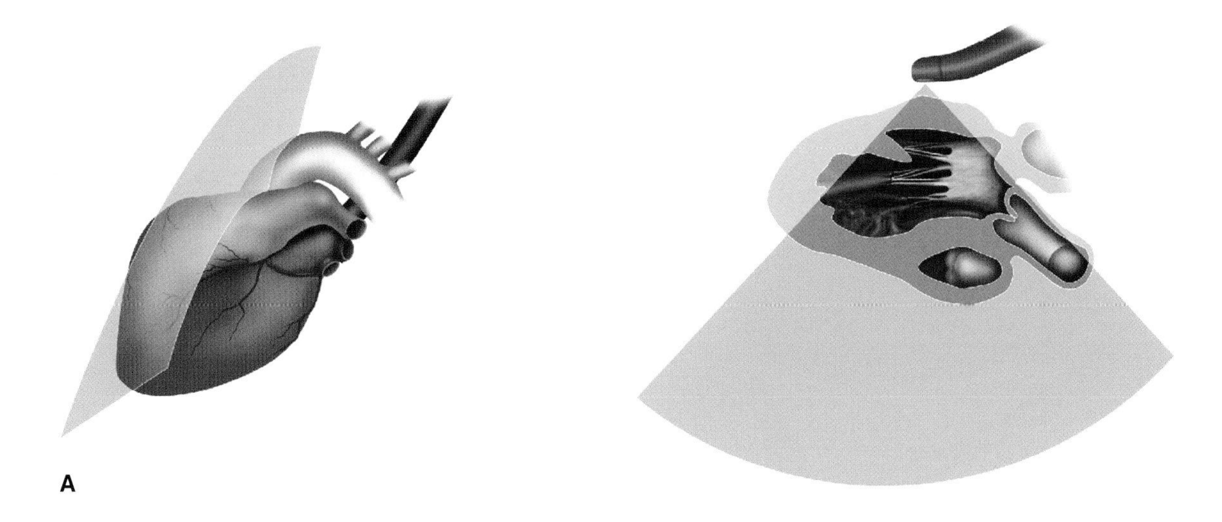

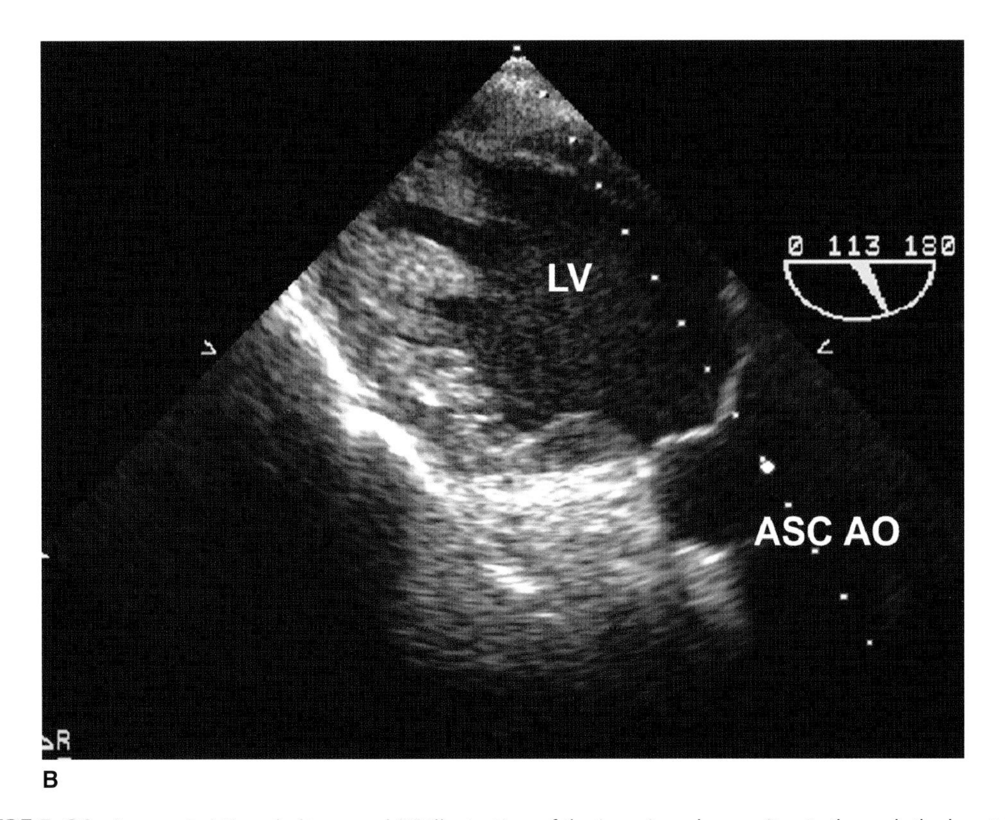

FIGURE 5–21. Anatomic **(A)** and ultrasound **(B)** illustration of the imaging plane as it cuts through the heart for the transgastric long-axis view. (LV, left ventricle; ASC AO, ascending aorta.)

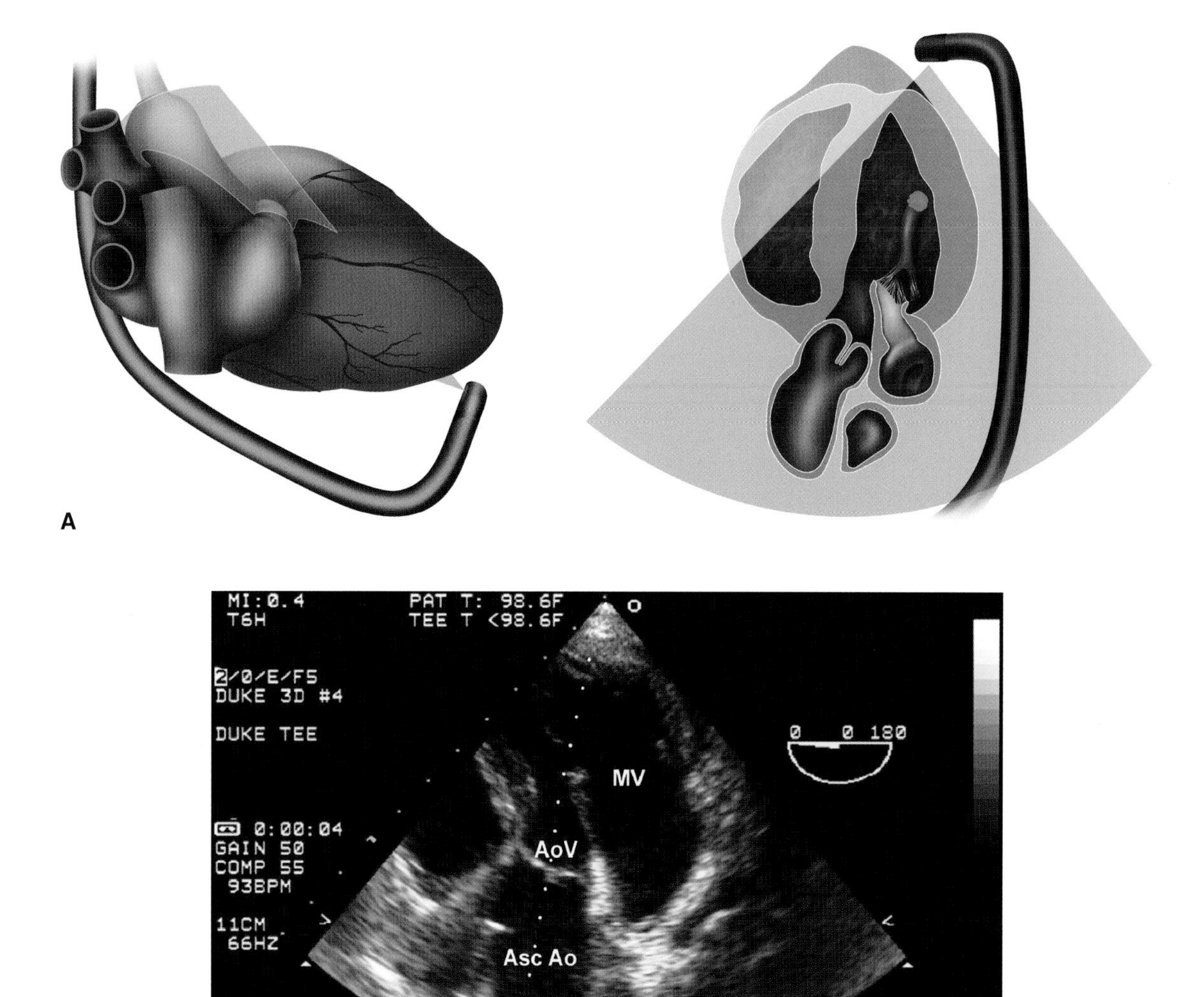

FIGURE 5–22. Anatomic **(A)** and ultrasound **(B)** illustration of the imaging plane as it cuts through the heart for the deep transgastric long-axis view. (MV, mitral valve; AoV, aortic valve; Asc Ao, ascending aorta.)

evidence of interatrial communication through a patent foramen ovale or atrial septal defect by using color-flow Doppler. Because the blood flow velocity is low between the two low-pressure atria, it is useful to turn down the Nyquist limit on the color-flow settings by reducing the scale. This technique generates more aliasing, which sometimes enables the detection of a small low-velocity jet across the interatrial septum. Reduction of the color scale to the point where all color appears aliased, however, can impair the diagnostic process. A more definitive demonstration of interatrial communication requires an injection of agitated saline solution into the right atrium at a time when the right atrial pressure is greater than the left. This is

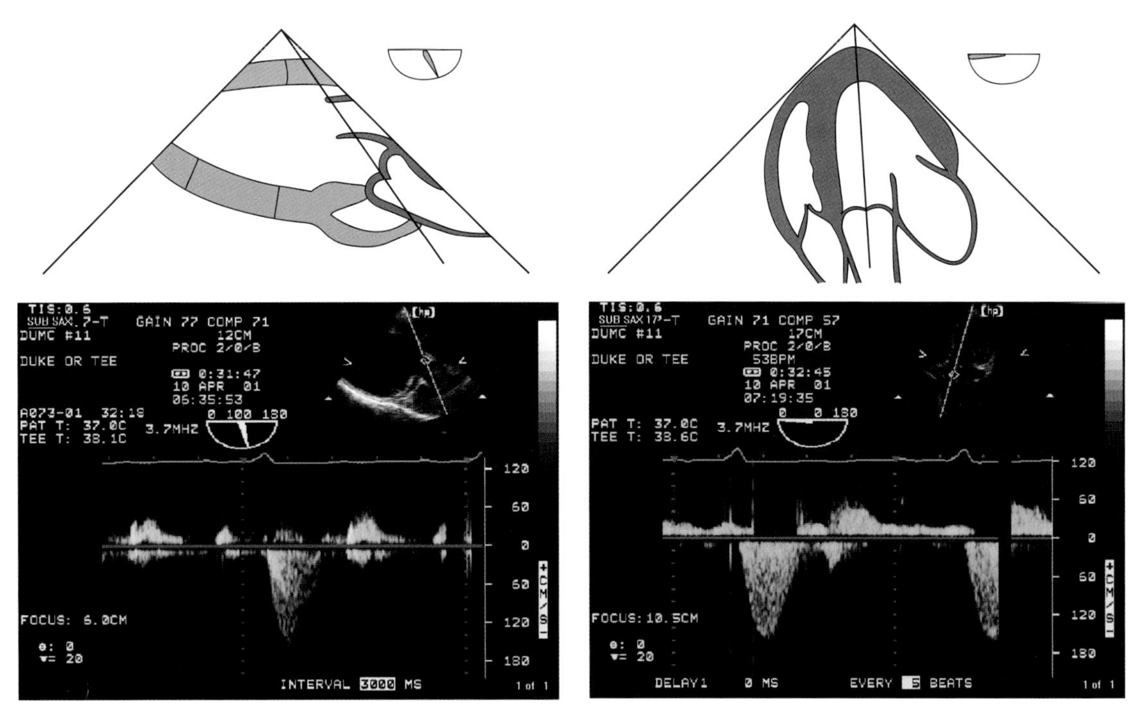

FIGURE 5–23. Transgastric and deep transgastric long-axis views demonstrate that the blood flow stream is more parallel with the Doppler beam in these views.

accomplished by using a Valsalva maneuver, which can be created in the ventilated patient by holding a positive pressure breath for 10 seconds to compromise venous return and thus lower atrial pressures. Upon abrupt release of the positive pressure, the initial filling of the right atrium will temporarily make right atrial pressure greater than left atrial pressure and create the opportunity to see agitated saline solution entering the left atrium through any interatrial communication. Timing of pressure release and saline injection must be coordinated (Valsalva is released just when the agitated saline solution enters the right atrium); if the Valsalva maneuver is successful, the interatrial septum should bow into the left atrium, thereby confirming that right atrial pressure is higher than left atrial pressure.

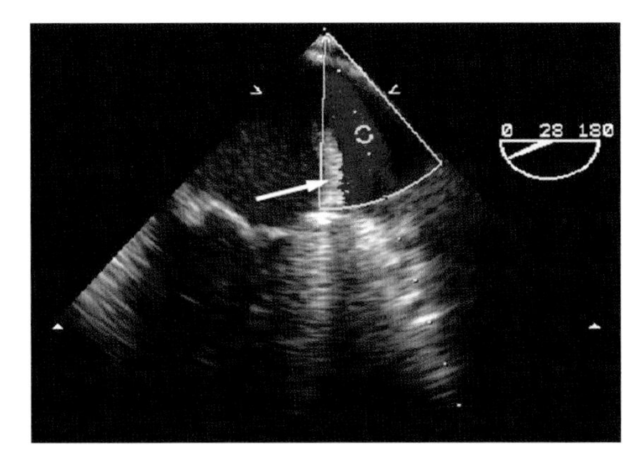

FIGURE 5–24. Color-flow Doppler demonstrating flow into the left atrium and toward the transducer in the left upper pulmonary vein. This vein enters the atrium just above the appendage and a ridge of tissue commonly referred to as the *coumadin ridge (arrow).*

Another, and often more favorable view of the interatrial septum is obtained with the bicaval view (Figure 5–25); the multiplane angle is rotated to about 90° and the probe is turned to the right until the superior vena cava comes into view at the right side of the image. The inferior vena cava (IVC) is then on the left side of the image. This view is also useful for a better view of the right superior pulmonary vein; the probe is turned slightly to the right until a large vessel is seen entering the left atrium at its superior and anterior side (approximately 4 o'clock). The bicaval view is preferred for identifying sinus venosus defects (between the superior vena cava and the left atrium) and often is the best way to see the IVC and its eustachian valve (a fold of endocardium that arises from the lower end of the

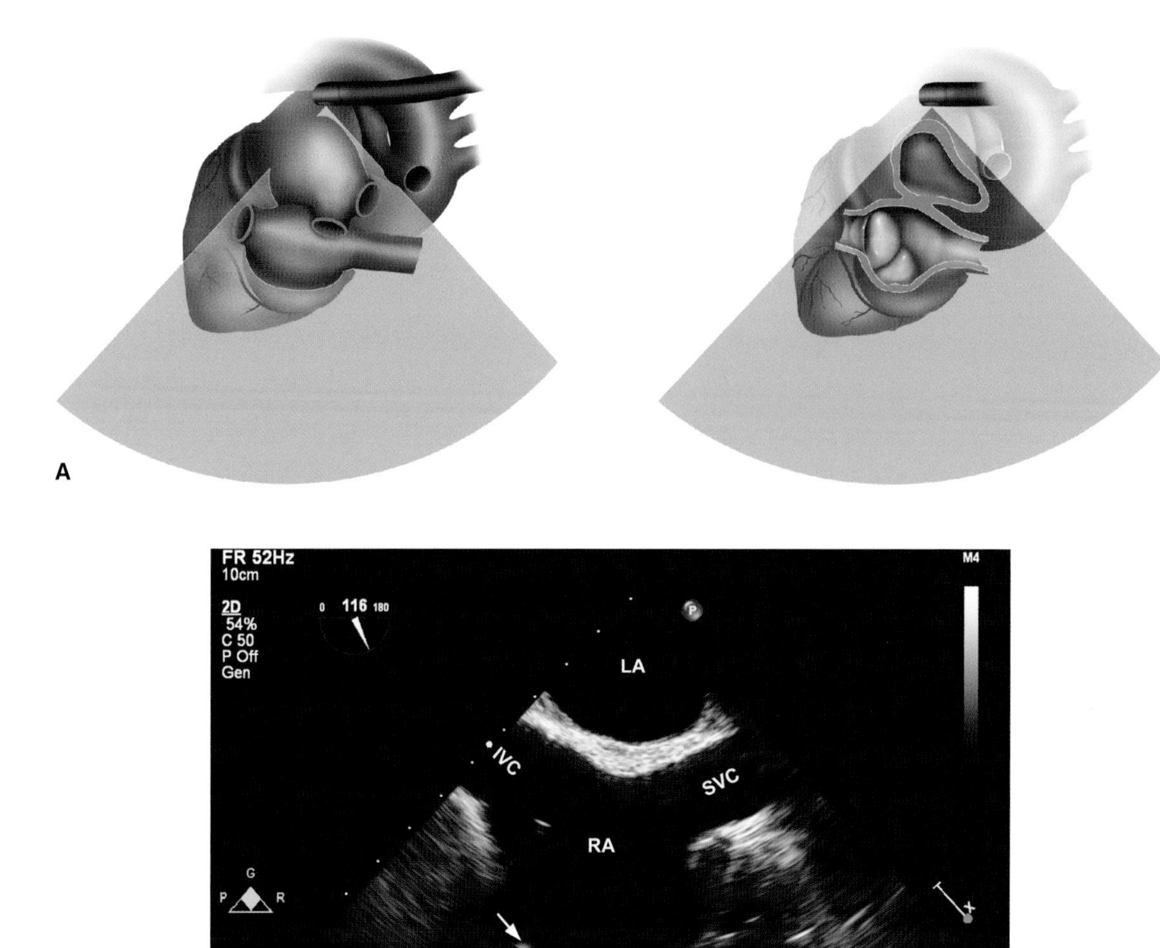

FIGURE 5–25. Anatomic **(A)** and ultrasound **(B)** illustration of the imaging plane as it cuts through the heart for the midesophageal bicaval view. Pectinate muscles *(arrow)* in the right atrial appendage can sometimes be seen in this view. (LA, left atrium; RA, right atrium; SVC, superior vena cava; IVC, inferior vena cava.)

crista terminalis and extends across the posterior margin of the IVC to merge with the border of the fossa ovalis; see Chapter 3).

The right atrium can be evaluated in the four-chamber view, but the bicaval view offers a better look at the pectinate muscles on the endocardial surface of the right atrium and the right atrial appendage, which is found at its superior and anterior border. In the inferior part of the right atrium, entering it immediately next to the IVC and the septal leaflet of the tricuspid valve is the coronary sinus. The coronary sinus can be followed, starting with the bicaval view from the right atrium medially into the left atrioventricular groove by turning the probe leftward and rotating the multiplane angle forward to 110° to 130° (Figure 5–26A). Rotating back to a two-chamber view presents the coronary sinus on the left side of the display screen, appearing as a vessel in cross section between the left atrium and the LV (see Figure 5–26B). The coronary sinus also can be seen in long axis by withdrawing the probe slightly from a transgastric basal short-axis view (see Figure 5–26C).

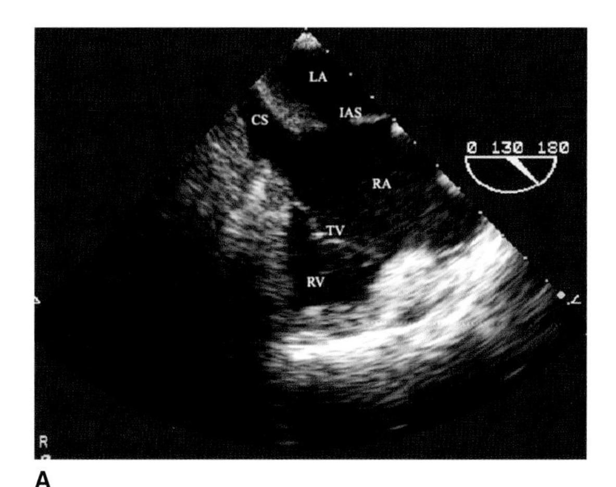

A

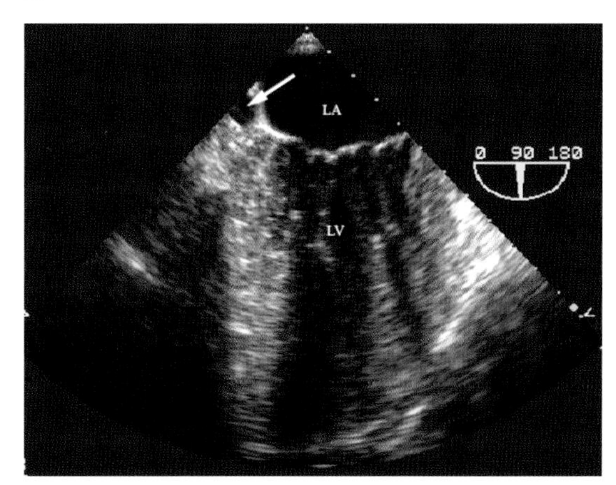

B

C

FIGURE 5–26. Imaging of the coronary sinus *(arrow)* in three different planes. (CS, coronary sinus; IAS, interatrial septum; LA, left atrium; LV, left ventricle; RA, right atrium; RV, right ventricle; TV, tricuspid valve.)

RIGHT VENTRICLE

- Views
  - Midesophageal four chamber and RV inflow and outflow
  - Transgastric basal short axis and RV inflow
- Assessment
  - Contractility (fractional area change)
  - Wall motion (subjective)
  - Chamber dimensions (enlargement and hypertrophy)
  - Masses and catheters

The right-side structures are farthest from the esophageal transducer, and their definition usually is not as good as for the left-side structures. The RV is first evaluated by turning to the right from the midesophageal four-chamber view until the tricuspid valve (TV) appears in the center of the screen. In this view, the basal and apical anterior free wall is seen with the septal leaflet of the TV on the right of the display and the posterior (usually) leaflet on the left. Because the RV is not symmetrical, estimation of chamber size and regional contractility is often difficult. One method to assess RV function examines the junction of the posterior leaflet and the RV free wall. This point of attachment of the leaflet appears to move anteriorly toward the apex of the heart during systole, a dimension (tricuspid annular plane systolic excursion) that shortens during systole and therefore can be used as an index of RV contractility. The RV typically appears as two-thirds the size of the LV, and an increase in this proportion with more of the apex including the RV is indicative of chamber enlargement. The RV free wall is also much thinner than the LV free wall, normally being thinner than 5 mm in diastole.

From the midesophageal four-chamber view, the multiplane angle is rotated forward to 60° to 90° to develop the midesophageal view of RV inflow and outflow (Figure 5–27). On this image, the RV outflow tract (RVOT) can be evaluated on the right side of the image display, and the inferior portion of the RV free wall is visible to the left. Another good view of the RV is obtained with the transgastric midpapillary short-axis view, where the RV appears as a crescent on the left side of the image (see Figure 5–11). A more circular-appearing RV is indicative of chamber enlargement. Rotating the multiplane angle to about 100° and turning the probe slightly to the right produces the final imaging plane used to evaluate the RV: the transgastric RV inflow view (Figure 5–28). This is roughly a long-axis view of the RV, with the inferior portion of the RV free wall visible at the top (near field) of the display.

TRICUSPID VALVE

- Views
  - Midesophageal four chamber and RV inflow and outflow
  - Transgastric RV inflow
- Assessment
  - Valve and annular morphology
  - Stenosis
  - Regurgitation
  - Tricuspid inflow
  - Hepatic vein flow

The TV is constituted by the right atrial and ventricular walls, chordae tendineae, papillary muscles, annulus, and three leaflets (anterior, posterior, and septal). Evaluation of the TV includes the midesophageal four-chamber view, with the TV positioned at the center of the display screen, where the septal leaflet is visible to the right of the display and the posterior or anterior (depending on the depth of the probe) leaflet is seen on the left. In the midesophageal view of RV inflow and outflow, the anterior leaflet is seen on the right and the posterior leaflet is visible on the left. Either of these views may be used to obtain a pulsed Doppler flow profile through the TV for the diagnosis of TV stenosis and RV diastolic function. Occasionally, the color jet of tricuspid regurgitation aligns with the Doppler beam best when examined from a modified midesophageal bicaval view (see Figure 5–26A). Continuous-wave Doppler assessment of tricuspid regurgitant flow is frequently used to estimate pulmonary artery pressures (see Chapter 4). The transgastric RV inflow view provides the best view of the subvalvular structures (see Figure 5–28). In this view, the posterior leaflet of the tricuspid valve is visualized in the near field, attached to the inferior wall, while the anterior leaflet is located in the far field, attached to the anterior wall of the right ventricle. Withdrawing the probe from the transgastric RV inflow view so that the TV annulus is in the center of the display and rotating the multiplane angle back to approximately 30° provide a cross section through the TV such that the anterior leaflet is to the left in the far field, the posterior leaflet is to the left in the near field, and the septal leaflet is to the right of the display screen. Each of these views should be examined with and without color to relate any abnormal flow jets to particular morphologic abnormalities. As with the mitral valve, the color-flow Doppler sector must include the right atrial portion to assess the regurgitant jet and the RV aspect of the valve to assess flow convergence.

Hepatic vein flow also should be interrogated with pulsed Doppler when assessing tricuspid regurgitation and RV diastolic function (see Chapter 12). The hepatic veins join the intrahepatic IVC tangentially and can be visualized by advancing and turning the TEE probe rightward from the midesophageal bicaval acoustic window.

PULMONARY VALVE AND PULMONARY ARTERY

- Views
  - Upper esophageal aortic arch short axis
  - Midesophageal RV inflow and outflow, and aortic valve short axis
  - Deep transgastric long axis
- Assessment
  - Valve and annular morphologies
  - Stenosis
  - Regurgitation
  - Pulmonary artery dimensions and embolus

In the midesophageal view of RV inflow and outflow, the pulmonary valve and the RVOT are on the right side of the image (Figure 5–29). Although it is difficult to discern the various leaflets of the pulmonary

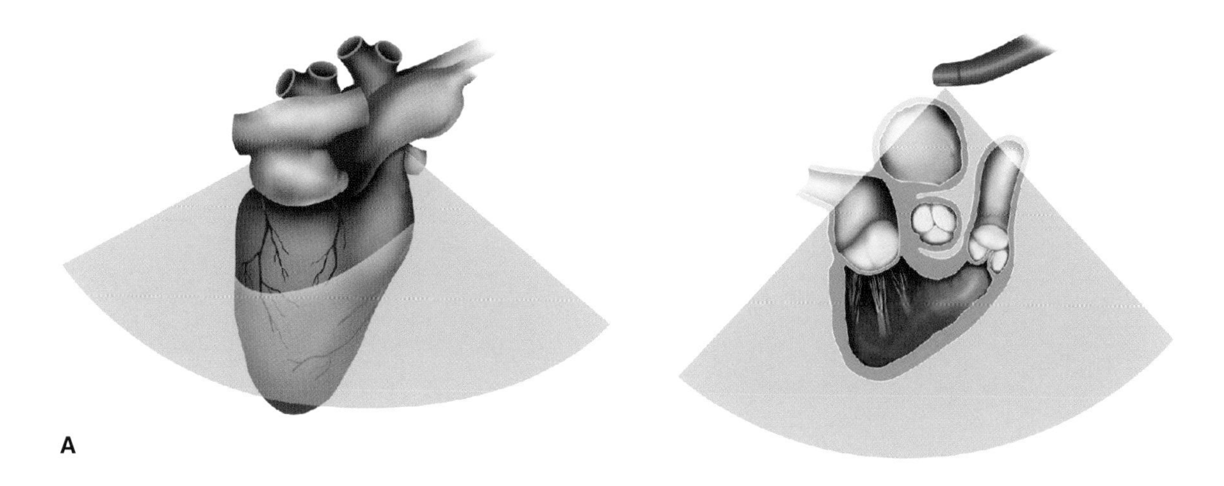

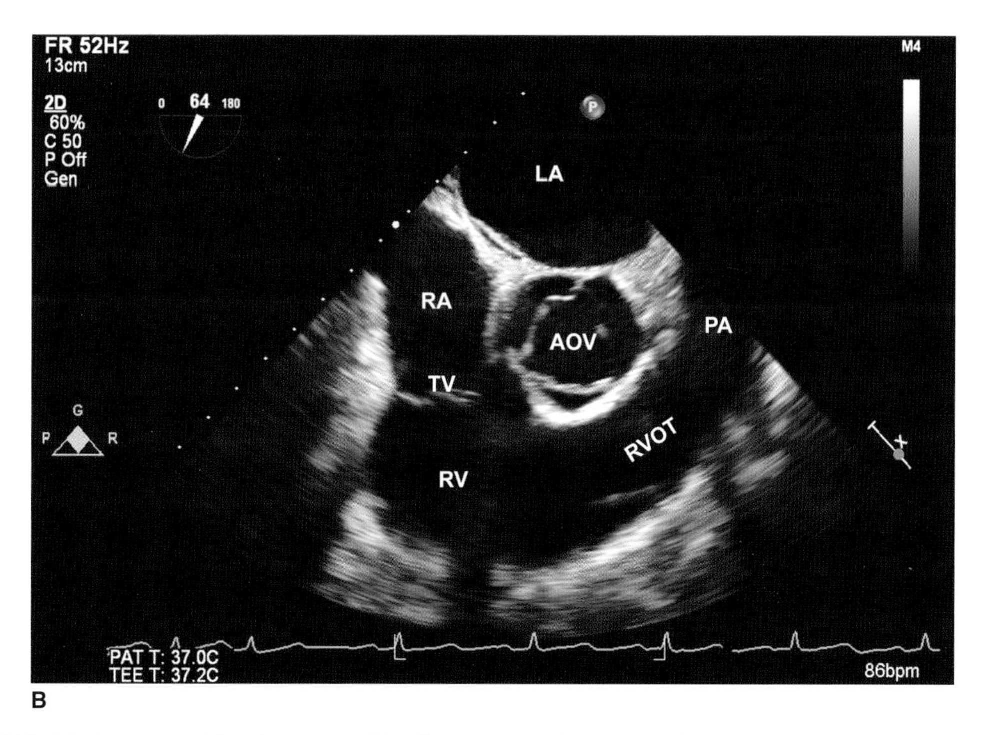

FIGURE 5–27. Anatomic **(A)** and ultrasound **(B)** illustration of the imaging plane as it cuts through the heart for the midesophageal right ventricular inflow-outflow view. (RA, right atrium; TV, tricuspid valve; RV, right ventricle; RVOT, right ventricular outflow tract; PA, pulmonary artery; AOV, aortic valve; LA, left atrium.)

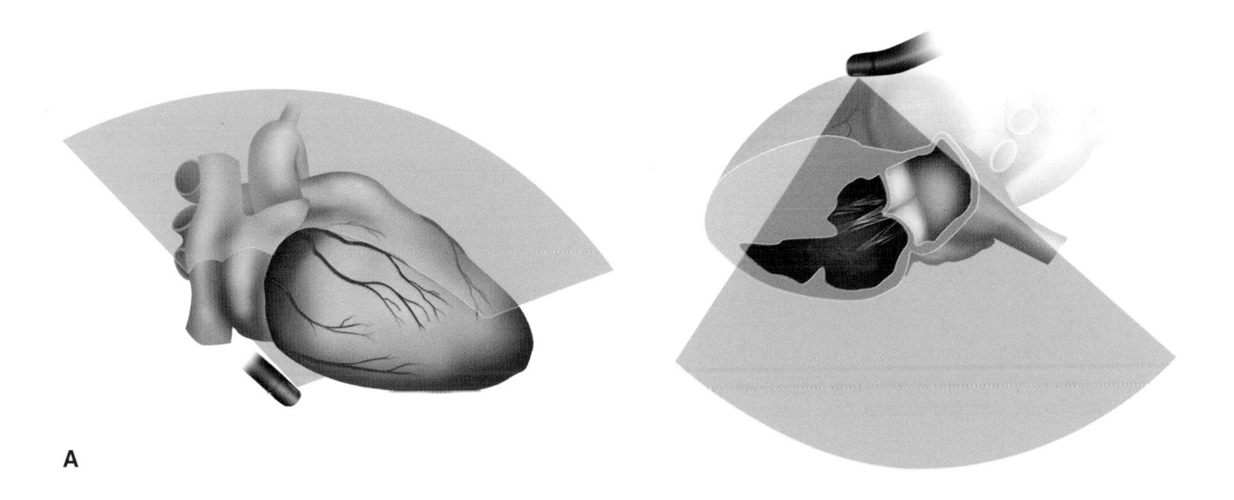

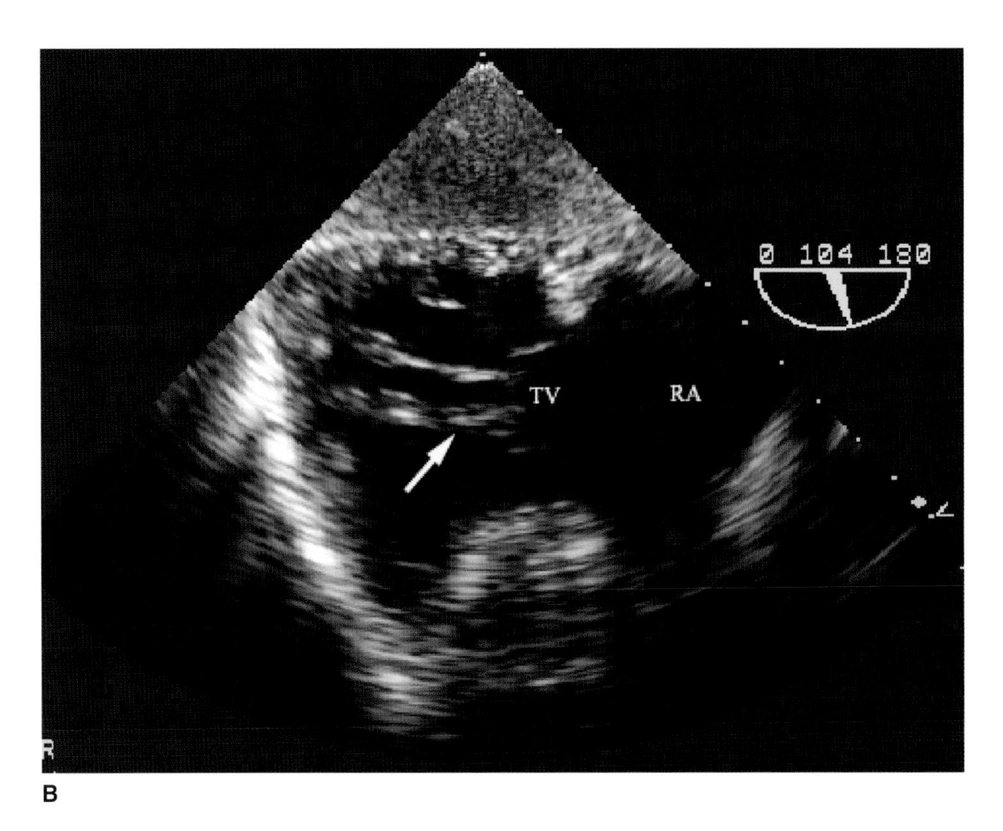

FIGURE 5–28. Anatomic **(A)** and ultrasound **(B)** illustration of the imaging plane as it cuts through the heart for the transgastric right ventricular inflow view. The inferior portion of the right ventricular free wall is seen at the top of the display. This is also an excellent view to evaluate the subvalvular structures *(arrow)* of the tricuspid valve. (RA, right atrium, TV, tricuspid valve.)

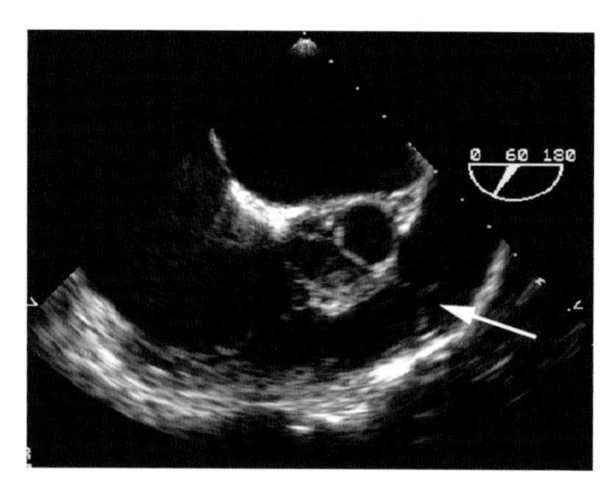

FIGURE 5–29. Midesophageal view of right ventricular inflow and outflow demonstrating the pulmonary valve *(arrow)*.

valve, seen now in long axis, this imaging plane is useful for detecting pulmonary regurgitation with color-flow Doppler. In this view, one may also see the pulmonary artery catheter as it passes through the RV into the main pulmonary artery. Rotating the multiplane angle back to about 30° from the midesophageal view of RV inflow and outflow obtains the atrioventricular short-axis view, where the pulmonary valve appears in short axis just to the right and below the aortic valve but is not clearly visualized. It may be necessary to anteflex or withdraw the probe slightly to identify the pulmonary valve leaflets. Rotating back to 0° and withdrawing the probe further will follow the main pulmonary artery superiorly and demonstrate the division into right and left main pulmonary arteries (Figure 5–30). The best view to image the pulmonary valve and the main pulmonary artery is often the upper esophageal aortic arch short axis. To obtain this window, the aortic arch is first imaged at 0° at a depth of 20 to 25 cm from the incisors (see below). With the aortic arch in the top center of the screen, the multiplane angle is rotated forward to 70° to 90°, producing an image where the aortic arch appears in cross section as a circle, the main pulmonary artery is usually seen just anteriorly in long axis, and the pulmonary valve is often visible in the far field (Figure 5–31). This can be an excellent view to assess stenosis or regurgitation through the pulmonary valve because the Doppler beam is aligned parallel to flow. On occasion, the RVOT also can be imaged in a deep transgastric long-axis view by turning the probe to the right.

THORACIC AORTA

- Views
  - Upper esophageal aortic arch short and long axis
  - Midesophageal ascending and descending aorta short and long axis
  - Epiaortic scanning
- Assessment
  - Atheromatous plaque
  - Calcification
  - Vessel dimensions (sinotubular junction, ascending aorta, and descending aorta)
  - Aneurysm
  - Dissection

TEE can be used to examine the proximal ascending aorta, the distal portion of the aortic arch, and the entire descending aorta. However, because of the interposition of the air-filled trachea, the distal ascending aorta and proximal arch aortic arch cannot be examined with TEE. Unfortunately, these portions of the aorta are those used most frequently for cannulation and for anastomosis of vein grafts for coronary bypass surgery. Delineation of atherosclerotic plaque and dissections in these regions therefore require epiaortic scanning (see Chapter 20).

Examination of the ascending aorta begins with a midesophageal short-axis view of the aortic valve. From this point, the probe is withdrawn to follow the aorta as far as possible (2 to 4 cm above the valve). Rotating the multiplane angle to 120° to 150° will provide the midesophageal ascending aortic long-axis view (Figure 5–32), which is useful for measuring the sinotubular and aortic root dimensions but not very useful for assessing atheromatous plaque.

The descending aorta is located by returning the multiplane angle to 0° and turning the probe leftward. The descending aorta lies just to the left of the left atrium and appears in cross section as a circle of about 2 cm in diameter in the descending aortic short-axis view (Figure 5–33). The descending aorta should be followed distally as far as possible while examining the wall for thickening and irregularity, indicating atheromatous plaque (see Figure 5–33). Descending aortic imaging is best accomplished by reducing the depth of field to 6 to 8 cm. Because the descending aorta gradually becomes more

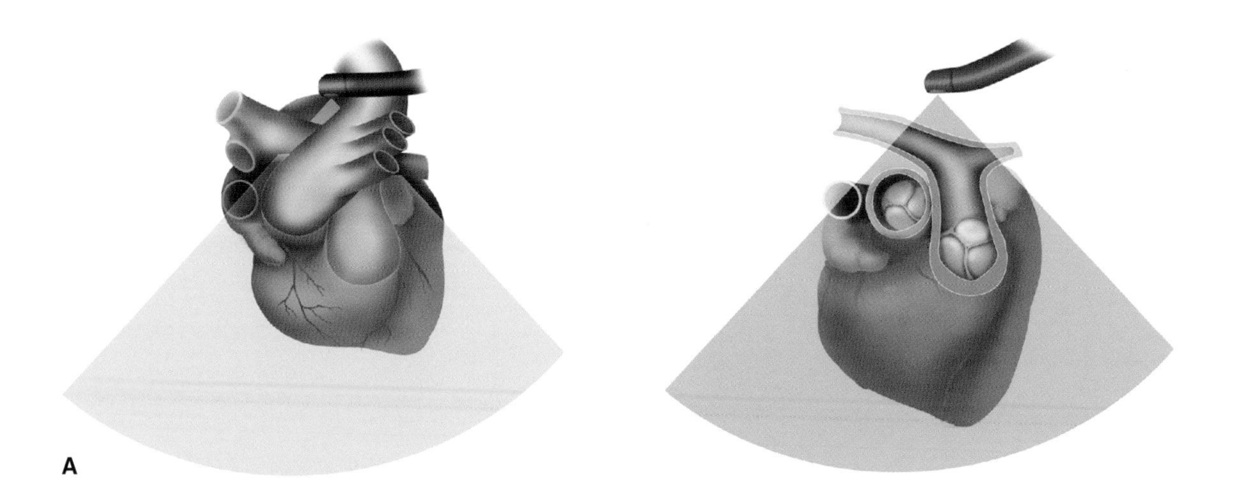

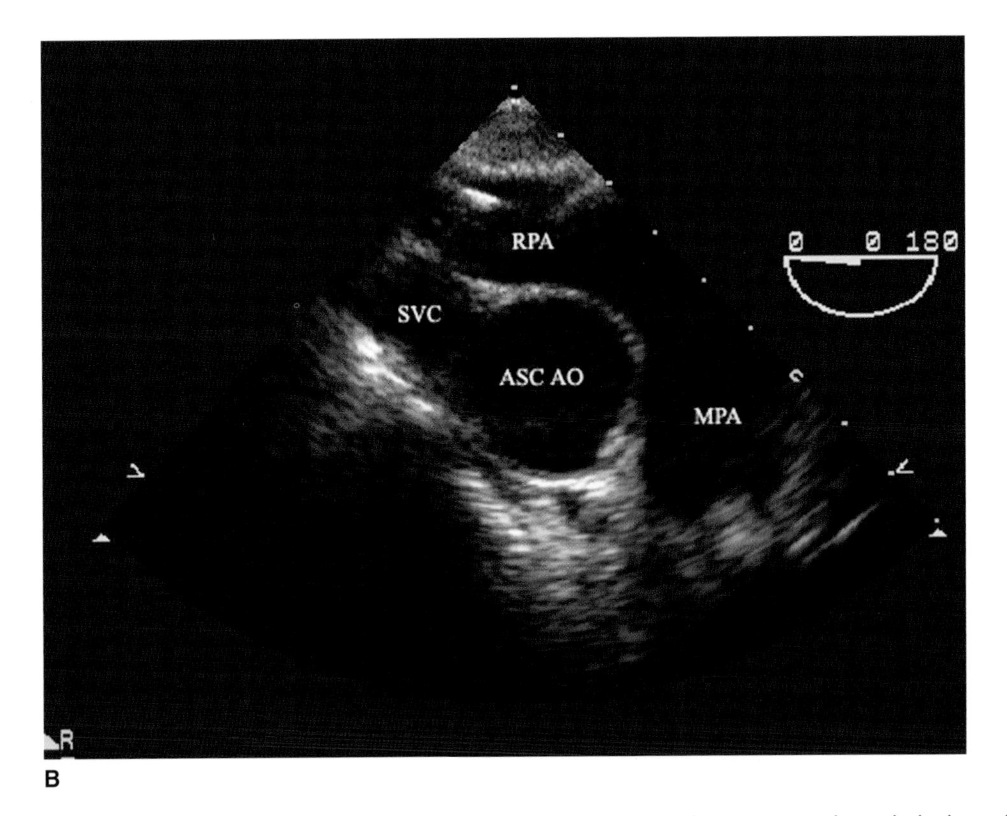

FIGURE 5–30. Anatomic **(A)** and ultrasound **(B)** illustration of the imaging plane as it cuts through the heart for the midesophageal ascending aortic short-axis view. (ASC AO, ascending aorta; MPA, main pulmonary artery; RPA, right pulmonary artery; SVC, superior vena cava.)

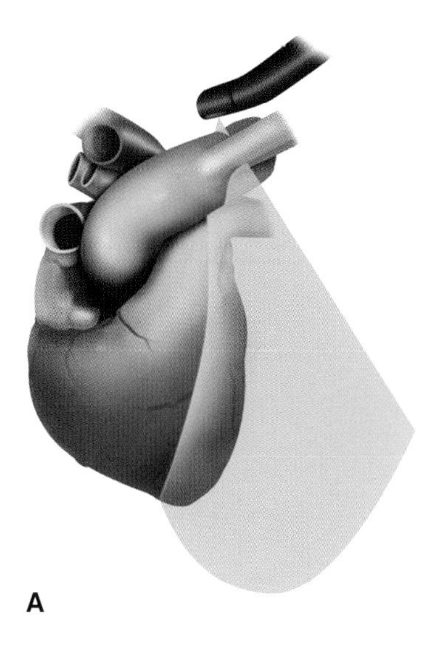
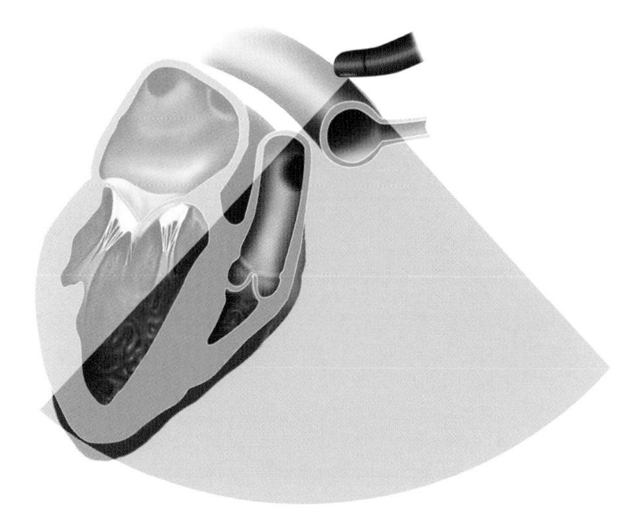
A

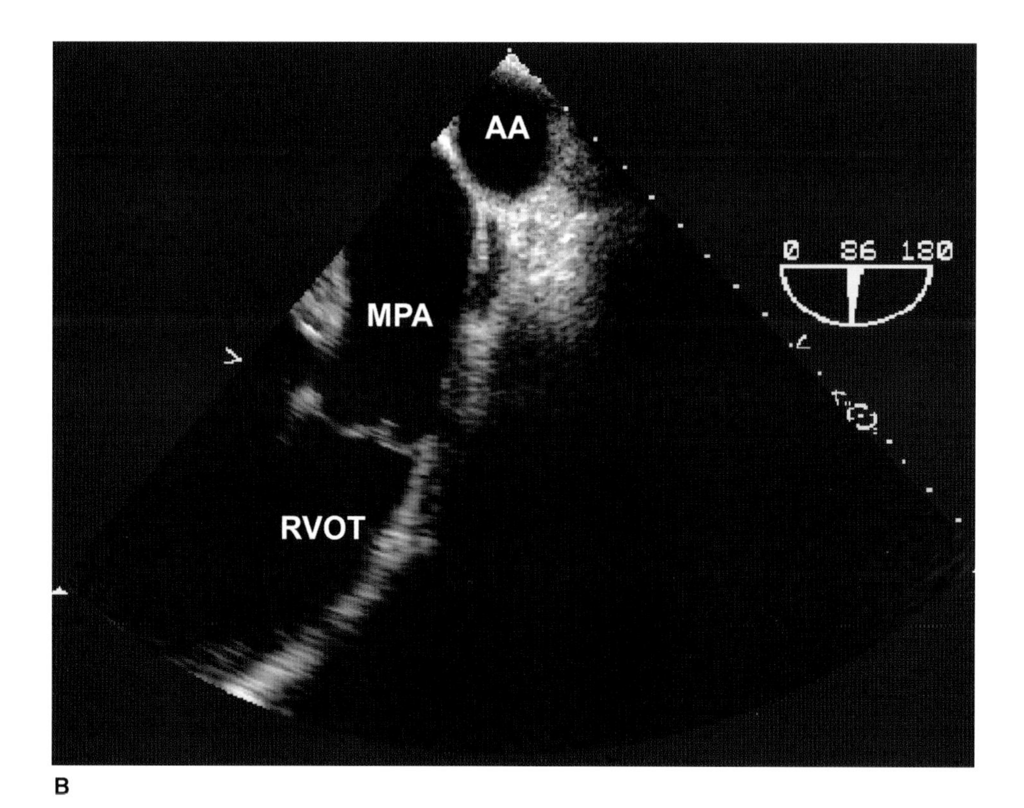

B

FIGURE 5–31. Anatomic **(A)** and ultrasound **(B)** illustration of the imaging plane as it cuts through the heart for the upper esophageal aortic arch short-axis view. (RVOT, right ventricular outflow tract; MPA, main pulmonary artery; AA, aortic arch.)

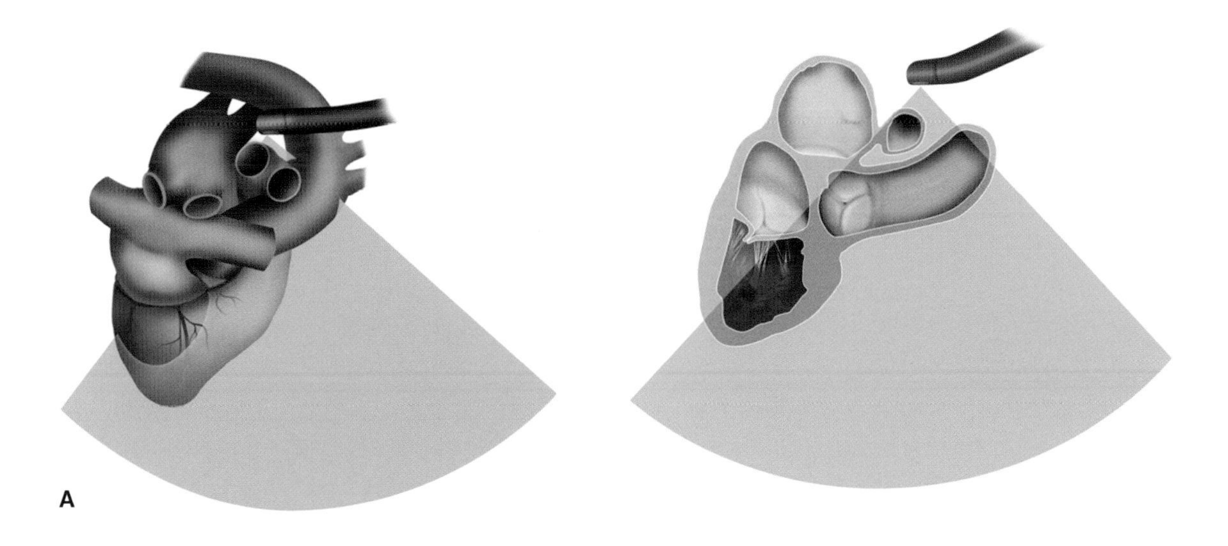

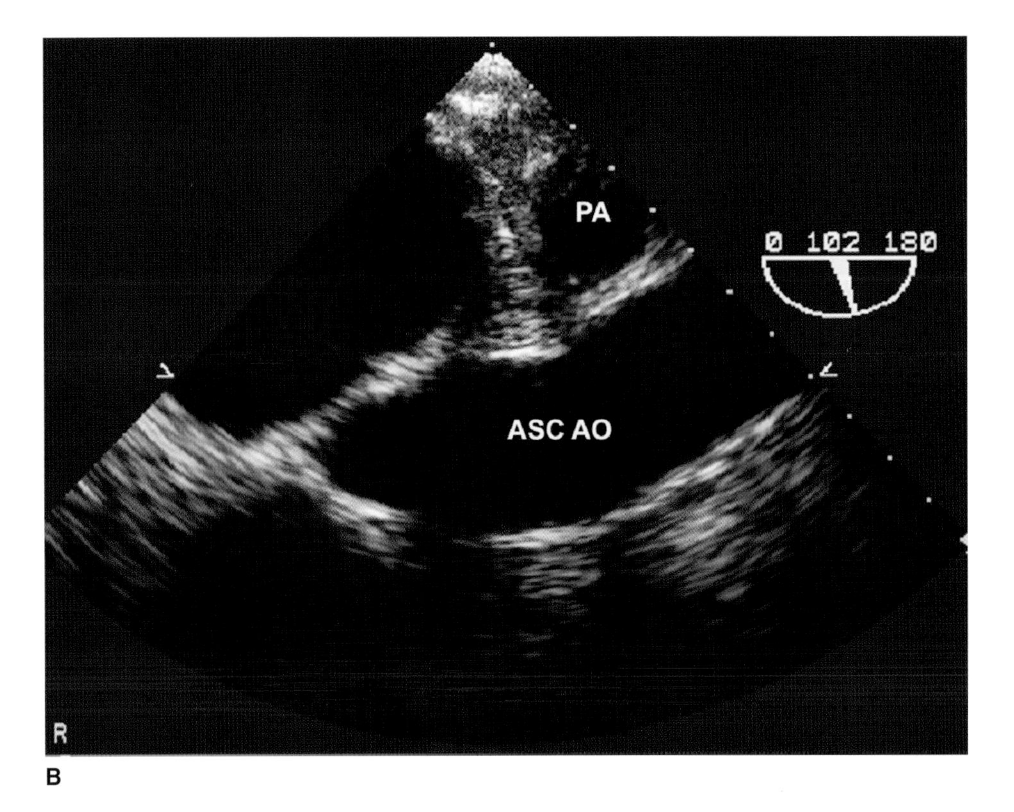

FIGURE 5–32. Anatomic **(A)** and ultrasound **(B)** illustration of the imaging plane as it cuts through the heart for the midesophageal ascending aortic long-axis view. (ASC AO, ascending aorta; PA, pulmonary artery.)

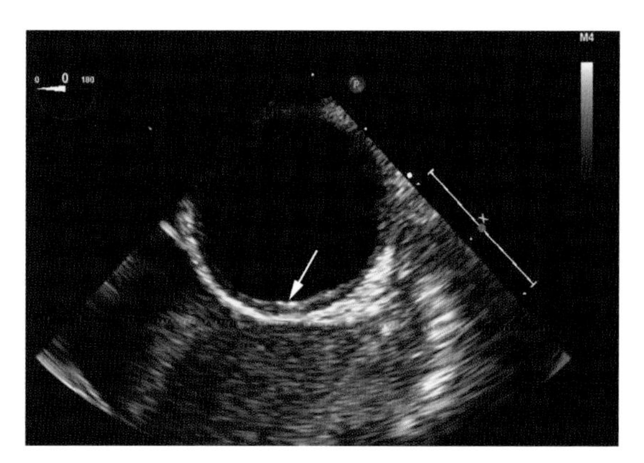

FIGURE 5–33. Descending aorta short-axis view showing an atheromatous plaque *(arrow)*.

posterior as the diaphragm is approached, only about 20 to 25 cm of descending aorta is easily seen with the TEE probe, and the abdominal aorta usually disappears from view. The location of lesions in the aorta can be described by the distance of the probe from the incisors or by relating the lesion to the level of the left atrium or left subclavian artery. At the distal limit of short-axis imaging, forward rotation of the multiplane angle to 90° generates the descending aorta long-axis view (see Figure 5–6). At this point, the probe is withdrawn toward the transition of the aorta from a tubular to a circular shape, which indicates cross-sectional imaging of the distal arch. Often, the subclavian and common carotid artery can be imaged at this transition point, a view that is particularly useful in the positioning of an intraaortic balloon pump. Rotation back to 0° generates the upper esophageal aortic arch long-axis view (Figure 5–34). Further withdrawal of the probe from the upper esophageal window can be used on occasion to image the origin of the arch vessels.

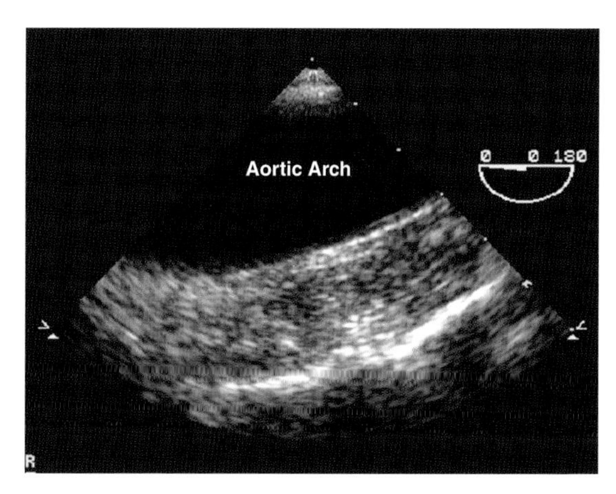

FIGURE 5–34. Upper esophageal aortic arch long-axis view.

ACKNOWLEDGMENTS

The authors gratefully acknowledge Heartworks (Inventive Medical Ltd, UK) for allowing the use of their TEE simulator as a guide for developing many of the images shown in this chapter. We would also like to acknowledge the contributions of Dr Fiona Clements from the previous edition.

REFERENCES

1. Shanewise JS, Cheung AT, Aronson S, et al. ASE/SCA guidelines for performing a comprehensive intraoperative multiplane transesophageal echocardiography examination: recommendations of the American Society of Echocardiography Council for Intraoperative Echocardiography and the Society of Cardiovascular Anesthesiologists Task Force for Certification in Perioperative Transesophageal Echocardiography. *Anesth Analg.* 1999;89(4):870-884.
2. Practice Guidelines for Perioperative Transesophageal Echocardiography. An Updated Report by the American Society of Anesthesiologists and the Society of Cardiovascular Anesthesiologists Task Force on Transesophageal Echocardiography. *Anesthesiology* 2010;112:1084-1096.
3. Na S, Kim CS, Kim JY, Cho JS, Kim KJ. Rigid laryngoscope-assisted insertion of transesophageal echocardiography probe reduces oropharyngeal mucosal injury in anesthetized patients. *Anesthesiology.* 2009;110(1):38-40.
4. Cerqueira MD, Weissman NJ, Dilsizian V, et al. Standardized myocardial segmentation and nomenclature for tomographic imaging of the heart: a statement for healthcare professionals from the Cardiac Imaging Committee of the Council on Clinical Cardiology of the American Heart Association. *Circulation.* 2002;105(4):539-542.
5. Voci P, Bilotta F, Caretta Q, Mercanti C, Marino B. Papillary muscle perfusion pattern. A hypothesis for ischemic papillary muscle dysfunction. *Circulation.* 1995;91(6):1714-1718.
6. Glenn WWL, Baue A. *Glenn's Thoracic and Cardiovascular Surgery.* 6th ed. Stamford, CT: Appleton & Lange; 1996.

REVIEW QUESTIONS

Select the *one best* answer for each item.

1. The most versatile "window" for transesophageal imaging is:
   a. Upper esophageal
   b. Midesophageal
   c. Transgastric
   d. Deep transgastric

2. The best single view for assessing adequacy of coronary perfusion is:
   a. Midesophageal four chamber

b. Deep transgastric LV long axis
c. Transgastric LV midpapillary short axis
d. Midesophageal LV long axis

3. LV segment 17 usually receives its coronary perfusion from the:
a. Posterior descending
b. Left anterior descending
c. Left circumflex
d. Obtuse marginal #1

4. The junction between the superior vena cava and the right atrium is best seen with the:
a. Midesophageal view of RV inflow and outflow
b. Midesophageal bicaval view
c. Midesophageal great vessel
d. Upper esophageal aortic arch long-axis view

5. The three segments of the anterior wall of the LV are best seen in the:
a. Midesophageal LV two-chamber view
b. Midesophageal LV long-axis view
c. Midesophageal four-chamber view
d. Deep transgastric long-axis view

6. The midesophageal "window" is normally found at approximately:
a. 25 cm from the teeth
b. 35 cm from the teeth
c. 40 cm from the teeth
d. 45 cm from the teeth

7. The best view for finding a patent foramen ovale would be:
a. View of RV inflow and outflow
b. Midesophageal four-chamber view
c. Midesophageal bicaval view
d. Midesophageal two-chamber view

8. The eustachian valve is seen best in a:
a. Midesophageal four-chamber view
b. Midesophageal view of the RV inflow and outflow tracts
c. Midesophageal bicaval view
d. Deep transgastric long-axis view

9. A foreshortened four-chamber view of the LV can be improved by:
a. Left lateral tilt of the probe tip
b. Rotation of the probe
c. Anteflexion of the probe
d. Retroflexion of the probe

10. A two-chamber view of the LV shows:
a. Anterior and inferior walls
b. Anteroseptal and posterior walls
c. Septal and lateral walls
d. Anterior and posterior walls

11. An aortic valve long-axis view would be obtained with a multiplane angle of approximately:
a. 30°
b. 70°
c. 120°
d. 150°

12. The upper esophageal window is usually found at a probe depth (from the teeth) of approximately:
a. 15 cm
b. 25 cm
c. 35 cm
d. 45 cm

13. A deep transgastric long-axis view is frequently the single best view for assessing:
a. Regional wall motion
b. Left atrial thrombus
c. Aortic valve gradient
d. Mitral valve area

14. A midesophageal short-axis view of the aortic valve shows the noncoronary cusp to be:
a. Closest to the interatrial septum
b. Most anterior
c. Closest to the RVOT
d. Toward the right side of the image

15. A midesophageal view of RV inflow and outflow tracts is obtained with a multiplane angle of approximately:
a. 20°
b. 70°
c. 110°
d. 150°

16. A midesophageal view of RV inflow and outflow tracts usually shows the aortic valve:
a. Anterior to the TV
b. Anterior to the pulmonary valve
c. Infrequently
d. In short axis

17. The left atrial appendage is located close to the:
a. Coronary sinus
b. Posteromedial commissure of the mitral valve
c. Anterolateral commissure of the mitral valve
d. Right coronary cusp of the aortic valve

18. A bicaval view usually shows the coronary sinus orifice to be:
    a. Anteromedial to the IVC orifice
    b. Posterolateral to the IVC orifice
    c. Anterior to the TV
    d. Next to the crista terminalis

19. In a transgastric basal short-axis view of the LV, the LV segment closest to the transducer is usually the:
    a. Basal inferior segment
    b. Basal inferolateral segment
    c. Basal anterolateral segment
    d. Basal inferoseptal segment

20. In a transgastric basal short-axis view of the LV, the portion of the mitral valve closest to the transducer is usually the:
    a. A2 region
    b. P1 region
    c. Anterolateral commissure
    d. Posteromedial commissure

21. In a midesophageal mitral commissural view, the portion of the mitral valve appearing closest to the coronary sinus is the:
    a. P1 region
    b. P2 region
    c. P3 region
    d. A2 region

22. In a midesophageal two-chamber view, the pulmonary vein usually seen adjacent to the left atrial appendage is the:
    a. Right upper pulmonary vein
    b. Left upper pulmonary vein
    c. Right lower pulmonary vein
    d. Left lower pulmonary vein

23. The portion of the aorta seen least well by TEE echocardiographic imaging is the:
    a. Sinotubular ridge
    b. Innominate artery take-off
    c. Left carotid take-off
    d. High descending thoracic aorta

24. A midesophageal long-axis view shows the aortic and mitral valves next to each other. The portions of these valves in closest proximity are:
    a. The posterior mitral valve leaflet and the left coronary cusp of the aortic valve
    b. The anterior mitral valve leaflet and the right coronary cusp of the aortic valve
    c. The posterior mitral valve leaflet and the non-coronary cusp of the aortic valve
    d. The anterior mitral valve leaflet and the non-coronary cusp of the aortic valve

25. A bicaval view often demonstrates the right pulmonary artery situated:
    a. Just cephalad of the left atrium and medial to the superior vena cava
    b. Just caudad of the right superior pulmonary vein
    c. Passing just anterior to the proximal superior vena cava
    d. Passing just anterior of the crista terminalis

26. The view most helpful in assessing for a sinus venosus defect is:
    a. Midesophageal four chamber
    b. Transgastric basal short axis
    c. Midesophageal bicaval
    d. Midesophageal long axis

27. A long-axis view of the coronary sinus is best acquired starting with which view?
    a. Transgastric basal short axis
    b. Midesophageal long axis
    c. Aortic valve short axis
    d. Midesophageal two chamber

28. The tricuspid valve leaflet seen on the left of the display in a right ventricular inflow-outflow view is most likely the:
    a. Septal leaflet
    b. Posterior leaflet
    c. Anterior leaflet
    d. Posterior or anterior leaflet

29. The aortic valve cusp farther from the transducer in the aortic valve long-axis view is most likely the:
    a. Septal cusp
    b. Left coronary cusp
    c. Right coronary cusp
    d. It depends on the imaging plane

30. The structure interposed between the transducer and the ascending aorta in the ascending aorta short-axis view is the:
    a. Superior vena cava
    b. Main pulmonary artery
    c. Left pulmonary artery
    d. Right pulmonary artery

31. CW Doppler interrogation of the pulmonic valve is best performed in this view:
    a. Deep transgastric long axis
    b. Midesophageal RV inflow-outflow

c. Upper esophageal aortic arch short axis
d. Transgastric RV inflow

32. If the deep transgastric view is unobtainable, this view can be used for CW Doppler of the aortic valve:
    a. Midesophageal AV short axis
    b. Midesophageal AV long axis
    c. Midesophageal bicaval
    d. Transgastric long axis

33. The mitral valve cusps most commonly seen in this imaging plane from left to right on the screen are:

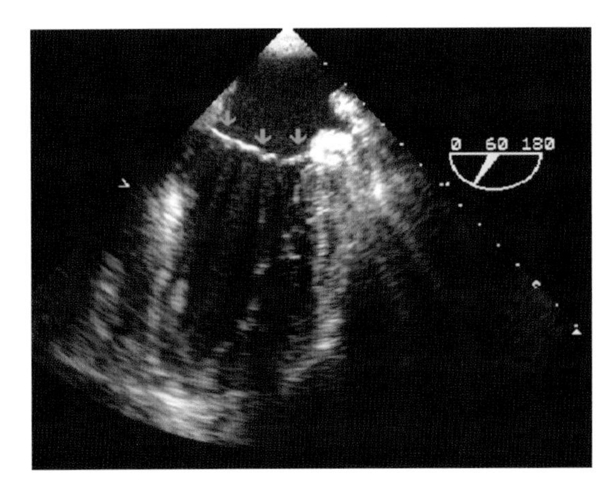

    a. P3, A2, P1
    b. P1, A1, P3
    c. P3, A3, P1
    d. P1, A2, P3

34. When testing for a patent foramen ovale with the agitated saline test, the Valsalva maneuver should be released:
    a. As soon as the saline is injected
    b. When the bubbles enter the right atrium
    c. When the bubbles cross the septum
    d. When the septum bows to the left

35. Hepatic vein flow can best be quantified starting with which view?
    a. Midesophageal four chamber
    b. Midesophageal bicaval
    c. Transgastric short axis
    d. Deep transgastric

36. The commissure pointed to by the arrow is:

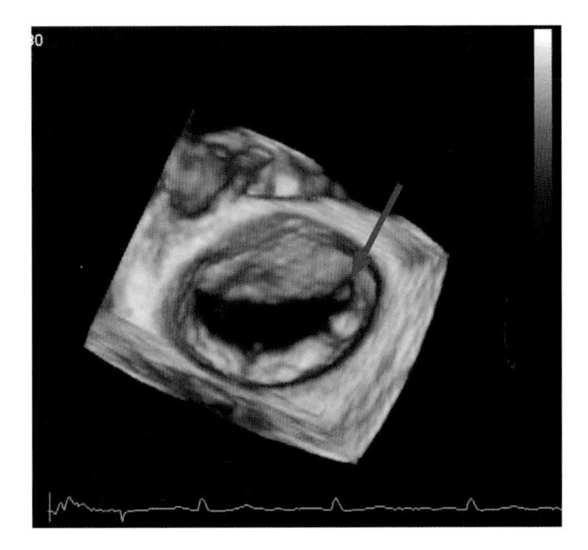

    a. Anterolateral
    b. Anterior
    c. Posteromedial
    d. Posterior

Assessment of Left Ventricular Systolic Function

6

Linda D. Gillam and Laura Ford-Mukkamala

The assessment of ventricular systolic performance is one of the most important roles of perioperative echocardiography. Ventricular function is a key determinant of cardiac output, and global or regional dysfunction may be present before surgery or develop de novo perioperatively. Patients with coronary disease are particularly at risk. The ability of the echocardiographer to recognize such abnormalities is critical to optimal patient care.

In most clinical settings, the assessment of ventricular systolic function is performed qualitatively and relies heavily on the scanning ability and trained interpretive eye of the echocardiographer.[1,2] The ability to accurately assess global and regional ventricular systolic function is one of the most difficult transesophageal echocardiographic (TEE) skills to acquire, and there is no shortcut to supervised training, ideally with access to an independent gold standard. Paradoxically, whereas quantitative methods may require more time for image acquisition and processing, interpretation of the results of such approaches may be relatively straightforward.

All the methods presented in this chapter were first described using transthoracic imaging methods and have been extrapolated to the transesophageal approach. However, it is worth noting that, in some situations, studies directly validating TEE-based applications have not been performed. Since right ventricular (RV) performance is arguably equally important, methods of assessing RV function are discussed in Chapter 13.

THE PHYSIOLOGY OF VENTRICULAR FILLING AND CONTRACTION: PRESSURE-VOLUME RELATIONS

A basic understanding of ventricular physiology, in particular pressure-volume relations, is essential to appropriate utilization of available methods of assessing left ventricular (LV) systolic performance.

The cardiac cycle includes three basic phases: ventricular contraction, relaxation, and filling. LV contraction is initiated when, as a result of rising cytosol calcium levels, the actin and myosin filaments increase the degree to which they overlap, resulting in sarcomere shortening. As more and more cardiomyocytes are activated, the left ventricle begins to contract and LV pressure rises. The LV pressure continues to rise until it overcomes the left atrial pressure, at which point the mitral valve closes. During *isovolumic contraction*, the period between mitral closure and aortic opening, the LV pressure continues to rise. When it exceeds the aortic pressure, the aortic valve opens and blood is ejected. As ejection continues, LV pressure peaks and begins to decrease. When it decreases below the aortic pressure, the aortic valve closes and ejected blood continues to be propagated through the systemic circulation. On a cellular level, calcium is taken up by the sarcoplasmic reticulum, and the myofilaments enter a state of relaxation. Because the mitral and aortic valves are in a closed position, ventricular volume remains constant. This period is known as *isovolumic relaxation*. With continued relaxation, LV pressure decreases further and the mitral valve opens. LV filling occurs in response to the gradient between the left atrium and the ventricle. This first period of filling is known as the *early diastolic filling period*. A second, later component occurs after atrial contraction. One method of displaying the phases of the cardiac cycle is by plotting pressure versus volume, thus creating pressure-volume loops (Figure 6–1).

It might appear that indices of systolic performance should focus exclusively on isovolumic contraction and ejection. However, the diastolic filling portion of the pressure-volume loops is also relevant because it addresses the concept of preload, which, as described below, is an important determinant of many of the most commonly used indices of systolic function. A discussion of diastolic function itself may be found in Chapter 12.

ASSESSMENT OF GLOBAL VENTRICULAR SYSTOLIC PERFORMANCE

Load Dependence

Overall cardiac performance is perhaps best measured by cardiac output or stroke volume (cardiac output/heart rate). These reflect not only ventricular systolic and diastolic function, but also function of the cardiac valves and

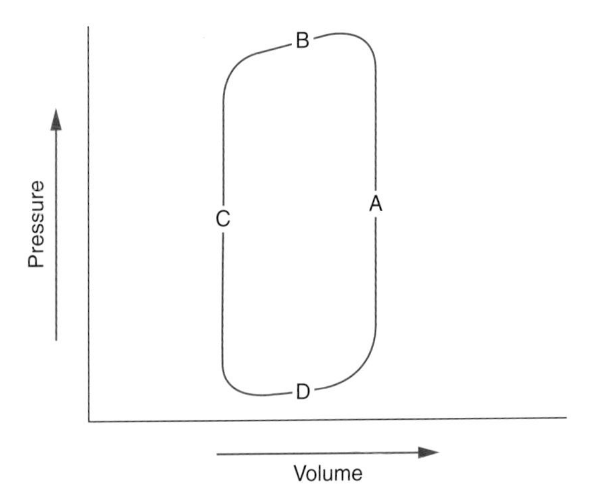

FIGURE 6–1. Left ventricular pressure-volume loop. Pressure is plotted along the y-axis and volume along the x-axis. The four sides of the loop correspond to the following: A—isovolumic contraction, B—systolic ejection, C—isovolumic relaxation, and D—diastolic filling.

pericardium. Ventricular systolic performance in turn is a function of intrinsic myocardial contractility and loading conditions. Thus, in discussing measures of ventricular systolic function, it is important to recognize that many of these are load dependent and that only a few are pure indices of myocardial contractility.

Preload is defined as the wall stress at end-diastole or the load the ventricle experiences before contraction is initiated. It is a function of venous return. Afterload is the wall stress during ventricular contraction or the load against which the ventricle ejects. In the absence of mechanical obstruction to ventricular emptying, such as aortic stenosis, it is a function of the systolic blood pressure.

An appreciation of the effect of loading conditions is particularly important in the intraoperative setting, where dynamic changes in loading typically occur. Preoperatively, preload may be reduced due to the patient's fasting status or, perhaps, from aggressive diuresis as treatment for the patient's underlying heart disease. In the noncardiac setting, an acute event associated with blood loss or fluid shifts may have led to hypovolemia. Induction of anesthesia typically is associated with vasodilation that may further reduce preload. In cardiac surgical patients, preload may be reduced after cardiopulmonary bypass if underlying shunts or regurgitant valve lesions have been corrected. This is compounded by the significant vasodilation that is typical of the period immediately after cardiopulmonary bypass.

Abrupt shifts in afterload also typically occur in the perioperative period. Anesthetic agents may reduce afterload, and surgical correction of outflow tract obstruction, such as aortic valve replacement for aortic stenosis, also may have a major effect. These changes do not invalidate the use of load-dependent indices of systolic function, but their effect must be understood if one is to use these measures appropriately.

In simple terms, load dependence refers to the fact that, for the same degree of intrinsic ventricular contractility, the index of systolic function will vary with the degree to which the ventricle is filled and/or the pressure against which it ejects. For example, in the presence of severe mitral regurgitation, a ventricle with normal contractility will have an LV ejection fraction (LVEF; a load-dependent index) that would be considered elevated in a normally loaded heart. Conversely, in the same setting, an LVEF that would be considered normal for a normally loaded heart would, in fact, indicate depressed function. Table 6–1 lists indices of ventricular systolic performance that can be derived with echocardiography.

Chamber Dimensions

The normal shape of the LV is symmetric with two relatively equal short axes and with the long axis running from the base through the mitral annulus to the apex. In the long-axis views, the apex is rounded, so the apical half of the ventricle resembles a hemiellipse. The basal half, however, is more cylindrical.

Initial evaluation of global systolic performance includes measurement of the linear dimensions of the LV cavity. Chamber dilation or hypertrophy often provides the first diagnostic clues of the underlying pathophysiology. The major long-axis measurement of ventricular dimension is made from the apical endocardium to the plane of the mitral valve by using a midesophageal four-chamber view (see Chapter 4). The minor short axis is measured perpendicular to a point one-third of the length of the long axis, moving from the base to the apex. Short-axis dimensions are often easier to obtain accurately with TEE and involve measurement of the end-diastolic anterior-posterior or medial-lateral diameter at the midpapillary level. A diameter larger than 5.4 cm is considered enlarged, but care must be taken to ensure that the papillary muscles are excluded from the line of measurement.

LV wall thickness is best determined from a transgastric long-axis or midpapillary short-axis view using M-mode or two-dimensional (2D) imaging. An end-diastolic wall thickness greater than 1.1 cm is considered increased. Although increased wall thickness is often viewed as being synonymous with left ventricular hypertrophy, this is incorrect, as left ventricular hypertrophy refers to increased left ventricular mass and LV mass may increase without an increase in thickness. LV

Table 6–1. Load-Dependent and -Independent Indices of Ventricular Function

Load-Dependent Indices	Load-Independent Indices
Cardiac output	End-systolic elastance
Ejection Phase Indices	Preload recruitable stroke work
Fractional shortening	Preload adjusted maximal power
Fractional area change	Strain rate
Ejection fraction	
Velocity of circumferential fiber shortening	
Doppler tissue imaging: peak systolic velocity	
Isovolumetric Phase Indices	
Maximum dP/dt (afterload insensitive, preload sensitive)	
Wall stress	

dP/dt, rate of rise of left ventricular pressure during systole.

mass is the total weight of the myocardium and is equal to the product of the volume of the myocardium and the specific density of cardiac muscle. LV mass can be derived from the transgastric midpapillary short-axis view by using a simple geometric cube formula:

$$\text{LV Mass} = \{1.04 \times [(\text{LVID} + \text{PWT} + \text{IVST})^3 - \text{LVID}^3]\} \times 0.8 + 0.6 \text{ g}$$

where LVID is the end-diastolic internal dimension (diameter), PWT is the inferolateral (posterior) wall thickness, IVST is the interventricular septal thickness, 1.04 is the specific density of the myocardium, and 0.8 and 0.6 are correction factors. Calculation of LV mass by TEE is comparable with transthoracic echocardiography (TTE); however, TEE measurements are higher by an average of 6 gm/m^2 (see Table 4–2).[3]

Cardiac Output

Cardiac output is the product of stroke volume and heart rate. Whereas right heart catheterization using Swan-Ganz catheters is common in the perioperative period and provides the most widely used method for deriving cardiac output, the thermodilution method may be invalid in the setting of tricuspid regurgitation. Further, the devices are expensive, and placement may be risky in some patients, such as those with right side cardiac masses. Echocardiographic methods are not used routinely for cardiac output determinations, in large part for logistic reasons. However, they are well validated and may provide an alternative or adjunct to thermodilution methods.

Echocardiographic measures of cardiac output are based on the continuity equation, which states that in the absence of valve dysfunction or shunting, blood flow is constant throughout the heart. Thus, cardiac output is equal to the forward flow across each of the cardiac valves. For a given valve, this assumption will be invalid if there is significant regurgitation or if valve flow reflects the augmented flow of a shunt lesion. Because of the circular and relatively fixed geometry of the ventricular outflow tracts and semilunar valves, and the relative ease of echocardiographic imaging of these sites, stroke volume calculations typically are derived by measuring forward flow across the LV outflow tract,[4,5] aortic valve,[6,7] or, less commonly, RV outflow tract.[8] Although several methods have been proposed for measuring transmitral and transtricuspid flows, the complex dynamic geometry of the orifices of these valves makes them less desirable.

The measurement of the stroke volume starts with the velocity time integral, the integrated area under the curve of a pulsed Doppler spectrum. This represents the length of a column of blood moving through the targeted point in the heart per beat and has units of distance. Multiplying the velocity time integral by the cross-sectional area of the sampling site yields stroke volume. Cross-sectional area is calculated by using the formula for the area of a circle (πr^2), where r is the cross-sectional diameter divided by 2. The product of stroke volume and heart rate is cardiac output. Although these methods were originally validated with transthoracic imaging, they have been successfully transposed to the transesophageal approach.

The most widely used method is shown in Figure 6–2. The velocity-time integral is recorded from a deep transgastric view of the LV outflow tract, and the LV outflow tract diameter is measured by using a midesophageal long-axis view.[4,5] Ideally, the diameter should be measured at the same location as the velocity-time integral.

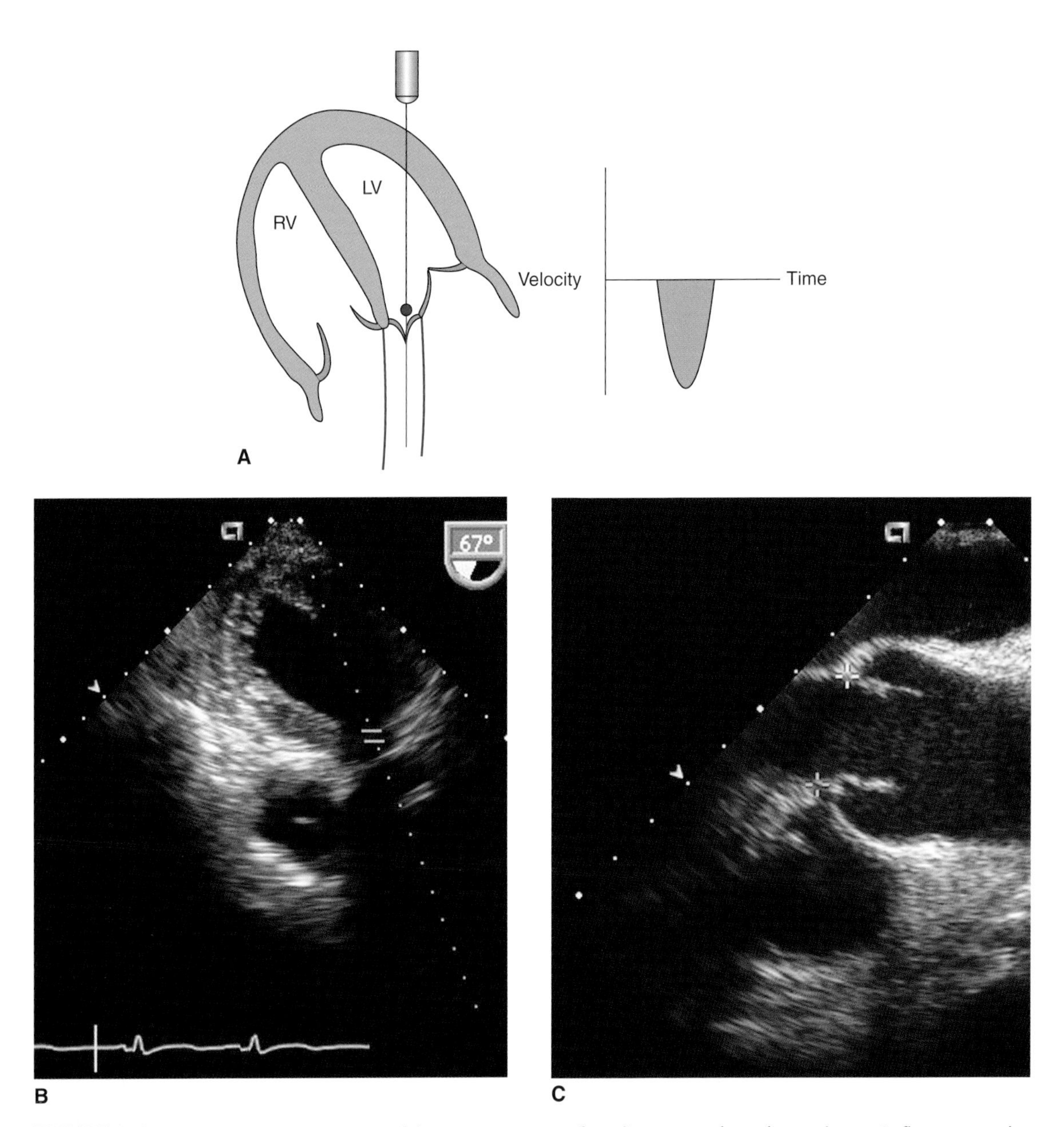

FIGURE 6–2. Schematic representation of the measurement of cardiac output based on volumetric flow across the left ventricular outflow tract. *Note*: This method should not be used in the setting of significant aortic valve disease. **A:** Using the deep transgastric view, the sample volume is placed in the left ventricular (LV) outflow tract just proximal to the aortic valve. This yields the spectral tracing shown to the right. The shaded area represents the velocity-time integral. (RV, right ventricle.) **B:** Representative transesophageal image demonstrates alignment of the image so that the line of Doppler interrogation is parallel to blood flow. **C:** The diameter of the left ventricular outflow tract is measured by using a midesophageal long-axis view. These measurements are analogous to those used in calculating aortic valve area with the continuity equation.

Measurement of the LV outflow tract diameter from a transgastric view is less desirable because it relies on the lateral resolution of the image rather than on the superior axial resolution used when the measurement is taken from a midesophageal window. Once the stroke volume is calculated (cross-sectional area × velocity-time integral), multiplication by the heart rate yields cardiac output.

Commercially available echocardiographic systems have software packages designed to facilitate these calculations, typically included in the more extended analysis needed for Qp/Qs shunt calculations. However, it must be understood that, although shunts or valve regurgitation do not invalidate this calculation as a measure of flow at the site being interrogated, these flows may no longer simply reflect forward systemic cardiac output. For example, in the presence of aortic regurgitation, LV outflow tract flow will include the forward flow (cardiac output) and the regurgitant flow. Another caveat relates to the presence of valvular stenosis, where prestenotic accelerated flow signals and signals at or distal to the stenosis must be avoided.

A potential alternative to the Doppler imaging approach is to determine LV volumes at end-systole and end-diastole. The difference between the two measurements is the stroke volume (equal to LV end-diastolic volume minus LV end-systolic volume), which, when multiplied by heart rate, yields cardiac output. Echocardiographic methods for determining LV volume are described at greater length in subsequent sections dealing with LVEF.

Ejection Phase Indices

Echocardiographic images provide a series of methods for measuring the reduction in chamber dimension that occurs with systole, typically expressed as:

$$\frac{\text{(End-Diastolic Value)} - \text{(End-Systolic Value)}}{\text{End-Diastolic Value}} \times 100\%$$

These ejection phase indices of systolic function include fractional shortening, fractional area change, and ejection fraction.

Fractional Shortening and Velocity of Circumferential Fiber Shortening

The simplest ejection phase index is fractional shortening, defined as:

$$\frac{\text{(End-Diastolic Diameter)} - \text{(End-Systolic Diameter)}}{\text{End-Diastolic Diameter}} \times 100\%$$

This method dates back to the M-mode era of transthoracic echocardiography. Although theoretically of value in the symmetrically contracting heart, its ability to provide a sense of global ventricular function is limited when there is regional dysfunction. Thus, its use is waning. For reference, the lower limit of normal when using a transthoracic approach is 25% in men and 27% in women.[3] Normal values using transesophageal views are reportedly similar but were derived from a smaller series of anesthetized patients.[9]

A variant of fractional shortening is the velocity of circumferential fiber shortening, defined as:

$$\text{Fractional Shortening} \times \text{Ejection Time}$$

Ejection time can be measured on M-mode or LV outflow tract spectral Doppler. The lower limit of normal is 1.1 circumferences/second. Although it has been suggested that this is less preload dependent than ejection fraction,[10] it is rarely used in the clinical setting.

Fractional Area Change (Area Ejection Fraction)

The tomographic slices of the left ventricle provided by 2D echocardiography provide another easily derived ejection phase index: fractional area change or area ejection fraction. This is defined as:

$$\frac{\text{(End-Diastolic Area)} - \text{(End-Systolic Area)}}{\text{End-Diastolic Area}} \times 100\%$$

Originally described using transthoracic short-axis or apical views of the left ventricle, this index can be derived with transesophageal echocardiography by using transgastric short-axis views. Due to the apical foreshortening that is inherent in the TEE midesophageal four-chamber view, this parameter is not generally derived through this window. Although ventricular areas typically are outlined and measured by manual planimetry, systems with automatic boundary detection can automate the process and provide real-time displays of area and calculated fractional area change. Fractional area change derived from TEE and manual planimetry has been shown to correlate with ejection fraction when using nuclear methods in a variety of clinical settings,[11-13] as has TEE-derived fractional area change assisted with automated boundary detection.[14] Acceptable inter- and intra-observer variabilities also have been demonstrated,[14] although Bailey and associates, in a study of pediatric patients with congenital heart disease, suggested an error of approximately 10% under optimal conditions.[15] In symmetrically contracting ventricles, values were shown to be similar at multiple short-axis levels (60 ± 6%, mean ± standard deviation).[16]

It must be emphasized that although such approaches may be valid in patients with symmetric ventricular contraction, they have limited value in patients with regional wall motion abnormalities. Further, the presence of an excellent correlation between fractional area change and LVEF does not mean that the two values are identical. Thus, although it may be conceded that determinations of fractional area change are the most widely used means of quantitating ventricular function with TEE, the reader is encouraged to use the terms *fractional area change* or *area ejection fraction* rather than simply *ejection fraction* when referring to these calculations. The term *ejection fraction* should be reserved for calculations based on ventricular volumes (see below).

VOLUME MEASUREMENT AND EJECTION FRACTION

The universal language for assessing LV systolic performance is ejection fraction (LVEF). Indeed, LVEF is measured routinely in invasive angiographic studies and with noninvasive echocardiographic, nuclear cardiologic, computed tomographic, and magnetic resonance methods. Although there are several quantitative echocardiographic approaches for calculating LVEF, a semiquantitative visual assessment is most widely applied in clinical transthoracic and transesophageal echocardiographic studies. This requires a trained eye. Although less desirable for research applications, this approach works well in the clinical setting in the hands of an operator with good scanning and interpretive skills.[17]

Quantitative Approaches

Quantitative approaches mandate excellent images with good endocardial definition and no apex-base foreshortening. Although the former is rarely a problem with TEE, the latter is common. Apex-base displays are typically optimized by using a midesophageal window with the transducer held in a retroflexed position, but it may be impossible to obtain an image that is not foreshortened. This may account, in part, for the fact that TEE-derived volumes generally underestimate those derived with other approaches. In using the midesophageal window, it may be necessary to move the imaging focus toward the apex and/or reduce the transducer frequency in order to optimally define the apical endocardium.

While this section will focus on 2D approaches, it is followed by an overview of newer three-dimensional (3D) approaches.

MODIFIED SIMPSON'S RULE METHOD (2D)

The Simpson's rule method is generally conceded to be the best method for deriving ventricular volumes, particularly in irregularly shaped ventricles.[13] It is based on modeling the left ventricle as a series of stacked cylindrical disks capped by an elliptical disk apex. The volume for each cylindrical disk is quantified by using the equation:

$$V = (\pi \times D_1/2 \times D_2/2) \times H$$

where D_1 and D_2 are orthogonal diameters of the cylinder, and H is the height of the cylinder.

The elliptical disk calculation uses a different equation:

$$V = Ah/2 + a^2/b^2 \times \pi \times h^3/6$$

where A is the area of the ellipsoid segment, h is the height of the ellipsoid segment, and a and b are radii of the total ellipsoid.

The disks are summed for systole and diastole to yield diastolic and systolic volumes. The difference in volumes is then divided by the end-diastolic volume to calculate ejection fraction:

$$\text{Ejection Fraction} = \frac{(\text{End-Diastolic Volume}) - (\text{End-Systolic Volume})}{\text{End-Diastolic Volume}} \times 100\%$$

Fortunately, the operator can rely on ultrasound system software to make these calculations; otherwise, these calculations would be a laborious process (Figure 6–3). These methods have been validated in vivo using TEE,[13,18] and the major advantage of this approach is that it makes no assumptions concerning LV geometry.

AREA-LENGTH METHOD (2D)

There are several echocardiographic methods for calculating LV volume based on modeling the left ventricle as one or more geometric figures.[19] One of the most common, the area-length approach, models the left ventricle as a *cylinder–hemiellipsoid.* It is traditionally obtained on transthoracic images from the apical four-chamber and parasternal short-axis (papillary muscle) views. With TEE, a midesophageal view at 0° (four chamber) is used to determine the major axis length, and the area is planimetered by using a short-axis view at the level of the mitral valve.

$$\text{Volume} = (5 \times \text{Area} \times \text{Length})/6$$

The area-length method has been validated extensively with the transthoracic approach and, to a lesser degree, TEE.[13,18]

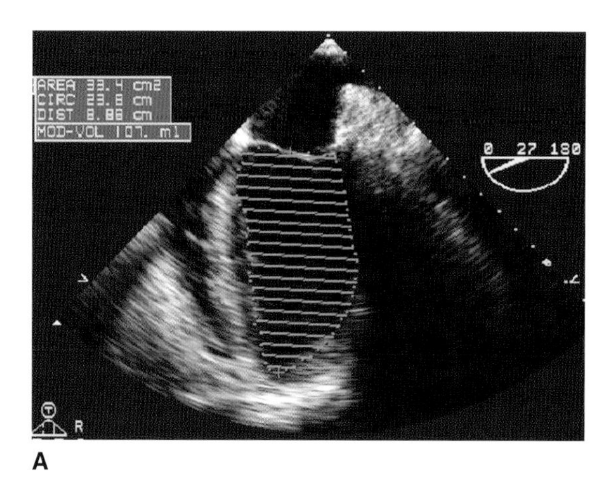

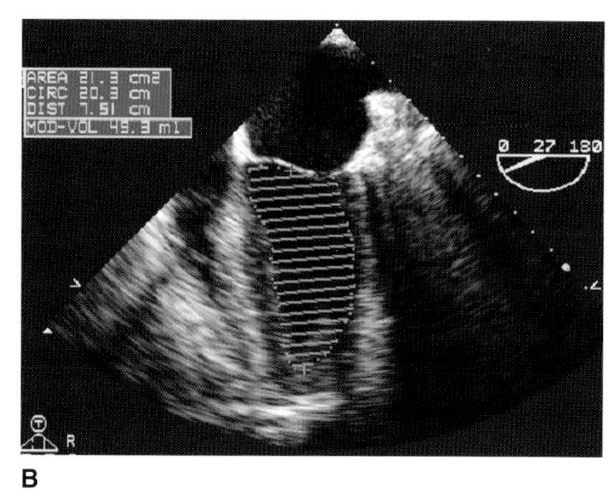

FIGURE 6–3. Illustration of the ultrasound system calculation of end-diastolic and end-systolic volumes using the Simpson method of disks. In this case, **(A)** end-diastolic volume was 107 mL and **(B)** end-systolic volume was 49.3 mL, yielding an ejection fraction of 53.9%.

A similar approach, the diameter-length method, models the left ventricle as a *prolate ellipsoid*:

$$\text{Volume} = (\pi \times D1 \times D2 \times \text{Length})/6$$

where *D*1 and *D*2 are orthogonal short-axis diameters.[18] In both approaches, it is important to avoid oblique short-axis images.

Quantitative Determination of Ejection Fraction

Each of the previously cited methods for deriving ventricular volume can be extrapolated to yield quantitative assessments of ejection fraction. The equation is as follows:

$$\text{LVEF} = \frac{(\text{LV End-Diastolic Volume}) - (\text{LV End-Systolic Volume})}{\text{LV End-Diastolic Volume}} \times 100\%$$

Isovolumetric Indices (dP/dt)

A more load-independent index of LV systolic performance is peak dP/dt, or the maximum rate of rise of LV pressure during systole. The echocardiographic method for deriving this parameter is based on the continuous-wave Doppler recording of the mitral regurgitant spectrum. This method is illustrated in Figure 6–4. As originally reported by Chen and colleagues,[20] the time for velocity to rise from 1 m/s to 3 m/s is measured, and dP/dt is calculated with the following equation:

$$dP/dt = 32 \times 1000/dt$$

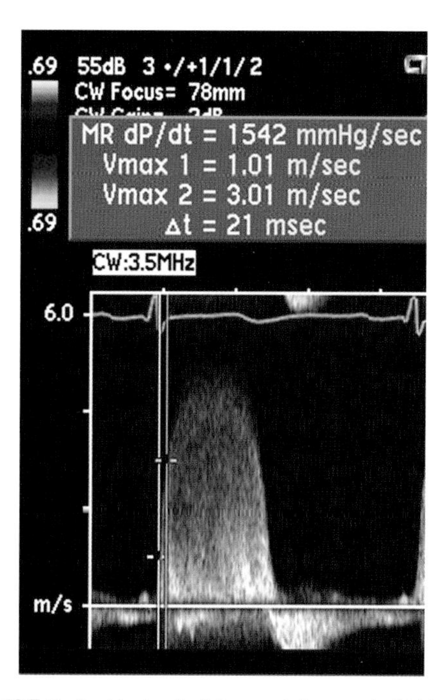

FIGURE 6–4. Method of determining peak dP/dt using the mitral regurgitant spectrum.

Normal values for this parameter are 1610 ± 290 mm Hg/s.[21] This calculation, which is automated in the analysis packages of many commercial ultrasound systems, is easy to perform but requires the presence of well-defined mitral regurgitant spectra. Although relatively afterload independent, dP/dt is preload dependent.

Wall Stress

The common measures of LV systolic function discussed above do not differentiate between abnormalities of contractility and alterations in afterload or preload. LV wall stress, defined as the load opposing ejection, is therefore sometimes used to describe systolic function. Wall stress is dependent on cavity dimensions, wall thickness, and pressure, and can be described as meridional (longitudinal), circumferential, or radial (not used clinically). Meridional stress is calculated from an end-systolic midpapillary short-axis view as:

$$\sigma_m = 1.33 \times P\,(A_c/A_m) \times 10^3 \text{ dyne/cm}^2$$

where P represents LV peak pressure, A_c is LV cavity area, and A_m represents LV myocardial area (area of the muscle in the short-axis view). Normal values for meridional stress are $86 \pm 16 \times 10^3$ dyne/cm^2.

Circumferential stress is calculated from a midesophageal four-chamber view as:

$$\sigma_c = \left[\frac{(1.33P\sqrt{A_c})}{(\sqrt{A_m + A_c} - \sqrt{A_c})}\right] \times \left[1 - \frac{(4A_c\sqrt{A_c}/\pi L^2)}{(\sqrt{A_m + A_c} + \sqrt{A_c})}\right] \text{dyne/cm}^2$$

where the additional variable L represents the LV long-axis length. Normal values for end-systolic circumferential stress are $213 \pm 29 \times 10^3$ dyne/cm^2

Load-Independent Methods of Assessing LV Contractility

LV contractility is an intrinsic property of the cardiomyocytes and an important determinant of overall ventricular systolic function. As initially reported by Suga and Sagawa,[22] the best and most load-independent index of left contractility is end-systolic elastance, which is calculated from pressure-volume loops.

As shown in Figure 6–5, elastance is determined by plotting pressure-volume loops under variable loading conditions. In the invasive or intraoperative setting, such families of curves typically are created by abruptly reducing preload through caval occlusion. A similar but less dramatic decrease in preload can be achieved with the intravenous administration of nitroglycerin. End-systolic elastance is defined by the slope of the line joining the end-systolic points.

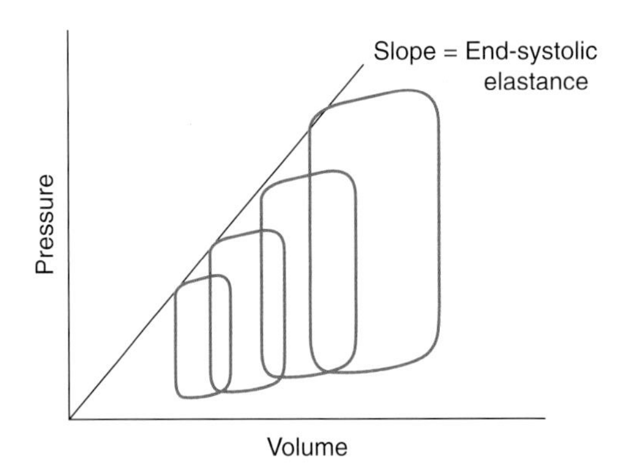

FIGURE 6–5. Calculation of time-varying elastance based on variably loaded pressure-volume loops. A family of loops is created by abruptly changing preload, typically with inferior vena caval occlusion. End-systolic elastance is the slope of the line connecting the end-systolic points of each loop and is a load-independent index of contractility.

An extension of this approach is the determination of preload-recruitable stroke work. Stroke work is the integrated area within a pressure-volume loop. It is possible to calculate stroke work for the variably loaded loops and to plot this as a function of end-diastolic volume. The slope of this linear relation is preload-recruitable stroke work, another relatively load-independent index of contractility.

Values for end-systolic elastance and preload-recruitable work can be approximated with echocardiographic short-axis images and automatic boundary-tracking algorithms. In these approaches,[23,24] area becomes a surrogate for volume. Pressure must be recorded invasively, typically by transmitral placement of a high-fidelity catheter. Specialized computer analysis capabilities are needed to plot the pressure-area loops and calculate elastance or preload-recruitable work. Values for end-systolic elastance and preload-recruitable stroke work are dependent on the size of the left ventricle, so it is impossible to precisely define a normal range.

To study the effect of volatile anesthetic agents on myocardial contractility, Declerck and coworkers[24] evaluated 23 patients undergoing bypass surgery with TEE by using several indices of cardiac performance derived by automatic boundary-tracking technology. These included fractional area change, velocity of circumferential shortening, end-systolic elastance, and preload-recruitable stroke work. They reported that fractional area change and velocity of circumferential fiber shortening had poor sensitivity in detecting changes in contractility when compared with end-systolic elastance and preload-recruitable stroke work. Similar observations were made by Gorcsan and associates.[25]

Another variant of these methods is the measurement of preload-adjusted maximal power (stroke work/end-diastolic volume^2) validated by Mandarino and colleagues.[26] Stroke work is the area within the pressure-volume loop. When echocardiographically derived pressure-area loops are substituted, the formula becomes:

$$\text{Preload-Adjusted Maximal Power Index} = \frac{\text{Integrated Area within Pressure-Area Loop}}{(\text{End-Diastolic Area})^{3/2}}$$

To date, none of these pressure-area approaches have been used clinically. However, they provide essential research tools in studies of dynamically changing contractility. This is particularly true in settings where changing loading conditions invalidate load-dependent indices, as is typically the case perioperatively.

ASSESSMENT OF REGIONAL LV FUNCTION

Because coronary revascularization is one of the primary indications for cardiac surgery and coronary disease is frequently present in patients undergoing noncardiac procedures, an understanding of the coronary vascular bed and the recognition of regional wall motion abnormalities is an important element of perioperative echocardiography. Regional dysfunction may be present preoperatively, develop de novo during surgery, or resolve intraoperatively after revascularization.[27,28] Worsening wall motion after coronary artery bypass graft (CABG) surgery should be considered a prognostic indicator of adverse cardiovascular outcome. Swaminathan et al[29] demonstrated in 1412 CABG surgery patients that subjects with worse regional wall motion immediately after surgical coronary revascularization had a twofold increased risk of death, myocardial infarction, or need for additional revascularization within the subsequent 2 years after surgery.

The echocardiographic manifestation of myocardial ischemia is impaired regional contraction, typically measured in terms of reduced wall thickening and/or abnormal endocardial excursion. The latter typically is assessed visually and described in semiquantitative terms: hypokinesis (mild, moderate, or severe), akinesis, or dyskinesis. Hypokinesis is defined as reduced endocardial excursion, akinesis as the absence of endocardial excursion, and dyskinesis as outward systolic endocardial motion. The term *aneurysm* is used to describe segments in which there is diastolic deformity and dyskinesis, a frequent association.

Normally, the myocardium thickens by at least 30% ((end-systolic thickness − end-diastolic thickness)/end-diastolic thickness) × 100. Thickening of 10% to 30% is considered mildly reduced, and less than 10% thickening is considered severely impaired.

Recognition of regional dysfunction is facilitated by the presence of at least one normally contracting and thickening segment, which serves as a reference; however, because diffuse coronary disease may create the situation in which there is regionally variable dysfunction with no truly normal segment (ie, all segments are abnormal but to different degrees) identification of abnormal contraction patterns based solely on a comparison to adjacent ventricular segments can be misleading.

A complete assessment of LV regional performance requires multiple views that incorporate midesophageal and transgastric views (see Chapter 5). A complete echocardiographic evaluation of regional function is intrinsically redundant in the sense that each segment and each vascular bed is seen in more than one view. The apparent presence of a wall motion abnormality in a single view should prompt a careful reevaluation of the images to ensure that there has not been an interpretive error due to translation of the heart or suboptimal views (off-axis or apically foreshortened). Measurements of systolic wall thickening may be useful supplements to the visual assessment of endocardial excursion.

With TEE, the most difficult area to image is the LV apex. This is best seen with midesophageal views, typically with the probe in a retroflexed position and focus moved to the far field. Transgastric short- and long-axis views also may be used, with an emphasis on avoiding oblique imaging planes and ensuring that the imaging planes reach the apex rather than simply the base of the papillary muscles.

Assessment of the septum and inferior wall may be difficult when septal contour is distorted by primarily right-sided disease. Septal flattening that occurs exclusively in diastole occurs with RV volume overload, whereas *systolic* septal flattening is a manifestation of RV pressure overload. RV hypertension is generally associated with tricuspid regurgitation and RV dilation, so pure RV pressure overload is uncommon in the adult heart; a pattern of septal flattening throughout the cardiac cycle is more common. This may falsely create the appearance of septal and adjacent inferior wall hypokinesis.

Another secondary abnormality of the septum is the dyssynchrony that occurs in the setting of left bundle branch block, whether intrinsic or secondary to RV pacing. This creates a contraction pattern in which the septum appears to writhe, thus making it difficult to determine whether its excursion is normal. In these settings, the assessment of wall thickening may provide a better method of excluding an abnormality of regional contraction.

Seventeen-Segment Model

To standardize the nomenclature for LV segmentation across imaging modalities, the American Society of Echocardiography, with other subspecialty imaging societies, has adapted a 17-segment model.[30] This replaces the 16-segment model previously used by echocardiographers, the differences being the addition of an apical cap as the 17th segment and renaming the posterior, lateral, and septal segments. This scheme is provided for reference in Figure 6–6, and Figure 6–7 provides a schematic assignment of each segment to a coronary vascular bed.

A semiquantitative approach to segmental function is the wall motion score in which each segment is assigned a score of 1 to 4 (1 = normal, 2 = hypokinetic, 3 = akinetic, and 4 = dyskinetic). These may be averaged to give a wall motion score index. Accounting for the severity of hypokinesis transforms this scoring system to: 1 = normal, 2 = mildly hypokinetic, 3 = severely hypokinetic, 4 = akinetic, and 5 = dyskinetic.

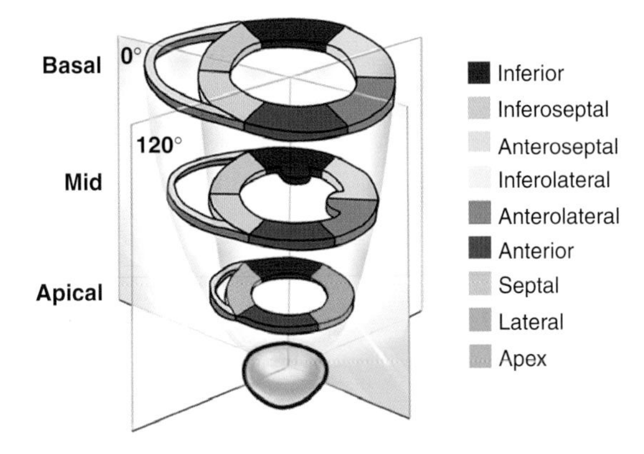

FIGURE 6–6. The 17-segment model of the left ventricle showing the basal, mid, and apical segments. *(Courtesy of F. Clements, MD.)*

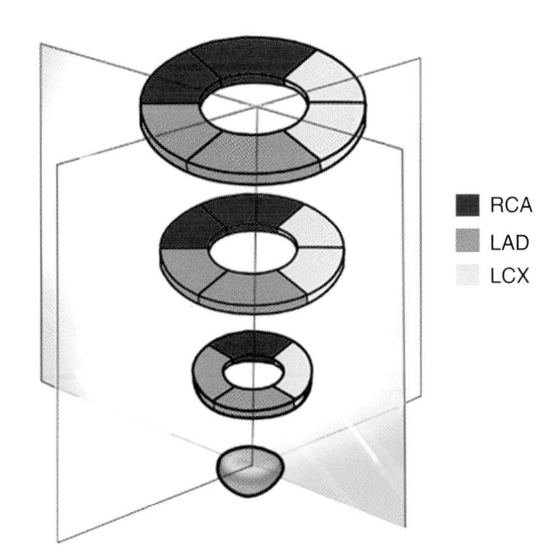

FIGURE 6–7. Typical perfusion beds of the epicardial coronary arteries. *Note*: There may be overlap between the beds of the left circumflex and right coronary arteries. (RCA, right coronary artery; LAD, left anterior descending artery; LCX, left circumflex artery.) *(Courtesy of F. Clements, MD.)*

NEW APPROACHES TO THE ECHOCARDIOGRAPHIC ASSESSMENT OF VENTRICULAR FUNCTION

Although the methods discussed in this section currently are not available with all TEE systems and are used primarily with transthoracic imaging, they are included both to provide a framework for interpreting information from transthoracic echocardiograms and in anticipation of their more widespread incorporation into transesophageal studies (see Chapter 24).

Doppler Tissue Imaging

Doppler tissue imaging (DTI) is a form of pulsed Doppler that focuses on the low-frequency, high-amplitude signals that return from tissue. Because the temporal resolution of DTI is better than that of standard two-dimensional echocardiography, DTI has been reported to be better able to identify subtle differences in regional wall motion than two-dimensional echocardiography alone.[31]

DTI information may be displayed by color-coding the Doppler information and superimposing it over an M-mode or two-dimensional real-time scan (Figure 6–8) or as a velocity-versus-time spectral display of information originating from a specific sample

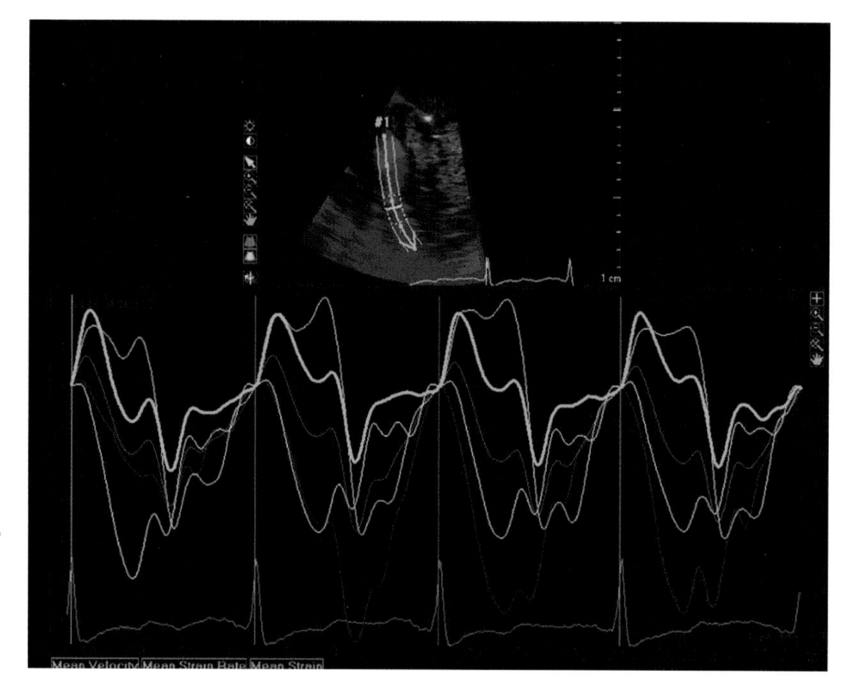

FIGURE 6–8. Doppler tissue imaging of the septal wall demonstrating measurement of mean (lime green color) and segmental strain.

volume within the heart. These display options are analogous to those for pulsed Doppler data originating from red blood cells.

The major limitation of these methods is the fact that they are influenced by translation of the heart. Thus, Doppler tissue imaging is unable to distinguish active motion of the heart based on myocardial contraction from passive motion due to translation. A second limitation derives from the angle dependence of tissue Doppler. Thus, as for blood-cell-derived Doppler data, tissue velocities are underestimated when the direction of motion is not parallel to the line of interrogation.

When the annulus rather than any particular myocardial segment is sampled in a four-chamber view, the technique provides indices of global LV performance. Although these methods have the potential to provide useful information concerning systolic and diastolic performances, their routine clinical use currently is limited largely to the assessment of diastolic function.

Nonetheless, the application of DTI intraoperatively has been reported,[32] and it has been suggested that the technique may be useful in tracking systolic function in this setting. However, overlap between values for normal and abnormal segments make it impossible for this to be used as the only method of assessing ventricular function. Importantly, DTI provides one approach to sophisticated analyses of systolic function along with strain and strain rate determinations and assessment of myocardial twist/torsion.

Speckle Tracking Imaging

The behavior of ultrasound in myocardium (scattering, reflection, and interference) results in 2D images where the myocardium is characterized by speckles. These speckles can be tracked from frame to frame throughout the cardiac cycle, and when their motion is analyzed, it can provide an angle- and translation-independent tool for measuring strain and strain rate as well as measures of ventricular twist/torsion (Figure 6–9).

Strain and Strain Rate Imaging

Strain is a dimensionless quantity defined as the fractional change in length produced by the application of stress:

$$\text{Strain} = \frac{\text{Length} - \text{Length}_0}{\text{Length}_0}$$

where length_0 is the initial length.

$$\text{Strain Rate} = \frac{\text{Strain}}{\text{Time}}$$

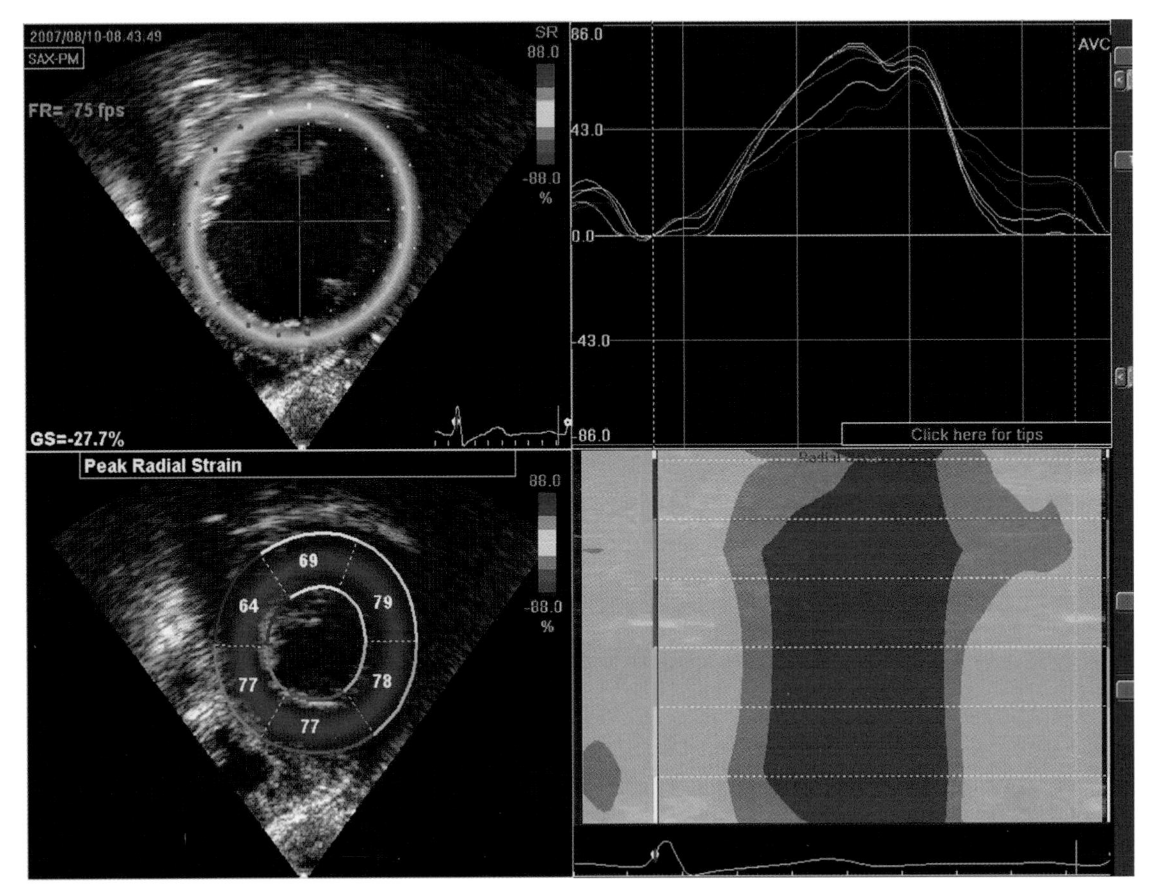

FIGURE 6–9. Speckle tracking imaging demonstrating measurement of radial strain in a transgastric short-axis image. *(Courtesy of C. Marcucci, MD.)*

The capability of deriving strain and strain rate echocardiographically from Doppler tissue imaging is available in most ultrasound systems (Figure 6–8).[33] DTI-derived strain rate is approximated by the ratio of the difference in velocities recorded at two targets over the distance between the two targets:

$$\text{Strain Rate} \cong \frac{\text{Velocity}_a - \text{Velocity}_b}{\text{Distance}}$$

Because strain and strain rate assess the *relative* length and motion of adjacent targets within the heart, they theoretically should be exempt from the influence of translation.[34] Strain rate has been reported to provide a load-independent assessment of myocardial contractility that correlates well with end-systolic elastance,[35] and peak systolic strain may provide an index of regional LV function.[36,37] However, when derived from DTI, the measurements are angle dependent, as demonstrated by Urheim and colleagues,[33] For this reason, and because it provides a means of deriving circumferential and radial strain, methods based on speckle tracking have gained popularity. Regardless of the approach (DTI or speckle tracking), strain rate determinations are limited by noise.[38] Nonetheless, this evolving technology appears to be a valuable tool in the assessment of ventricular function both preoperatively and perioperatively.

Color Kinesis

Color kinesis, an echocardiographic technique based on automated border detection, compares tissue backscatter values between successive acoustic frames, detects pixel

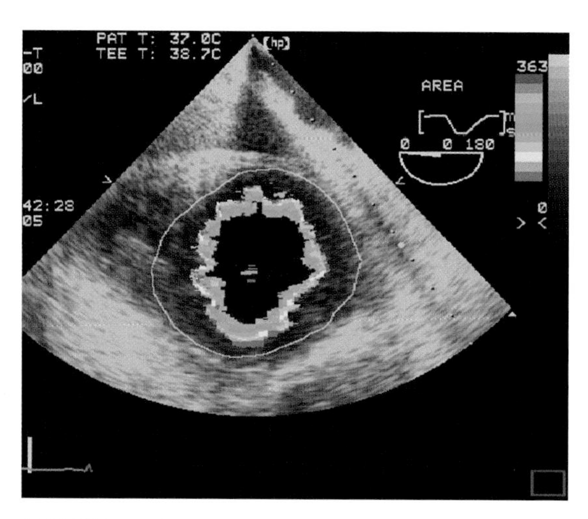

FIGURE 6–10. Color kinesis image of the left ventricle in the short axis. A decrease in color in any wall segment indicates decreased endocardial excursion.

transitions between blood and myocardium, and color encodes these transitions in real time. Segmental analysis of color kinesis images thus provides an objective method for quantifying the spatio-temporal aspects of regional and global LV endocardial motion (Figure 6–10). It may be interpreted semiquantitatively by visual estimation or quantitatively with specially developed off-line analysis systems.[39]

In a study of patients undergoing minimally invasive coronary artery bypass grafting, Kotoh and colleagues[40] suggested that color kinesis is a more sensitive marker of intraoperative ischemia than concurrent electrocardiographic monitoring. Further, Podgoreanu and coworkers[41] demonstrated that quantitative color kinesis analysis of intraoperative LV function agrees more closely with expert analysis than interpretation of gray-scale images by less experienced readers. They concluded that quantitative color kinesis may be a useful adjunct to visual assessment, especially with less experienced reviewers. Despite its apparent merits, color kinesis is not widely available and is infrequently used.

Torsion/Twist

Recently there has been renewed interest in the apex-to-base rotational (twisting/untwisting) characteristics of left ventricular contraction and relaxation. These become particularly important in understanding the response to isolated abnormalities of afterload and preload as occur with valve disease, as well as more common ischemic heart disease. It is notable that the capability exists for performing these analyses with TEE using speckle tracking (Figure 6–11) or more cumbersome DTI-based approaches.

Contrast Echocardiography

Echocardiographic contrast agents capable of left heart opacification after an intravenous injection are valuable tools in transthoracic echocardiography because of their ability to improve endocardial definition. In general, transesophageal images provide excellent images that render contrast enhancement unnecessary. However, in patients in whom TEE images are suboptimal, particularly those who are obese or in whom there is

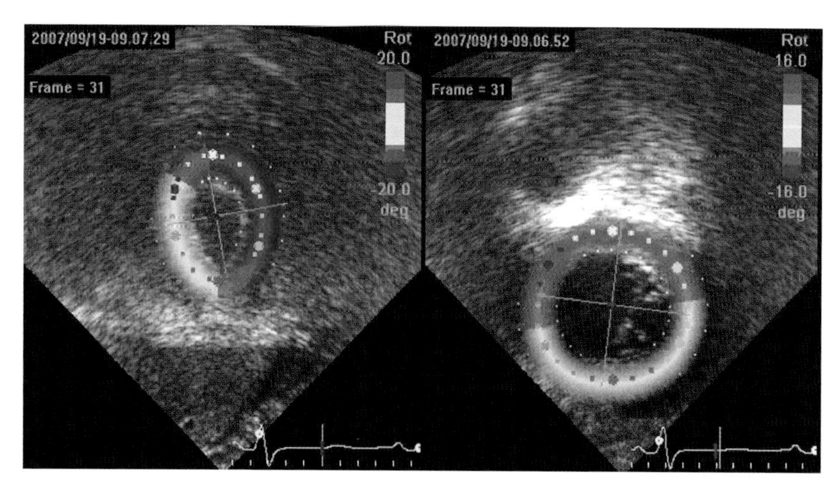

FIGURE 6–11. Speckle tracking imaging demonstrating differential torsion between the base and apex of the heart. *(Courtesy of C. Marcucci, MD.)*

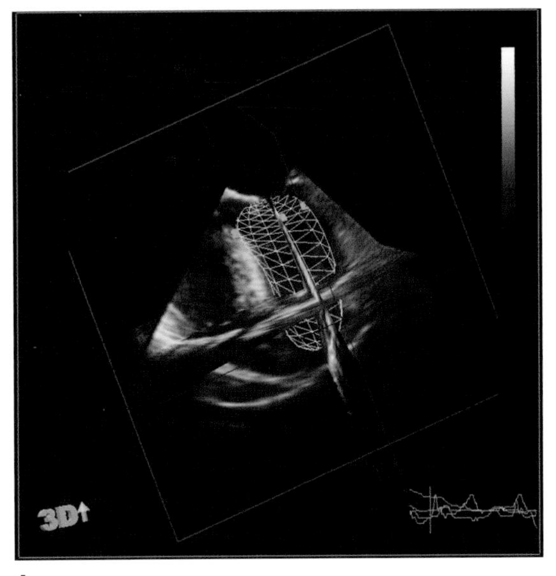

A

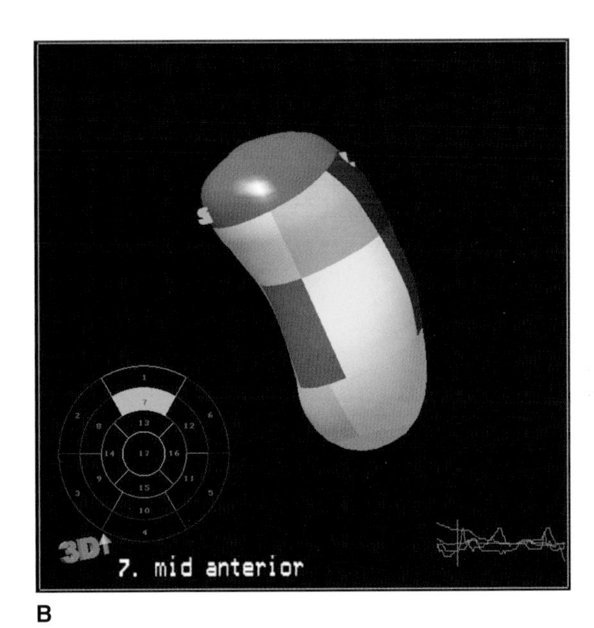

B

FIGURE 6–12. Three-dimensional image of the left ventricle demonstrating volumetric assessment **(A)** and segmentation for assessment of wall motion **(B)**. In this still frame, the mid–anterior segment is highlighted in yellow.

interference by subdiaphragmatic air, contrast may facilitate endocardial border delineation. In addition, contrast may help delineate masses, enhance Doppler spectra, and define myocardial perfusion. It has been shown that contrast administration has no effect on intraoperative hemodynamics.[42] If contrast is used, it is important that machine settings optimized for contrast be employed. These include harmonic imaging (available on newer TEE systems) and low mechanical index (power). Ideally, a preset for contrast imaging should be created for the system.

THREE-DIMENSIONAL APPROACHES

Recently, three-dimensional (3D) and real-time three-dimensional (4D or RT3D) echocardiography has become available on TEE probes. Arguably this has revolutionized the TEE assessment of mitral pathology and has become increasingly important in providing guidance for interventional cardiology procedures such as device repair of congenital defects. These techniques may also be used to assist in the qualitative assessment of ventricular systolic function, since multiple 2D images can be derived by post-acquisition cropping and rotation of single full-volume acquisitions and 3D slices of the ventricle can be obtained using conventional 2D windows (Figure 6–12). For the time being, however, full ventricular volumes are too large to be captured in truly real-time display using a transesophageal approach, and only semigated methods that create a full volume by electronically "stitching" together partial volumes exist. Similarly, while current off-line analysis tools can create detailed quantitative assessments of global and regional volumes and function using transthoracic 3D data, these methods have not yet been validated with TEE. However such tools should soon be available with the caveat that the difficulty of imaging the LV apex with TEE may ultimately limit the accuracy of volume and LVEF determinations.

REFERENCES

1. Picano E, Lattanzi F, Orlandini A, Marini C, L'Abbate A. Stress echocardiography and the human factor: the importance of being expert. *J Am Coll Cardiol.* 1991;17(3):666-669.
2. Martin RP. Real time ultrasound quantification of ventricular function: has the eyeball been replaced or will the subjective become objective. *J Am Coll Cardiol.* 1992;19(2): 321-323.
3. Lang RM, Bierig M, Devereux RB, et al. Recommendations for chamber quantification: a report from the American Society of Echocardiography's Guidelines and Standards Committee and the Chamber Quantification Writing Group, developed in conjunction with the European Association of Echocardiography, a branch of the European Society of Cardiology. *J Am Soc Echocardiogr.* 2005;18(12):1440-1463.
4. Stoddard MF, Prince CR, Ammash N, Goad JL, Vogel RL. Pulsed Doppler transesophageal echocardiographic determination of cardiac output in human beings: comparison with thermodilution technique. *Am Heart J.* 1993;126(4):956-962.

5. Descorps-Declere A, Smail N, Vigue B, et al. Transgastric, pulsed Doppler echocardiographic determination of cardiac output. *Intensive Care Med.* 1996;22(1):34-38.
6. Perrino AC Jr, Harris SN, Luther MA. Intraoperative determination of cardiac output using multiplane transesophageal echocardiography: a comparison to thermodilution. *Anesthesiology.* 1998;89(2):350-357.
7. Darmon PL, Hillel Z, Mogtader A, Mindich B, Thys D. Cardiac output by transesophageal echocardiography using continuous-wave Doppler across the aortic valve. *Anesthesiology.* 1994;80(4):796-805; discussion 725A.
8. Maslow A, Comunale ME, Haering JM, Watkins J. Pulsed wave Doppler measurement of cardiac output from the right ventricular outflow tract. Anesth Analg. 1996;83(3):466-471.
9. Skarvan K, Lambert A, Filipovic M, Seeberger M. Reference values for left ventricular function in subjects under general anaesthesia and controlled ventilation assessed by two-dimensional transoesophageal echocardiography. *Eur J Anaesthesiol.* 2001;18(11):713-722.
10. Colan SD, Borow KM, Neumann A. Left ventricular end-systolic wall stress-velocity of fiber shortening relation: a load-independent index of myocardial contractility. *J Am Coll Cardiol.* 1984; 4(4):715-724.
11. Clements FM, Harpole DH, Quill T, Jones RH, McCann RL. Estimation of left ventricular volume and ejection fraction by two-dimensional transoesophageal echocardiography: comparison of short axis imaging and simultaneous radionuclide angiography. *Br J Anaesth.* 1990;64(3):331-336.
12. Urbanowicz JH, Shaaban MJ, Cohen NH, et al. Comparison of transesophageal echocardiographic and scintigraphic estimates of left ventricular end-diastolic volume index and ejection fraction in patients following coronary artery bypass grafting. *Anesthesiology.* 1990;72(4):607-612.
13. Ryan T, Burwash I, Lu J, et al. The agreement between ventricular volumes and ejection fraction by transesophageal echocardiography or a combined radionuclear and thermodilution technique in patients after coronary artery surgery. *J Cardiothorac Vasc Anesth.* 1996;10(3):323-328.
14. Cahalan MK, Ionescu P, Melton HE Jr, Adler S, Kee LL, Schiller NB. Automated real-time analysis of intraoperative transesophageal echocardiograms. *Anesthesiology.* 1993;78(3):477-485.
15. Bailey JM, Shanewise JS, Kikura M, Sharma S. A comparison of transesophageal and transthoracic echocardiographic assessment of left ventricular function in pediatric patients with congenital heart disease. *J Cardiothorac Vasc Anesth.* 1995;9(6):665-669.
16. Domanski MJ, Cunnion RE, Roberts WC. Analysis of fractional area change at various levels in the normal left ventricle. *Am J Cardiol.* 1992;70(15):1367-1368.
17. Stamm RB, Carabello BA, Mayers DL, Martin RP. Two-dimensional echocardiographic measurement of left ventricular ejection fraction: prospective analysis of what constitutes an adequate determination. *Am Heart J.* 1982;104(1):136-144.
18. Smith MD, MacPhail B, Harrison MR, Lenhoff SJ, DeMaria AN. Value and limitations of transesophageal echocardiography in determination of left ventricular volumes and ejection fraction. *J Am Coll Cardiol.* 1992;19(6):1213-1222.
19. Wyatt HL, Heng MK, Meerbaum S, et al. Cross-sectional echocardiography. II. Analysis of mathematic models for quantifying volume of the formalin-fixed left ventricle. *Circulation.* 1980;61(6):1119-1125.
20. Chen C, Rodriguez L, Guerrero JL, et al. Noninvasive estimation of the instantaneous first derivative of left ventricular pressure using continuous-wave Doppler echocardiography. *Circulation.* 1991;83(6):2101-2110.
21. Little W, Braunwald E. Assessment of cardiac function. In: *Heart Disease: A Textbook of Cardiovascular Medicine.* 5th ed. Braunwald E, ed. Philadelphia: Saunders; 1997.
22. Suga H, Sagawa K, Shoukas AA. Load independence of the instantaneous pressure-volume ratio of the canine left ventricle and effects of epinephrine and heart rate on the ratio. *Circ Res.* 1973;32(3):314-322.
23. Gorcsan J 3rd, Romand JA, Mandarino WA, Deneault LG, Pinsky MR. Assessment of left ventricular performance by on-line pressure-area relations using echocardiographic automated border detection. *J Am Coll Cardiol.* 1994;23(1): 242-252.
24. Declerck C, Hillel Z, Shih H, Kuroda M, Connery CP, Thys DM. A comparison of left ventricular performance indices measured by transesophageal echocardiography with automated border detection. *Anesthesiology.* 1998;89(2): 341-349.
25. Gorcsan J 3rd, Gasior TA, Mandarino WA, Deneault LG, Hattler BG, Pinsky MR. Assessment of the immediate effects of cardiopulmonary bypass on left ventricular performance by on-line pressure-area relations. *Circulation.* 1994;89(1): 180-190.
26. Mandarino WA, Pinsky MR, Gorcsan J 3rd. Assessment of left ventricular contractile state by preload-adjusted maximal power using echocardiographic automated border detection. *J Am Coll Cardiol.* 1998;31(4):861-868.
27. Topol EJ, Weiss JL, Guzman PA, et al. Immediate improvement of dysfunctional myocardial segments after coronary revascularization: detection by intraoperative transesophageal echocardiography. *J Am Coll Cardiol.* 1984;4(6): 1123-1134.
28. Beaupre PN, Kremer PF, Cahalan MK, Lurz FW, Schiller NB, Hamilton WK. Intraoperative detection of changes in left ventricular segmental wall motion by transesophageal two-dimensional echocardiography. *Am Heart J.* 1984;107(5 Pt 1): 1021-1023.
29. Swaminathan M, Morris RW, De Meyts DD, et al. Deterioration of regional wall motion immediately after coronary artery bypass graft surgery is associated with long-term major adverse cardiac events. *Anesthesiology.* 2007;107(5):739-745.
30. Cerqueira MD, Weissman NJ, Dilsizian V, et al. Standardized myocardial segmentation and nomenclature for tomographic imaging of the heart: a statement for healthcare professionals from the Cardiac Imaging Committee of the Council on Clinical Cardiology of the American Heart Association. *Circulation.* 2002;105(4):539-542.
31. Bolognesi R, Tsialtas D, Barilli AL, et al. Detection of early abnormalities of left ventricular function by hemodynamic, echo-tissue Doppler imaging, and mitral Doppler flow techniques in patients with coronary artery disease and normal ejection fraction. *J Am Soc Echocardiogr.* 2001;14(8): 764-772.
32. Skarvan K, Filipovic M, Wang J, Brett W, Seeberger M. Use of myocardial tissue Doppler imaging for intraoperative monitoring of left ventricular function. *Br J Anaesth.* 2003;91(4): 473-480.

33. Urheim S, Edvardsen T, Torp H, Angelsen B, Smiseth OA. Myocardial strain by Doppler echocardiography. Validation of a new method to quantify regional myocardial function. *Circulation.* 2000;102(10):1158-1164.
34. Weidemann F, Kowalski M, D'Hooge J, Bijnens B, Sutherland GR. Doppler myocardial imaging. A new tool to assess regional inhomogeneity in cardiac function. Basic Res *Cardiol.* 2001;96(6):595-605.
35. Greenberg NL, Firstenberg MS, Castro PL, et al. Doppler-derived myocardial systolic strain rate is a strong index of left ventricular contractility. *Circulation.* 2002;105(1):99-105.
36. Armstrong G, Pasquet A, Fukamachi K, Cardon L, Olstad B, Marwick T. Use of peak systolic strain as an index of regional left ventricular function: comparison with tissue Doppler velocity during dobutamine stress and myocardial ischemia. *J Am Soc Echocardiogr.* 2000;13(8):731-737.
37. Edvardsen T, Urheim S, Skulstad H, Steine K, Ihlen H, Smiseth OA. Quantification of left ventricular systolic function by tissue Doppler echocardiography: added value of measuring pre- and postejection velocities in ischemic myocardium. *Circulation.* 2002;105(17):2071-2077.
38. D'Hooge J, Heimdal A, Jamal F, et al. Regional strain and strain rate measurements by cardiac ultrasound: principles, implementation and limitations. *Eur J Echocardiogr.* 2000;1(3):154-170.
39. Lang RM, Vignon P, Weinert L, et al. Echocardiographic quantification of regional left ventricular wall motion with color kinesis. *Circulation.* 1996;93(10):1877-1885.
40. Kotoh K, Watanabe G, Ueyama K, et al. On-line assessment of regional ventricular wall motion by transesophageal echocardiography with color kinesis during minimally invasive coronary artery bypass grafting. *J Thorac Cardiovasc Surg.* 1999;117(5):912-917.
41. Podgoreanu MV, Djaiani GN, Davis E, Phillips-Bute B, Mathew JP. Quantitative echocardiographic assessment of regional wall motion and left ventricular asynchrony with color kinesis in cardiac surgery patients. *Anesth Analg.* 2003;96(5):1294-1300, table of contents.
42. Erb JM, Shanewise JS. Intraoperative contrast echocardiography with intravenous optison does not cause hemodynamic changes during cardiac surgery. *J Am Soc Echocardiogr.* 2001;14(6):595-600.

REVIEW QUESTIONS

Select the *one best* answer for each item.

1. Which of the following describes the diastolic filling phase of the LV pressure-volume loop?
   a. Volume remains constant, pressure falls.
   b. Volume remains constant, pressure rises.
   c. Volume and pressure remain constant.
   d. Volume rises, pressure falls.
   e. Volume and pressure rise.

2. Which of the following describes the isovolumic contraction phase of the LV pressure-volume loop?
   a. Volume remains constant, pressure falls.
   b. Volume remains constant, pressure rises.
   c. Volume and pressure remain constant.
   d. Volume rises, pressure falls.
   e. Volume and pressure rise.

3. Which of the following is the most load-independent index of ventricular contractility?
   a. Fractional area change
   b. Ejection fraction
   c. Peak dP/dt
   d. End-systolic elastance
   e. Fractional shortening

4. For each of the following conditions, indicate whether LV preload is:
   A. Increased
   B. Decreased
   C. Unchanged
   a. Mitral regurgitation
   b. Ventricular septal defect
   c. Aortic regurgitation
   d. Aortic stenosis
   e. Acute blood loss

5. For each of the following conditions, indicate whether LV afterload is:
   A. Increased
   B. Decreased
   C. Unchanged
   a. Mitral regurgitation
   b. Peri-infarction ventricular septal defect
   c. Aortic stenosis
   d. Systemic hypertension

6. Relative to the preinduction resting state, which of the following best describes the typical change in LV loading conditions after the induction of general anesthesia before cardiac surgery?
   a. Afterload increased, preload increased
   b. Afterload increased, preload decreased
   c. Afterload decreased, preload increased
   d. Afterload decreased, preload decreased

7. A 26-year-old patient with critical aortic stenosis undergoes successful aortic valve replacement. Preoperative LVEF is 45%. Immediate postoperative LVEF is 65%. What is the most likely explanation for the improvement in LVEF?
   a. Intrinsic myocardial contractility has acutely improved.
   b. Intrinsic myocardial contractility has acutely worsened.
   c. Afterload has acutely decreased.
   d. Afterload has acutely increased.
   e. Preload has acutely increased.

8. Which of the following is *not* required to calculate cardiac output when using the continuity equation as applied to LV outflow?
   a. LV outflow tract velocity-time integral
   b. Heart rate
   c. Diameter of the LV outflow tract
   d. Nyquist limit (aliasing velocity) of the LV outflow tract pulsed Doppler spectrum

9. A patient with severe aortic regurgitation undergoes measurement of volumetric flow per minute across the LV outflow tract by using continuity-based methods. This will provide a measure that is:
   a. Identical to true forward output
   b. An overestimation of true forward output
   c. An underestimation of true forward output

10. Which of the following is the most appropriate method for determining the ejection fraction of a left ventricle with a large apical aneurysm?
   a. Area-length (prolate ellipsoid)
   b. Area-length (cylinder–hemiellipsoid)
   c. Summation of disks (Simpson's rule)
   d. Fractional area change

11. Automated boundary tracking facilitates measurement of all of the following except:
   a. Fractional shortening
   b. LVEF
   c. Fractional area change
   d. Strain rate

12. A family of pressure-volume loops is created during transient inferior vena caval occlusion. What is the slope of the line connecting the end-systolic points?
   a. Elastance
   b. Preload-recruitable stroke work
   c. dP/dt
   d. Preload-adjusted maximal power

13. The measurement of peak LV dP/dt requires which of the following Doppler spectra?
   a. Continuous wave, LV outflow
   b. Pulsed wave, LV outflow
   c. Continuous wave, descending thoracic aorta
   d. Pulsed wave, mitral inflow
   e. Continuous wave, mitral regurgitant jet

14. Doppler tissue imaging is used to record signals from the LV myocardium. These are typically:
   a. High velocity, high amplitude
   b. High velocity, low amplitude
   c. Low velocity, high amplitude
   d. Low velocity, low amplitude

15. Strain and strain rate measurements are derived from:
   a. Pulsed Doppler measurements of LV outflow
   b. Continuous-wave Doppler measurements of LV outflow
   c. Automatic boundary detection: short-axis view
   d. Myocardial Doppler tissue imaging

16. Regional wall motion abnormalities are the hallmark of LV dysfunction due to:
   a. Hypertensive heart disease
   b. Dilated cardiomyopathy
   c. Chronic severe mitral regurgitation
   d. Coronary artery disease

17. Using the 17-segment model of the left ventricle, akinesis of the inferoseptal segments is most likely to correspond to occlusion in which of the following coronary arteries?
   a. Right
   b. Left anterior descending
   c. Left circumflex

18. Using the 17-segment model of the left ventricle, akinesis of the lateral wall segments is most likely to correspond to occlusion in which of the following coronary arteries?
   a. Right
   b. Left anterior descending
   c. Left circumflex

19. Using the 17-segment model of the left ventricle, akinesis of the apical cap is most likely to correspond to occlusion in which of the following coronary arteries?
   a. Right
   b. Left anterior descending
   c. Left circumflex

20. Difficulty in imaging the left ventricle from the midesophageal views is reflected most commonly in:
   a. Oblique short-axis views
   b. Foreshortening of the apex
   c. Endocardial drop-out of the base

21. Which of the following does *not* typically alter motion of the interventricular septum?
   a. Left bundle branch block
   b. Right ventricular pacing
   c. Right bundle branch block
   d. Right ventricular hypertension

22. Echocardiographic contrast agents may be used to optimize delineation of:
   a. Left ventricular endocardium
   b. Left ventricular apical thrombus

c. Continuous-wave Doppler spectra recorded in the setting of aortic stenosis
d. All of the above
e. None of the above

23. Stunned myocardium is defined as:
 a. Myocardium after cardioversion for atrial fibrillation
 b. Myocardium that is hibernating
 c. Reperfused viable myocardium that is not functioning
 d. Myocardium that is functional at rest but not with exercise

24. Scarred myocardium after chronic myocardial infarction is characterized by all of the following *except*:
 a. Thinning of the wall
 b. More echogenic than the surrounding healthy myocardium
 c. Akinesis
 d. Speckled appearance

25. LV aneurysm formation is most commonly associated with anterior infarction.
 a. True
 b. False

Mitral Valve

7

Johannes van der Westhuizen and Justiaan Swanevelder

The evaluation of valvular heart disease has become increasingly dependent on echocardiography. Since its introduction to the operating room, transesophageal echocardiography (TEE) has played a major role in surgical decision making and anesthetic management of patients undergoing mitral valve surgery. Mitral valve replacement has its own implications and is not free of risk, leading surgeons to develop techniques for mitral valve repair, which are becoming more and more intricate as our understanding of valve function expands. Recent outcome literature indicates strong support for repair relative to replacement in patients with organic, nonischemic mitral valve pathology,[1] and the role of intraoperative TEE in mitral valve repair[2] and replacement surgery[3] is well established. A good knowledge of mitral valve anatomy and its assessment by TEE is therefore vital to any successful intraoperative echocardiographer.

ANATOMY AND FUNCTION OF THE MITRAL VALVE[4]

The mitral valve is located between the left atrium and the left ventricle and allows unidirectional flow of blood towards the left ventricle, prevents backward flow of blood into the left atrium during left ventricular systole, and allows unobstructed flow of blood to the left ventricle during diastole, maintaining low left atrial pressures. The anterior mitral valve leaflet also forms part of the left ventricular outflow tract and allows for unimpeded left ventricular ejection during systole. For the mitral valve to function normally, it relies on the integrated function of a number of structures, which are collectively referred to as the mitral valvar complex. This complex consists of the anterior (aortic) and posterior (mural) leaflets, together with the annulus, chordae tendineae, papillary muscles, and left ventricle. Abnormalities of any of these structures can result in valvular dysfunction, and should therefore be included in the comprehensive evaluation of the mitral valve.

Mitral Valve Leaflets and Commissures

Two leaflets separated by two commissural areas cover the mitral valve area during systole. The anterior or aortic leaflet is situated anteriorly and to the right, adjacent to and in continuum with the aortic valve, and occupies approximately one-third of the annular circumference. Both the aortic and mitral valves contribute to the so-called fibrous skeleton of the heart, and the connection between the two is sometimes described as the aortomitral continuity. The posterior or mural leaflet occupies the remaining two-thirds of the annular circumference and is much narrower than the anterior leaflet. Although the posterior leaflet appears to have less height than the anterior leaflet, they are similar in surface area. The posterior leaflet is subdivided into three scallops by clefts. The scallop adjacent the anterolateral commissure is named P1, with P3 situated on the other end of the posterior leaflet in close relation to the posteromedial commissure. P2 is the middle scallop in between P1 and P3. Even though the anterior leaflet is not anatomically divided into scallops, the areas opposing the posterior leaflet are correspondingly referred to as the A1, A2, and A3 segments (Figure 7–1).[5] Closure of the valve requires apposition and coaptation of the two leaflets, and this occurs along a single semilunar coaptation line. The ends of this coaptation line do not extend all the way to the annulus and are known as commissures. These commissural areas are situated anterolaterally and posteromedially, in relation to their papillary muscles.

Mitral Annulus

Anatomically, the annulus is formed by lateral extensions of fibroelastic tissue, originating from the left and right fibrous trigones. The amount of fibrous tissue decreases towards the inferolateral aspect of the annulus until only myocardium is present, making the inferolateral annulus most susceptible to dilatation. The aortomitral fibrous continuity, another area where the annulus is not well defined, is situated between the two trigones. Left atrial implantation serves as an indicator of the mitral annulus in this region. Undulations in the mitral annulus results in a saddle shape, with the commissural areas located more towards the ventricle and the intertrigonal and posterolateral areas located more towards the left atrium. The annulus is oval shaped,

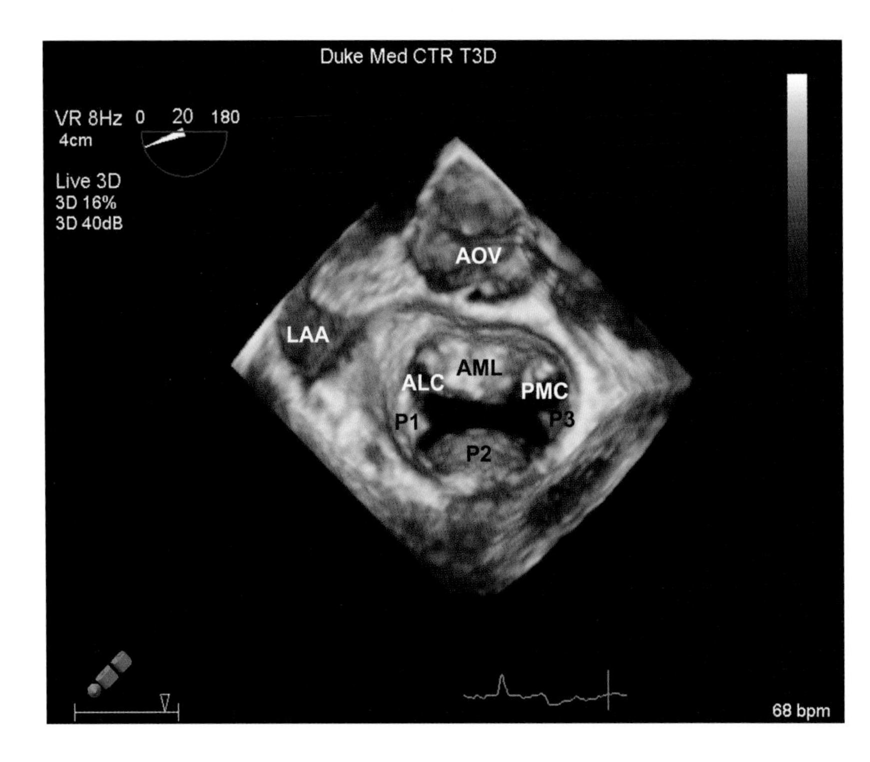

FIGURE 7–1. This full-volume 3D dataset of the heart demonstrates the mitral valve during diastole. The anterior leaflet, scallops of the posterior leaflet (P1, P2, P3), and both anterolateral and posteromedial commissures are clearly visible. (AOV, aortic valve; LAA, left atrial appendage; ALC, anterolateral commissure; PMC, posteromedial commissure; AML, anterior mitral leaflet.)

with the intercommissural (intertrough) distance greater than the aortic to mural (interpeak) distance. The valve is slightly tilted in the chest, with the anterior part superior to the more inferiorly positioned inferolateral part.

Papillary Muscles and Chordae Tendineae

The subvalvular apparatus consists of two papillary muscles supporting the mitral valve leaflets by means of multiple chordae tendineae. The posteromedial papillary muscle is found in close relation to the posteromedial commissure and the interventricular septum. In the case of the mitral valve, there is no direct leaflet connection to the interventricular septum as occurs with the tricuspid valve septal leaflet. This is a distinguishing feature allowing identification of the tricuspid or mitral valve where transposition is suspected. Blood supply to the posteromedial papillary muscle is usually provided by a single coronary artery. Depending on dominance of the circulation, it can be either a branch from the posterior descending artery, or a branch from the obtuse marginal artery. The anterolateral papillary muscle is found in relation to the anterolateral commissure and receives blood supply from both the left anterior descending artery via the first marginal artery, and from the circumflex artery via the first obtuse marginal artery. This dual supply makes dysfunction of the anterolateral papillary muscle less likely.[6]

Primary chordae tendineae stretch from the papillary muscles and attach to the tips of the mitral valve leaflets. Secondary and tertiary chordae also attach to the body and base of the leaflets, respectively. Separate chordae also originate from the left ventricular free wall and attach to the ventricular surface of the posterior leaflet, in particular. During ventricular systole, contraction of the papillary muscles and left ventricular free wall therefore prevents the mitral valve leaflets from prolapsing into the left atrium. Dysfunction of the papillary muscles or chordae can cause mitral valve dysfunction by either allowing excessive motion of the leaflets or by restricting movement of the leaflets and thus preventing proper coaptation.

Left Ventricular Myocardium

The left ventricular myocardium determines the position of the papillary muscles relative to the mitral coaptation point. Left ventricular dilatation alters the spatial relation of the papillary muscles and attachment of tertiary chordae to the leaflets, thus moving the coaptation point deeper into the ventricle. The result is tethering of the leaflets with inadequate coaptation and valvular dysfunction.

Left Atrium

The role of the left atrium in normal mitral valve function is not clearly defined. However, left atrial tissue is continuous with the mural leaflet and may potentially interfere with normal leaflet motion when left atrial dilatation occurs.[7] The atrial attachment to the aortomitral fibrous continuity is also the hinge point of the aortic leaflet, and atrial dilatation may therefore affect the function of the aortic leaflet.

TRANSESOPHAGEAL ECHOCARDIOGRAPHIC ASSESSMENT OF THE MITRAL VALVE[8]

Complete and accurate two-dimensional (2D) echocardiographic assessment of mitral valve morphology requires the examiner to obtain multiple tomographic two-dimensional views and mentally reconstruct a three-dimensional interpretation (Figure 7–2). Three-dimensional imaging, when it is available on all ultrasound systems, will make such mental reconstruction unnecessary (Figure 7–3). The following views, included in the American Society of Echocardiography (ASE)/Society of Cardiovascular Anesthesiologists (SCA) guidelines for performing a comprehensive intraoperative TEE exam, allow systematic assessment of the mitral valve.

Midesophageal Four-Chamber View (ME 4 CH)

This view is achieved by gently retroflexing the probe in the midesophageal position, directing the imaging sector towards the cardiac apex through the mitral valve. In the classical ME 4 CH view, which is obtained at 20° to 30°, the imaging plane transects the mitral valve in an oblique plane relative to the valve commissures, thus showing the A3 segment of the aortic or anterior leaflet to the left of the display and the P1 scallop of the posterior leaflet to the right of the display (see Figures 7–2 and 7–3). By withdrawing or anteflexing the probe

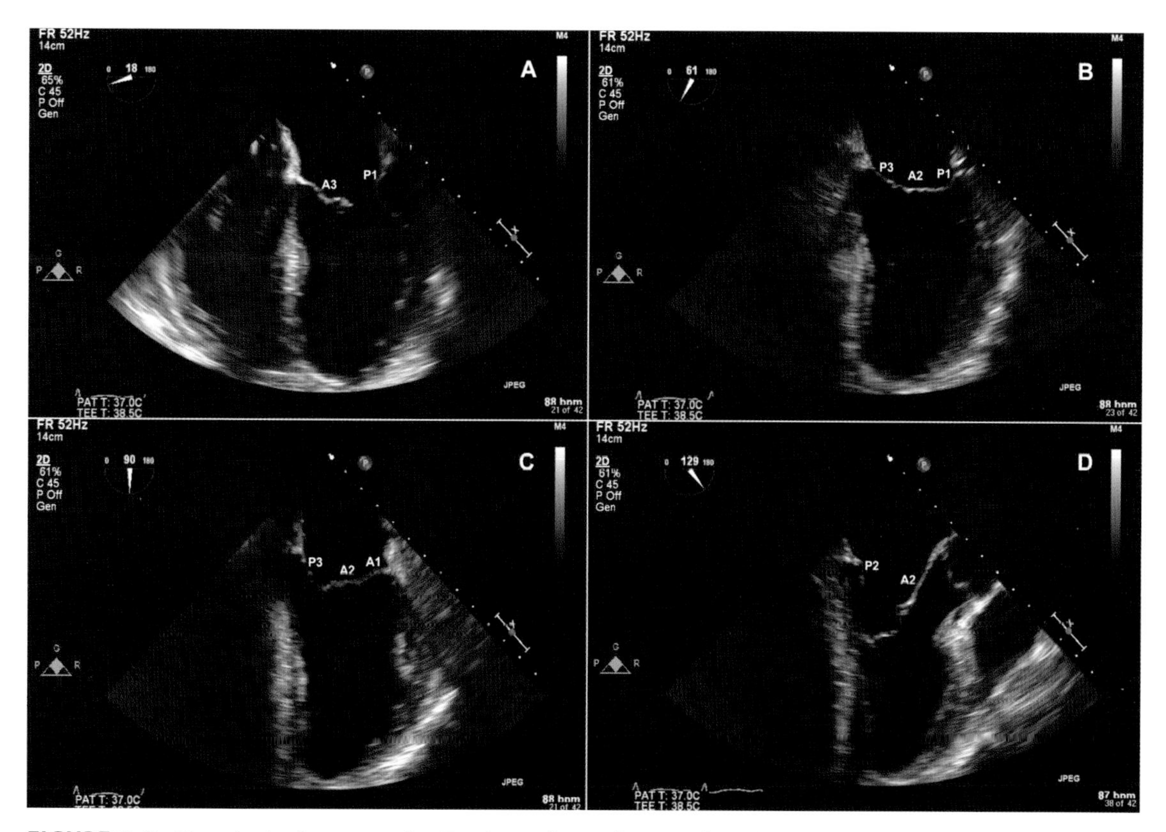

FIGURE 7–2. The mitral valve as seen in 2D echocardiography. **A:** Midesophageal four-chamber view. **B:** Midesophageal mitral commissural view. **C:** Midesophageal two-chamber view. **D:** Midesophageal long-axis view.

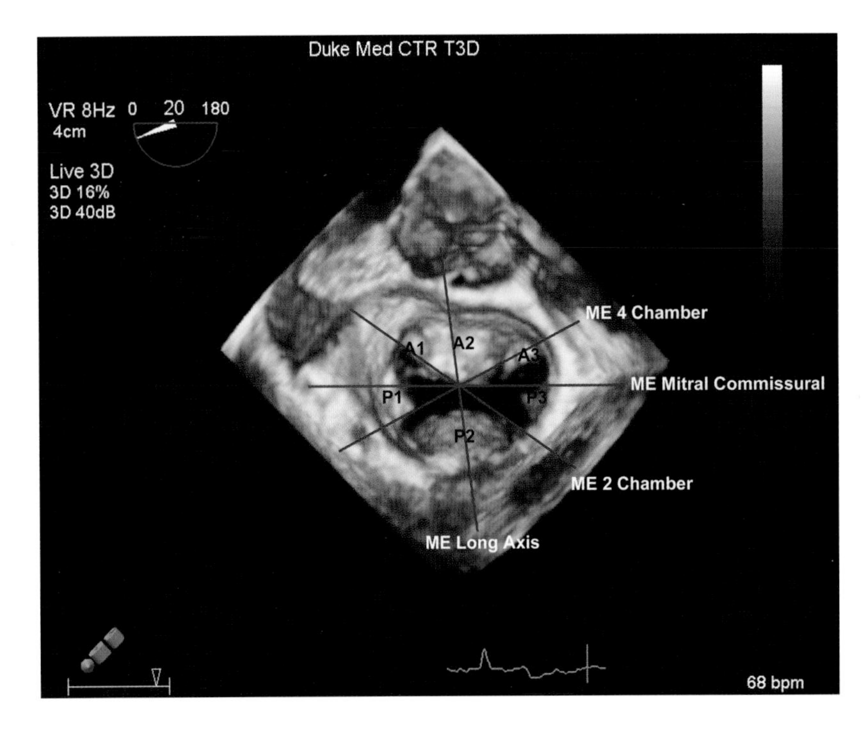

FIGURE 7–3. Three-dimensional image of the mitral valve seen from the left atrium illustrating how the valve is transected by the midesophageal (ME) two-dimensional views.

slightly, the tomographic plane will transect the valve closer to the anterolateral commissure, bringing the left ventricular outflow tract (LVOT) into view, while advancing or retroflexing the probe slightly transects the valve more toward the posteromedial commissure. When the ME 4 CH imaging plane is at 0° (often the five-chamber rather than four-chamber view), the middle part of the aortic leaflet (A2 segment) and the more anterior part of P2 are seen. Any subvalvular or LVOT pathology can be visualized in this view.

Midesophageal Mitral Commissural View (ME COMM)

From the ME 4 CH view, the multiplane angle of the probe is electronically rotated forward to approximately 60°, aligning the tomographic sector with the mitral valvar commissures. In this view, the P1 scallop is viewed to the right of the screen, and the P3 scallop to the left of the image. In the middle will be the A2 segment moving in and out of view as the valve opens and closes (see Figures 7–2 and 7–3). P2 will be behind A2 (into the screen), but is usually not visible unless it is prolapsing. Applying color Doppler imaging to the valve and rotating the probe in small increments allows one to accurately identify the origin of any mitral regurgitation jet.

Midesophageal Two-Chamber View (ME 2 CH)

Further rotation of the multiplane angle to approximately 90° displays this view. Once again, the imaging sector cuts through the mitral valve at an oblique angle relative to the commissures, showing the more anterior parts of the aortic leaflet (A2, A1) to the right of the image and the more posterior parts of the mural leaflet (P3) to the left of the image (see Figures 7–2 and 7–3).

Midesophageal Long-Axis View (ME LAX)

With the multiplane angle between 120° and 140°, the aortic valve should appear in its long axis together with the mitral valve. This imaging plane cuts through the mitral valve perpendicular to the coaptation line, and in diastole clearly demonstrates the aortomitral continuity and the unfolded length/height of A2, together with P2 (see Figures 7–2 and 7–3). Turning the probe to the right will show the more posterior part of the mitral valve (A3/P3), and leftwards the more anterior parts of the mitral valve (A1/P1). Since the midesophageal long-axis view intersects the mitral valve perpendicular to the coaptation line, it is the best view to measure the interpeak distance of the annulus (Figure 7–4) or the diameter of a mitral regurgitant jet vena contracta in systole (Figure 7–5). The left ventricular outflow tract is

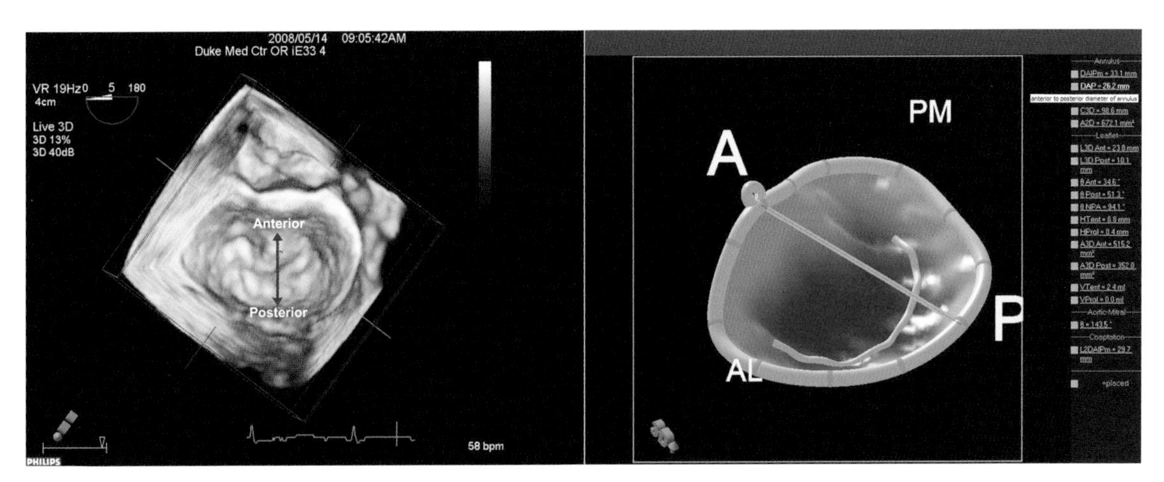

FIGURE 7–4. This 3D animation of the MV annulus (*right*) is reconstructed from a real-time 3D image of the MV (*left*). It demonstrates the anterior-posterior or interpeak distance, which is also measured in the 2D midesophageal long-axis view.

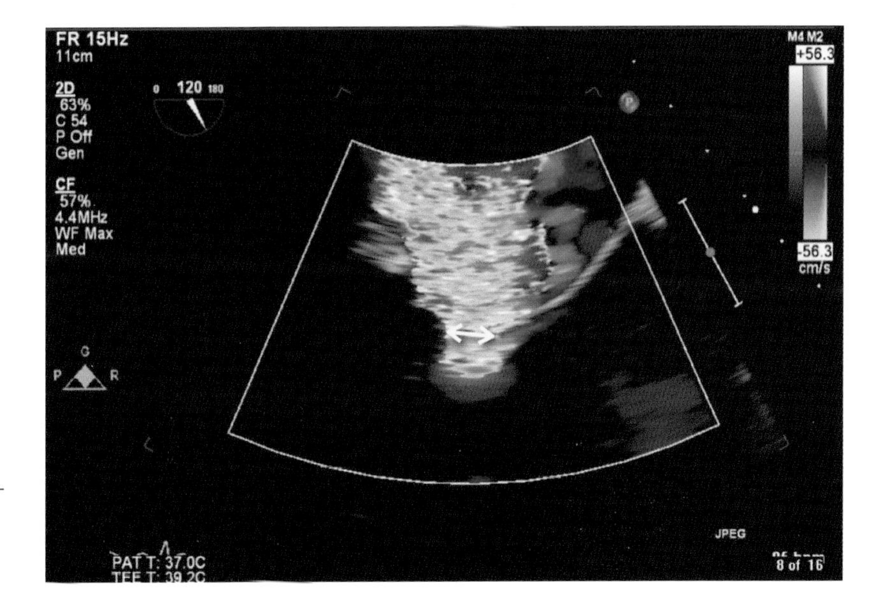

FIGURE 7–5. Midesophageal long-axis view of mitral regurgitation demonstrating where the vena contracta should be measured.

also clearly visualized to assess any subaortic valve or outflow tract pathology.

Transgastric Two-Chamber View (TG 2 CH)

Advancing the probe into the stomach and rotating the multiplane angle forward to approximately 90° demonstrates this view (Figure 7–6). Here, the subvalvar apparatus can be assessed, with the posteromedial papillary muscle in the near field and the anterolateral papillary muscle in the far field. Chordal pathology can also be identified and located.

Transgastric Basal Short-Axis View

From the transgastric two-chamber view, the probe is slowly withdrawn until the mitral valve is in the middle of the image and perpendicular to the tip of the probe.

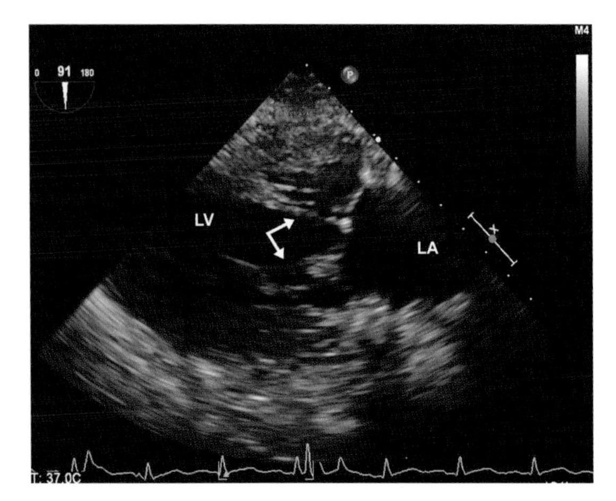

FIGURE 7–6. In the transgastric two-chamber view, the subvalvular apparatus can be readily assessed. In this view, the chordae (*arrows*) are easily seen, and the posteromedial papillary muscle is seen in the near field while the anterolateral papillary muscle is seen in the far field. (LA, left atrium; LV, left ventricle.)

The multiplane angle is reduced to 0°, and the mitral valve will now be seen in short axis. The anterolateral commissure together with A1/P1 will be in the far field and to the right of the image, while the posteromedial commissure and A3/P3 are in the near field and to the left of the image (Figure 7–7). Although quantification of mitral valve pathology with color Doppler is not possible in this view, it is helpful to identify the origin of mitral regurgitation. One should be careful not to confuse the color jet of aortic regurgitation with a color jet originating from mitral regurgitation.

It is important to complete a 2D evaluation of the mitral valve before color Doppler is applied in order to establish mechanisms of mitral valve disease as well as its hemodynamic consequences. Chamber enlargement and indirect signs of pulmonary hypertension are indicators of severe degrees of mitral valve disease, as well as long-standing pathology.

Doppler Assessment

After a comprehensive 2D examination of the valve, color Doppler is applied to all of the midesophageal views. In order to achieve good temporal resolution, it is necessary to keep the two-dimensional and color Doppler sectors as small as possible, but still big enough to include the whole mitral valve area of interrogation. A frame rate of at least 15 frames per second is considered adequate. With color Doppler the presence of mitral regurgitation (in systole) or mitral stenosis (in diastole) can be demonstrated. Pulsed-wave and continuous-wave Doppler should be applied across the valve to quantify the degree of mitral valve disease severity, and will be discussed below under specific headings.

Three-Dimensional Echocardiography

Considerable experience is usually required to mentally integrate a number of two-dimensional views of the mitral valve into a three-dimensional structure and then present a clear description to the surgeon. The recent

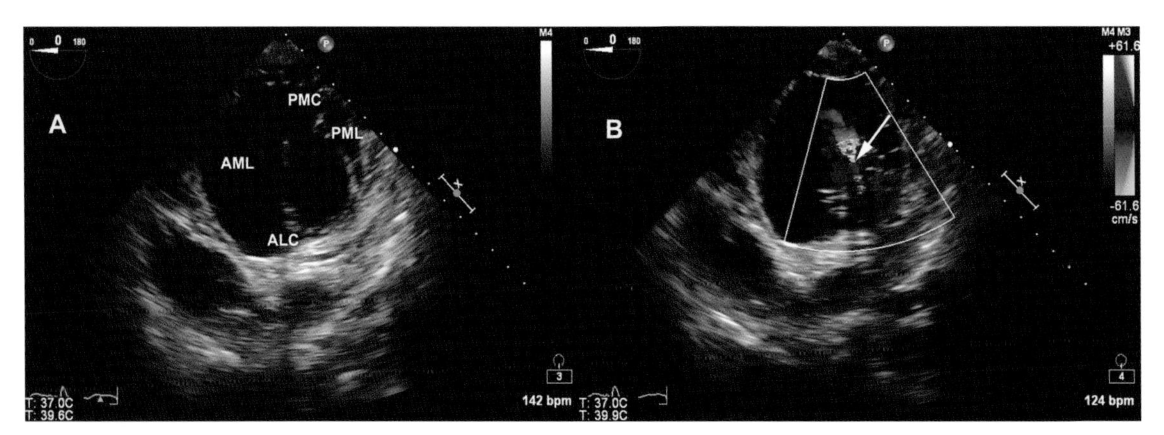

FIGURE 7–7. In the transgastric basal short-axis view **(A)**, the mitral valve is seen with the anterolateral commissure (ALC) in the far field and to the right of the image, while the posteromedial commissure (PMC) is in the near field and to the left of the image. In this patient with a dilated cardiomyopathy, the ventricle is more spherical and a central mitral regurgitant jet (*arrow*) is identified with color Doppler **(B)**. (AML, anterior mitral leaflet; PML, posterior mitral leaflet.)

introduction of real-time three-dimensional (3D) transesophageal echocardiography into clinical practice is proving to add incremental value in localizing and demonstrating mitral valve pathology during repair procedures.[9,10] The spatial and temporal resolution of the currently available matrix array transesophageal transducer allows three-dimensional views of unparalleled quality at acceptable frame rates (see Figure 7–3). A single 3D volume acquisition allows a comprehensive 2D evaluation in any plane extracted from the dataset. It significantly reduces the number of steps required to complete a comprehensive examination of the mitral valve, thus reducing the examination time.[11] The feasibility of intraoperative geometric analysis using integrated 3D mitral valve assessment software has been confirmed, providing much greater quantitative assessment of the mitral valve within the operative environment than has ever been possible.[12] Postoperatively, it also provides excellent views of both bioprosthetic and mechanical valves and annuloplasty rings or bands (see Chapter 24).[13] It is expected that a combined 2D and 3D transesophageal echocardiography examination will in the foreseeable future become routine for preoperative surgical planning and guidance during mitral valve procedures.

MITRAL VALVE PROLAPSE

Mitral valve prolapse (MVP) is characterized by the displacement of an abnormally thickened mitral valve leaflet into the left atrium during systole. Thickening of the mitral leaflets greater than 5 mm and leaflet displacement greater than 2 mm indicates classic MVP. In severe cases of classic MVP, complications include mitral regurgitation, infective endocarditis, congestive heart failure, and in rare circumstances, cardiac arrest, usually resulting in sudden death. Early studies estimated a prevalence of 38% among healthy teenaged males, but with improved echocardiographic techniques and clear diagnostic criteria, the true prevalence of MVP is estimated at 2% to 3% of the population.[14]

MITRAL REGURGITATION

Mitral regurgitation results from the incomplete closure of the mitral valve leaflets during left ventricular systole, resulting in backflow of blood into the left atrium. The amount of backflow will determine the hemodynamic consequences of the mitral regurgitation and appears to be mostly affected by the area of the regurgitant orifice. Other factors that influence the amount of regurgitation include the duration of systole and the pressure gradient between the left ventricle and atrium.

Normal size and function of the left atrium, left ventricle, mitral annulus, and leaflets is required to ensure a competent mitral valve complex. Dysfunction of any of these components can result in mitral regurgitation. Typically, leaflet motion will be altered in a way to prevent adequate coaptation and apposition. A functional classification of mitral regurgitation was proposed by Carpentier in the 1980s,[15] whereby valvular pathology is described in terms of the opening and closing motion of the leaflet (Figure 7–8). This allows a better understanding of the etiology and type of valvular dysfunction. In mitral valve repair, this classification also helps in deciding whether repair is feasible or not and which type of surgical procedure will be best suited for the specific lesion.

Type I lesions are characterized by normal leaflet motion, and mitral regurgitation is caused by annular dilatation or leaflet perforation. The resultant mitral regurgitation jet is usually centrally directed (Figure 7–9A).

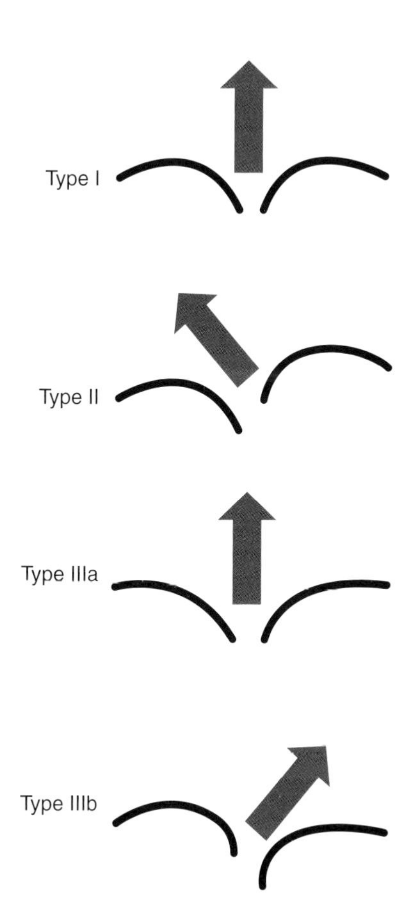

FIGURE 7–8. Schematic representation of the functional classification of mitral incompetence as proposed by Carpentier.

Type II lesions result from increased leaflet motion. This results from elongated or ruptured chordae allowing the affected leaflet to move beyond the coaptation point and level of the annulus. The direction of the mitral regurgitation jet is directed away from the pathological leaflet (Figure 7–9B).

Type III lesions are the result of restricted leaflet motion. This category is differentiated into *type IIIa* and *type IIIb* lesions. In *type IIIa* lesions, leaflet motion is restricted during systole and diastole and is usually the consequence of rheumatic heart disease. This type of mitral regurgitation is seldom seen in isolation as the diastolic restriction causes varying degrees of stenosis as well. The usually eccentric mitral regurgitation jet is more likely to be in the direction of the pathological restricted leaflet (Figure 7–9C). When both leaflets are equally involved in the disease process, the jet may be centrally directed. In *type IIIb* lesions, leaflet motion is restricted during systole and is the result of displacement of either one or both of the papillary muscles, or any segment of the ventricular wall, as found in ischemic mitral regurgitation. The posterior leaflet is typically involved, and the regurgitant

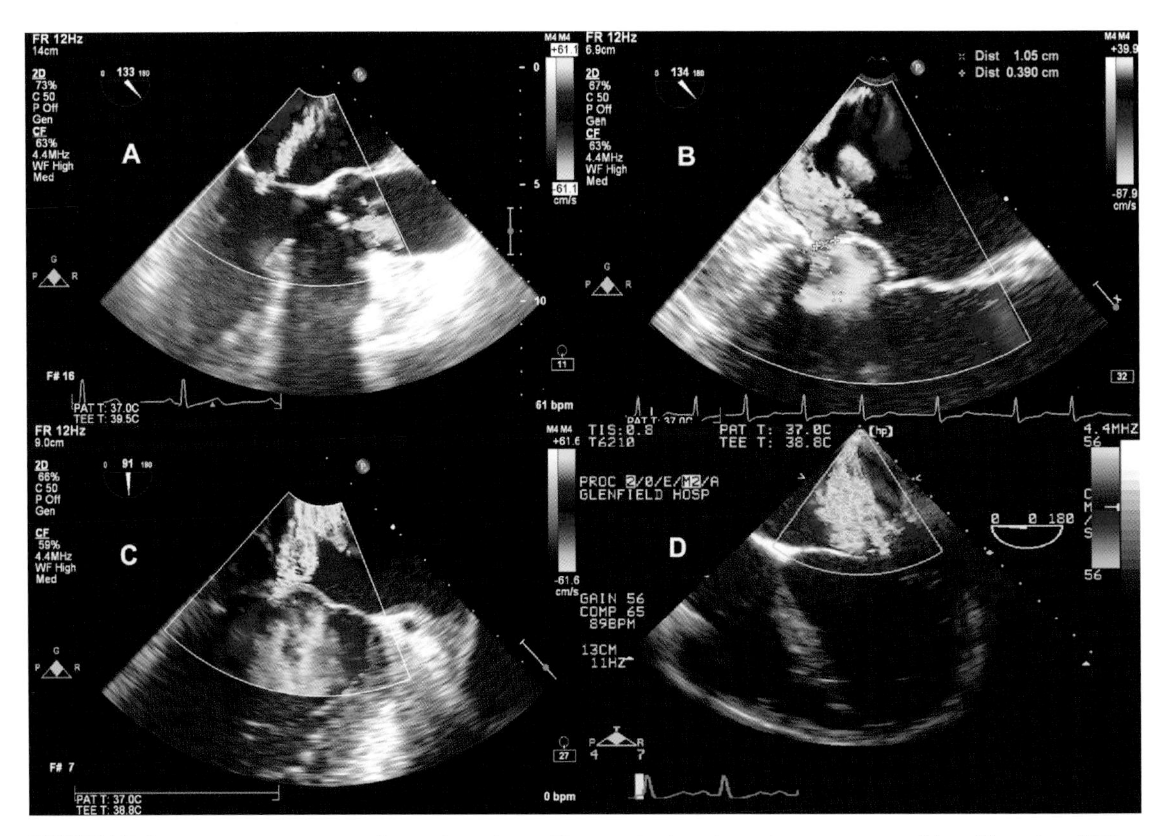

FIGURE 7–9. **A:** Carpentier type I: This midesophageal long-axis view demonstrates a central jet of functional MR because of a high ventricular pressure and annular dilatation, due to concurrent aortic valve stenosis. The MV is morphologically normal. **B:** Carpentier type II: The color Doppler study demonstrates the eccentric incompetence jet directed away from the pathological anterior leaflet in a posterolateral direction. **C:** Carpentier type IIIa: This patient has rheumatic heart disease with movement of the posterior leaflet restricted during systole and diastole. The eccentric regurgitant jet is directed towards the pathological posterior leaflet. **D:** Carpentier type IIIb: This midesophageal four-chamber view demonstrates restricted MV leaflet motion as found with global ventricular dysfunction. Both leaflets are pulled out of position by the chordae and dilated ventricle, leading to tenting and poor coaptation, with a central MR jet.

jet is directed towards the restricted leaflet. It can also be due to a global ventricular dysfunction as found in dilated cardiomyopathy. In this condition both leaflets are tethered and pulled out of position by the chordae and dilated ventricle, leading to tenting and poor coaptation, with the coaptation point displaced into the ventricle (Figure 7–9D). A *type IIIb* lesion is a ventricular problem and the leaflets themselves are not abnormal. *Type IIIb* is also usually accompanied by a dilated annulus.

PATHOLOGY INVOLVED IN MITRAL REGURGITATION

Abnormalities of the Leaflets

Rheumatic heart disease results in thickening and deformation of the mitral leaflets (Figure 7–10) with subsequent insufficient coaptation (almost always associated with mitral stenosis). Infective endocarditis can result in direct destruction of valvar tissue, preventing closure, or even perforation, of the leaflets. Furthermore, the presence of large vegetations can also interfere with proper closure of the valve.

Abnormalities of the Mitral Annulus

The intercommissural annular dimension (intertrough distance) is greater than the dimension measured perpendicular to the mitral coaptation surface (interpeak distance), resulting in an oval-shaped mitral annulus. Furthermore, the inferolateral mitral annulus is almost devoid of fibrous support and is the area most likely to be involved in annular dilatation. Thus, when annular dilatation occurs, the ratio of interpeak to intertrough distance is altered. The result is an inability of the mitral leaflets to coapt sufficiently to prevent the backflow of blood to the left atrium during systole.

Annular calcification can also result in improper leaflet motion and subsequent mitral regurgitation. Degenerative calcification is accelerated by conditions such as systemic hypertension, aortic stenosis, and diabetes. Intrinsic abnormalities of the fibrous skeleton of the heart, such as is found in patients with Marfan and Hurler syndromes, as well as other connective tissue diseases, may result in accelerated calcification as well as annular dilatation. Patients with hyperparathyroidism secondary to renal disease may suffer from early calcification of the mitral annulus. Annular calcification can also result in mitral stenosis, and mixed valvular disease is common.

The presence of mitral regurgitation of hemodynamic significance results in a volume overload of the left ventricle with subsequent dilatation. During systole this ventricle offloads into the left atrium and therefore experiences a falsely low afterload, resulting in apparent hyperdynamic ventricular function. Ventricular dilatation is often accompanied by mitral annular dilatation, which is a compounding factor in other mechanisms of mitral regurgitation.[16] For this reason one will often hear that "mitral valve regurgitation begets mitral valve regurgitation."

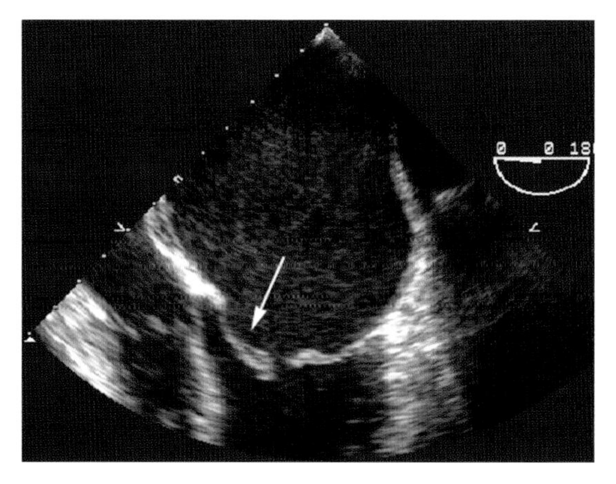

FIGURE 7–10. Mitral stenosis due to rheumatic heart disease showing doming (*arrow*) of the anterior leaflet of the mitral valve.

Abnormalities of the Chordae Tendineae

Disruption of chordae leads to excessive motion of the involved mitral leaflet and subsequent regurgitation. This typically presents as a flail leaflet with rather sudden onset of symptoms. Ruptured chordae can result from infective endocarditis, chest trauma, and fibroelastic deficiency of mitral valve tissue. Mitral regurgitation secondary to chord rupture is more likely to be severe (Figure 7–11). Prolongation of the chordae, as occurs in myxomatous degeneration of the mitral valve, results in prolapse of the affected leaflet (Figure 7–12). The onset of symptoms in these patients is typically gradual over time. Certain diseases can result in fibrosis and shortening of the chordae. The result is retraction of the mitral valve leaflets from the coaptation point and restricted motion of leaflets. This typically occurs in rheumatic heart disease where the chordal involvement can be severe.

Abnormalities of the Papillary Muscles

The posteromedial papillary muscle is more prone to ischemic events, as blood is supplied by the terminal part of a single coronary artery in the majority of

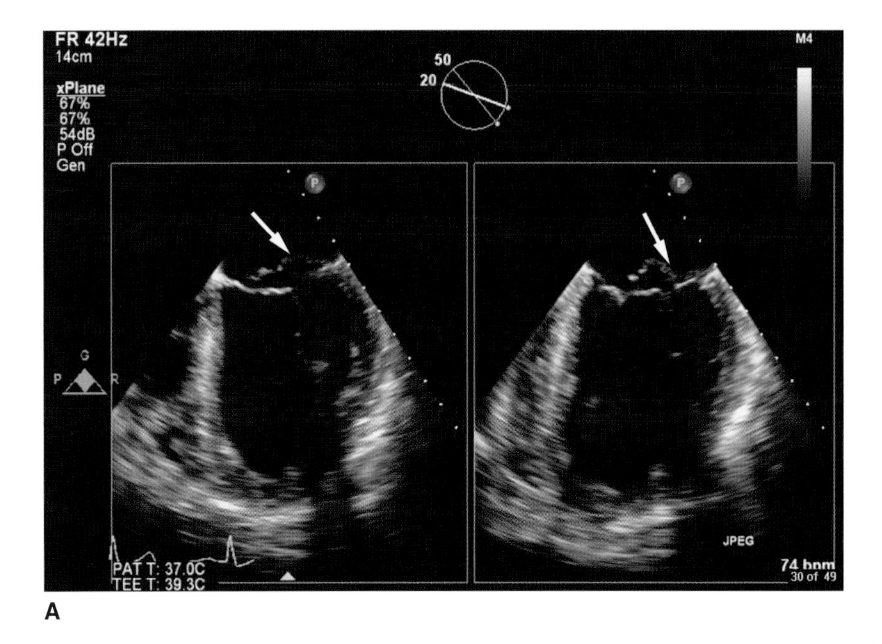

A

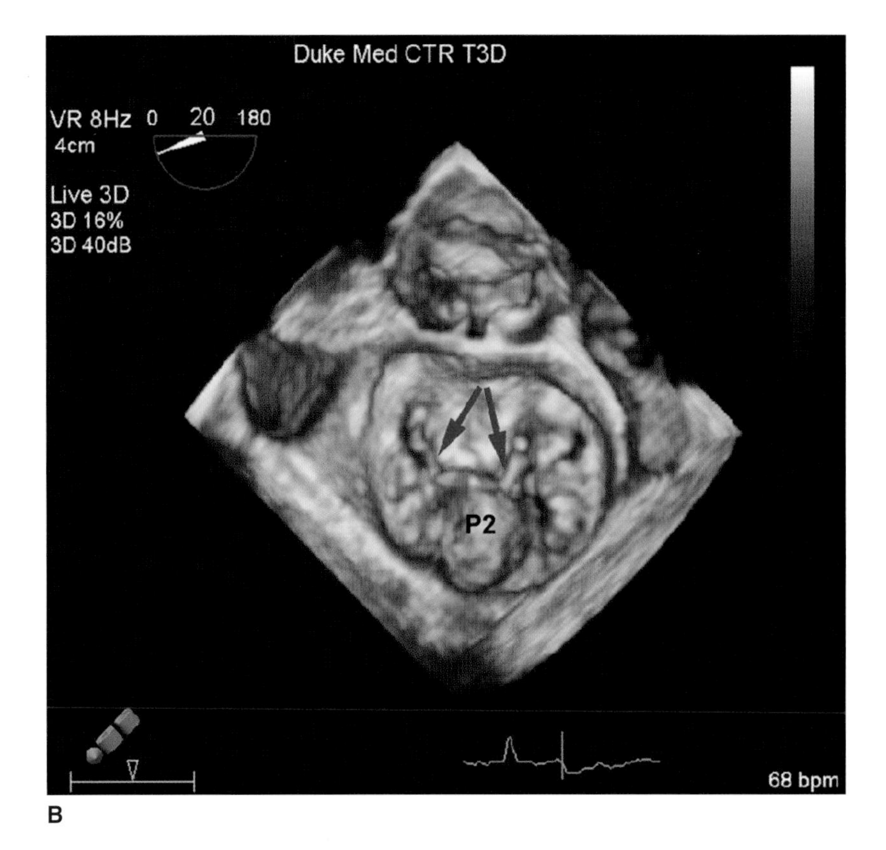

B

FIGURE 7–11. Flail (*arrows*) P2 leaflet seen with **(A)** 2D and **(B)** 3D imaging.

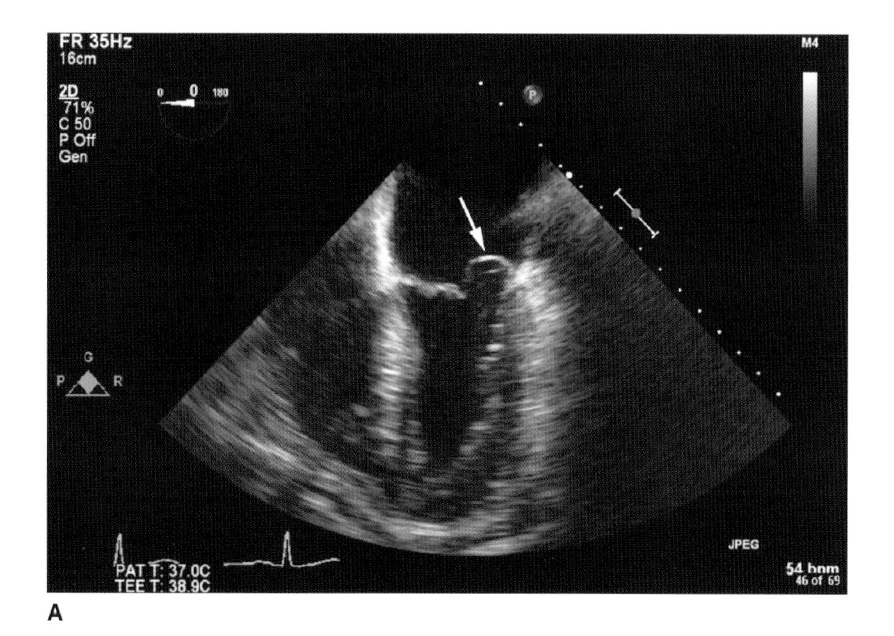

A

B

FIGURE 7–12. Prolapsing (*arrows*) P2 leaflet seen with **(A)** 2D and **(B)** 3D imaging.

patients.[6] Necrosis of the papillary muscle after myocardial infarction is not uncommon, but acute rupture is a rare occurrence. Ischemic dysfunction of the papillary muscle can result in inadequate leaflet coaptation with mitral regurgitation. Alteration in the papillary muscle structure or its spatial relation to the rest of the mitral valve apparatus, such as occurs in ventricular dilation and remodeling, can also result in restricted motion of especially the posterior leaflet.

Abnormal Left Ventricular Function and Structure

Ventricular dilatation alters the orientation of the papillary muscle relative to the valvular apparatus (Figure 7–13). The chordae arising from the inferolateral free wall to the posterior mitral leaflet is also pulled down, and subsequent tethering of especially the posterior leaflet occurs. This commonly occurs in ventricular dilation secondary to ischemia or dilated cardiomyopathy. Asymmetric hypertrophy of the left ventricle with dynamic left ventricular outflow tract obstruction can also result in mitral regurgitation. Flow phenomena caused by forceful left ventricular ejection through a narrowed left ventricular outflow tract results in systolic anterior motion of the anterior mitral valve leaflet with inadequate coaptation (Figure 7–14).

As evident from the mechanisms discussed above, it is important to assess all parts of the mitral valvar apparatus as more than one mechanism of regurgitation can be present at the same time.

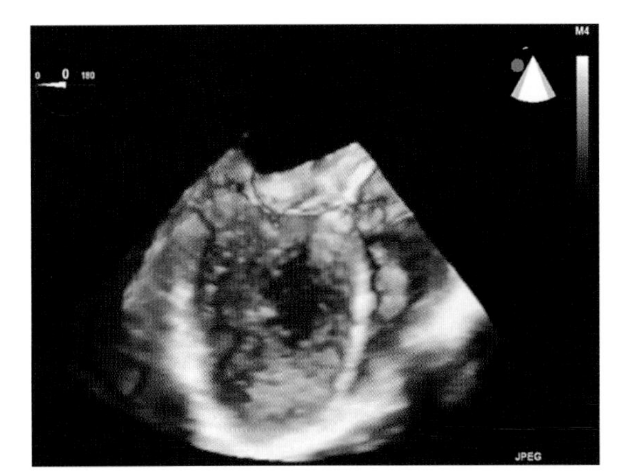

FIGURE 7–13. This cropped 3D dataset demonstrates the tethering of the subvalvular apparatus (especially on the inferolateral side) due to a globally dilated left ventricle.

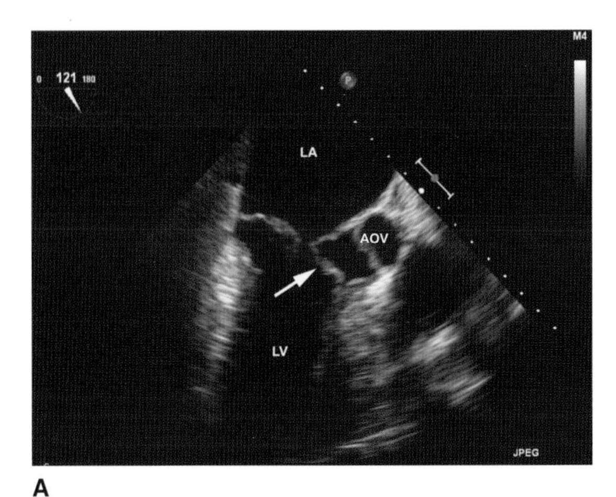

A

B

FIGURE 7–14. **A:** This midesophageal long-axis view shows asymmetric hypertrophy of the left ventricular outflow tract with dynamic obstruction. Systolic anterior motion of the anterior mitral valve leaflet (*arrow*) leads to inadequate coaptation and subsequent mitral regurgitation. The color Doppler image **(B)** shows turbulence in the left ventricular outflow tract (LVOT) and a dynamic mitral regurgitation jet (*arrow*). (LA, left atrium; LV, left ventricle; AOV, aortic valve.)

GRADING THE SEVERITY OF MITRAL REGURGITATION

Two-Dimensional Imaging

Dysfunction of any of the components of the mitral valve apparatus can result in mitral regurgitation and should prompt a comprehensive 2D evaluation of the valve. When mitral valve disease is to be addressed by means of surgery, the 2D evaluation of the mechanism of pathology plays an important role in deciding whether either valve repair or replacement is indicated, and in the case of repair, which technique will be more appropriate.[17] Mitral regurgitation results in volume overload of the left-sided cardiac chambers with subsequent dilatation.[18] The right ventricle and atrium may also be affected secondary to the development of pulmonary hypertension. Chamber dilatation is usually seen in long-standing hemodynamic significant mitral regurgitation, but might not be present in the case of sudden-onset severe mitral regurgitation. When mitral valve morphology is abnormal on 2D examination, the chances of dealing with a more severe degree of mitral regurgitation are much greater than when the valve appears normal. Indications of more severe mitral regurgitation on 2D evaluation include flail leaflets such as in chordal or papillary muscle rupture, severe prolapse as in myxomatous degeneration of the valve, leaflet perforation, or the presence of leaflet tenting with a large coaptation defect.

Doppler Imaging

Color-Flow Doppler

With the aliasing velocity set to between 50 and 60 cm/s and the color gain settings adjusted to eliminate noise, a midesophageal four chamber view is obtained. Position the color Doppler sector to include the whole of the mitral valve. If mitral regurgitation appears to be present, reduce the size of the Doppler sector to the smallest size that still includes the entire mitral regurgitation jet. This will help to improve temporal resolution by increasing frame rate. After recording a number of cardiac cycles, scroll back and forth and identify the frame where the jet area appears at its biggest. Using the trace function, planimeter the surface area of the regurgitant jet and the surface area of the left atrium. Keep in mind that only the mosaic area of the regurgitation jet should be included when determining jet area. For grading of mitral regurgitation using jet area, see Table 7–1.

In the case of eccentric jets, the greatest surface area may fall outside the tomographic plain imaged and may result in underestimation of the severity of mitral regurgitation. Eccentric wall-hugging jets (Coanda effect) also lead to underestimation of the severity of mitral regurgitation. On the other hand, conditions that cause excessive pressures in the left ventricle such as severe systemic hypertension and aortic stenosis can lead to overestimation of mitral regurgitation due to a very high-velocity jet extending far into the left atrium. For these reasons, it is recommended that jet area not be used as the sole method for quantification of mitral regurgitation.[19]

Vena Contracta[20]

Visualize the mitral valve in the ME LAX view and zoom in to optimize image size. With the aliasing velocity (Nyquist limit) set to between 50 and 60 cm/s and color gain settings adjusted to reduce background noise, position the color Doppler sector over the mitral valve and visualize the regurgitant jet. When the tomographic plane is aligned with the regurgitant orifice, color Doppler should display an area of systolic flow convergence proximal to the valve, a color jet into the left atrium, and a narrow neck of color as the jet passes through the regurgitant orifice. This narrowest part as it *emerges* from the coaptation site of the leaflets is referred to as vena contracta, and its width, measured perpendicular to the direction of regurgitation, correlates well with mitral regurgitation severity determined by means of regurgitant volume and effective regurgitant orifice area. The maximal diameter during any portion of systole is recorded (Figure 7–15). Once again, the color Doppler sector should be kept as small as possible to obtain maximal temporal resolution. Measurement of the vena contracta should be made perpendicular to the coaptation line formed by the anterior and posterior leaflets in order to avoid a false increase in vena contracta from a tangential imaging plane. Thus, the midesophageal long-axis view, which transects the mitral valve perpendicular to the line of coaptation, is the optimal view to measure vena contracta. Repeating the measurement over several cardiac cycles will also increase the accuracy of this method. Vena contracta was proposed to be a load-independent measure of mitral regurgitation, but subsequent data have proven that alterations in afterload can affect the apparent severity in an unpredictable fashion.[21] It is therefore recommended that hemodynamic parameters be adjusted during measurement to approximate awake conditions.

Regurgitant Volume, Regurgitant Fraction, and Effective Regurgitant Orifice Area

Flow across an incompetent valve is always greater than the effective forward stroke volume. In mitral regurgitation, the difference between forward stroke volume and flow across the mitral valve is equal to regurgitant volume. The effective forward stroke volume can be measured in the left ventricular outflow tract or across the pulmonic valve in the absence of significant regurgitation of the aortic or pulmonic valves.

$$\mathrm{RVol}_{\mathrm{Mitral}} = \mathrm{SV}_{\mathrm{MV}} - \mathrm{SV}_{\mathrm{LVOT}}$$

$$\mathrm{SV}_{\mathrm{MV}} = \text{MV Annulus Area} \times \mathrm{VTI}_{\mathrm{MV}}$$

(at the level of the MV annulus)

Table 7–1. Parameters for the determination of the severity of mitral regurgitation.

	Mild	Moderate	Severe
Structural Parameters			
LA size	Normal[a]	Normal or dilated	Usually dilated[b]
LV size	Normal[a]	Normal or dilated	Usually dilated[b]
Mitral leaflets or support apparatus	Normal or abnormal	Normal or abnormal	Abnormal or flail leaflet, or ruptured papillary muscle
Doppler Parameters			
Color flow jet area[c]	Small, central jet (usually <4 cm^2 or <20% of LA area)	Variable	Large central jet (usually >10 cm^2 or >40% of LA or variable size wall-impinging jet swirling in LA
Mitral inflow: PWD	A-wave dominant[d]	Variable	E-wave dominant[d] (E usually >1.2 m/s)
Jet density: CWD	Incomplete or faint	Dense	Dense
Jet contour: CWD	Parabolic	Usually parabolic	Early peaking, triangular
Pulmonary vein flow	Systolic dominance	Systolic blunting[e]	Systolic flow reversal[f]
Quantitative Parameters[g]			
VC width (cm)	<0.3	0.3-0.69	≥0.7
RVol (mL/beat)	<30	30-44/45-59	≥60
RF (%)	<30	30-39/40-49	≥50
EROA (cm^2)	<0.20	0.20-0.29/0.30-0.39	≥0.40

[a]Unless there were other reasons for LA or LV dilation.
[b]An exception is acute mitral regurgitation.
[c]At a Nyquist limit of 50 to 60 cm/s.
[d]Usually in patients older than 50 years or in conditions of impaired relaxation, in the absence of mitral stenosis or other causes of elevated LA pressure.
[e]Unless other reasons for systolic blunting (eg, atrial fibrillation or elevated left atrial pressure).
[f]Pulmonary venous systolic flow reversal is specific but not sensitive for severe mitral regurgitation.
[g]Quantitative parameters can help subclassify the moderate regurgitation group into mild-to-moderate and moderate-to-severe groups as shown.
CWD, continuous-wave Doppler; LA, left atrial; ERO, effective regurgitant orifice area; LV, left ventricular; PWD, pulsed-wave Doppler; RF, regurgitant fraction; RVol, regurgitant volume; VC, vena contracta.
Source: Zoghbi WA, Enriquez-Sarano M, Foster E, et al. Recommendations for evaluation of the severity of native valvular regurgitation with two-dimensional and Doppler echocardiography. *J Am Soc Echocardiogr.* 2003;16:777.

and

$$\text{MV Annulus Area} = \pi r^2$$

or, more practically,

$$(\text{Mitral Annulus Diameter})^2 \times 0.785$$

Another method used to calculate the MV annulus area is based on the fact that the mitral valve annulus is elliptical in shape rather than circular. Determination of the area requires that 2 measurements of the mitral annulus are made in perpendicular planes in mid-diastole:

$$\text{MV Annulus Area} = \pi/4 \times AB$$

A = annular diameter in one plane (cm)

B = annular diameter in a plane perpendicular to plane A (cm)

$$SV_{LVOT} = \text{LVOT Area} \times VTI_{LVOT}$$

and

$$\text{LVOT Area} = \pi r^2$$

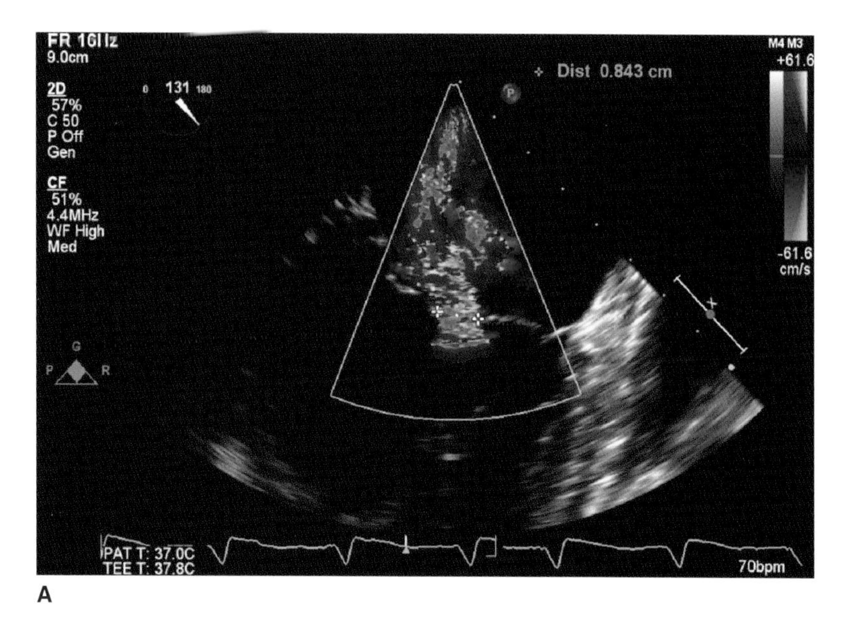

A

B

FIGURE 7–15. Vena contracta seen with two-dimensional **(A)** and three-dimensional **(B)** imaging. In the 3D image, the *en face* view (*right panel*) revealed a wider vena contracta than that seen with 2D imaging.

or, more practically,

$$(\text{LVOT Diameter})^2 \times 0.785$$

$$RF_{Mitral} = \frac{RVol_{Mitral}}{SV_{Mitral}} \times 100$$

$$EROA_{Mitral} = \frac{RVol_{Mitral}}{\text{VTI of the MR Jet}}$$

Where SV = Stroke volume
MV = Mitral valve
LVOT = Left ventricular outflow tract
VTI = Velocity-time integral

RF = Regurgitant fraction
RVol = Regurgitant volume
EROA = Effective regurgitant orifice area
MR = Mitral regurgitation

The result must be carefully interpreted because a small operator error in measurement will have a major impact on the squared calculation. For quantitative parameters of mitral regurgitation as determined through the above formulae, refer to Table 7–1.

PROXIMAL ISOVELOCITY SURFACE AREA (PISA)[22]

In mitral regurgitation, flow accelerates when approaching the regurgitant orifice. This results in concentric hemispheric shells of increasing velocity as the valve is approached. The area of one such hemisphere is referred to as proximal isovelocity surface area (Figure 7–16). By applying color Doppler to the mitral valve in the midesophageal views, the regurgitant jet can be displayed. As determined by convention, flow towards the mitral valve in the ME LAX view will be displayed as differing intensities of red. When the Nyquist limit is reached, as invariably happens with high velocities achieved in mitral regurgitation, the direction of flow apparently reverses, a phenomenon referred to as aliasing. This apparent reversal is not a true reversal, but rather an inability to measure high velocities. By adjusting the baseline of the color Doppler scale upwards (in the direction of regurgitant flow), the velocity at which aliasing will occur can be adjusted in order to alter the radius of the aliasing hemisphere. It is recommended that the color Doppler baseline be adjusted in order to achieve an aliasing contour with a radius of 11 to 15 mm. Smaller radii result in flattening of the aliasing hemisphere and larger radii result in a cone-shaped aliasing contour.[23] The radius of the hemisphere should be measured from the narrowest part of the jet to the contour where aliasing occurs first, and the velocity of blood at the aliasing contour is obtained from the top of the color Doppler scale (see Figure 7–16). The area of the hemisphere is then calculated with the following formula:

$$\text{Surface Area of Hemisphere (cm}^2) = 2\pi r^2$$

where π = 3.14 and r is the radius of the aliasing contour, measured from the narrowest part of the color jet.

The flow at the surface area where aliasing occurs can then be calculated using the following formula:

$$2\pi r^2 \times V_a$$

where V_a is aliasing velocity from the top of the color legend.

The maximal isovelocity surface area should occur at the instant of maximal velocity through the regurgitant orifice. This can be measured by applying continuous-wave Doppler to the regurgitant jet and measuring the peak velocity (Figure 7–17). The principle of conservation of mass states that flow in a closed system should be equal at all points; therefore, flow rate at the effective regurgitant orifice area (EROA) should equal the flow

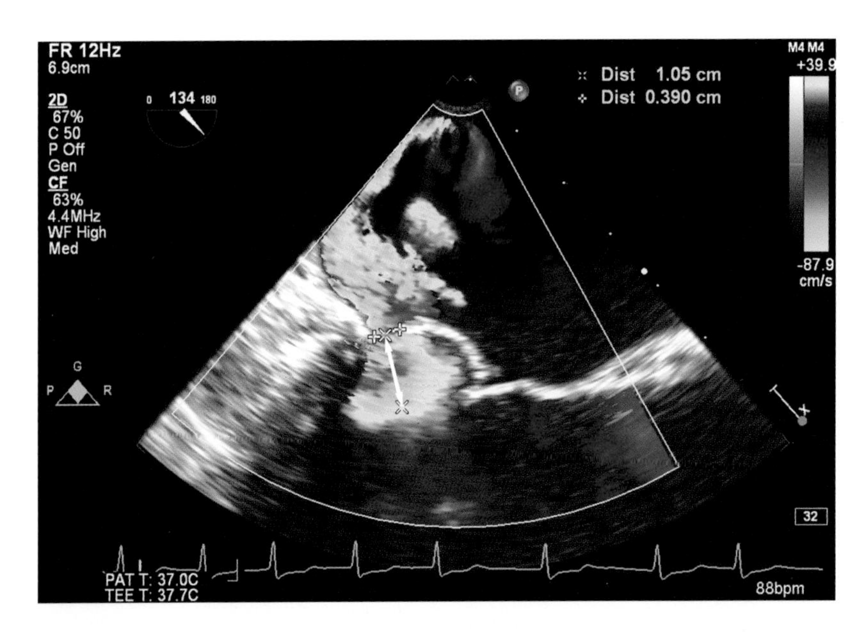

FIGURE 7–16. Flow acceleration in the region proximal to a regurgitant orifice forming concentric hemispheres of increasing velocity. The radius of the hemisphere should be measured from the narrowest part of the jet to the contour where aliasing occurs.

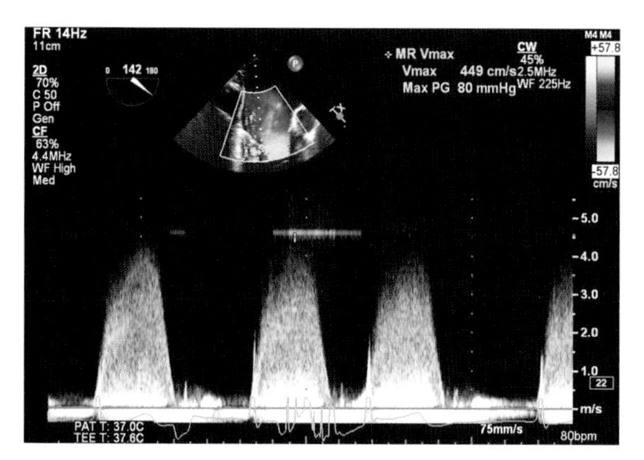

FIGURE 7–17. The maximal systolic velocity through the regurgitant orifice can be measured by applying continuous-wave Doppler to the regurgitant jet. Together with the area of the PISA hemisphere, it is used to calculate the effective regurgitant orifice area and subsequently the regurgitant volume.

rate at any given isovelocity surface area. Thus, the effective regurgitant orifice area can be calculated by the following equation:

$$\text{PISA} \times V_a = \text{EROA} \times V_{max}$$

$$\text{EROA} = \frac{2\pi r^2 \times V_a}{V_{max}}$$

where r is the radius of the first contour of aliasing, V_a is the aliasing velocity, EROA is the effective regurgitant orifice area, and V_{max} is the maximal regurgitant velocity obtained with continuous-wave (CW) Doppler.

Once the effective regurgitant orifice area has been determined, regurgitant volume can also be calculated by using the velocity time integral of the mitral valve regurgitant jet.

$$R_{Vol} = \text{EROA} \times \text{VTI}_{\text{Mitral Regurgitant Jet}}$$

where R_{Vol} is the regurgitant volume and $\text{VTI}_{\text{Mitral Regurgitant Jet}}$ is the velocity-time integral of the mitral regurgitant jet as measured with CW Doppler trace.

The examiner should keep in mind that the proximal isovelocity surface area method assumes a flat surface area proximal to the regurgitant orifice. In the case of an angled ventricular surface area of the mitral valve, a correction factor should be used to improve the accuracy of this method. The effective regurgitant orifice area should be multiplied by $\alpha/180$, where α is the angle of the proximal converging surfaces (Figure 7–18).

In spite of relatively low frame rates, 3D color Doppler imaging allows for a more accurate determination of the proximal isovelocity surface area (Figure 7–19).[24] For instance, in functional mitral regurgitation the proximal isovelocity surface area is not hemispherical but a hemiellipsoid. Three-dimensional color Doppler may avoid underestimation of severity of mitral disease using the proximal isovelocity surface area method.

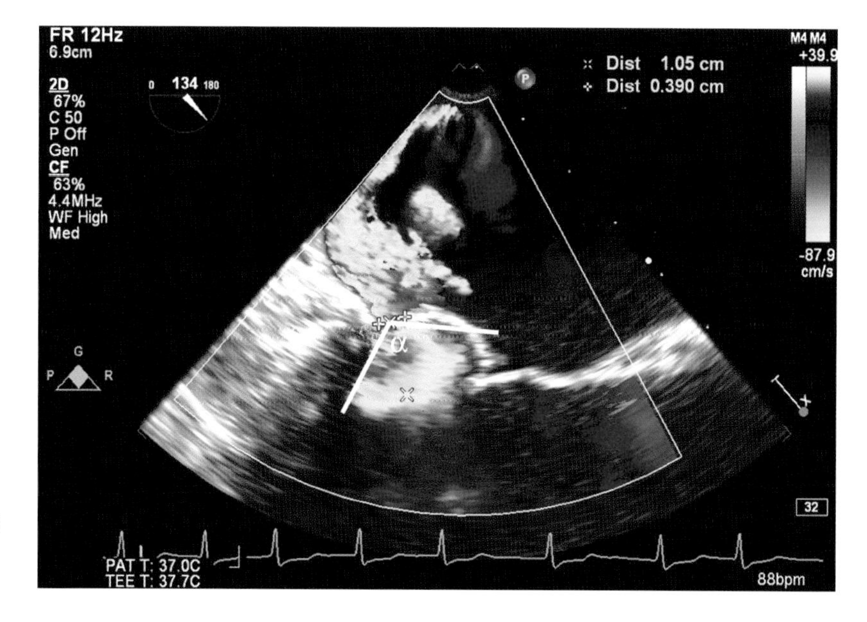

FIGURE 7–18. Image demonstrating the determination of the angle α in a patient with a regurgitant jet that has eccentric convergence.

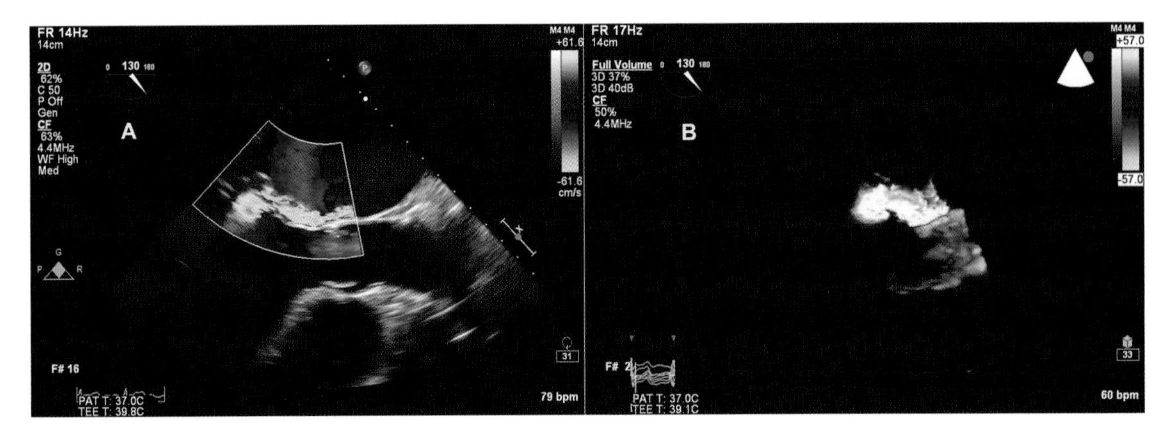

FIGURE 7–19. Two-dimensional **(A)** and three-dimesional **(B)** imaging of the proximal isovelocity surface area. Three-dimensional color Doppler imaging allows for a more accurate determination of the proximal isovelocity surface area and avoids underestimation of EROA and regurgitant volume.

Pulmonary Venous Flow Patterns

Pulsed-wave (PW) Doppler can be used to assess pulmonary venous flow patterns in order to quantify mitral valve regurgitation. In order to visualize the left upper pulmonary vein, the probe is pulled back and turned to the left from the midesophageal four-chamber view until the left atrial appendage is observed. The left upper pulmonary vein will be superior and posterior to the left atrial appendage, and parallel alignment for Doppler analysis could be optimized by rotating the multiplane angle forward to between 20° and 60°. The right upper pulmonary vein can be visualized by obtaining the bicaval view and then rotating the probe towards the right, beyond the aortic root. Slight withdrawal of the probe will allow visualization of the right upper pulmonary vein. Placement of the color Doppler cursor over the pulmonary veins showing flow predominantly towards the probe will help to correctly identify these vessels. Pulmonary venous flow patterns are obtained by placing the cursor of the pulsed-wave Doppler approximately 1 cm into the pulmonary vein under interrogation.

A normal pulmonary venous flow pattern has a large forward systolic component (S-wave), a slightly smaller forward diastolic component (D-wave), and a small reversed component (A-wave) caused by atrial contraction. Should reversal of the systolic component occur, severe mitral regurgitation can be diagnosed with a specificity of 100% and sensitivity of 90% (Figure 7–20).[25] However, systolic blunting of flow (S < D), as seen with atrial fibrillation or diastolic dysfunction, is diagnostic only of an elevation in left atrial pressure.[26] In the case of severe eccentric mitral regurgitation, the wall-hugging jet may cause systolic flow reversal in only some of the pulmonary veins. It is therefore important to assess pulmonary venous flow in both left- and right-sided pulmonary veins.

Other Doppler Measures for Determining MR Severity

Pulsed-wave Doppler assessment of transmitral inflow patterns can also aid in the grading of mitral regurgitation. In the midesophageal four-chamber view, the

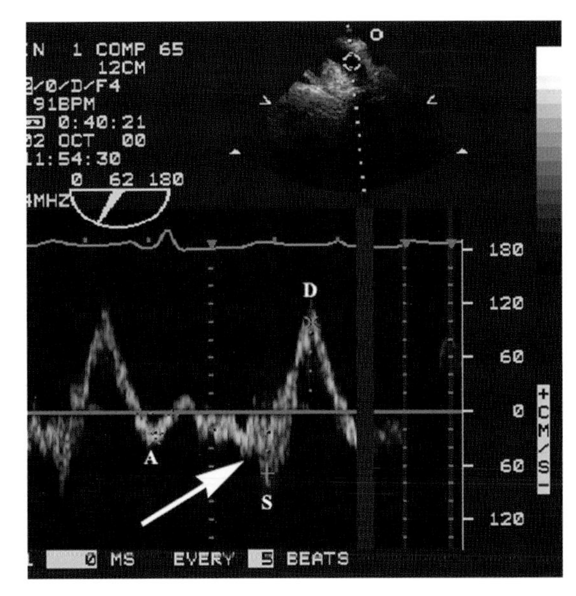

FIGURE 7–20. Pulsed-wave Doppler interrogation of pulmonary venous flow exhibiting systolic reversal *(arrow)* in a patient with severe mitral regurgitation. (A, atrial contraction flow; S, systolic flow; D, diastolic flow.)

pulsed-wave Doppler cursor should be positioned at the level of the leaflet tips during ventricular filling. A spectral Doppler trace of the transmitral inflow pattern should then be recorded. Large regurgitant volumes such as in severe mitral regurgitation result in increased left atrial pressures at the end of systole. The subsequent high diastolic gradient between left atrium and left ventricle results in an E-wave dominant inflow pattern, with the E-wave velocity typically exceeding 1.2 m/s.[27,28] In the case of the transmitral inflow pattern being dominated by the A-wave, severe mitral regurgitation can be excluded.[28]

Continuous-wave (CW) Doppler interrogation of the mitral regurgitant jet also contributes to the grading of mitral regurgitation. The normal spectral Doppler trace of lesser degrees of mitral regurgitation is parabolic in shape and follows the pressure gradient between the left ventricle and left atrium during systole. Large regurgitant volumes result in a rise in the left atrial pressure during systole and also results in an inability of the left ventricle to achieve normal peak systolic pressures. The resultant decrease in pressure gradient between the left ventricle and atrium causes an early peaking, truncated spectral Doppler trace seen in severe mitral regurgitation (Figure 7–21). The quality of spectral Doppler trace is also helpful. In mild mitral regurgitation the jet is faint, but in severe mitral regurgitation a very dense spectral Doppler trace can be obtained. A faint trace results from small numbers of red blood cells passing through the regurgitant orifice, but large regurgitant volumes cause a dense representation of the jet.[27]

When grading mitral regurgitation with TEE under general anesthesia, one should consider the effect of altered loading conditions on the circulation and the effect it will have on the indices used to grade mitral regurgitation. Reduction in ventricular filling, systemic vascular resistance, and blood pressure typically occurs in anesthetized patients and can decrease the apparent degree of mitral regurgitation compared to preoperative assessments. In order to gain more reliable information it may be necessary to simulate awake loading conditions by maintaining preload or increasing afterload through the administration of a vasopressor.[29] Cancellation of mitral valve surgery based on intraoperative findings after preoperative assessment indicated a need for surgery should therefore be made with great caution.

MITRAL STENOSIS

The normal mitral valve area is 4 to 5 cm^2. Reduction of the mitral valve area to less than 2.5 cm^2 requires an increase in the atrioventricular pressure gradient to maintain an adequate cardiac output and often marks the onset of symptoms during exercise.[30] An increase in left atrial pressure results in atrial enlargement and eventually the onset of atrial dysrhythmias, uaually atrial fibrillation.[31] New-onset atrial fibrillation typically leads to an acute worsening of symptoms as a result of loss of atrial contribution to left ventricular filling and the rapid ventricular rates. Elevated left atrial pressures also result in pulmonary hypertension and eventually alterations in right ventricular function and tricuspid regurgitation.[32] As mitral stenosis progresses further, the presence of low cardiac output and atrial fibrillation is a common cause of left atrial thrombi and embolic events (Figure 7–22). Echocardiographic evaluation of patients with mitral stenosis should therefore aim to exclude the presence of intracardiac thrombi, especially when there is a history of embolic events.[33] In rheumatic mitral stenosis, left ventricular function can

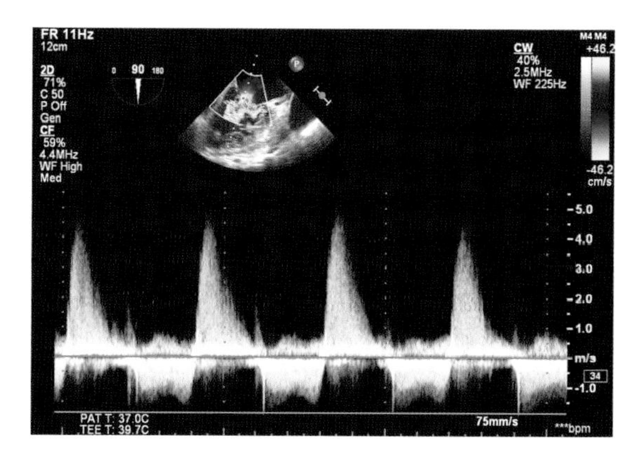

FIGURE 7–21. The continuous-wave Doppler trace contributes to the grading of mitral regurgitation. A large regurgitant volume results in this dense jet pattern which is early peaking and truncated.

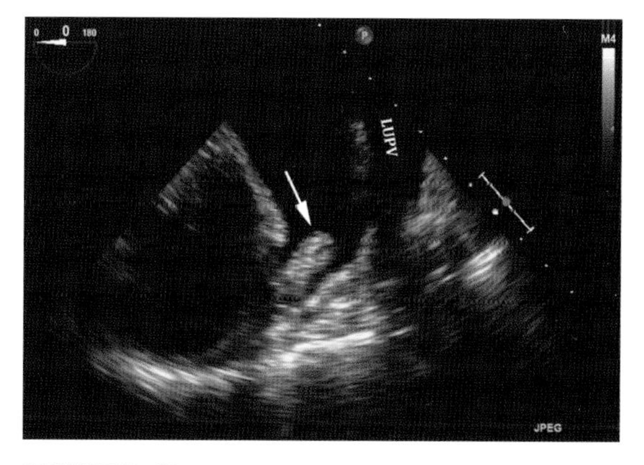

FIGURE 7–22. A thrombus (*arrow*) in the left atrial appendage. (LUPV, left upper pulmonary vein.)

be reduced secondary to scarring of the basal inferolateral wall of the ventricle and by impaired diastolic function in patients with pulmonary hypertension as a consequence of septal displacement.[34] Acute attacks of rheumatic heart disease can result in a pancarditis with subsequent ventricular dysfunction.

ETIOLOGY

The most common cause of mitral stenosis is rheumatic heart disease.[35] Progressive inflammatory reaction in valve tissue results in thickening of the leaflet tips and fusion of anterior and posterior leaflets in the commissural areas, with subsequent reduction in valve opening. In long-standing rheumatic heart disease or after recurrent episodes, varying degrees of thickening and calcification of the leaflet bodies and bases can also occur. Chordae tendineae are typically thickened and shortened, leading to reduced movement of the mitral leaflets. Mitral regurgitation commonly occurs with rheumatic mitral stenosis.

Degenerative calcification of the mitral annulus is a rare cause of mitral stenosis and mostly occurs in the presence of other diseases that accelerate calcification. These diseases include certain connective tissue abnormalities, hyperparathyroidism, systemic lupus erythematosis, rheumatoid arthritis, systemic carcinoid disease, amyloid deposition, mediastinal radiation therapy, systemic hypertension, and aortic stenosis.

Congenital mitral stenosis presents in childhood and is rarely seen. One rare congenital anomaly responsible for mitral stenosis is a parachute mitral valve. In this condition, all the chordae originate from a single papillary muscle, and mitral stenosis is the result of impaired leaflet motion during diastole.[36] Other developmental anomalies, such as cor triatriatum or a supravalvular membrane, can also simulate mitral stenosis even though the mitral valve apparatus is usually normal.

Atrial myxoma, an intracardiac tumor, typically causes left ventricular inflow obstruction, and the patient may present with intermittent signs of mitral stenosis.

ECHOCARDIOGRAPHIC ASSESSMENT IN MITRAL STENOSIS

Two-Dimensional Imaging

In early rheumatic mitral stenosis, thickening of the leaflet tips is commonly seen while the bases of the leaflets are still pliable. This results in bowing of the leaflets during diastole, which gives a typical hockey stick appearance to the anterior mitral leaflet (see Figure 7–10). As the disease process progresses, calcification of the leaflets and annulus becomes apparent and involvement of the subvalvular apparatus can be seen in the transgastric two-chamber view. The chordae tendineae may be thickened, calcified, and shortened. These pathological changes of the mitral valve apparatus pose important limitations on the suitability of certain interventions to address mitral stenosis. As a consequence, various scoring systems have been proposed to grade severity and aid selection of the most appropriate intervention. Among others, the Wilkins and Cormier scores are commonly used to predict the potential success of closed mitral commissurotomy.[37,38]

In the transgastric mitral valve short-axis view, mitral valve area can be determined by means of planimetry. This method shows good correlation with the actual mitral valve area as measured on excised valves when used in transthoracic echocardiography.[39] However, the fact that the mitral valve is cone shaped during diastole could lead to inaccuracies in measurement of mitral valve area by means of planimetry. The tomographic plane should therefore be carefully aligned with the mitral valve orifice, and mitral valve area planimetry should be performed at the level of the leaflet tips. The lowest gain settings to allow visualization of the whole mitral valve area should be selected to avoid underestimation. For grading of mitral stenosis severity based on mitral valve area, refer to Table 7–2.

Left atrial enlargement occurs as a consequence of the increased left atrial pressure in mitral stenosis. With transesophageal echocardiography, left atrial size can be assessed in the midesophageal long-axis or four-chamber

Table 7–2. Classification of mitral stenosis severity

	Mild	Moderate	Severe
Mean pressure gradient (mm Hg)	<5	5-10	>10
Pressure half-time (ms)	90-150	150-219	>220
Mitral valve area (cm^2)	>1.5	1.0-1.5	<1.0
Pulmonary artery pressure (mmHg)	<30	30-50	>50
Mitral valve resistance ($dyne.s.cm^{-5}$)			>85

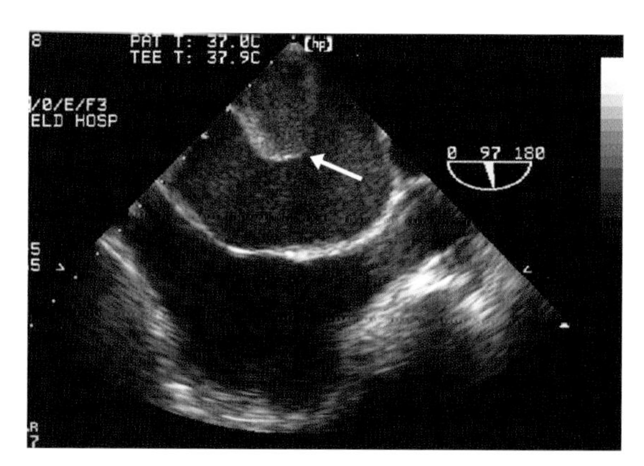

FIGURE 7–23. A thrombus *(arrow)* on the posterior wall of the left atrium in a patient with severe mitral stenosis, as seen in the midesophageal bicaval view.

views; however, left atrial measurements have been validated only in the parasternal long-axis view on transthoracic echocardiography.[40] In the presence of left atrial enlargement and especially atrial fibrillation, echocardiographic evaluation of patients with mitral stenosis should aim to exclude the presence of intracardiac thrombi (Figure 7–23). The presence of spontaneous echo contrast should also be noted, as this indicates sluggish flow with a very high risk for the development of thrombi.[41] Finally, in the midesophageal four-chamber view, bowing of the interatrial septum towards the right is an indication of elevated left atrial pressures.

Significant long-standing mitral stenosis initially results in pulmonary venous hypertension and subsequently pulmonary arterial hypertension. This is followed by right ventricular hypertrophy and right ventricular and atrial enlargement. In the presence of functional tricuspid regurgitation, continuous-wave Doppler of the tricuspid regurgitant jet can be used to calculate systolic right ventricular and pulmonary artery pressures. Acute right ventricular pressure overload with an under-filled left ventricle can cause the interventricular septum to move towards the left, resulting in a D-shaped appearance of the left ventricle in the transgastric midpapillary short-axis view (Figure 7–24). The presence of pulmonary hypertension is an important consideration in the management of mitral stenosis. The degree of pulmonary hypertension, however, helps little in the determination of mitral valve area, as a wide range of pulmonary pressures can be found for the same degree of mitral stenosis.[42]

Rheumatic heart disease seldom affects the mitral valve only. The aortic and tricuspid valves can also be affected, and careful examination of these valves is indicated.[43] Furthermore, structurally abnormal valves are

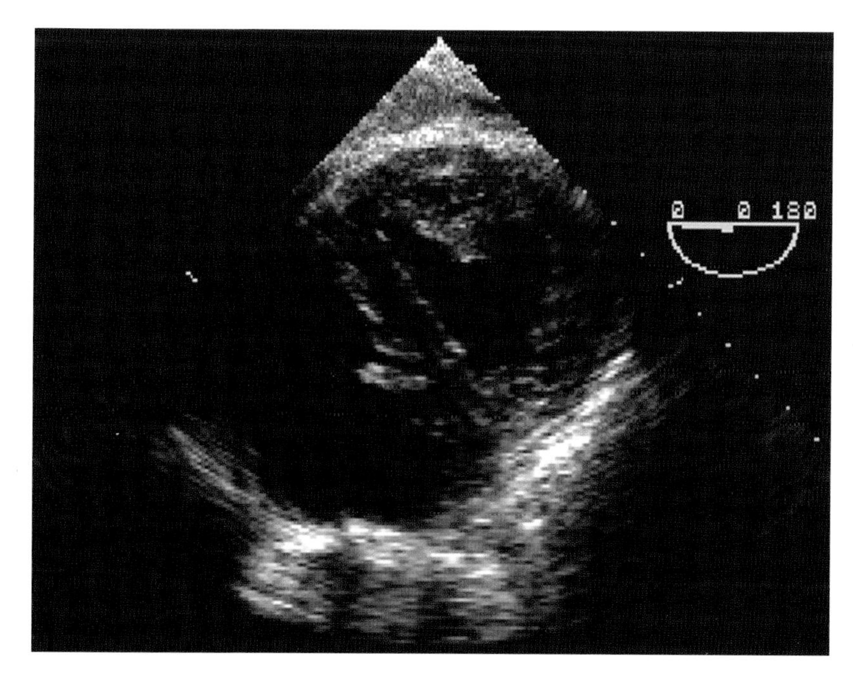

FIGURE 7–24. Pressure overload of the right ventricle producing right ventricular enlargement and flattening of the interventricular septum (D-shaped left ventricle).

predisposed to infective endocarditis. Affected valves should therefore be carefully examined for the presence of vegetations and signs of infection.[44]

Doppler Measurements

Pressure Gradient

Left atrial pressure increases as mitral stenosis progresses. The result is an increase in transvalvular pressure gradient with a subsequent increase in flow velocity across the mitral valve. This velocity can be used to calculate the pressure drop from left atrium to left ventricle by applying the simplified Bernoulli equation.

$$\Delta P = 4v^2$$

where ΔP is the pressure gradient and v is the velocity.

In significant mitral stenosis, velocities resulting from the pressure gradient are often higher than what can be recorded with pulsed-wave Doppler, and therefore continuous-wave Doppler is used to ensure that the accurate maximum velocity is measured. In the midesophageal long-axis view that allows best alignment with direction of transmitral inflow, the continuous-wave Doppler cursor is applied across the mitral valve and a spectral Doppler trace is recorded with sweep speed set to 75 cm/s or more. Increasing sweep speed improves visual discrimination between 2 points and thus, improves accuracy of measurements. In severely deformed valves, the use of color Doppler imaging will help to identify the position and direction of mitral valve inflow. A single spectral Doppler profile is selected, and the trace function used to follow the outline from the beginning of the E-wave to the end of the A-wave. Automated software available on most ultrasound systems will calculate maximum velocity, velocity-time integral, and mean and peak gradients (Figure 7–25). For grading of mitral stenosis according to pressure gradients, refer to Table 7–2. In a patient with atrial fibrillation, the spectral Doppler profile should be traced in five cardiac cycles where the heart rate is close to being regular to obtain an average transvalvular gradient.[45]

Situations that result in alterations of cardiac output will affect flow across the valve and hence the measured pressure gradient. Increases in cardiac output will result in an increased flow across the valve and an increase in calculated gradient, whereas decrease in cardiac output will result in the opposite. Other factors that influence measured gradients include heart rate and the presence of severe mitral regurgitation.[46]

Mitral Valve Area by Pressure Half Time Method[47]

Diastole causes the left ventricular pressure to drop below left atrial pressure. This pressure gradient opens the mitral valve and causes rapid early left ventricular filling, resulting in a relative quick decline in flow as the left atrial pressure becomes equal to left ventricular pressure. This mid-diastolic cessation of flow is referred to as diastases. In the presence of mitral stenosis, left ventricular filling occurs slower due to obstruction caused by the stenotic valve, and the pressure gradient

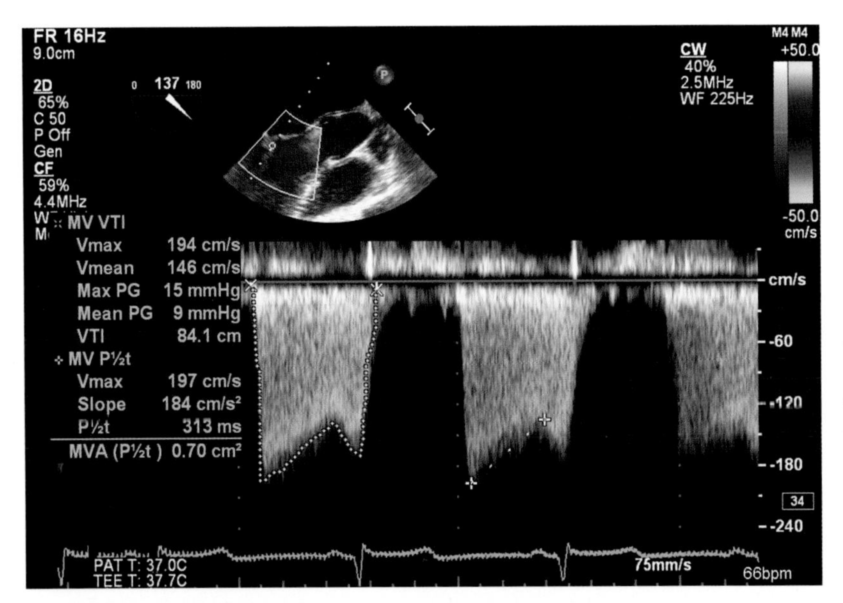

FIGURE 7–25. This spectral Doppler image demonstrates an increased flow velocity across a stenotic mitral valve (peak 194 cm/s, mean 146 cm/s). This velocity is then used to calculate the transvalvular pressure gradient (peak 15 mm Hg, mean 9 mm Hg).

between left atrium and left ventricle persists during diastole. The more severe the stenosis, the longer it takes for transmitral pressure gradient and flow velocities to decline.

To assess the time required for transmitral gradient to decline, a spectral Doppler trace of the transmitral inflow velocities should be obtained. In this instance, the caliper function is selected and the first cursor is placed on the peak velocity measured by spectral Doppler trace. The second cursor is positioned on the slope of the early velocity, immediately before the onset of the A-wave, resulting in a line connecting the two cursors, which represents the deceleration slope (see Figure 7–25). This deceleration slope may in some cases appear as two slopes, with the initial decline being more rapid than the decline during the latter part of diastole. In these cases it is recommended that the pressure decline slope during the latter part of diastole be used.[48] The ultrasound system will automatically calculate the time it takes for the pressure gradient to decline to half of what it was at the beginning of diastole, a variable known as the pressure half time ($P_{1/2t}$) that is inversely related to mitral valve area. Mitral valve area (MVA) can be calculated from the $P_{1/2t}$ with the following equation:

$$\text{MVA (cm}^2\text{)} = 220/P_{1/2t}$$

The accuracy of the $P_{1/2t}$ method for determining mitral valve area also depends on the compliance of the left atrium and the left ventricle. Conditions that result in altered compliance of either chamber, such as left ventricular diastolic dysfunction, will make the mitral valve area calculated from the $P_{1/2t}$ inaccurate.[45] The presence of aortic regurgitation may have an influence on the calculated mitral valve area by this method as well. If an aortic regurgitation jet is directed onto the ventricular surface of the anterior mitral valve leaflet, the opening of the mitral valve may be limited, with subsequent overestimation of mitral stenosis severity. On the other hand, significant aortic regurgitation will result in a more rapid rise in left ventricular pressure than can solely be attributed to filling through the mitral valve. The decline in pressure gradient between left ventricle and left atrium will be more rapid, and hence result in underestimation of the severity of mitral stenosis.[49,50]

An irregular heart rate as in atrial fibrillation may result in significant differences in $P_{1/2t}$ mitral valve area determinations when different beats are traced. Therefore, similar to when transvalvular pressure gradients are obtained, it is recommended that $P_{1/2t}$ be measured in a number of cardiac cycles and averaged.[51] Rapid heart rates result in fusion of the A- and E-waves, making it hard to accurately confirm the deceleration slope with the caliper function.

Using the $P_{1/2t}$ method for determining mitral valve area has only been validated in natural valves. In the case of degenerate or malfunctioning bioprosthetic or mechanical valves, use of this method results in inaccurate grading of inflow obstruction.[52]

MITRAL VALVE AREA BY DECELERATION TIME[53]

Similar to the $P_{1/2t}$ method described above, the time that it would take for the gradient across a stenotic mitral valve to decline to zero can also be used to determine mitral valve area. This measurement is referred to as deceleration time. By using the caliper function in the same fashion as described for the $P_{1/2t}$ method, software integrated into the ultrasound systems will calculate the deceleration time. This measurement, however, requires the second cursor to be placed on the baseline in such a way that the line connecting the two cursors runs along the slope of the early velocity before the A-wave. An inverse ratio between mitral valve area and deceleration time exists, and mitral valve area can be calculated by the following equation:

$$\text{MVA (cm}^2\text{)} = 759/\text{DT(ms)}$$

The limitations to using this measurement are the same as described above for $P_{1/2t}$.

MITRAL VALVE AREA BY CONTINUITY EQUATION[54]

In a closed system, flow (cm^3/s) will be equal in all parts at any given time. For this to be valid, velocity of flow has to increase in areas where the cross-sectional area of the system is reduced. This principle is referred to as the conservation of flow and is mathematically represented by the continuity equation (Figure 7–26).

In mitral stenosis, the continuity equation can be used in two ways to calculate mitral valve area. The first method requires transmitral flow to be equal to left ventricular stroke volume; in other words, there can be no aortic or mitral regurgitation.[54] As a second method, the proximal isovelocity surface area can be used. This

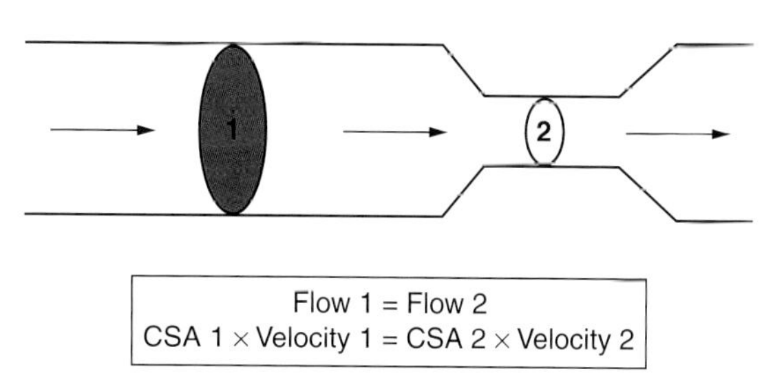

Flow 1 = Flow 2
CSA 1 × Velocity 1 = CSA 2 × Velocity 2

FIGURE 7–26. Diagrammatic representation of the continuity equation.

method is unaffected by the presence of valvular regurgitation.

With competent left-sided valves and mitral stenosis, the continuity equation is applied as follows:

1. According to the conservation of flow principle, forward stroke volume (SV) in the left ventricular outflow tract (LVOT) will be equal to the forward stroke volume across the mitral valve.
2. Forward stroke volume in the left ventricular outflow tract is calculated as follows: In deep transgastric long-axis or transgastric long-axis views, pulsed-wave Doppler is applied to obtain a spectral Doppler trace of left ventricular outflow tract flow velocity. By using the trace function, a single spectral Doppler envelope is outlined and velocity-time integral (VTI; in cm) is obtained. In the midesophageal aortic valve long-axis view, left ventricular outflow tract diameter is measured during ejection, ie, with open aortic valve. This measurement should be made in systole within 1 cm from the coaptation point of aortic valve leaflets. Accuracy is improved by using zoom to enlarge the image as much as possible, and by performing more than one measurement and using the largest obtained. Stroke volume can then be calculated as follows:

$$SV_{LVOT} = CSA_{LVOT} \times VTI_{LVOT}$$

$$CSA_{LVOT} = \pi r^2$$

$$\begin{aligned} SV_{LVOT} &= \pi(d/2)^2 \times VTI_{LVOT} \\ &= \pi\,(d^2/4) \times VTI_{LVOT} \\ &= \pi/4 \times d^2 \times VTI_{LVOT} \\ &= 0.785 \times d^2 \times VTI_{LVOT} \end{aligned}$$

Where π = 3.14
LVOT = Left ventricular outflow tract
VTI = Velocity-time integral of the LVOT in centimeters
d = Diameter of the LVOT, and the assumption is made that the LVOT cross-sectional area is circular

3. Next, in the midesophageal four-chamber view, continuous-wave Doppler is placed through the mitral valve opening with the sweep speed set to 75mm/s or more. A spectral Doppler trace of transmitral inflow is recorded. Again the trace function is used to obtain the velocity-time integral of transmitral inflow, and measurement of several cardiac cycles is averaged to improve accuracy. The continuity equation is then used to calculate mitral valve area:

$$SV_{LVOT} = SV_{Transmitral}$$

where

$$0.785 \times D^2_{LVOT} \times VTI_{LVOT} = MVA \times VTI_{MV}$$

Thus,

$$MVA = \frac{0.785 \times D^2_{LVOT} \times VTI_{LVOT}}{VTI_{MV}}$$

Where D_{LVOT} = Left ventricular outflow tract diameter
MVA = Mitral valve area
VTI = Velocity-time integral
SV = Stroke volume
MV = Mitral valve

To use this method accurately, one should consider beat-to-beat variation in stroke volume with ventilation. Various measurements made during different cardiac cycles may result in inaccurate calculations. To reduce error, a number of measurements should be averaged, and if possible, ventilation stopped when spectral Doppler tracings are recorded. Arrhythmias such as atrial fibrillation can result in significant differences in stroke volume from beat to beat, and will have a significant impact on the mitral valve area determined by this method. Furthermore, forward flow is always greater across incompetent valves than forward flow across competent valves. This discrepancy makes the above-described method inappropriate in mixed mitral valve disease or in aortic regurgitation.[45]

The second application of continuity equation uses the proximal isovelocity surface area method[55] in a similar way as that described for determination of effective regurgitant orifice area in mitral regurgitation (Figure 7–27A). The mitral valve is visualized in midesophageal four-chamber view, and color Doppler sector is applied over the mitral valve. The transducer and color Doppler sector are oriented to display maximum transmitral flow velocity. The baseline on the color scale is adjusted downward towards the direction of flow. A Nyquist limit of 21 cm/s is recommended as mitral valve area is progressively underestimated with higher aliasing velocities.[56] Flow away from the transducer appears blue by convention, but as the accelerating color hemispheres reach aliasing velocity, the color will alias and change to yellow. The hemisphere radius is measured from the aliasing (blue to yellow) contour to the narrowest part of mitral valve inflow. Using the color-suppress mode will help to accurately determine the narrowest part of mitral valve opening. Once again, it is important to accurately determine the hemispheric radius as this value is squared during calculation, resulting in exaggeration of any errors.

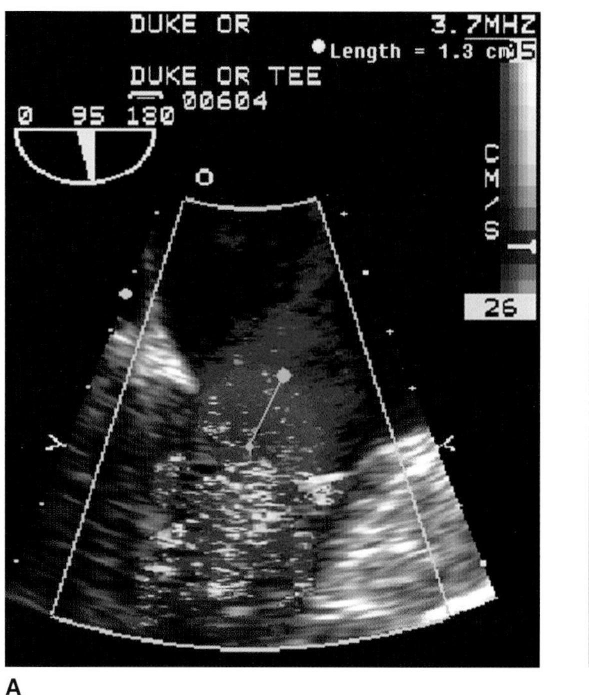

A

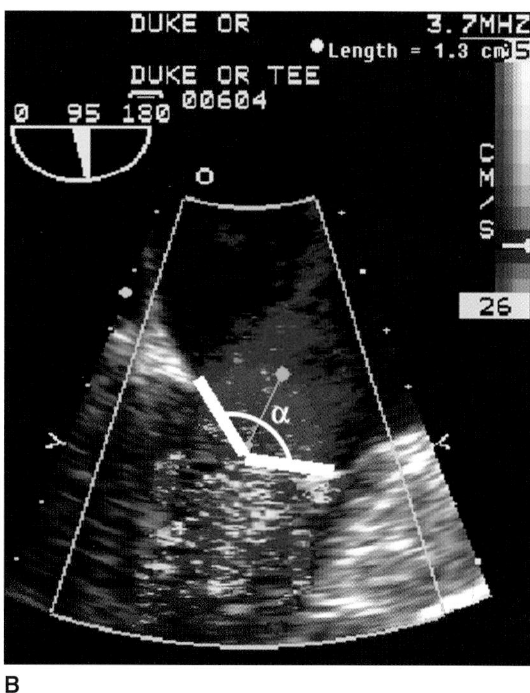

B

FIGURE 7–27. Color-flow Doppler examination of transmitral flow in mitral stenosis. **A:** Velocity acceleration as flow approaches the stenotic orifice is demonstrated by aliasing of color flow and a shell of proximal isovelocity surface area. The edge of the proximal isovelocity surface area is defined by the transition from blue to red color. In this case, the aliasing velocity is 26 cm/s and the radius of the hemisphere is 1.3 cm. **B:** The angle (α) subtended by the mitral leaflets is shown.

Where temporal resolution (frame rate) is low, the biggest radius over a number of cardiac cycles should be measured. Continuous-wave Doppler is then applied across the valve to obtain a spectral Doppler trace of the transmitral inflow and the maximum velocity is measured. Mitral valve area can be calculated as follows:

$$\text{PISA} \times V_a = \text{MVA} \times V_{max}$$

$$2\pi r^2 \times V_a - \text{MVA} \times V_{max}$$

$$\text{MVA} = \frac{2\pi r^2 \times V_a}{V_{max}}$$

Where PISA = Proximal isovelocity surface area
r = Radius of proximal isovelocity contour
V_a = Aliasing velocity obtained from the bottom of the color Doppler scale
V_{max} = Maximum velocity measured across mitral valve during diastole

Since the maximum PISA radius occurs at the same time as maximum transmitral inflow velocity, and since measurements are commonly not taken during the same cardiac cycle, they should be repeated over several cardiac cycles to increase accuracy. In the presence of atrial fibrillation where stroke volume varies between cardiac cycles, determination of mitral valve area with the proximal isovelocity surface area method is inaccurate. Furthermore, true hemispheric shells require a flat surface area, and since the mitral valve surface area is often not flat, an angle correction factor should be used to improve accuracy (Figure 7–27B). In such cases, the mitral valve area should be multiplied by α/180, where α is the angle subtended by the mitral leaflets.[55]

Mitral Valve Resistance

Most indices used to quantify the severity of mitral stenosis are influenced by flow across the valve at time of measurement. Therefore, significant variations in measurements can occur in the same patient subsequent to changes in cardiac output. This has led to the use of valve resistance as a flow-independent index of the hemodynamic burden of stenosed valves, as both pressure gradient and flow are incorporated in its calculation.

$$VR = \frac{1333 \times TMG_{mean}}{Q}$$

Where

VR = Valve resistance in dyne.s.cm^{-5}
TMG_{mean} = Mean transmitral pressure gradient
Q = Transmitral flow rate in cm^3/s calculated as stroke volume/diastolic filling period
1333 = Conversion factor to metric units

Mitral valve resistance was found to be the best predictor of resting and stressed pulmonary artery pressures in patients with mitral stenosis, when compared with mitral valve area and mean transmitral pressure gradient. This is considered important, as a stressed pulmonary artery pressure is the only independent predictor of exercise capacity.[57] It has, however, become apparent that valve resistance does increase as flow increases, and its unpredictability makes the use of this index contentious.[58]

Three-Dimensional Echocardiographic Assessment of Mitral Stenosis

The introduction of real-time 3D echocardiography (RT3D) adds to the evaluation of mitral stenosis (Figure 7–28). Mitral valve pathology, and especially affected subvalvular apparatus, can be clearly visualized from any desired orientation. Three-dimensional imaging allows for accurate planimetry of the mitral valve area. Good correlation was found between mitral valve area measured by planimetry in 3D imaging and mitral valve area calculated by means of pressure half time and proximal isovelocity surface area.[59] There is better interobserver agreement with RT3D than 2D for the assessment of pre-valvuloplasty Wilkins score. After balloon valvuloplasty, the pressure half time method for calculating mitral valve area becomes inaccurate,[60] and RT3D has been shown to be superior in quantifying mitral valve area in the immediate post-valvuloplasty period. During this time there is good correlation between mitral valve area measured with planimetry in 3D and the Gorlin method as applied during cardiac catheterization.[61] The large number of recent publications on RT3D imaging reflects the rapidly growing body of knowledge on this exciting new development and the enthusiasm for it (see Chapter 24).

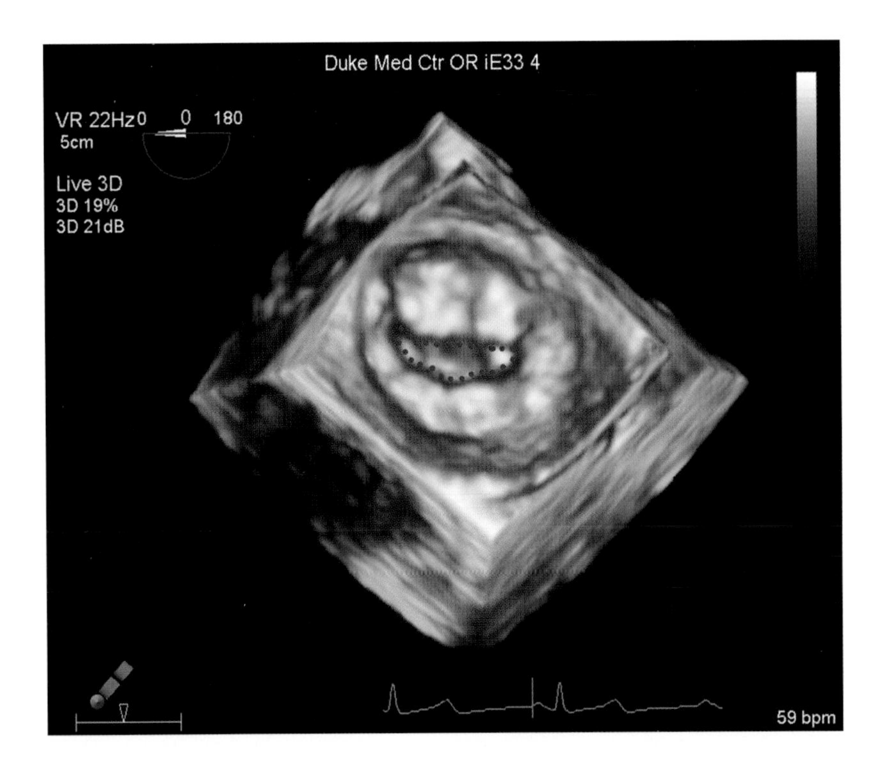

FIGURE 7–28. Three-dimensional image of a stenotic mitral valve. A dotted red line has been added to highlight the mitral valve opening.

REFERENCES

1. Shuhaiber J, Anderson RJ. Meta-analysis of clinical outcomes following surgical mitral valve repair or replacement. *Eur J Cardiothorac Surg.* 2007;31(2):267-275.
2. Cheitlin MD, Armstrong WF, Aurigemma GP, et al. ACC/AHA/ASE 2003 guideline update for the clinical application of echocardiography—summary article: a report of the American College of Cardiology/American Heart Association Task Force on Practice Guidelines (ACC/AHA/ASE Committee to Update the 1997 Guidelines for the Clinical Application of Echocardiography). *J Am Coll Cardiol.* 2003;42(5):954-970.
3. Shapira Y, Vaturi M, Weisenberg DE, et al. Impact of intraoperative transesophageal echocardiography in patients undergoing valve replacement. *Ann Thorac Surg.* 2004;78(2):579-583; discussion 583-574.
4. Muresian H. The clinical anatomy of the mitral valve. *Clin Anat.* 2009;22(1):85-98.
5. Carpentier A, Deloche A, Dauptain J, et al. A new reconstructive operation for correction of mitral and tricuspid insufficiency. *J Thorac Cardiovasc Surg.* 1971;61(1):1-13.
6. Voci P, Bilotta F, Caretta Q, Mercanti C, Marino B. Papillary muscle perfusion pattern. A hypothesis for ischemic papillary muscle dysfunction. *Circulation.* 1995;91(6):1714-1718.
7. Levy MJ, Edwards JE. Anatomy of mitral insufficiency. Prog Cardiovasc Dis. 1962;5:119-144.
8. Shanewise JS, Cheung AT, Aronson S, et al. ASE/SCA guidelines for performing a comprehensive intraoperative multiplane transesophageal echocardiography examination: recommendations of the American Society of Echocardiography Council for Intraoperative Echocardiography and the Society of Cardiovascular Anesthesiologists Task Force for Certification in Perioperative Transesophageal Echocardiography. *J Am Soc Echocardiogr.* 1999;12(10):884-900.
9. Fabricius AM, Walther T, Falk V, Mohr FW. Three-dimensional echocardiography for planning of mitral valve surgery: current applicability? *Ann Thorac Surg.* 2004;78(2):575-578.
10. Grewal J, Mankad S, Freeman WK, et al. Real-time three-dimensional transesophageal echocardiography in the intraoperative assessment of mitral valve disease. *J Am Soc Echocardiogr.* 2009;22(1):34-41.
11. Sugeng L, Weinert L, Thiele K, Lang RM. Real-time three-dimensional echocardiography using a novel matrix array transducer. *Echocardiography.* 2003;20(7):623-635.
12. Mahmood F, Karthik S, Subramaniam B, et al. Intraoperative application of geometric three-dimensional mitral valve assessment package: a feasibility study. *J Cardiothorac Vasc Anesth.* 2008;22(2):292-298.
13. Shernan SK. Intraoperative three-dimensional echocardiography: ready for primetime? *J Am Soc Echocardiogr.* 2009; 22(1):27A-28A.
14. Playford D, Weyman AE. Mitral valve prolapse: time for a fresh look. *Rev Cardiovasc Med.* 2001;2(2):73-81.
15. Carpentier A. Cardiac valve surgery—the "French correction." *J Thorac Cardiovasc Surg.* 1983;86(3):323-337.
16. Carabello BA, Crawford FA Jr. Valvular heart disease. *N Engl J Med.* 1997;337(1):32-41.
17. Stewart WJ, Salcedo EE, Cosgrove DM. The value of echocardiography in mitral valve repair. *Cleve Clin J Med.* 1991; 58(2):177-183.
18. Szymczyk E, Wierzbowska-Drabik K, Drozdz J, Krzeminska-Pakula M. Mitral valve regurgitation is a powerful factor of left ventricular hypertrophy. *Pol Arch Med Wewn.* 2008;118(9): 478-483.
19. Sahn DJ. Instrumentation and physical factors related to visualization of stenotic and regurgitant jets by Doppler color flow mapping. *J Am Coll Cardiol.* 1988;12(5):1354-1365.
20. Roberts BJ, Grayburn PA. Color flow imaging of the vena contracta in mitral regurgitation: technical considerations. *J Am Soc Echocardiogr.* 2003;16(9):1002-1006.
21. Kizilbash AM, Willett DL, Brickner ME, Heinle SK, Grayburn PA. Effects of afterload reduction on vena contracta width in mitral regurgitation. *J Am Coll Cardiol.* 1998;32(2):427-431.
22. Lambert AS. Proximal isovelocity surface area should be routinely measured in evaluating mitral regurgitation: a core review. *Anesth Analg.* 2007;105(4):940-943.
23. Utsunomiya T, Doshi R, Patel D, et al. Calculation of volume flow rate by the proximal isovelocity surface area method: simplified approach using color Doppler zero baseline shift. *J Am Coll Cardiol.* 1993;22(1):277-282.
24. Matsumura Y, Saracino G, Sugioka K, et al. Determination of regurgitant orifice area with the use of a new three-dimensional flow convergence geometric assumption in functional mitral regurgitation. *J Am Soc Echocardiogr.* 2008;21(11):1251-1256.
25. Castello R, Pearson AC, Lenzen P, Labovitz AJ. Effect of mitral regurgitation on pulmonary venous velocities derived from transesophageal echocardiography color-guided pulsed Doppler imaging. *J Am Coll Cardiol.* 1991;17(7):1499-1506.
26. Pu M, Griffin BP, Vandervoort PM, et al. The value of assessing pulmonary venous flow velocity for predicting severity of mitral regurgitation: a quantitative assessment integrating left ventricular function. J Am Soc Echocardiogr. 1999;12(9):736-743.
27. Zoghbi WA, Enriquez-Sarano M, Foster E, et al. Recommendations for evaluation of the severity of native valvular regurgitation with two-dimensional and Doppler echocardiography. J *Am Soc Echocardiogr.* 2003;16(7):777-802.
28. Thomas L, Foster E, Schiller NB. Peak mitral inflow velocity predicts mitral regurgitation severity. *J Am Coll Cardiol.* 1998;31(1):174-179.
29. Mihalatos DG, Gopal AS, Kates R, et al. Intraoperative assessment of mitral regurgitation: role of phenylephrine challenge. *J Am Soc Echocardiogr.* 2006;19(9):1158-1164.
30. Gorlin R, Gorlin SG. Hydraulic formula for calculation of the area of the stenotic mitral valve, other cardiac valves, and central circulatory shunts. *I. Am Heart J.* 1951;41(1):1-29.
31. Levy S. Factors predisposing to the development of atrial fibrillation. *Pacing Clin Electrophysiol.* 1997;20(10 Pt 2): 2670-2674.
32. Remetz MS, Cleman MW, Cabin HS. Pulmonary and pleural complications of cardiac disease. *Clin Chest Med.* 1989;10(4): 545-592.
33. Agmon Y, Khandheria BK, Gentile F, Seward JB. Echocardiographic assessment of the left atrial appendage. *J Am Coll Cardiol.* 1999;34(7):1867-1877.
34. Gaasch WH, Folland ED. Left ventricular function in rheumatic mitral stenosis. *Eur Heart J.* 1991;12(suppl B):66-69.
35. Iung B, Baron G, Butchart EG, et al. A prospective survey of patients with valvular heart disease in Europe: the Euro Heart Survey on Valvular Heart Disease. *Eur Heart J.* 2003; 24(13): 1231-1243.

36. Chauvaud S. Surgery of congenital mitral valve disease. *J Cardiovasc Surg (Torino).* 2004;45(5):465-476.
37. Wilkins GT, Weyman AE, Abascal VM, Block PC, Palacios IF. Percutaneous balloon dilatation of the mitral valve: an analysis of echocardiographic variables related to outcome and the mechanism of dilatation. *Br Heart J.* 1988;60(4):299-308.
38. Iung B, Cormier B, Ducimetiere P, et al. Immediate results of percutaneous mitral commissurotomy. A predictive model on a series of 1514 patients. *Circulation.* 1996;94(9):2124-2130.
39. Faletra F, Pezzano A Jr, Fusco R, et al. Measurement of mitral valve area in mitral stenosis: four echocardiographic methods compared with direct measurement of anatomic orifices. *J Am Coll Cardiol.* 1996;28(5):1190-1197.
40. Pearlman JD, Triulzi MO, King ME, Abascal VM, Newell J, Weyman AE. Left atrial dimensions in growth and development: normal limits for two-dimensional echocardiography. *J Am Coll Cardiol.* 1990;16(5):1168-1174.
41. Black IW. Spontaneous echo contrast: where there's smoke there's fire. *Echocardiography.* 2000;17(4):373-382.
42. Vahanian A, Baumgartner H, Bax J, et al. Guidelines on the management of valvular heart disease: the Task Force on the Management of Valvular Heart Disease of the European Society of Cardiology. *Eur Heart J.* 2007;28(2):230-268.
43. Han QQ, Xu ZY, Zhang BR, Zou LJ, Hao JH, Huang SD. Primary triple valve surgery for advanced rheumatic heart disease in Mainland China: a single-center experience with 871 clinical cases. *Eur J Cardiothorac Surg.* 2007;31(5):845-850.
44. Cetinkaya Y, Akova M, Akalin HE, et al. A retrospective review of 228 episodes of infective endocarditis where rheumatic valvular disease is still common. *Int J Antimicrob Agents.* 2001;18(1):1-7.
45. Baumgartner H, Hung J, Bermejo J, et al. Echocardiographic assessment of valve stenosis: EAE/ASE recommendations for clinical practice. *Eur J Echocardiogr.* 2009;10(1):1-25.
46. Rahimtoola SH, Durairaj A, Mehra A, Nuno I. Current evaluation and management of patients with mitral stenosis. *Circulation.* 2002;106(10):1183-1188.
47. Thomas JD, Weyman AE. Doppler mitral pressure half-time: a clinical tool in search of theoretical justification. *J Am Coll Cardiol.* 1987;10(4):923-929.
48. Gonzalez MA, Child JS, Krivokapich J. Comparison of two-dimensional and Doppler echocardiography and intracardiac hemodynamics for quantification of mitral stenosis. *Am J Cardiol.* 1987;60(4):327-332.
49. Bonow RO, Carabello BA, Kanu C, et al. ACC/AHA 2006 guidelines for the management of patients with valvular heart disease: a report of the American College of Cardiology/American Heart Association Task Force on Practice Guidelines (Writing Committee to Revise the 1998 Guidelines for the Management of Patients With Valvular Heart Disease): developed in collaboration with the Society of Cardiovascular Anesthesiologists: endorsed by the Society for Cardiovascular Angiography and Interventions and the Society of Thoracic Surgeons. *Circulation.* 2006;114(5):e84-231.
50. Bonow RO, Carabello BA, Chatterjee K, et al. 2008 Focused update incorporated into the ACC/AHA 2006 guidelines for the management of patients with valvular heart disease: a report of the American College of Cardiology/American Heart Association Task Force on Practice Guidelines (Writing Committee to Revise the 1998 Guidelines for the Management of Patients With Valvular Heart Disease): endorsed by the Society of Cardiovascular Anesthesiologists, Society for Cardiovascular Angiography and Interventions, and Society of Thoracic Surgeons. *Circulation.* 2008;118(15):e523-661.
51. Kim HK, Kim YJ, Chang SA, et al. Impact of cardiac rhythm on mitral valve area calculated by the pressure half time method in patients with moderate or severe mitral stenosis. *J Am Soc Echocardiogr.* 2009;22(1):42-47.
52. Chambers JB. Mitral pressure half-time: is it a valid measure of orifice area in artificial heart valves? *J Heart Valve Dis.* 1993;2(5):571-577.
53. Mathew JP, Ayoub CM. *Clinical Manual and Review of Transesophageal Echocardiography.* New York: McGraw-Hill, Medical Pub Division; 2005.
54. Nakatani S, Masuyama T, Kodama K, Kitabatake A, Fujii K, Kamada T. Value and limitations of Doppler echocardiography in the quantification of stenotic mitral valve area: comparison of the pressure half-time and the continuity equation methods. *Circulation.* 1988;77(1):78-85.
55. Rodriguez L, Thomas JD, Monterroso V, et al. Validation of the proximal flow convergence method. Calculation of orifice area in patients with mitral stenosis. *Circulation.* 1993;88(3): 1157-1165.
56. Deng YB, Matsumoto M, Wang XF, et al. Estimation of mitral valve area in patients with mitral stenosis by the flow convergence region method: selection of aliasing velocity. *J Am Coll Cardiol.* 1994;24(3):683-689.
57. Izgi C, Ozdemir N, Cevik C, et al. Mitral valve resistance as a determinant of resting and stress pulmonary artery pressure in patients with mitral stenosis: a dobutamine stress study. *J Am Soc Echocardiogr.* 2007;20(10):1160-1166.
58. Blais C, Pibarot P, Dumesnil JG, Garcia D, Chen D, Durand LG. Comparison of valve resistance with effective orifice area regarding flow dependence. *Am J Cardiol.* 2001;88(1):45-52.
59. Perez de Isla L, Casanova C, Almeria C, et al. Which method should be the reference method to evaluate the severity of rheumatic mitral stenosis? Gorlin's method versus 3D-echo. *Eur J Echocardiogr.* 2007;8(6):470-473.
60. Messika-Zeitoun D, Meizels A, Cachier A, et al. Echocardiographic evaluation of the mitral valve area before and after percutaneous mitral commissurotomy: the pressure half-time method revisited. *J Am Soc Echocardiogr.* 2005;18(12):1409-1414.
61. Zamorano J, Perez de Isla L, Sugeng L, et al. Non-invasive assessment of mitral valve area during percutaneous balloon mitral valvuloplasty: role of real-time 3D echocardiography. *Eur Heart J.* 2004;25(23):2086-2091.

REVIEW QUESTIONS

Select the *one best* answer for each item.

1. With regard to the mitral valve leaflets, which of the following statements is true?
   a. The anterior mitral leaflet is divided into three scallops by clefts
   b. The posterior leaflet occupies approximately two-thirds of the mitral annulus

c. The posterior leaflet is associated with the aortic valve
d. The commissures extend all the way to the mitral annulus

2. Which of the following statements related to the function of the mitral valve is false?
   a. It keeps the left atrial pressure low in order to prevent pulmonary hypertension
   b. It allows unobstructed flow to the left ventricular outflow tract during diastole
   c. It prevents the backflow of blood to the left atrium during systole
   d. It offers little resistance to ventricular filling during diastole

3. Which of the following structures is not included in the mitral valvar complex?
   a. Mitral valve leaflets
   b. Chordae tendineae
   c. Left atrial appendage
   d. Mitral valvar annulus
   e. Aortomitral fibrous continuity

4. Papillary muscle dysfunction:
   a. Is more commonly limited to the anterolateral papillary muscle
   b. Often leads to muscle rupture after an ischemic event
   c. Is seen more commonly in the posteromedial papillary muscle
   d. Is seldom a cause of mitral regurgitation

5. Which of the following views does not allow complete visualization of the mitral valve?
   a. Midesophageal four chamber
   b. Midesophageal mitral commissural
   c. Midesophageal aortic valve short axis
   d. Transgastric two chamber
   e. Deep transgastric long axis

6. Which combination of mitral valve segments is demonstrated by the midesophageal four-chamber view (20° to 30°)?
   a. A1 and P1
   b. P3 and P4
   c. A2 and P2
   d. P1 and A3

7. Which mitral valve segments are seen in the far field in the transgastric mitral valve short-axis view?
   a. A1 and P1
   b. A2 and P2
   c. A3 and P3
   d. A1 and A2

8. Which of the following structures does not appear in the far field of the transgastric two-chamber view?
   a. Left atrial appendage
   b. Anterior mitral valve leaflet
   c. Posteromedial papillary muscle
   d. Anterior ventricular free wall

9. The vena contracta in mitral regurgitation correlates best with other measures of severity when measured in which of the following views?
   a. Midesophageal long axis
   b. Midesophageal four chamber
   c. Midesophageal mitral commissural
   d. Transgastric two chamber

10. In the midesophageal mitral commissural view, which one of the following mitral valve segments is typically seen?
   a. P2
   b. A2
   c. A1
   d. A3

11. Which of the following views allows for the best assessment of the subvalvar apparatus?
   a. Midesophageal four chamber
   b. Midesophageal long axis
   c. Transgastric two chamber
   d. Deep transgastric long axis

12. In which area or dimension is mitral annular dilatation most likely to occur?
   a. The dimension perpendicular to the leaflet coaptation
   b. The intercommisural dimension
   c. The intertrigonal dimension
   d. The intertrough dimension

13. Which statement with regard to the mechanism of mitral regurgitation is true?
   a. Carpentier type I lesions are typically seen in rheumatic heart disease.
   b. Dilated cardiomyopathy results in abnormal mitral valve leaflets.
   c. In patients with ventricular ischemia, the mitral regurgitation jet is mostly directed in an inferolateral direction.
   d. Mitral valve leaflet perforation results in a Carpentier type II lesion.

14. Chordal rupture is least likely to be the mechanism of mitral regurgitation in:
    a. Barlow's disease
    b. Fibroelastic deficiency
    c. Blunt chest trauma
    d. Infective endocarditis

15. Which of the following is not a consequence of long-standing hemodynamically significant mitral regurgitation?
    a. Eccentric hypertrophy of the left ventricle
    b. Left atrial dilatation
    c. Right ventricular hypertrophy
    d. Bulging of the interatrial septum to the left

16. In a patient with mitral regurgitation secondary to myocardial ischemia:
    a. Using the PISA method during 2D evaluation overestimates the effective regurgitant orifice area.
    b. The proximal isovelocity surface area usually assumes a perfect hemisphere.
    c. The PISA method results in an underestimation of the effective regurgitant orifice area.
    d. The regurgitation jet is typically directed in the direction of the aortic valve.

17. Dilatation of the mitral annulus never results in an increase in the intertrigonal distance.
    a. True
    b. False

18. In a patient with a flail posterior mitral valve leaflet, which of the following is not expected to be found?
    a. Systolic reversal of flow in the pulmonary veins
    b. Transmitral inflow velocity greater than 120 cm/s
    c. A centrally directed mitral regurgitation jet
    d. E-wave–dominated transmitral inflow pattern on Doppler interrogation

19. In mild mitral regurgitation, which of the following findings can be expected?
    a. Early peaking flow pattern on continuous-wave Doppler interrogation of the mitral regurgitation jet
    b. Severe dilatation of the left atrium
    c. Normal-appearing mitral valve leaflets
    d. Significant prolapse of the mitral valve leaflets above the annular plane

20. According to Carpentier, how would you classify the mitral regurgitation resulting from left ventricular dilatation?
    a. Type I
    b. Type II
    c. Type IIIa
    d. Type IIIb

21. Which of the following statements would not correlate with severe mitral regurgitation?
    a. Vena contracta of 0.8 cm
    b. Effective regurgitant orifice area of 0.45 cm^2
    c. Systolic dominance in pulmonary venous flow
    d. Regurgitant fraction of 55%

22. Which of the following would be most consistent with moderate mitral regurgitation?
    a. Left atrial diameter of 4.5 cm
    b. Vena contracta of 0.71 cm
    c. Faint continuous-wave Doppler trace of the mitral regurgitation jet
    d. Normal mitral valve apparatus on 2D examination

23. Which of the following indices is the best measure of the severity of mitral regurgitation?
    a. Jet surface area on color-flow mapping
    b. Jet area expressed as a percentage of left atrial area on color-flow mapping
    c. Pulsed-wave Doppler interrogation of the pulmonary venous flow pattern
    d. Vena contracta

24. If the aliasing contour radius in the left ventricle is greater than 1 cm with a Nyquist limit of 40 cm/s, what is the degree of mitral regurgitation?
    a. Mild
    b. Moderate
    c. Severe
    d. Not enough information to quantify mitral regurgitation

25. The correct Nyquist limit for color Doppler interrogation of mitral regurgitation and measurement of the vena contracta is:
    a. 30-40 cm/s
    b. 40-50 cm/s
    c. 50-60 cm/s
    d. 60-70 cm/s

26. The initial pathology of rheumatic mitral valve disease is:
    a. Calcification of the mitral annulus
    b. Calcification and shortening of the chordae tendineae
    c. Fusion of the mitral valve commissures
    d. Thickening of the leaflet tips

27. Mitral stenosis in long-term dialysis-dependent renal failure is very amenable to percutaneous mitral valvotomy.
    a. True
    b. False

28. When do patients with mitral stenosis start to develop symptoms during exercise?
    a. Mitral valve area less than 1.5 cm^2
    b. Mitral valve area less than 2.5 cm^2
    c. Pulmonary artery pressures greater than 25 mm Hg
    d. Pulmonary artery pressures greater than 30 mm Hg

29. What common complication of mitral stenosis marks the sudden worsening of symptoms in patients with mitral stenosis?
    a. Left atrial enlargement
    b. Left ventricular failure
    c. Onset of atrial fibrillation
    d. Development of left atrial appendage thrombus

30. What is the most common cause of mitral stenosis in developing countries?
    a. Chronic renal failure
    b. Congenital mitral valve abnormalities
    c. Parachute mitral valve
    d. Rheumatic heart disease

31. In rheumatic heart disease, which of the following statements is false?
    a. Rheumatic mitral stenosis seldom occurs as isolated stenosis only.
    b. The tricuspid valve is most commonly affected after the mitral valve.
    c. Rheumatic heart valves are prone to the development of infective endocarditis and careful evaluation for vegetations is indicated.
    d. Chordal involvement is often severe.

32. The presence of spontaneous echo contrast in the left atrium should prompt careful examination for which of the following?
    a. Severe mitral regurgitation
    b. Abnormal hemostasis in a patient with mitral stenosis
    c. The presence of a mural thrombus in the left ventricle
    d. The presence of a left atrial appendage thrombus

33. Which of the following is not a component of the Wilkins score used to predict the success rate of percutaneous mitral valvotomy?
    a. Leaflet mobility
    b. Calcification of valvar apparatus
    c. Peak transmitral pressure gradient
    d. Leaflet thickening

34. Which of the following is consistent with a moderate degree of mitral stenosis?
    a. Mean transmitral pressure gradient of 10 mm Hg
    b. Mitral valve area of 2.1 cm^2
    c. Left atrial enlargement
    d. Pressure half time of 240 milliseconds

35. Mitral valve area determined by the pressure half time method is unaffected by:
    a. Aortic regurgitation
    b. Aortic stenosis
    c. Atrial fibrillation
    d. None of the above

36. In the presence of significant aortic regurgitation, the degree of mitral stenosis is overestimated when using the pressure half-time or deceleration time methods.
    a. True
    b. False

37. Which of the following methods used to determine mitral valve area applies the principle of the conservation of flow?
    a. Modified Bernoulli method
    b. Proximal isovelocity surface area
    c. Mitral valve resistance
    d. Pressure half time method

38. Which is the correct formula to use for the calculation of mitral valve area by means of the continuity equation?
    a. $MVA = 2\pi r^2 \times V_{Aliasing}/V_{max}$
    b. $MVA = 0.785 \times D^2/V_{max}$
    c. $MVA = (2\pi r^2 \times V_{Aliasing}/V_{max}) \times \alpha/180$
    d. $MVA = (4\pi r^2 \times V_{Aliasing}/V_{max}) \times \alpha/180$

39. The proximal isovelocity surface area method for the determination of mitral valve area assumes:
    a. A flat surface proximal to the stenosis and a circular orifice
    b. An angle of 150° degrees proximal to the mitral valve
    c. A perfectly hemispherical isovelocity surface area and an ellipsoid orifice
    d. That the maximal radius of the aliasing contour occurs at the end of diastole

40. The following values were obtained during echocardiographic evaluation in a patient with mitral stenosis: $LVOT_{Diameter}$ = 20 mm; $LVOT_{VTI}$ = 23.86 cm; $transmitral_{VTI}$ = 80 cm; aortic $valve_{VTI}$ = 45 cm.

   A. What is the forward stroke volume?
      a. 75 cm/s
      b. 75 cm^3
      c. 141.3 cm^2
      d. 141.3 cm^3

   B. The $LVOT_{VTI}$ is measured with continuous-wave Doppler.
      a. True
      b. False

   C. What is the mitral valve area?
      a. 1.89 cm^2
      b. 1.66 cm^2
      c. 0.94 cm^2
      d. 3.14 cm^2

   D. What is the severity of mitral stenosis in this patient based on the available information?
      a. Mild
      b. Moderate
      c. Severe
      d. No stenosis

41. The following values were obtained during echocardiographic assessment in a patient with mitral stenosis: $PISA_{Radius}$ = 10 mm; aliasing velocity = 21 cm/s; maximum transmitral gradient = 16 mm Hg; $transmitral_{VTI}$ = 113 cm.

   A. In which direction should the color scale baseline be adjusted when the PISA method is employed to determine the mitral valve area?
      a. In the opposite direction of flow
      b. Towards the apex of the heart
      c. Towards the left atrium
      d. Adjusting the color scale baseline is never necessary

   B. What is the calculated mitral valve area in this patient?
      a. 0.14 cm^2
      b. 1.17 cm^2
      c. 0.66 cm^2
      d. 0.88 cm^2

   C. What is the stroke volume?
      a. 75 cm^3
      b. 132 cm^3
      c. 100 cm^3
      d. 75 cm^2

   D. How would you grade the severity of mitral stenosis in this patient?
      a. No stenosis
      b. Mild
      c. Moderate
      d. Severe

42. Which of the following statements is true?
   a. Mitral valve resistance is the most important factor determining pulmonary artery pressure during exercise.
   b. Mitral valve resistance is measured in dyne.s.cm^5.
   c. Pulmonary artery pressure can be closely related to mitral valve area.
   d. Indirect determination of mitral valve area is independent of cardiac output.

43. During the calculation of mitral valve resistance, the transvalvular flow is accounted for, making this a flow-independent index of the severity of mitral stenosis.
   a. True
   b. False

44. A patient with MR has a radius of the proximal isovelocity contour of 9 mm at a Nyquist limit of the color-flow Doppler at 0.69 m/s, and a CWD velocity of the MR of 5 m/s. The CWD VTI of the MR jet is 130 cm. Tricuspid regurgitant jet peak velocity is 4 m/s. PWD assessment of the hepatic veins shows a systolic forward flow velocity of 40 cm/s and a diastolic forward flow velocity of 40 cm/s.

   A. The calculated effective regurgitant orifice area of the mitral valve is:
      a. 2.70 cm^2
      b. 0.35 cm^2
      c. 0.70 cm^2
      d. 0.90 cm^2

   B. The mitral regurgitant volume is:
      a. 101 mL
      b. 50 mL
      c. 91 mL
      d. 61 mL

Mitral Valve Repair

8

Ghassan Sleilaty, Issam El Rassi, and Victor Jebara

The superiority of mitral valve repair over replacement in patients with mitral valve disease is now widely accepted. This is mainly due to better preservation of left ventricular (LV) function, greater regression of left heart dimensions, resistance to endocarditis, avoidance of long-term anticoagulation (mechanical valves) or reoperation (bioprosthetic valves), fewer valve-related complications (mechanical and bioprosthesis), and improved survival.[1-4]

FUNCTIONAL ANATOMY OF THE MITRAL VALVE

The mitral valve is comprised of three distinct components: the mitral annulus, the subvalvar apparatus, and the mitral leaflets.

Mitral Annulus

Two structures from the cardiac skeleton form part of the mitral valve ring: the right and the left fibrous trigones. The most prominent is the right fibrous trigone, also known as the *central fibrous body*, which is located between the mitral (left), tricuspid (right), and aortic (anterior) orifices in a triangular form that justifies its name. The left fibrous trigone has a similar structure but is less prominent and is situated ventrally and to the left, between the left margins of the mitral and aortic valves. The two fibrous trigones are interconnected to form the "curtain" of fibrous tissue between the aortic valve and the anterior leaflet of the mitral valve (mitral-aortic fibrous continuity). In this region, the left fibrous trigone extends superiorly to form part of the scalloped aortic root. This concentration of fibrous tissue helps prevent dilatation of the correspondent segment of the mitral annulus. Laterally, bands of connective tissue (the left filum coronarium) extend from the two fibrous bodies but fade out progressively and leave the posterior third of the mitral annulus completely devoid of collagen fibers. This segment of the annulus is therefore ill defined and without true anatomical substance. The two fibrous bodies act as the fixed points on which the contraction of the myocardial fibers is based. Thus, the annulus is dynamic, and its motion is coordinated by the cardiac cycle. Mitral annular dysfunction occurs mainly in the posterior and medial portions of the valve.[3]

Chordae Tendineae

The chordal system is the most extensively studied component of the mitral apparatus, yet it remains the most controversial because of the wide variations of number and form of the chordae and their attachments. As the name indicates, the chordae tendineae are tendinous structures that originate from the tip of the papillary muscles on one side and insert into the valve leaflets on the other. However, chordae originating directly from the ventricular wall, and muscular chordae (chorda muscularis) have been described in a number of normal hearts. After a short but variable course, the chordae tendineae usually branch before insertion, but a small number of unbranched chordae may insert directly into the leaflet. The insertion into the posterior leaflet occurs at any point between the free edge and the base. The mode of insertion into the anterior leaflet is different, with most descriptions referring to the ventricular surface of the anterior leaflet as being devoid of chordae beyond the marginal rough zone. However, thick chordae originating from either papillary muscle, inserting well beyond the rough zone, have been reported. The significance of recognizing them during reconstruction of the mitral valve is discussed later (see section Chordae Transposition).

It is also important to distinguish between commissural chordae and leaflet chordae (Figure 8–1).

COMMISSURAL CHORDAE

A single chord branches in a fan-like manner into five to seven small chordae, which then insert into the free edge of the commissural segment of each leaflet. The arrangement is similar for both commissures, but with a wider lateral spread in the posteromedial commissural area. The average length of the chordae of the anterolateral commissure is 1.2 to 1.4 cm and that of the posteromedial commissural chordae is 1.4 to 1.7 cm. Knowledge of the commissural chordae is essential to understanding the pathophysiology and management of ischemic mitral regurgitation.

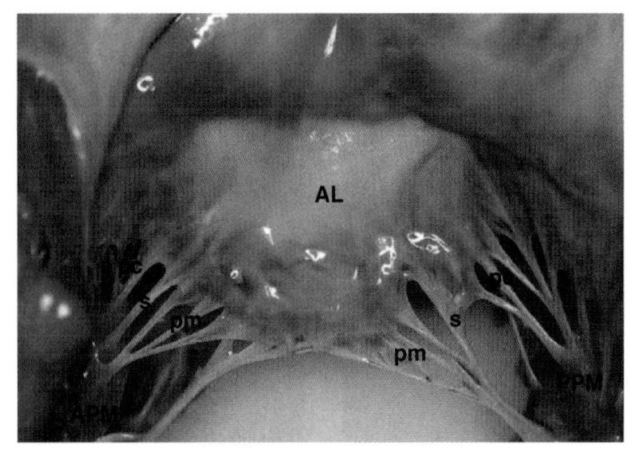

A

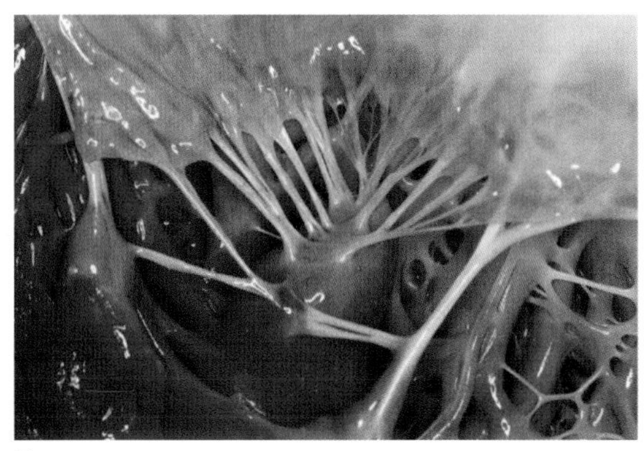

B

FIGURE 8–1. **A:** Anatomy of the anterior leaflet and its chordae tendineae. **B:** Commissural chordae tendineae. A single chord branches in a fan-like manner to insert into the free edge of the commissural portion of each leaflet. The arrangement is similar for both commissures. (AL, anterior leaflet; APM, anterior papillary muscle; pc, paracommissural chordae tendineae; pm, paramedial chordae tendineae; PPM, posterior papillary muscle; s, strut chordae tendineae.) *(Reproduced with permission from Antunes, Mitral valve repair, R. S. Schulz, 1989.)*

LEAFLET CHORDAE

From each papillary muscle three groups of chordae insert in an oblique manner into the corresponding half of the anterior leaflet, on either side of the midline: paramedial, central (strut), and paracommissural. The strut chordae are the thickest, and arise at the very summit of the papillary muscle and insert into the ventricular surface of the rough zone, usually away from the edge of the leaflet. They appear to constitute the "cornerstone" of the chordal system of the anterior leaflet, whereas the paramedial and paracommissural chordae play an accessory role in the support of the leaflet. Typically, each of them divides into three branches that insert directly or, after further branching, into the free edge, limit of the rough zone, and intermediate area of the leaflet, respectively, and act together as a functional unit. Chordae similar to those described for the anterior leaflet reach the free edge and the ventricular surface of the posterior leaflet in a parallel alignment. However, the basal and cleft chordae are unique to this leaflet. The former originate in the papillary muscles or ventricular wall and attach into the base (annular region) of the central scallop of the posterior leaflet. The latter always originate from the papillary muscle and insert into the margins and adjacent areas of the central and lateral scallops. The typical fan-shape attachment of the chordae to the ventricular surface of the posterior leaflet has pathologic and surgical implications that are discussed later. The mitral valve has an average of 25 primary chordae. Nine of these insert into the anterior leaflet, 14 into the posterior leaflet, and two into the commissures. Most of the "variations from normal" are characterized by the absence of one or a group of chordae, leaving a portion of the leaflet unsupported.

Papillary Muscles

The left ventricle has two papillary muscles: anterior (or anterolateral) and posterior (or posteromedial). Both originate from the ventricular free wall, at or near the junction between the apical and middle thirds. The anterior papillary muscle is attached to the anterior wall of the ventricle, close to its lateral border. The posterior papillary muscle originates from the posterior wall, near the junction with the ventricular septum. Both papillary muscles have equal anatomic and functional importance and have the same volume. However, there are also notable variations of form. Acar and coworkers established a classification based on the ways that the papillary muscles relate to the leaflets via the chordae.[5] Four types are described (Figure 8–2). In type I, the papillary muscle is single. In type II, the papillary muscle has two heads, one of which sends chordae exclusively to the posterior leaflet. In type III, the papillary muscle is also divided, with one head supporting the commissural area exclusively. Type IV papillary muscle resembles but is distinct from type III in that the head supporting the commissure is very short. In type IV, the different heads also originate at different levels on the ventricular wall from the apex to the base.

The blood supply to the papillary muscles is provided by septal branches of the right and left coronary arteries. The anterior papillary muscle usually is supplied by several branches of the left coronary artery, including the second septal branch of the anterior descending (interventricular) artery and branches of the circumflex artery.

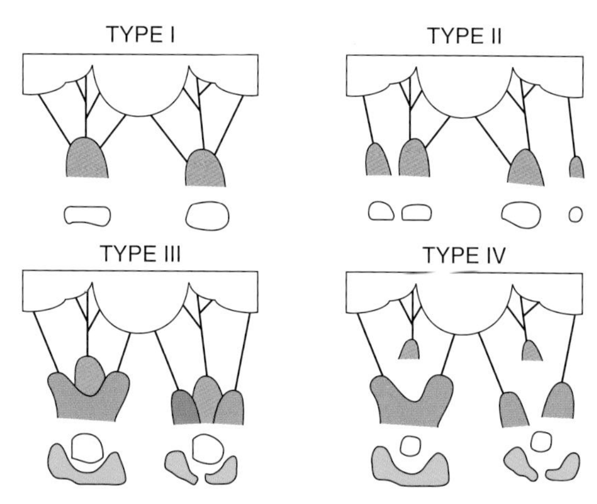

FIGURE 8–2. Anatomic classification of papillary muscles. *(Reproduced with permission from Acar C, Tolan M, Berrebi A, et al. Homograft replacement of the mitral valve. Graft selection, technique of implantation, and results in forty-three patients. J Thorac Cardiovasc Surg. 1996;111:367.)*

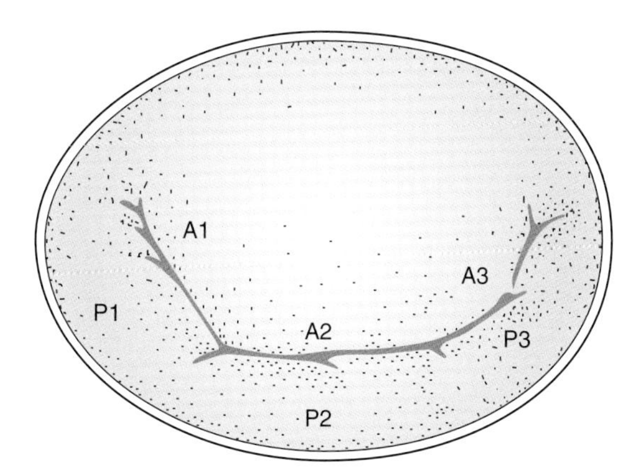

FIGURE 8–3. The posterior leaflet segments are designated as P1, P2, and P3. P1 is adjacent to the anterolateral commissure, P2 is the middle scallop, and P3 is adjacent to the posteromedial commissure. The anterior leaflet has less clearly defined segments designated as A1, A2, and A3, corresponding to the adjacent posterior leaflet segments.

Conversely, the posterior papillary muscle receives its supply from one of the septal branches of the posterior descending artery and/or another branch directly from the circumflex artery. In approximately two-thirds of the population, the posterior papillary muscle is perfused by only one vessel. Within the papillary muscles, each artery divides into two branches that course centrally and subendocardially throughout the length of the muscle and usually are interconnected by multiple anastomoses. However, the supply may be from a single central artery. The highly variable anatomy of the posterior descending artery renders the posterior papillary muscle more susceptible to rupture, secondary to occlusion of the right coronary artery, circumflex artery, or both. Although the major contribution is from the intramural arteries, the most peripheral portions of the papillary muscles are perfused by oxygen diffusion from intracavitary blood.

Mitral Leaflets

The normal mitral valve has two leaflets: the anterior leaflet (AML), which covers 80% of the orifice area, and the posterior leaflet (PML), which covers the remaining 20% of the orifice area. Disease of the mitral valve leading to mitral regurgitation (MR) rarely involves the whole leaflet, but is usually confined to specific segments. To unify the language between cardiologists and surgeons and among the surgeons themselves, Carpentier proposed a nomenclature that would allow clear identification of the anatomic segment(s) involved. He designated the posterior leaflet segments as P1, P2, and P3. P1 is adjacent to the anterolateral commissure, P2 is the middle scallop, and P3 is adjacent to the posteromedial commissure. The anterior leaflet has less clearly defined segments designated as A1, A2, and A3, corresponding to the adjacent posterior leaflet segments (Figure 8–3). The transesophageal echocardiographic (TEE) transgastric basal short-axis view of the left ventricle, with some anteflexion, provides the "fishmouth" view of the mitral valve (MV), in which the A3 and P3 segments are at the top of the screen and the A1 and P1 segments are at the bottom (anterior leaflet to the left). In the surgeon's view, A3 and P3 are to the right, and A1 and P1 are to the left (anterior leaflet superior).

FUNCTIONAL CLASSIFICATION OF MR

One of the most important breakthroughs in the management of MR was the introduction by Carpentier in the early 1980s of the functional classification of MR.[6] This classification describes mitral valve disease in terms of the pathophysiologic triad of type of valve dysfunction, lesion, and etiology. It is based on the opening and closing motions of the mitral leaflets (Figure 8–4):

Type I has normal motion of the leaflets and MR is due to leaflet perforation (endocarditis) or to annular dilatation (LV dysfunction).

Type II has increased leaflet motion with the free edge of the leaflet traveling above the plane of the mitral annulus during systole (leaflet prolapse). This

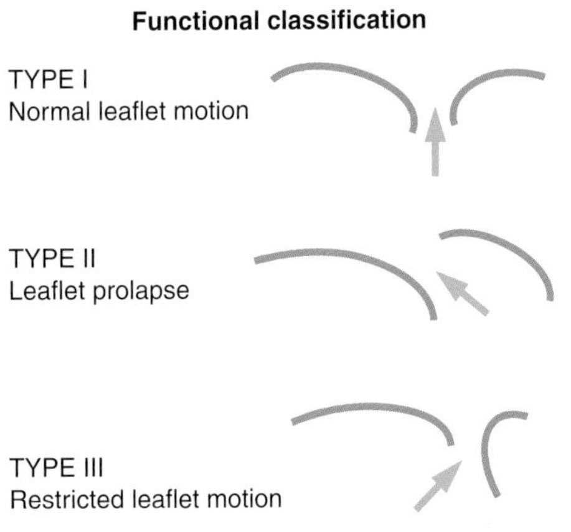

Functional classification

TYPE I
Normal leaflet motion

TYPE II
Leaflet prolapse

TYPE III
Restricted leaflet motion

FIGURE 8–4. Functional classification proposed by Carpentier based on the opening and closing motions of the mitral leaflets.

is due to chordal elongation or rupture as seen in degenerative valve disease.

Type III has restricted leaflet motion.

Type IIIa dysfunction implies restricted leaflet motion during diastole and systole due to rheumatic changes.

Type IIIb dysfunction correlates to restricted leaflet motion during systole secondary to papillary muscle displacement in ischemic or dilated cardiomyopathy.

ETIOLOGY OF MR

Diseases of the mitral valve responsible for MR are numerous. The most common causes of MR include degenerative mitral valve disease, ischemic mitral regurgitation, endocarditis, and dilated cardiomyopathy. Other less frequent causes include rheumatic heart disease, traumatic MR, and systemic inflammatory diseases.

Degenerative Mitral Valve Disease

Although the most common cause of MR is degenerative disease, it is interesting to note the confusing terminology, typical of the literature, used to define degenerative mitral valve disease (eg, "myxomatous degeneration," "floppy leaflets," "billowing leaflets," "Barlow's disease," "flail leaflets," and "leaflet prolapse"). Patients with degenerative mitral valve disease most commonly have type II dysfunction, which corresponds to the overriding of the free edge of the leaflet above the plane of the mitral annulus during systole (leaflet prolapse). This is usually related to chordal elongation or chordal rupture. Associated annular dilation is a common finding in these patients; however, isolated annular dilatation (type I dysfunction) with normal motion of both leaflets has been reported. Of note is the fact that leaflet restriction (type III dysfunction) is not observed in patients with degenerative disease.

Controversy continues as to the pathologic types of degenerative mitral valve. Some investigators have claimed that this is a single disease diagnosed at different stages, and others have described multiple subtypes. For the sake of clarity, we distinguish three types of degenerative mitral valve disease: fibroelastic deficiency (first described by Carpentier), Barlow's disease (characterized by myxoid degeneration with excess leaflet tissue), and Marfan's disease.

Fibroelastic deficiency is most common in elderly patients with a relatively short history of valve dysfunction. Intraoperative analysis typically shows transparent leaflets with no excess tissue except in the prolapsing segment, and elongated, thin, frail, and often ruptured chordae. The annulus is often dilated and may be calcified. In contrast, *Barlow's disease* appears early in life, and patients typically have a long history of a systolic murmur. The valve leaflets are typically thick with marked excess tissue. The chordae are thickened, elongated, and may be ruptured. Papillary muscles also are occasionally elongated. The annulus is dilated and sometimes calcified. *Marfan's disease* with MR is characterized by excess leaflet tissue, which may be thickened (without myxoid degeneration), and a dilated annulus that is rarely calcified. In some patients with degenerative mitral valve disease, the exact etiology of valvular regurgitation remains undetermined. The most common lesions encountered in all types of degenerative mitral valve disease are posterior leaflet prolapse secondary to elongation and rupture of the corresponding chordae, and annular dilatation and deformation.

Ischemic Mitral Valve Disease

In the acute phase after myocardial infarction, massive ischemic MR usually is secondary to a ruptured papillary muscle, a catastrophic event that in most cases requires emergency replacement of the mitral valve. However, in the vast majority of patients, MR can develop after a myocardial infarction without papillary muscle rupture as a consequence of LV remodeling, due to the apical and inferior displacement of the papillary muscles producing incomplete coaptation of leaflets. In these cases, ischemic MR may be due to one of the following reasons:

1. Simple annular dilatation (secondary to LV enlargement), which causes incomplete mitral leaflet coaptation associated with type I (normal) leaflet motion.
2. Local LV remodeling with papillary muscle displacement producing apical tethering or tenting of the leaflets (with type IIIb restricted systolic leaflet motion).
3. Both mechanisms.

4. Recent studies show that mitral leaflets in functional MR are stiffer than normal leaflets with altered extracellular matrix composition.[7]

Endocarditis

In the setting of bacterial endocarditis, MR can develop due to:

1. Leaflet prolapse secondary to rupture or destruction of marginal chordae
2. Leaflet perforation due to abscess formation
3. Leaflet destruction with giant vegetations

Dilated Cardiomyopathy

Mitral valve regurgitation is a common finding in end-stage cardiomyopathy caused by dilatation of the mitral annulus (type I) and of the left ventricle (type IIIb). Mitral insufficiency leads to a vicious circle, with increasing volume overload of the dilated left ventricle, leading to further annular and ventricular dilatation, worsening of mitral valve regurgitation, and volume overload. The resulting mitral valve insufficiency is often refractory to medical therapy and predicts poor survival in this patient group. Surgical correction of MR can interrupt this vicious cycle.

Rheumatic Valve Disease

Once the most frequent cause of mitral valve disease, rheumatic disease has been almost eradicated in the Western world. However, physicians practicing in Africa and in some parts of Asia still face the difficult problem of rheumatic mitral valves in children and young adults.

Rheumatic fever causes severe changes in all components of the mitral valve. The chordae are thickened, fused, and shortened; the leaflets become rigid and calcified; the commissures are fused; and with time, the annulus and the entire valve calcify.

SURGICAL TECHNIQUES

Since the mid-1970s considerable efforts have been made to develop and standardize surgical techniques for mitral valve reconstruction. Techniques of mitral valve repair were developed and adapted to treat specific anatomic lesions leading to MR. There is no doubt that Carpentier pioneered a large number of these advances, and hence deserves the paternity of mitral valve repair. However, other groups from around the world have brought considerable insight into mitral valve pathology, its treatment, and the results of surgical repair.

Annuloplasty

Annuloplasty is used to treat annular dilation or deformation (type I MR), which is often encountered in association with other anatomic lesions. Annuloplasty is therefore used as an adjunct to other surgical techniques. It has been demonstrated that annuloplasty is an indispensable technique to ensure long-term durability of the repair in the vast majority of cases. Several techniques and prosthetic devices have been used to perform annuloplasty, but there is some evidence showing the superiority of prosthetic rings (complete or incomplete) over stitch reduction of the annulus or localized reinforcements.

Leaflet Resection

Leaflet resection is used to treat leaflet prolapse, most frequently at the level of the PML. In fact, quadrangular resection of the posterior leaflet is the most common technique used in degenerative mitral valve disease (Figure 8–5). It is the most predictable technique,

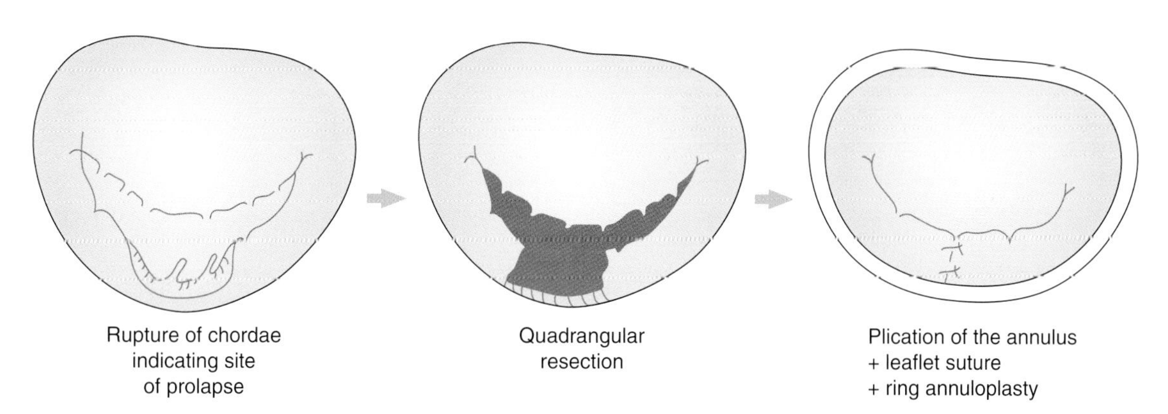

FIGURE 8–5. Quadrangular resection technique. *(Reproduced with permission from Acar J, Acar C. Cardiopathies Valvulaires Acquises. Paris: Flammarion; 2000.)*

yielding the best results postoperatively and in the long term. Triangular resections with less extensive resections at the level of the annulus of the PML offer equivalent results without the need for a wide plication of the posterior annulus to prevent kinking or damage of a dominant circumflex artery. Results of leaflet resection of the anterior leaflet are less favorable than those observed with posterior leaflet resection. Therefore, resection of the AML should be avoided and replaced by alternative techniques. However, in rare cases with excessive leaflet tissue (Barlow's disease), localized resections have been used with good results.

Sliding Leaflet Technique

This technique is a variation of the quadrangular resection of the posterior leaflet. It was introduced in 1989 by Carpentier to address the problem of systolic anterior motion (SAM) of the AML after mitral valve repair.[8] The rationale behind this technique resides in the understanding of the pathophysiology of SAM in this setting. The sliding leaflet technique aims to reduce the height of a tall posterior leaflet, which is one of the major risk factors for SAM. Results with this technique (Figure 8–6) have been extremely favorable, with virtually total eradication of significant SAM after mitral repair.[8,9]

Chordae Transposition

Chordal transposition is the technique of choice to treat prolapse of the anterior leaflet. Chordae transposition (Figure 8–7A) from the PML to the diseased segment of the AML has replaced chordal shortening techniques (see Figure 8–7B). Shortened chordae tend to rupture at the site of insertion into the papillary muscle trench and should be avoided whenever possible, but transposition is not associated with an increase in the rate of reoperation.[10-13] Chordae transposition is also known as the "flip-over" technique and usually requires resection of a corresponding segment of the PML. However, in some cases, secondary chordae of the AML can be transposed to the free margin to replace elongated or ruptured chordae (see Figure 8–7C). This latter technique is particularly helpful to reinforce fragile chords or bare margins of the anterior and posterior leaflets.

Shortening of the Papillary Muscle

A group of elongated chordae arising from one papillary muscle or, more often, from one of the heads of a papillary muscle can be treated by shortening of the head of the papillary muscle, by incomplete resection of a segment of the culprit head, or by tilting the head and suturing it to the base of the papillary muscle. Papillary muscle repositioning for repair of anterior leaflet prolapse caused by chordal elongation is a variant described by Dreyfus and colleagues.[14]

Artificial Chordae

Use of expanded polytetrafluoroethylene sutures to reinforce or replace chordae tendineae was described in 1985 by David and associates and has been used by many surgeons with satisfactory results.[15] However, in cases in which a large number of chords have to be replaced, care should be taken to find the exact length of the new chords. In our personal experience, we rarely use artificial chordae because repair is always possible with more conventional techniques.

Patch Closure of Leaflet Perforation

When the defect is on the body of the AML, it is easily corrected by debridement and patch closure with autologous pericardium (Figure 8–8).[16] If the free margin or the commissure is involved, more exhaustive techniques usually are required, including leaflet resection and reconstruction using autologous pericardium and chordae transposition. In more extensive cases, a partial homograft can be used to replace the damaged segments and avoid mitral valve replacement, as advocated by Acar and colleagues.[5,17]

"Bow-Tie" Repair or Alfieri Stitch

This procedure, also known as the *double orifice mitral valve*, consists of anchoring the free edge of the anterior leaflet to the posterior leaflet (Figure 8–9).[18] It is an alternative technique used to treat leaflet prolapse and to restore the area of coaptation. In our experience, the Alfieri stitch is particularly helpful in treating commissural regurgitation due to prolapse or to restriction. This technique has also been advocated as a "bailout" to reduce residual leaks at the completion of a mitral repair procedure.

Commissurotomy

Commissurotomy is the oldest technique used to repair the mitral valve. It aims to relieve mitral stenosis secondary to rheumatic heart disease. In the absence of calcification, interventional cardiologists using a specially designed balloon can perform mitral commissurotomy.

Leaflet Extension

Leaflet extension with autologous pericardium is a technique used to increase leaflet height and restore the area of coaptation (Figure 8–10). Leaflet extension of the

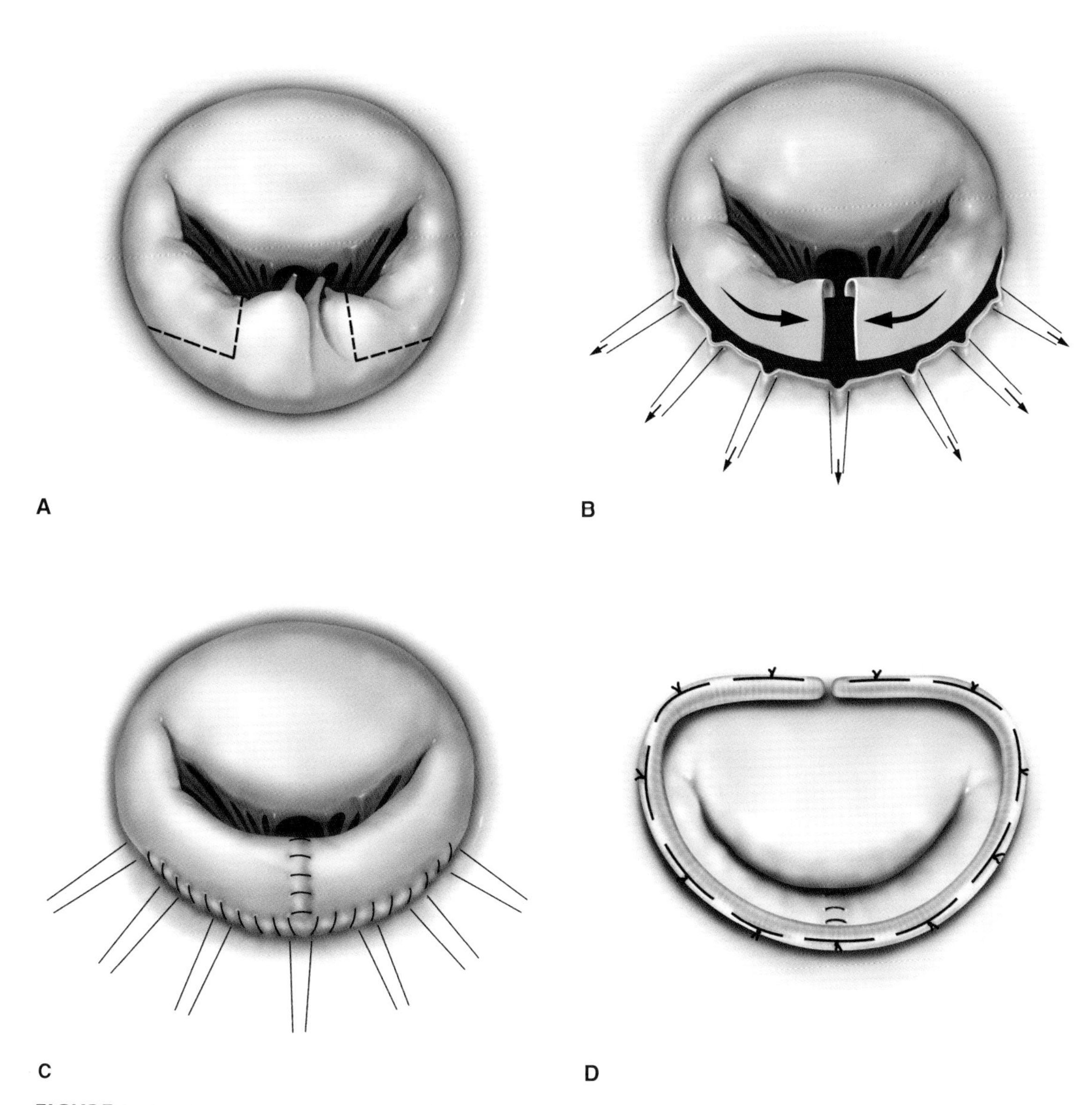

FIGURE 8–6. Sliding leaflet technique. **A:** Resection of excess tissue and prolapsed segment of the posterior leaflet. **B:** Medial translation of remnants of the posterior leaflet. **C:** Completed repair. **D:** Ring insertion.

PML was first described by Duran and associates[19,20] to treat type IIIa restricted leaflets observed in rheumatic heart disease.[21] Acar and coworkers described extension of the AML by using a very large pericardial patch that results in a twofold increase in the surface of the AML.[5,17] Results of this technique have been very encouraging.

Resection of Secondary Chordae Tendineae

This technique was described initially to increase leaflet motion in rheumatic heart disease. Recently, chord resection has been used in ischemic MR at the level of the AML to resect tethered secondary chordae (gull sign).

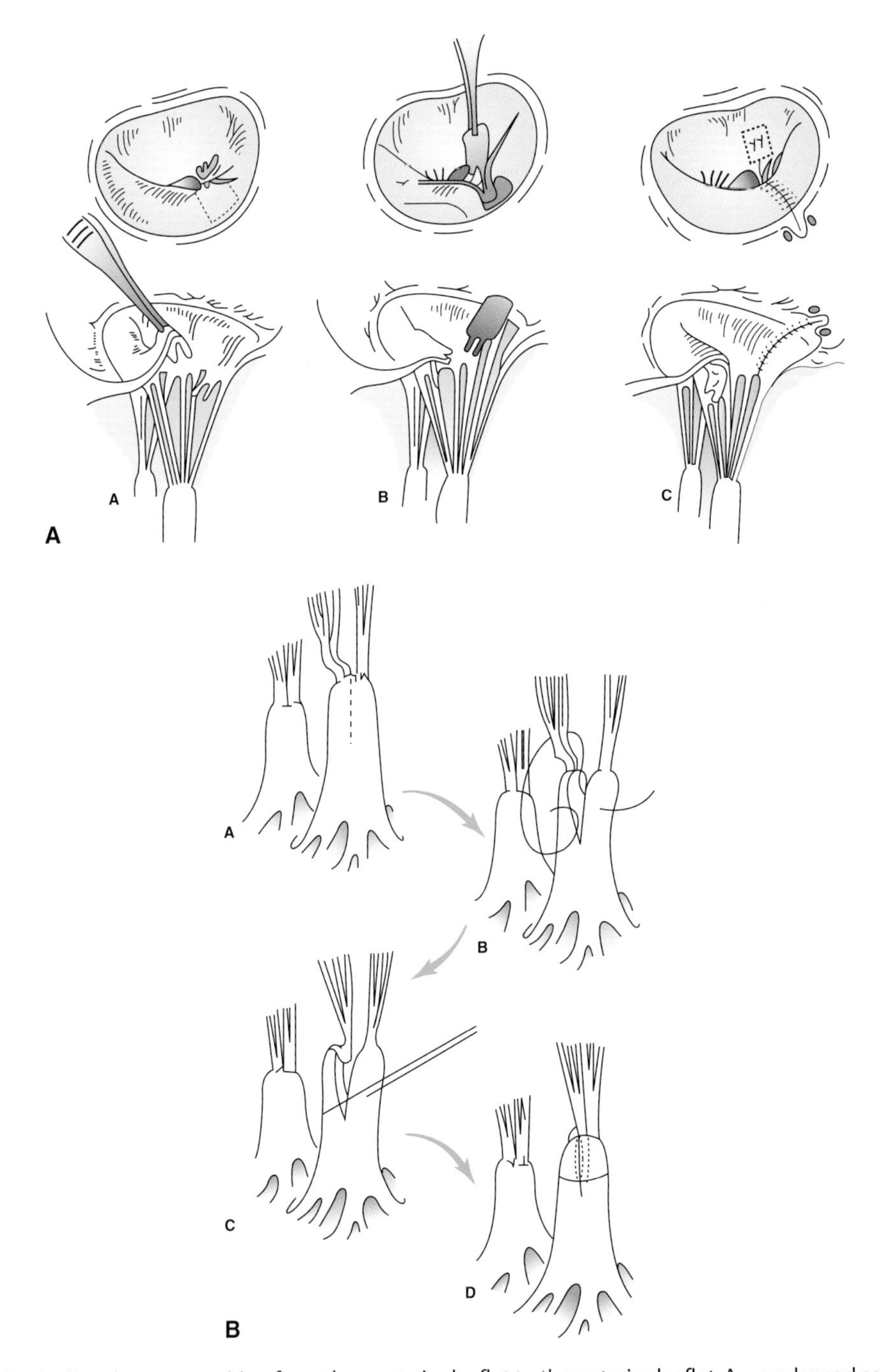

FIGURE 8–7. **A:** Chordae transposition from the posterior leaflet to the anterior leaflet. A—prolapsed segment of the anterior leaflet due to rupture chords; B—resection of a localized segment of the posterior leaflet with its chords; C—flip over to the anterior leaflet and suturing of the posterior leaflet. **B:** Chordae shortening technique. A—trench created in the head of the papillary muscle; B and C—elongated chords are buried inside the trench; D—trench is closed. **C:** Repair of ruptured chords. A—prolapsed segment of the anterior leaflet due to ruptured chords; B—resection of a secondary chord; C—translation to the free margin. *(Reproduced with permission from Edmunds LH. Cardiac Surgery in the Adult. New York: McGraw-Hill; 1997.)*

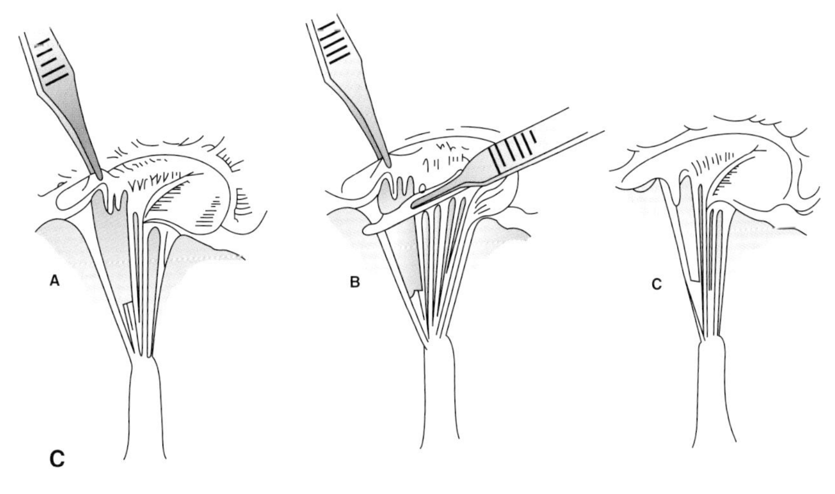

FIGURE 8–7. *(Continued)*

INDICATIONS FOR MITRAL VALVE REPAIR

Traditionally, surgery for MR was indicated only in symptomatic patients with overt signs of deterioration of LV function. However, reports from the Mayo Clinic on the natural history of the disease and the effect of LV dysfunction on surgical outcome have resulted in a widespread evolution toward earlier surgical intervention.[10,22-24] Enriquez-Sarano and coworkers analyzed the natural history of MR caused by flail leaflets.[10,22-25] They observed, in comparison with the expected survival rate, a higher mortality rate (6.3% yearly). In addition, they found 10-year incidences of 30% for atrial fibrillation and 63% for heart failure. Further, at 10 years, 90% of patients were dead or had undergone surgery, which means that the operation is inevitable. Patients with New York Heart Association functional class III or IV symptoms, even transient, displayed a considerable mortality (34% yearly) if not operated on. In addition, patients with class I or II had a notable mortality (4.1% yearly). Patients with ejection fraction less than 60% also displayed a higher mortality rate as compared with those with ejection fraction greater than 60%. Sudden death is responsible for approximately 25% of the deaths occurring under medical treatment and, although the rate of sudden death increases with severe clinical symptoms and with reduced ejection fraction, most sudden death occurred in patients with no or minimal symptoms and with normal LV function. The rate of sudden death is 1.8% per year overall; even in patients without risk factors, it is 0.8% per year. These data underscore the serious prognostic implication of severe MR, suggesting that surgery should be considered early in the course of the disease.[26] In 2003, the Euro Heart Survey found that around 50% of patients with MR receive a valve

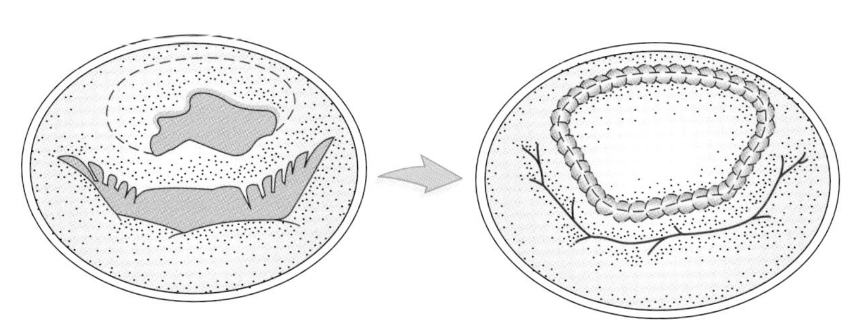

FIGURE 8–8. Patch closure of leaflet perforation. Endocarditis with abscess and perforation of the anterior leaflet is seen in the left panel. Debridement *(dotted line)* is initially carried out followed by placement of a pericardial patch *(right panel).*

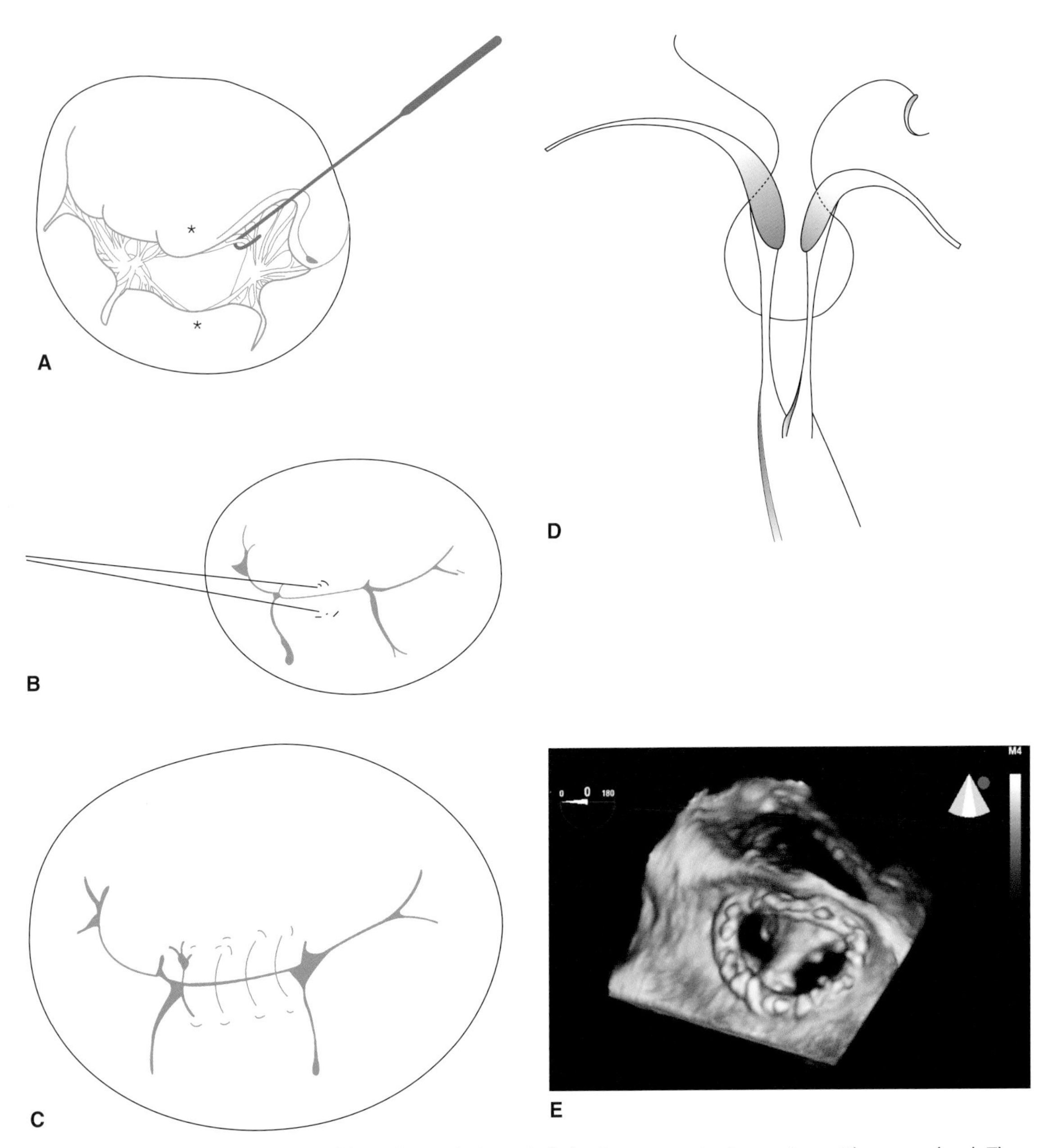

FIGURE 8–9. Alfieri repair: the double-orifice technique. **A:** Subvalvar apparatus inspection with a nerve hook. The middle portion of the leaflets is identified (*). **B:** The central stitch is used to check the symmetry of the orifices. **C:** A running suture along the free edge of the leaflets is sewn. **D:** Deep bites through the rough zone of the leaflets are placed to avoid tearing of the suture. **E:** Three-dimensional echocardiographic image in a patient who has undergone an annuloplasty and Alfieri repair. The double orifice created by the central stitch between A2 and P2 is clearly visible. *(Reproduced with permission from Maisano F, Schreuder JJ, Oppizzi M, et al. The double-orifice technique as a standardized approach to treat mitral regurgitation due to severe myxomatous disease: surgical technique. Eur J Cardiothorac Surg. 2000;17:201.)*

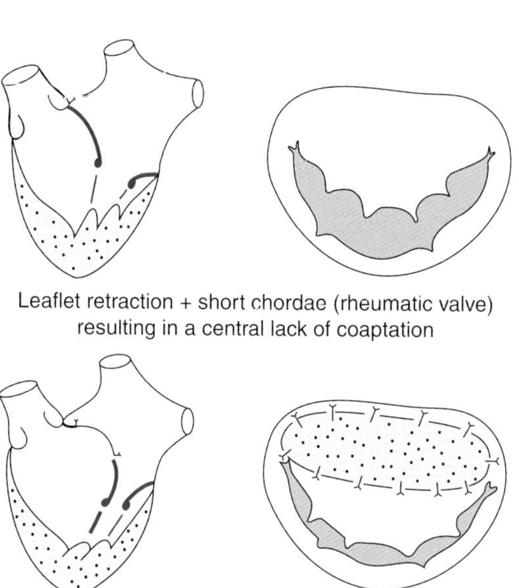

FIGURE 8–10. Leaflet extension technique. *(Reproduced with permission from Acar J, Acar C. Cardiopathies Valvulaires Acquises. Paris: Flammarion; 2000.)*

replacement rather than a repair.[27] The figure is not much different in the United States where about one-third of the patients benefit from MV repair.[28]

REPAIR DURABILITY

Since the introduction of standardized techniques for mitral valve reconstruction, mitral valve repair has become the surgical treatment of choice for MR. Numerous retrospective studies have demonstrated important advantages of mitral valve repair over mitral valve replacement. Mitral valve repair is most applicable to patients with degenerative mitral valve disease, with successful valvuloplasty in more than 95% of these patients. Further, it is in patients with degenerative mitral valve disease that repair has been shown to have the greatest durability. With the longest follow-up to date, Deloche, Braunberger, and associates[29,30] found that 93% of patients with degenerative disease did not require reoperation 15 years after their initial mitral valve repair. Gillinov and colleagues[12] analyzed 1072 patients undergoing mitral valve repair for degenerative disease at the Cleveland Clinic. This study corroborated the excellent long-term results of Deloche and coworkers (92.9% at 10 years). Using propensity score adjustment, Jokinen and colleagues[31] confirmed once more the superiority of MV repair over replacement. Despite these excellent results in patients with degenerative disease, some patients may require reoperation for recurrent mitral valve dysfunction. Causes of failed mitral valve repair may be classified as related to procedure (rupture of previously shortened chordae, suture dehiscence, or incomplete initial operation) or to the valve (progressive disease or endocarditis). Previous studies have noted a high proportion of procedure-related repair failures in patients with degenerative disease, suggesting that modification of the operative technique might increase repair durability.[11,24,32]

Other risk factors for failure of mitral valve repair include advanced myxomatous changes of leaflets, chordal shortening procedures, failure to perform an annuloplasty, residual MR at the completion of repair, New York Heart Association functional class III or IV, and performance of concomitant cardiac procedures. Patients with the most common pathologic finding, namely posterior leaflet prolapse caused by chordal rupture, have the lowest risk of late reoperation. In addition, the "standard" mitral valve repair of posterior leaflet quadrangular resection and annuloplasty has the greatest durability. Failure to add an annuloplasty to posterior leaflet resection or performing an annuloplasty alone increases the risk of late reoperation.[32] Of interest, the type of annuloplasty ring used (Cosgrove-Edwards, Carpentier-Edwards, or pericardial band) did not influence repair durability.[11] As previously discussed, chordal shortening increases the risk of reoperation because shortened chordae tend to rupture at the site of insertion into the papillary muscle. Moreover, the need for additional leaflet sutures to increase local leaflet coaptation increases the risk of reoperation. Intraoperative TEE guidance also decreases the risk of reoperation.

INFERENCES CONCERNING REPAIR OF DEGENERATED MITRAL VALVES

1. Intraoperative echocardiography should be routinely used to assess the mechanism of valve dysfunction and the results of valve repair.
2. Posterior leaflet quadrangular resection should be accompanied by an annuloplasty.
3. Anterior leaflet prolapse should be corrected by techniques other than chordal shortening.
4. Chordal transfer does not increase the risk of repair failure, and this procedure is considered a

durable technique for the treatment of anterior leaflet prolapse.[7]

5. Other techniques for correction of anterior leaflet prolapse might include the use of artificial chordae and anchoring the free edge of the anterior leaflet to the posterior leaflet. Data comparing these techniques to chordal transfer are currently unavailable. Therefore, we currently favor chordal transfer for correction of anterior leaflet prolapse.

Clinical Decisions In Ischemic MR

Patients requiring surgical revascularization for suspected ischemic MR should be assessed carefully with preoperative echocardiography to determine the severity of the MR. More recently, Song et al[33] used real-time 3D echocardiography to show that geometrical determinants of ischemic MR depend on the location of the prior myocardial infarction, implying that MV repair differs between ischemic and dilated MR. Although intraoperative TEE can be very helpful in more precisely assessing anatomic details, the severity of MR will be underestimated in most patients, and provocative testing with increased preload and afterload may be necessary. Coronary artery bypass grafting (CABG) alone will leave many patients with moderate or severe (3 to 4+) residual MR, and therefore may not be the optimal therapy. Wider application of mitral annuloplasty may be warranted in this group of patients, but more detailed analysis is necessary to determine preoperative factors that predict residual MR after CABG alone. Long-term follow-up is also necessary to determine the effect of residual MR on late symptoms and survival. Prospective, randomized studies are currently under way through the Cardiothoracic Surgical Trials Network to assess the role of mitral valve repair in patients with ischemic or "functional" MR.

Effect of CABG on MR

Aklog and associates[34] addressed the question of whether CABG alone could correct moderate ischemic MR. In their study, 40% of the patients who underwent postoperative transthoracic echocardiography showed no improvement with CABG alone and were left with moderate or severe (3 to 4+) residual MR. Approximately 50% of patients had some improvement and were left with mild (2+) residual MR. Only a few patients (fewer than 10%) had significant improvement, with no more than trace (0 to 1+) residual MR. These results suggest that CABG alone has an inconsistent and relatively weak effect on moderate ischemic MR.

Only a few studies have addressed this issue directly, with contradictory conclusions.[35] Three reports have suggested that CABG alone can correct ischemic MR. Balu and colleagues,[36] in a report from 1982, presented preoperative and postoperative ventriculography data on a heterogeneous group of 12 patients with ischemic MR and suggested that CABG alone improves MR and functional status. However, this study was limited by the heterogeneity and small number of patients enrolled. In a more recent report, Christenson and associates[37] reviewed data from 56 patients with severe LV dysfunction (ejection fraction less than 25%) and various degrees of MR on preoperative echocardiography who underwent CABG alone. On postoperative echocardiography, 93% of the patients had no more than trace (0 to 1+) MR, and the remaining patients had mild (2+) MR. The investigators concluded that "moderate co-existing MR seems to normalize after myocardial revascularization and should not be surgically corrected therefore at the primary operation." However, this study also had several limitations that, in our opinion, make it difficult to interpret and do not justify this broad recommendation. Most importantly, only seven patients (13%) in the study had moderate (3+) preoperative MR, and 40% had trace (1+) MR. In addition, nearly 10% of these patients underwent concomitant LV aneurysm repair, which can improve MR by decreasing ventricular dimensions. This fact may explain the unusually large increase in mean ejection fraction (18% to 44%) as compared with most reports on CABG in severe LV dysfunction. Kang et al[38] assigned 107 patients with moderate to severe ischemic MR to CABG with concomitant MV repair (n = 50) or CABG alone (n = 57). The operative mortality in the combined CABG and MVR group was 12%, compared to 2% in the CABG-alone group. On follow-up, the 5-year survival rate was similar in both groups and approximated 88%. However, among the patients with severe MR, ischemic MR was improved in all patients of the repair group and in 67% of patients in the CABG group ($P < .001$), whereas improvement rates in patients with moderate MR were similar in the two groups. This study has several limitations: mainly, this was a nonrandomized study, implying an inherent selection bias. The series also included seven patients who underwent concomitant LV aneurysm repair for apical aneurysm, and the repair group had a higher percentage of patients with atrial fibrillation or severe MR than the CABG group. Moreover, on inspecting the survival curves, one sees that the repair-associated mortality occurs strictly in the early postoperative period, then the survival curves remain horizontal despite the higher risk profile in this group.

SIMRAM, an ongoing, large, prospective, multicenter, nonrandomized registry, is currently evaluating the effects of surgery on ischemic MR at rest and on its dynamic component at exercise.[39] The SIMRAM registry is also designed to define the place of pre- and postoperative exercise testing in these settings along with the predictive factors affecting outcome. Prospective, randomized studies are also currently under way through the Cardiothoracic Surgical Trials Network (http://www.ctsurgerynet.org/) to assess the role of mitral valve repair in patients with ischemic or "functional" MR.

Clinical Implications

Whether more liberal use of mitral annuloplasty is indicated depends on the answers to the following questions:

1. Can mitral annuloplasty reliably and predictably correct moderate ischemic MR, and what is the additional operative risk of this procedure?
2. What is the long-term effect of residual MR on functional status and survival?

Success Rate and Operative Risk of Mitral Annuloplasty

Although it has been our impression that nearly all cases of Carpentier type I or IIIb moderate ischemic MR can be corrected with a restrictive annuloplasty and posterior commissuroplasty, few reports have addressed this issue specifically. Czer and coworkers[40] and Bolling[41] and associates found that ring annuloplasty is successful at correcting functional ischemic MR in nearly all patients. Dion and colleagues[42] reported some residual MR in only 15% of patients undergoing ring annuloplasty alone for ischemic MR. The additional operative risk with concomitant mitral annuloplasty was evaluated by Aklog and colleagues, who reported a 3.7% operative mortality rate in their most recent cohort of patients with moderate ischemic MR.[34] Other studies have reported similar mortality rates of 4% to 6%, but none have addressed this patient population specifically.[40,41] Results from studies reporting a relatively high operative mortality rate (8% to 15%) are difficult to extrapolate because they include a heterogeneous group of patients, including those undergoing complex repairs or replacement, those from the remote past, and those with significant residual MR after repair.

Based on the review of existing literature, we recommend annuloplasty associated with closure of the posterior commissure in patients with ischemic MR.

Calcified Mitral Annulus

The presence of annular calcification considerably increases the risk of complications with mitral valve regurgitation by increasing the risk of ventricular rupture, damage to the circumflex coronary artery, and postoperative residual MR. Calcification is seen most commonly in the posterior annulus, but can extend into the leaflet tissue or the ventricular myocardium, although it rarely affects the anterior annulus. It is distinguished from the calcifications occurring with rheumatic heart disease, in which primary leaflet calcification may extend to the annulus with concomitant calcification of subchordal structures. Annular calcification in association with MR occurs most frequently in the elderly and in patients with Marfan's syndrome or Barlow's disease.[15,43,44] Annular calcification must be identified preoperatively, because its presence influences the type and timing of the surgical procedure to be performed. Localized calcification to a short segment of the annulus (usually facing P1) is rather easy to treat and does not require special modifications of the management strategies. Conversely, if the posterior annulus is massively calcified, with calcium extruding behind the PML and into the left ventricle, mitral valve repair becomes more challenging to perform. Carpentier and colleagues[43] reported successful en bloc resection of the entire calcium deposit with subsequent repair. Once the calcium is resected, the atrioventricular groove is repaired with vertical mattress sutures. The posterior leaflet (or its remnants in the case of a P2 resection) is then reattached. However, this technique has not gained wide popularity due to its complexity and to the potential hazard of ventricular rupture. Alternative solutions in patients with massively calcified mitral annulus include conservative medical treatment or mitral valve replacement with an undersized bioprosthesis attached to the posterior leaflet itself.

LV Outflow Tract Obstruction after Mitral Valve Repair

LV outflow tract (LVOT) obstruction (LVOTO) is observed in 4% to 8% of all patients after mitral valve repair.[8,9,11,45] Although LVOTO is reversible in most cases with a combination of intravascular volume expansion and stopping inotropic drugs and/or beta-blockade, valve re-repair or replacement may be necessary in a few instances.[46,47] After careful analysis of the mechanism of LVOTO with transthoracic echocardiography and TEE in correlation with intraoperative anatomic observations, SAM of the anterior leaflet was found in all cases and was considered responsible for the obstruction. Contrary to prior belief, these studies have demonstrated that SAM is not due to the somewhat rigid nature of the prosthetic ring, but rather to the discrepancy between the ventricular cavity and the amount of mitral valve tissue. Normally, a wide mitral-aortic angle will keep the inflow compartment away from the outflow region. At the end of diastole and in the isovolumic contraction period, mitral leaflets will coapt in a region where flow is at a low velocity, away from the region of LV ejection through the LVOT. This maintains two distinct functional compartments and prevents obstruction.

The critical reduction in the size of the mitral annulus and the implantation of a prosthetic ring during valve repair produce an anterior displacement (toward the aorta) of the posterior ventricular wall. Thus, the filling compartment of the ventricle becomes part of the subaortic region. In addition, a significant narrowing of the mitral-aortic angle occurs, which is responsible for an abnormal positioning of the mitral leaflets into the ejection region. This will result in a clear inversion and overlapping of the usually distinct functional compartments: the inflow and the outflow compartments. Thus, filling of the left ventricle is altered in such a fashion that, during ejection, the posterior leaflet is pushed anteriorly, causing SAM of the anterior leaflet (Figure 8–11). A Venturi

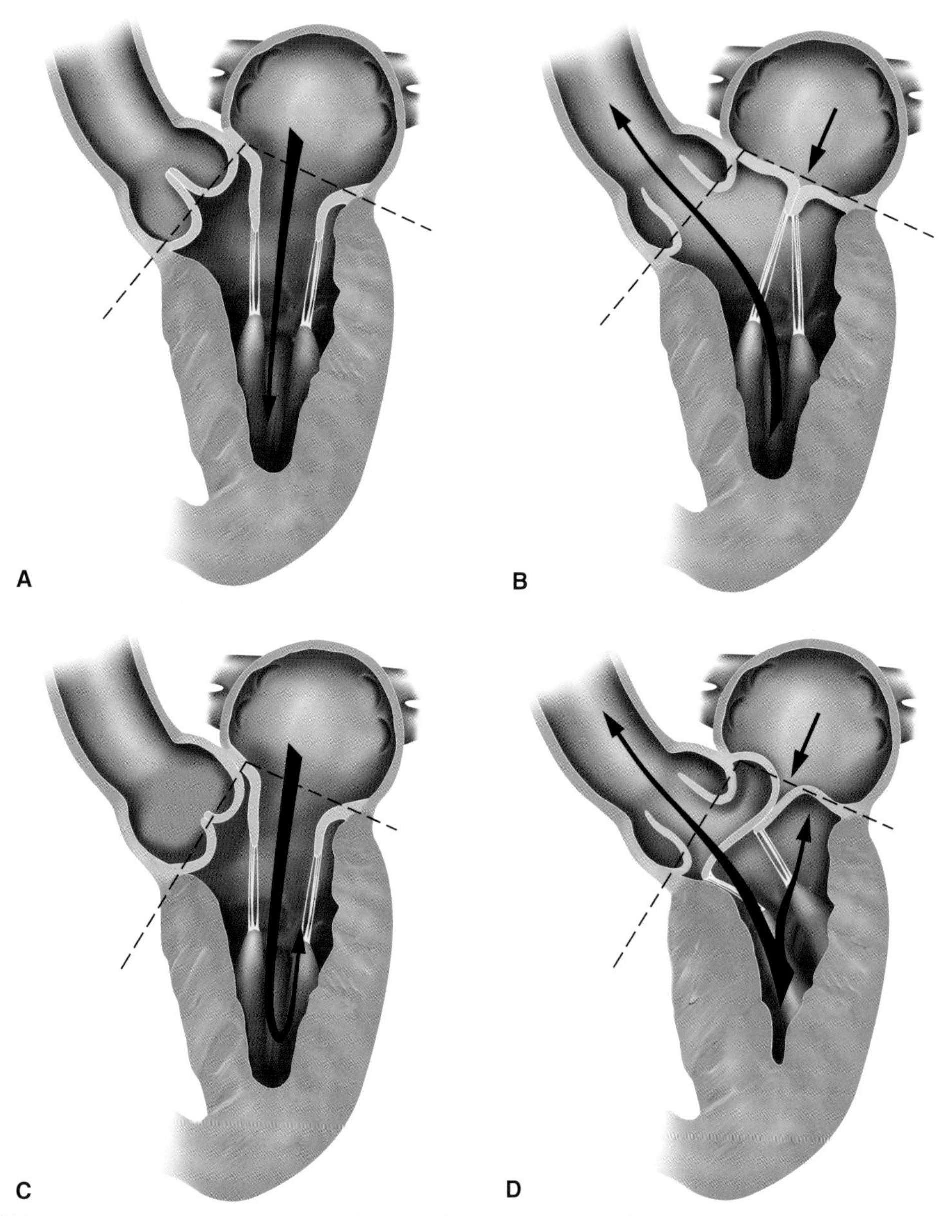

FIGURE 8–11. **A:** Normal mitral-aortic angle and inflow. **B:** Normal outflow. **C:** Acute mitral-aortic angle with overlapping inflow and outflow. **D:** The posterior leaflet is pushed anteriorly by the flow, causing systolic anterior motion of the anterior leaflet. **E:** Wide posterior leaflet. **F:** Midesophageal four-chamber transesophageal echographic image shows systolic anterior motion of the anterior mitral leaflet *(arrow)* in a patient with hypertrophic obstructive cardiomyopathy. (LA, left atrium; RV, right ventricle; LV, left ventricle.)

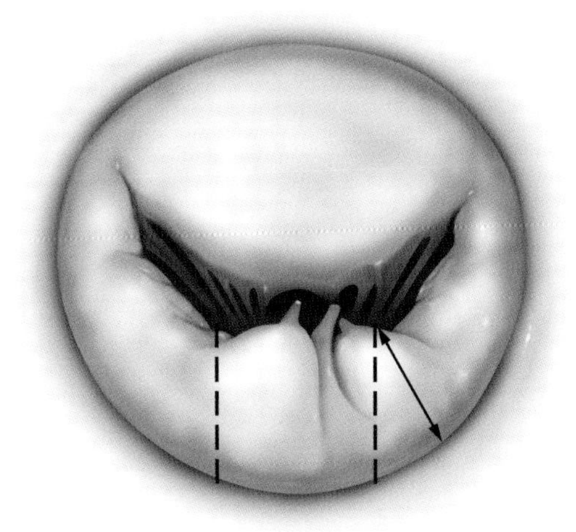

E

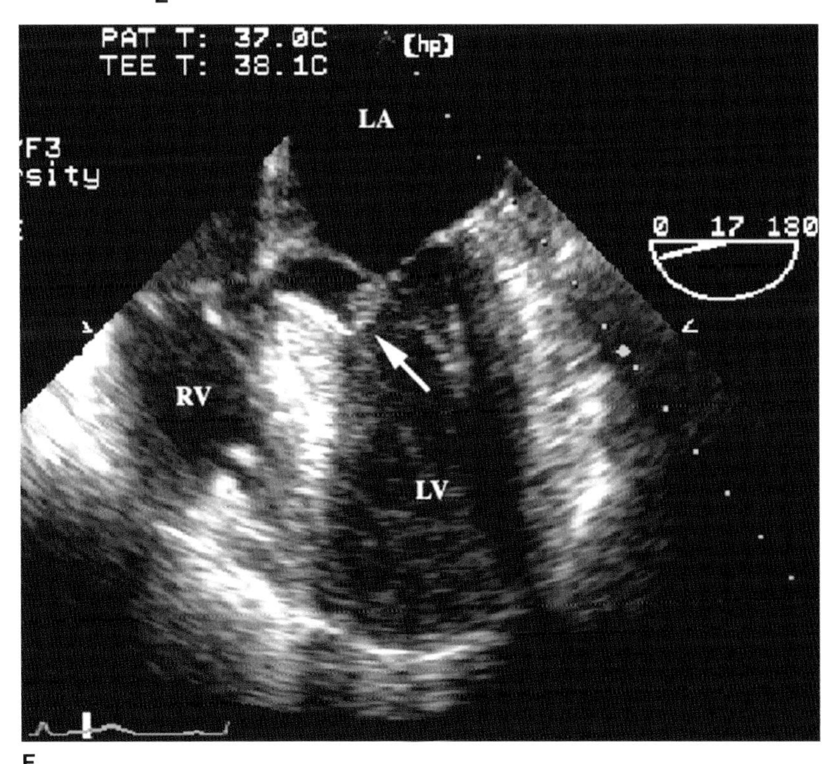

F

FIGURE 8–11. *(Continued)*

or vacuum effect on the anterior leaflet during ejection through the LVOT is also thought to contribute to the narrowing of the LVOT. The incidence of SAM increases in patients with a more anterior position of the mitral coaptation point (ie, greater contribution of the posterior leaflet to the coaptation point). Maslow and coworkers[48] showed that when the ratio of the heights of the anterior leaflet (from the anterior annulus to the coaptation point) and the posterior leaflet (from the posterior annulus to the coaptation point) is less than or equal to 1.3, or when the distance between the coaptation point and the ventricular septum is less than or equal to 2.5 cm, the risk of SAM is increased after mitral valve repair.

Previous studies have demonstrated that the incidence of significant LVOTO in a *high-risk* population presenting with one or more of the predisposing factors for SAM is as high as 14%.[8] The use of the sliding leaflet technique, by decreasing the height of the posterior leaflet, transferring both remnants toward the midline, and avoiding extensive annular plication, may decrease the occurrence of significant LVOTO. In fact, among 82 patients with high risk for SAM who underwent mitral valve repair using the sliding leaflet technique, no significant LVOTO was noted.[8] In two patients, however, mild gradients below 20 mm Hg were recorded immediately after the operation, without clinical significance. These gradients disappeared spontaneously at 3 months postoperatively. Of note is the fact that in all study patients, a prosthetic ring annuloplasty was performed, contradicting the hypothesis that a remodeling annuloplasty ring is the cause of SAM and LVOTO after mitral valve repair. Further, the sliding leaflet technique tackled the intrinsic pathologic basis for the occurrence of SAM via two mechanisms: reduction of the leaflet surface with respect to ventricular cavity and by leaving a physiologic predominance to the anterior leaflet for initiating the systolic closure.

Other Complications after Mitral Valve Repair

In addition to LVOTO from SAM of the AML, a few other complications of mitral valve repair deserve mention. The circumflex artery can be injured during annular suture placement, leading to wall motion abnormalities in the anterolateral and inferolateral walls. Similarly, suture placement in the anterior annulus can damage the non- and left coronary cusps of the aortic valve. Moreover, disruption of the atrioventricular groove may be rarely seen, particularly in patients undergoing extensive annular decalcification. These patients frequently demonstrate continual entrainment of intracardiac air and may require endocardial patch placement for successful repair of the disruption. Low cardiac output syndrome requiring inotropic and/or mechanical support has been reported after MV repair in approximately 6% but a decreasing incidence in the modern era has also been described.[49] The incidence of low cardiac output may be increased in older patients, in female patients, in patients with preoperative left ventricle dysfunction, or in complex surgery requiring a prolonged aortic cross-clamping time and hypothermic bypass.

Concomitant Functional Mitral Regurgitation at the Time of Aortic Valve Replacement

Not infrequently, moderate functional MR is encountered in patients with severe aortic valve disease requiring aortic valve replacement (AVR). In the majority of these patients, MR improves after AVR, but the evidence supporting this intuitive clinical reasoning is sparse.[10,50] However, few studies have addressed the impact of significant functional MR on the aortic valve surgery outcome. In one large study (n = 848) with a mean follow-up of 5.4 ± 3.4 years, Ruel et al[51] found that functional 2+ MR was associated with crude late mortality in patients undergoing AVR for aortic stenosis (AS) or aortic regurgitation (AR), but its effect disappeared after adjusting for comorbid conditions. Furthermore, in AS patients with functional 2+ MR, several factors—describing advanced diastolic dysfunction—placed the patients at risk for heart failure symptoms, heart failure death, or subsequent mitral valve repair/replacement. These included a left atrial size greater than 5 cm, a preoperative peak aortic valve gradient less than 60 mm Hg or preoperative mean aortic valve gradient less than 40 mm Hg, and chronic atrial fibrillation. AR patients with functional 2+ MR and a preoperative LV end-systolic diameter less than 45 mm were also at increased risk.

REFERENCES

1. Enriquez-Sarano M, Akins CW, Vahanian A. Mitral regurgitation. *Lancet.* 2009;373(9672):1382-1394.
2. Russo A, Grigioni F, Avierinos JF, et al. Thromboembolic complications after surgical correction of mitral regurgitation incidence, predictors, and clinical implications. *J Am Coll Cardiol.* 2008;51(12):1203-1211.
3. Fedak PW, McCarthy PM, Bonow RO. Evolving concepts and technologies in mitral valve repair. *Circulation.* 2008; 117(7):963-974.
4. Schaff HV, Suri RM, Enriquez-Sarano M. Indications for surgery in degenerative mitral valve disease. *Semin Thorac Cardiovasc Surg.* 2007;19(2):97-102.
5. Acar C, Tolan M, Berrebi A, et al. Homograft replacement of the mitral valve. Graft selection, technique of implantation, and results in forty-three patients. *J Thorac Cardiovasc Surg.* 1996;111(2):367-378; discussion 378-380.
6. Carpentier A. Cardiac valve surgery—the "French correction". *J Thorac Cardiovasc Surg.* 1983;86(3):323-337.

7. Grande-Allen KJ, Borowski AG, Troughton RW, et al. Apparently normal mitral valves in patients with heart failure demonstrate biochemical and structural derangements: an extracellular matrix and echocardiographic study. *J Am Coll Cardiol.* 2005;45(1):54-61.
8. Jebara VA, Mihaileanu S, Acar C, et al. Left ventricular outflow tract obstruction after mitral valve repair. Results of the sliding leaflet technique. *Circulation.* 1993;88(5 Pt 2):II30-34.
9. Perier P, Clausnizer B, Mistarz K. Carpentier "sliding leaflet" technique for repair of the mitral valve: early results. *Ann Thorac Surg.* 1994;57(2):383-386.
10. Absil B, Dagenais F, Mathieu P, et al. Does moderate mitral regurgitation impact early or mid-term clinical outcome in patients undergoing isolated aortic valve replacement for aortic stenosis? *Eur J Cardiothorac Surg.* 2003;24(2):217-222; discussion 222.
11. Gillinov AM, Cosgrove DM, Lytle BW, et al. Reoperation for failure of mitral valve repair. *J Thorac Cardiovasc Surg.* 1997;113(3):467-473; discussion 473-465.
12. Gillinov AM, Cosgrove DM, Blackstone EH, et al. Durability of mitral valve repair for degenerative disease. *J Thorac Cardiovasc Surg.* 1998;116(5):734-743.
13. Sousa Uva M, Grare P, Jebara V, et al. Transposition of chordae in mitral valve repair. Mid-term results. *Circulation.* 1993;88(5 Pt 2):II35-38.
14. Dreyfus GD, Souza Neto O, Aubert S. Papillary muscle repositioning for repair of anterior leaflet prolapse caused by chordal elongation. *J Thorac Cardiovasc Surg.* 2006;132(3):578-584.
15. David TE, Omran A, Armstrong S, Sun Z, Ivanov J. Long-term results of mitral valve repair for myxomatous disease with and without chordal replacement with expanded polytetrafluoroethylene sutures. *J Thorac Cardiovasc Surg.* 1998;115(6): 1279-1285; discussion 1285-1276.
16. Dreyfus G, Serraf A, Jebara VA, et al. Valve repair in acute endocarditis. *Ann Thorac Surg.* 1990;49(5):706-711; discussion 712-703.
17. Acar C, Farge A, Ramsheyi A, et al. Mitral valve replacement using a cryopreserved mitral homograft. *Ann Thorac Surg.* 1994;57(3):746-748.
18. Alfieri O, Maisano F, De Bonis M, et al. The double-orifice technique in mitral valve repair: a simple solution for complex problems. *J Thorac Cardiovasc Surg.* 2001;122(4):674-681.
19. Duran CM, Gometza B, De Vol EB. Valve repair in rheumatic mitral disease. *Circulation.* 1991;84(5 Suppl):III125-132.
20. Duran CM. Pericardium in valve operations. *Ann Thorac Surg.* 1993;56(1):1-2.
21. Chauvaud S, Jebara V, Chachques JC, et al. Valve extension with glutaraldehyde-preserved autologous pericardium. Results in mitral valve repair. *J Thorac Cardiovasc Surg.* 1991;102(2):171-177; discussion 177-178.
22. Enriquez-Sarano M. Timing of mitral valve surgery. *Heart.* 2002;87(1):79-85.
23. Enriquez-Sarano M, Nkomo V, Mohty D, Avierinos JF, Chaliki H. Mitral regurgitation: predictors of outcome and natural history. *Adv Cardiol.* 2002;39:133-143.
24. Enriquez-Sarano M, Schaff HV, Frye RL. Mitral regurgitation: what causes the leakage is fundamental to the outcome of valve repair. *Circulation.* 2003;108(3):253-256.
25. Ling LH, Enriquez-Sarano M. Long-term outcomes of patients with flail mitral valve leaflets. *Coron Artery Dis.* 2000;11(1):3-9.
26. Sousa Uva M, Dreyfus G, Rescigno G, et al. Surgical treatment of asymptomatic and mildly symptomatic mitral regurgitation. *J Thorac Cardiovasc Surg.* 1996;112(5):1240-1248; discussion 1248-1249.
27. Iung B, Baron G, Butchart EG, et al. A prospective survey of patients with valvular heart disease in Europe: The Euro Heart Survey on Valvular Heart Disease. *Eur Heart J.* 2003;24(13): 1231-1243.
28. Savage EB, Ferguson TB Jr, DiSesa VJ. Use of mitral valve repair: analysis of contemporary United States experience reported to the Society of Thoracic Surgeons National Cardiac Database. *Ann Thorac Surg.* 2003;75(3):820-825.
29. Braunberger E, Deloche A, Berrebi A, et al. Very long-term results (more than 20 years) of valve repair with Carpentier's techniques in nonrheumatic mitral valve insufficiency. *Circulation.* 2001;104(12 Suppl 1):I8-11.
30. Deloche A, Jebara VA, Relland JY, et al. Valve repair with Carpentier techniques. The second decade. *J Thorac Cardiovasc Surg.* 1990;99(6):990-1001; discussion 1001-1002.
31. Jokinen JJ, Hippelainen MJ, Pitkanen OA, Hartikainen JE. Mitral valve replacement versus repair: propensity-adjusted survival and quality-of-life analysis. *Ann Thorac Surg.* 2007;84(2):451-458.
32. Perier P, Stumpf J, Gotz C, et al. [Isolated prolapse of the posterior leaflet of the mitral valve. Results of reconstructive surgery]. *Arch Mal Coeur Vaiss.* 1998;91(7):831-836.
33. Song JM, Qin JX, Kongsaerepong V, et al. Determinants of ischemic mitral regurgitation in patients with chronic anterior wall myocardial infarction: a real time three-dimensional echocardiography study. *Echocardiography.* 2006;23(8):650-657.
34. Aklog L, Filsoufi F, Flores KQ, et al. Does coronary artery bypass grafting alone correct moderate ischemic mitral regurgitation? *Circulation.* 2001;104(12 Suppl 1):I68-75.
35. Gillinov AM. Is ischemic mitral regurgitation an indication for surgical repair or replacement? *Heart Fail Rev.* 2006; 11(3):231-239.
36. Balu V, Hershowitz S, Zaki Masud AR, Bhayana JN, Dean DC. Mitral regurgitation in coronary artery disease. *Chest.* 1982;81(5):550-555.
37. Christenson JT, Simonet F, Bloch A, Maurice J, Velebit V, Schmuziger M. Should a mild to moderate ischemic mitral valve regurgitation in patients with poor left ventricular function be repaired or not? *J Heart Valve Dis.* 1995;4(5):484-488; discussion 488-489.
38. Kang DH, Kim MJ, Kang SJ, et al. Mitral valve repair versus revascularization alone in the treatment of ischemic mitral regurgitation. *Circulation.* 2006;114(1 Suppl):I499-503.
39. Lancellotti P, Donal E, Cosyns B, et al. Effects of surgery on ischaemic mitral regurgitation: a prospective multicentre registry (SIMRAM registry). *Eur J Echocardiogr.* 2008; 9(1):26-30.
40. Czer LS, Maurer G, Bolger AF, DeRobertis M, Chaux A, Matloff JM. Revascularization alone or combined with suture annuloplasty for ischemic mitral regurgitation. Evaluation by color Doppler echocardiography. *Tex Heart Inst J.* 1996; 23(4):270-278.
41. Bolling SF. Mitral reconstruction in cardiomyopathy. *J Heart Valve Dis.* 2002;11 Suppl 1:S26-31.
42. Dion R, Benetis R, Elias B, et al. Mitral valve procedures in ischemic regurgitation. *J Heart Valve Dis.* 1995;4 Suppl 2:S124-129; discussion S129-131.

43. Carpentier AF, Pellerin M, Fuzellier JF, Relland JY. Extensive calcification of the mitral valve anulus: pathology and surgical management. *J Thorac Cardiovasc Surg*. 1996;111(4):718-729; discussion 729-730.
44. Fuzellier JF, Chauvaud SM, Fornes P, et al. Surgical management of mitral regurgitation associated with Marfan's syndrome. *Ann Thorac Surg*. 1998;66(1):68-72.
45. Brown ML, Abel MD, Click RL, et al. Systolic anterior motion after mitral valve repair: is surgical intervention necessary? *J Thorac Cardiovasc Surg*. 2007;133(1):136-143.
46. George KM, Gillinov AM. Posterior leaflet shortening to correct systolic anterior motion after mitral valve repair. *Ann Thorac Surg*. 2008;86(5):1699-1700.
47. Kudo M, Yozu R, Kokaji K, Kimura N. A simple method of prevention for systolic anterior motion in mitral valve repair by loop technique method. *Ann Thorac Surg*. 2009;87(1):324-325.
48. Maslow AD, Regan MM, Haering JM, Johnson RG, Levine RA. Echocardiographic predictors of left ventricular outflow tract obstruction and systolic anterior motion of the mitral valve after mitral valve reconstruction for myxomatous valve disease. *J Am Coll Cardiol*. 1999;34(7):2096-2104.
49. Detaint D, Sundt TM, Nkomo VT, et al. Surgical correction of mitral regurgitation in the elderly: outcomes and recent improvements. *Circulation*. 2006;114(4):265-272.
50. Wan CK, Suri RM, Li Z, et al. Management of moderate functional mitral regurgitation at the time of aortic valve replacement: is concomitant mitral valve repair necessary? *J Thorac Cardiovasc Surg*. 2009;137(3):635-640 e631.
51. Ruel M, Kapila V, Price J, Kulik A, Burwash IG, Mesana TG. Natural history and predictors of outcome in patients with concomitant functional mitral regurgitation at the time of aortic valve replacement. *Circulation*. 2006;114(1 Suppl):I541-546.

REVIEW QUESTIONS

Select the *one* best answer for each of the following questions.

1. Which of the following statements concerning the insertion of the anterior leaflet to the mitral annulus is true?
   a. It inserts into the posterior annulus.
   b. It inserts into one-third of the annulus.
   c. It inserts into two-thirds of the annulus.
   d. It inserts into half of the annulus.
   e. Its insertion covers the entire annulus.

2. Concerning the papillary muscles of the mitral valve, which of the following statements is *true*?
   a. The anterior papillary muscle is much larger than the posterior papillary muscle.
   b. The chordae of the AML are attached to the anterior papillary muscle, whereas those of the PML are attached to the posterior papillary muscle.
   c. Their morphology may vary among individuals.
   d. The anterior papillary muscle arises from the septum.
   e. They are tendinous structures with little or no blood supply.

3. Concerning the mitral leaflets, all the following statements are true *except*:
   a. The AML is much larger than the PML.
   b. Each leaflet has its own papillary muscle.
   c. The AML has a small annular attachment when compared with that of the PML.
   d. The AML is attached to the annulus between the two fibrous trigones of the heart.
   e. The commissures are the areas of continuity between both mitral leaflets.

4. Echocardiographic findings in patients with chronic ischemic MR include:
   a. Type I MR
   b. Type II MR
   c. Type III MR
   d. Type I and III MR
   e. Type I, II, and III MR

5. Prolapse of the posterior leaflet can be due to all of the following *except*:
   a. Ruptured chordae
   b. Elongated chordae
   c. Endocarditis
   d. Dilated left ventricle
   e. Myocardial infarction with ruptured papillary muscle

6. With regard to degenerative mitral valve disease, which of the following statements is *true*?
   a. It is always encountered after age 60 years.
   b. It is the leading cause of MR in developing countries.
   c. It usually results in type II MR.
   d. The mitral valve is often globally affected and cannot be repaired.
   e. MR is usually due to restricted motion (type III).

7. All of the following are risk factors for LVOTO after mitral valve repair *except*:
   a. Septal bulge
   b. Acute (closed) mitral-aortic angle
   c. Wide (large) posterior leaflet
   d. Dilated left ventricle
   e. Small-size ring annuloplasty

8. Complications occurring after mitral valve repair include all of the following *except*:
   a. Aortic regurgitation
   b. Aortic stenosis
   c. Myocardial infarction

d. Rupture of the left ventricle
e. SAM of the AML

9. MR due to posterior leaflet prolapse is best treated with:
   a. Mitral valve replacement
   b. Annuloplasty alone
   c. Chordae shortening
   d. Chordae transposition
   e. Leaflet resection

10. Alternative techniques to treat prolapse of the anterior leaflet include all of the following *except*:
    a. Double-orifice technique (Alfieri)
    b. Use of artificial chords
    c. Chordae transposition
    d. Shortening of the papillary muscle
    e. Annuloplasty alone

11. Which of the following statements is *true* regarding the midterm results after surgical treatment of symptomatic patients (New York Heart Association classes III and IV) with moderate to severe (3+, 4+) ischemic MR?
    a. They are identical if CABG is performed alone or in association with mitral valve repair.
    b. They are better when CABG is associated with mitral valve repair.
    c. They are better when CABG is performed alone.
    d. They are better when mitral valve repair is performed alone.
    e. They are independent of the surgical technique used.

12. Which statement is *true* concerning the "double-orifice technique"?
    a. It requires the insertion of a specially designed "figure-of-8" ring.
    b. It is used to treat posterior leaflet prolapse.
    c. It is used to treat anterior leaflet prolapse.
    d. Long-term results (longer than 20 years) are excellent.
    e. It often results in secondary mitral stenosis.

13. In patients with MR and a massive calcified posterior mitral annulus, which of the following statements is *correct*?
    a. Calcification does not modify the surgical strategy.
    b. The calcifications can be easily removed with no additional complications.
    c. Ring annuloplasty should be performed without touching the calcifications.
    d. Mitral valve replacement with a large mechanical prosthesis is indicated.
    e. None of the above.

14. The superiority of mitral valve repair over replacement in patients with mitral valve disease is now widely accepted, mainly due to:
    a. Better preservation of LV function
    b. Avoidance of long-term anticoagulation (mechanical valves)
    c. Avoidance of reoperation (bioprosthetic valves)
    d. Avoidance of valve-related complications (mechanical and bioprosthesis)
    e. All of the above

15. Which of the following statements is *true* concerning the mitral valve?
    a. Diseases of the mitral valve leading to MR usually involve an entire leaflet.
    b. Diseases of the mitral valve leading to MR are rather confined to specific segments.
    c. The anterior leaflet has clearly defined segments designated as A1, A2, and A3.
    d. Type I MR denotes MR resulting from restriction of leaflet movement, which tends to limit the incriminated leaflet excursion toward the annulus plane, thereby prohibiting leaflet coaptation.
    e. Type II MR designates MR with normal leaflet movement, ie, a functional MR without leaflet abnormality.

16. The pathophysiology of chronic MR after myocardial infarction includes which of the following mechanisms?
    a. Acutely ruptured papillary muscle as a consequence of acute myocardial infarction involving the papillary muscle
    b. Simple annular dilatation (secondary to LV enlargement), which causes incomplete mitral leaflet coaptation associated with type I (normal) leaflet motion
    c. Local LV remodeling with papillary muscle displacement producing apical tethering or tenting of the leaflets
    d. Type IIIb restricted systolic leaflet motion
    e. All the mechanisms described in b to d

17. In the setting of bacterial endocarditis, MR can develop secondary to:
    a. Leaflet prolapse secondary to rupture or destruction of marginal chords.
    b. Leaflet perforation due to abscess formation and secondary perforation.
    c. Leaflet destruction with giant vegetations observed in severe cases.
    d. All the aforementioned mechanisms are true.
    e. All the aforementioned mechanisms are false.

18. Which of the following statements best describes mitral valve leaflet resection?
    a. It is used to treat leaflet prolapse most frequently at the level of the AML.
    b. Quadrangular resection of the posterior leaflet is the most common technique used in degenerative mitral valve.
    c. Extensive resections at the level of the annulus of the PML associated with a wide plication of the posterior annulus offer the best results, with no kinking or damage to a dominant circumflex artery.
    d. Results of leaflet resection of the anterior leaflet are more favorable than those observed with posterior leaflet resection.
    e. Annuloplasty should not be combined with quadrangular resection.

19. All of the following statements regarding chordae transposition and chordae shortening are true *except*:
    a. Chordae transposition is the technique of choice to treat prolapse of the anterior leaflet.
    b. Chordae transposition from the PML to the diseased segment of the AML is less efficient then chordal shortening techniques.
    c. Shortened chordae tend to rupture at the site of insertion into the papillary muscle trench.
    d. Chordae shortening should be avoided whenever possible.
    e. Chordae transposition, also known as the "flip-over" technique, usually requires resection of a corresponding segment of the PML.

20. All of the following techniques can be applied for the repair of a defect in the body of the AML *except*:
    a. Debridement and patch closure with autologous pericardium
    b. Leaflet resection and reconstruction using autologous pericardium
    c. Chordae transposition if the free margin or the commissure is available
    d. Partial homograft can be used to replace the destroyed segments in more extensive cases
    e. "Bow-tie" repair or Alfieri stitch

21. Surgery should be considered early in the course of mitral valve disease due to which of the following reasons:
    a. In comparison to the expected survival, an excess mortality is noted in patients with degenerative MR.
    b. In patients with MR, the 10-year incidence of atrial fibrillation is 30% and that of heart failure is 63%.
    c. At 10 years, 90% of patients would be dead or have undergone surgery.
    d. Sudden deaths occur in patients with no or minimal symptoms and normal LV function.
    e. All of the above.

22. All of the following are risk factors for failure of mitral valve repair *except*:
    a. Advanced myxomatous changes of both leaflets
    b. Chordal transposition procedures
    c. Failure to perform an annuloplasty
    d. Residual MR at the completion of repair
    e. Performance of concomitant cardiac procedures

23. Which of the following statements concerning the surgical technique for repair of a degenerative mitral valve is *incorrect*?
    a. Posterior leaflet quadrangular resection should be accompanied by an annuloplasty.
    b. Anterior leaflet prolapse must be corrected by chordal shortening.
    c. Chordal transfer does not increase the risk of repair failure.
    d. Chordal transfer is a durable technique for treatment of anterior leaflet prolapse.

24. The presence of annular calcification considerably complicates mitral valve repair because it:
    a. Increases the risk for ventricular rupture
    b. Increases the risk of damaging the circumflex coronary artery
    c. Leaves postoperative residual MR
    d. Interferes with the type of surgical procedure to be used and with the timing of the operation
    e. All of the above

25. Treatment of hypotension secondary to SAM of the AML shortly after separating from CPB may include all of the following *except*:
    a. Fluid administration
    b. Discontinuation of vasodilators
    c. Beta-blocker therapy
    d. Initiation of inotropic support
    e. Decreasing the temporary pacing rate from 90 to 70 beats per minute

Aortic Valve

9

Mark A. Taylor and Christopher A. Troianos

Aortic valve replacement (AVR) is the most common valve replacement procedure and the second most common cardiac operation following coronary artery bypass grafting (CABG) in the United States. Intraoperative transesophageal echocardiography (TEE) alters the surgical plan in 13% of patients undergoing aortic valve surgery.[1] Furthermore, a consensus statement from the American College of Cardiology, American Heart Association, and American Society of Echocardiography gave intraoperative TEE a class I designation ("evidence and/or general agreement that a given procedure or treatment is useful and effective") in patients undergoing surgical repair of valvular lesions.[2] Thus, a comprehensive TEE evaluation of the aortic valve should be performed in all patients, particularly those undergoing aortic valve procedures.

Intraoperative transesophageal echocardiography is utilized to evaluate aortic valve anatomy, valve function, and hemodynamics. A comprehensive exam includes an evaluation of valvular architecture using two- (2D) and three-dimensional (3D) imaging techniques. Stenotic and regurgitant valvular lesions and their associated hemodynamic perturbations are assessed with pulsed-wave and continuous-wave Doppler echocardiography. TEE evaluation of left ventricular function and ventricular filling yields accurate and rapid assessment in patients with altered left ventricular compliance due to long-standing aortic valve pathology. The immediate post-bypass examination provides rapid assessment of the adequacy of the valve repair/replacement and any associated cardiac complications. Intraoperative examination thus aids surgical decision making, and is especially helpful in determining the feasibility of aortic valve repair versus aortic valve replacement.

AORTIC VALVE FUNCTION

A thorough understanding of the anatomy and function of the aortic valve apparatus is necessary to obtain the optimal benefit from transesophageal echocardiographic interrogation of the aortic valve. The aortic valve apparatus is comprised of the left ventricular outflow tract (LVOT), valve cusps, sinuses of Valsalva, and proximal ascending aorta (Figure 9–1). The LVOT consists of the inferior or ventricular surface of the anterior mitral leaflet, the interventricular septum, and the posterior left ventricular free wall.

A normally functioning aortic valve apparatus allows unrestricted blood flow from the left ventricle to the ascending aorta during systole and prevents retrograde blood flow from the aorta to left ventricle during diastole. Stresses during diastole are distributed across the leaflets to the commissures and into the sinuses of Valsalva. The sinuses of Valsalva also play a critical role in systole by allowing the aortic valve to open fully without contacting the walls of the aorta. Disruption in this normal anatomy or mechanisms leads to valve dysfunction. In late diastole and associated LV filling, a 12% expansion of the aortic root is observed immediately prior to aortic valve opening,[3-5] which actually initiates leaflet opening prior to ventricular contraction.[3,6]

AORTIC VALVE ANATOMY

Tomographic Views

The proximity of the aortic valve to the upper esophagus yields detailed and high-resolution TEE images. The American Society of Echocardiography and the Society of Cardiovascular Anesthesiologists have published guidelines on obtaining the necessary tomographic views for performing a comprehensive transesophageal echocardiographic examination and are further discussed in the chapter on tomographic views (see Chapter 5). There are four recommended views for evaluation of the aortic valve.[7]

Midesophageal Short-Axis View

The midesophageal aortic valve short-axis (ME AV SAX) view permits detailed 2D, 3D and color-flow Doppler (CFD) interrogation of the aortic valve and associated root structures. The ME AV SAX view is obtained by anteflexing the TEE probe and rotating the transducer forward to between 30° and 60° in the midesophagus.[7]

The normal valve consists of three cusps suspended from an associated sinus of Valsalva. The cusps are of similar shape and size with fine, feathery leaflet edges that open fully, creating the appearance of an outwardly

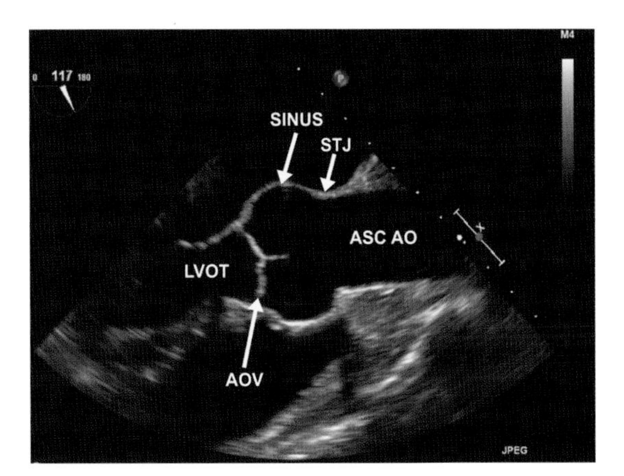

FIGURE 9–1. Midesophageal long-axis imaging plane demonstrating the left ventricular outflow tract (LVOT), aortic valve (AOV), sinus of Valsalva (SINUS), sinotubular junction (STJ), and ascending aorta (ASC AO).

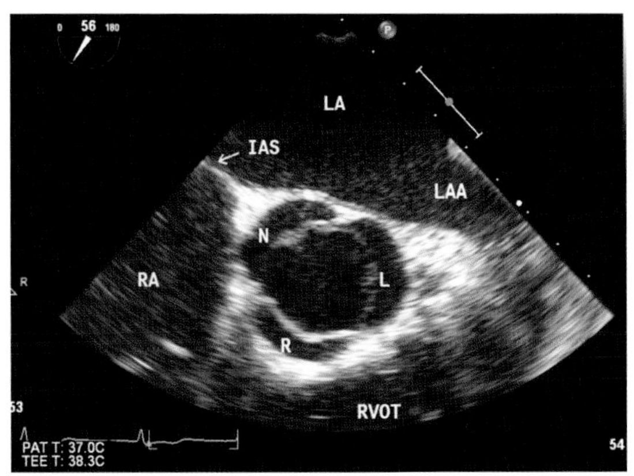

A

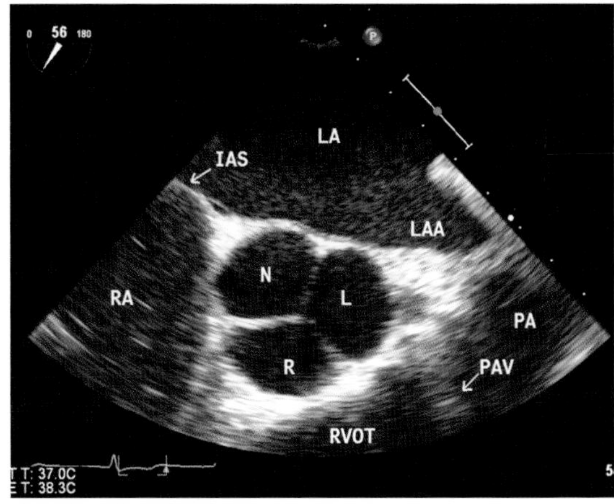

B

FIGURE 9–2. Midesophageal aortic valve short-axis view during systole **(A)** and diastole **(B)**. Note that all three aortic valve cusps are similar in size and appearance, indicating a true short-axis cross section. The aortic valve is identified by the right (R), left (L), and noncoronary (N) cusps. (LA, left atrium; LAA, left atrial appendage; RA, right atrium; IAS, interatrial septum; RVOT, right ventricular outflow tract; PAV, pulmonic valve; PA, pulmonary artery.)

bulging equilateral triangle. During diastole the valve leaflets should close or coapt completely. The aortic valve axis is obliquely orientated to the esophageal axis with the right coronary cusp anterior and superior to the noncoronary cusp but inferior to the left coronary cusp. Two-dimensional examination in the ME AV SAX view permits evaluation of individual leaflet architecture and range of motion throughout the systolic (opening) and diastolic (closing) cycle. Since the right coronary cusp is the most anterior cusp, it is displayed below the noncoronary and left cusps on the image display (Figure 9–2). The interatrial septum attaches to the aortic wall near the noncoronary cusp, and the left main coronary artery orifice can frequently be visualized in the left coronary sinus. Thickening, calcification, commissural fusion, and decreased mobility of the leaflets are observed with valvular aortic stenosis. Bicuspid aortic valves have an eccentric circular or "fish mouth" orifice, and often a thickening or raphe that extends from the leaflet edge to the aortic wall. This raphe can be misleading in that it creates the appearance of a fused commissure, suggesting a tricuspid valve. Insertion of the leaflets to the aortic annulus differentiates a bicuspid from a tricuspid valve as the anatomic relationship between the commissures and aortic root are typically altered. Unicuspid and quadricuspid valves can also be identified easily with 2D and 3D imaging in the ME AV SAX view.

The degree of valve opening can be measured by planimetry of the orifice by using the trackball and the caliper and trace functions of the machine (Figure 9–3). Although this method is simple and rapid, it is subject to error, with poor reliability between observers. Overestimation of the valve area by planimetry may occur, particularly in patients with pliable leaflets if the ultrasound beam intersects the leaflets below their tips (Figure 9–4). In addition, in many patients, the leaflets may be so calcified that the orifice cannot be identified. Color-flow Doppler in this view assesses leaflet coaptation and the severity of any associated aortic regurgitation in a semiquantitative fashion.

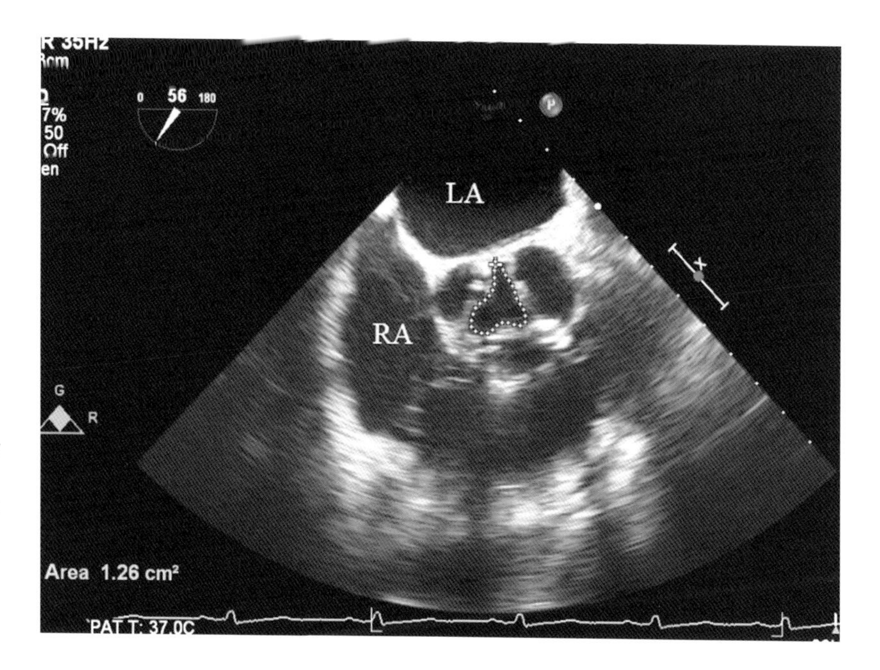

FIGURE 9–3. Midesophageal aortic valve short-axis view used for planimetry of the aortic valve orifice in a patient with moderate aortic stenosis as indicated by the measured area of 1.26 cm^2. (LA, left atrium; RA, right atrium.)

Midesophageal Long-Axis View

The midesophageal aortic valve long-axis (ME AV LAX) view is perpendicular to the ME AV SAX view and allows imaging of all the components of the aortic valve apparatus, including the left ventricular outflow tract, aortic valve, sinuses of Valsalva, sinotubular junction, and proximal ascending aorta. From the ME AV SAX view, the transducer is rotated forward to 120° to 150° while keeping the aortic valve in the center of view.[7] A normal aortic valve appears as two thin lines that open parallel to the aortic walls during systole. The right coronary cusp, being the most anterior cusp, is displayed along the anterior surface of the aortic wall during systole (lower on the image display). The cusp seen at the top of the display is either the noncoronary or left coronary cusp depending upon probe orientation (see Figure 9–4).[7]

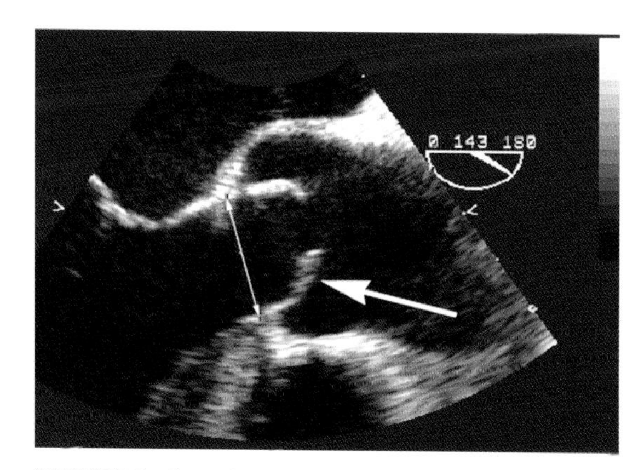

FIGURE 9–4. Midesophageal aortic valve long-axis view during systole demonstrating the characteristic doming of a stenotic bicuspid aortic valve with pliable leaflets *(arrow)*. Planimetry can overestimate aortic valve area in this patient if the ultrasound beam does not intersect the leaflet tips. The annulus diameter is measured from the hinge point of one leaflet to the hinge point of the opposing leaflet during systole.

The ME AV LAX view is used to examine leaflet morphology, mobility, thickening, and calcification, and to detect subaortic pathology (eg, subaortic membrane). During systole, normal leaflets move freely, parallel to the axis of flow, and return to the plane of the annulus during diastole. Doming is the characteristic bowing appearance of the leaflets during systole as a result of calcification of the tips but not the bodies of the leaflets (see Figure 9–4). With membranous subaortic stenosis, the LVOT should be examined for the presence of a thin fibrous band or ring stretching from a hypertrophied interventricular septum to the base of the anterior leaflet of the mitral valve (MV) (Figure 9–5), which also may be thickened and stiff. Systolic anterior motion of the anterior leaflet of the MV causing dynamic LVOT obstruction in hypertrophic obstructive cardiomyopathy or after MV repair often is detected in this view. The ME AV LAX view is also used to measure the aortic annulus, sinus of Valsalva, sinotubular junction, and ascending

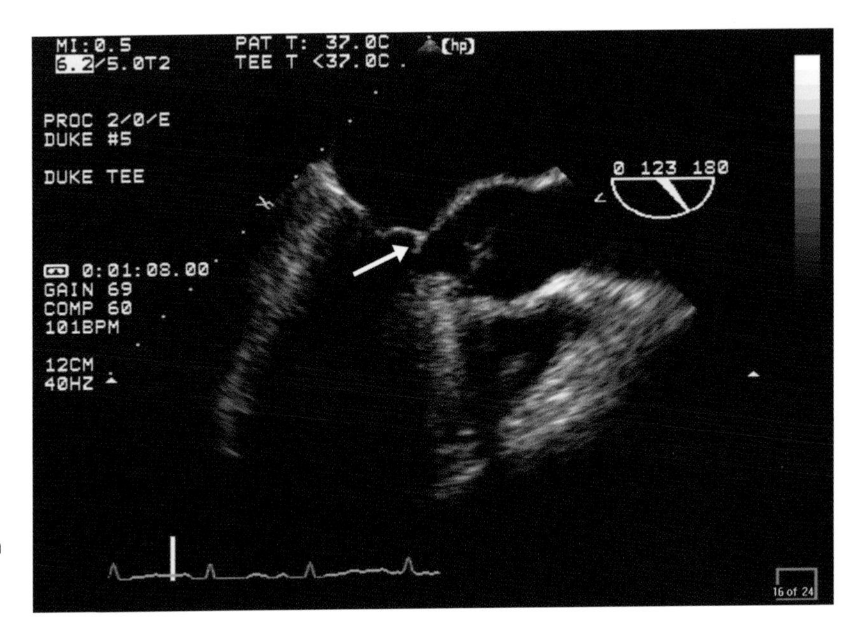

FIGURE 9–5. Membranous subaortic stenosis. The arrow points to the membrane seen below the aortic valve in the left ventricular outflow tract.

aorta diameters when determining the appropriate size of prosthesis during valve replacement surgery. These measurements are particularly important in homograft implantations where size and geometry have tremendous implications on the success of the procedure.[8] Annulus measurement in a normal valve is made from the hinge point of one leaflet to the hinge point of the opposite leaflet of the opened valve during systole (see Figure 9–4; Figure 9–6). However, in heavily diseased valves, better estimations can be made at the junction of the aortic annulus and the LVOT. To improve the estimate, multiple measurements should be made at slightly different scan angles and averaged.

Color-flow Doppler evaluation in the ME AV LAX view identifies systolic blood flow disturbances in the ascending aorta due to aortic stenosis or in the left ventricular outflow tract due to left ventricular outflow tract obstruction (LVOTO) and diastolic flow disturbances due to aortic regurgitation. M-mode measurements also can be made in the ME AV LAX view to examine leaflet mobility, thickness, and tip separation.

Transgastric Long-Axis View

The transgastric long-axis (TG LAX) view is obtained by starting with the transgastric short-axis (TG SAX) view of the left ventricle at the midpapillary level and rotating the transducer forward to 90° to 110°. The mitral valve is visualized on the right side of the display in the near field while the aortic valve is displayed in the far field (Figure 9–7). The far field position of the aortic valve in this view often leads to attenuation of the ultrasound beam, thus limiting 2D imaging. However, parallel alignment of the continuous- or pulsed-wave Doppler beam through the LVOT, aortic valve, and ascending aorta is often possible and allows for the

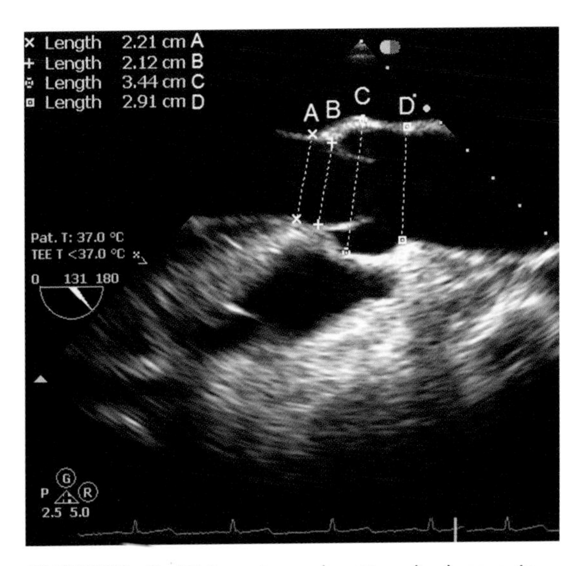

FIGURE 9–6. Midesophageal aortic valve long-axis view during systole with the four recommended measurements, including the left ventricular outflow tract (A), aortic valve annulus (B), sinus of Valsalva (C), and sinotubular junction (D).

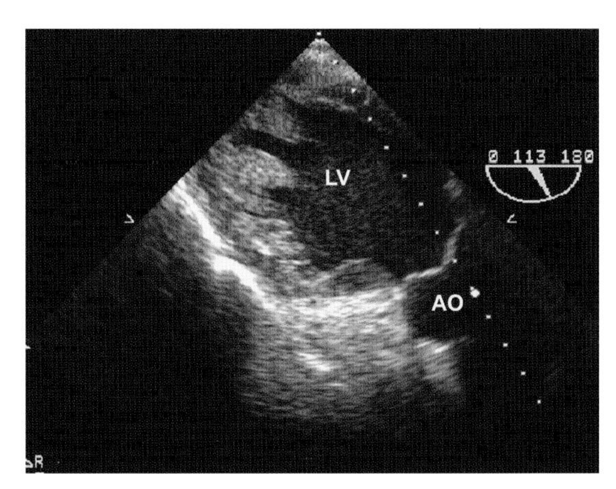

FIGURE 9–7. Transgastric long-axis view of the aortic valve. (AO, ascending aorta; LV, left ventricle.)

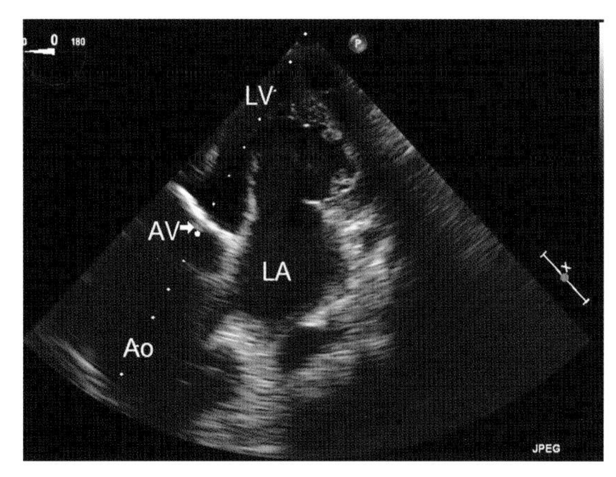

FIGURE 9–8. Deep transgastric long-axis view of the aortic valve, which allows parallel orientation between aortic valve (AV) flow and the continuous-wave Doppler beam. (LA, left atrium; LV, left ventricle; Ao, ascending aorta.)

determination of velocities in the outflow tract and through the aortic valve. Acoustic shadowing in the LVOT can also be avoided using this view, making this and the deep TG LAX views invaluable in assessing prosthetic valve function.

Deep Transgastric Long-Axis View

A second view that consistently affords parallel alignment of the Doppler beam with aortic valve blood flow is the deep transgastric long-axis (deep TG LAX) view. This view is developed from the TG SAX view by advancing the probe and utilizing slight leftward flexion and anteflexion. Commonly, the probe is slowly withdrawn until the image is developed. In the deep TG LAX view, the left ventricular apex is located in the near field (top of the screen), the mitral inflow is on the right of the screen, the left atrium is located in the lower right-hand corner, and the aortic valve apparatus is seen in the lower left-hand corner of the display (far field) (Figure 9–8). As with the TG LAX view, the far-field location of aortic valve structures leads to ultrasound attenuation and 2D image degradation. Color-flow Doppler is useful during probe manipulation in order properly align the left ventricular outflow tract, aortic valve, and ascending aorta with the Doppler beam. In aortic stenosis, the continuous-wave Doppler cursor is aligned with the narrow, turbulent, high-velocity jet and the spectral Doppler display is activated. Accurate localization provides a distinctive audible sound and high-velocity (greater than 3 m/s) spectral Doppler recording that exhibits a fine feathery appearance and a midsystolic peak. Planimetry of the spectral envelope yields the velocity-time integral (VTI) and an estimate of mean aortic valve gradient. Transgastric velocity measurements obtained with Doppler imaging correlate well with data obtained by both transthoracic echocardiography (TTE) and cardiac catheterization.[9]

Skill and practice are necessary to obtain the deep transgastric long-axis and transgastric long-axis views. Stoddard et al demonstrated a significant increase in successful deep transgastric image acquisition with increasing experience (53% feasibility in the first 43 patients, 88% feasibility in the latter 43 patients).[10]

PATHOPHYSIOLOGY

Aortic Stenosis

Normal aortic valve area is 3 to 4 cm^2.[11] Obstruction of LVOT flow into the ascending aorta can occur at three distinct anatomical sites: valvular, subvalvular, or supravalvular. Valvular obstruction is discussed in this chapter with a brief introduction to dynamic subvalvular obstruction, while subvalvular and supravalvular obstruction is discussed in the chapters on cardiomyopathies (see Chapter 14) and congenital heart disease (see Chapter 18). Valvular obstruction accounts for the vast majority of LVOT obstruction and is therefore the primary focus of this chapter.

The most common cause of aortic stenosis in the United States is calcific aortic stenosis of the elderly (Figure 9–9), followed by congenital abnormalities, including bicuspid and rarely unicuspid or quadricuspid valves (Figure 9–10). Bicuspid aortic valves account for approximately 50% of the aortic valve replacements performed in the United States and Europe, while progressive calcification of a tricuspid valve accounts for

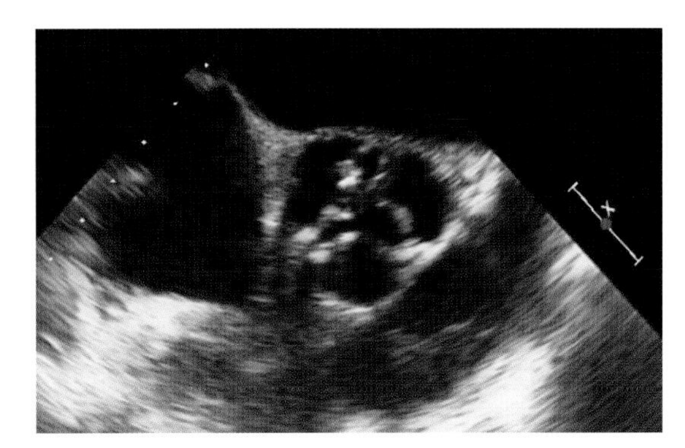

FIGURE 9–9. Transesophageal echocardiogram of the midesophageal aortic valve short-axis view during systole in a patient with aortic stenosis.

the remainder.[12] The mechanism of aortic stenosis in the elderly and in congenital cases is distorted flow through the diseased valve leading to degenerative changes in the cusps, which predisposes the valve to calcification. The rate of calcification and stenosis varies widely, although elderly men with associated coronary artery disease and individuals with a history of smoking, hypercholesterolemia, and elevated serum creatinine levels demonstrate a more rapid disease progression.[13-15] Many experts believe that the development of aortic stenosis is an active process, which involves chronic inflammation fueled by atherosclerotic risk factors.[16] An infrequent cause of aortic stenosis in the United States is rheumatic disease, which produces commissural fusion; however, rheumatic disease remains a common cause of aortic stenosis worldwide.

Calcific aortic stenosis of the elderly characteristically occurs in patients greater than the age of 65, while patients between the ages of 35 and 55 with aortic stenosis typically have a congenital bicuspid aortic valve. Four percent of the elderly U.S. population has significant aortic stenosis,[17] and approximately 1% to 2% of the population has a bicuspid aortic valve.[18] Patients with a bicuspid aortic valve may also have coarctation of the aorta, dilation of the aortic root, or aortic dissection. In patients with a bicuspid aortic valve, aortic root dilation can develop irrespective of hemodynamics and age, and has been shown to continue after valve repair, suggesting a common developmental defect.[19] Concomitant replacement of the ascending aorta should be considered if the ascending aortic diameter is greater than or equal to 4.5 cm, given the tendency for progressive aortic root dilation even after aortic valve replacement.[20]

The European Association of Echocardiography and the American Society of Echocardiography recently published guidelines and standards regarding the echocardiographic assessment of valve stenosis.[11] Methods graded as appropriate and recommended for all patients (level 1) with aortic stenosis (AS) include measurement of:

- AS jet velocity
- Mean transaortic gradient
- Valve area by continuity equation (utilizing velocity-time integrals)

Methods considered reasonable when additional information is needed in select patients (level 2) include:

- Simplified continuity equation (utilizing maximum velocities)
- Velocity ratio or dimensionless index
- Aortic valve area planimetry

Two-Dimensional Measures

Two-dimensional imaging of a stenotic aortic valve in the ME AV SAX and ME AV LAX views will typically

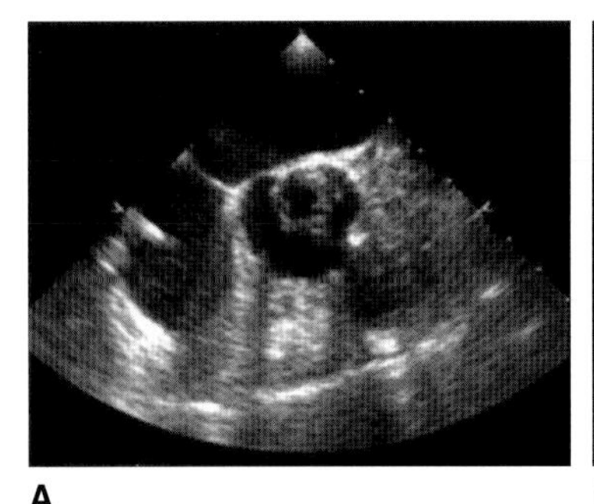

A

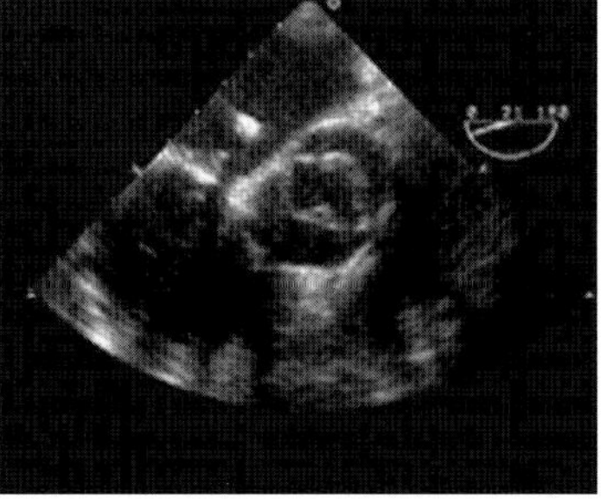

B

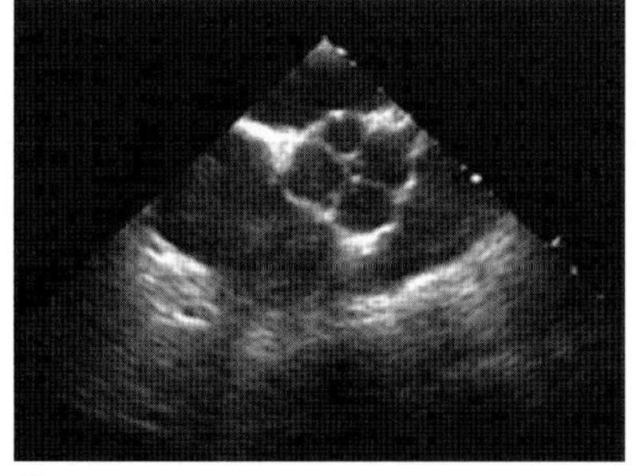

C

FIGURE 9–10. Transesophageal echocardiogram of the midesophageal aortic valve short-axis view in a patient with a unicuspid **(A)**, bicuspid **(B)**, and quadricuspid **(C)** aortic valve.

demonstrate leaflet restriction, calcification, commissural fusion, and failed leaflet coaptation. The ME AV SAX view can be used for measuring the aortic valve orifice area by planimetry, which has been shown to correlate well with other quantitative methods,[21] but is also subject to error in the presence of highly pliable or heavily calcified leaflets.[22] A cross section that is oblique or inferior to the leaflet tips overestimates the orifice size (see Figure 9–4). It is important, therefore, to develop an image with the smallest orifice size to ensure that the imaging plane transects the leaflet tips. To do so, the aortic valve is first imaged in the ME AV LAX, and the smallest orifice seen on the long axis is centered on the image display screen. The transducer position is then stabilized within the esophagus as the multiplane angle is rotated backward to the short-axis view. In a true short-axis cross section, the valve should appear relatively circular and all three cusps appear equal in shape. Planimetry for aortic valve area is a level 2 recommendation by expert consensus and is considered reasonable when additional information is needed in selected patients.[11]

The ME AV LAX view provides imaging of the left ventricular outflow tract, aortic valve, and aortic root, and is useful in differentiating valvular from subvalvular and supravalvular pathology. Reduced leaflet separation and doming with the curvature towards the aortic wall are sufficient for the qualitative diagnosis of aortic stenosis. Maximal cusp separation of less than 8 mm in a long-axis view suggests critical stenosis, whereas greater than 12 mm separation suggests noncritical disease.[23] Measurements of aortic valve separation can be made with M-mode techniques where a characteristic "box car" pattern is seen on M-mode display when the aortic valve is open, with leaflet separation represented by the width of the box car. In patients with membranous subaortic stenosis, M-mode assessment may show early systolic closure of the valve (Figure 9–11).

PRESSURE GRADIENTS

The primary echocardiographic technique used to quantify the severity of aortic stenosis is Doppler echocardiography for determination of pressure gradient and aortic valve area. Valvular stenosis produces a decrease in pressure distal or downstream from the stenosis. This pressure gradient or pressure drop across the valve stenosis is proportional to the velocity of flow as described by the Bernoulli equation:

$$\Delta P = 4\,(V_2^2 - V_1^2) + \text{Local Acceleration} + \text{Viscous Losses}$$

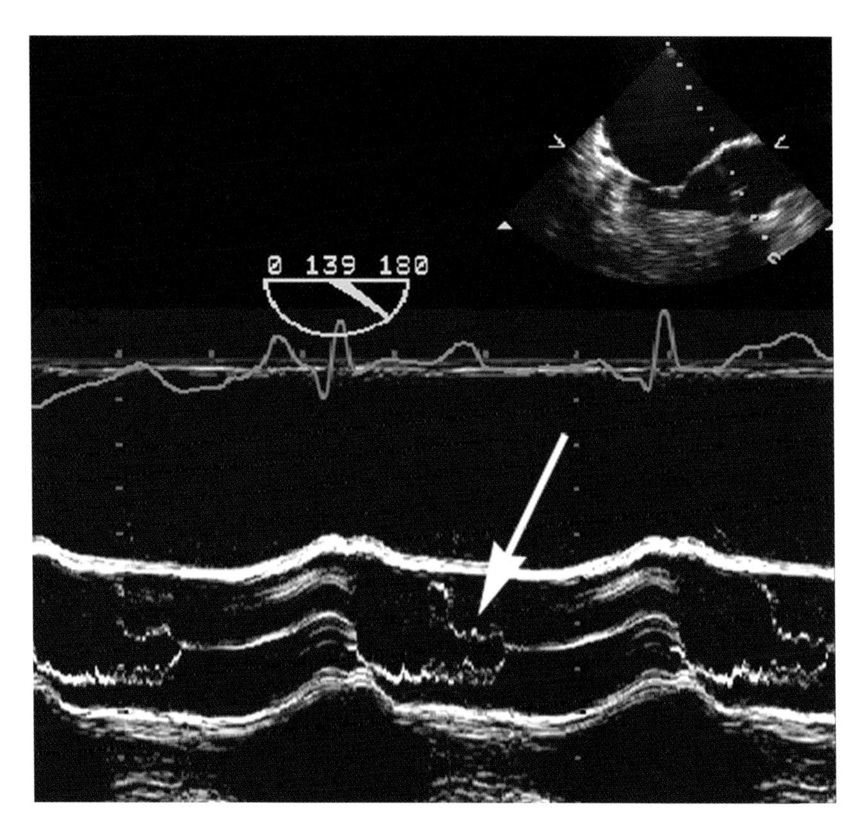

FIGURE 9–11. M-mode of the aortic valve in a patient with membranous subaortic stenosis demonstrating early closure *(arrow)* of the valve.

Where ΔP = Pressure gradient (mm Hg)
V_2 = Velocity of flow (m/s) distal to the stenosis (aortic valve)
V_1 = Velocity of flow (m/s) proximal to the stenosis (LVOT)

Given that local acceleration is only significant for long tubular lesions, and viscosity losses are only important when hematocrit is extremely high, these factors can be disregarded in clinical practice. Typically, V_1 or the LVOT velocity is less than 1 m/s and therefore can be disregarded as well. This yields the commonly applied *simplified* Bernoulli equation:

$$\Delta P = 4\,(V_2)^2$$

$$\Delta P = 4\,(V_{\text{Aortic Valve}})^2$$

When V_1 exceeds 1.5 m/s (eg. LVOT flow acceleration or obstruction), the *modified* Bernoulli equation should be utilized:

$$\Delta P = 4\,(V_2^{\,2} - V_1^{\,2})$$

V_1 is commonly elevated in the presence of aortic regurgitation, volume overload, or other high output states. Failure to use the modified Bernoulli equation in these conditions when LVOT velocity exceeds 1.5 m/s will overestimate the pressure gradient and the severity of aortic stenosis.

In order to measure transvalvular blood velocity, continuous-wave Doppler (CWD) is used in either the TG LAX or deep TG LAX view. The CWD cursor is aligned with the narrow, turbulent, high-velocity jet and the spectral Doppler display is activated. Accurate localization provides a distinctive high-velocity (>3 m/s) spectral Doppler recording that exhibits a fine feathery appearance and a midsystolic peak (Figure 9–12). Planimetry of the spectral envelope yields the velocity-time integral and an estimate of mean aortic valve gradient. The mean gradient is a derived measurement obtained by all ultrasound systems by averaging the instantaneous gradients over the entire ejection period. The peak pressure gradient (also provided by all ultrasound systems) can be estimated from the peak velocity measurement using the simplified Bernoulli equation:

$$\text{Peak Aortic Valve Pressure Gradient } (PG_{AV}) = 4\,(\text{Aortic Valve Velocity})^2$$

Peak gradients are calculated from velocity information and therefore do not provide additional clinical information in comparison to peak velocity. A peak velocity greater than 4 m/s and a mean gradient greater than 40 mm Hg are suggestive of severe aortic stenosis (Table 9–1).

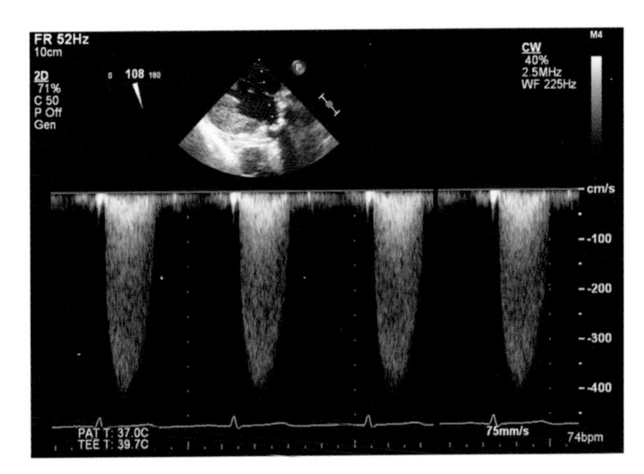

FIGURE 9–12. Continuous-wave spectral Doppler velocities through a stenotic aortic valve. The fine feathery appearance of the high velocities with a mid-systolic peak indicates flow through a stenotic aortic valve. The denser lower velocities near the baseline indicate flow through the left ventricular outflow tract.

Gradients derived in the operating room may be significantly different from those obtained during preoperative echocardiographic studies or in the cardiac catheterization laboratory. Stenotic orifice gradients are flow dependent, and an increase in cardiac output across the aortic valve will increase the gradient. Conditions that increase systolic blood flow through the aortic valve such as hyperdynamic left ventricular function, sepsis, severe aortic regurgitation, and hyperthyroidism will also increase the pressure gradient. Conversely, conditions that decrease systolic blood flow through the aortic valve such as severe LV dysfunction, severe mitral regurgitation, mitral stenosis, and a left to right shunt will decrease the aortic transvalvular pressure gradient (Table 9–2). Thus, pressure gradients should be measured under constant and optimal loading conditions, and cardiac output should be determined whenever possible to ensure estimation of true gradients. If necessary, the cardiac output should be increased to the normal range by using an agent such as dobutamine (start at 2.5 or 5 mcg/kg/min and increase every 3 to 5 minutes to a maximum of 10 to 20 mcg/kg/min). Further, in the presence of irregular heart rhythms, such as premature ventricular contractions and atrial fibrillation, an averaged VTI from at least five consecutive beats should be used for all calculations. If patients are being mechanically ventilated,

Table 9–1. Parameters for the Determination of the Severity of Aortic Stenosis

Indicator	Mild	Moderate	Severe
Peak jet velocity (m/s)	<3.0	3.0-4.0	>4.0
Mean gradient (mm Hg)	<20	20-40	>40
Valve area (cm^2)	1.5	1.0-1.5	<1.0
Dimensionless index	>0.50	0.25-0.50	<0.25
Indexed AVA (cm^2/m^2)	>0.85	0.60-0.85	<0.6

From Baumgartner H, Hung J, Bermejo J, et al. Echocardiographic assessment of valve stenosis: EAE/ASE recommendations for clinical practice. J Am Soc Echocardiogr. 2009;22(1):1-23; quiz 101-102; and Bonow RO, Carabello BA, Chatterjee K, et al. ACC/AHA 2006 guidelines for the management of patients with valvular heart disease: a report of the American College of Cardiology/American Heart Association Task Force on Practice Guidelines (writing Committee to Revise the 1998 guidelines for the management of patients with valvular heart disease) developed in collaboration with the Society of Cardiovascular Anesthesiologists endorsed by the Society for Cardiovascular Angiography and Interventions and the Society of Thoracic Surgeons. J Am Coll Cardiol. 2006;48(3):e1-148.

measurements should be made at the end of exhalation. In heavily calcified and stenotic valves, the VTI can be difficult to obtain, and peak velocities may be underestimated if the CWD beam does not pass through the orifice. Color-flow Doppler can be helpful in aligning the CWD beam by identifying the location of the flow through the valve. Aortic stenosis jets also can be confused with mitral regurgitant jets when measured in the deep TG LAX view. Differentiating the two jets involves recognition that the aortic stenosis jet begins later (after isovolumic contraction: mid to latter portions of the QRS complex) and ends earlier than the mitral regurgitant jet and that the peak velocity of a mitral regurgitant jet is always higher than that of an AS jet. When subvalvular velocities exceed 1.5 m/s, the *modified* rather than the simplified Bernoulli equation must be used to avoid overestimating the true pressure gradient.

Differences in gradients between the intraoperative echocardiography examination and catheterization data are also commonly seen. It should be remembered that catheterization reports frequently present *peak-to-peak* gradients, which is the difference between the peak LV pressure and the peak aortic pressure (Figure 9–13). Because the peak aortic pressure is attained (a fraction of a second) later than the peak LV pressure, it is not an actual physiologic measurement, whereas Doppler measurements reflect peak *instantaneous* gradients.

Table 9–2. Limitations to Assessing the Severity of Aortic Stenosis by Transvalvular Velocity Measurement

Etiology of Limitation	Consequence
Decreased transvalvular flow	
• Severe left ventricular dysfunction	Decreased pressure gradient
• Severe mitral regurgitation	
• Mitral stenosis	
• Left-to-right intracardiac shunt	
• Low cardiac output	
Increased transvalvular flow	
• Hyperdynamic left ventricular function	Increased pressure gradient
• Sepsis	
• Hyperthyroidism	
• Severe aortic regurgitation	

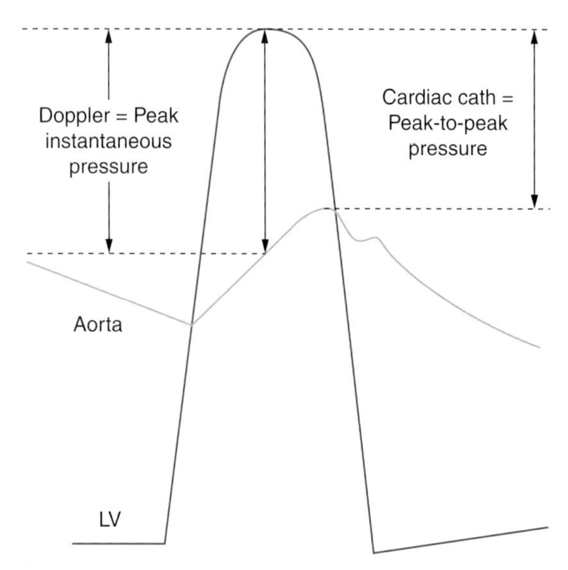

FIGURE 9–13. Illustration of the pressure tracings obtained during cardiac catheterization in a patient with aortic stenosis. The pressure gradient obtained with Doppler echocardiography is reflective of the peak instantaneous gradient. The cardiac catheterization gradient is the difference between the peak left ventricular (LV) and peak aortic pressures. *(From Troianos CA. Perioperative echocardiography. In: Troianos CA, ed. Anesthesia for the Cardiac Patient. St. Louis: Mosby; 2002, with permission.)*

Thus, Doppler-derived gradients may be greater than catheter-derived gradients when peak-to-peak gradients are reported. Doppler-derived gradients may also be greater than catheter-derived gradients when the phenomenon of pressure recovery (reconversion of kinetic energy not completely dissipated as turbulence back to pressure energy distal to a stenosis, resulting in decrease in the pressure gradient) is present. Pressure recovery appears to be clinically relevant only in patients with a small (<3 cm) aorta or a small (<19 mm) bileaflet tilting disk prosthesis.

Nonvalvular Stenosis Left ventricular outflow tract gradients can also occur from subvalvular or supravalvular pathology. Subvalvular stenosis may present as a fixed or a dynamic (different degrees of obstruction during systole) lesion. In membranous subaortic stenosis (also discussed in Chapter 18), there is a fibrous band or ring just below the AV causing obstruction to LV outflow that remains fixed (unchanged) throughout systole. In hypertrophic obstructive cardiomyopathy (also discussed in Chapter 14), hypertrophy of the basal segment of the interventricular septum produces dynamic LVOT obstruction, typically peaking late in systole. Thus, valvular aortic stenosis produces a rounded spectral Doppler pattern with a midsystolic peak, while dynamic left ventricular outflow tract obstruction produces a late systolic peak with a "dagger-shaped" or "shark's tooth" spectral pattern (Figure 9–14). Turbulent flow in the LVOT on color-flow Doppler imaging is usually the first clue of the existence of subvalvular obstruction.

Low-Gradient Aortic Stenosis A particularly challenging perioperative dilemma is the evaluation of the patient with aortic stenosis and low cardiac output, or "low-flow, low-gradient aortic stenosis." Patients with low-gradient aortic stenosis typically have a valve area less than 1.0 cm^2, impaired systolic function, and a mean transvalvular pressure gradient less than 30 mm Hg. Mortality rates for aortic valve replacement in this setting are as high as 18% if the ejection fraction is less than 30% to 35%,[24-26] but the 4-year survival without intervention is less than 20%.[27,28] Intraoperative echocardiography combined with dobutamine stress testing plays an important role in assessing perioperative risk by determining contractile reserve. A 20% stroke volume increase from baseline to peak dobutamine dose identifies the existence of contractile reserve,[29] and operative mortality is reported to be 5% and 32%, respectively, in patients with or without contractile reserve.[28] In addition to assessing risk, dobutamine administration normalizes cardiac output for a more accurate estimation

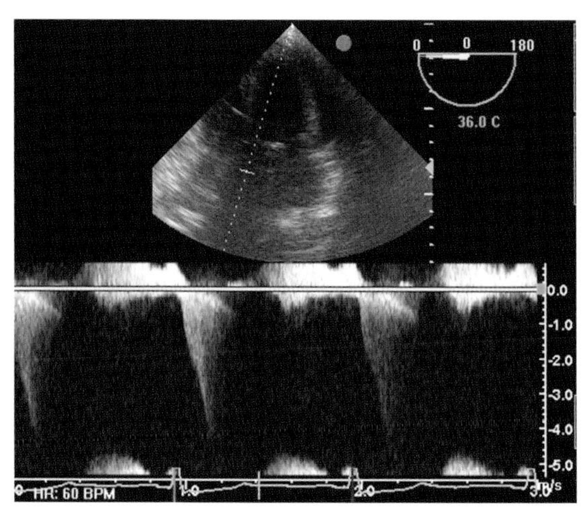

FIGURE 9–14. Continuous-wave spectral Doppler display of left ventricular outflow tract and aortic valve flow velocities in a patient with left ventricular outflow tract obstruction. The characteristic "dagger" or "shark tooth" appearance indicates increased jet acceleration as velocity increases.

of transvalvular gradients.[30] Alternatively, aortic valve area in patients with low ejection fraction and cardiac output can be estimated using the continuity equation method or the dimensionless index (see below).

Aortic Valve Area—Continuity Equation

The continuity equation method to calculate aortic valve area is based upon the concept of conservation of mass and continuity of flow. The flow of blood through the left ventricular outflow tract must equal flow through the aortic valve into ascending aorta:

$$SV_{AV} = SV_{LVOT}$$

$$SV_{AV} = CSA_{Aortic\ Valve} \times VTI_{Aortic\ Valve}$$

$$SV_{LVOT} = CSA_{LVOT} \times VTI_{LVOT}$$

Where SV = Stroke volume

CSA = Cross-sectional area

Thus,

$$CSA_{Aortic\ Valve} \times VTI_{Aortic\ Valve} = CSA_{LVOT} \times VTI_{LVOT}$$

Aortic valve area is then calculated as:

$$\text{Aortic Valve Area} = \frac{CSA_{LVOT} \times VTI_{LVOT}}{VTI_{Aortic\ Valve}}$$

Assuming that the LVOT is circular:

$$CSA_{LVOT} = \pi \times (d/2)^2$$

$$CSA_{LVOT} = \pi/4 \times d^2$$

$$CSA_{LVOT} = 0.785 \times d^2$$

Where d = LVOT diameter

The valve area calculated with the continuity equation is the effective orifice area or the cross-sectional flow area of blood as it passes through the valve. It should be remembered that this effective orifice area is smaller than the anatomic valve area due to contraction of the flow stream, but the calculated effective orifice area is accepted as a measure of aortic valve area and is the primary predictor of clinical outcome.[11]

To obtain the three measurements required to solve the continuity equation for aortic valve area, one must utilize three different echocardiographic techniques and tomographic views:

Technique	Tomographic View
Aortic valve velocity by CWD	TG LAX or deep TG LAX
LVOT velocity with PWD or CWD	TG LAX or deep TG LAX
LVOT diameter by 2D with calipers	ME AV LAX

In the setting of stenosis, CWD is used to measure aortic valve velocity because velocities encountered are usually greater than 2 m/s. Proper alignment of the Doppler beam with flow through the aortic valve is essential as any deviation from a parallel intercept angle leads to velocity underestimation. Orientation of the CWD beam using color-flow Doppler and audible signaling may be helpful. If the intercept angle is within 20° of parallel, the degree of underestimation is 6% or less and clinically acceptable. The resulting CWD spectral envelope is solid or shaded in character, reflecting nonlaminar flow, and demonstrates a high-velocity midsystolic peak. Planimetry is then utilized to trace the spectral envelope and obtain the aortic valve velocity-time integral (VTI) and peak velocity. Although both VTI and peak velocity are considered acceptable by some experts, a recent consensus statement indicated that the utilization of peak velocities may be less reliable for determination of aortic valve area using the continuity equation.[11,31]

The LVOT VTI is determined by placing the pulsed-wave Doppler sample volume in the LVOT just proximal to the aortic valve and tracing the spectral Doppler envelope. The pulsed-wave sample volume should first be placed at the level of the valve and slowly withdrawn into the LVOT until a smooth spectral pattern without aliasing is obtained. In patients with AS, the sample volume may need to be withdrawn 0.5 to 1.0 cm apically to obtain a laminar flow curve due to the flow acceleration in close proximity to the valve.[11] The spectral profile should demonstrate laminar flow as demonstrated by a hollow or unshaded spectral envelope. Normal peak velocities in the LVOT range from 0.8 to 1.5 m/s.

An accurate determination of aortic valve area using the continuity method requires that the LVOT diameter be measured at the same point in the LVOT as where the LVOT spectral velocity was recorded. This measurement is usually obtained with the ME AV LAX view, because 2D imaging is optimal when the ultrasound beam intersects its target perpendicularly. The LVOT annular diameter is obtained during midsystole with electronic calipers placed along the inner edges of the endocardium. Normal values for the LVOT diameter are a mean of 2.0 cm with a range of 1.8 to 2.2 cm.

Accurate measurement of the LVOT diameter is essential because this measurement is squared to determine CSA_{LVOT} and is the greatest source for error in determining aortic valve area with the continuity equation. Underestimation of LVOT diameter will result in underestimation of the aortic valve area. A second source of error is introduced when the LVOT diameter and the LVOT velocity are not measured in the same location. A technical limitation of TEE is that the best view for 2D imaging of the LVOT (ME AV LAX) is not the best view for Doppler interrogation of LVOT velocity (TG LAX or deep TG LAX). Similarly, the LVOT and aortic valve velocity measurements should be acquired from the same heartbeat to minimize the effect of beat-to-beat variability in stroke volume. The most common clinical scenario of beat-to-beat variability is the patient with an irregular cardiac rhythm, eg, atrial fibrillation. In patients with atrial fibrillation, it is recommended that at least five consecutive beats be analyzed and averaged. Alternatively, CWD through both the aortic valve and the left ventricular outflow tract often yields two spectral envelopes, the higher velocity related to the aortic valve and a lower, denser pattern consistent with the left ventricular outflow tract velocity (Figure 9–15). This "double-envelope" technique circumvents the problem of different stroke volumes by allowing both velocity-time integrals to be determined on the same beat.[32] Another potential source of error is the inability to align the Doppler beam to be parallel with flow. Ensuring that axial alignment deviates less than 20° from parallel minimizes this error. A final limitation is the inability to obtain adequate tomographic views, leading to an inability to estimate aortic valve area in up to 6% of patients.[33,34] Epicardial echocardiography (see Chapter 20) can overcome this limitation in 100% of patients and demonstrates excellent correlation with TEE, TTE, and cardiac catheterization–derived measures.[35]

VELOCITY RATIO OR DIMENSIONLESS INDEX

The ratio of the LVOT velocity-time integral to the aortic valve velocity-time integral is termed the dimensionless index (DI) and is used as an estimate of aortic stenosis severity.

$$\text{Dimensionless Index (DI)} = \frac{\text{LVOT}_{\text{VTI}}}{\text{Aortic Valve}_{\text{VTI}}}$$

The continuous-wave VTI of a normal aortic valve will equal the VTI of the LVOT, and therefore the DI will equal 1. With progression of aortic stenosis, the aortic valve velocity increases while the left ventricular outflow tract velocity remains unchanged. Severe aortic stenosis is present when the DI is less than 0.25.[36] Patients with a normal LVOT diameter of 2.0 cm, have a calculated LVOT area of $3.14 \times (1)^2 = 3.14\ \text{cm}^2$. A DI less than 0.25 thus corresponds to an aortic valve area that is 25% of the LVOT area or approximately $0.25(3.14) = 0.8\ \text{cm}^2$ (see Table 9–1).

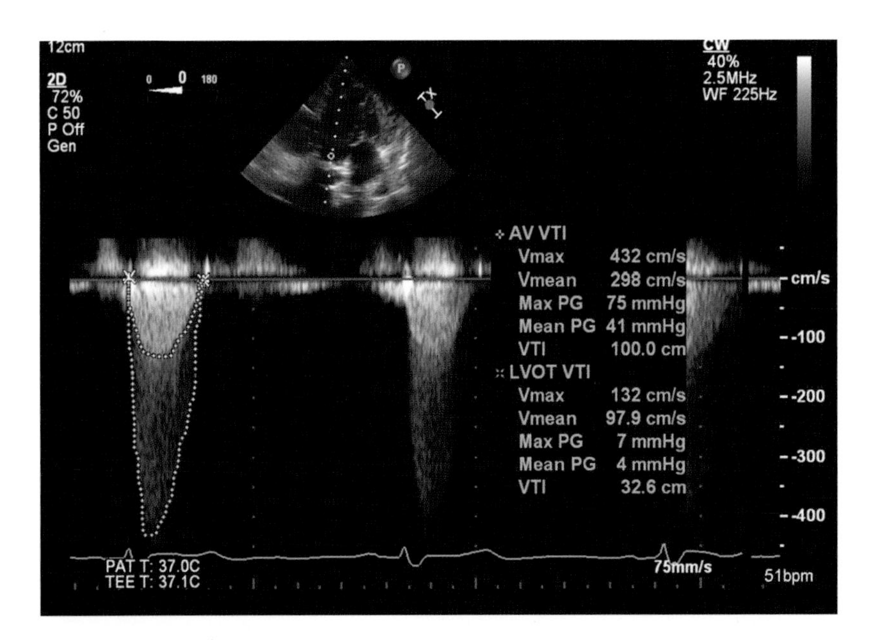

FIGURE 9–15. The aortic valve and left ventricular outflow tract velocities are seen on the same cardiac beat using continuous-wave spectral Doppler and the double-envelope technique. The ratio of LVOT velocity to aortic valve velocity is known as the dimensionless index.

ASSOCIATED ECHOCARDIOGRAPHIC FINDINGS

Pressure overload from the increased resistance to ejection initially results in concentric hypertrophy of the LV, thus allowing the ventricle to preserve SV by increasing the contractile mass. Posterior wall thickness should be measured in aortic stenosis using the caliper function in the TG SAX view, at end-diastole (excluding the papillary muscles). Wall thickness 1.0 cm or greater in women and 1.1 cm or greater in men is considered abnormal. Septal hypertrophy as a consequence of aortic stenosis can lead to the development of systolic anterior motion (SAM) of the mitral valve after AVR (see Chapters 8 and 14). Diastolic dysfunction also is commonly seen in these patients because relaxation is impaired in the hypertrophied ventricle and optimal ventricular filling becomes dependent to a greater degree on atrial contraction. Mitral inflow velocities typically demonstrate a decrease in the velocity of early diastolic inflow (decrease in E-wave amplitude), an increase in the velocity of late diastolic inflow due to atrial contraction (increase in A-wave amplitude), a decrease in E/A velocity ratio, and a prolonged deceleration time (see Chapter 12). Early in aortic stenosis, LV end-systolic volume and end-diastolic volume remain unchanged; however, an increase in LV end-diastolic pressure may be present from abnormal relaxation and stiffness of the hypertrophied ventricle. Chronic increases in LV end-diastolic pressure result in elevated left atrial (LA) pressures and LA enlargement, predisposing to the development of atrial fibrillation. Loss of the atrial contraction can then further impair LV filling, thus producing dramatic decreases in SV and cardiac output. Ventricular dilatation, resulting in an elevated LV end-diastolic volume and LV end-systolic volume, occurs late in the disease. Dilation of the ascending aorta may be a consequence of long-standing aortic stenosis from an adaptive mechanism promoting left ventricular ejection, or may be due to intrinsic disease within the aortic wall. A comprehensive examination of the ascending aorta, including epiaortic scanning, is recommended to determine the need for surgical repair and to guide cannulation and perfusion strategies. Finally, mitral regurgitation is common in patients with aortic stenosis and is related to either LV pressure overload or intrinsic mitral disease. In the majority of patients without intrinsic mitral disease, mitral regurgitation improves after aortic valve replacement, but the evidence supporting this intuitive clinical reasoning is sparse.

Aortic Regurgitation

Aortic regurgitation is caused by intrinsic disease of the aortic valve leaflets or diseases that affect the integrity of the ascending aorta. Intrinsic disease of the aortic cusps includes calcific, rheumatic, myxomatous, congenital, infectious, and traumatic abnormalities. Conditions that alter the structural support of the aortic annulus include annular dilatation, aortic dissection, and aneurysmal disease. Assessment of aortic regurgitation by TEE requires determination of the etiology of valve dysfunction, classification of the severity of aortic regurgitation, and associated cardiovascular changes. El Khoury et al have proposed a classification system describing the mechanism of aortic regurgitation.[37] This classification system, similar to the Carpentier classification system for mitral regurgitation,[38] was developed to provide insight into the mechanism of aortic regurgitation, guide repair techniques, and provide a framework for the assessment of long-term outcomes. Type I lesions are associated with normal leaflet motion and are subclassified according to the segment of the aortic root that is dilated or by the presence of cusp perforation. Type Ia lesions are caused by dilation of the sinotubular junction and ascending aorta; type Ib lesions are caused by dilation of the sinus of Valsalva and sinotubular junction; and type Ic lesions are caused by isolated dilation of the aortic annulus. Type Id lesions have normal leaflet mobility and normal aortic root dimensions, but are characterized by leaflet perforation. Type II lesions are caused by leaflet prolapse secondary to excessive cusp tissue or commissural disruption, and type III lesions are caused by leaflet restriction (Figure 9–16).[37]

TWO-DIMENSIONAL MEASURES

The four standard TEE views of the aortic valve (ME AV SAX, ME AV LAX, TG LAX, and deep TG LAX) are also utilized to evaluate an insufficient aortic valve. The ME AV LAX view will identify prolapsing aortic valve cusps, an aortic aneurysm, or aortic dissection with loss of aortic valve cusp suspension from the aortic annulus. Leaflet perforations secondary to endocarditis may be visible in both the ME AV SAX and ME AV LAX views. The ME AV SAX view allows for planimetric assessment of the end-diastolic gap between the aortic cusps as an estimate of the severity of aortic regurgitation. A gap area less than 0.2 cm^2 (small), 0.2 to 0.4 cm^2 (moderate), and greater than 0.4 cm^2 (large) demonstrates good angiographic correlation with mild, moderate, and severe aortic regurgitation, respectively.[39]

DOPPLER COLOR-FLOW MAPPING

Doppler echocardiography provides several quantitative estimates of the severity of aortic regurgitation (Table 9–3). The ME AV SAX view allows visualization of all aortic valve cusps during interrogation with color-flow Doppler and is useful for identifying the location of regurgitant flow. Color-flow Doppler applied to the ME AV LAX view allows assessment of the width of the AR jet relative to the LVOT during diastole. Central jets are more common with aortic annular dilatation, whereas an eccentric jet implies underlying leaflet

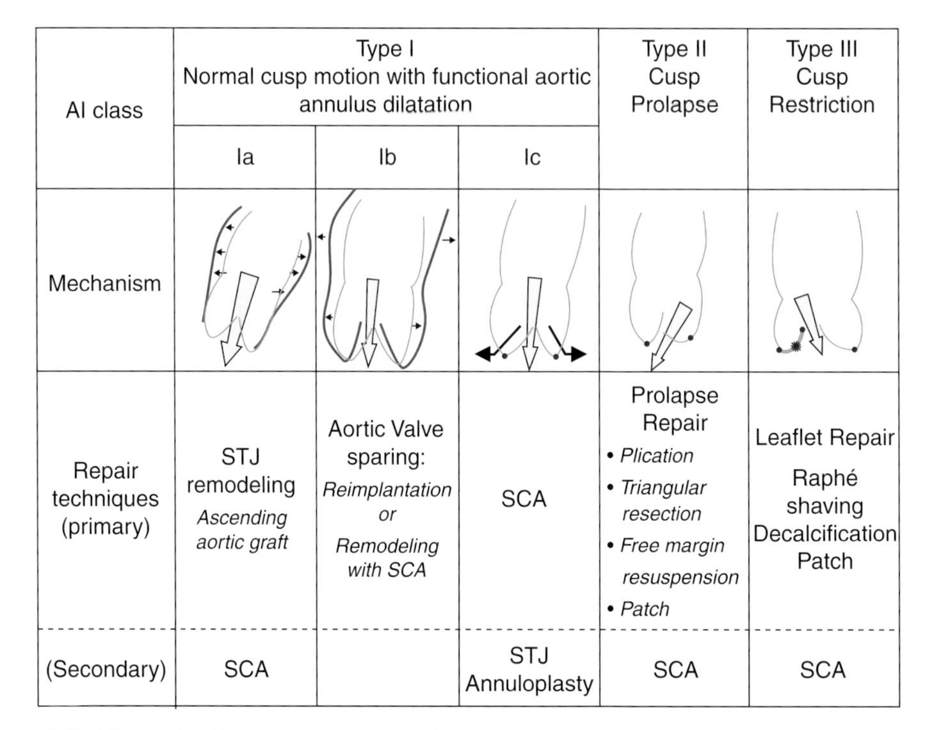

AI class	Type I Normal cusp motion with functional aortic annulus dilatation			Type II Cusp Prolapse	Type III Cusp Restriction
	Ia	Ib	Ic		
Mechanism					
Repair techniques (primary)	STJ remodeling *Ascending aortic graft*	Aortic Valve sparing: *Reimplantation or Remodeling with SCA*	SCA	Prolapse Repair • *Plication* • *Triangular resection* • *Free margin resuspension* • *Patch*	Leaflet Repair Raphé shaving Decalcification Patch
(Secondary)	SCA		STJ Annuloplasty	SCA	SCA

FIGURE 9–16. El Khoury classification of aortic regurgitation. Type Ia—dilation of the sinotubular junction and ascending aorta; Type Ib—dilation of the sinus of Valsalva and sinotubular junction; Type Ic—isolated dilation of the aortic annulus; Type Id—leaflet perforation (not shown); Type II—leaflet prolapse secondary to excessive cusp tissue or commissural disruption; Type III—leaflet restriction. (AI, aortic insufficiency; STJ, sinotubular junction; SCA, subcommissural annuloplasty.) *(Modified from Boodhwani M, de Kerchove L, Glineur D, et al. Repair-oriented classification of aortic insufficiency: impact on surgical techniques and clinical outcomes. J Thorac Cardiovasc Surg. 2009;137:286-94, with permission.)*

pathology, whether intrinsic to the valve or secondary to disruption of the valve suspension mechanism (Figures 9–17 through 9–19).

One method for estimating aortic regurgitation that demonstrates good correlation with angiographic determinants of aortic regurgitation is the ratio of the jet width measured at the *origin of the jet* (within 1 cm of the aortic valve) to the width of the LVOT.[31] A jet width/LVOT width ratio of less than 0.25 is mild AR, while a ratio greater than 0.64 is indicative of severe AR. An alternative estimate for the severity of aortic regurgitation is based upon the ratio of the cross-sectional area of the regurgitant jet (within 1 cm of the valve) to the cross-sectional area of the LVOT. A ratio of jet area–to–LVOT area less than 5% represents mild AR, while a ratio greater than 60% represents severe AR.[40] It is important to remember that the length of the aortic regurgitation jet into the left ventricle does not correlate with severity because of the dependence of this measure upon loading conditions and ventricular compliance.

VENA CONTRACTA WIDTH

The vena contracta is the narrowest portion of the regurgitant jet and is located at or just proximal to the orifice. It is obtained in the ME LAX view with the imaging depth reduced to optimize imaging size. The largest diameter of the vena contracta during any portion of diastole should be measured. Vena contracta width correlates well with the severity of AR by angiography; a width greater than 6.0 mm is severe, while a width less than 3.0 mm represents mild aortic regurgitation (Figure 9–20).[41] Vena contracta width is a load-independent determinant of AR severity, as it is not affected by changes in afterload or volume loading.

Table 9-3. Parameters for the Determination of the Severity of Aortic Regurgitation

	Mild	Moderate	Severe
Structural Parameters			
LV size	Normal[a]	Normal or dilated	Usually dilated[b]
Aortic leaflets	Normal or abnormal	Normal or abnormal	Abnormal or flail, or wide coaptation defect
Doppler Parameters			
Jet width in LVOT: color flow[c]	Small in central jets	Intermediate	Large in central jets; variable in eccentric jets
Jet density: CWD	Incomplete or faint	Dense	Dense
Jet deceleration rate: CWD (PHT; ms)[d]	Slow: >500	Medium: 500-200	Steep: <200
Diastolic flow reversal in descending aorta: PWD	Brief, early diastolic reversal	Intermediate	Prominent holodiastolic reversal
Quantitative Parameters[e]			
Angiographic grade	1+	2+/3+	4+
VC width (cm)[c]	<0.3	0.3-0.60	>0.6
Jet width/LVOT width (%)[c]	<25	25-45/46-64	≥65
Jet CSA/LVOT CSA (%)[c]	<5	5-20/21-59	≥60
RVol (mL/beat)	<30	30-44/45-59	≥60
RF (%)	<30	30-39/40-49	≥50
EROA (cm^2)	<0.10	0.10-0.19/0.20-0.29	≥0.30

[a]Unless there were other reasons for LV dilation.
[b]An exception would be acute AR, in which chambers have not had time to dilate.
[c]At a Nyquist limit of 50 to 60 cm/s.
[d]PHT is shortened with increasing LV diastolic pressure and vasodilator therapy and may be lengthened in chronic adaptation to severe AR.
[e]Quantitative parameters can subclassify the moderate regurgitation group into mild-to-moderate and moderate-to-severe regurgitation as shown.
From Bonow RO, Carabello BA, Chatterjee K, et al. ACC/AHA 2006 guidelines for the management of patients with valvular heart disease: a report of the American College of Cardiology/American Heart Association Task Force on Practice Guidelines (writing Committee to Revise the 1998 guidelines for the management of patients with valvular heart disease) developed in collaboration with the Society of Cardiovascular Anesthesiologists endorsed by the Society for Cardiovascular Angiography and Interventions and the Society of Thoracic Surgeons. J Am Coll Cardiol. 2006;48(3):e1-148; and Zoghbi WA, Enriquez-Sarano M, Foster E, et al. Recommendations for evaluation of the severity of native valvular regurgitation with two-dimensional and Doppler echocardiography. J Am Soc Echocardiogr. 2003;16(7):777-802.

Pressure Half-Time and Deceleration Slope

Continuous-wave Doppler is utilized to determine the severity of aortic regurgitation by measuring the pressure half-time (PHT) and the deceleration slope of the regurgitant jet. A parallel intercept between the regurgitant jet and Doppler beam is typically obtained using the deep TG LAX or TG LAX views. Color Doppler is then used to identify the location and direction of the AR jet, and the Doppler cursor is placed within the jet to obtain the continuous-wave spectral Doppler velocity profile. A large regurgitant orifice allows for a more rapid equalization of the aortic and left ventricular pressures, yielding a more rapid decline in the regurgitant jet velocity, thus generating a steep deceleration slope and a short pressure half-time (time for the diastolic pressure gradient to fall to half its initial value) (Figure 9–21). A deceleration slope greater than 3 m/s^2 or a pressure half-time shorter than 200 milliseconds is indicative of severe (3 to 4+) aortic regurgitation.[42] A pressure half-time of greater than 500 milliseconds is indicative of mild aortic regurgitation (Figure 9–22). In patients with elevated LV end-diastolic pressure (e.g. ischemia, cardiomyopathy, chronic AR) the use of PHT may overestimate the true severity of regurgitation because the elevated ventricular pressure will decrease the time required for equalization of pressures between the aorta and the left ventricle. Similarly, decreased SVR (e.g. sepsis, post-CPB) results in a steeper deceleration slope.

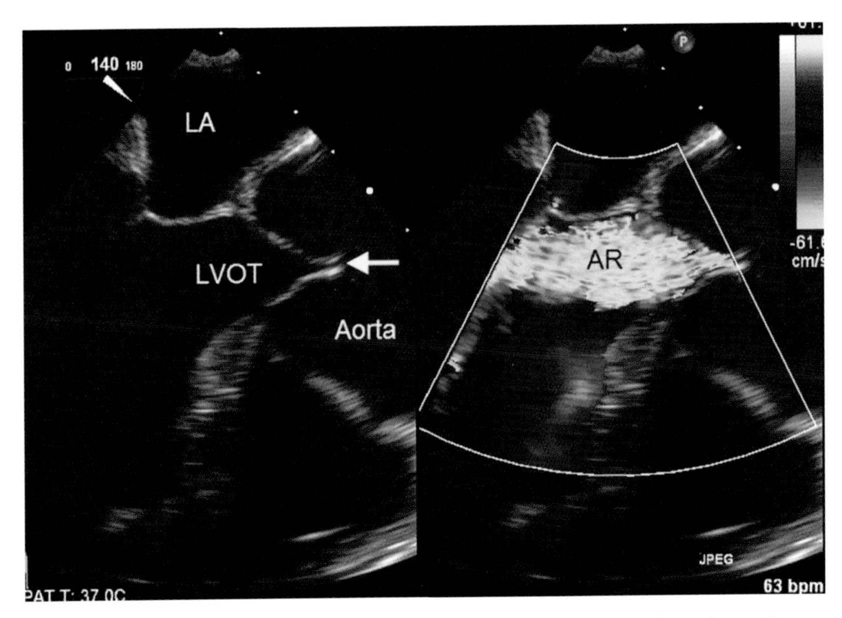

FIGURE 9–17. *Left*: Transesophageal echocardiogram of the midesophageal aortic valve long-axis view in a patient with aortic root dilation leading to incomplete closure of the aortic valve *(arrow)*. (LA, left atrium; LVOT, left ventricular outflow tract; Aorta, ascending aorta.) *Right*: Color comparison of the same image with color-flow Doppler showing the incomplete valve closure leading to severe aortic regurgitation (AR).

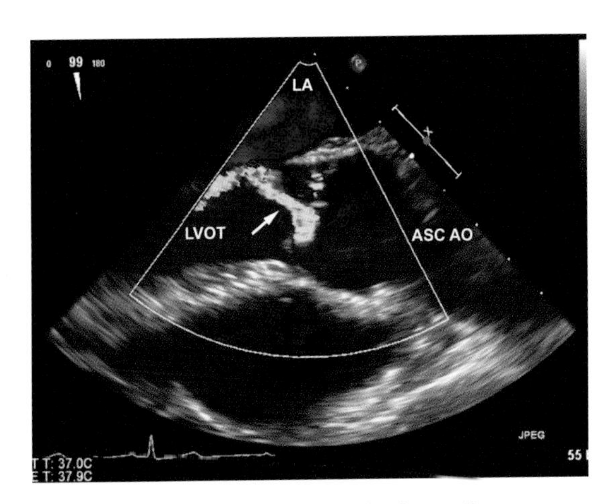

FIGURE 9–18. Transesophageal echocardiogram with color-flow Doppler in a patient with eccentric aortic regurgitation. The aortic regurgitation is identified by the color-flow disturbance *(arrow)* that originates from the aortic valve and is directed towards the anterior mitral valve leaflet. (LA, left atrium; LVOT, left ventricular outflow tract; ASC AO, ascending aorta.)

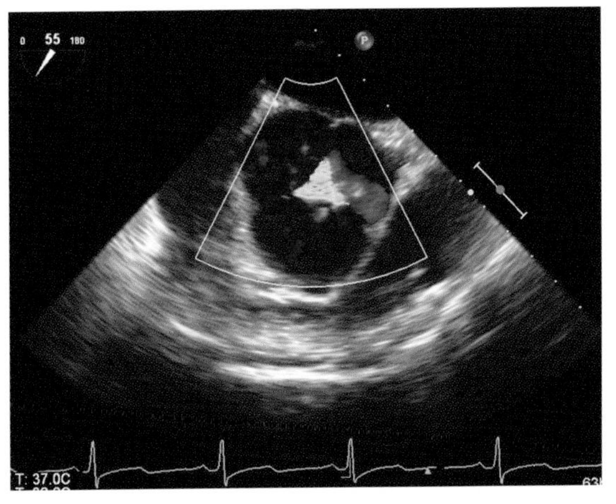

FIGURE 9–19. Midesophageal aortic valve short-axis view and color-flow Doppler in a patient with aortic regurgitation. The origin of the aortic regurgitation is predominantly central.

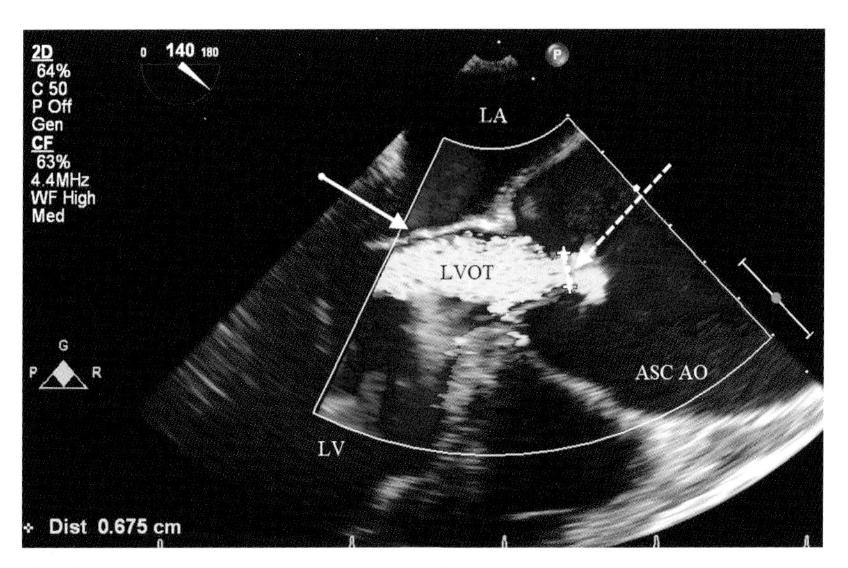

FIGURE 9–20. Transesophageal echocardiogram of the midesophageal aortic valve long-axis view with color-flow Doppler in a patient with aortic regurgitation. The vena contracta at the aortic valve *(dashed arrow)* measuring 0.675 cm indicates severe aortic regurgitation. (LA, left atrium; LV, left ventricle; LVOT, left ventricular outflow tract; ASC AO, dilated ascending aorta; *solid arrow*, anterior leaflet of the mitral valve.)

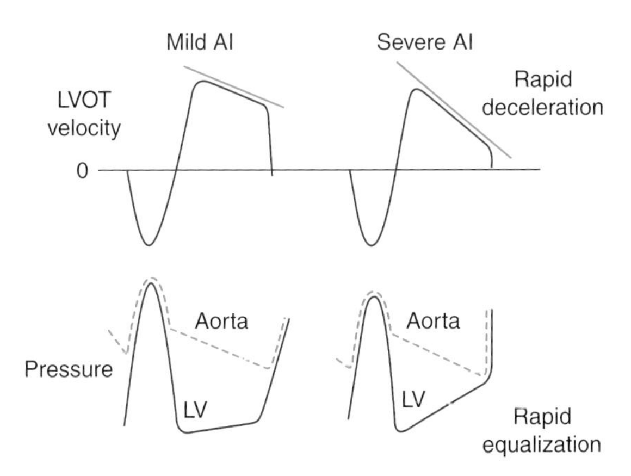

FIGURE 9–21. Illustration of the association between the left ventricular outflow tract (LVOT) deceleration slope and the pressure difference between the aorta and left ventricle (LV) during diastole. The deceleration slope is steeper and approaches zero velocity more rapidly with severe aortic regurgitation (AI) as the pressures in the aorta and left ventricle equalize more rapidly. *(Troianos CA. Perioperative echocardiography. In: Troianos CA, ed. Anesthesia for the Cardiac Patient, St. Louis: Mosby; 2002, with permission, and adapted from Feigenbaum H. Echocardiography. 5th ed. Philadelphia: Lea & Febiger; 1994:286, with permission.)*

DESCENDING AORTIC FLOW REVERSAL

The presence of holodiastolic flow reversal on pulsed-wave Doppler (PWD) examination of the descending aorta indicates severe AR (Figure 9–23). The PWD sample is placed in the descending aorta, just beyond the aortic arch, in the longitudinal plane of the descending aorta (multiplane angle at 90°), with the sample volume in the center of the aorta. However, better alignment with aortic flow may be obtained in the distal descending aorta. Holodiastolic flow reversal in the proximal descending aorta is sensitive but not specific for detection of severe AR, whereas flow reversal in the abdominal aorta is sensitive and specific for AR.[43,44] False-positive results in the proximal aorta can be due to the presence of a patent ductus arteriosus, Blalock-Taussig shunt, or a descending aortic aneurysm.

REGURGITANT VOLUME, REGURGITANT FRACTION, AND EFFECTIVE REGURGITANT ORIFICE AREA

Patients with mild aortic regurgitation as determined by jet width, vena contracta size, and pressure half-time require no further assessment of AR severity. However, if any of these parameters suggest more than mild AR, other quantitative measures such as regurgitant volume, regurgitant fraction, and effective regurgitant orifice area should

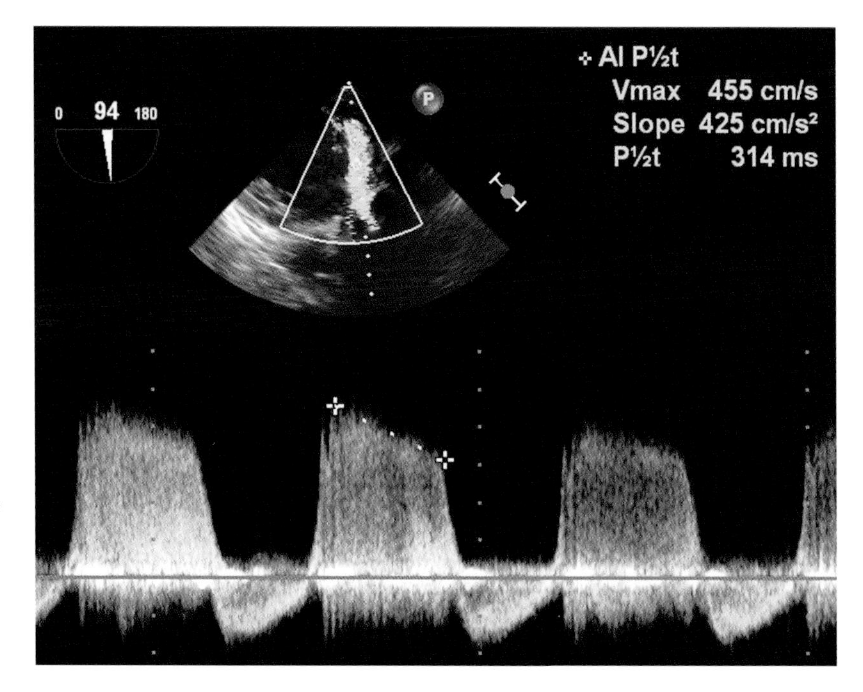

FIGURE 9–22. Continuous-wave spectral Doppler velocities within the left ventricular outflow tract of a patient with aortic regurgitation. The slope of the velocity deceleration (AR slope, 4.25 m/s^2) and the pressure half time (314 milliseconds) indicates the severity of the aortic regurgitation.

be assessed (see Table 9–3).[40] Regurgitant volume is the difference between the volume of blood flowing antegrade through the regurgitant valve compared to the volume of blood flowing antegrade through a different but nonregurgitant cardiac valve. For example, in the absence of intracardiac shunts and mitral regurgitation, the aortic valve regurgitant volume is the difference between aortic valve systolic flow and systolic flow through the pulmonic valve or diastolic flow through the mitral valve.

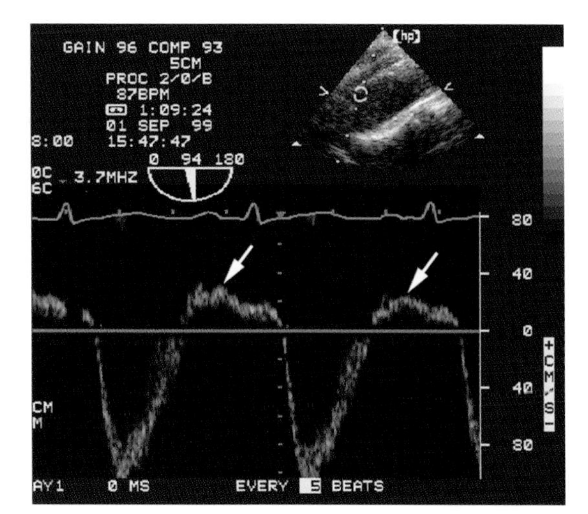

FIGURE 9–23. Pulsed-wave Doppler spectral velocity of blood flow in the descending thoracic aorta. The retrograde flow throughout diastole *(arrows)* is termed holodiastolic and is associated with severe aortic regurgitation.

$$\text{Regurgitant Volume (RV)} = SV_{\text{Regurgitant Valve}} - SV_{\text{Competent Valve}}$$

$$RV_{\text{Aortic Valve}} = SV_{\text{Aortic Valve}} - SV_{\text{Pulmonic or Mitral Valve}}$$

$$RV_{\text{Aortic Valve}} = (VTI_{\text{Aortic Valve}} \times CSA_{\text{Aortic Valve}}) - (VTI_{\text{Pulmonic or Mitral Valve}} \times CSA_{\text{Pulmonic or Mitral Valve}})$$

Pulmonary artery blood flow is reliably measured with TEE and is typically favored over mitral inflow because the mitral valve annulus is saddle shaped and not circular as required for the calculation of CSA. In the absence of aortic stenosis, SV_{LVOT} can be substituted for $SV_{\text{Aortic Valve}}$.

Regurgitant fraction is the proportion of aortic flow that is regurgitant and equals the aortic valve regurgitant volume divided by the aortic valve systolic volume.

$$\text{Regurgitant Fraction (RF)} = \frac{\text{Regurgitant Volume}}{\text{Total Forward Stroke Volume}}$$

$$\text{Regurgitant Fraction (RF)} = \frac{SV_{\text{Regurgitant Valve}} - SV_{\text{Competent Valve}}}{SV_{\text{Regurgitant Valve}}}$$

Regurgitant fraction (RF) =

$$\frac{(VTI_{Aortic\ Valve} \times CSA_{Aortic\ Valve}) - (VTI_{Pulmonic\ Valve} \times CSA_{Pulmonic\ Valve})}{(VTI_{Aortic\ Valve} \times CSA_{Aortic\ Valve})}$$

Effective regurgitant orifice area (EROA) is calculated by dividing the regurgitant volume by the velocity-time integral of the regurgitant jet recorded by continuous-wave Doppler.[41]

$$EROA = \frac{Regurgitant\ Volume_{Aortic\ Valve}}{VTI_{Aortic\ Regurgitant\ Jet}}$$

ASSOCIATED ECHOCARDIOGRAPHIC FINDINGS

The size of the left ventricle is an indirect indicator of the severity of aortic regurgitation in patients with chronic AR. A dilated ventricle usually excludes mild AR, instead favoring moderate to severe chronic aortic regurgitation. In cases of acute aortic regurgitation, a normal-sized ventricle does not exclude severe AR because the left ventricle has not had the time to remodel and dilate. Late in the disease course after long-standing dilation, left ventricular systolic function will irreversibly deteriorate; therefore, surgical intervention is recommended before LV systolic function declines. An aortic regurgitation jet may also cause a diastolic fluttering and premature closure of the anterior mitral leaflet. An eccentric AR jet may cause diastolic doming of the mitral valve towards the left atrium.

EFFECT OF AR ON ASSOCIATED VALVULAR LESIONS

As described earlier, AS severity may be overestimated in patients with AR if elevated subvalvular velocities are ignored by applying the simplified instead of the modified Bernoulli equation. Patients with both moderate aortic stenosis and moderate aortic regurgitation are considered to have severe valvular disease.[11] Similarly, mitral valve area (MVA) is overestimated in patients with both mitral stenosis and aortic regurgitation when the pressure half-time (PHT) method is used. The PHT method utilizes the deceleration of mitral valve inflow to estimate mitral valve area. Deceleration is based on the equalization of pressure between the left atrium and left ventricle, and deceleration time increases (shallow slope) as mitral valve area decreases. In the absence of aortic insufficiency, left ventricular pressure rise occurs from diastolic mitral inflow alone. With aortic insufficiency, however, left ventricular pressure rise occurs more rapidly, leading to a steeper mitral inflow slope and an overestimation of mitral valve area (Table 9–4).

NOVEL IMAGING TECHNIQUES

The introduction of three-dimensional echocardiography into clinical practice has allowed a more detailed evaluation of the left ventricular outflow tract and aortic valve apparatus, compared with two-dimensional echocardiography (Figures 9–24 through 9–26). Incorporation of a three-dimensional LVOT area produces less deviation from invasively or planimetrically measured aortic valve areas than conventionally (2D) calculated areas using the continuity equation.[45] Real-time intraoperative three-dimensional echocardiography is also useful for identifying aortic valve abnormalities that may be missed with two-dimensional echocardiography.[46]

The technique of geometric aortic valve analysis, which employs pattern recognition to generate a dynamic analysis of the aortic valve area, LVOT diameter, sinotubular junction, and ascending aorta, has also recently been introduced into clinical practice (Figure 9–27) and may offer greater quantification of aortic valve function.

Table 9–4. Aortic Regurgitation and Echocardiographic Assessment of Other Valvular Abnormalities

Aortic Regurgitation Associated With:	Consequence
Aortic stenosis	• Overestimates systolic pressure gradient due to increased transaortic flow • Use modified Bernoulli equation when LVOT flow exceeds 1.5 m/s
Mitral stenosis	• Shortens mitral inflow pressure half-time • Steeper deceleration slope • Underestimates severity of mitral stenosis • Overestimates MVA

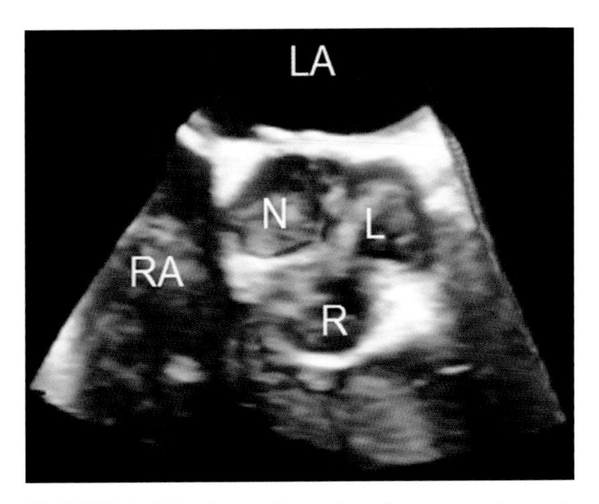

FIGURE 9–24. Three-dimensional transesophageal echocardiogram of the midesophageal aortic valve short-axis view of a normal aortic valve during diastole. The aortic valve is identified by the right (R), left (L), and noncoronary (N) cusps. (RA, right atrium; LA, left atrium.)

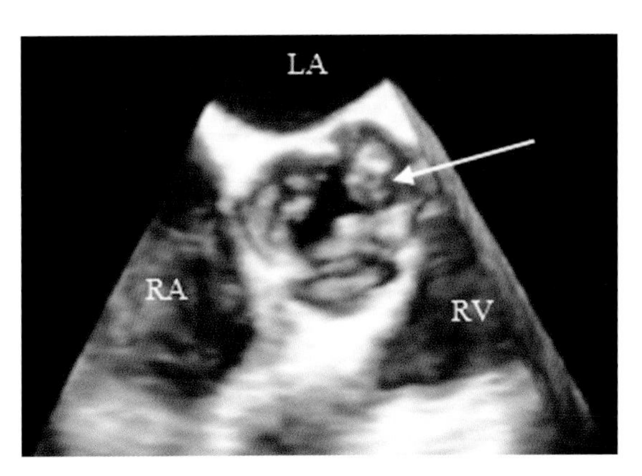

FIGURE 9–26. Three-dimensional transesophageal echocardiogram of the midesophageal aortic valve short-axis view during systole in a patient with moderate aortic stenosis. The arrow points to a calcified aortic valve leaflet. (LA, left atrium; RA, right atrium; RV, right ventricle.)

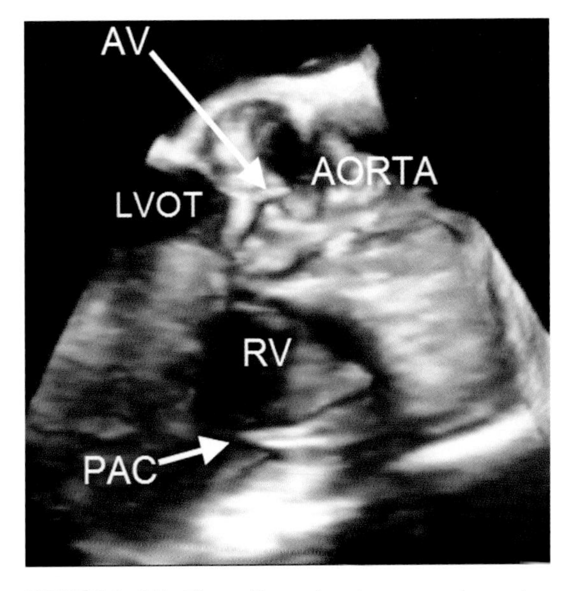

FIGURE 9–25. Three-dimensional transesophageal echocardiogram of the midesophageal aortic valve long-axis view during diastole with the AV arrow indicating the aortic valve leaflet tips during diastole. (LVOT, left ventricular outflow tract; RV, right ventricle; AORTA, ascending aorta; PAC, pulmonary artery catheter.)

AORTIC REGURGITATION AND SURGICAL TECHNIQUES

Aortic Valve Repair Versus Replacement

Just as with the mitral valve, aortic valve repair techniques are always preferred when feasible, as compared to replacement procedures. The vast majority of aortic valves suitable for repair, however, have regurgitant rather than stenotic lesions. Aortic regurgitation that results from aortic dissection is easily repaired by resuspension of the cusps and is highly successful in the absence of additional leaflet pathology. Unfortunately, calcific aortic stenosis is rarely amenable to repair. Boodhwani et al evaluated a series of 264 patients presenting for aortic valve repair for greater than moderate aortic regurgitation. Sixty-four percent of patients in this study had a single type of AR as classified by El Khoury et al,[37] 30% had two types, and 6% had three different types. The majority of patients had type I or functional aortic annular dilation, 35% had type II or leaflet prolapse, and 15% had restricted leaflet mobility or type III AR (see Figure 9–16). Patients with type III AR had a higher risk for recurrent AR at follow-up, and therefore these patients need to be considered for valve replacement rather than repair.[47] Data from the Cleveland Clinic also suggest that repair of regurgitant bicuspid aortic valves is superior (0% immediate replacement rate after repair) to that of a tricuspid aortic regurgitant valve (15% immediate post-repair replacement

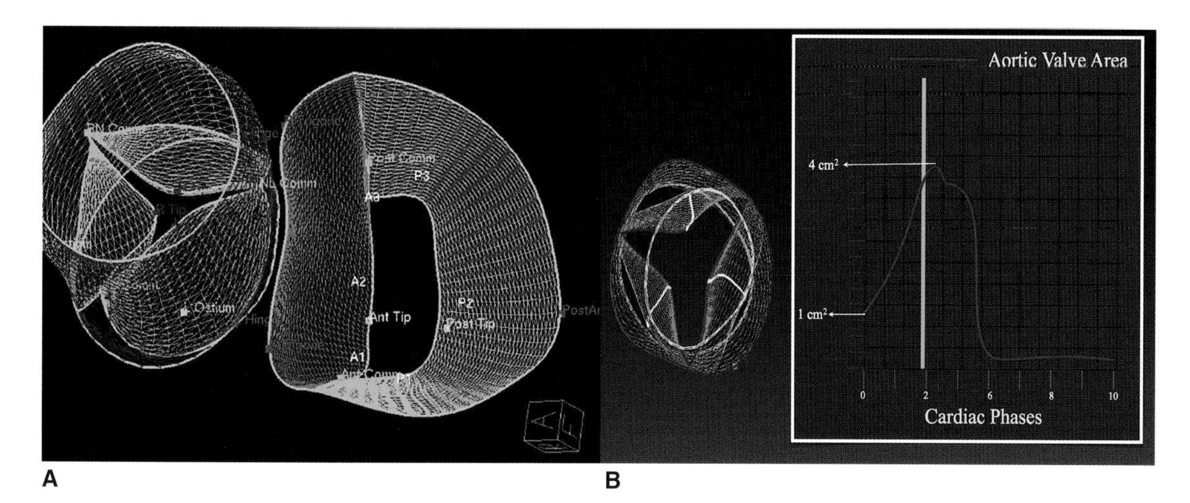

FIGURE 9–27. Geometric aortic valve analysis demonstrating the relationship between aortic and mitral leaflets **(A)** and change in aortic valve area over time **(B)**. *(Courtesy of F. Mahmood, MD.)*

rate).[48] Compared to mitral valve repair, the aortic valve repair failure rate is higher (14% vs 6.6%) due to the greater technical difficulty of aortic valve repair.[49]

Cardioplegia Delivery

Moderate to severe aortic regurgitation necessitates an altered myocardial perfusion strategy during aortic cross clamping to keep the LV empty and avoid the increase in wall tension and oxygen demand during cardioplegic arrest. Milder degrees of aortic regurgitation have also been described on occasion to produce greater than expected degrees of incompetence during cardiopulmonary bypass, perhaps from an alteration of the three-dimensional architecture of the valve when the LV is decompressed. Cardioplegia is most often provided in this setting via selective antegrade delivery into each coronary ostia or retrograde through the coronary sinus.

FUTURE DIRECTIONS

Aortic valve disease will become more prevalent as our population ages. Intraoperative TEE has been demonstrated to be safe, effective, and instrumental in the management of patients undergoing aortic valve surgery. TEE confirms the preoperative diagnosis, evaluates the severity of aortic valve disease, determines the feasibility of aortic valve repair versus replacement, and evaluates the success of surgical correction. Two-dimensional imaging combined with pulsed-wave, continuous-wave, and color Doppler allow for quantitative evaluation of stenotic and regurgitant lesions, as well as identification of the etiology of valve dysfunction. The recent introduction of real-time three-dimensional TEE will undoubtedly enhance the ability of the echocardiographer to better define aortic valve pathology, communicate a more accurate description of the valve dysfunction to the surgeon, and provide for safer deployment of percutaneous valves (see Chapter 11).

ACKNOWLEDGMENTS

The authors would like to thank Drs. Stephen R. Strelec and Saket Singh for their insight, review, and recommendations regarding this chapter.

REFERENCES

1. Nowrangi SK, Connolly HM, Freeman WK, Click RL. Impact of intraoperative transesophageal echocardiography among patients undergoing aortic valve replacement for aortic stenosis. *J Am Soc Echocardiogr.* 2001;14(9):863-866.
2. Cheitlin MD, Armstrong WF, Aurigemma GP, et al. ACC/AHA/ASE 2003 guideline update for the clinical application of echocardiography—summary article: a report of the American College of Cardiology/American Heart Association Task Force on Practice Guidelines (ACC/AHA/ASE Committee to Update the 1997 Guidelines for the Clinical Application of Echocardiography). *J Am Coll Cardiol.* 2003;42(5):954-970.
3. Mihaljevic T, Paul S, Cohn LH, Wechsler A. Pathophysiology of aortic valve disease. In: Cohn LH, Edmunds LH, eds. *Cardiac Surgery in the Adult.* 2nd ed. New York: McGraw-Hill, Medical Pub Division; 2003:791-810.
4. Deck JD, Thubrikar MJ, Schneider PJ, Nolan SP. Structure, stress, and tissue repair in aortic valve leaflets. *Cardiovasc Res.* 1988;22(1):7-16.

5. Thubrikar M, Harry R, Nolan SP. Normal aortic valve function in dogs. *Am J Cardiol.* 1977;40(4):563-568.
6. Gnyaneshwar R, Kumar RK, Balakrishnan KR. Dynamic analysis of the aortic valve using a finite element model. *Ann Thorac Surg.* 2002;73(4):1122-1129.
7. Shanewise JS, Cheung AT, Aronson S, et al. ASE/SCA guidelines for performing a comprehensive intraoperative multiplane transesophageal echocardiography examination: recommendations of the American Society of Echocardiography Council for Intraoperative Echocardiography and the Society of Cardiovascular Anesthesiologists Task Force for Certification in Perioperative Transesophageal Echocardiography. *Anesth Analg.* 1999; 89(4):870-884.
8. Oh CC, Click RL, Orszulak TA, Sinak LJ, Oh JK. Role of intraoperative transesophageal echocardiography in determining aortic annulus diameter in homograft insertion. *J Am Soc Echocardiogr.* 1998;11(6):638-642.
9. Blumberg FC, Pfeifer M, Holmer SR, Kromer EP, Riegger GA, Elsner D. Transgastric Doppler echocardiographic assessment of the severity of aortic stenosis using multiplane transesophageal echocardiography. *Am J Cardiol.* 1997;79(9):1273-1275.
10. Stoddard MF, Hammons RT, Longaker RA. Doppler transesophageal echocardiographic determination of aortic valve area in adults with aortic stenosis. *Am Heart J.* 1996;132(2 Pt 1):337-342.
11. Baumgartner H, Hung J, Bermejo J, et al. Echocardiographic assessment of valve stenosis: EAE/ASE recommendations for clinical practice. *J Am Soc Echocardiogr.* 2009;22(1):1-23; quiz 101-102.
12. Roberts WC, Ko JM. Frequency by decades of unicuspid, bicuspid, and tricuspid aortic valves in adults having isolated aortic valve replacement for aortic stenosis, with or without associated aortic regurgitation. *Circulation.* 2005;111(7):920-925.
13. Peter M, Hoffmann A, Parker C, Luscher T, Burckhardt D. Progression of aortic stenosis. Role of age and concomitant coronary artery disease. *Chest.* 1993;103(6):1715-1719.
14. Bahler RC, Desser DR, Finkelhor RS, Brener SJ, Youssefi M. Factors leading to progression of valvular aortic stenosis. *Am J Cardiol.* 1999;84(9):1044-1048.
15. Palta S, Pai AM, Gill KS, Pai RG. New insights into the progression of aortic stenosis: implications for secondary prevention. *Circulation.* 2000;101(21):2497-2502.
16. Mohler ER 3rd. Are atherosclerotic processes involved in aortic-valve calcification? *Lancet.* 2000;356(9229):524-525.
17. Brown JM, O'Brien SM, Wu C, Sikora JA, Griffith BP, Gammie JS. Isolated aortic valve replacement in North America comprising 108,687 patients in 10 years: changes in risks, valve types, and outcomes in the Society of Thoracic Surgeons National Database. *J Thorac Cardiovasc Surg.* 2009;137(1):82-90.
18. Hoffman JI, Kaplan S. The incidence of congenital heart disease. *J Am Coll Cardiol.* 2002;39(12):1890-1900.
19. Hahn RT, Roman MJ, Mogtader AH, Devereux RB. Association of aortic dilation with regurgitant, stenotic and functionally normal bicuspid aortic valves. *J Am Coll Cardiol.* 1992;19(2):283-288.
20. Borger MA, Preston M, Ivanov J, et al. Should the ascending aorta be replaced more frequently in patients with bicuspid aortic valve disease? *J Thorac Cardiovasc Surg.* 2004; 128(5): 677-683.
21. Hoffmann R, Flachskampf FA, Hanrath P. Planimetry of orifice area in aortic stenosis using multiplane transesophageal echocardiography. *J Am Coll Cardiol.* 1993; 22(2): 529-534.
22. Bernard Y, Meneveau N, Vuillemenot A, et al. Planimetry of aortic valve area using multiplane transoesophageal echocardiography is not a reliable method for assessing severity of aortic stenosis. *Heart.* 1997;78(1):68-73.
23. Godley RW, Green D, Dillon JC, Rogers EW, Feigenbaum H, Weyman AE. Reliability of two-dimensional echocardiography in assessing the severity of valvular aortic stenosis. *Chest.* 1981;79(6):657-662.
24. Tarantini G, Buja P, Scognamiglio R, et al. Aortic valve replacement in severe aortic stenosis with left ventricular dysfunction: determinants of cardiac mortality and ventricular function recovery. *Eur J Cardiothorac Surg.* 2003;24(6):879-885.
25. Vaquette B, Corbineau H, Laurent M, et al. Valve replacement in patients with critical aortic stenosis and depressed left ventricular function: predictors of operative risk, left ventricular function recovery, and long term outcome. *Heart.* 2005;91 (10):1324-1329.
26. Powell DE, Tunick PA, Rosenzweig BP, et al. Aortic valve replacement in patients with aortic stenosis and severe left ventricular dysfunction. *Arch Intern Med.* 2000;160(9): 1337-1341.
27. Pereira JJ, Lauer MS, Bashir M, et al. Survival after aortic valve replacement for severe aortic stenosis with low transvalvular gradients and severe left ventricular dysfunction. *J Am Coll Cardiol.* 2002;39(8):1356-1363.
28. Monin JL, Quere JP, Monchi M, et al. Low-gradient aortic stenosis: operative risk stratification and predictors for long-term outcome: a multicenter study using dobutamine stress hemodynamics. *Circulation.* 2003;108(3):319-324.
29. Bermejo J, Yotti R. Low-gradient aortic valve stenosis: value and limitations of dobutamine stress testing. *Heart.* 2007; 93(3):298-302.
30. Bonow RO, Carabello BA, Chatterjee K, et al. ACC/AHA 2006 guidelines for the management of patients with valvular heart disease: a report of the American College of Cardiology/American Heart Association Task Force on Practice Guidelines (writing Committee to Revise the 1998 guidelines for the management of patients with valvular heart disease) developed in collaboration with the Society of Cardiovascular Anesthesiologists endorsed by the Society for Cardiovascular Angiography and Interventions and the Society of Thoracic Surgeons. *J Am Coll Cardiol.* 2006;48(3):e1-148.
31. Quinones MA, Otto CM, Stoddard M, Waggoner A, Zoghbi WA. Recommendations for quantification of Doppler echocardiography: a report from the Doppler Quantification Task Force of the Nomenclature and Standards Committee of the American Society of Echocardiography. *J Am Soc Echocardiogr.* 2002;15(2):167-184.
32. Maslow AD, Mashikian J, Haering JM, Heindel S, Douglas P, Levine R. Transesophageal echocardiographic evaluation of native aortic valve area: utility of the double-envelope technique. *J Cardiothorac Vasc Anesth.* 2001;15(3): 293-299.
33. Blumberg FC, Pfeifer M, Holmer SR, Kromer EP, Riegger GA, Elsner D. Quantification of aortic stenosis in mechanically ventilated patients using multiplane transesophageal Doppler echocardiography. *Chest.* 1998;114(1):94-97.

34. Hilbcrath JN, Shernan SK, Segal S, Smith B, Eltzschig HK. The feasibility of epicardial echocardiography for measuring aortic valve area by the continuity equation. *Anesth Analg* 2009;108(1):17-22.
35. Reeves ST, Glas KE, Eltzschig H, et al. Guidelines for performing a comprehensive epicardial echocardiography examination: recommendations of the American Society of Echocardiography and the Society of Cardiovascular Anesthesiologists. *Anesth Analg.* 2007;105(1):22-28.
36. Oh JK, Taliercio CP, Holmes DR Jr, et al. Prediction of the severity of aortic stenosis by Doppler aortic valve area determination: prospective Doppler-catheterization correlation in 100 patients. *J Am Coll Cardiol.* 1988;11(6):1227-1234.
37. El Khoury G, Glineur D, Rubay J, et al. Functional classification of aortic root/valve abnormalities and their correlation with etiologies and surgical procedures. *Curr Opin Cardiol.* 2005;20(2):115-121.
38. Carpentier A. Cardiac valve surgery—the "French correction". *J Thorac Cardiovasc Surg.* 1983;86(3):323-337.
39. Ozkan M, Ozdemir N, Kaymaz C, Kirma C, Deligonul U. Measurement of aortic valve anatomic regurgitant area using transesophageal echocardiography: implications for the quantitation of aortic regurgitation. *J Am Soc Echocardiogr.* 2002;15(10 Pt 2):1170-1174.
40. Zoghbi WA, Enriquez-Sarano M, Foster E, et al. Recommendations for evaluation of the severity of native valvular regurgitation with two-dimensional and Doppler echocardiography. *J Am Soc Echocardiogr.* 2003;16(7):777-802.
41. Tribouilloy CM, Enriquez-Sarano M, Bailey KR, Seward JB, Tajik AJ. Assessment of severity of aortic regurgitation using the width of the vena contracta: a clinical color Doppler imaging study. *Circulation* 2000;102(5):558-564.
42. Grayburn PA, Handshoe R, Smith MD, Harrison MR, DeMaria AN. Quantitative assessment of the hemodynamic consequences of aortic regurgitation by means of continuous wave Doppler recordings. *J Am Coll Cardiol.* 1987;10(1):135-141.
43. Sutton DC, Kluger R, Ahmed SU, Reimold SC, Mark JB. Flow reversal in the descending aorta: a guide to intraoperative assessment of aortic regurgitation with transesophageal echocardiography. *J Thorac Cardiovasc Surg.* 1994;108(3):576-582.
44. Takenaka K, Sakamoto T, Dabestani A, Gardin JM, Henry WL. [Pulsed Doppler echocardiographic detection of regurgitant blood flow in the ascending, descending and abdominal aorta of patients with aortic regurgitation]. *J Cardiol.* 1987;17(2):301-309.
45. Khaw AV, von Bardeleben RS, Strasser C, et al. Direct measurement of left ventricular outflow tract by transthoracic real-time 3D-echocardiography increases accuracy in assessment of aortic valve stenosis. *Int J Cardiol.* 2009;136(1):64-71.
46. Armen TA, Vandse R, Bickle K, Nathan N. Three-dimensional echocardiographic evaluation of an incidental quadricuspid aortic valve. *Eur J Echocardiogr.* 2008;9(2):318-320.
47. Boodhwani M, de Kerchove L, Glineur D, et al. Repair-oriented classification of aortic insufficiency: impact on surgical techniques and clinical outcomes. *J Thorac Cardiovasc Surg.* 2009; 137(2):286-294.
48. Faber CN, Smedira NG. Surgical considerations in aortic valve surgery. In: Savage RM, Aronson S, eds. *Comprehensive Textbook of Intraoperative Transesophageal Echocardiography.* Philadelphia: Lippincott Williams and Wilkins; 2005:537.
49. Grimm RA, Stewart WJ. The role of intraoperative echocardiography in valve surgery. *Cardiol Clin.* 1998;16(3):477-489.

REVIEW QUESTIONS

Select the *one* best answer for each of the following questions.

1. The recommended transesophageal views of the aortic valve include which of the following:
   a. ME AV SAX
   b. ME AV LAX
   c. TG LAX
   d. Deep TG
   e. All of the above

2. Regarding the use of Doppler techniques in the evaluation of the aortic valve, which of the following is true?
   a. The evaluation is limited only for the ME AV SAX view as the Doppler cursor is perpendicular to the aortic valve.
   b. The evaluation is limited for the ME AV LAX view as the Doppler cursor is parallel to the aortic valve.
   c. The evaluation is limited for the TG LAX view as the Doppler cursor is perpendicular to the aortic valve.
   d. The evaluation is limited for both the ME AV SAX and ME AV LAX views as the Doppler cursor is perpendicular to the aortic valve.
   e. No limitations are encountered in any of the views.

3. The preferred views to measure velocities in the LVOT and through the aortic valve include which of the following:
   a. ME AV SAX and deep TG
   b. ME AV LAX and ME AV SAX
   c. TG LAX and ME AV LAX
   d. TG LAX and deep TG LAX

4. The most common site of obstruction from the LVOT to the ascending aorta is:
   a. Subvalvular
   b. Valvular
   c. Supravalvular
   d. Dynamic

5. The most frequent type of aortic stenosis in the United States is:
   a. Calcific
   b. Bicuspid
   c. Rheumatic
   d. Congenital

6. In a 40-year-old male who presents with aortic stenosis for an aortic valve replacement, the most likely diagnosis is:
   a. Fixed subvalvular obstruction
   b. Dynamic subaortic obstruction
   c. Supravalvular stenosis
   d. Bicuspid aortic valve

7. Aortic abnormalities associated with bicuspid aortic valves include which of the following:
   a. Coarctation of the aorta
   b. Aortic aneurysms
   c. Aortic dissections
   d. All of the above

8. In patients with bicuspid aortic valves, replacement should be considered when the aortic root diameter exceeds:
   a. 3.5 cm
   b. 4.5 cm
   c. 5.5 cm
   d. 6.5 cm

9 The normal aortic valve area is:
   a. 2 to 3 cm^2
   b. 3 to 4 cm^2
   c. 4 to 5 cm^2
   d. 5 to 6 cm^2

10. Which of the following methods in the evaluation of aortic stenosis is recommended in all patients?
   a. Velocity ratio
   b. Peak transaortic gradient
   c. Aortic valve area by continuity equation
   d. Planimetry

11. Which of the following methods in the evaluation of aortic stenosis is recommended when additional information is needed?
   a. Velocity ratio
   b. Mean transaortic gradient
   c. Aortic valve area by continuity equation
   d. AS jet velocity

12. In contrast to the continuity equation, the simplified continuity equation utilizes which of the following velocity measurements?
   a. VTI.
   b. V_{max}.
   c. V_{mean}.
   d. Both utilize the same velocity measurement.

13. Which is the simplified Bernoulli equation?
   a. $\Delta P = 4\,V_2^2$
   b. $\Delta P = 2\,V_2^2$
   c. $\Delta P = 4\,(V_2^2 - V_1^2)$
   d. $\Delta P = 2\,(V_2^2 - V_1^2)$

14. Which is the modified Bernoulli equation?
   a. $\Delta P = 4\,V_2^2$
   b. $\Delta P = 2\,V_2^2$
   c. $\Delta P = 4\,(V_2^2 - V_1^2)$
   d. $\Delta P = 2\,(V_2^2 - V_1^2)$

15. The velocity in the LVOT (V_1) exceeds 1.5 m/s in which of the following conditions?
   a. Aortic stenosis
   b. Volume depletion
   c. High output states
   d. Mitral stenosis

16. Which of the following statements is true?
   a. Mean gradient is superior to peak gradient as mean gradients are derived by averaging the instantaneous gradient over the entire ejection period.
   b. Mean gradient is inferior to peak gradient as mean gradients are derived by averaging the instantaneous gradient over the entire ejection period.
   c. Peak gradient is superior to mean gradient as mean gradients are derived by averaging the instantaneous gradient over the entire ejection period.
   d. Peak gradient is inferior to mean gradient as peak gradients are derived by averaging the instantaneous gradient over the entire ejection period.

17. Which of the following statements is true?
   a. Gradients obtained in the cardiac catheterization lab tend to be higher than echocardiographic-obtained gradients.
   b. Gradients obtained in the cardiac catheterization lab tend to be lower than echocardiographic-obtained gradients.
   c. Gradients obtained in the cardiac catheterization lab are equal to echocardiographic-obtained gradients.
   d. Gradients obtained by echocardiography are peak-to-peak gradients.

18. Which of the following statements is true?
   a. Gradients obtained by echocardiography are peak-to-peak gradients.
   b. Gradients obtained in the cardiac catheterization lab are peak-instantaneous gradients.

c. Gradients obtained by echocardiography are mean-instantaneous gradients.
d. Gradients obtained by echocardiography are peak-instantaneous gradients.

19. Which of the following statements is true regarding aortic valve gradients?
a. They are independent of flow.
b. They tend to decrease with sepsis and severe aortic insufficiency.
c. They tend to increase with severe mitral regurgitation and severe mitral stenosis.
d. They tend to increase in hyperthyroidism and decrease in left to right shunt.

20. Which of the following is most helpful in determining the site of obstruction in the ME AV LAX view?
a. Combining 2D imaging and pulsed-wave Doppler
b. Combining 2D imaging and color-flow Doppler
c. Combining 2D imaging and continuous-wave Doppler
d. Combining 2D imaging and tissue Doppler

21. Which of the following is true regarding the spectral doppler evaluation in dynamic subvalvular aortic obstruction?
a. A rounded, mid-systolic wave is seen.
b. A rounded, late-systolic wave is seen.
c. A dagger-shaped, early-systolic wave is seen.
d. A dagger-shaped, late-systolic wave is seen.

22. To differentiate mitral regurgitation from aortic stenosis on the spectral display when using the deep TG view:
a. The AS jet spans systole, while the MR jet begins later in systole.
b. The AS jet spans systole, while the MR jet appears early in systole.
c. The MR jet spans systole, while the AS jet begins later in systole.
d. The MR jet begins later in systole, while the AS jet appears early in systole.

23. Which of the following statements regarding the continuity equation is true?
a. It is based on the concept of velocity acceleration.
b. The greatest source of error in the continuity equation arises from the measurement of the cross-sectional area (CSA) of the LVOT.
c. The greatest source of error in the continuity equation arises from the measurement of the peak velocity in the LVOT.
d. The following three variables are needed: CSA_{LVOT}, peak $velocity_{LVOT}$, and peak $velocity_{aortic\ valve}$

24. If the LVOT diameter is 2.0 cm, the LVOT cross-sectional area is:
a. 2.0 cm^2
b. 3.14 cm^2
c. 6.28 cm^2
d. 12.56 cm^2

25. Which of the following statements regarding normal peak velocities in the LVOT is correct?
a. Normal peak velocity is 0.8 to 1.5 m/s.
b. Normal peak velocity should be less than 1.0 m/s when using the simplified Bernoulli equation.
c. LVOT velocity should be measured with continuous-wave Doppler.
d. LVOT velocity should be measured in the ME LAX.

26. Assuming the LVOT is circular, the formula for the calculation of the LVOT area is:
a. LVOT Area = $\pi \times d$
b. LVOT Area = $\pi \times d^2$
c. LVOT Area = $2 \pi \times r^2$
d. LVOT Area = $\pi \times r^2$

27. Which of the following statements regarding the measurement of velocities is correct?
a. The intercept angle between blood flow and the Doppler beam should be more than 20°.
b. The Doppler shift is directly proportional to the transmitted frequency.
c. The maximal measurable velocity increases as θ increases.
d. The Doppler shift is independent of the angle of beam incidence.

28. Velocity ratio or dimensionless index is:
a. A ratio of LVOT VTI to aortic valve VTI
b. A ratio of aortic valve VTI to LVOT VTI
c. Obtained with pulsed-wave Doppler
d. Obtained from the ME LAX view

29. Severe aortic stenosis is defined with a velocity ratio of:
a. 0.4
b. 0.35
c. 0.3
d. 0.24

30. Severe aortic stenosis is defined when:
    a. Peak velocity exceeds 3.0 m/s.
    b. Mean gradient exceeds 40 mm Hg.
    c. Valve area is less than 1.0 cm^2.
    d. Peak instantaneous pressure gradient is 40 mm Hg.

31. Which of the following statements is true regarding the El Khoury classification of aortic insufficiency?
    a. Type I AI is associated with normal aortic leaflet mobility.
    b. Type II AI is due to leaflet restriction.
    c. Type III AI is due to leaflet prolapse.
    d. Type IV AI is due to dilatation of the ventriculoaortic junction.

32. Which of the following statements is true regarding type I aortic insufficiency in the El Khoury classification?
    a. Type Ia results from dilatation of the ventriculoaortic junction.
    b. Type Ib results from sinotubular junction enlargement and dilatation of the ascending aorta.
    c. Type Ic results from dilatation of the sinuses of Valsalva and the sinotubular junction.
    d. Type Id results from cusp perforation without a primary functional aortic annular lesion.

33. Which of the following statements is true?
    a. Vena contracta width greater than 6.0 mm is indicative of severe aortic insufficiency.
    b. Vena contracta width is a load-dependent measure.
    c. A jet width/LVOT width ratio greater than 0.5 is indicative of severe aortic insufficiency.
    d. Effective regurgitant orifice area (EROA) of 0.2 cm^2 is indicative of severe aortic insufficiency.

34. Which of the following is consistent with severe acute aortic insufficiency?
    a. A pressure half-time less than 300 milliseconds
    b. A pressure half-time less than 350 milliseconds
    c. A pressure half-time less than 200 milliseconds
    d. A pressure half-time less than 250 milliseconds

35. Which of the following is consistent with severe acute aortic insufficiency?
    a. A deceleration slope greater than 1.5 m/s^2
    b. A deceleration slope greater than 2 m/s^2
    c. A deceleration slope greater than 2.5 m/s^2
    d. A deceleration slope greater than 3 m/s^2

36. In patients with mitral stenosis and aortic insufficiency, calculation of mitral valve area by pressure half-time will tend to:
    a. Underestimate the severity of mitral stenosis when using pressure half- time.
    b. Overestimate the severity of mitral stenosis when using pressure half-time.
    c. The presence of aortic insufficiency does not affect the estimation of mitral stenosis.
    d. The deceleration time should be used in this setting.

37. In patients with mitral stenosis and aortic insufficiency, calculation of mitral valve area when using the formula MVA = PHT/220 will tend to:
    a. Underestimate the mitral valve area.
    b. Overestimate the mitral valve area.
    c. The estimation is accurate.
    d. Overestimate the severity of mitral stenosis.

38. Which of the following is most suggestive of severe aortic regurgitation?
    a. Vena contracta (cm) = 0.4
    b. Regurgitant volume (cc/beat) = 62
    c. Regurgitant fraction (%) = 45
    d. Regurgitant orifice area (cm^2) = 0.2

39. Aortic valve replacement rather than repair should be considered for:
    a. Type Ia lesions
    b. Type Ib lesions
    c. Type II lesions
    d. Type III lesions

40. Which of the following helps differentiate between LVOT obstruction and aortic stenosis?
    a. Aortic stenosis creates a larger pressure gradient between the LV and the aorta.
    b. LVOT obstruction is influenced by loading conditions.
    c. Systolic anterior motion of the anterior mitral leaflet is seen in aortic stenosis.
    d. The obstruction in aortic stenosis is dynamic.

41. Which of the following is an indirect echocardiographic sign of aortic valve regurgitation?
    a. Late closure of the mitral valve
    b. Left ventricle dyskinesis
    c. Apparent hypokinesis of the left ventricle
    d. Fluttering of the mitral valve leaflets
    e. Abnormal pattern of mitral inflow demonstrating an increased deceleration time and a decreased E/A ratio

42. This continuous wave Doppler spectrum of the aortic valve corresponds to which of the following clinical conditions:

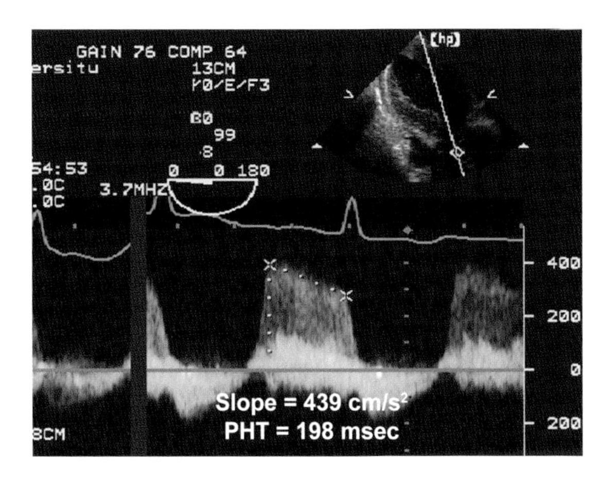

a. Mild aortic regurgitation
b. Moderate aortic regurgitation
c. Severe aortic regurgitation
d. Mild aortic stenosis
e. Moderate aortic stenosis

43. Which of the following regarding the anatomy of the aortic valve is true?
a. Each leaflet attaches to the aortic wall in a curvilinear fashion beginning at one commissure and ending at another, after descending approximately 1 cm from the midpoint.
b. There is a significant leaflet overlap above the line of coaptation, which creates a zone of redundancy called the "the zone of Arantius."
c. At the center of each leaflet, there is a nodule of Valsalva; this nodule is important in maintaining diastolic competence.
d. The noncoronary cusp of the aortic valve is located laterally.

44. Identify the cusps in this short-axis view of the aortic valve (RCC, right coronary cusp; LCC, left coronary cusp; NCC, noncoronary cusp):
a. 1 = RCC, 2 = NCC, 3 = LCC
b. 1 = RCC, 2 = LCC, 3 = NCC
c. 1 = LCC, 2 = NCC, 3 = RCC
d. 1 = NCC, 2 = RCC, 3 = LCC
e. 1 = LCC, 2 = RCC, 3 = NCC

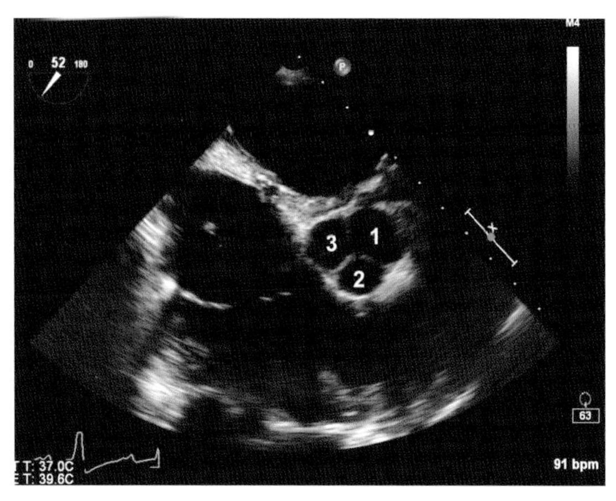

45. The cusp pointed to by the arrow is:

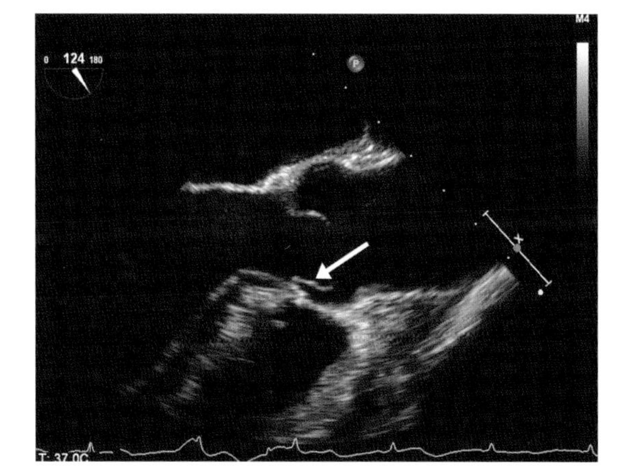

a. Anterior
b. Posterior
c. Noncoronary
d. Right coronary
e. Left coronary

Tricuspid and Pulmonic Valves 10

George V. Moukarbel and Antoine B. Abchee

A detailed transesophageal echocardiographic (TEE) examination of the right-sided heart valves can provide accurate diagnosis of valvular diseases; define anatomic, functional, and perivalvular abnormalities; and guide appropriate management. Integration of this information with the evaluation of the cardiac chambers is necessary to assess the degree of the pathology and determine its impact on cardiac function. In a review of 1918 cases undergoing intraoperative TEE prior to cardiac surgery, discrepant findings at the time of surgical inspection were present in only 48 patients, of which five involved the tricuspid and pulmonic valves.[1] Therefore, this modality should yield adequate diagnostic accuracy when the exam is conducted appropriately. This chapter discusses the main pathologies involving the tricuspid and pulmonic valves leading to regurgitation and/or stenosis, and their assessment by two-dimensional TEE (Table 10–1). Even with the advent of three-dimensional matrix array probes allowing the acquisition of real-time images, optimal visualization of the tricuspid and pulmonary valves is seldom feasible[2]; therefore, their three-dimensional evaluation will depend on future improvements of this technology.

TRICUSPID VALVE

Relevant Anatomical Landmarks

The tricuspid valve, the largest of the four cardiac valves, lies slightly below the plane of the mitral valve, and is in close proximity to the aortic valve. The three leaflets of the tricuspid valve are named anterior, posterior (inferior), and septal (medial) based on their relative positions (Figure 10–1). The septal leaflet's insertion point at the septum is more apically displaced than that of the anterior mitral leaflet. The two major papillary muscles, the anterior and posterior, are located on the corresponding walls of the right ventricle. Through their chordae tendineae, they attach to the anterior and posterior cusps, and the posterior and septal cusps, respectively. When present, a smaller septal papillary muscle attaches to the septal and anterior cusps.[3] The three leaflets of the valve can be imaged using different angulations of the imaging plane together with flexion of the probe tip (see Figure 10–1).

Tomographic Views

Midesophageal Four-Chamber View

From the midesophageal four-chamber view, rightward rotation of the probe can help position the tricuspid valve in the center of the image. This view will show the septal leaflet to the right of the display and the nonseptal (anterior or posterior) leaflet to the left of the display, depending on the amount of anteflexion or retroflexion of the probe (Figure 10–2).

Midesophageal Right Ventricular Inflow-Outflow View

Starting from the midesophageal four-chamber view, rotating the angle forward to approximately 60° will yield a cross-sectional view of the aortic valve, with a transverse section of the right ventricular inflow and outflow tracts. Slight turning of the probe to the right might be needed for better visualization of the structures. In this view, the anterior leaflet of the tricuspid valve is seen next to the aortic valve. The posterior leaflet of the tricuspid valve is seen to the left of the display attached to the right ventricular wall (Figure 10–3).

Transgastric Right Ventricular Inflow View

Turning the probe to the right in the transgastric short-axis view of the left ventricle will bring the right ventricle to the center of the display. A long-axis view of the right ventricle is then obtained by rotating the multiplane angle to about 120°. The chordae tendineae and papillary muscles are well seen, since they are perpendicular to the ultrasound beam. In this view, the posterior leaflet of the tricuspid valve is visualized in the near field, attached to the inferior wall, while the anterior leaflet is located in the far field, attached to the anterior wall of the right ventricle (Figure 10–4).

Transgastric Tricuspid Short-Axis View

Starting from the transgastric right ventricular inflow view, the tricuspid annulus is centered in the image by slightly withdrawing the probe. Rotating the angle back to about 30° will generate a short-axis view of the tricuspid valve. The septal leaflet is visualized to the right of the display. The anterior and posterior leaflets are seen in the left-sided far and near fields, respectively (Figure 10–5).

Table 10–1. Conditions causing tricuspid and pulmonic valve dysfunction

	Tricuspid Valve		Pulmonic Valve	
	Regurgitation	Stenosis	Regurgitation	Stenosis
Congenital				
Predominant leaflet problem				
Prolapse	+			
Congenital stenosis		+		+
Ebstein anomaly	+			
Dysplasia	+	+	+	+
Cleft leaflet	+			
Predominant annulus problem				
Marfan syndrome	+		+	
Acquired				
Predominant leaflet problem				
Endocarditis	+	+	+	+
Rheumatic heart disease	+	+	+	+
Carcinoid heart disease	+	+	+	+
Hypereosinophilic syndrome	+	+		
Radiation therapy	+	+		
Drugs (Fen-Phen, methysergide)	+	+/–		
Predominant annulus problem				
Pulmonary hypertension	+		+	
Other				
Trauma	+		+	
Right ventricular infarction	+			
Tumor (eg, myxoma)	+	+		

TRICUSPID REGURGITATION

Common Causes

Trivial or very mild degrees of tricuspid regurgitation can frequently be present in normal individuals, and in the absence of abnormalities of the valvular structures or cardiac chambers, it should be regarded as a normal variant. Pathologic tricuspid regurgitation can be either congenital or acquired. Ebstein's anomaly is one of the important causes of congenital tricuspid regurgitation, and echocardiography plays a major role in the diagnosis and surgical planning. More commonly, however, tricuspid regurgitation is the result of right ventricular dilatation and/or dysfunction secondary to pulmonary hypertension or right ventricular infarction. Rheumatic heart disease (less frequently encountered in developed countries) and carcinoid heart disease result in thickening, restricted mobility, and/or malcoaptation of the leaflets, leading to incompetence of the valve. In patients with endocarditis, vegetations that tend to form on the atrial surface of the leaflets can lead to destruction of the leaflets and/or chordae, causing significant degrees of regurgitation in advanced cases. Annular dilatation can be seen in some cases of Marfan's syndrome, and tricuspid valve prolapse with or without associated mitral valve prolapse is another cause of tricuspid regurgitation. Occasionally, tumors such as right atrial myxomas can interfere with the normal coaptation of the leaflets, therefore causing regurgitation.

Two-Dimensional Evaluation

Two-dimensional examination of the tricuspid valve apparatus provides significant information regarding the underlying cause and mechanism of tricuspid regurgitation. The identification of anatomic abnormalities (eg, Ebstein's anomaly), abnormal masses, annular dilatation, and noncoaptation (see Figure 10–3) are all essential to make a correct diagnosis. Pacemaker wires or catheters passing through the tricuspid orifice are

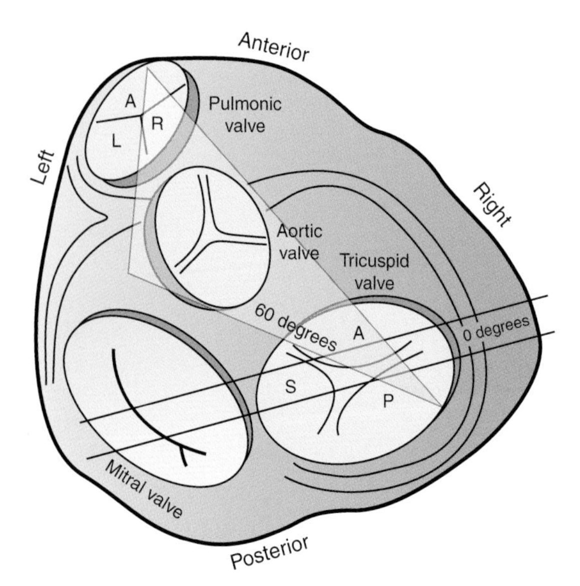

FIGURE 10–1. Schematic diagram of the heart that shows the spatial relationships of the valves. Note that the aortic valve plane is almost perpendicular to that of the pulmonic valve, so that when the imaging plane is along the short axis of the aortic valve (imaging at 60°, *shaded triangle*), the pulmonic valve is imaged in its long axis. When imaging at 0° to obtain the four-chamber view *(solid straight lines)*, anteflexion and retroflexion will move the imaging plane anteriorly and posteriorly to allow imaging of the anterior and posterior leaflets of the tricuspid valve, respectively. (A, anterior; P, posterior; S, septal; L, left; R, right.)

readily visualized (Figure 10–6), and although uncommonly encountered with the right-sided valves,[4] TEE is highly sensitive for the detection of vegetations.[5] Movement of any of the leaflets beyond the plane of the tricuspid annulus inside the right atrium indicates the presence of tricuspid prolapse (Figure 10–7).[6] Additionally, in patients with tricuspid valve prolapse, the leaflets and chordae are usually redundant and myxomatous. Features characteristic of Ebstein's anomaly include apical displacement or "off-setting" of the hinge point attachment of the septal leaflet relative to that of the anterior mitral leaflet. A displacement index is easily produced by measuring the distance between the two hinge points and indexing to body surface area. This can be done in the midesophageal four-chamber view, and different angulations of the probe will help obtain the maximal difference. An indexed value greater than 8 mm/m squared[7,8] or a nonindexed value of greater than 15 mm in children and 20 mm in adults,[9] together with elongation of the anterior leaflet (the so-called "sail-like" or "curtain-like" appearance),[10,11] tethering, and restricted leaflet motion,[7] distinguish this congenital anomaly from other causes of tricuspid regurgitation. Additional echocardiographic features of Ebstein's anomaly include apical displacement of the other leaflets, absence or fenestration of any of the leaflets, and "atrialization" of a part of the right ventricle.

Carcinoid heart disease in patients with carcinoid syndrome results from fibrous deposits on the endocardium of the right-sided valves and chambers. This leads to thickening and rigidity of the leaflets, with the valves fixed in an open position, and associated stenosis is common. Involvement of the left-sided valves should

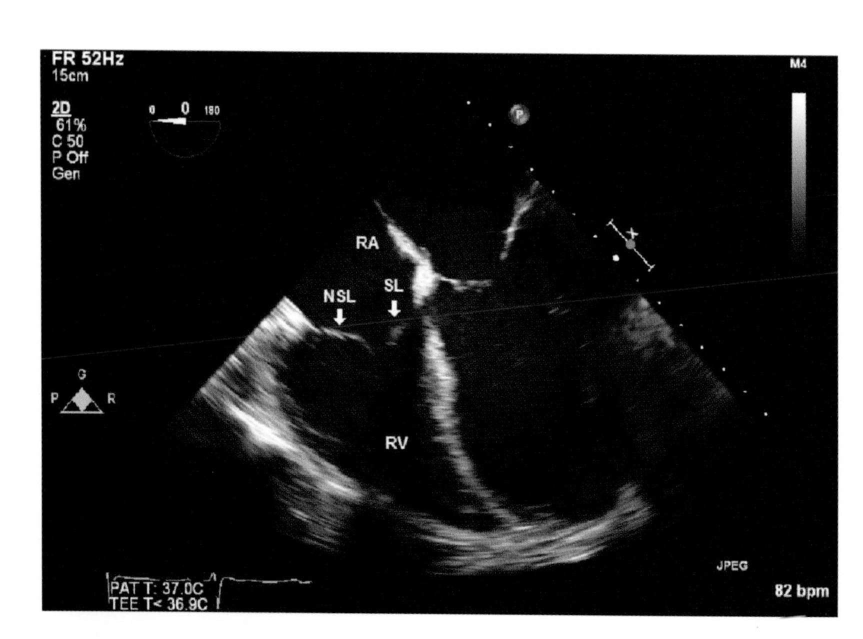

FIGURE 10–2. Midesophageal four-chamber view showing the septal and nonseptal leaflets of the tricuspid valve. The degree of anteflexion or retroflexion determines if the anterior or posterior leaflet is imaged. (NSL, nonseptal leaflet; SL, septal leaflet; RA, right atrium; RV, right ventricle.)

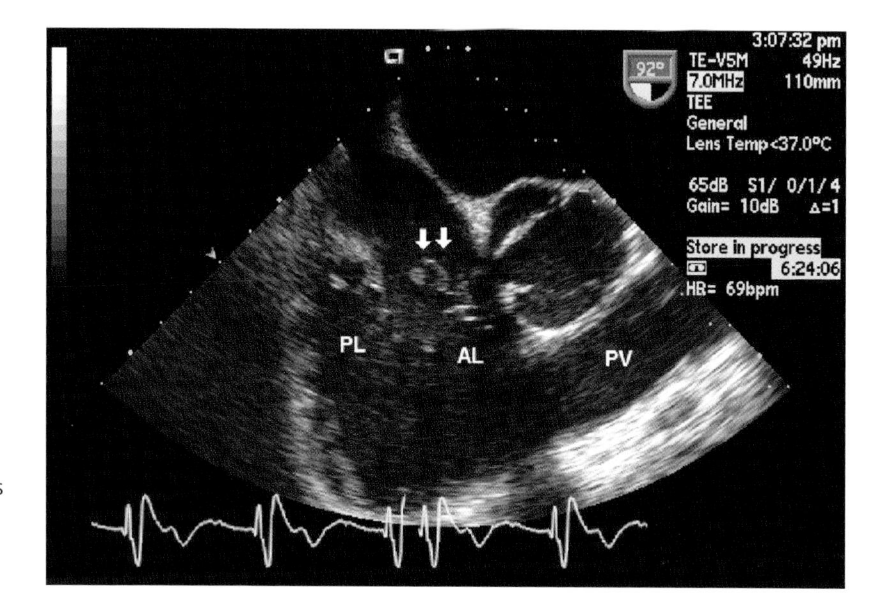

FIGURE 10–3. Midesophageal right ventricular inflow-outflow view. In this patient, a flail septal leaflet is seen *(double arrows)*. (AL, anterior leaflet; PL, posterior leaflet; PV, pulmonic valve.)

prompt a careful evaluation for right-to-left shunting.[12] Thickening, shortening, and restricted mobility of the leaflets are all characteristics of rheumatic involvement of the valve. The presence of malcoaptation of the leaflets usually indicates severe regurgitation, as does a large tricuspid annulus (>2.1 cm/m^2 of body surface area).[13] Although measurement of the tricuspid annulus should be performed in multiple views during diastole, using the frame that shows maximal distance between the insertion points of the leaflets, the measurement from the transgastric right ventricular (RV) inflow view correlates best with surgical measures.[14] Moreover, the dimensions of the right-sided chambers can provide clues to the severity of regurgitation. In contrast to mild regurgitation, chronic moderate and severe tricuspid regurgitation are usually associated with a dilated right atrium and ventricle. This is, however, not true in cases of acute moderate or severe tricuspid regurgitation where the chambers do not have time to remodel.

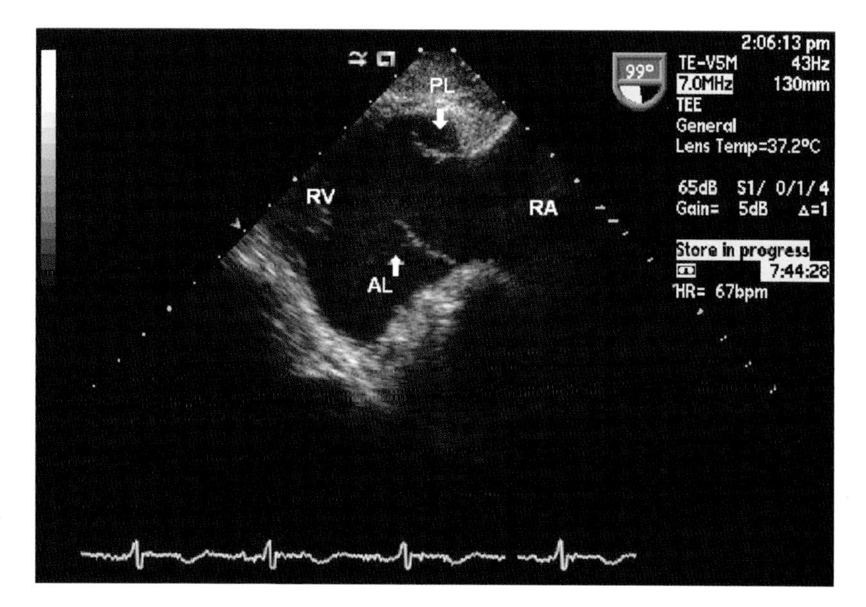

FIGURE 10–4. Transgastric right ventricular inflow view. (AL, anterior leaflet; PL, posterior leaflet; RA, right atrium; RV, right ventricle.)

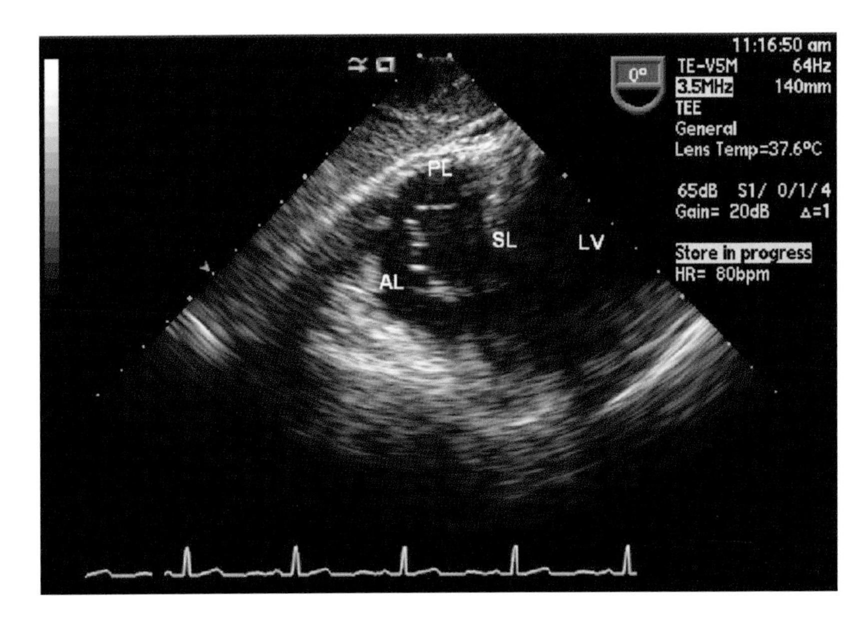

FIGURE 10–5. Transgastric short-axis view showing all three leaflets of the tricuspid valve. (AL, anterior leaflet; SL, septal leaflet; PL, posterior leaflet; LV, left ventricle.)

Doppler Evaluation

Color Doppler mapping can detect and provide a degree of quantification of the severity of tricuspid regurgitation. When applied, the multiplane angle should be changed and the probe tip manipulated in order to demonstrate the largest possible jet of regurgitation (Figure 10–8). Doppler principles similar to those used in the assessment of mitral regurgitation can be used to assess tricuspid regurgitation (Table 10–2). Measuring the vena contracta, which is the narrowest portion of the jet at the orifice of the valve, is easy to perform in the midesophageal four-chamber view; the cutoff for severe regurgitation is considered to be 7 mm.[15,16] In centrally directed regurgitation, measurement of the jet area can be helpful; an area of greater than 10 cm^2 is indicative of severe insufficiency.[16] Doppler parameters that indicate increased severity of tricuspid regurgitation include a tricuspid inflow velocity higher than 1 m/s, and a dense, triangular, and early-peaking continuous-wave (CW) Doppler signal of the tricuspid valve. The proximal isovelocity surface area (PISA) method can be applied for more quantitative assessment (Figure 10–9). A simplified approach has been suggested, whereby measuring the PISA radius at a Nyquist limit of about 28 cm/s can provide an estimate of the severity of the regurgitation; a radius of 5 mm or less usually identifies mild degrees, and a radius greater than 9 mm is found in severe cases.[16]

In addition, severe tricuspid regurgitation is associated with systolic flow reversal in the hepatic veins and/or the coronary sinus, similar to what is seen in the pulmonary veins in the case of severe mitral regurgitation.

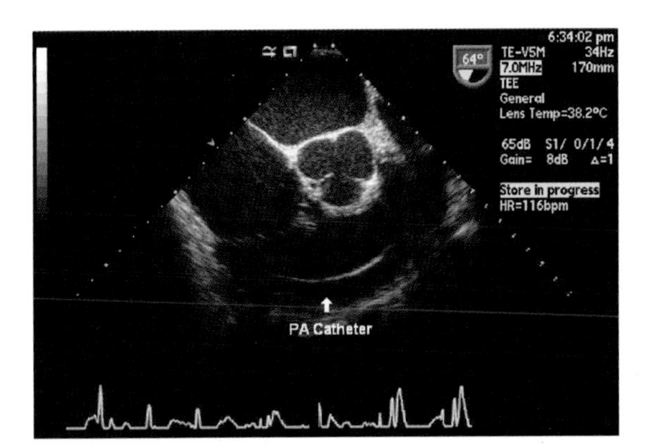

FIGURE 10–6. Midesophageal right ventricular inflow-outflow view showing a pulmonary artery catheter crossing the tricuspid valve and coursing through the outflow tract. (PA, pulmonary artery.)

Hepatic Venous Flow Patterns

Imaging of the hepatic veins can be performed from the stomach by withdrawing the probe and rotating it to the right to visualize liver parenchyma in the transverse plane. The hepatic veins can be identified with the help of color Doppler (Figure 10–10) at a reduced Nyquist limit (<40 cm/s). Pulsed-wave (PW) Doppler is used to assess flow patterns in the largest hepatic vein identified. A normal flow pattern consists of larger systolic and smaller diastolic forward-flow waves. In addition, two

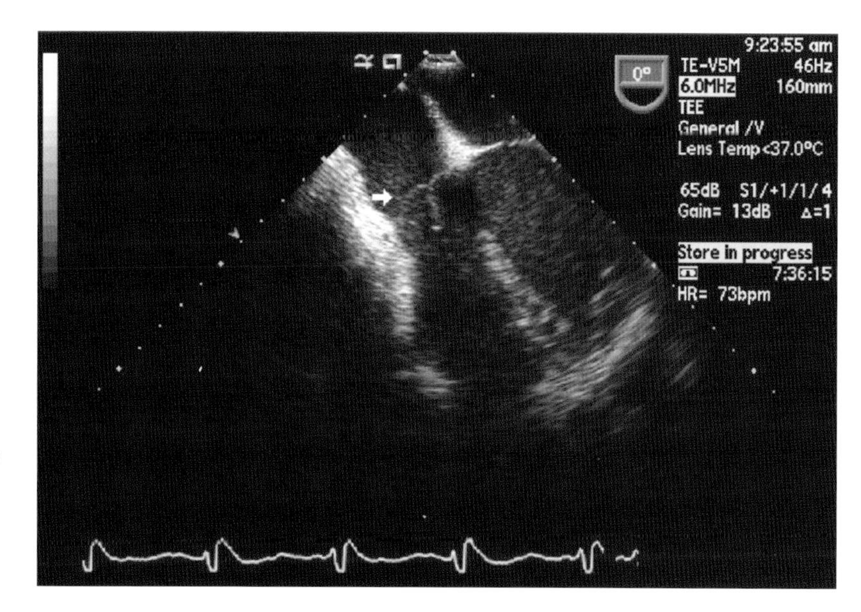

FIGURE 10–7. Midesophageal four-chamber view of a patient with Marfan syndrome showing mild prolapse of the tricuspid leaflets *(arrow)*.

flow-reversal waves may be noted: one in late diastole (which is the result of atrial contraction) and another in late systole. A blunted or reversed systolic wave is seen in patients with severe tricuspid regurgitation.[17] Patients with elevated right atrial pressures or atrial fibrillation can exhibit blunting of the systolic wave.

CORONARY SINUS FLOW PATTERNS

PW Doppler sampling of the coronary sinus flow is best performed in the transverse view of the coronary sinus, obtained from the midesophageal four-chamber view by advancing the probe slightly and retroflexing it. This will visualize the coronary sinus in its long axis in the atrioventricular groove (Figure 10–11). In normal individuals with absent or mild degrees of tricuspid regurgitation, two negative waves are noted: a late systolic wave and a diastolic wave with higher velocity and longer duration. When severe tricuspid regurgitation is present, reversal of the systolic wave is seen. This finding has a high sensitivity and a good specificity for the detection of severe tricuspid regurgitation.[18]

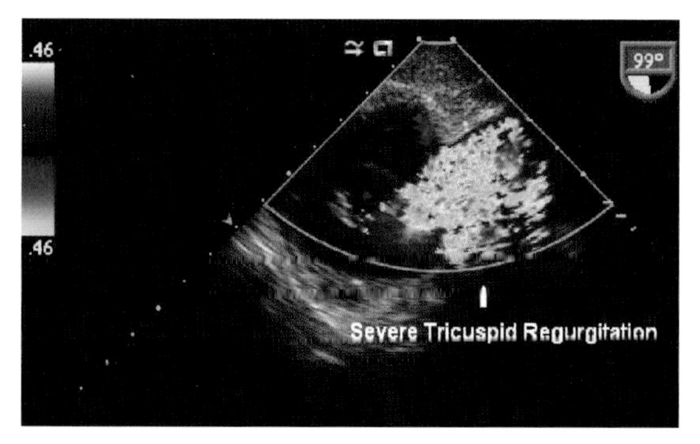

FIGURE 10–8. Transgastric right ventricular inflow view showing severe tricuspid regurgitation.

ESTIMATION OF SYSTOLIC PULMONARY ARTERY PRESSURE

Using CW Doppler, measurement of the peak tricuspid regurgitation jet velocity can be performed. Usually, the midesophageal right ventricular inflow-outflow view provides good alignment of the regurgitation jet with the Doppler signal. Localization of the jet is assisted by color Doppler flow mapping, and angulation of the probe with adjustment of the multiplane angle should be performed in order to identify the maximal velocity jet (Figure 10–12). Based on the simplified Bernoulli equation, the pressure gradient between the right ventricle and atrium is given by:

$$\text{Pressure Gradient (mm Hg)} = 4 \times [\text{Peak Regurgitant Velocity (m/s)}]^2$$

When added to an estimate of the right atrial pressure, this gradient provides an approximation of the right ventricular systolic pressure, which in the absence of right ventricular outflow obstruction is equivalent to the systolic pulmonary artery pressure. Right atrial pressure

Table 10–2. Echocardiographic findings in tricuspid regurgitation

	Regurgitation Severity		
	Mild	**Moderate**	**Severe**
Two-dimensional findings			
Leaflet morphology	Usually normal	Can be normal	Abnormal
Leaflet coaptation	Normal		Malcoaptation ± flail
Right-side chambers	Usually normal	Can be normal	Dilated (unless acute)
Tricuspid annulus diameter			>2.1 cm/m^2
Doppler findings			
Area of the jet (cm^2)[a,b]	<5	5-10	>10
Vena contracta width (mm)[b]			>7
PISA radius (mm)[c]	≤5	6-9	>9
CW Doppler signal	Soft and parabolic	Dense, variable contour	Dense, triangular with early peaking
Coronary sinus flow	Forward in systole		Systolic reversal
Hepatic venous flow	Systolic dominance	Systolic blunting	Systolic reversal

[a]Cannot be applied to eccentric jets.
[b]At a Nyquist limit of 50 to 60 cm/s.
[c]At a Nyquist limit of 28 cm/s.
CW, continuous-wave; PISA, proximal isovelocity surface area.

is commonly assessed by examining the respirophasic changes in the diameter of the inferior vena cava (IVC) (Figure 10–13). A greater than 50% change in the diameter of the IVC with inspiration indicates a right atrial pressure of less than 10 mm Hg, while a less marked change is associated with a pressure that is above 10 mm Hg.[19] This, however, is not reliable in patients on mechanical ventilation, or in those who do not mount a good inspiratory effort. In these patients, right atrial pressure can be assessed by examining the

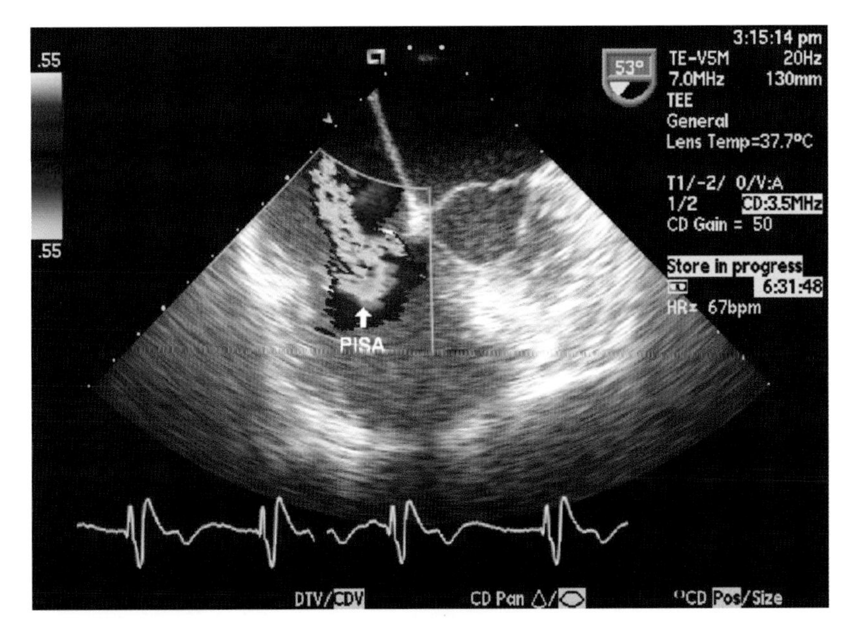

FIGURE 10–9. Modified midesophageal view showing flow acceleration and the proximal isovelocity surface area (PISA) contour.

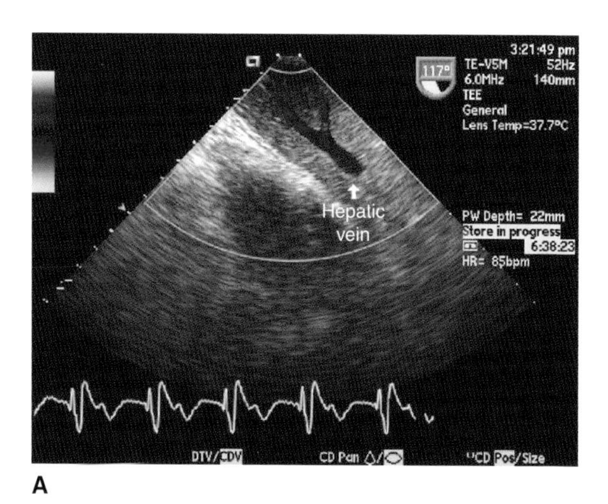

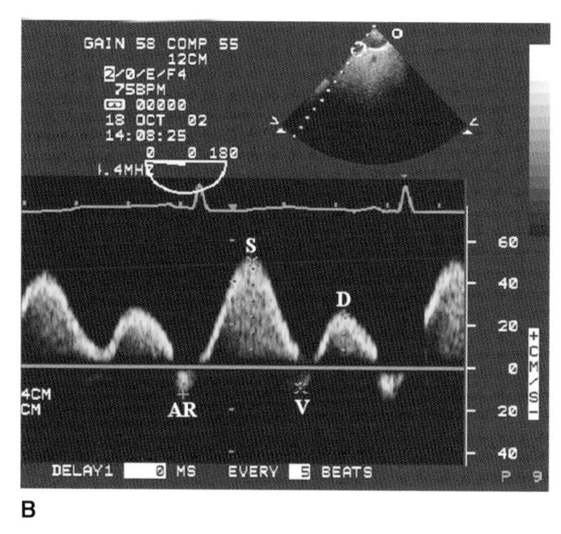

FIGURE 10–10. Color Doppler visualization of hepatic venous flow **(A)**. Normal hepatic vein Doppler profile **(B)** characterized by a small reversal of flow after atrial contraction (AR wave), an antegrade systolic phase during atrial filling from the superior and inferior vena cavae (S wave), a second small flow reversal at end-systole (V wave), and a second antegrade diastolic filling phase (D wave).

PW Doppler pattern of the hepatic veins, based on the following formula[20]:

Mean Right Atrial Pressure (mm Hg) = 21.6 – (24 × SFF)

where SFF is systolic filling fraction of the hepatic venous flow, which is obtained by dividing the hepatic vein systolic velocity-time integral (VTI) by the sum of systolic and diastolic VTIs. For the purpose of simplification, peak velocities can be used in lieu of VTIs.[20] This method, however, has not been validated in patients with severe tricuspid regurgitation; instead, the right atrial pressure can be estimated in these patients at a constant of 20 mm Hg, especially in the presence of other indicators of

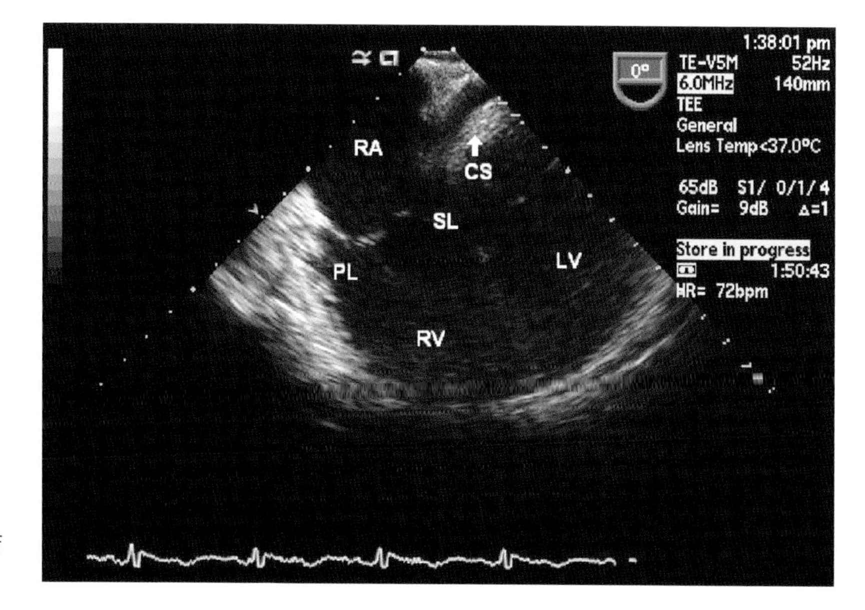

FIGURE 10–11 Long axis view of the coronary sinus. (CS, coronary sinus; LV, left ventricle; RV, right ventricle; RA, right atrium; SL, septal leaflet; PL, posterior leaflet of the tricuspid valve.)

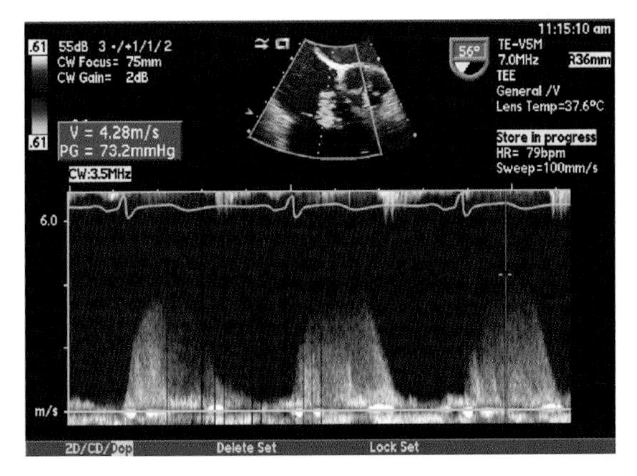

FIGURE 10–12. Continuous-wave Doppler measurement of the peak tricuspid regurgitation jet velocity from the midesophageal inflow-outflow view. Color Doppler is used to guide the placement of the CW Doppler cursor. In this patient, the peak systolic gradient across the tricuspid valve was 73 mm Hg, indicating significant pulmonary hypertension (there was no right ventricular outflow tract obstruction or pulmonary stenosis present).

elevated right atrial pressure (eg, significantly distended jugular veins).[21]

More recently, Arthur et al[22] found that measurement of the IVC diameter by TEE can provide an estimate of the central venous pressure (CVP) in mechanically ventilated patients. In their study, the IVC diameter was measured in the bicaval view (at 110°) at the level of the cavo-atrial junction and at the end of the T-wave of the electrocardiogram. The ventilator was turned off at time of the measurement to eliminate the effect of intrathoracic pressure changes. The linear regression–derived equation to calculate the CVP based on the IVC diameter *[CVP = (IVC diameter − 4.004)/0.751]* showed a good correlation with catheter-measured CVP. Based on their findings, we propose the following simplified formula for estimating the CVP based on the IVC diameter:

$$\text{CVP (mm Hg)} = 4/3 \times [\text{IVC diameter (mm)} - 4]$$

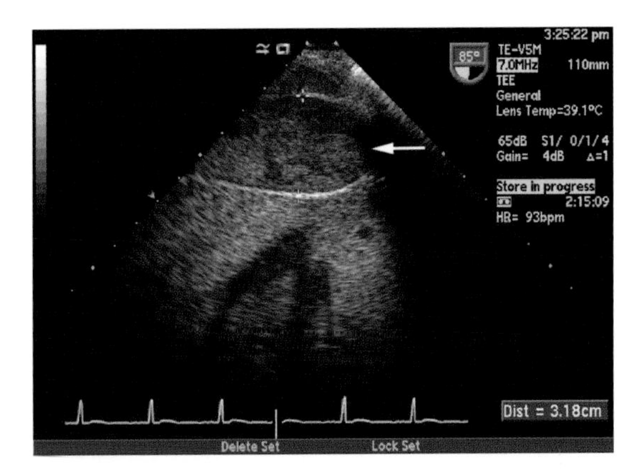

FIGURE 10–13. Significantly dilated vena cava *(arrow)*, with spontaneous echocontrast, indicative of low flow. There were no respiratory variations in the diameter of the vessel, indicating elevated right atrial pressures.

TRICUSPID STENOSIS

Common Pathophysiology

Tricuspid stenosis is less frequently found in the community given the low incidence of rheumatic heart disease, the most common cause of this valvular lesion. In areas where rheumatic heart disease is still prevalent, tricuspid stenosis is usually associated with involvement of other valves, namely the mitral valve. In addition, it is frequently coupled with tricuspid regurgitation. Rheumatic disease leads to thickening of the leaflets and commissural fusion as well as involvement of the subvalvular apparatus.[23] Other causes of tricuspid stenosis include endomyocardial fibrosis and carcinoid heart disease, in which fibrous deposits on the endocardium lead to thickening of the valve and leaflets that are fixed in a semi-open position. This is invariably associated with regurgitation. When present, the increased flow from the regurgitation will lead to higher gradients across the valve. Patients with tricuspid stenosis usually have a significantly dilated right atrium. Dilatation of the right ventricle is a function of the severity of the associated tricuspid regurgitation.

Two-Dimensional Evaluation

Careful examination of the tricuspid leaflets is needed to assess for thickening and/or calcifications, and for the presence of restricted mobility with or without doming in diastole (Figure 10–14). Planimetry of the valvular orifice in the transgastric short-axis view can be attempted, but is difficult and unlikely to yield accurate results. Lesions (tumors, large vegetations, etc) causing mass obstruction of the valvular inlet can be identified. Information from the assessment of the other valves and chambers can help in the determination of the underlying etiology of stenosis, such as involvement of the mitral valve in patients with rheumatic heart disease or the pulmonic valve in patients with carcinoid disease. The presence of left ventricular dysfunction and

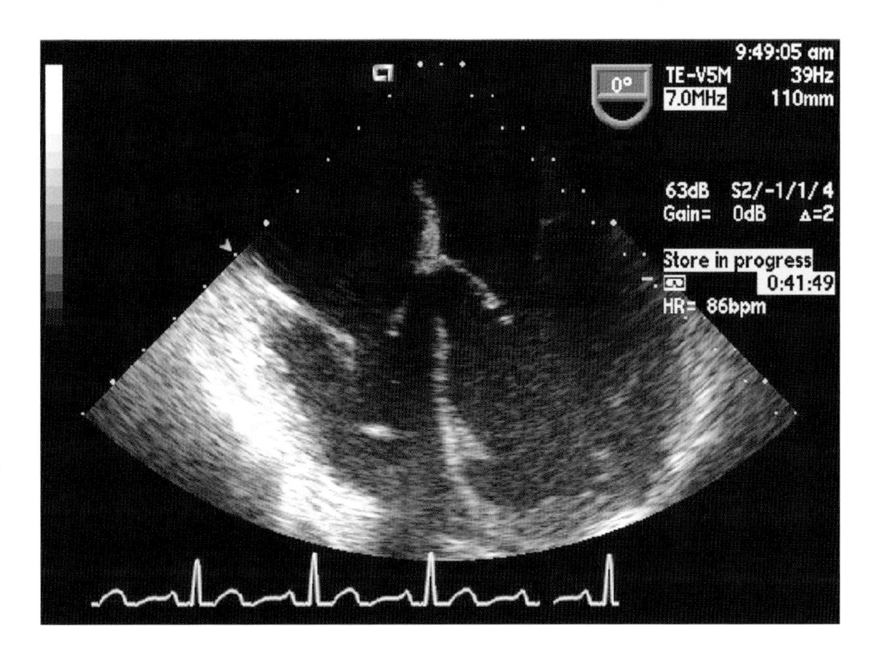

FIGURE 10–14. In this patient with carcinoid heart disease, thickening of the tricuspid leaflets along with restricted opening in diastole is noted on the midesophageal four-chamber view.

apical thrombus raises the possibility of endomyocardial fibrosis as a cause for tricuspid stenosis. In general, the right atrium and inferior vena cava are dilated, especially in chronic and more severe cases.

Doppler Evaluation

Color Doppler usually reveals evidence of turbulent, high-velocity flow. Using PW Doppler with the sample volume placed at the tip of the leaflets, the RV inflow velocities can be shown to be increased (>0.7 m/s).[24] This is typically performed in the midesophageal right ventricular inflow-outflow view where the Doppler beam can be aligned with the blood flow. Assessment of the diastolic pressure gradients using CW Doppler can be performed while increasing the sweep speed (100 mm/s) for better accuracy of measurements (Figure 10–15). Also, it is recommended to average at least five cycles to account for respiratory variations, or changing cycle length in patients with atrial fibrillation. As with the other valves, the pressure gradient across the tricuspid depends on both the valvular orifice area and the flow across it, which is increased in the presence of concomitant regurgitation. However, current assessment of severity of tricuspid stenosis is mainly based on the gradient alone, with a mean gradient of more than 5 mm Hg considered reflective of severe stenosis.[24] The pressure half-time (PHT) method using a constant of 190 (i.e. 190/PHT) can be used to estimate the orifice area,[25] but is not as well validated as for mitral stenosis, and is of limited usefulness in clinical practice. Finally, in the absence of regurgitation, dividing the stroke volume measured at either the left or right ventricular outflow tract by the tricuspid inflow VTI from the CW Doppler recording (continuity equation) can be used to calculate the stenotic orifice area.[26] An area of 1 cm^2 or less is consistent with significant tricuspid stenosis (Table 10–3).[24]

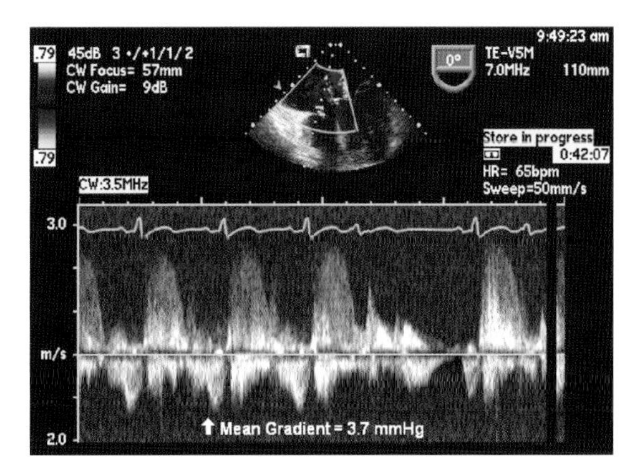

FIGURE 10–15. Continuous-wave Doppler measurement of the tricuspid valve diastolic gradient reveals a mean gradient of 3.7 mm Hg in this patient, consistent with moderate tricuspid stenosis.

Table 10–3. Echocardiographic findings in tricuspid stenosis

	Stenosis Severity		
	Mild	**Moderate**	**Severe**
Two-dimensional findings			
Leaflet morphology	Usually normal	Thickening	Thickening ± calcifications
Leaflet mobility	Normal	Moderately restricted	Severely restricted; doming
Right-side chambers[a]	Can be normal	Dilated	Significantly dilated
Doppler findings			
Color Doppler			Turbulent inflow
Inflow velocity (m/s)	<0.7	>0.7	>>0.7
Mean diastolic gradient	≤2		≥5
Pressure half-time			≥190 ms
Area by continuity equation			≤1 cm^2

[a]Mostly the right atrium and the inferior vena cava. Right ventricular dilatation is present when there is associated insufficiency.

PULMONIC VALVE

Relevant Anatomical Landmarks

The three cusps of the pulmonic valve are labeled as the anterior, right, and left cusps. The names of the cusps are derived from their developmental origin from the truncus arteriosus.[3] The plane of the opening of the pulmonic valve faces superiorly and to the left (see Figure 10–1).[27] Due to its anatomical position away from the esophagus, the pulmonic valve is frequently difficult to image by TEE.

Tomographic Views

Midesophageal Short-Axis View

The short-axis view of the aortic valve is first obtained from the midesophageal position with the multiplane angle set between 35° and 50°. Withdrawing the probe slightly along with minor rotation will bring up a long-axis view of the pulmonic valve (Figure 10–16). In this view, the pulmonary valve and the proximal segment of the main pulmonary artery are located to the right of the display. The anterior pulmonary cusp is seen in the far field and the right cusp is seen in the proximity of the aortic valve.[28]

Midesophageal Right Ventricular Inflow-Outflow View

In this view, the pulmonic valve can be visualized along its long axis to the right of the display (see Figure 10–3). Color-flow Doppler can be used to assess for the presence of pulmonary insufficiency (Figure 10–17). In some patients with heavy aortic valve calcifications or a prosthetic aortic valve, acoustic shadowing can prohibit adequate visualization of the pulmonic valve. In addition, the direction of the pulmonary blood flow is almost perpendicular to the Doppler beam, making assessment of velocities and gradients unreliable in this view.

Upper Esophageal Aortic Arch Short-Axis View

This imaging plane provides a long-axis view of the pulmonic valve and pulmonary artery with the ultrasound beam being almost parallel to the direction of blood flow. It is obtained from the upper esophageal window with the multiplane angle at approximately 90°, along with rotation of the probe to the left. The pulmonic valve and pulmonary artery are seen to the left of the display (Figure 10–18). Slight retroflexion of the probe and an increased imaging depth are often needed to better visualize the pulmonic valve.

Transgastric Right Ventricular Inflow-Outflow View

This view is obtained from the transgastric position at the midpapillary muscle level, by turning the probe to the patient's left and forward rotation of the multiplane angle to 110° to 140°. The right ventricular outflow tract (RVOT) and pulmonic valve (PV) will appear in the mid-far field, parallel to the beam, often in optimal position for color and spectral Doppler analysis (see Chapter 13).

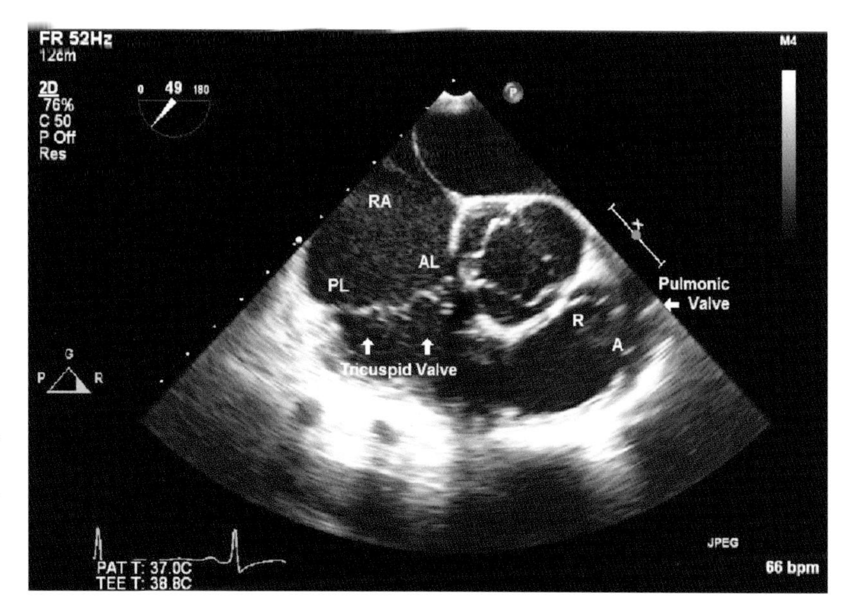

FIGURE 10–16. Midesophageal aortic valve short-axis view, with the pulmonic valve clearly seen in the right-side far field. The right (R) and anterior (A) cusps of the valve are seen in this view. (RA, right atrium; AL, anterior leaflet; PL, posterior leaflet.)

Deep Transgastric Right Ventricular Outflow View

This image is obtained by advancing the probe to the deep transgastric position, flexing the tip to identify the deep-transgastric images of the left ventricle (LV), and turning the probe slightly towards the patient's right side (see Chapter 13).

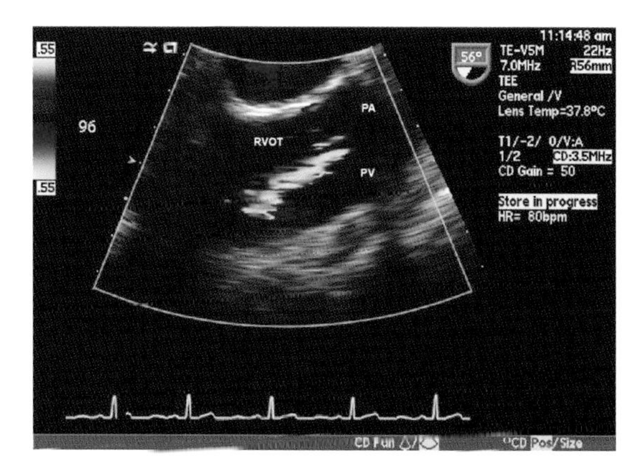

FIGURE 10–17. Midesophageal view with zoom on the pulmonic valve. Color Doppler shows the presence of mild regurgitation. (RVOT, right ventricular outflow tract; PV, pulmonic valve; PA, pulmonary artery.)

PULMONIC REGURGITATION

Common Causes

In the adult population, pulmonary hypertension leading to pulmonary artery and annular dilatation is the most common cause of pulmonary regurgitation.

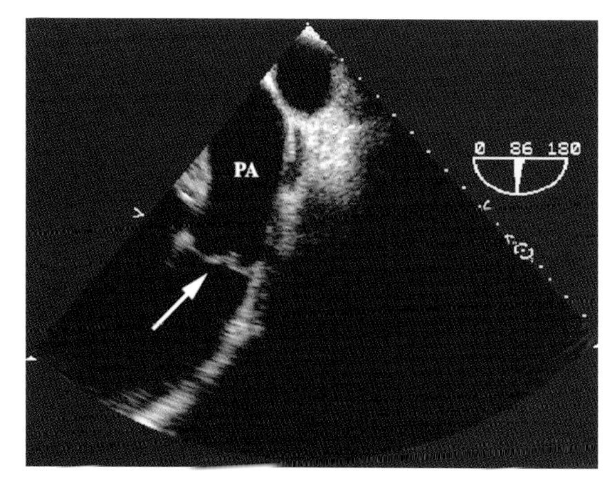

FIGURE 10–18. Upper esophageal aortic arch short-axis view, showing the pulmonary artery along its long axis. This view is useful because it aligns the Doppler beam with the flow of blood. The arrow points to the pulmonic valve. (PA, pulmonary artery.)

Connective tissue disorders, such as Marfan's syndrome, can also lead to dilatation and insufficiency. Carcinoid and rheumatic heart disease cause restricted leaflet mobility and malcoaptation. Additional etiologies include endocarditis, trauma, congenital malformations, and complications of surgical interventions (repair of pulmonary stenosis or tetralogy of Fallot).

Two-Dimensional Evaluation

Two-dimensional echocardiography is essential in defining the anatomy of the pulmonic valve. Lesions such as annular dilatation, valve prolapse, vegetations, congenital malformations, and rheumatic involvement are frequently easily identified. Thickening and restricted mobility, malcoaptation (Figure 10–19), along with narrowing of the annulus can be seen in patients with carcinoid heart disease.[12] The presence of right ventricular dilatation in the absence of other etiologies is usually indicative of severe chronic pulmonary insufficiency.

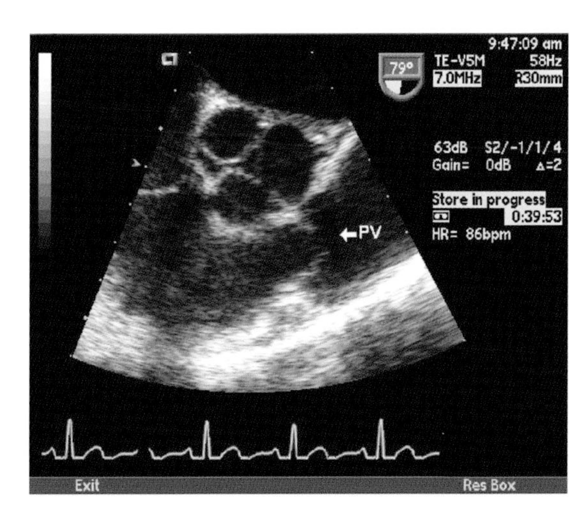

FIGURE 10–19. Midesophageal view with zoom showing malcoaptation of the pulmonic valve leaflets in a patient with carcinoid heart disease. (PV, pulmonic valve.)

Doppler Evaluation

There is no validated quantitative grading of pulmonary regurgitation using TEE. Assessment of pulmonary regurgitation is commonly performed qualitatively (Table 10–4).[29] Transthoracic echocardiography has relied on jet width and jet length. A ratio of the jet width to the right ventricular outflow tract diameter of no greater than 38% indicates mild to moderate pulmonary regurgitation; a ratio of 39% to 74% indicates moderate to severe regurgitation; and a ratio of at least 75% indicates severe regurgitation.[30] A jet length shorter than 10 mm has been found in normal subjects with no cardiopulmonary disease, whereas a jet length longer than 20 mm has been associated with pulmonic insufficiency murmur.[31] As with aortic regurgitation, it should be remembered that jet length is dependent on loading conditions and ventricular compliance.

Table 10–4. Echocardiographic findings in pulmonic regurgitation

	Regurgitation Severity		
	Mild	**Moderate**	**Severe**
Two-dimensional findings			
Leaflet morphology	Usually normal	Can be normal	Abnormal
Leaflet coaptation	Normal		Malcoaptation
Right-side chambers	Usually normal	Can be normal	Dilated (unless acute)
Pulmonic annulus	Usually normal		Dilated
Doppler findings			
Jet length by color Doppler[a]	Usually <10 mm	Intermediate	>20 mm
Jet width/RVOT diameter ratio[a]	≤0.38	≥0.39-0.74	≥0.75
CW Doppler signal	Soft; slow deceleration	Dense; variable deceleration	Dense; steep deceleration (PHT <100 ms)

[a]At a Nyquist limit of 50 to 60 cm/s.
RVOT, right ventricular outflow tract; CW, continuous-wave; PHT, pressure half-time.

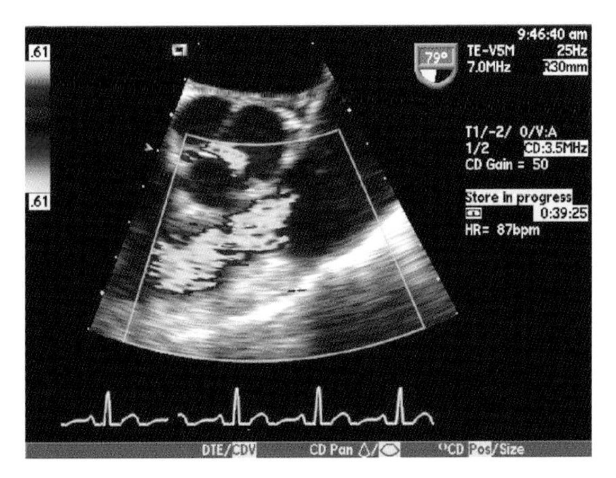

FIGURE 10–20. Moderate to severe pulmonic regurgitation is seen by color Doppler.

Figure 10–20 displays the color Doppler signal of moderate to severe regurgitation in a patient with carcinoid syndrome.

CW Doppler interrogation of the pulmonic regurgitation jet in the upper esophageal aortic arch short-axis view, the *transgastric* right ventricular inflow-outflow view, or the deep transgastric *right* ventricular outflow view allows estimation of the end-diastolic flow velocity, and therefore the end-diastolic gradient (using the simplified Bernoulli equation) between the pulmonary artery and the right ventricle. This gradient can be used to estimate the pulmonary artery diastolic pressure by adding an estimate of the right atrial pressure,[32] and is equal to that of the right ventricle at end-diastole, if there is no pulmonic valve stenosis (see Chapter 4). Furthermore, the slope of the Doppler envelope can provide information about the severity of the pulmonic regurgitation, with steeper slopes being associated with significant degrees of regurgitation.[33] Recently, a pressure half-time of the pulmonary insufficiency jet of less than 100 milliseconds was found to reliably identify patients with adult congenital heart disease who had angiographically confirmed severe regurgitation.[34]

PULMONIC STENOSIS

Common Pathophysiology

Pulmonic stenosis is mostly a congenital lesion, with the abnormal valve having abnormal leaflet number or morphology. Sometimes, associated abnormalities of the right ventricular outflow tract are noted. In the adult population, pulmonic stenosis can result from rheumatic heart disease or carcinoid syndrome wherein involvement of other valves is usually evident.[23] Right ventricular outflow tract obstruction can result from hypertrophy of the infundibular septum, protrusion of the right sinus of Valsalva of the aortic valve into the right ventricular outflow tract, aneurysm of membranous ventricular septum, and the presence of mass lesions such as sarcoma. Congenital conditions such as tetralogy of Fallot can be recognized from the presence of associated malformations (Figure 10–21; see Chapter 18). The presence of pulmonic stenosis and/or right ventricular outflow tract obstruction leads to increased afterload and consequently hypertrophy of the right ventricle. In advanced cases, right ventricular failure and dilatation may ensue, leading to the development of tricuspid regurgitation.

Two-Dimensional Evaluation

Examination of the leaflets and their mobility in the long axis can be performed in most of the views defined above. The presence of thickening, calcifications, and doming in systole should be noted. Abnormalities of the outflow tract can be detected in the midesophageal views, whereas the upper esophageal aortic short-axis view provides good imaging of the proximal part of the pulmonary artery. Direct planimetry of the pulmonic valve cannot be performed since the valve is not imaged well in cross section by TEE. Examination of the right ventricular chamber size and function is helpful for the assessment of the severity of the stenosis.

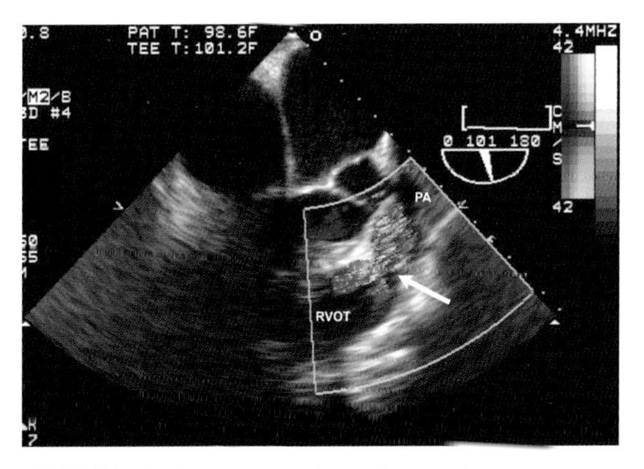

FIGURE 10–21. Midesophageal view of a patient with tetralogy of Fallot showing turbulent flow secondary to pulmonary stenosis *(arrow)*. (PA, pulmonary artery; RVOT, right ventricular outflow tract.)

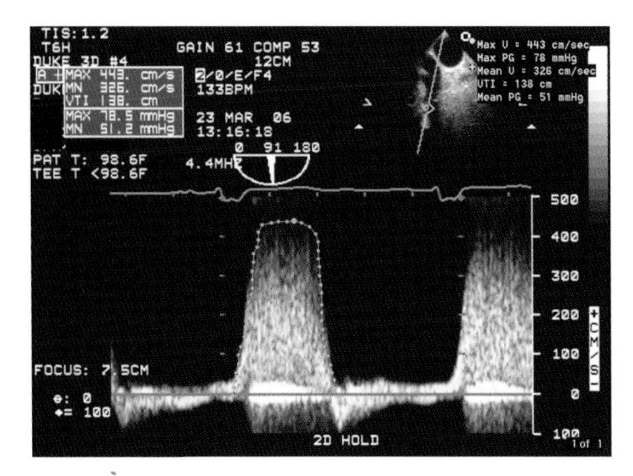

FIGURE 10–22. Assessment of the pulmonary gradients using CW Doppler in the upper esophageal aortic arch short-axis view in the same patient with tetralogy of Fallot as in Figure 10–21.

Doppler Evaluation

Using color-flow Doppler, the pattern of flow across the valve can be assessed; the presence of aliasing indicating turbulent flow should alert the examiner to the possibility of outflow obstruction. Also, color-flow Doppler can help guide the appropriate positioning of the CW Doppler cursor for optimal measurement of mean and peak gradients. This is readily performed in the upper esophageal aortic arch short-axis view (Figure 10–22), or occasionally in the *transgastric* right ventricular inflow-outflow or deep transgastric *right* ventricular outflow views, where the blood flow across the valve is almost parallel to the Doppler signal. Assessment of the VTI of the right ventricular outflow tract and measurement of the diameter of the right ventricular outflow tract during early systole can be used to assess flow through the right ventricular outflow tract.[35,36] Combined with VTI of the pulmonic valve, the area of the valve can potentially be calculated using the continuity equation. A late-peaking, "dagger-shaped" Doppler envelope should alert the operator to the presence of dynamic outflow tract obstruction. Since there is lack of validated methods to accurately assess valvular area, grading of pulmonic stenosis relies largely on the gradients across the valve, with cutoffs for moderate and severe stenosis being a velocity of 3 m/s (gradient of 36 mm Hg) and 4 m/s (gradient of 64 mm Hg), respectively (Table 10–5).[15,24]

CONCLUSIONS

TEE can provide accurate evaluation of the right-side cardiac valves. Details of the anatomy of the leaflets, subvalvular apparatus, and associated lesions can be readily appreciated. Complete assessment requires combining two-dimensional and Doppler data together with information about the cardiac chambers. This will provide the necessary information to make accurate diagnoses and guide appropriate management. Further technological advances are needed before three-dimensional evaluation of the tricuspid and pulmonic valves becomes a routine part of a comprehensive TEE examination.

Table 10–5. Echocardiographic findings in pulmonic stenosis

	Stenosis Severity		
	Mild	**Moderate**	**Severe**
Two-dimensional findings			
Leaflet morphology	Usually normal	Thickening	Thickening ± calcifications
Leaflet mobility	Normal	Moderately restricted	Severely restricted; doming
RV hypertrophy	Usually absent		Usually present
Doppler findings			
Color Doppler			Turbulent outflow
Peak velocity (m/s)	<3	3-4	>4
Peak gradient (mm Hg)	<36	36-64	>64

REFERENCES

1. Chaliki HP, Click RL, Abel MD. Comparison of intraoperative transesophageal echocardiographic examinations with the operative findings: prospective review of 1918 cases. *J Am Soc Echocardiogr.* 1999;12(4):237-240.
2. Sugeng L, Shernan SK, Salgo IS, et al. Live 3-dimensional transesophageal echocardiography initial experience using the fully-sampled matrix array probe. *J Am Coll Cardiol.* 2008; 52(6):446-449.
3. Agur AMR, Dalley AF. *Grant's Atlas of Anatomy.* 12th ed. Philadelphia: Wolters Kluwer Health/Lippincott Williams & Wilkins; 2009.
4. Tariq M, Smego RA Jr, Soofi A, Islam N. Pulmonic valve endocarditis. *South Med J.* 2003;96(6):621-623.
5. Reynolds HR, Jagen MA, Tunick PA, Kronzon I. Sensitivity of transthoracic versus transesophageal echocardiography for the detection of native valve vegetations in the modern era. *J Am Soc Echocardiogr.* 2003;16(1):67-70.
6. Zaroff JG, Picard MH. Transesophageal echocardiographic (TEE) evaluation of the mitral and tricuspid valves. *Cardiol Clin.* 2000;18(4):731-750.
7. Shiina A, Seward JB, Edwards WD, Hagler DJ, Tajik AJ. Two-dimensional echocardiographic spectrum of Ebstein's anomaly: detailed anatomic assessment. *J Am Coll Cardiol.* 1984;3(2 Pt 1):356-370.
8. Ammash NM, Warnes CA, Connolly HM, Danielson GK, Seward JB. Mimics of Ebstein's anomaly. *Am Heart J.* 1997;134(3):508-513.
9. Gussenhoven EJ, Stewart PA, Becker AE, Essed CE, Ligtvoet KM, De Villeneuve VH. "Offsetting" of the septal tricuspid leaflet in normal hearts and in hearts with Ebstein's anomaly. Anatomic and echographic correlation. *Am J Cardiol.* 1984; 54(1):172-176.
10. Warnes CA, Williams RG, Bashore TM, et al. ACC/AHA 2008 guidelines for the management of adults with congenital heart disease: a report of the American College of Cardiology/ American Heart Association Task Force on Practice Guidelines (Writing Committee to Develop Guidelines on the Management of Adults With Congenital Heart Disease). Developed in Collaboration With the American Society of Echocardiography, Heart Rhythm Society, International Society for Adult Congenital Heart Disease, Society for Cardiovascular Angiography and Interventions, and Society of Thoracic Surgeons. *J Am Coll Cardiol.* 2008;52(23):e1-121.
11. Paranon S, Acar P. Ebstein's anomaly of the tricuspid valve: from fetus to adult: congenital heart disease. *Heart.* 2008;94(2):237-243.
12. Pellikka PA, Tajik AJ, Khandheria BK, et al. Carcinoid heart disease. Clinical and echocardiographic spectrum in 74 patients. *Circulation.* 1993;87(4):1188-1196.
13. Colombo T, Russo C, Ciliberto GR, et al. Tricuspid regurgitation secondary to mitral valve disease: tricuspid annulus function as guide to tricuspid valve repair. Cardiovasc *Surg.* 2001;9(4):369-377.
14. Maslow AD, Schwartz C, Singh AK. Assessment of the tricuspid valve: a comparison of four transesophageal echocardiographic windows. *J Cardiothorac Vasc Anesth.* 2004;18(6): 719-724.
15. Bonow RO, Carabello BA, Chatterjee K, et al. ACC/AHA 2006 guidelines for the management of patients with valvular heart disease: a report of the American College of Cardiology/ American Heart Association Task Force on Practice Guidelines (writing Committee to Revise the 1998 guidelines for the management of patients with valvular heart disease) developed in collaboration with the Society of Cardiovascular Anesthesiologists endorsed by the Society for Cardiovascular Angiography and Interventions and the Society of Thoracic Surgeons. *J Am Coll Cardiol.* 2006;48(3):e1-148.
16. Zoghbi WA, Enriquez-Sarano M, Foster E, et al. Recommendations for evaluation of the severity of native valvular regurgitation with two-dimensional and Doppler echocardiography. *J Am Soc Echocardiogr.* 2003;16(7):777-802.
17. Nomura T, Lebowitz L, Koide Y, Keehn L, Oka Y. Evaluation of hepatic venous flow using transesophageal echocardiography in coronary artery bypass surgery: an index of right ventricular function. *J Cardiothorac Vasc Anesth.* 1995;9(1):9-17.
18. Zamorano J, Almeria C, Alfonso F, et al. Transesophageal Doppler analysis of coronary sinus flow: a new method to assess the severity of tricuspid regurgitation. *Echocardiography.* 1997;14(6 Pt 1):579-588.
19. Kircher BJ, Himelman RB, Schiller NB. Noninvasive estimation of right atrial pressure from the inspiratory collapse of the inferior vena cava. *Am J Cardiol.* 1990;66(4):493-496.
20. Nagueh SF, Kopelen HA, Zoghbi WA. Relation of mean right atrial pressure to echocardiographic and Doppler parameters of right atrial and right ventricular function. *Circulation.* 1996; 93(6):1160-1169.
21. Currie PJ, Seward JB, Chan KL, et al. Continuous wave Doppler determination of right ventricular pressure: a simultaneous Doppler-catheterization study in 127 patients. *J Am Coll Cardiol.* 1985;6(4):750-756.
22. Arthur ME, Landolfo C, Wade M, Castresana MR. Inferior vena cava diameter (IVCD) measured with transesophageal echocardiography (TEE) can be used to derive the central venous pressure (CVP) in anesthetized mechanically ventilated patients. *Echocardiography.* 2009;26(2):140-149.
23. Freeman WK. *Transesophageal Echocardiography.* Boston: Little, Brown; 1994.
24. Baumgartner H, Hung J, Bermejo J, et al. Echocardiographic assessment of valve stenosis: EAE/ASE recommendations for clinical practice. *J Am Soc Echocardiogr.* 2009;22(1):1-23; quiz 101-102.
25. Fawzy ME, Mercer EN, Dunn B, al-Amri M, Andaya W. Doppler echocardiography in the evaluation of tricuspid stenosis. *Eur Heart J.* 1989;10(11):985-990.
26. Karp K, Teien D, Eriksson P. Doppler echocardiographic assessment of the valve area in patients with atrioventricular valve stenosis by application of the continuity equation. *J Intern Med.* 1989;225(4):261-266.
27. Moore KL, Dalley AF, Agur AMR. *Clinically Oriented Anatomy.* 5th ed. Philadelphia: Lippincott Williams & Wilkins; 2006.
28. Shively BK. Transesophageal echocardiographic (TEE) evaluation of the aortic valve, left ventricular outflow tract, and pulmonic valve. *Cardiol Clin.* 2000;18(4):711-729.
29. Mulhern KM, Skorton DJ. Echocardiographic evaluation of isolated pulmonary valve disease in adolescents and adults. *Echocardiography.* 1993;10(5):533-543.

30. Nanda NC, Domanski MJ. *Atlas of Transesophageal Echocardiography.* Baltimore: Williams & Wilkins; 1998.
31. Takao S, Miyatake K, Izumi S, et al. Clinical implications of pulmonary regurgitation in healthy individuals: detection by cross sectional pulsed Doppler echocardiography. *Br Heart J.* 1988;59(5):542-550.
32. Schiller NB. Hemodynamics derived from transesophageal echocardiography (TEE). *Cardiol Clin.* 2000;18(4): 699-709.
33. Lei MH, Chen JJ, Ko YL, Cheng JJ, Kuan P, Lien WP. Reappraisal of quantitative evaluation of pulmonary regurgitation and estimation of pulmonary artery pressure by continuous wave Doppler echocardiography. *Cardiology.* 1995;86(3): 249-256.
34. Yang H, Pu M, Chambers CE, Weber HS, Myers JL, Davidson WR Jr. Quantitative assessment of pulmonary insufficiency by Doppler echocardiography in patients with adult congenital heart disease. *J Am Soc Echocardiogr.* 2008;21 (2):157-164.
35. Maslow A, Comunale ME, Haering JM, Watkins J. Pulsed wave Doppler measurement of cardiac output from the right ventricular outflow tract. *Anesth Analg. 1996;83(3): 466-471.*
36. Zhao X, Mashikian JS, Panzica P, Lerner A, Park KW, Comunale ME. Comparison of thermodilution bolus cardiac output and Doppler cardiac output in the early post-cardiopulmonary bypass period. *J Cardiothorac Vasc Anesth.* 2003;17(2):193-198.

REVIEW QUESTIONS

Select the best answer.

1. Tricuspid regurgitation can occur:
   a. In the absence of other valvular diseases
   b. In association with mitral valve prolapse
   c. Secondary to pulmonary hypertension
   d. With a structurally normal tricuspid valve
   e. With all of the above

2. Which of the following statements about the tricuspid valve is *false*?
   a. Mild tricuspid regurgitation on transesophageal echocardiography is a common finding in normal, healthy individuals.
   b. Systolic pulmonary artery pressure can be estimated by studying the tricuspid regurgitation jet velocity.
   c. In a patient with pulmonic stenosis, estimation of the right ventricular systolic pressure can be obtained from Doppler study of the tricuspid regurgitant jet.
   d. In a patient with tricuspid regurgitation, color Doppler study of the regurgitant jet is always enough to decide on its severity.

3. The three leaflets of the tricuspid valve can be assessed in which of the following tomographic views?
   a. Midesophageal RV inflow-outflow view
   b. Midesophageal four-chamber view
   c. Transgastric RV inflow view
   d. Transgastric short-axis view

4. Which of the following does not indicate the presence of severe tricuspid regurgitation?
   a. Systolic reversal of the coronary sinus flow
   b. Presence of noncoaptation of the tricuspid leaflets
   c. Dense CW Doppler signal of the tricuspid regurgitation jet
   d. Systolic dominance of hepatic vein flow

5. Estimation of the systolic pulmonary artery pressure is best done in which of the following views?
   a. Midesophageal two-chamber view
   b. Midesophageal four-chamber view
   c. Transgastric RV inflow view
   d. Transgastric short-axis view

6. Assessment of pulmonic insufficiency using color-flow Doppler cannot be done in which of the following tomographic views?
   a. Midesophageal RV inflow-outflow view
   b. Midesophageal aortic short-axis view
   c. Upper esophageal aortic short-axis view
   d. Transgastric short-axis view

7. Assessment of the severity of pulmonic insufficiency relies on:
   a. Jet length and width
   b. Jet timing
   c. Jet shape
   d. Jet area

8. In a patient with severe tricuspid regurgitation, the PW Doppler study of the hepatic veins will show:
   a. A large forward systolic wave and a reversed diastolic wave
   b. A large atrial reversal wave with a forward systolic wave
   c. A small forward systolic wave with a large forward diastolic wave
   d. A large systolic reversal wave and a forward diastolic wave

9. The most common cause of pulmonic insufficiency is:
   a. Rheumatic heart disease
   b. Pulmonary hypertension
   c. Marfan syndrome
   d. Endocarditis

10. The best tomographic view for the CW Doppler interrogation of pulmonic insufficiency is the:
    a. Midesophageal RV inflow-outflow view
    b. Upper esophageal aortic arch short-axis view
    c. Midesophageal short-axis view
    d. Transgastric short-axis view

11. The best tomographic view for the assessment of tricuspid valve gradient is the:
    a. Transgastric short-axis view
    b. Midesophageal two-chamber view
    c. Midesophageal RV inflow-outflow view
    d. Transgastric RV inflow view

12. The most common cause of tricuspid stenosis worldwide is:
    a. Rheumatic heart disease
    b. Endomyocardial fibrosis
    c. Carcinoid heart disease
    d. Congenital

13. The following indicates significant tricuspid stenosis:
    a. Mean diastolic gradient of 3 mm Hg
    b. Calculated area by continuity equation of 1.5 cm^2
    c. Pressure half-time of 235 milliseconds
    d. Pliable leaflets

14. In patients with pulmonic stenosis:
    a. Right ventricular hypertrophy is always present.
    b. A peak gradient of 56 mm Hg indicates severe stenosis.
    c. Calcifications of the valve leaflet are always present.
    d. It is important to rule out the presence of right ventricular outflow tract obstruction.

15. The following can provide a reliable estimation of the degree of pulmonic stenosis:
    a. The amount of thickening of the leaflets
    b. The presence of doming in systole
    c. The presence of calcifications
    d. The degree of mobility of the leaflets
    e. None of the above

Prosthetic Valves

11

Blaine A. Kent, Madhav Swaminathan, and Joseph P. Mathew

Over the past three decades, significant advances have been made with respect to the evolution of prosthetic heart valves and the manner in which they are evaluated in vivo. New materials and configurations of mechanical and biologic valves have improved the quality of life for patients around the world. However, despite the benefits they confer by replacing a diseased valve, all prosthetic valves have inherent limitations and possible complications that may develop in the immediate or late post-implantation period. This chapter provides an overview of (1) the clinical indications for implantation of prosthetic heart valves; (2) the major types of prostheses and (3) their evaluation using transesophageal echocardiography (TEE); (4) some inherent limitations of echocardiography; and (5) common prosthetic pathology.

Similar to the assessment of native cardiac valves (see Chapters 7, 9, and 10), TEE can provide a detailed evaluation of the structure, function, and integrity of prosthetic valves using two-dimensional (2D), color-flow Doppler (CFD), continuous-wave Doppler (CWD), pulsed-wave Doppler (PWD), and three-dimensional (3D) imaging modalities. However, several features unique to the intraoperative environment such as dynamic changes to preload, myocardial contractility, and afterload can create challenges for the TEE assessment of prosthetic valves. In addition, prosthesis malfunction can affect adjacent valves and chambers, and this must be considered in the assessment. Nevertheless, the integration of information from the TEE examination can provide a comprehensive assessment of the patient's overall cardiac status.

CLINICAL INDICATIONS FOR PROSTHETIC VALVE PLACEMENT

A diseased native valve that is symptomatic will ultimately require intervention (repair or replacement) by percutaneous or surgical means. The most commonly replaced valves are those in the aortic and mitral positions commensurate with the high prevalence of diseases that involve these valves. Recently, with significant improvements in mitral valve repair, the numbers of valves implanted for mitral regurgitation have been decreasing and stenosis has become a more common indication for mitral valve replacement. In addition, with a large number of prosthetic valves already implanted, pathologies involving these replaced valves are increasing the frequency of repeat surgery. Often presenting as new or increased valvular regurgitation in the setting of a systemic infection, endocarditis of the native valve or prosthetic grafts is an infrequent yet important indication for placement of a new prosthesis. In addition, inadequate anticoagulation can lead to acute or chronic stenosis of previously placed valves. The myriad of systemic diseases that can cause valvular dysfunction are comprehensively discussed in the ACC/AHA guidelines for evaluation of patients with valve disease.[1]

TYPES OF PROSTHETIC VALVES

When faced with a patient who needs a valve replacement, cardiologists and cardiac surgeons have a wide variety of valves from a number of manufacturers to select from. The decision as to which prosthesis should be implanted depends on a number of factors including the patient's age, gender (women of child-bearing age), life expectancy, comorbidities, location and size of the diseased valve, surgical expertise or preference, and considerations regarding anticoagulation (noncompliance or likely loss to follow-up).[2] A detailed description of the process of valve selection is beyond the scope of this text and is discussed elsewhere.[1]

All valves can be classified as mechanical or biologic depending on the predominant material of composition. While mechanical valves are further classified according to the occlusion device, biologic valves are subclassified according to the presence of synthetic support structures (stented or stentless) and by the origin of the valve tissue (xenografts, homografts, or autografts).[2-4]

Mechanical Valves

Mechanical valves are available in a variety of sizes and designs. All mechanical valves are comprised of a sewing ring (used to secure the valve in the patient) and an occluding device (designed to provide one-way flow through the prosthesis). The design of the occluding device is used to further subclassify this type of prosthesis into one of three major categories: (1) ball-in-cage, (2) tilting disk, and (3) bileaflet.

BALL-IN-CAGE

The first successful prosthetic heart valve implantation in the early 1960s was of the ball-in-cage design. The Starr-Edwards valve was the most widely used, with more than 200,000 prostheses placed since its introduction into clinical practice in 1965.[3,5] Although it has undergone several modifications, the basic design remains unchanged, with a silastic ball constrained within a sewing ring comprised of Teflon or polypropylene cloth and two stellite alloy U-shaped arches that form a cage (Figure 11–1). The ball travels forward into the cage during antegrade flow, with the blood passing between the sewing ring and under the trailing edge of the ball between the struts. The occluder then moves back to seat snugly against the sewing ring when pressures equalize between the two chambers. There is no regurgitant flow during elevation of pressures in the receiving chamber.

Their bulky design and flow characteristics (the smaller the valve, the more obstructive in nature the valve becomes) limit their use to the mitral position. They are also not typically implanted in individuals with small left ventricular cavities or with small aortic annular diameters. Although durable and therefore still seen in patients presenting for repeat surgery, these valves are no longer implanted, having been supplanted by valves with a better hemodynamic profile.

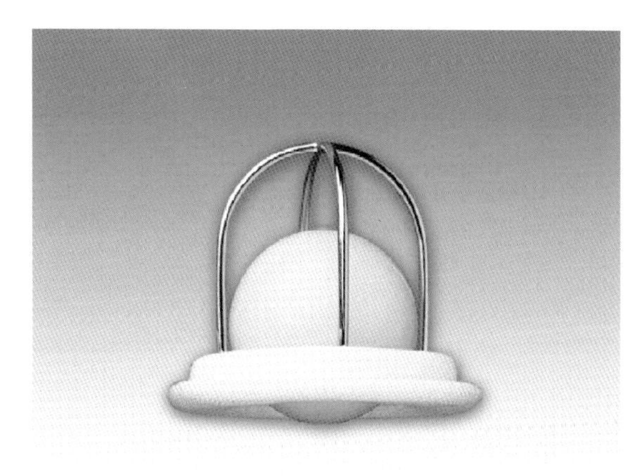

FIGURE 11–1. Starr-Edwards ball-in-cage valve. *(Reproduced with permission from Edwards LifeSciences.)*

TILTING DISK

Representatives of this design include the Medtronic-Hall (Medtronic, Minneapolis, MN), OmniScience (MedicalCV Inc., Inver Grove Heights, MN), and the Bjork-Shiley valves (Figure 11–2). Although each of these valves has its own distinctive design features, a typical tilting disk valve is comprised of a circular sewing ring and an eccentrically hinged or pivoting disk occluder. The pyrolytic carbon disk opens to show two

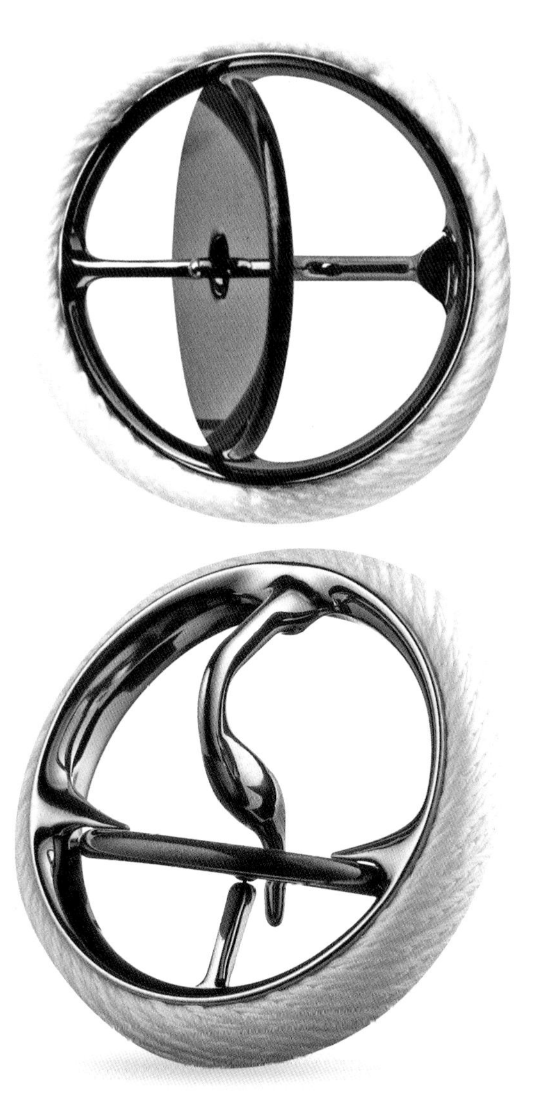

FIGURE 11–2. Single tilting disk designs of mechanical Medtronic-Hall prostheses. *(Reproduced with permission from Medtronic, Inc.)*

unequal (major and minor) orifices during antegrade blood flow. With reversal of pressures, retrograde flow against the larger leading portion of the disk results in closure by rotation on its hinge or pivot.

The Medtronic-Hall valve, first used clinically in 1977, is the most commonly implanted tilting disk valve and is second only to the St. Jude bileaflet valve as the most frequently implanted mechanical prosthesis. The pyrolytic carbon disk has a small central orifice through which the eccentrically placed hinge mechanism passes. The disk and struts are enclosed within a titanium housing that is attached to the native valve annulus with a Teflon sewing ring. The maximum opening angle of an aortic Medtronic-Hall valve is 75°, whereas a mitral prosthesis generally opens no more than 70°.[3,6] The fact that the occluder disk opens less than 90° generates resistance to forward flow and small eddies of stagnant flow proximally that predispose to thrombus development. The small hole in the occluder mechanism results in a characteristic central regurgitant jet that is visible with CFD.

The OmniScience valve also consists of a pyrolytic carbon disk suspended within a titanium housing; however, the sewing ring is comprised of polyester knit rather than of Teflon. Unlike the Medtronic-Hall valve, the OmniScience prosthesis does not have a central hinge; rather, the motion of the disk is restricted by a series of struts. Because there is no central hinge and prerequisite hole, the OmniScience valve does not have a central regurgitant jet when in the closed position. The maximum opening angle of this design is approximately 80°.[2]

The Bjork-Shiley prosthesis, the first successful low-profile tilting disk design (1969), is no longer available in the United States because of problems with strut fracture. However, more than 360,000 valves of this type were implanted, so one occasionally may encounter a patient with this design in situ. The disk of this design has a convex-concave design, with a maximum opening angle of 70°.[2]

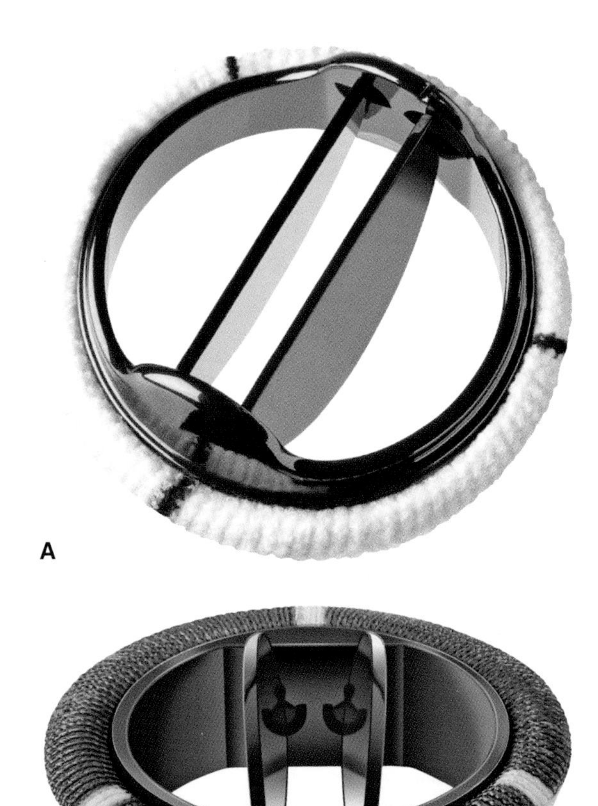

FIGURE 11–3. Bileaflet tilting disk design prosthetic valves. **A:** St. Jude Medical. **B:** Sulzer Carbomedics. *(Reproduced with permission from St. Jude Medical and Sulzer Carbomedics.)*

BILEAFLET

The major representatives of the bileaflet design are the St. Jude (St. Jude Medical, St. Paul, MN), the Carbomedics (Sulzer Carbomedics, Austin, TX) and the On-X (On-X LTI, Austin, TX) prostheses (Figure 11–3). The St. Jude bileaflet prosthesis is the most widely used mechanical valve in the world, with more than 600,000 implantations since its introduction in 1977. Each of these prostheses has two semicircular pyrolytic carbon occluders attached by small midline hinges to a support ring (pyrolytic carbon ring in St. Jude) and a Dacron sewing cuff. The manner in which the two occluder disks are hinged means they require no supporting struts, and therefore have an extremely favorable flow profile with lower transvalvular gradients as compared with the ball-in-cage and single tilting disk designs at similar annular diameters.[3] With antegrade flow, both leaflets open to a maximum angle of 85°, resulting in two large, semicircular lateral orifices and a much smaller central rectangular orifice. With sufficient back pressure, the leaflets rotate on their hinges to close with an angle of approximately 25° to the plane of the supporting ring.[2]

The Carbomedics prosthesis is similar to the St. Jude in design; however, it has an adjustable titanium housing that can be rotated to position the leaflets in such a manner that they avoid contact with subvalvular tissue. The On-X valve is a newer valve made of pure pyrolitic carbon with a longer flow channel and an inlet that is flared outward to improve the flow dynamics through the valve. In addition, two leaflet guards are present to limit pannus encroachment onto the leaflets.[7]

Biologic Valves

Biologic tissue valves may be stented or stentless, depending on the presence of synthetic support structures. They may also be composed of either porcine or bovine leaflet tissue (xenografts), human cadaveric tissue (homografts), or native human tissue (autografts, as in the Ross procedure). Some biologic valves contain a mix of synthetic and natural biological materials (heterografts). Frequently, xenografts or homografts, especially for the aortic position, will include surrounding aortic tissue for improved natural structural support (composite grafts). The principal advantage of biologic over mechanical valves is related to the need for anticoagulation: mechanical valves require long-term anticoagulation, whereas biologic valves require only a short period (8 to 12 weeks) during endothelialization of the sewing ring.

STENTED BIOLOGIC PROSTHESES

Stented biologic valves combine synthetic structural and supporting elements, with leaflets comprised of porcine valve leaflets (Hancock [Medtronic, Minneapolis, MN] and Carpentier-Edwards [Edwards Lifesciences, Irvine, CA] valves) or shaped pericardial tissue (Ionescu-Shiley [discontinued] and Carpentier-Edwards Perimount [Edwards Lifesciences, Irvine, CA] valves; Figure 11–4). The biologic elements of these valves are treated with glutaraldehyde to reduce antigenicity and increase tissue strength. However, this same process renders the tissue less pliable than native human valves and can promote calcification and degeneration in the long term.

The porcine valve leaflets in the Carpentier-Edwards prosthesis are mounted on a flexible Elgiloy frame, with stents manufactured from a single piece of wire attached to a Dacron sewing ring. The individual leaflets are mounted above the sewing ring, which allows for a larger orifice area and an improved hemodynamic profile as compared with valves with a similar ring size. However, the addition of the supporting struts (stents) does reduce the effective orifice area (EOA) as compared with a native human valve.[8] The Hancock valve has many similarities to the Carpentier-Edwards valve on gross visual inspection. Nevertheless, each has a distinctive radiographic shape, with the Carpentier-Edwards valve appearing as a crown and the Hancock valve appearing as a circular ring because its stents are constructed from polypropylene, which is not radiopaque. During antegrade flow, the valve leaflets assume a somewhat irregular cone shape secondary to the slight restriction in opening caused by the valve stents. With pressure reversal, the leaflets coapt

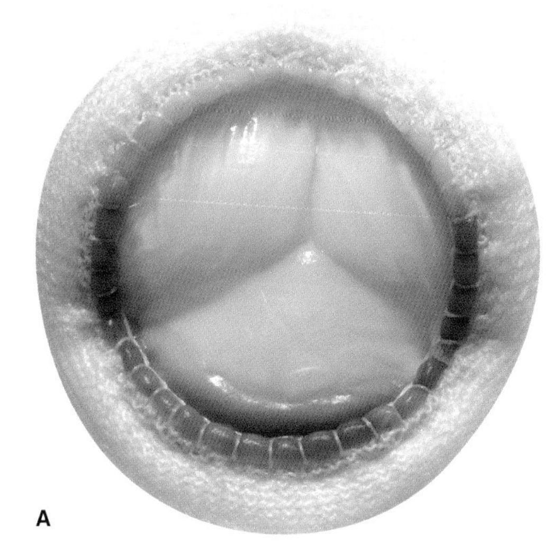

A

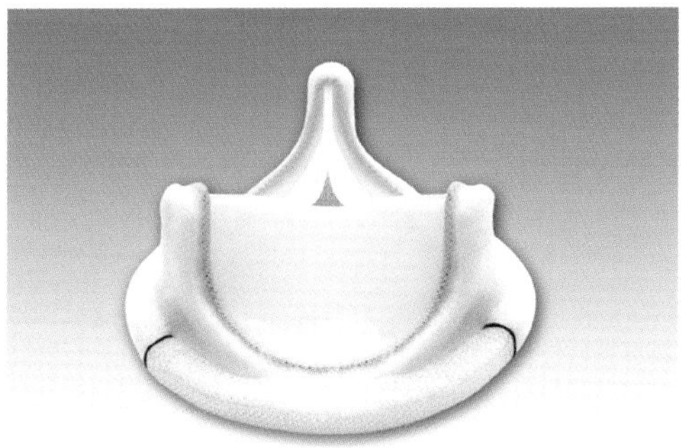

B

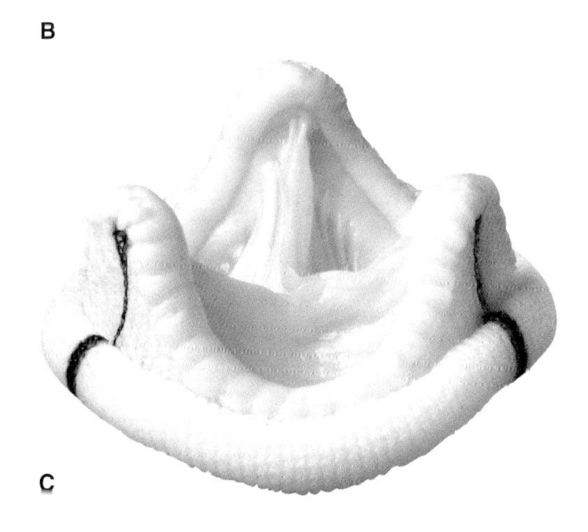

C

FIGURE 11–4. Stented bioprostheses. **A:** Hancock valve (porcine; Medtronic). **B:** Carpentier-Edwards Perimount pericardial valve (bovine; Baxter Healthcare). **C:** St. Jude Epic (porcine; St. Jude Medical). *(Reproduced with permission from Medtronic, Inc; Baxter Healthcare; and St. Jude Medical.)*

and commonly show a small central regurgitant jet, even in a normally functioning biologic valve.

Pericardial biologic valves (Ionescu-Shiley and Carpentier-Edwards Perimount) are not restricted by the physiologic size of the donor valve leaflets, thus allowing for the construction of larger valves. The Ionescu-Shiley valve was a low-profile prosthesis with three bovine pericardial cusps mounted to a Dacron-covered titanium frame using retention sutures. This prosthesis had difficulties with leaflet dehiscence and was discontinued after 10 years. The Perimount valve by Carpentier-Edwards has its pericardial leaflets mounted within the stent to maximize leaflet opening and to reduce abrasion between the leaflet and the stent.[8]

Stentless Biologic Prostheses

The development of stentless bioprostheses progressed with the desire to improve hemodynamics and long-term durability and preserve the benefits afforded by a tissue valve. The removal of the stent and sewing cuff permit the implantation of a relatively larger valve as compared with a stented biologic or mechanical valve of the same circumference. In addition, removal of the stent appears to significantly reduce stress at the base of the leaflets, which reduces calcification and slows valve degeneration. These valves are used only in the aortic position in which the patient's annulus and aortic root provide support and flexibility to the implanted materials. The typical stentless valve is comprised of an intact porcine aortic valve with an outer layer of polyester fabric to lend support and to facilitate implantation (Figure 11–5). Prior to the addition of the fabric, the valves are processed at very low fixation pressures to maintain collagen pliability. In addition, the Medtronic Freestyle valve is treated with amino-oleic acid to decrease calcium deposition. Several stentless valves are currently available, including the Toronto SPV (St. Jude Medical, St. Paul, MN), Medtronic Freestyle (Medtronic, Minneapolis, MN), and the CryoLife-O'Brien (CryoLife, Kennesaw, GA). These valves are technically more challenging to implant, and the exact surgical technique depends on how much of the recipient's aortic root and native sinus tissue are used in the process (full root technique with reimplantation of the coronary arteries, the root inclusion technique with preservation of the native coronary arteries, or a complete subcoronary or modified subcoronary technique).

The operative mortality rate for the stentless valves is slightly higher than that for other biologic valves (3% to 6%) partly due to the increased complexity of surgical technique. However, stentless valves have a very favorable 12-month complication rate (low rates of endocarditis, thrombosis, and hemorrhage) and survival rate of 91 ± 4% at 6 years. Currently, the engineered durability has held true, with no reported structural failures.[9]

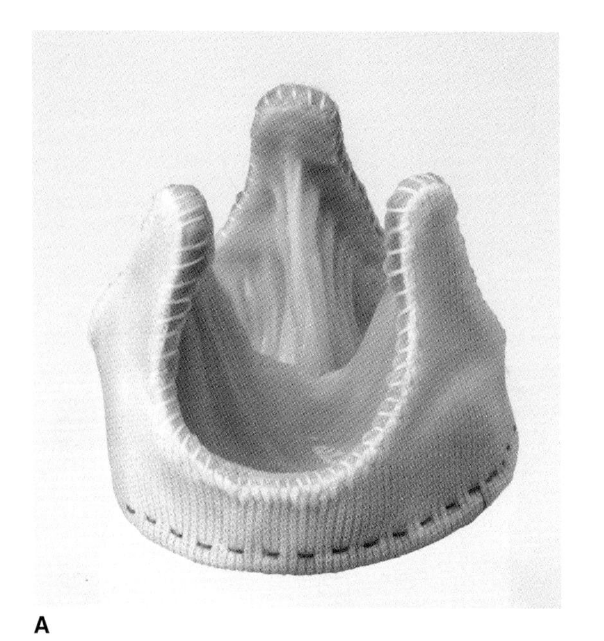
A

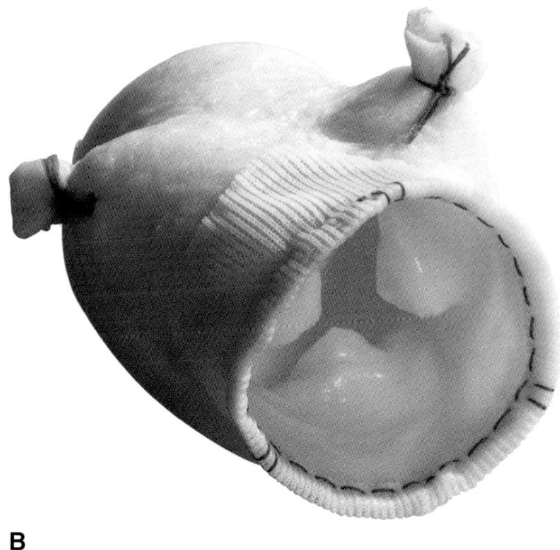
B

FIGURE 11–5. Stentless bioprostheses. **A:** Toronto SPV valve (St. Jude Medical). **B:** Medtronic Freestyle valve (Medtronic). *(Reproduced with permission from St. Jude Medical and Medtronic, Inc.)*

HOMOGRAFTS AND AUTOGRAFTS

Homografts (human cadaveric tissue) are collected from the aortic and pulmonic positions within 24 hours of donor death and are treated with antibiotics before sterilization and preservation in liquid nitrogen at −196°C. These valves provide excellent hemodynamics, have low rates of thrombogenesis, are relatively resistant to infection, and are therefore ideal for use in the setting of acute native or prosthetic endocarditis.[10,11] However, these cryopreserved valves are subject to accelerated degeneration as compared with native and mechanical valves. In addition, they require ongoing cryopreservation, have limited availability (most institutions carry a limited number of sizes, if at all), and require additional surgical time if the valve is not sized and thawed until the annulus is directly measured after arrest of the heart rather than relying on TEE valve sizing.[12] The implantation of a homograft requires a highly skilled surgeon. Mitral homografts have been attempted in the past, but are no longer common.

Pulmonary autograft for aortic valve replacement (Ross procedure) uses the patient's native pulmonic valve and proximal main pulmonary artery to replace the diseased aortic valve and ascending aorta, with reimplantation of the native coronary arteries into the neo-ascending aorta. A stentless homograft (or other bioprosthesis) is usually placed in the pulmonic position so that anticoagulation is not required in the long term. Autografts are used most commonly in children, adolescents, adults with a longer than 20-year life expectancy, and those individuals in whom long-term anticoagulation is contraindicated or unwanted because of lifestyle factors.[2,3] These valves have excellent hemodynamic profiles and are extremely durable with the "life expectancy" of a native valve. Limitations to its use include a technically more complex operation with the necessary replacement of two heart valves and the degeneration and/or obstruction of the new "pulmonic" valve and proximal pulmonary artery necessitating reoperation.

Transcatheter Aortic Valves

Endovascular transcatheter aortic valve implantation (TAVI) has recently become an option for those patients with calcific aortic stenosis who were previously deemed to be too high risk for a conventional valve replacement. The combination of advanced age with multiple comorbidities including renal, pulmonary, and cerebrovascular dysfunction increases the operative risk to over 2[illegible]%.[10] Following the first successful human implant in 2002, several different techniques have been developed (antegrade–transapical, and retrograde–transarterial) to more safely position and deploy the expandable bovine pericardial valves.

Currently there are two types of TAVI valves. The balloon expandable bovine pericardial "Sapien" valve (Figure 11–6) (Edwards Lifesciences, Irvine, California) is mounted onto a stainless steel stent and comes in two sizes (23 and 26 mm). The 23-mm valve is preferred for annular diameters of 18 to 21 mm, and the larger 26-mm valve for larger annular diameters up to 24 mm. The CoreValve (Medtronic, Minneapolis, MN) is also manufactured using bovine pericardium, but it is mounted on a self expanding Nitinol stent and is available in two sizes: a 26-mm valve for an annulus diameter of 20 to 23 mm, and a 29-mm valve for a 23- to 27-mm annulus. The valve chosen must be larger than the annulus diameter to reduce the risk of paravalvular leaks while allowing adequate anchoring of the valve system.

Proper positioning of these valves is critical. Incorrect positioning can lead to embolization into the left ventricular cavity or anywhere along the aorta, paravalvular leaks, coronary ostial obstruction, or interference with the mitral valve (native or prosthetic). Both fluoroscopy and TEE are utilized in many centers, with TEE becoming the preferred imaging modality because of its versatility. TEE allows for a full assessment of ventricular function, a complete evaluation of all valves, sizing of the annulus and other structures, measurement of gradients, and quantification of trans- or paravalvular regurgitant jets. Echocardiography can also be

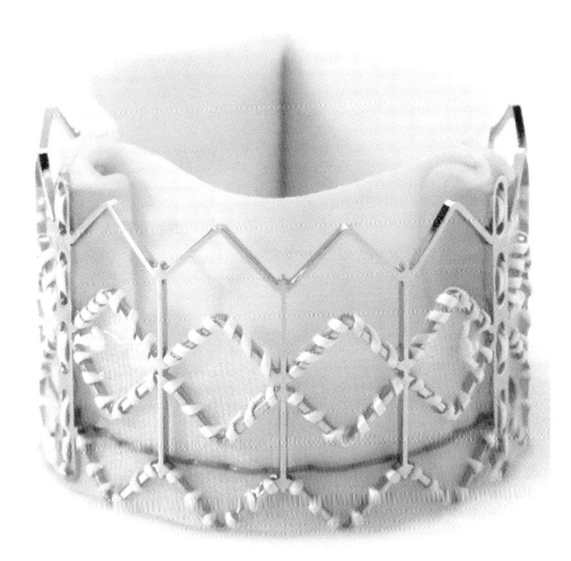

FIGURE 11–6. Sapien Transcatheter Aortic Valve Replacement bioprostheses (Edwards Lifesciences). *(Reproduced with permission from Edwards Lifesciences Inc.)*

utilized to direct the advancement of guidewires and delivery devices prior to and during the placement and delivery of the valve.[14]

TEE EVALUATION OF PROSTHETIC HEART VALVES

The evaluation of patients with prosthetic valves begins with an understanding of the patient's symptoms, which often provide clues to the expected pathology. It is also important to record the blood pressure, heart rate, and cardiac output (when available) since Doppler-derived gradients are dependent upon flow and diastolic filling time. Finally, the height, weight, and body surface should be noted in order to assess patient-prosthesis mismatch and cardiac chamber size.[15]

Evaluation of prosthetic heart valves using TEE can be technically challenging, but it provides a vitally important means to image and interrogate the normal and abnormal structure and function of an implanted valve prosthesis. Rather than being a "standalone" technique, TEE often complements methods such as fluoroscopy, magnetic resonance imaging, transthoracic echocardiography (TTE), and catheterization studies in the evaluation and routine follow-up of patients with prosthetic heart valves.[1] TEE is minimally invasive, especially in the intraoperative setting, and provides superior 2D images as compared with traditional TTE because of the use of higher-frequency probes, the proximity of the ultrasound beam to the area of interest, and the lack of intervening structures to absorb or interfere with the beam. The development of real-time three-dimensional TEE (RT3DTEE) has also been shown to be beneficial in the assessment of indwelling prostheses.[16,17]

Synthetic materials (metals, plastics, fabrics, and pyrolytic carbon) on prosthetic valves present distinct challenges to a thorough echocardiographic examination. Interference with ultrasound transmission and reflection can produce several types of artifacts that make comprehensive assessment challenging. While mechanical valves are more prone to imaging artifacts, biologic valves also include synthetic components that can generate similar difficulties. Ultrasound artifacts are directly related to the reflective and absorptive properties of the prosthetic materials employed. In addition, the speed of sound through the synthetic materials may be faster or slower than that through human tissue, which can lead to alterations in the displayed size and location of the image. One must always keep these artifacts and imaging limitations in mind to avoid the misinterpretation of information that can result in false or missed diagnoses.

Reverberation artifact and acoustic shadowing (see Chapter 3) can conceal anatomic structures distal to the reflector and often render CFD evaluation impossible. The ability to place the transducer directly posterior to the left atrium with TEE allows for an unobstructed view of the mitral surface of the prosthesis and a comprehensive Doppler evaluation. From the midesophageal position, all shadowing and reverberation artifacts reside on the ventricular aspect of the valve. Similarly, the transgastric and deep transgastric views usually allow for the evaluation of the ventricular aspect of the valve, with the artifacts now located within the atria.

TEE imaging of prosthetic valves is not different from regular ultrasound imaging. The best 2D images are generated when the reflector is perpendicular to the ultrasound beam, whereas accurate Doppler studies require an angle of interrogation of less than 20° from parallel to the jet or flow. The measurement of transprosthetic gradients and flows using Doppler ultrasound follows the same limitations and caveats described in Chapters 7, 9, and 10, namely that it may be difficult to obtain the proper position or angle to locate the maximal jet or flow. The multiplane transducer frequently needs to be rotated to adjust the ultrasound beam so that imaging artifacts are minimized and proper identification of normal and pathologic structures can be elucidated. The acquisition of 3D images is described in Chapter 24.

Normal TEE Findings in Prosthetic Valves

While all prosthetic valves are obstructive by the nature of their design, each class and subclass of valve has unique echocardiographic structural characteristics that can be used to identify the specific type, and subsequently the proper function, of the valve. Regardless of the type of valve undergoing evaluation, a complete examination includes imaging the area in question with a variety of views to obtain an accurate assessment. Although usually not immediately available in the operating room setting, comparisons with previous studies can be invaluable in the evaluation of a prosthetic valve. Flow patterns and transvalvular gradients can change over time and new findings should be compared with previous measurements.[18,19]

Additionally, there are special considerations unique to the intraoperative setting. Loading conditions often fluctuate in the immediate post-CPB phase, making transvalvular gradients difficult to quantify. Moreover, frequent changes in inotrope levels and pacing strategies also result in changing hemodynamics. These must all be considered while interpreting the results of Doppler-based measurements.[15]

2D Imaging

The sewing ring (if any) should be examined for movement. A rocking motion is suggestive of valve dehiscence, loose or fractured sutures, or a perivalvular abscess. The periannular area is often somewhat obscured by calcification or artifacts from the valve itself. However, it is important to check for small periannular or perivalvular echolucent areas that may indicate fistula or abscess formation. Frequently, the aortic root can appear thickened as a result of hematoma or edema after surgery. This appearance may be prone to misinterpretation and should be distinguished from an abscess.[15] Next, valve leaflet or occluding device motion is evaluated. Mechanical occluders should move rapidly and extend to the full limit of the design specifications. Restricted or incomplete opening is suggestive of primary valve dysfunction or of an obstructing material or object (suture material, perivalvular tissue, pannus, thrombus, endocarditis, vegetations, or masses). In addition, residual periannular materials may interfere with the proper closure of the occluders of mechanical prostheses resulting in significant regurgitation through the valve (Figure 11–7). The leaflets on a biologic valve should be thin and have the same appearance as native nondiseased leaflets. A close inspection for tears, perforations, thickening, and calcification should be carried out. Information from the rest of the TEE examination should be incorporated into the assessment of the prosthetic valve. Left atrial "smoke," or thrombus, is suggestive of a functionally stenotic mitral prosthesis. Similarly, LV dilation or LV hypertrophy with new native mitral regurgitation could be suggestive of prosthetic aortic regurgitation or stenosis, respectively.

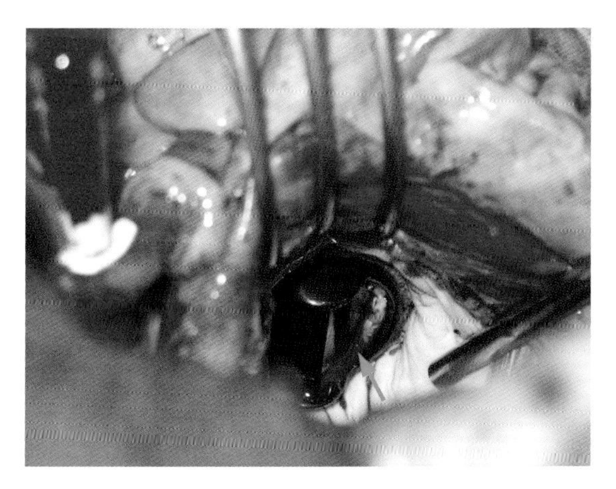

FIGURE 11–7. Periannular tissue (remnant of posterior leaflet; *arrow*) trapped between sewing ring and occluder of a dual tilting disk mechanical prosthesis. The patient had moderate mitral regurgitation within the sewing ring on TEE immediately following the termination of CPB. Subsequent excision of the redundant tissue resulted in no regurgitation other than the washing jets.

Epicardial Echocardiography

Infrequently an intraoperative TEE exam cannot be performed because either a TEE probe could not be inserted or there was a contraindication to probe insertion. In these circumstances, the evaluation of prosthetic valves can be performed using epicardial echocardiography (EE). The performance of a complete EE exam is discussed further in Chapter 20 and in the guidelines published by the American Society of Echocardiography and the Society of Cardiovascular Anesthesiologists.[20] Although not specifically outlined in these guidelines, the majority of normal cardiac structures (including prosthetic materials) can be visualized using a high-frequency epicardial ultrasound probe.

3D Imaging

The sequential evaluation of prosthetic valves using 3D TEE is similar to that of the 2D examination (see Chapter 24). The evaluation of both the prosthesis and the peri-prosthetic structures using 3D echocardiography may facilitate interrogation of structures that are difficult and/or impossible with regular 2D imaging alone. The ability to take a large volume sample, and crop then rotate the image frequently provides improved visualization of structures opposite the transducer, small perivalvular leaks, leaflet/occluder problems, and thrombi/vegetations. Evaluation of both biologic and mechanical prostheses by 3D echocardiography is both feasible and accurate (96% correlation with surgical findings), especially in the presurgical assessment. However, 3D TEE is subject to the same limitations of 2D TEE with regard to ultrasound artifacts.[16,17]

Color-Flow and Spectral Doppler

A full color-flow and spectral Doppler examination should be carried out on all prosthetic valves. Care should be taken to properly align the transducer and use appropriate machine settings to ensure that the results are truly representative of the actual in vivo flows and gradients. Normally functioning tissue valves typically have no regurgitation. However, trivial to mild central regurgitant jets are visible about 10% of the time and are considered normal.[3] Rarely, trace jets may originate from the commissures. New, significant regurgitant jets in tissue valves may signal leaflet degeneration. A moderate to severe regurgitant jet immediately after separation from cardiopulmonary bypass (CPB) may suggest a leaflet tethered by an annular suture (Figure 11–8) or an improperly sized, stentless prosthesis.

All mechanical valves, except for the Starr-Edwards, have normal "washing jets" that originate from between the occluder device and the support ring, which are

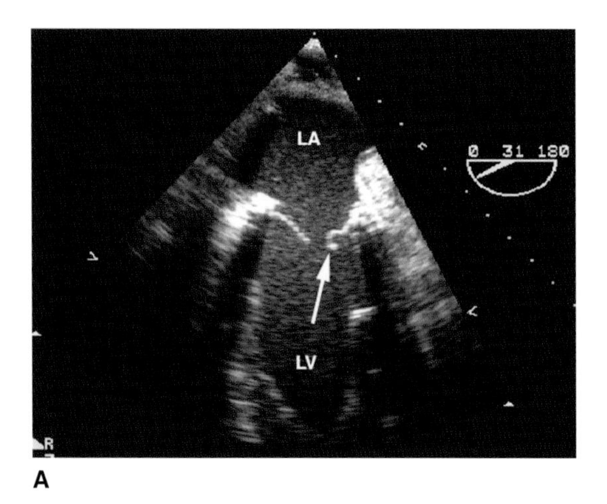

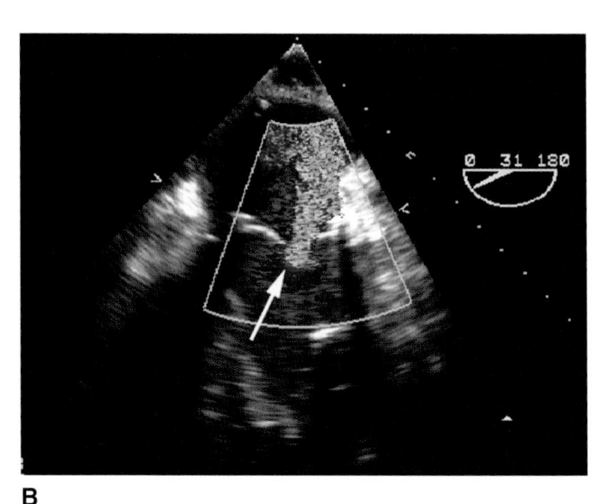

FIGURE 11–8. Mitral prosthetic leaflet tethered by an annular suture *(arrow)* leading to severe regurgitation *(arrow)*. **A:** Tethered leaflet. **B:** Severe regurgitation. (LA, left atrium; LV, left ventricle.)

designed to help reduce the incidence of thrombus formation on the underside of the prosthesis (Figure 11–9). These jets are considered normal if they are shorter than 2.5 cm and are trivial to mild in nature.[1,19] An exception to this rule is the Medtronic-Hall single tilting disk valve in which the central regurgitant jet can be as long as 5 cm. The number of these jets is variable, depending on the angle of interrogation; however, one to two jets are most commonly seen, but up to five have been reported. Depending on the type of valve in question, up to a 10% to 15% regurgitant fraction is considered within the design limits. Moderate to severe

FIGURE 11–9. Normal "washing jets" *(arrows)* in a bileaflet tilting disk (St. Jude) valve originating at the leaflet hinge points. (MV, mitral valve.)

regurgitant flow can be seen in mechanical valves with malfunctioning or restricted occluding devices. In addition, mechanical valves exhibit what is referred to as *closure backflow*. This is the small volume of retrograde flow that forces the occluding device(s) closed. It is considered a normal finding and appears as a very brief regurgitant flash immediately within the area of the valve. With mechanical valves, a few microbubbles (microcavitations) may also be seen in the LV. Mechanical and tissue prostheses can exhibit perivalvular leaks, which are suggestive of valve ring or annular dehiscence or endocarditis.

Spectral Doppler assessment of prosthetic valves is mandatory following implantation. Routine evaluation of prostheses should include an estimation of valve gradients using the Bernoulli equation and calculation of the effective orifice area (EOA) using the continuity equation:

$$\text{EOA} = \frac{Q}{\text{VTI}}$$

where Q represents stroke volume through a reference site proximal or distal to the valve and VTI refers to the velocity-time integral across the valve. The label size of the prosthetic valve is not considered a valid substitute for the cross-sectional area of the annulus.[15] Using the *simplified* Bernoulli equation (peak pressure gradient equals four times the square of the peak velocity: $\Delta P = 4V^2$) can yield high trans-prosthesis pressure gradients. It must be remembered that this equation does not account for the velocity proximal to the valve, which can be elevated, especially for prosthetic valves in the aortic position. Higher left ventricular outflow tract (LVOT) velocities should be accounted for by using the *modified* Bernoulli equation to obtain an accurate gradient [$\Delta P = 4(V_2^2 - V_1^2)$, where V_1 is the peak LVOT velocity and V_2 is the peak transvalvular velocity].[15]

TEE ASSESSMENT OF VALVES BY TYPE

The standard 2D, color-flow, and spectral Doppler findings for each type of prosthesis are described in detail in the following sections.

Mechanical Valves

BALL-IN-CAGE

The silastic ball of the Starr-Edwards valve may demonstrate one or several intense echoes generated from its leading edge, which frequently obliterate or mask the other prosthetic components. It is uncommon to be able to visualize the U-shaped struts, whereas the sewing or support ring can almost always be seen. This valve is identified most easily by the detection of a large, rapidly moving, echo-dense structure that passes in and out of the imaging plane, casting a broad distal acoustic shadow. When color-flow Doppler is applied, highly turbulent blood flow is seen to originate from the lateral edges of the support ring as the blood circumnavigates the high-profile ball (Figure 11–10). Small retrograde eddies at the periphery also may be seen. With pressure equalization and valve closure, a trivial to small amount of central closure backflow (2 to 5 mL) can be appreciated with CFD. Once seated, the snug fit of the ball into the supporting ring limits further retrograde backflow.

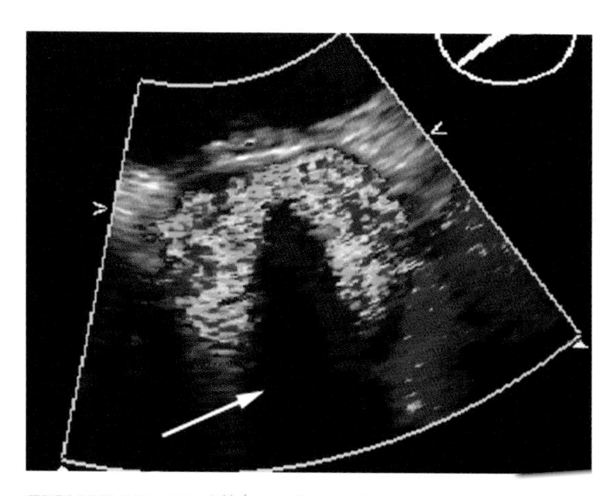

FIGURE 11–10. Midesophageal aortic valve short-axis view of a ball-in-cage (Starr-Edwards) valve in the aortic position shows the highly turbulent blood flow emanating from the lateral edges of the support ring as the blood circumnavigates the high-profile ball. The silastic ball in turn leaves a broad acoustic shadow *(arrow)*.

Spectral Doppler interrogation shows moderately high antegrade pressure gradients along the edges of the prosthesis as compared with tilting disk and bileaflet valves.[5]

TILTING DISK

All single tilting disk prostheses have an occluder with an asymmetrical opening pattern. Identification of particular subtypes can be extremely difficult when using 2D TEE because all have an identical pattern of motion and overall appearance. The echocardiographer must be methodical in attempts to image the prosthesis by using the long- and short-axis views with fine adjustments of the multiplane transducer to provide a satisfactory evaluation of occluder motion. M-mode evaluation may be helpful because the 2D frame rate is almost always too slow to accurately represent the pattern of occluder motion. In case of difficulties in identifying the actual number of disk occluders, it is helpful to know that tilting disks travel farther into the antegrade side than bileaflet occluders. Prostheses in the mitral position are frequently oriented with the major orifice facing the lateral wall. Tilting disk prostheses in the aortic position are placed in a manner such that the antegrade flow through the major orifice is directed toward the greater curvature of the aortic arch.

Color-flow Doppler allows differentiation between the Medtronic-Hall valve and the Bjork-Shiley and OmniScience valves. The Medtronic-Hall valve has been engineered with a central hinge and perforation in the occluder that results in a narrow central regurgitant jet (Figure 11–11) with the prosthesis in the closed position, whereas the other valves do not. With the valve in the open position, major and minor orifices often can be visualized, with the minor orifice possessing a more turbulent flow pattern. Spectral Doppler demonstrates

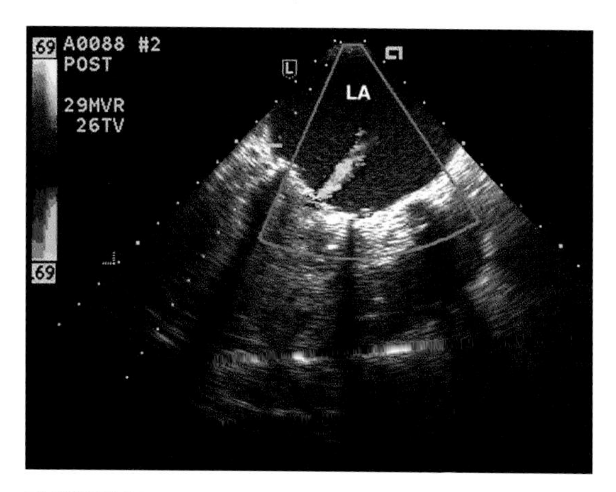

FIGURE 11–11. Narrow central regurgitant jet seen in a normal Medtronic-Hall valve in the closed position. (LA, left atrium.)

a lower peak and mean gradient as compared with the ball-in-cage design because the disk occluder is less of an obstruction to antegrade flow.[6] The average gradient for each valve type is dependent on the size and location of the prosthesis, and on the compliance and function of the left ventricle (see Appendix F and G for a more detailed listing). Spectral CWD should be directed through the lateral orifices of these valves.

Bileaflet

Two-dimensional evaluation of bileaflet prostheses (St. Jude, Carbomedics, On-X) is similar to that described for tilting disk prostheses. One must ensure that all available imaging planes are used to properly evaluate the prosthesis and keep the valve centered on the screen with the beam bisecting the support ring. When imaging in the long axis, rapid simultaneous oscillating hemidisks with variably shaped, distal acoustic shadows are seen.[12,18] For mitral valve replacement, surgeons generally position these valves in an "anatomic" orientation, with the occluder pivot points located where the anterolateral and posteromedial commissures previously resided in the mitral position. In the aortic position, one pivot point is usually located at the junction of the left and noncoronary sinuses of Valsalva with the other positioned opposite to it in the mid–right sinus. Alternatively, others attempt to position the valve so that flow from the outflow tract is evenly divided between the two major orifices.

When the ultrasound beam is perpendicular to the plane of the sewing ring, a distinctive V pattern is generated by the occluding disks on 2D imaging (Figure 11–12). It is from this orientation that color-flow and spectral analyses are best performed. Color flow demonstrates a reasonably laminar antegrade flow pattern through the two major orifices. Upon disk closure, two regurgitant jets that converge to form a "V" on the low-pressure side of the valve (see Figure 11–9) are commonly seen at the periphery between the occluders and the sewing ring. All regurgitant jets are generally short and are of a low velocity. The CWD beam should be directed along the major orifices toward the lateral edge of the prosthesis. Spectral Doppler consistently demonstrates that the bileaflet valves have the lowest gradient (flow velocities in the 2 m/s range) for any comparably sized mechanical valve. Three-dimensional imaging, especially in the mitral position, clearly identifies the two disks and enables assessment of disk motion with ease (Figure 11–13). The On-X valve has a unique echocardiographic appearance that can lead to misinterpretation of normal echo findings. The leaflet guards in this valve are commonly seen on a short-axis image (Figure 11–14) and should not be confused with the leaflets themselves.

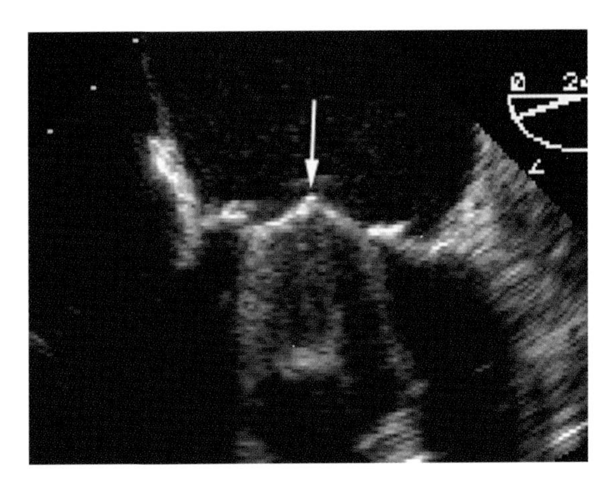

FIGURE 11–12. Characteristic V pattern produced by the occluding disks of a bileaflet tilting disk valve. The arrow points to the hinge point of the V.

Furthermore, the profile of the inlet flare can cause extensive shadowing in the LVOT, and the diastolic washing jets are directed away from the central axis of the valve and towards the walls of the LVOT (see Figure 11–14).[7] In contrast, the washing jets in the St. Jude bileaflet valve are typically directed inward, towards the central axis of the valve.

Biologic Valves

Stented Valves

Hancock and Carpentier-Edwards valves appear similar on 2D imaging. At each commissure, a strut is usually visible, appearing as a narrow echogenic structure. All three struts are usually visible within the same view (Figure 11–15). A strong reflective signal is obtained from the support ring when the beam is directed through the annulus. In long-axis views, the leaflets appear similar to native leaflets. The struts now appear as linear reflectors arising from the highly reflective support ring. In general, one can view only two struts at a time due to the finite thickness of the ultrasound beam. Acoustic shadowing and reverberation artifact from the support ring interferes with the acquisition of usable information from the area immediately distal to the ring.

Color-flow Doppler usually demonstrates nonturbulent antegrade flow, with little to no central regurgitation after valve closure. Different interrogation angles may be necessary to remove imaging artifacts out of the area of interest. These valves generally have a low to moderate peak and mean gradients, which are inversely related to prosthesis size. Three-dimensional imaging

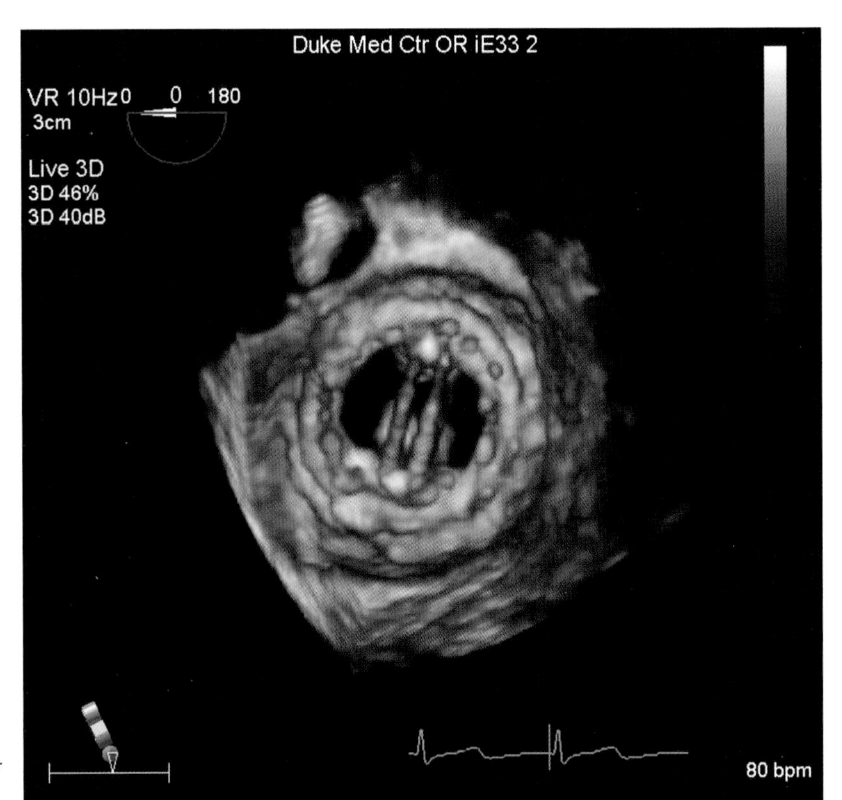

FIGURE 11–13. Three-dimensional image of a bileaflet valve clearly demonstrating the sewing ring, two disks, and the minor and major orifices.

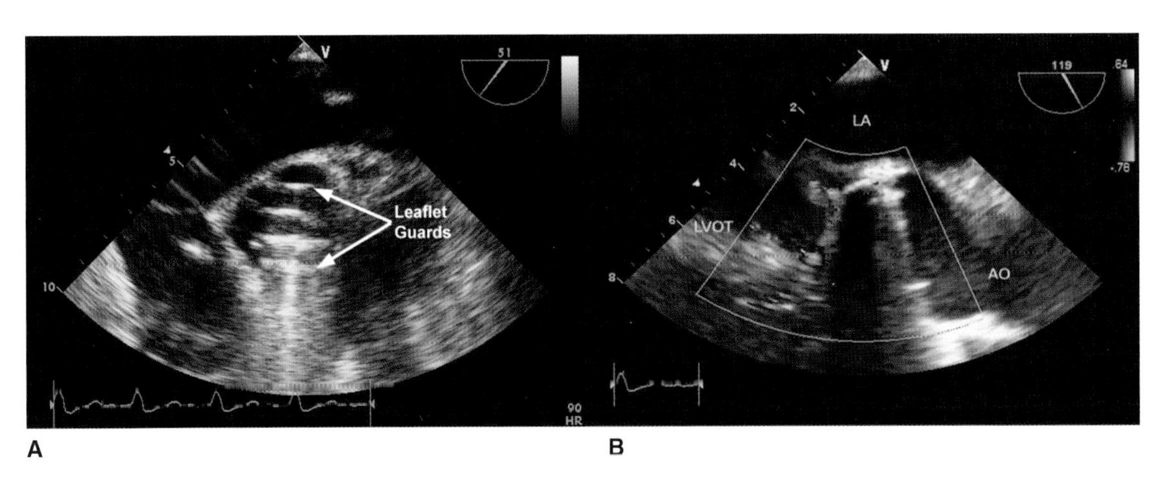

FIGURE 11–14. Two-dimensional image **(A)** of an On-X valve in short axis demonstrating the leaflet guards *(arrows)* with the two disks in between the guards. Color-flow Doppler imaging **(B)** demonstrating the outwardly directed washing jets. (LA, left atrium; LVOT, left ventricular outflow tract; AO, aorta.) *(Courtesy of Dr. Aman Mahajan.)*

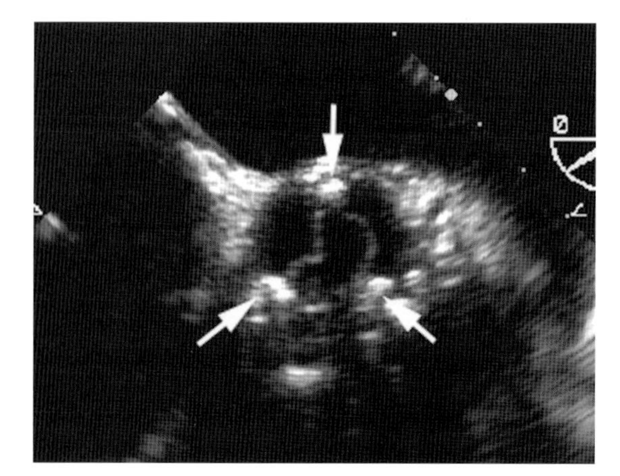

FIGURE 11–15. Midesophageal aortic valve short-axis view of a stented biologic valve in the aortic position. The struts *(arrows)* and the partly open leaflets often are seen clearly in this view.

again provides superior imaging in the mitral position (Figure 11–16).

STENTLESS VALVES

These valves are usually difficult to distinguish from native valves, except for an increase in echo signal from the annulus and around the base of the leaflets. Other 2D findings depend on the surgical technique used to implant the valve. When the root inclusion technique is used, the ascending aorta often can appear to be thicker in the area of the aortic root and proximal ascending aorta because the wall now contains layers from the prosthesis and the native aorta (a tube within a tube; Figure 11–17). In the immediate postoperative period, blood, fluid, or thrombus may occupy the potential space between these two layers, and very rarely has caused problems with valve function. This potential space usually disappears within the first few postoperative months.[3,9] Color-flow and spectral Doppler signals from stentless prostheses are similar to those from native valves.[6]

HOMOGRAFTS AND AUTOGRAFTS

These valves can also be very difficult to distinguish from native valves. A small to moderate increase in echogenicity is frequently noted at the annulus from suture material and accelerated calcification. Doppler signals are comparable to stentless prostheses and should be similar to that of native valves.

PERCUTANEOUS AORTIC VALVES

Prior to the placement of an expandable biologic valve in the aortic position, a complete echocardiographic exam is mandatory. Assessment of LV and valvular function should be comprehensive, and LVOT/annular dimensions, aortic valve areas, and gradients should be recorded. During the positioning of the valve, TEE can be used to monitor advancement of guidewires and the delivery device, evaluate the location of the prosthesis, determine complications (tamponade, dissection, device malposition) and observe the LV for dilation/overload following balloon valvuloplasty of the native aortic valve.

Following the deployment of the valve, both long- and short-axis midesophageal aortic valve views should

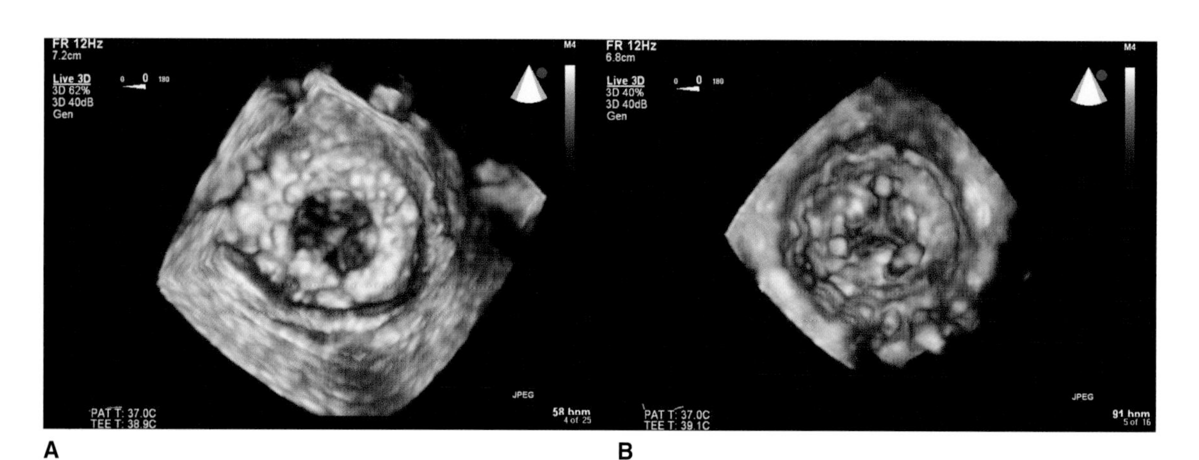

FIGURE 11–16. Three-dimensional image of a stented bioprosthetic valve in the mitral position viewed from the left atrium **(A)** and left ventricle **(B)**.

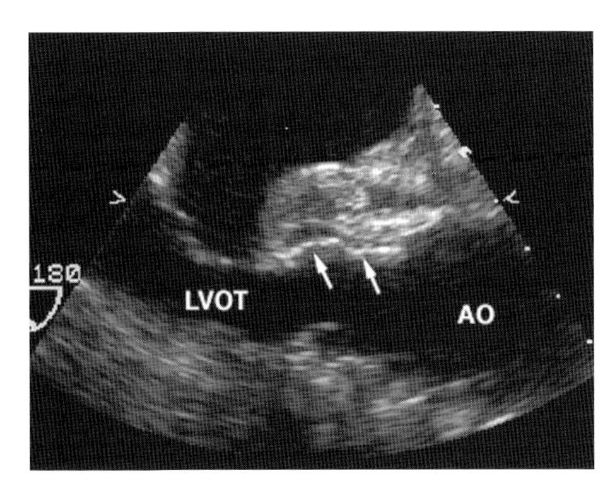

FIGURE 11–17. Stentless aortic valve. The area of the aortic root and proximal ascending aorta appear thicker *(arrows)* because the wall now contains layers from the prosthesis and the native aorta. (LVOT, left ventricular outflow tract; AO, aorta.)

be obtained to assess the final position of the device. The assessment of these valves (Sapien and CoreValve) is similar to that of biologic valves with respect to the leaflets. Significant artifact from the metal stents in which they are housed may require multiple angles and views for a thorough assessment (Figure 11–18). Other important features of a complete evaluation include assessment of leaflet function using 2D or 3D imaging, measurement of transvalvular gradients using CWD,

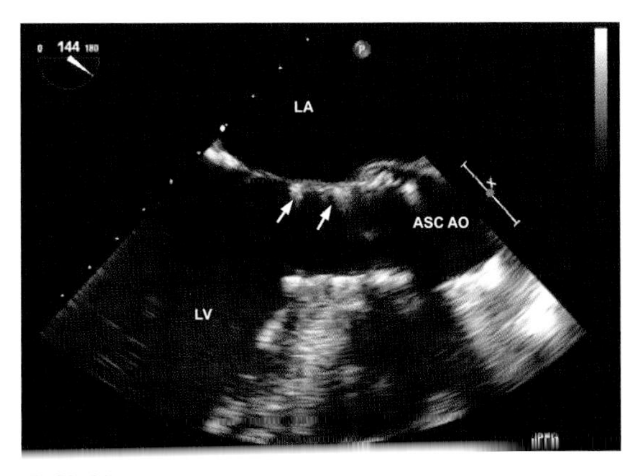

FIGURE 11–18. Two-dimensional image of a percutaneous aortic valve (CoreValve) demonstrating the acoustic shadowing *(arrows)* from the Nitinol stent. (LV, left ventricle; LA, left atrium; ASC AO, ascending aorta.) *(Courtesy of Dr. Johan Bence and Dr. Justiaan Swanevelder.)*

and an evaluation of any transvalvular (within the stent) or paravalvular (around the stent) leaks.

SITE-SPECIFIC QUALITATIVE AND QUANTITATIVE ANALYSES

The various techniques for assessment of stenotic or regurgitant native valves described in Chapters 7, 9, and 10 can be used or modified to evaluate prosthetic valves. The physical principles of the continuity equation, modified Bernoulli equation, mean gradients, velocity-time integral (VTI) ratios, pressure half-times (PHTs), and specific flow characteristics are also applicable to implanted valves. Readers are encouraged to refer to the aforementioned chapters for a complete discussion on the qualitative and quantitative assessments of regurgitant or stenotic lesions.

Mitral Position

TEE is particularly suited for the complete imaging and interrogation of prostheses in the mitral position. Midesophageal views allow for unobstructed imaging of the left atrial side for assessment of regurgitation, paravalvular leaks, and mechanical occluder motion.[21] Transgastric and deep transgastric views generally afford views of the ventricular aspects of prostheses, thus enabling confirmation of previously gleaned information.

EOA is derived for a prosthetic mitral valve as the stroke volume through the valve divided by the VTI of the transmitral flow:

$$\text{EOA (cm}^2) = \frac{\text{Stroke Volume}}{\text{VTI}_{\text{Valve}}}$$

where, in the absence of significant mitral or aortic regurgitation, stroke volume can be measured at the LVOT. EOA can be underestimated in bileaflet mechanical valves since the peak velocity measured with CWD includes the higher velocity seen in the smaller central orifice.

Use of the pressure half-time constant of 220 milliseconds in the assessment of a stenotic prosthetic valve overestimates the EOA because this number was derived from studies in native stenotic valves and not validated in prosthetic valves.[22] However, a single pressure half-time value greater than 200 milliseconds or a consistent value in excess of 130 milliseconds may indicate pathologic obstruction.

When interpreting velocities across prosthetic valves in the mitral position, one must differentiate an increase in transvalvular velocity due to mitral regurgitation from prosthetic valve stenosis and high output states. The absence of a regurgitant jet or presence of appropriately moving leaflets would obviously suggest a high output state. Another measurement that has been proposed to help in this differentiation is the ratio of VTI across the mitral valve to the VTI across the LVOT (VTI_{MV}/VTI_{LVOT}). A normal ratio suggests a high output state since the velocity is increased across the MV and the LVOT, while a high ratio indicates either prosthetic mitral stenosis or regurgitation. A value greater than 2.2 should prompt the search for pathology.[15] Significant prosthetic mitral stenosis is suggested by (1) peak transmitral velocity of 2.5 m/s or greater, (2) mean gradient greater than 10 mm Hg, (3) VTI_{MV}/VTI_{LVOT} greater than 2.5, (4) EOA less than 1 cm^2, and (5) PHT greater than 200 milliseconds.[15]

In the absence of significant mitral regurgitation, the continuity equation is a valid and better method than using pressure half-time for determining the area of the mitral prosthesis. This may be explained by the fact that most prostheses, with the exception of the annuloplasty rings, are circular in nature. Thus, the assumption of mitral annular circularity in the calculation of the continuity equation is satisfied. Comparisons with previous studies and knowledge of the normal parameters are extremely important in distinguishing a normal from a dysfunctional valve. Indicators of severe mitral prosthetic regurgitation include (1) increased inflow velocities with normal pressure half-time, (2) dense regurgitant CWD signal, (3) pulmonary vein systolic flow reversal, (4) regurgitant jet greater than 40% of the left atrial area or a jet area greater than 8 cm^2, (5) regurgitant volume 60 mL or greater, (6) regurgitant fraction 50% or greater, (7) effective regurgitant orifice 0.5 cm^2 or greater, and (8) vena contracta greater than 0.6 cm.[2,6,15,23] Since regurgitant lesions may involve a dehiscence of the valve suture line, it is imperative to examine the valve from all possible angles with 2D and CFD to determine the origin of the jet.

Aortic Position

A full and accurate evaluation of aortic prostheses usually can be obtained with TEE. Proper interrogation using 2D, 3D, color-flow, and spectral Doppler sometimes can be challenging, even for experienced echocardiographers, because of artifact interference and image acquisition. In the midesophageal planes, the sewing or support ring and/or stents from prosthetic valves are interposed between the transducer and the valve orifice, resulting in unavoidable artifacts in the area of interest. When attempting to evaluate the prosthesis for regurgitation or paravalvular leaks, or for spectral Doppler interrogation, the transgastric long-axis (110° to 130°) and deep transgastric long-axis views are often very helpful. These views remove the echo artifacts out of the region of the LVOT and provide for a more parallel alignment between the CWD or PWD beam and transvalvular flow. However, this places the sample volume in the far field, which predisposes to aliasing and sampling errors. Small manipulations of the probe tip and fine adjustments of the multiplane transducer in all views generally allows for visualization of most, if not all, relevant structures.

Prosthetic aortic valve replacement requires measurement of the aortic annulus. The echocardiographer first obtains a midesophageal long-axis view of the aortic valve and LVOT with the depth setting set so that the structures in question fill the screen. The image is frozen and the frames are advanced sequentially until maximal valve opening is visualized (usually mid-systole on electrocardiography), and the calipers are placed at the junction of the aortic valve leaflet and the LVOT on each side. Several measurements should be made to ensure an accurate assessment; the LVOT is a three-dimensional structure shaped like a cylinder and care should be taken that the measurement is taken at the widest part of the cylinder. When a stentless biologic valve is to be placed, the diameter of the sinotubular junction (STJ) also needs to be carefully measured (Figure 11–19).[5] This usually can be accomplished in the same view used for the measurement of the aortic annulus. The STJ diameter is generally about 80% of the annular diameter. If the STJ is dilated, the stentless valve leaflets will have a tendency to separate centrally during diastole secondary to a lack of lateral support from the dilated proximal ascending aorta. If the STJ or ascending aorta is significantly dilated, the surgeon should consider a composite prosthesis that incorporates the ascending aorta. The Ross procedure deserves special mention because the TEE-derived measurements of the aortic annulus, pulmonic annulus, and STJ may determine whether the surgery actually proceeds or whether an alternative prosthetic valve type is selected. If there is a significant mismatch between the pulmonic valve (which is to become the neo-aortic valve) and the aortic annulus or STJ, the valve likely will be incompetent because of distortion of the valve and its leaflets. Post-bypass regional wall motion abnormalities may also be present in these patients, especially in the basal anteroseptal region, due to compromise of the septal perforator branch as it arises from the left ascending descending artery (LAD) in close proximity to the pulmonic valve.

Use of the continuity equation in aortic prostheses has been validated and can be useful to measure the EOA. Applied to the aortic position, the equation is expressed as:

$$\text{EOA (cm}^2\text{)} = \frac{(\text{VTI}_{\text{LVOT}} \times \text{Area}_{\text{LVOT}})}{\text{VTI}_{\text{Valve}}}$$

An EOA of less than 0.8 cm^2 usually suggests stenosis. However, this value may be considered normal for some

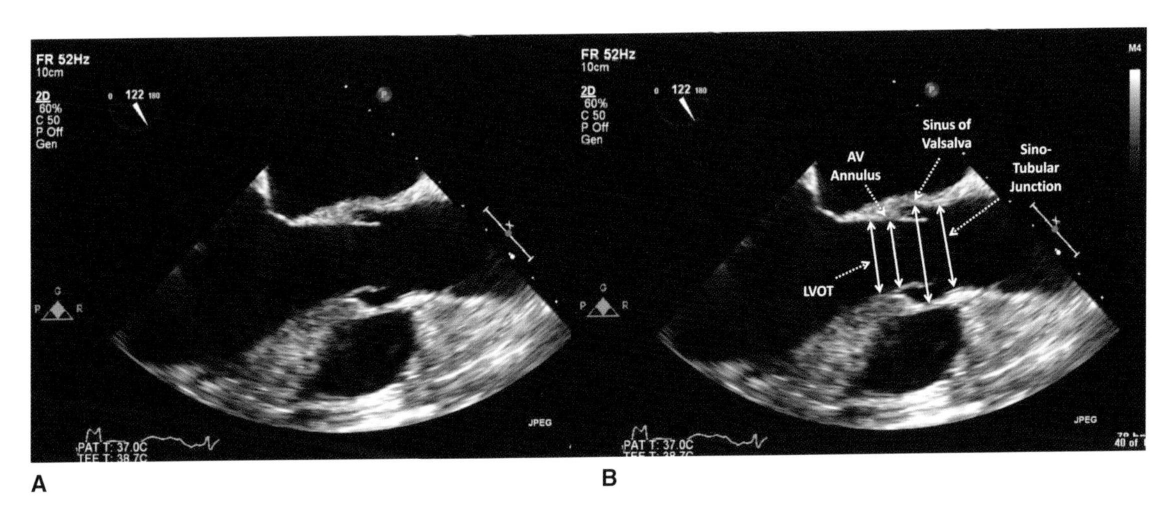

FIGURE 11–19. Midesophageal aortic valve long-axis view shown as a mid-systolic frame (panel **A**) and with relevant measurements (panel **B**). (AV, aortic valve; LVOT, left ventricular outflow tract.)

mechanical valves. Bileaflet valves usually have higher velocities across their central orifice compared to the larger lateral orifices. Since CWD does not distinguish between the two velocities, and measures the highest values, the calculated peak gradients are often high, leading to an underestimation of EOA.[15] This is especially true in high flow situations and with smaller valves. Many centers report mean valve gradients rather than peak gradients because there is less variability over time. The phenomenon of pressure recovery (reconversion of kinetic energy not completely dissipated as turbulence back to pressure energy distal to a stenosis, resulting in decrease in the pressure gradient) should also be considered in patients with a small (<3 cm) aorta or a small (<19 mm) bileaflet tilting disk prosthesis.

The Doppler velocity index (DVI), a ratio of the peak velocity in the outflow tract to that through the prosthesis, is a useful tool in the assessment of prosthetic aortic valves:

$$DVI = \frac{V_{LVOT}}{V_{AVR}}$$

where V_{AVR} is velocity through the aortic valve prosthesis.

It may be particularly useful during TEE assessment since it does not need to account for LVOT diameter, which can be difficult to measure with a prosthetic device in situ. In addition, since the implanted valve size is usually proportional to the LVOT size at the time of surgery, DVI is less dependent on valve size. Due to higher velocities across the prosthesis, the DVI is always less than one, but a DVI value less than 0.25 suggests severe prosthetic stenosis.[15]

The contour of the jet tracing can provide valuable clues to the presence of underlying stenosis. With progressive stenosis, the jet contour changes from a triangular shape with a short acceleration time (AT, time from start of flow to peak velocity) to a smoother contour with a prolonged AT. An AT beyond 100 milliseconds indicates stenotic flow, while an AT to-ejection time ratio greater than 0.4 also indicates obstruction.[15] In summary, significant aortic prosthetic stenosis is suggested by (1) peak transvalvular velocity greater than 4 m/s; (2) mean gradient greater than 35 mm Hg; (3) DVI less than 0.25; (4) EOA less than 0.8 cm^2; (5) rounded, symmetrical contour of the jet velocity through the valve; and (6) AT greater than 100 milliseconds.

Pathologic regurgitation in aortic prostheses may be more difficult to quantify than native valves. Acoustic shadows from the prosthetic valve may render quantification attempts more difficult. However, criteria used for native valves may be reasonably applied to prostheses, especially spectral Doppler parameters such as the pressure half-time of the regurgitant jet (see Chapter 9).[15] Additionally, the qualitative evaluation of the nature of regurgitant jets with CFD and 2D examination is more valuable. Identification of the origin of the regurgitant jet with CFD may help determine pathology such as pannus, endocarditis, or prosthetic valve leaflet dysfunction.

Tricuspid and Pulmonic

Placement of prosthetic valves on the right side of the heart is much less common than on the left. Patients are often able to tolerate significant regurgitation without major signs and symptoms because pressures are lower in the right heart. Replacement of the pulmonic valve is performed most commonly secondary to congenital malformations of the valve or outflow tract (usually done in infancy) or as part of the Ross procedure for aortic valve pathology. Frequently, tricuspid pathology is amenable to valve repair with sutures alone (De Vega annuloplasty) or with a ring. When valve replacement is necessary, biologic valves are almost always placed because of the higher risk of thrombosis with mechanical valves and the fact that low right-side pressures cannot reliably open and close the occluders of mechanical valves.[2,3] After tricuspid replacement, it is not uncommon to see a small paravalvular jet emanating from the septal portion of the ring because surgeons frequently leave a small gap in the fixation sutures so as not to interfere with the bundle of His and thereby reduce the rate of iatrogenic third-degree heart block. Pathologic regurgitation or stenosis of the tricuspid prosthesis is difficult to quantify but conventional techniques as applied to native valves or prosthetic mitral valves may be used with reasonable confidence. It is important to use an averaged measurement of at least five beats for the tricuspid prosthesis. A pressure half time of 230 milliseconds or greater, a peak E velocity of greater than 1.7 m/s, and a mean gradient 6 mm Hg or greater suggest prosthetic tricuspid stenosis.[15] Other than CFD patterns indicating severe tricuspid regurgitation (TR) (jet area >10 cm^2, vena contracta [VC] >0.7 cm), secondary signs suggestive of prosthetic regurgitation include a dilated right atrium and holosystolic flow reversal in the hepatic veins. Calculation of the EOA should not be performed using the pressure half-time algorithm applied to the mitral valve since this technique has not been validated in the tricuspid position. However, estimation of EOA using a combination of Doppler techniques such as trans-tricuspid VTI and LVOT stroke volume is reasonable as long as significant aortic and tricuspid regurgitation do not coexist.

The pulmonic valve position can be difficult to examine even in the absence of a prosthetic valve because it is the valve farthest from the TEE probe. Nevertheless, one usually is able to identify the type of prosthetic valve and any associated pathology. The best views for assessing the pulmonic valve include the upper esophageal aortic arch short-axis view (approximately 70°) with the depth adjusted to 10 to 12 cm, which shows the valve and the main pulmonary artery trunk, and allows for measurement of transvalvular gradients and color-flow assessment; and the right ventricular inflow–outflow view at approximately 60°, which provides satisfactory windows for valve identification and qualitative assessment of regurgitant jets. Color-flow Doppler will usually indicate turbulent flows in prosthesis regurgitation or stenosis, while 2D examination will reveal leaflet thickening or obstructive lesions. Peak velocities greater than 3 m/s for prosthetic valves or 2 m/s for homografts are considered suspicious for prosthetic stenosis, while a prosthetic pulmonary valve regurgitant jet that exceeds 50% of the pulmonary annulus diameter is suggestive of severe regurgitation.[15] There are limited data validating these techniques with TEE, and careful inspection of the valve using all available modalities is mandatory for a complete assessment.

MULTIVALVE REPLACEMENT

It is not uncommon for surgeons to have to replace more than one valve, at the same time or sequentially. Diseases such as rheumatic fever and myxomatous degeneration frequently affect more than one valve in the same individual. Surgical implantation of multiple prosthetic valves is an added technical challenge. Combined aortic and mitral valve replacement carries a 70% higher risk and poorer survival rate than replacement of either valve alone. The Society of Thoracic Surgeons national database committee (STS National Database Fall 2008—Executive Summary) gives an operative mortality of 9.6% for all multiple valve surgeries, compared with 3.2% and 5.7% for aortic and mitral valves alone, respectively. Long-term survival depends on preoperative functional status.

TEE evaluation of prosthetic valve structure and function with multiple valves in situ also provides a challenge to the echocardiographer. Imaging artifacts from one valve frequently obscure the examination of the other, sometimes making a complete examination impossible.

PROSTHETIC MITRAL RINGS

See Chapter 8 for a full discussion of mitral valve repair. One method of repairing a leaking mitral valve uses prosthetic materials to reestablish anatomic coaptation of the anterior and posterior mitral leaflets. Rings also are used frequently to rectify mitral regurgitation secondary to annular dilation (cardiomyopathy or end-stage coronary heart failure) or leaflet prolapse. Different prosthetic rings are available with different amounts of flexibility and overall shapes. Many are complete D-shaped rings, whereas others are shaped like a C or even attempt to reproduce the saddle-shape of the mitral annulus. Surgical preference usually dictates the type of prosthesis placed. The ring itself is visible around the periphery of the native mitral valve, as are the sutures used to secure it in place (Figure 11–20). Prosthetic mitral rings do not require long-term anticoagulation.

PROSTHETIC VALVE PATHOLOGY

Patient-Prosthesis Mismatch

Patient-prosthesis mismatch (PPM) is best characterized using EOA indexed to body surface area. PPM in the aortic position is considered to be hemodynamically insignificant if EOA is greater than 0.85 cm^2/m^2, moderately significant at 0.65 to 0.85 cm^2/m^2, and severe at less than 0.65 cm^2/m^2. In the mitral position, EOA should be greater than 1.2 cm^2/m^2 to avoid high postoperative gradients and persistent pulmonary hypertension. PPM has also been associated with reduced short- and long-term survival.[15]

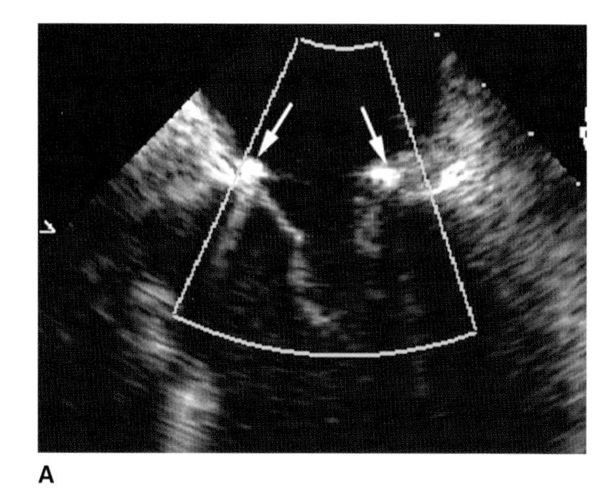

A

B

FIGURE 11–20. Prosthetic mitral ring *(arrows)* is easily seen after mitral valve repair in the midesophageal TEE views. **B:** Three-dimensional image after a mitral repair demonstrating the sutured prosthetic ring.

Endocarditis

Bacterial infections of implanted prosthetic materials are problematic regardless of their location, and infection of prosthetic heart valves can lead to significant mortality, with reported rates as high as 70% for acute (<6 months of implantation) and 45% in late (>6 months) endocarditis.[10,11] Prosthetic valves are at an increased risk for endocarditis for two reasons: abnormal flow patterns and foreign material. The annual rate for late endocarditis is approximately 0.5%, with no significant difference between mechanical and stented biologic valves.[10,11] Compared with native valves, prosthetic valves are more likely to have ring abscesses, conduction abnormalities, and fistulae, and have a poorer prognosis. Endocarditis has two common appearances on mechanical valves: vegetations on leaflets, occluders, or support material; and echolucent ring abscesses with or without fistulae. Tissue valves most frequently develop new stenotic or regurgitant lesions but also can develop vegetations (Figure 11–21) and/or abscesses. New or worsening periprosthetic leaks are highly suggestive of endocarditis and are a particularly ominous sign.

TEE is vastly superior to TTE for the evaluation and diagnosis of prosthetic endocarditis, with significantly greater sensitivity and specificity (TTE sensitivity is 60% to 80% and specificity is 98%; TEE sensitivities are 100% for native valves and 86% to 94% for prosthetic valves, with a specificity of 88% to 100%).[11] TEE better characterizes vegetations, abscesses (Figure 11–22), and fistulae, thereby providing important diagnostic information related to medical versus surgical intervention. The recent introduction of real-time three-dimensional echocardiography has shown significant promise in imaging infected prosthetic valves because of the ability to crop and rotate a volumetric sample of echocardiographic information.[24] This can allow the operator to generate views that may not be feasible using conventional 2D imaging. Endocarditis should be suspected in all patients with prosthetic valves who develop septicemia. Perivalvular abscess formation should be considered in those who do not respond to aggressive antibiotic therapy. Other

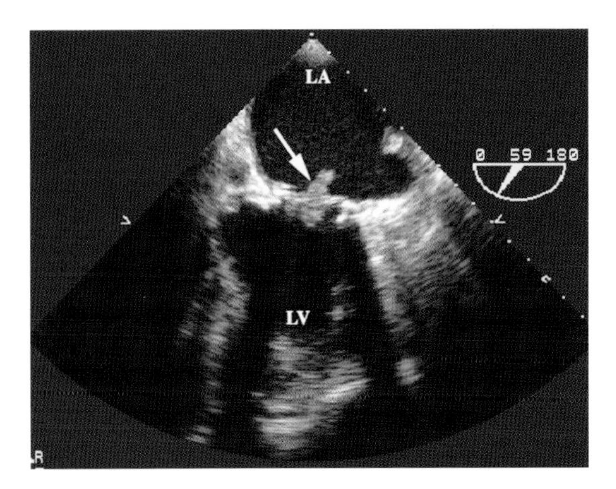

FIGURE 11–21. Endocarditis *(arrow)* on a porcine biologic valve in the mitral position. The acoustic shadow cast by the struts of the prosthesis is seen extending into the left ventricle. (LA, left atrium; LV, left ventricle.)

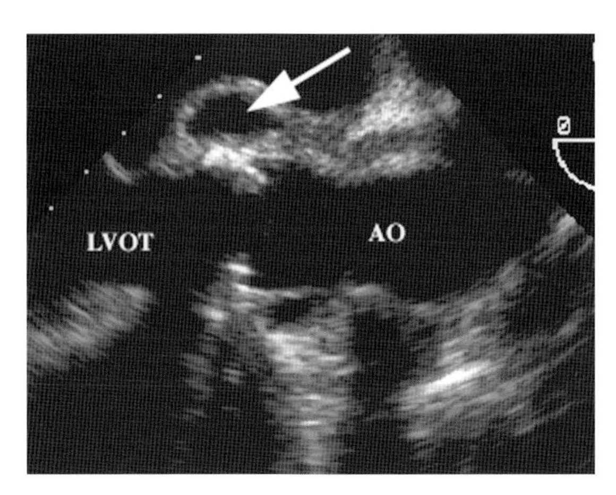

FIGURE 11–22. Echolucent abscess cavity *(arrow)* at the aortic root in a patient with a prosthetic aortic valve. (AO, aorta; LVOT, left ventricular outflow tract.)

clinical indicators prompting a thorough TEE "hunt" for an abscess include new conduction abnormalities and worsening heart failure (possible fistula formation). Findings commonly associated with abscess formation on a 2D study include dehiscence manifested as a rocking of the valve (Figure 11–23), perivalvular lucency, and periaortic root thickening.[4,10,11] Abnormal color-flow patterns can be suggestive of fistulas and blood flow into abscess cavities. Abscess ruptures into the LVOT, right atrium, left atrium, ascending aorta, pericardial space, and main pulmonary artery have been described in the literature.

Thrombosis and Hemorrhage

Thrombosis and hemorrhage account for more than 50% of all reported complications in left-side biologic valves and nearly 75% of all mechanical prostheses.[2] Maintenance of therapeutic anticoagulation levels continues to be one of the most daunting challenges related to valve replacement. Even "perfect" anticoagulation levels do not guarantee freedom from these serious and potentially deadly complications. The early detection of periprosthetic thrombosis has been improved significantly with TEE, which can help guide management, be it medical (thrombolytic therapy) or surgical. However, previously described imaging artifacts and limitations can interfere with the proper diagnosis.[25] Furthermore, differentiating a thrombus from a pannus can be difficult but is often critical to directing therapy. In general, pannus formation is more common in the aortic position and is characterized by a small, dense mass, whereas thrombi are larger, have a soft ultrasound density similar to myocardium, and are more likely to be associated with abnormal prosthetic valve motion.[15]

All mechanical valves carry approximately the same incidence of thrombosis and require long-term anticoagulation and/or aspirin administration to help prevent clot formation (the greatest incidence is during the first postoperative year). Even with therapeutic levels of anticoagulation, the rate of thrombosis is 0.6% to 1.8% per patient-year for bileaflet valves.[5] The risk of spontaneous thromboembolism is three to six times higher if anticoagulation is not administered or is sub-therapeutic. When placed in the tricuspid position, thrombosis of a mechanical valve is seen in more than 20% of patients because of the lower pressures in the right heart. Thrombus adherent to prosthetic materials usually can be visualized, but sometimes the only indication of thrombosis is inappropriate occluder motion with failure to completely open or close (Figure 11–24). Faulty occluder motion can be visualized directly with 2D echo or 3D echo (particularly in the mitral position), or be surmised by new obstructive or regurgitant lesions on color flow and/or spectral Doppler.

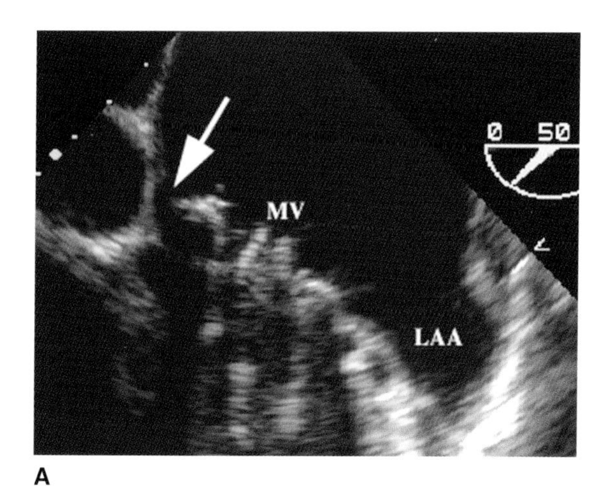

A

B

FIGURE 11–23. **A:** Complete dehiscence of a St. Jude valve in the mitral position. A rocking motion of the valve was visible at this site of discontinuity *(arrow)* accompanied by severe regurgitation. (LAA, left atrial appendage; MV, mitral valve.) **B:** Three-dimensional image of a mitral valve prosthetic ring showing clear dehiscence from the annulus *(arrow)*.

Thromboembolism

Embolic events in patients with mechanical valves have been reduced to 1% to 4% per patient-year with strict anticoagulation protocols. However, the risk of a serious bleed while on anticoagulants is 1% to 5% per patient-year.[26]

Fibrin Strands

Occasionally, thin filamentous strands can appear to be attached to the atrial side of mitral, and the ventricular side of aortic, mechanical prostheses (and occasionally tissue valves). These strands are comprised of fibrin and are usually a few millimeters in length. Their motion is

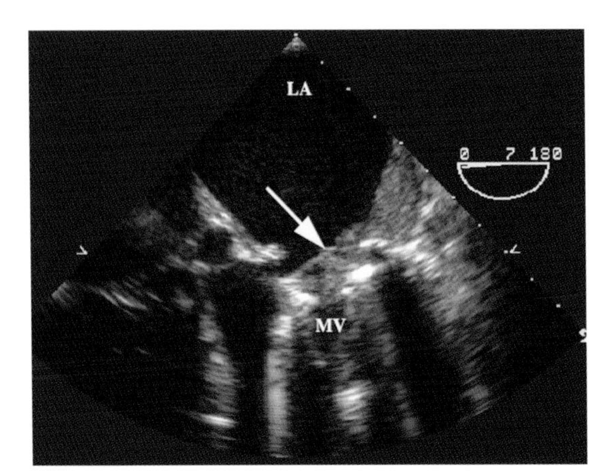

FIGURE 11–24. Thrombus *(arrow)* occluding a prosthetic mitral valve and extending into the left atrium. In this case, the thrombus is grossly visible, but sometimes the only indication of thrombosis is inappropriate occluder motion with failure to completely open or close. (LA, left atrium; MV, mitral valve.)

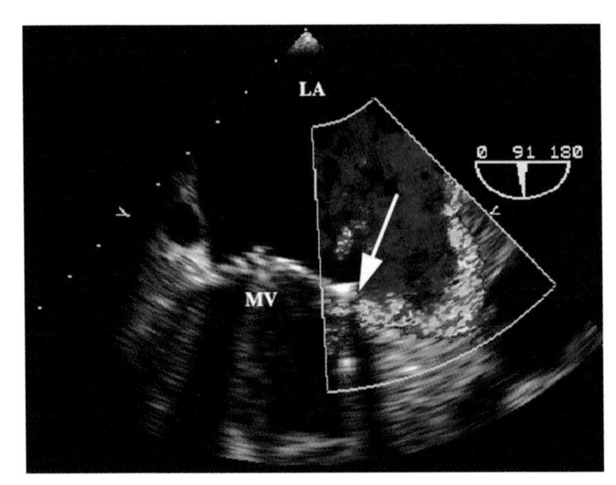

FIGURE 11–25. Paravalvular regurgitation in a patient with a bileaflet tilting disk mitral valve. The jet is seen originating lateral to the sewing ring *(arrow)* and "hugging" the wall of the left atrium. (LA, left atrium; MV, mitral valve.)

unrelated to that of the valve itself, and they can be distinguished from vegetations and thrombi by their movement in and out of the imaging plane. Several studies have suggested higher rates of systemic embolization when these strands are present.[2]

Primary Prosthesis Failure

Fortunately, a primary failure of mechanical prosthetic valves is a rare occurrence. Case reports of occluder device and strut embolization have been published for most available valves. An uncommon complication with the Starr-Edwards valve was "ball variance," in which small cracks would develop in the silastic occluder ball, leading to thrombosis within the stellite cage and subsequent valve obstruction.

Prosthesis failure in tissue valves usually is related to calcific degeneration of the leaflets themselves, leading to restricted cusp motion (stenosis) and, more commonly, regurgitation secondary to tears and malocclusion. All non-autograft tissue valves will eventually degenerate to the point of requiring replacement in the long term. However, the newer stentless biologic valves appear to have a much slower degeneration rate.

Paravalvular Regurgitation

Paravalvular regurgitation appears as one or more regurgitant jets that originate from outside the prosthetic valve annulus (Figure 11–25). Mechanical failures, suture fracture, inadequate approximation and fixation of the prosthetic valve annulus, valve dehiscence, a heavily calcified annulus, and endocarditis may result in paravalvular leaks. In addition to the CFD findings, valves with large paravalvular leaks often appear to have a "rocking" motion of the valve sewing ring on the 2D examination. Identification of one finding should lead to a search for the other.

LVOT Obstruction

Although quite rare, obstruction of the LVOT has been described after implantation of prosthetic mitral valves or mitral annular rings.[21] Obstruction can be caused by residual submitral valvular tissue (leaflets or chordae), strut or tissue leaflets in the case of stented bioprostheses, or the native leaflets themselves in the case of mitral valve ring annuloplasty. The presence of LVOT obstruction should be considered in all cases, especially in situations of poor hemodynamics after cessation of CPB in a previously normal ventricle (see Chapters 8 and 14). This is most easily assessed from the transgastric long-axis or deep transgastric long-axis views. Residual subvalvular tissues also may interfere with the valve function, resulting in mitral regurgitation rather than outflow tract obstruction.[27]

Obstruction Secondary to Tissue Adhesives or Glues

The last several years have seen a dramatic increase in the use of a variety of sealants, glues, and other materials that are either directly applied to or sprayed on the surgical field for the purpose of controlling bleeding at suture lines or repairs of cardiac tissues. Unfortunately, from time to time some of these materials can make their way into a cardiac chamber or vessel and pose the risk of embolization or interference with the proper function of native or prosthetic valves.[28] A thorough examination following the separation from CPB should demonstrate the presence of foreign materials.

SUMMARY

The evaluation of prosthetic valves is a necessary tool in the armamentarium of a transesophageal echocardiographer. Whether evaluating a new valve immediately after CPB or assessing a prosthesis that has been in situ longer than 10 years, echocardiography provides critical information that allows clinical decisions to be made solely on the basis of echo findings. The evaluation of prosthetic valves does not stop at successfully identifying the type and location of the valve. A comprehensive interrogation by using all modalities available should be carried out so that significant pathology is not overlooked.

REFERENCES

1. Bonow RO, Carabello BA, Kanu C, et al. ACC/AHA 2006 guidelines for the management of patients with valvular heart disease: a report of the American College of Cardiology/American Heart Association Task Force on Practice Guidelines (writing committee to revise the 1998 Guidelines for the Management of Patients With Valvular Heart Disease): developed in collaboration with the Society of Cardiovascular Anesthesiologists: endorsed by the Society for Cardiovascular Angiography and Interventions and the Society of Thoracic Surgeons. *Circulation.* 2006;114(5):e84-231.
2. Zabalgoitia M. Echocardiographic assessment of prosthetic heart valves. *Curr Probl Cardiol.* 2000;25(3):157-218.
3. Bach DS. Transesophageal echocardiographic (TEE) evaluation of prosthetic valves. *Cardiol Clin.* 2000;18(4):751-771.
4. Van den Brink RB. Evaluation of prosthetic heart valves by transesophageal echocardiography: problems, pitfalls, and timing of echocardiography. *Semin Cardiothorac Vasc Anesth.* 2006;10(1):89-100.
5. Godje OL, Fischlein T, Adelhard K, Nollert G, Klinner W, Reichart B. Thirty-year results of Starr-Edwards prostheses in the aortic and mitral position. *Ann Thorac Surg.* 1997;63(3):613-619.
6. MacKenzie GS, Heinle SK. Echocardiography and Doppler assessment of prosthetic heart valves with transesophageal echocardiography. *Crit Care Clin.* 1996;12(2):383-409.
7. Yezbick AB, Ho JK, Crowley R, Sanchez E, Mahajan A. Echocardiographic signature of the On-X valve. *Echocardiography.* 2008;25(9):1016-1018.
8. Jamieson WR, Munro AI, Miyagishima RT, Allen P, Burr LH, Tyers GF. Carpentier-Edwards standard porcine bioprosthesis: clinical performance to seventeen years. *Ann Thorac Surg.* 1995;60(4):999-1006; discussion 1007.
9. Mohr FW, Walther T, Baryalei M, et al. The Toronto SPV bioprosthesis: one-year results in 100 patients. *Ann Thorac Surg.* 1995;60(1):171-175.
10. Karchmer AW, Longworth DL. Infections of intracardiac devices. *Infect Dis Clin North Am.* 2002;16(2):477-505, xii.
11. Ryan EW, Bolger AF. Transesophageal echocardiography (TEE) in the evaluation of infective endocarditis. *Cardiol Clin.* 2000;18(4):773-787.
12. Oh CC, Click RL, Orszulak TA, Sinak LJ, Oh JK. Role of intraoperative transesophageal echocardiography in determining aortic annulus diameter in homograft insertion. *J Am Soc Echocardiogr.* 1998;11(6):638-642.
13. Cheung A, Ree R. Transcatheter aortic valve replacement. *Anesthesiol Clin.* 2008;26(3):465-479.
14. Rodes-Cabau J, Dumont E, De LaRochelliere R, et al. Feasibility and initial results of percutaneous aortic valve implantation including selection of the transfemoral or transapical approach in patients with severe aortic stenosis. *Am J Cardiol.* 2008;102(9):1240-1246.
15. Zoghbi WA, Chambers JB, Dumesnil JG, et al. Recommendations for evaluation of prosthetic valves with echocardiography and doppler ultrasound: a report from the American Society of Echocardiography's Guidelines and Standards Committee and the Task Force on Prosthetic Valves, developed in conjunction with the American College of Cardiology Cardiovascular Imaging Committee, Cardiac Imaging Committee of the American Heart Association, the European Association of Echocardiography, a registered branch of the European Society of Cardiology, the Japanese Society of Echocardiography and the Canadian Society of Echocardiography, endorsed by the American College of Cardiology Foundation, American Heart Association, European Association of Echocardiography, a registered branch of the European Society of Cardiology, the Japanese Society of Echocardiography, and Canadian Society of Echocardiography. *J Am Soc Echocardiogr.* 2009;22(9):975-1014.
16. Jungwirth B, Mackensen GB. Real-time 3-dimensional echocardiography in the operating room. *Semin Cardiothorac Vasc Anesth.* 2008;12(4):248-264.
17. Sugeng L, Shernan SK, Weinert L, et al. Real-time three-dimensional transesophageal echocardiography in valve disease: comparison with surgical findings and evaluation of prosthetic valves. *J Am Soc Echocardiogr.* 2008;21(12):1347-1354.
18. Burstow DJ, Nishimura RA, Bailey KR, et al. Continuous wave Doppler echocardiographic measurement of prosthetic valve gradients. A simultaneous Doppler-catheter correlative study. *Circulation.* 1989;80(3):504-514.
19. Grunkemeier GL, Starr A, Rahimtoola SH. Prosthetic heart valve performance: long-term follow-up. *Curr Probl Cardiol.* 1992;17(6):329-406.
20. Reeves ST, Glas KE, Eltzschig H, et al. Guidelines for performing a comprehensive epicardial echocardiography examination: recommendations of the American Society of Echocardiography and the Society of Cardiovascular Anesthesiologists. *J Am Soc Echocardiogr.* 2007;20(4):427-437.
21. Gallet B, Berrebi A, Grinda JM, Adams C, Deloche A, Hiltgen M. Severe intermittent intraprosthetic regurgitation after mitral valve replacement with subvalvular preservation. *J Am Soc Echocardiogr.* 2001;14(4):314-316.
22. Fernandes V, Olmos L, Nagueh SF, Quinones MA, Zoghbi WA. Peak early diastolic velocity rather than pressure half-time is the best index of mechanical prosthetic mitral valve function. *Am J Cardiol.* 2002;89(6):704-710.
23. Zoghbi WA, Enriquez-Sarano M, Foster E, et al. Recommendations for evaluation of the severity of native valvular regurgitation with two-dimensional and Doppler echocardiography. *J Am Soc Echocardiogr.* 2003;16(7):777-802.

24. Kort S. Real-time 3-dimensional echocardiography for prosthetic valve endocarditis: initial experience. *J Am Soc Echocardiogr.* 2006;19(2):130-139.
25. Kodali S, Vivas Y, Jakub C, et al. Continuous transesophageal monitoring for thrombolytic therapy of an acute prosthetic mitral valve thrombosis. *J Am Soc Echocardiogr.* 2007;20(8): 1009 e1001-1003.
26. Cannegieter SC, Rosendaal FR, Briet E. Thromboembolic and bleeding complications in patients with mechanical heart valve prostheses. *Circulation.* 1994;89(2):635-641.
27. Thomson LE, Chen X, Greaves SC. Entrapment of mitral chordal apparatus causing early postoperative dysfunction of a St. Jude mitral prosthesis. *J Am Soc Echocardiogr.* 2002;15(8):843-844.
28. Sidhu S, Goyer C, Hatzakorzian R, et al. Transesophageal echocardiographic detection of intracardiac BioGlue postmitral valve replacement. *Anesth Analg.* 2007;105(6):1572-1573.

REVIEW QUESTIONS

Select the single *MOST LIKELY* answer for the following questions.

1. How much "rocking" motion is allowed in an implanted mechanical valve support ring?
   a. None
   b. Minimal (<5°) just after separation from CPB
   c. <5° of angulation
   d. <10° of angulation
   e. <15° of angulation

2. What is the maximal opening angle of the occluder disk in a Medtronic-Hall mechanical valve in the mitral position?
   a. 90°
   b. 80°
   c. 70°
   d. 60°
   e. 50°

3. The constant of 220 milliseconds with the pressure half-time method of valve area calculation can overestimate the effective orifice area of a mitral prosthetic valve.
   a. True
   b. False

4. Over time, stenosis is more common with bioprosthetic valves than regurgitation.
   a. True
   b. False

5. Measurement of the STJ is critical during implantation of a stentless aortic biologic valve because of the need to:
   a. Assess maximal valve diameter.
   b. Assess for proper prosthesis length.
   c. Ensure proper prosthesis geometry.
   d. Satisfy the surgeon's curiosity.
   e. Assess for post-stenotic dilation and possible aortic root replacement.

6. The primary advantage of tissue valves is:
   a. Durability
   b. Ease of implantation
   c. Silence (patient cannot hear or feel the occluder click on closure)
   d. Does not require long-term anticoagulation
   e. Less expensive

7. The annual rate of thromboembolism with bioprosthetic valves is:
   a. <1% per patient-year
   b. 1% to 2% per patient-year
   c. 2% to 4% per patient-year
   d. 4% to 6% per patient-year
   e. 6% to 8% per patient-year

8. Pressure recovery is a reason for the Doppler-derived gradient to be greater than the catheter gradient.
   a. True
   b. False

9. The EOA of a stented or mechanical valve is the same as the size of the sewing ring orifice.
   a. True
   b. False

10. Calcific degeneration is less common in stentless valves than in stented valves.
    a. True
    b. False

11. Thrombosis of prosthetic valves in the right heart is more common than thrombosis of left-side prosthetic valves.
    a. True
    b. False

12. The rate of late endocarditis for mechanical valves is less than that for biologic valves.
    a. True
    b. False

13. TEE can reliably differentiate between thrombus and vegetation in mechanical prostheses.
    a. True
    b. False

14. What is the normal mean gradient across a St. Jude valve in the aortic position?
    a. 5 mm Hg
    b. 10 mm Hg

c. 15 mm Hg
d. 20 mm Hg
e. 25 mm Hg

15. What is the normal mean gradient across a St. Jude valve in the mitral position?
a. 2 mm Hg
b. 4 mm Hg
c. 6 mm Hg
d. 8 mm Hg
e. 10 mm Hg

16. What is the normal mean gradient across a homograft in the aortic position?
a. 2 mm Hg
b. 4 mm Hg
c. 6 mm Hg
d. 7 mm Hg
e. 10 mm Hg

17. In the mitral position, what is the maximal normal regurgitation jet length of prosthetic valves other than the Medtronic-Hall tilting disk valve?
a. <0.5 cm
b. <1.0 cm
c. <1.5 cm
d. <2.0
e. <2.5 cm

18. Are the peripheral "washing jets" convergent or divergent in a Starr-Edwards prosthesis?
a. Convergent
b. Divergent
c. Both
d. Neither

19. During which period of the cardiac cycle are "washing jets" visualized with bileaflet valves in the aortic position?
a. Early diastole
b. Mid-diastole
c. Late systole
d. Throughout systole
e. Throughout diastole

20. Trace to mild regurgitation is seen in what percentage of "normal" biologic valves?
a. <2.5%
b. 5%
c. 7.5%
d. 10%
e. 15%

21. How are the pivot points of a dual tilting disk mechanical prosthesis (St. Jude Medical, Carbomedics) oriented in the mitral position?
a. Perpendicular to the line of the old commissures.
b. 45° to the line of the old commissures.
c. Superimposed over the old commissures.
d. Orientation does not matter.
e. 120° to the line of the old commissures.

22. Toward which portion of the aortic arch is the major orifice of a single tilting disk mechanical prosthesis oriented?
a. Toward the lesser curvature of the arch.
b. Directly posterior.
c. Directly anterior.
d. Toward the greater curvature of the arch.
e. Orientation does not matter.

23. What is the most common TEE presentation of endocarditis with mechanical prosthetic valves?
a. Vegetations on the occluder surfaces
b. New regurgitant lesions
c. New stenotic lesions
d. Increased attenuation artifact from the sewing ring
e. Ring or myocardial abscesses

24. What portion of a mechanical or stented bioprosthesis is most difficult to image with 2D TEE?
a. Anterior portion.
b. Posterior portion.
c. Lateral portions.
d. All portions are seen equally well.
e. Inferior surface.

25. All the following are primary advantages of homografts *EXCEPT*:
a. Favorable hemodynamic profile
b. Resistance to infection
c. Does not require long-term anticoagulation
d. Low cost

26. Which of the following methods overestimates the effective orifice area in patients with stenotic prosthetic valves?
a. Pressure gradients
b. Continuity equation
c. Doppler velocity index (DVI)
d. Pressure half-time

27. TEE is a better modality than TTE for assessment of the mitral valve because:
a. There is less interference with imaging.
b. It uses lower-frequency imaging.

c. Transducer is positioned more anteriorly.
d. Transducer is positioned farther from the valve.

28. Which of the following is true regarding "washing jets"?
a. A narrow central jet is characteristic of the Medtronic-Hall valve.
b. St. Jude valves have two centrally divergent jets.
c. Ball-in-cage valves have two centrally convergent jets.
d. Single leaflet tilting disks do not have washing jets.

29. The major orifice of a single tilting disk mechanical mitral valve is typically directed toward which LV wall?
a. Posterior
b. Anterior
c. Lateral
d. Inferior

30. Which of the following is *NOT* an important anatomic measurement in the Ross procedure?
a. Aortic annulus diameter
b. Pulmonic annulus diameter
c. Sinotubular junction diameter
d. Main pulmonary artery diameter

31. Which of the following views provides a suitable angle and artifact-free view to measure the transaortic gradient with Doppler in the presence of mitral prosthesis?
a. Midesophageal aortic long axis
b. Deep transgastric long axis
c. Upper esophageal aortic arch short axis
d. Modified aortic inflow-outflow

32. All the following diameters are important anatomic measurements that should be taken before placement of a stented or stentless aortic biologic valve *EXCEPT*:
a. Aortic annulus
b. Sinotubular junction
c. Proximal ascending root
d. LVOT

33. What is the maximum opening angle of a 27-mm St. Jude bileaflet valve?
a. 75°
b. 80°
c. 85°
d. 90°

34. Which of the following material can obstruct or restrict a mechanical valve?
a. Thrombus
b. Pannus
c. Inflammatory material
d. Subvalvular tissue
e. All of the above

35. Which of the following is a major disadvantage of biologic valves and homografts?
a. Infinite lifespan for valve
b. Require long-term anticoagulation
c. Calcification of the leaflets secondary to fixation
d. Prone to thromboembolic events

36. All of the following are major advantages of stentless over stented bio-prosthetic valves *EXCEPT*:
a. Improved hemodynamics
b. No need for anticoagulation
c. Increased effective orifice area
d. Longer lasting

37. Which of the following statements is true regarding Doppler- and catheter-derived aortic valve gradients?
a. The Doppler-derived gradient is the peak-to-peak gradient.
b. The catheter gradient tends to be greater than the Doppler-derived gradient.
c. Catheter techniques measure maximal instantaneous gradient.
d. Peak-to-peak gradients are not true physiologic measures.

38. Which of the following statements regarding homografts and autografts is correct?
a. Autografts are harvested from human cadavers.
b. Homografts are treated with antibiotics and decalcifying agents before implantation.
c. Autografts degenerate over time because of the cryopreservation process.
d. Homografts last longer than autografts.

39. TEE is a better modality than TTE for assessment of endocarditis because:
a. Lower-frequency probes allow for better resolution.
b. Posterior probe position allows better visualization of valves.
c. Does not need clinical correlation.
d. TEE imaging can penetrate further than TTE.

40. Mechanical valves generally are not placed in the tricuspid position because:
a. Round mechanical prostheses do not fit well in the triangular tricuspid position.
b. Size limitations.
c. High incidence of endocarditis.
d. Inconsistent occluder movement secondary to low flows.

41. Which of the following statements regarding the difference between prosthetic valve and native valve endocarditis is true?
    a. Prosthetic valve endocarditis is more likely to result in abscess formation.
    b. Native valve endocarditis is more likely to be associated with conduction abnormalities.
    c. The prognosis after prosthetic valve endocarditis is better.
    d. Resistance to antibiotics is uncommon in prosthetic valve endocarditis.

42. When comparing endocarditis of a biologic valve with that of a mechanical valve, which of the following statements is correct?
    a. Stenosis is a common feature of both.
    b. Mechanical valve endocarditis typically presents as valve regurgitation.
    c. Biologic valve endocarditis typically presents as valve destruction.
    d. Ring abscesses are more likely with mechanical valves.

43. Which of the following echocardiographic clues is associated with a perivalvular abscess?
    a. Rocking motion of the heart
    b. Aortic root softening
    c. Perivalvular opacification
    d. Visualization of fistula tract

44. Which of the following clinical features supports the suspected echocardiographic diagnosis of a perivalvular abscess?
    a. Persistent sepsis despite adequate antibiotic treatment
    b. New or worsening heart failure
    c. New bundle branch block
    d. All of the above

45. TEE 2D findings that are suggestive of a malfunctioning (obstructive) mitral prosthesis include:
    a. Acute right atrial enlargement
    b. Increased occluder excursion
    c. Thickened cusps
    d. Overfilled left ventricle

46. Which of the following describes the TEE appearance of the proximal ascending aorta immediately after a root inclusion stentless aortic valve implantation?
    a. Three layers are seen in the proximal ascending aorta.
    b. Coronary ostia are visualized more easily.
    c. Peak velocities greater than 3 m/s are common.
    d. Small amounts of fluid may be present between the layers seen in the ascending aorta.

47. Common echocardiographic artifacts associated with mechanical or stented biologic valves include:
    a. Side lobes
    b. Attenuation
    c. Reverberation
    d. Mirror image
    e. All of the above

48. A 78-year-old female with multiple medical comorbidities is scheduled for an endovascular transcatheter aortic valve replacement. Multimodal preoperative imaging consistently measures the aortic annulus at 18 mm. Which of the currently available prostheses would be most appropriate?
    a. Small Sapien valve
    b. Large Sapien valve
    c. Small CoreValve prosthesis
    d. Large CoreValve prosthesis

49. The use of real-time 3D TEE for assessment of prosthetic valves has been shown to be:
    a. Very good for the evaluation of mechanical prostheses and occluder movement in the aortic position using the aortic perspective
    b. Highly reliable for evaluation of biologic sewing rings, leaflets, and struts in the mitral position using the left atrial or left ventricular perspectives
    c. Equally good at evaluating problems with the sewing ring and leaflet function in the tricuspid position
    d. Unreliable and should not be used for the assessment of biologic or mechanical prostheses

50. Regarding the use of intraoperative epicardial echocardiography for the assessment of aortic valve area using the continuity equation:
    a. It has never been validated and should not be used to calculate the aortic valve area.
    b. It has been demonstrated to consistently underestimate the aortic valve area by 18% and all measurements should multiplied by 1.18 to provide the true valve area.
    c. It has been validated against TEE, TTE, and cardiac catheterization methods and found to be a reliable technique for the assessment of AVA intraoperatively.
    d. It should only be used in patients who have a contraindication to TEE.

Assessment of Left Ventricular Diastolic Function

12

Alina Nicoara and Wanda M. Popescu

INTRODUCTION

In recent years diastolic function has received greater recognition for its impact on overall cardiac performance. Diastole is no longer regarded as a passive phase of the cardiac cycle, but rather as a complex sequence of interrelated events, which are dependent upon loading conditions, heart rate, and contractility, and ultimately influence the systolic function of the left ventricle (LV). Studies have suggested that patients with diastolic dysfunction presenting for cardiac surgery are prone to hemodynamic instability and potentially worse outcomes,[1] and that patients with diastolic heart failure are at increased risk for decompensation in the perioperative period.[2] Therefore, the perioperative echocardiographer should be familiar with the pathophysiology of diastolic heart failure and understand how to monitor and optimize diastolic function. Although advances in ultrasound technology have rendered Doppler echocardiography as the clinician's "Rosetta Stone" for diastolic function evaluation, this chapter will familiarize the readers with all the echocardiographic techniques routinely employed to assess LV diastolic function, explain the significance of these diastolic indices, and provide a diagnostic algorithm to evaluate diastolic dysfunction.

CLINICAL IMPORTANCE OF DIASTOLIC DYSFUNCTION

Diastolic dysfunction is defined as the inability of the LV to fill at normal left atrial (LA) pressure and represents a mechanical dysfunction of the LV, characterized by delayed LV relaxation and/or decreased compliance. Diastolic dysfunction may be present in the absence of signs and symptoms of heart failure, but when these symptoms occur, the diagnosis of diastolic heart failure can be made. Therefore, while diastolic dysfunction describes a cardiac mechanical abnormality, diastolic heart failure represents a clinical syndrome. Heart failure is the most common cause of hospital admission in patients over 65 years of age, accounting for approximately 1 million admissions annually in the United States and more then $15 billion in costs.[3] Nearly half of these patients, however, have a preserved ejection fraction and are defined as having diastolic heart failure.[4] The prevalence of diastolic heart failure is age dependent, increasing from less than 15% in patients younger than 45 years of age to 35% in those between the ages of 50 and 70 years, and more then 70% in patients older than 70 years.[5] The increased prevalence of diastolic dysfunction in the elderly appears to be related to the coexistence of diseases associated with aging such as hypertension, coronary artery disease, aortic stenosis, and cardiomyopathies that alter the normal LV structure and lead to deterioration of the LV diastolic properties. Morbidity from diastolic heart failure is high and the 1-year readmission rate approaches 50%.[5] The annual mortality rate for patients with diastolic heart failure (5% to 8%) is lower than that for those with systolic heart failure, except in patients 70 years or older, where the mortality rates are similar.[5]

DIASTOLIC PHYSIOLOGY

From a clinical standpoint, the cardiac cycle has been divided into systole and diastole. Systole starts with closure of the atrioventricular valves and encompasses isovolumic contraction and ejection, finishing with the closure of the semilunar valves. At this point, diastole ensues, which comprises four phases: isovolumic relaxation, early filling, diastasis, and atrial contraction (Figure 12–1).

1. *Isovolumic relaxation* begins with aortic valve (AV) closure and ends with mitral valve (MV) opening. During this interval, relaxation of cardiac muscle and a closed mitral valve cause a decline in pressure. Because of the lack of blood flow and the absence of interaction with other parameters of ventricular compliance, physiologic assessment of relaxation is best achieved during this isovolumic phase and extrapolated to the other phases of diastole. Under normal conditions, the duration of this phase varies from 90 to 120 milliseconds. Relaxation is influenced by the rate of inactivation of contractile proteins as a result of an active reentry of Ca^{2+} into the sarcoplasmic reticulum. Therefore, factors that affect intracellular

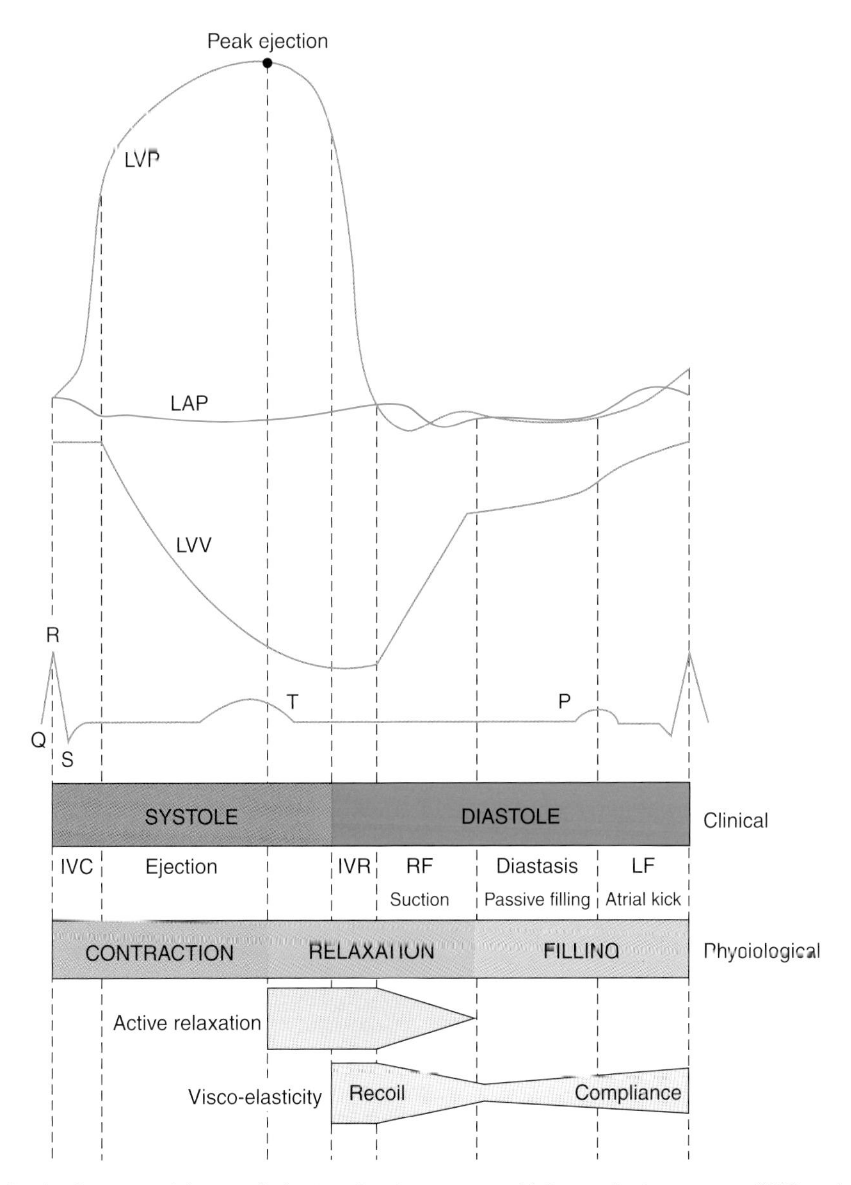

FIGURE 12–1. The first part of the graph depicts the time-course of left ventricular pressure (LVP) and volume (LVV) and left atrial pressure (LAP) during the cardiac cycle. According to the clinical definitions, the cardiac cycle is divided into the systolic and diastolic phases with their subdivisions: isovolumic contraction (IVC), ejection, isovolumic relaxation (IVR), rapid filling (RF), diastasis, and atrial contraction (LF). According to the physiological definitions, the cardiac cycle is divided into contraction, active relaxation, and filling phases. Note that the rapid filling phase is present in both the active relaxation and filling phases. See text for further explanations. The second part of the graph depicts the schematic representation of the determinants of intrinsic left ventricular diastolic function with respect to time. Note that active relaxation starts after peak ejection, in the second half of systole, and that the viscoelastic properties contribute to recoil during early diastole and to ventricular compliance during late diastole. *(Modified with permission from Claessens TE, et al. New echocardiographic applications for assessing global left ventricular diastolic function. Ultrasound Med Biol. 2007;33:823-841.)*

Ca^{2+} removal may cause a Ca^{2+} release-reuptake mismatch, and hence lead to impaired relaxation. The preceding systolic load and the nonuniform distribution in time of load on the ventricular wall also affect ventricular relaxation.

2. *Rapid filling phase* starts with MV opening and extends to the equalization of pressure between the LV and LA. Under normal conditions, this phase accounts for approximately 80% of the ventricular filling and lasts from 180 to 200 milliseconds. The persistence of myocardial relaxation and the elastic recoil of the myocardium during this phase create a drop in ventricular pressure, despite the initial increase in ventricular volume.[6] Filling of the ventricle is thus thought to be the result of a "suction" mechanism rather than of a passive flow of blood into the ventricle.[7] Equalization of atrial and ventricular pressures occurs at mid-diastole, when the rate of filling drops, representing the end of the rapid filling phase and the beginning of diastasis. The rapid filling phase coincides with and is dependant upon the continuous relaxation of the myocardium.
3. *Diastasis* contributes less than 5% of the diastolic filling of the ventricle. Since myocardial relaxation has ended, filling becomes dependent mainly on the passive compliance of the myocardium, and any further increase in ventricular volume will lead to an increase in ventricular pressure. Because of its small contribution to ventricular filling, pathologic changes affecting diastasis have little or no effect on overall filling.
4. *Atrial contraction* occurs at the end of diastole; the increased LA pressure surpasses the LV pressure and generates additional forward flow from the LA to the LV. Atrial systole contributes, under normal conditions, to approximately 20% to 25% of total ventricular filling. During this phase, any additional increase in ventricular volume is coupled with an increase in ventricular pressure. The increase in atrial pressure also leads to a retrograde flow toward the pulmonary veins. Therefore, the contribution of this phase to total cardiac output depends on ventricular compliance, intrinsic atrial contractility, and ventricular pressure at the onset of atrial contraction. Diastole ends when the pressure in the LV exceeds the LA pressure, leading to MV closure.

Nishimura and colleagues have proposed a physiologic division of the cardiac cycle based on the load-bearing characteristics of the myocardium. From this point of view, the cardiac cycle is divided into three phases—systolic contraction, relaxation, and diastolic filling.[8] The *contraction* phase consists of isovolumic contraction and the first half of ejection and is characterized by a pressure increase in the LV followed by myocardial fiber shortening that ultimately results in ejection of the blood into the ascending aorta. After the initial ejection, the myocardial fiber will respond differently to a changing load, signaling the transition from the contraction phase to the relaxation phase.[9] The *relaxation* phase consists of the second half of ejection, the isovolumic relaxation period, and most of the rapid filling phase. In a normal heart, active relaxation is thought to finish at the end of rapid filling. The *diastolic filling* phase then includes a small portion of the rapid filling phase, diastasis, and atrial contraction. The critical insight from Nishimura's proposal is that myocardial relaxation begins during the second part of *ejection* and continues during the isovolumic relaxation and rapid filling phase, illustrating the interdependency of systole and diastole (see Figure 12–1).

PATHOPHYSIOLOGY OF DIASTOLIC DYSFUNCTION

The hallmark of diastolic dysfunction is the increased resistance to ventricular filling that produces an upward shift of the pressure-volume curve and accounts for a disproportionate increase in pressure relative to the increase in volume (Figure 12–2).[10] This ultimately leads to signs and symptoms of congestion and, in severe cases, to a decrease in ventricular filling and stroke volume. Diastolic dysfunction can be caused by intrinsic myocardial factors (eg, alterations in calcium homeostasis, cytoskeleton, and extracellular matrix) or non-myocardial extrinsic factors (eg, afterload, pericardial effusion or restriction, and right ventricular [RV] dilation).

Intrinsic Myocardial Factors

Impaired calcium homeostasis is the main mechanism of impaired relaxation. Relaxation is an energy-dependent process that requires active removal of Ca^{2+} from the troponin C binding sites and from the cytoplasm by the sarcoplasmic reticulum.[6] Removal of intracellular Ca^{2+} also occurs by extrusion and exchange with extracellular Na^{+} through the sarcolemma, and ultimately results in dissociation of actinmyosin cross bridges while consuming adenosine triphosphate. Factors that affect intracellular Ca^{2+} removal may cause a Ca^{2+} release-reuptake mismatch, leading not only to impaired relaxation but also to increased passive stiffness.

Alterations in the extracellular matrix also affect diastolic function. Among the fibrillar proteins, proteoglycans, and basement membrane proteins that make up the extracellular matrix, fibrillar collagen is thought

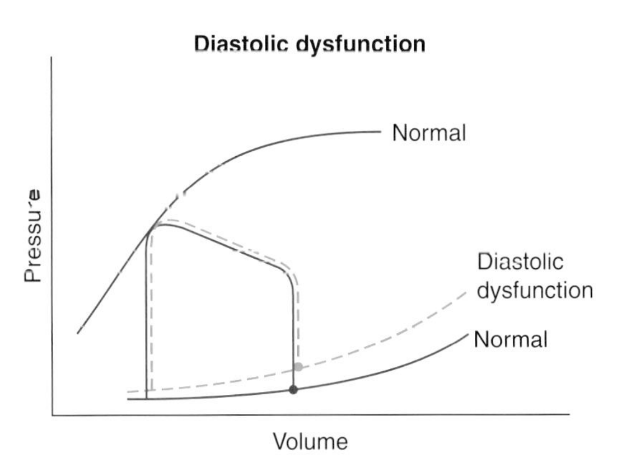

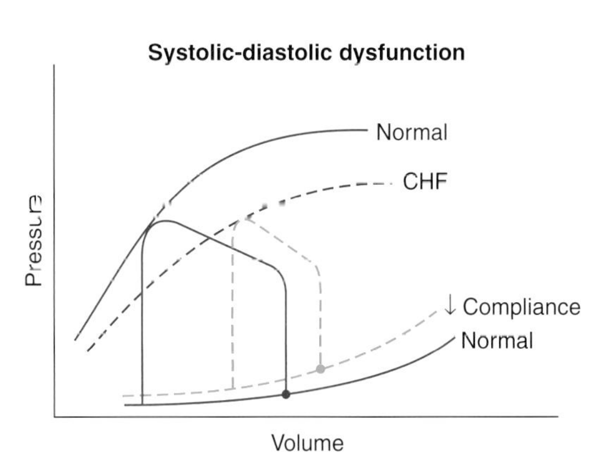

FIGURE 12–2. Pressure volume relation in patients with pure diastolic dysfunction *(left)* characterized by an upward shift of diastolic curve, and in patients with systolic-diastolic dysfunction *(right)* with a downward shift of the systolic portion of the curve. (CHF, congestive heart failure.) *(Modified with permission from Grossman W. Diastolic dysfunction and congestive heart failure. Circulation 1990; 81 (2 Suppl):III 1-7.)*

to contribute to the development of diastolic dysfunction by altering ventricular distensibility and increasing the resistance to filling. Alterations of collagen metabolism and fibrillar physical properties are determined by chronic changes in ventricular load, growth factors, and neurohormonal modulation, including the sympathetic nervous system and the renin-angiotensin system.[5] Acute and chronic neurohumoral activation and/or inhibition have variable effects on diastolic function. In contrast to the acute stimulation of the renin-angiotensin-aldosterone system, in which a rise in cardiac filling pressure is noted possibly by direct action on the cardiomyocyte, chronic renin-angiotensin-aldosterone activation induces an increase in extracellular fibrillar collagen with increased passive stiffness. The effect of angiotensin on diastolic cardiac performance may be related to changes in the mobilization and reuptake of cytosolic calcium.[11]

Non-Myocardial Extrinsic Factors

Extrinsic compression from lung or mediastinal masses and pericardial diseases, such as effusion or constriction, result in direct compression of the ventricles, thus restricting ventricular filling.[5] Moreover, RV enlargement shifts the interventricular septum to the left, leading to an increase in LV pressure and alteration of ventricular filling.[12] Engorgement of coronary veins secondary to elevated right atrial (RA) pressure also increases myocardial blood volume and reduces the capacity of the ventricle to distend during diastole.

Acute pressure or volume overload is another extrinsic cause of diastolic dysfunction. The increase in load tends to prolong ventricular contraction and to delay and shorten relaxation,[13] an effect that can be reproduced by catecholamines, angiotensin, and vasopressin. Acute hypertension is a primary cause of decompensation of pre-existing diastolic failure. Chronic overload as a consequence of chronic elevation of pressure (hypertension, aortic valve stenosis, or congenital disease) or chronic volume overload (valve incompetence or cardiomyopathy) produces myocardial cell hypertrophy as a compensatory mechanism.[14] Hypertrophy in turn increases the likelihood of diastolic dysfunction by impairing myocardial relaxation or by causing myocardial ischemia. Tachycardia also may produce diastolic dysfunction by increasing oxygen demand and by decreasing coronary perfusion and LV filling time, but it most often is an aggravating factor. Incomplete relaxation is a physiologic response to prolonged systolic contraction (delayed systole) and leads to increased dependence on the atrial contribution to ventricular filling in late diastole. The loss of atrial contraction is often a precipitating factor in diastolic heart failure in patients with relaxation abnormalities.

INVASIVE MEASURES OF DIASTOLIC FUNCTION

A physiologic description of diastolic function is classically based on the analysis of ventricular volume and pressure changes over the period of a cardiac cycle. The cycle typically begins at end-diastole, corresponding to the right lower corner of the pressure-volume loop (see Figure 12–2). Measurable parameters used to describe and study diastolic function include relaxation and compliance. The effect of relaxation predominates during the first phase of diastole, whereas compliance affects mainly late diastole. In pathologic situations, both parameters may interact, leading to diastolic dysfunction.

1. *Relaxation* can be assessed by the peak –dP/dt, the duration of the isovolumic relaxation period (IVRT), and the time constant of relaxation (τ).[15] Peak –dP/dt (mm Hg/s) is the maximum rate of LV pressure decline and is usually the lowest value of the first derivative of this pressure. The peak –dP/dt occurs at or around the time of aortic valve closure and appears to depend on aortic and LV pressures. Accurate calculation of –dP/dt necessitates invasive measurement of left intraventricular pressure. Like peak –dP/dt, IVRT is an index of pressure decline and can be assessed by Doppler echocardiography. IVRT is dependent on the timing of aortic valve closure and mitral valve opening. The time constant of relaxation (τ) is mathematically derived from peak –dP/dt and corresponds to the rate of decline of pressure from the peak –dP/dt to the end of the IVRT (mitral valve opening). The τ constant is relatively independent of preload but is affected by afterload. Impaired relaxation leads to a reduction in peak –dP/dt and prolongation of IVRT and τ.
2. *Compliance* is the ratio of change in volume to unit change in pressure (dV/dP) and depends on the intrinsic properties of the myocardium (myocardial compliance) and the geometric characteristics of the ventricular chamber (chamber compliance).[5] Stiffness is the opposite of compliance and reflects the ratio of change in pressure to a unit change in volume (dP/dV). Chamber stiffness is not constant but increases throughout ventricular filling. Thus dV/dP and dP/dV are global indices and cannot be used to compare different ventricles.[16] The relation between dP/dV and ventricular pressure, however, is linear with a slope (K_c) called the modulus of chamber stiffness that is proportional to ventricular chamber stiffness. The slope becomes steeper with increases in ventricular *chamber* stiffness, a relation that is independent of ventricular geometry, and therefore can be used to compare different patients.

Intrinsic myocardial stiffness can be assessed by examining the relation between stress (σ) and strain (ε) during diastole. Stress expresses the resisting force of the myocardium to increases in length, and strain is defined as the percentage change in muscle length during the application of a force (pressure change). The relation between $d\sigma/d\varepsilon$ and stress is also linear, and the slope of this relation (K_m) is the modulus of myocardial stiffness. The slope is steeper (K_m increases) when *myocardial* stiffness increases.

ECHOCARDIOGRAPHIC MEASURES OF DIASTOLIC FUNCTION

Diastolic dysfunction can be associated with normal or abnormal systolic function. Measurement of ejection fraction (EF) before assessing ventricular filling parameters is therefore necessary to differentiate systolic-diastolic dysfunction from pure diastolic dysfunction. Patients with normal EF and heart failure have isolated diastolic heart failure, whereas those with a decreased EF have combined systolic-diastolic dysfunction. Information on LV filling provided by echocardiography includes two-dimensional evaluation of cardiac chamber dimensions and Doppler recordings of mitral inflow and pulmonary venous flow (PVF). Most measured Doppler parameters are dependent on load or heart rate and may be difficult to interpret individually; thus, evaluating one parameter would be insufficient to evaluate and understand all aspects of diastolic function. The analysis of any given parameter should always be coupled with all other parameters measured simultaneously. One also should keep in mind that most studies in diastology were conducted using transthoracic echocardiography (TTE) on patients breathing spontaneously, thus making it hazardous to extrapolate the conclusions of such studies to intensive care or operative patients in whom load-dependent parameters can be altered by mechanical ventilation and/or general anesthesia. Color M-mode and tissue Doppler techniques may overcome many of these limitations by increasing the sensitivity and the precision of the evaluation.

TRANSMITRAL INFLOW

The transmitral velocity profile detected by pulsed-wave Doppler echocardiography reflects volumetric changes in LV filling and provides the initial basic information on LV diastolic properties.[17] Because the pressure gradient across the mitral valve determines the volume and velocity of mitral flow, mitral Doppler flow depends on left atrial pressure (LAP; pushing force) and the decrease of LV pressure by active relaxation to provide a "suction" effect (pulling force).

Normal Patterns and Basic Variables

Analogous to the different phases of diastole previously described, mitral inflow can be divided into four periods (Figure 12–3). Measured parameters from the transmitral velocity profile include:

1. IVRT, which represents the time needed for the LV myocardium to relax and for the left intraventricular pressure to decrease below the LAP. IVRT is determined primarily by the timing of MV opening, which is influenced by the rate of LV relaxation and left atrial pressure.

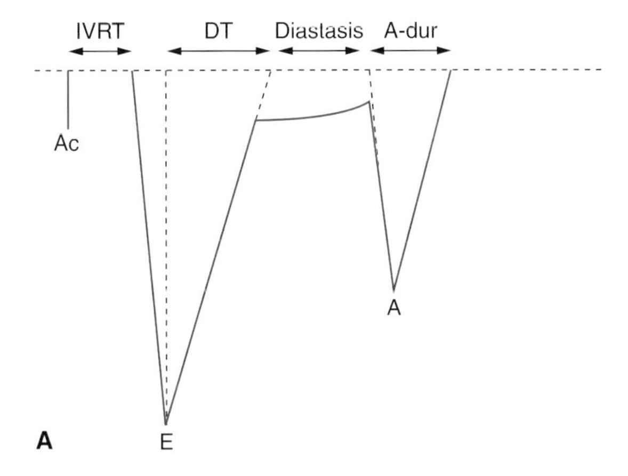

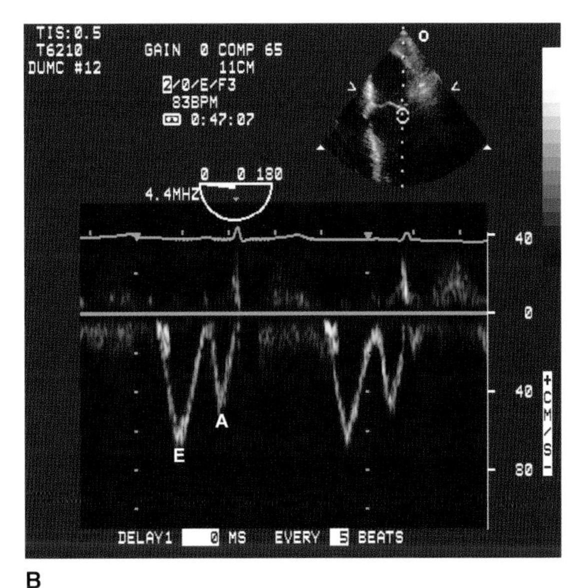

FIGURE 12–3. Schematic representation of mitral flow. **A:** Early diastolic rapid filling, diastasis and late diastolic atrial contraction follow the click of aortic valve closure. **B:** Mitral flow recorded with pulsed-wave Doppler from a four-chamber long-axis view by transesophageal echocardiography. (A, late diastolic atrial contraction flow; Ac, aortic valve closure; A-dur, duration of atrial systole; DT, deceleration time; E, early diastolic rapid filling flow; IVRT, isovolumic relaxation time.)

2. Peak E velocity, which depends on the left atrial pressure at MV opening, the relative driving force between the LA and LV, minimal LV diastolic pressure, compliance of the LA, and the rate of ventricular relaxation.[18]
3. The deceleration time (DT) of the E velocity, which is the interval from peak E to the point of intersection of the deceleration of flow with the baseline. DT correlates with time of pressure equalization between the LA and LV and is a measure of LV compliance.[19]
4. Peak A velocity, which is influenced by atrial contractility, residual atrial pressure, and LV compliance.
5. The duration of atrial systole (A-wave duration), which is important in assessing LV diastolic pressure and is measured as the interval from the beginning to the end of A wave.

Mitral velocity profiles change with age despite the absence of detectable cardiac diseases. This should not be interpreted as normal patterns, but rather as an age-related alteration in the physiologic properties of myocardial fibers. Normal values with regard to age are summarized in Table 12–1.[20] In young subjects, the rate of relaxation is vigorous, and LV filling occurs primarily during early diastole (80%). Therefore, mitral Doppler flow shows a high E velocity, high E/A ratio, and a short DT. However, with aging, there is a gradual decrease in the rate of myocardial relaxation, as well as in elastic recoil. Thus, the LV pressure decline and filling become slower, resulting in a prolonged IVRT and DT and a progressive decline in the E velocity. Since early LV filling is reduced, the contribution of atrial contraction to LV filling becomes more important. In most individuals, the peak E- and A-wave velocities become approximately equal during the seventh decade of life, with atrial filling contributing up to 35% to 40% of LV diastolic stroke volume (Figure 12–4).[2,20,21]

Technical Recommendations

IVRT is best acquired from a deep transgastric long-axis view, with a 3- to 4-mm pulsed sample volume placed in the area of the mitral leaflet tips until the onset of mitral flow is clearly seen.[22] The transducer beam is then angulated toward the LV outflow tract until an aortic valve closure click appears above and below the zero-velocity baseline. If aortic closure cannot be seen clearly, continuous-wave Doppler recording of simultaneous aortic and mitral flows can be used (Figure 12–5). Normal values for IVRT are provided in Table 12–1. Common pitfalls include mistaking wall motion artifacts for aortic valve closure clicks and angulating the beam too far toward the LV outflow tract, resulting in a delay in the recorded onset of mitral flow.

The most parallel alignment with mitral inflow usually is obtained on the midesophageal four-chamber view. Proper alignment of the ultrasound beam, with a near-zero angle of incidence to the atrioventricular

Table 12–1. Normal Transthoracic Echocardiography Values for Doppler-Derived Diastolic Measurements in Different Age Groups

Measurement	Age Group (y)			
	16-20	21-40	41-60	>60
IVRT (ms)	50 ± 9 (32-68)	67 ± 8 (51-83)	74 ± 7 (60-88)	87 ± 7 (73-101)
E/A ratio	1.88 ± 0.45 (0.98-2.78)	1.53 ± 0.40 (0.73-2.33)	1.28 ± 0.25 (0.78-1.78)	0.96 ± 0.18 (0.6-1.32)
DT (ms)	142 ± 19 (104-180)	166 ± 14 (138-194)	181 ± 19 (143-219)	200 ± 29 (142-258)
A duration (ms)	113 ± 17 (79-147)	127 ± 13 (101-153)	133 ± 13 (107-159)	138 ± 19 (100-176)
PV S/D ratio	0.82 ± 0.18 (0.46-1.18)	0.98 ± 0.32 (0.34-1.62)	1.21 ± 0.2 (0.81-0.61)	1.39 ± 0.47 (0.45-2.33)
PV Ar (cm/s)	16 ± 10 (1-36)	21 ± 8 (5-37)	23 ± 3 (17-29)	25 ± 9 (11-39)
PV Ar duration (ms)	66 ± 39 (1-144)	96 ± 33 (30-162)	112 ± 15 (82-142)	113 ± 30 (53-173)
Septal E′ (cm/s)	14.9 ± 2.4 (10.1-19.7)	15.5 ± 2.7 (10.1-20.9)	12.2 ± 2.3 (7.6-16.8)	10.4 ± 2.1 (6.2-14.6)
Septal E′/A′ ratio	2.4[a]	1.6 ± 0.5 (0.6-2.6)	1.1 ± 0.3 (0.5-1.7)	0.85 ± 0.2 (0.45-1.25)
Lateral E′ (cm/s)	20.6 ± 3.8 (13.0-28.2)	19.8 ± 2.9 (14.0-25.6)	16.1 ± 2.3 (11.5-20.7)	12.9 ± 3.5 (5.9-19.9)
Lateral E′/A′ ratio	3.1[a]	1.9 ± 0.6 (0.7-3.1)	1.5 ± 0.5 (0.5-2.5)	0.9 ± 0.4 (0.1-1.7)

Data are expressed as mean ± SD (95% confidence interval). Note that for E′ velocity in subjects aged 16 to 20 years, values overlap with those for subjects aged 21 to 40 years. This is because E′ increases progressively with age in children and adolescents. Therefore, the E′ velocity is higher in a normal 20-year-old than in a normal 16-year-old, which results in a somewhat lower average E′ value when subjects aged 16 to 20 years are considered.

[a]Standard deviations are not included because these data were computed, not directly provided in the original articles from which they were derived.

IVRT, isolvolumic relaxation time; E, early diastolic peak velocity; A, late diastolic peak velocity; E/A, ratio of early to late velocities; DT, deceleration time of early diastolic wave; PV S/D, ratio of systolic to diastolic peak pulmonary vein velocities; PV Ar, peak velocity of pulmonary vein reverse atrial flow; E′, early diastolic peak velocity by tissue Doppler imaging; A′, late diastolic peak velocity by tissue Doppler imaging.

From Nagueh SF, Appleton CP, Gillebert TC, et al. Recommendations for the evaluation of left ventricular diastolic function by echocardiography. J Am Soc Echocardiogr. 2009;22(2):107-133.

inflow, minimizes errors in peak velocity (6% error at 20°), helps place the sample volume in an area of laminar flow, and reduces the spectral broadening, which makes measurements of flow duration and deceleration time difficult. Typically, there is an angle of 20° between mitral inflow (normally directed toward the lateral wall) and the LV longitudinal axis. Cardiac chamber remodeling, as in patients with dilated cardiomyopathy, can increase this angle to 40°; in cases of asymmetric hypertrophic cardiomyopathy, the direction of the flow can be even more difficult to delineate (Figure 12–6; see Chapter 14).[22] In such instances, color Doppler imaging should be used to visualize the direction of the inflow in each patient and to obtain the best alignment with that flow. It is also important to recognize that velocity profiles change with the Doppler sample position within the mitral inflow tract. For accurate evaluation of diastolic function, the pulsed-wave Doppler sample volume typically is placed at the mitral leaflet tips. Moving from the mitral annulus to the tip of the leaflets produces an increase in E velocity and a decrease in DT (Figure 12–7). However, the duration of the mitral A wave may be best acquired by moving the sampling gate into the annular plane of the mitral valve.

Sample volume also should be reduced (1.5 to 2.0 mm) to obtain sharper limits of the spectral envelope and the most accurate DT. Further, the

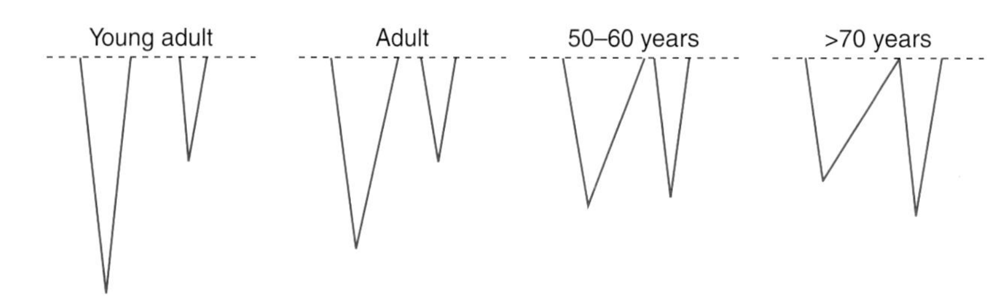

FIGURE 12–4. Schematic representation of the mitral velocity profile at different ages in a population with no cardiac disease.

aliasing limit should be maintained between 0.7 and 1 m/s, the velocity filter should be reduced (between 200 and 600 Hz) to improve visualization of low flows, a sweep speed of 50 to 100 mm/s should be implemented, and an average of three beats should be recorded.[22] The use of low-velocity filters is of particular importance for the measurement of time intervals, which can be masked by the numerous artifacts seen at zero baseline.

Abnormal Patterns

In diastolic dysfunction, three abnormal transmitral filling patterns have been described—impaired relaxation (grade I), pseudonormal (grade II), and restrictive

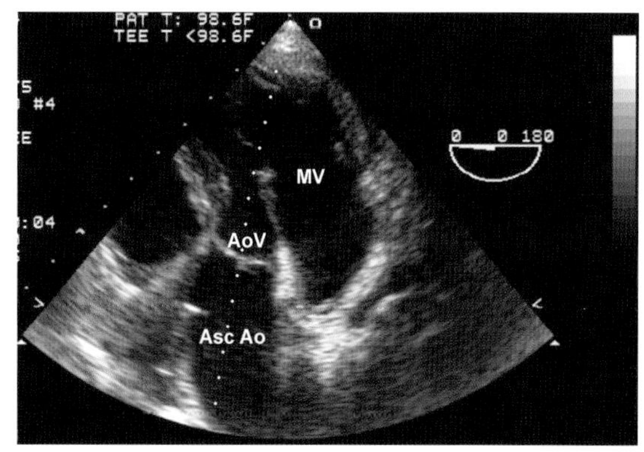

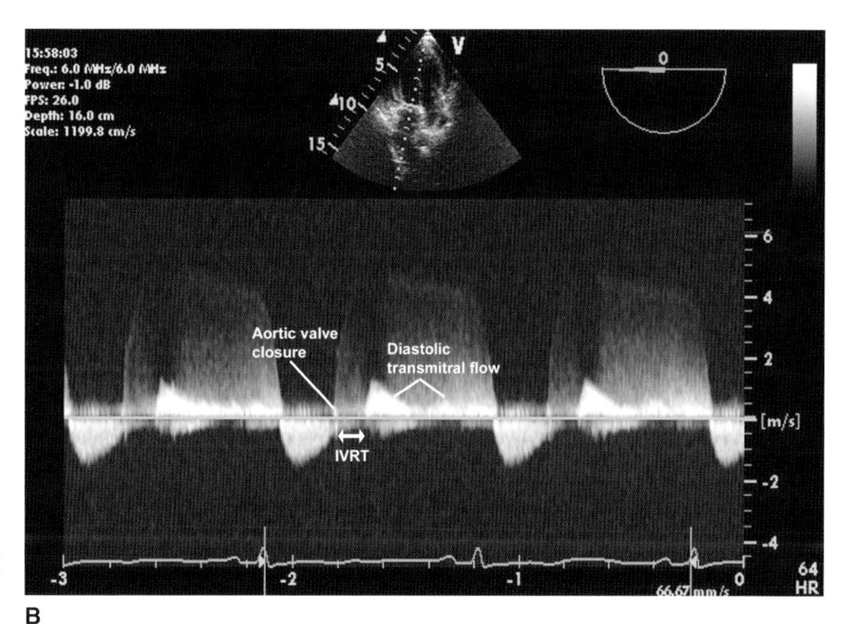

FIGURE 12–5. **A:** Deep transgastric long-axis view with the dotted line indicating a continuous-wave (CW) Doppler beam intercepting the aortic valve flow and the transmitral valve flow. (Asc Ao, ascending aorta; AoV, aortic valve; MV, mitral valve.) **B:** The velocity pattern obtained by applying CW Doppler as shown in panel **(A)**. The isovolumic relaxation time (IVRT) is measured from the aortic valve closure to the beginning of the transmitral diastolic flow.

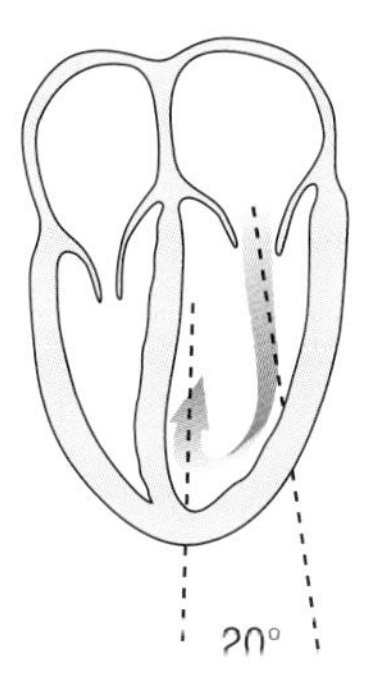

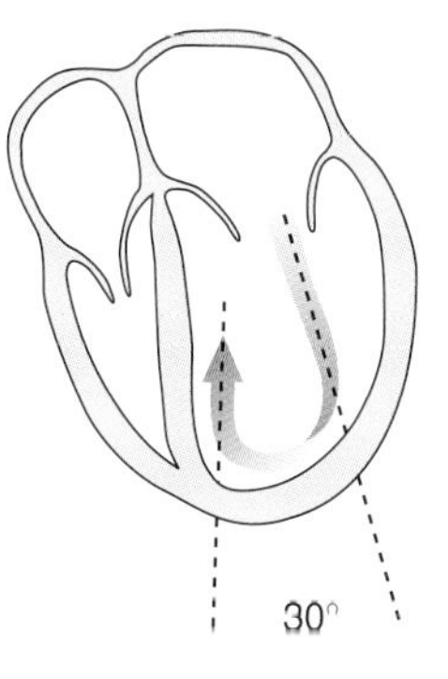

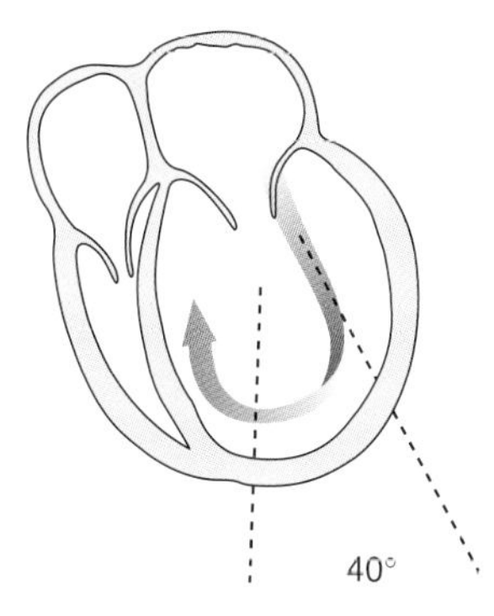

FIGURE 12–6. Alteration of mitral inflow with progressive cardiac dilation. Flow normally is directed approximately 20° laterally toward the apex. With severe left ventricular dilation, optimal beam alignment may be as much as 40° or more laterally from the apex.

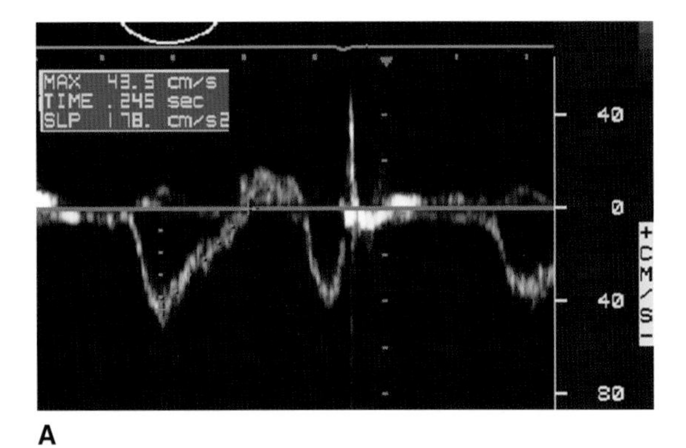

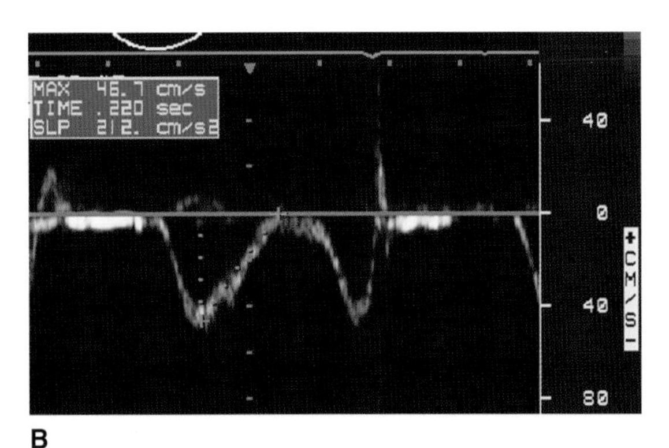

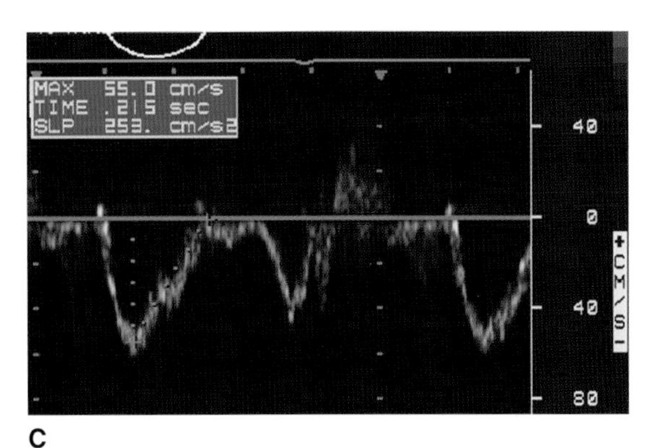

FIGURE 12–7. Doppler envelope at different levels of the atrioventricular valve apparatus: the annulus, midportion of the leaflets, and tips of leaflets. Moving from the mitral annulus to the tip of the leaflets produces an increase in peak velocity and a decrease of deceleration time. **A:** Annulus. **B:** Midportion of the leaflets. **C:** Tips of leaflets.

filling (grade III). The restrictive pattern is further categorized as reversible restrictive (grade IIIa) and irreversible restrictive (grade IIIb).

Grade I: Impaired Relaxation Pattern

The initial manifestation of diastolic dysfunction is abnormal relaxation and is often seen in patients with hypertension and coronary artery disease, and in the elderly. Abnormal relaxation is characterized by a lower rate of LV pressure decay during isovolumic relaxation causing a delay in MV opening, which translates into a prolonged IVRT. Since LV relaxation is prolonged, DT is lengthened and there is a compensatory increase in flow velocity during atrial contraction. Hence, grade I diastolic dysfunction is characterized by a decrease in peak E wave, an increase in peak A wave, an E/A ratio less than 1 and a prolonged DT (Figure 12–8A).

Grade II: Pseudonormal Pattern

As the disease progresses, an alteration in LV compliance ensues. Decreased LV compliance can be caused by an increase in LV stiffness (myocardial fibrosis or necrosis), an increased pericardial restraint (pericardial tamponade or constrictive pericarditis), or volume overload. In these pathophysiologic states an increase in LV volume will lead to a disproportionate increase of LV pressure, and ultimately to a compensatory increase of LA pressure. The increase of LA pressure reestablishes the normal LA-LV pressure gradient, and therefore improves LV filling during the rapid filling phase. However, the "normalization" of diastolic filling is obtained at the cost of increased LAP, which is associated with a host of detrimental effects (LA enlargement, possible atrial arrhythmias, and ultimately heart failure). These changes are represented on the mitral inflow velocity profile by a normal E/A ratio, DT, and IVRT.

The pseudonormal pattern represents a transition period between isolated relaxation abnormality and increased stiffness.[20,22] Since the pattern "normalizes" because of an increase in preload, preload reduction using a Valsalva maneuver, reverse Trendelenburg position, or nitroglycerin administration will unmask diastolic dysfunction by changing the pseudonormal pattern to an impaired relaxation pattern. In contrast, when diastolic function is normal, the decrease in preload will result in a decrease in both peak E and A velocities with an unchanged E/A ratio.[20] Methods used to distinguish a normal from a pseudonormal pattern are summarized in Table 12–2.

Grade III: Restrictive Pattern

In late stages of diastolic dysfunction, the LV compliance decreases drastically and causes increased mean intracavitary diastolic pressures and, as a compensatory mechanism, a severe increase of LA pressure.

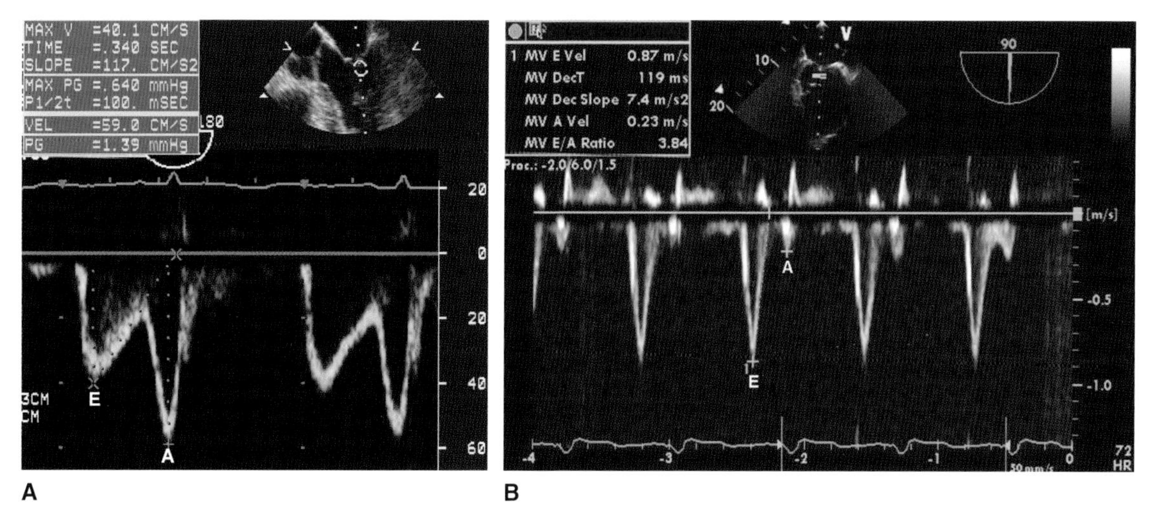

FIGURE 12–8. Examples of mitral inflow recorded with pulsed-wave Doppler. **A:** Impaired relaxation. **B:** Restrictive pattern. (E, early filling peak velocity; A, late filling peak velocity.)

Patients with this type of abnormality have isolated severe diastolic dysfunction (restrictive cardiomyopathy) or concomitant significant systolic dysfunction (dilated cardiomyopathy). The increased LA pressure results in an earlier mitral valve opening and higher initial transmitral pressure gradient, producing a fast acceleration of blood flow into the LV during the rapid filling phase. As the ventricle is very stiff, the LV pressure will rise rapidly to equalize with LAP and allow only a limited amount of blood to fill the cavity. Atrial contraction at the end of diastole will contribute very little to the filling of the noncompliant LV, as increased LV pressure will terminate mitral flow prematurely. This sequence of events will result in a shortened IVRT, an increased E velocity, a shorter E-wave deceleration time, a decreased A-wave velocity, and a decreased A-wave duration (Figure 12–8B).[20]

It is widely accepted that an increased early diastolic mitral velocity (E wave), a reduced atrial contribution (A wave), and an increased E/A ratio are reliable markers of increased filling pressure, particularly in patients with reduced ejection fraction.[18,23] The DT accurately predicts high filling pressures in patients with left ventricular systolic dysfunction, but is not as reliable in patients with normal ejection fraction.[23-25] Another sign of markedly elevated LV diastolic pressures is diastolic mitral regurgitation, which can be observed in patients with competent mitral valves. In patients with grade IIIa diastolic dysfunction, preload reduction (nitroglycerin administration, Valsalva maneuver) changes the restrictive filling pattern to one of impaired relaxation, whereas in patients with grade IIIb diastolic dysfunction the restrictive pattern is irreversible. Grade IIIb diastolic dysfunction is associated with a poor prognosis.[18,26]

Table 12–2. Different Methods to Differentiate the Pseudonormal from Normal Mitral Flow Pattern[a]

Clinical elements	Age >70 years; hypertrophic or ischemic cardiomyopathy
2D echocardiography evidence of LV remodeling	Hypertrophy, dilation, scars of myocardial infarction
2D echocardiography evidence of elevation of LA pressure	LA enlargement without history of atrial fibrillation or mitral valve disease
Preload reduction through dynamic maneuvers	Unmasked mitral inflow pattern of impaired relaxation
Doppler evidence of elevation of filling pressure using pulmonary venous flow	Systolic fraction <55%; increased velocity and duration of atrial flow
Color M-mode propagation velocity	Decreased propagation velocity
Mitral annulus tissue Doppler imaging	Decreased E′ velocity: E′/A′ <1

[a]Findings on the right side of the table are indicative of a pseudonormal pattern.
2D, two-dimensional; A′, atrial contraction; DTI, Doppler tissue imaging; E′, early diastolic relaxation; LA, left atrial; LV, left ventricular.

Limitations

Ventilation affects Doppler flow recording by altering the loading conditions induced by pleural pressure variations during the respiratory cycle. The increase in airway and pleural pressures during mechanical ventilation produces a constant decrease in LV impedance and thus can alter mitral flow profiles. During the inspiratory phase, LV filling changes according to pulmonary vein filling. When the pulmonary veins are dilated, an increase in airway pressure can produce a parallel increase in LA and LV filling flow. Conversely, when pulmonary veins are empty, an elevated airway pressure during the inspiratory phase can be an obstacle to atrial and ventricular filling. Positive end-expiratory pressure ventilation reduces global mitral flow with a relatively greater decrease in E wave, such that the E/A ratio is only moderately decreased. Therefore, Doppler flow recordings should be accomplished during apnea in patients breathing spontaneously or at end-expiration for mechanically ventilated patients.[27]

Mitral inflow velocities are determined by the transmitral pressure gradient and are highly dependent on age, heart rate, intrinsic properties of the myocardium, and loading conditions. Hypovolemia can mimic a relaxation abnormality even in young patients with normal cardiac function. Conversely, an increase in preload (fluid administration) in healthy subjects produces an increase in E velocity, a shortened IVRT, and a decrease in DT.[28] An increase in afterload (phenylephrine administration) also produces a significant decrease in E velocity and increase in DT.[29] In an experimental study on dogs, Choong et al found that peak E-wave velocity increased linearly with increasing LA pressure at constant LV systolic pressure and decreased with increasing LV systolic pressure at constant LA pressure.[30] Tachycardia leads to fusion of the E and A waves, a decrease in the E/A ratio, and an increase in the A velocity. Because of a shortened diastolic period associated with tachycardia, LV filling is incomplete when atrial contraction occurs, thus causing an elevation in the atrioventricular pressure gradient during late diastole.[29] An abnormally prolonged PR interval will result in a similar pattern. When the PR interval is abnormally short, the A wave will be terminated prematurely as a result of the beginning of the LV systole. This change may result in decreased diastolic filling, and thus decreased stroke volume and an increased diastolic filling pressure.[20] Evaluation of diastolic function in atrial fibrillation remains a clinical challenge due to the asynchrony of atrial contraction and variable cardiac cycle length. Multiple studies have shown that in the setting of atrial fibrillation, mitral E-wave deceleration time can provide an accurate assessment of LV filling pressures, especially in patients with depressed systolic function. In atrial fibrillation, a DT less than 130 milliseconds has been associated with restrictive filling, and less beat-to-beat variability in mitral inflow parameters has been associated with increased filling pressures.[31-33]

Mitral stenosis increases mitral velocities and causes a fusion of E and A waves, with an increase in DT. Mitral regurgitation strongly affects transmitral flow, especially peak E wave and DT. Increased LA pressures will result in a restrictive transmitral flow pattern in the absence of diastolic dysfunction.[34] In mitral regurgitation, end-diastolic Doppler parameters such as A-wave duration have been shown to be more reliable in assessing LV filling pressure.[23] Severe acute aortic regurgitation results in a restrictive transmitral flow pattern (increased E-wave velocity, decreased A-wave velocity, and decreased E-wave DT) due to rapid increase in the LV pressure, which often exceeds LA pressure in late diastole thus resulting in diastolic mitral regurgitation.[35,36] Chronic aortic insufficiency has less impact on the transmitral flow due to the development of increased LV compliance over time.[37]

PULMONARY VENOUS FLOW

Pulmonary venous (PV) flow profiles used in conjunction with transmitral flow velocities are useful in assessing LV filling pressures and grading the severity of LV diastolic dysfunction.

Normal Pattern and Basic Variables

Six variables can be derived from interrogation of PV flow (Figure 12–9)[38]:

1. The peak systolic flow velocity or S-wave velocity. The systolic forward flow sometimes has a biphasic pattern termed S_1 in early systole and S_2 in late systole.[39] S_1 occurs during early systole due to active atrial relaxation and a subsequent fall in LA pressure, which promotes forward flow from the PV to the LA. The S_2 wave is associated with an increase in PV forward flow caused by the continuing descent of the LV base during LV contraction, leading to a further decrease in LA pressure. S_2 maximum velocity and timing are influenced by RV function, the compliance relation between the pulmonary vasculature and the LA, LV contraction, and the presence of mitral regurgitation.[40]
2. The peak diastolic flow velocity or D-wave velocity. The D wave represents the PV forward flow during LV diastole. It occurs after MV opening when the LA serves as a conduit between the pulmonary veins and the LV. PVD coincides with, has a similar contour to, and is dependent on the same factors that influence the early transmitral flow (E wave).[18,41]

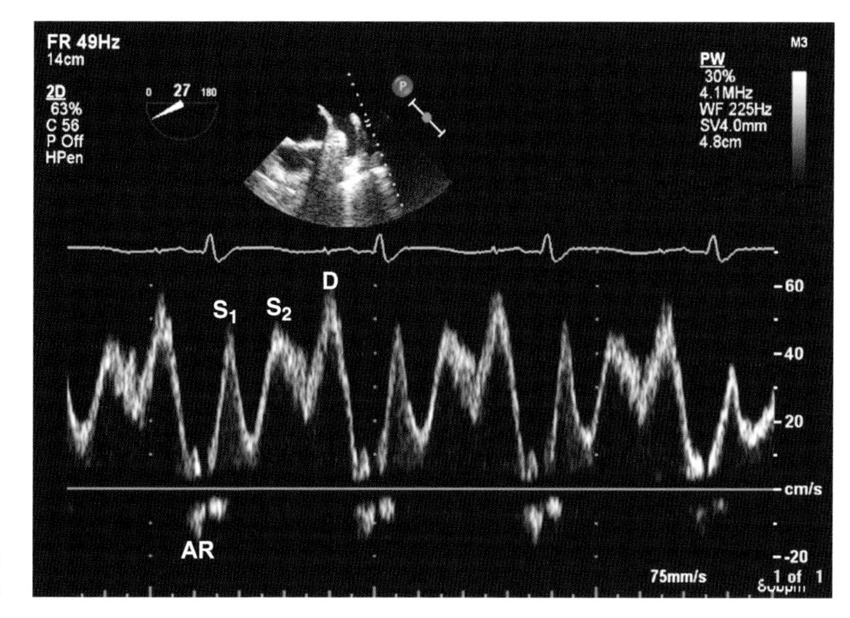

FIGURE 12–9. Normal pattern of pulmonary venous flow. There is an antegrade systolic flow with a biphasic pattern (S_1 and S_2), an antegrade diastolic flow (D), and a retrograde diastolic flow (AR).

3. The peak atrial reversal flow velocity or AR-wave velocity. The PV flow reversal in late diastole (PV AR) occurs due to atrial contraction and is dependent on LA contractility as well as the compliance of the pulmonary venous bed, LA, and LV.
4. The duration of the AR wave (AR-dur).
5. The time difference between the duration of PV AR wave (AR-dur) and mitral A wave (A-dur).
6. The deceleration time of the D wave, defined as the time interval from peak D velocity to zero baseline.

The normal PV flow pattern is characterized by predominance of the systolic waves in which the systolic velocities are slightly higher than the diastolic ones. As a consequence the systolic-to-diastolic ratio is more than 1 (S/D >1). The systolic filling fraction is the ratio of systolic time-velocity integral (TVI) to the sum of the systolic and diastolic time-velocity integrals, with normal values being greater than or equal to 55%.

Technical Recommendations

The PV flow velocity profile is obtained by pulsed-wave (PW) Doppler interrogation of the flow in the left or right upper pulmonary veins. Both upper pulmonary veins enter the atrium in an anterior-to-posterior direction and are thus suitable for Doppler interrogation, while the lower pulmonary veins typically course in a lateral-to-medial direction entering the atrium almost perpendicular to the Doppler beam, making them less than optimal for routine assessment of PV flow. The left upper pulmonary vein can be visualized lateral to the left atrial appendage by withdrawing the probe slightly from the midesophageal four-chamber (ME4C) view and then turning to the left. Depending on the orientation of the heart within the mediastinum, advancement of the multiplane angle between 30° and 60° may be necessary in order to align the Doppler beam parallel with the PV flow (Figure 12–10A). The right upper pulmonary vein can be visualized in a modified bicaval view by withdrawing the TEE probe and advancing the multiplane angle to 110° to 130° until the right upper pulmonary vein is seen lateral to the superior vena cava (Figure 12–10B). Color-flow Doppler with low-velocity settings is also useful in locating the pulmonary veins and assists in aligning the Doppler beam with the laminar blood flow. The PW Doppler sample is positioned 1 to 2 cm into the PV, beyond its insertion into the left atrium. As with mitral inflow recordings, the velocity filter should be reduced in order to improve visualization of low flows, a sweep speed of 50 to 100 mm/s should be implemented, and an average of 3 beats should be recorded. To minimize the impact of changes in intrathoracic pressures on PV flows, all measurements must be made at end-expiration or during apnea.

A small sample volume (1 to 2 mm) can produce a weak spectral signal containing excessive wall motion artifacts; therefore, increasing the sample volume from 2 mm to 3 to 5 mm may improve an inadequate signal. However, a large sample volume (>5 mm) as well as a Doppler gain set too high could result in a dense Doppler signal with indistinguishable spectral envelopes.

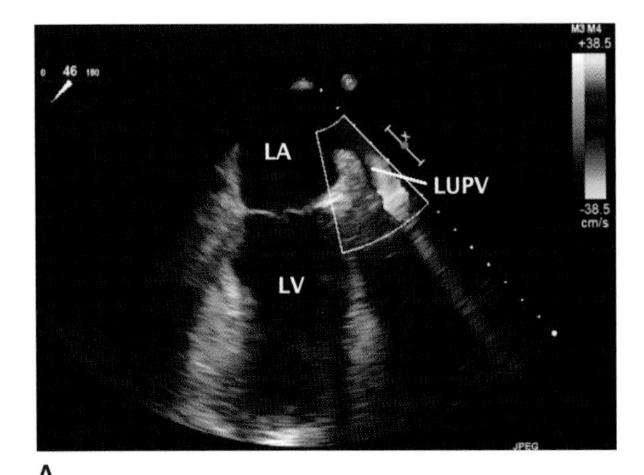

A

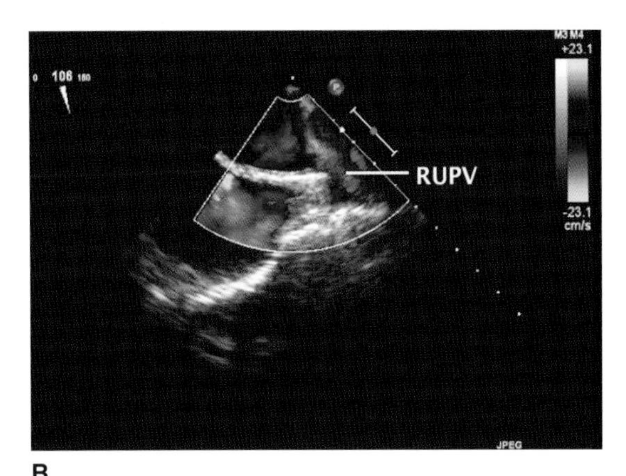

B

FIGURE 12–10. **A:** The left upper pulmonary vein (LUPV) is visualized at the midesophageal level as detailed in the text. (LA, left atrium; LV, left ventricle.) **B:** The right upper pulmonary vein (RUPV) is visualized in a modified midesophageal bicaval view. Color-flow Doppler can be used to identify the veins.

Wall motion artifacts are common in PV recordings and often mask the PV AR wave. Although these artifacts are difficult to eliminate completely, a slight angulation of the transducer beam or placing a larger sample volume (4 mm) farther into the PV may improve the flow velocity signal.[22] As the sample volume is moved into the pulmonary vein, the PV flow profile is influenced more by pulmonary arterial pressure.[40] Although the PV flow profile is a more sensitive index of LA pressure when the sampling volume is placed at the atriovenous junction, in order to obtain a clear Doppler signal, the sample volume has to be located 1 to 2 cm into the PV.[22]

Abnormal Patterns

The analysis of PV flow velocities complements the assessment of the transmitral flow velocity pattern but may not add substantial incremental value in the assessment of diastolic function, especially with the advent of tissue Doppler imaging, which can accurately detect underlying LV relaxation abnormalities.[42,43] As stated earlier, because the LA functions as a passive conduit for flow during early diastole, the PV diastolic flow velocity correlates well with the mitral E-wave velocity. Therefore, in an isolated relaxation abnormality (grade I diastolic dysfunction) the diastolic component of the PV flow is significantly diminished when compared with the systolic component (S>>D) (Figure 12–11A). As diastolic dysfunction progresses to the pseudonormal pattern (grade II diastolic dysfunction), the abnormally elevated LA pressure is associated with a decrease in forward systolic flow, and thus a more prominent diastolic velocity (S<D). In the late stages of diastolic dysfunction, the restrictive pattern (grade III diastolic dysfunction) is characterized on the PVF velocity curves by a dominant diastolic forward flow velocity and a diminished systolic forward flow (S<<D) (Figure 12–11B).[21,41]

Elevated LV filling pressures can be inferred from the PV flow velocities. A systolic filling fraction less than 40% and a deceleration time of the PV D wave less than 160 milliseconds are associated with LV end-diastolic pressure above 18 mm Hg in patients with impaired systolic function.[26,44,45] The relationship between the duration of PV AR wave and transmitral A wave (AR-dur and A-dur, respectively) is of special importance in the estimation of LV filling pressures. Under normal conditions, AR-dur is equal to or less than A-dur. In the presence of abnormal compliance of the LV and higher end-diastolic pressures there is more resistance to forward flow across the MV during atrial contraction, and AR wave increases both in duration as well as in amplitude. Studies have shown that an AR velocity greater than 35 cm/s, AR-dur greater than 30 milliseconds, and AR-dur longer than A-dur are indicative of an LV end-diastolic pressure greater than 15 mm Hg regardless of the systolic function.[44,46]

Limitations

The PV flow profile is influenced by age, respiration, heart rate, and loading conditions. Variations in PV flow velocities with aging are presented in Table 12–1. In normal young adults and athletes, in whom atrial contribution to LV filling is minimal and the LA behaves more as a "passive" conduit, predominant forward flow occurs in diastole resulting in a blunted systolic component, while in older aged adults predominant flow occurs in systole.[26,47] PV AR duration and

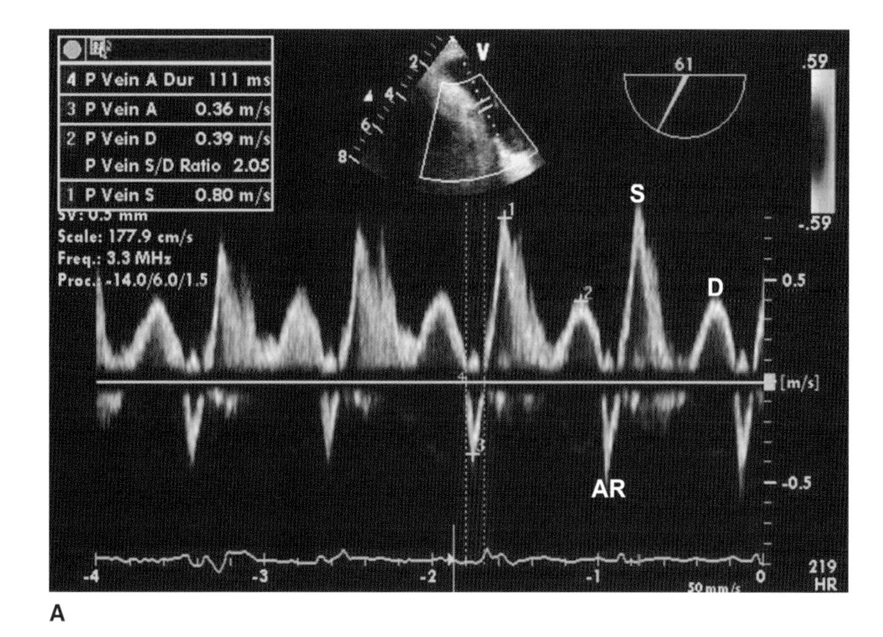

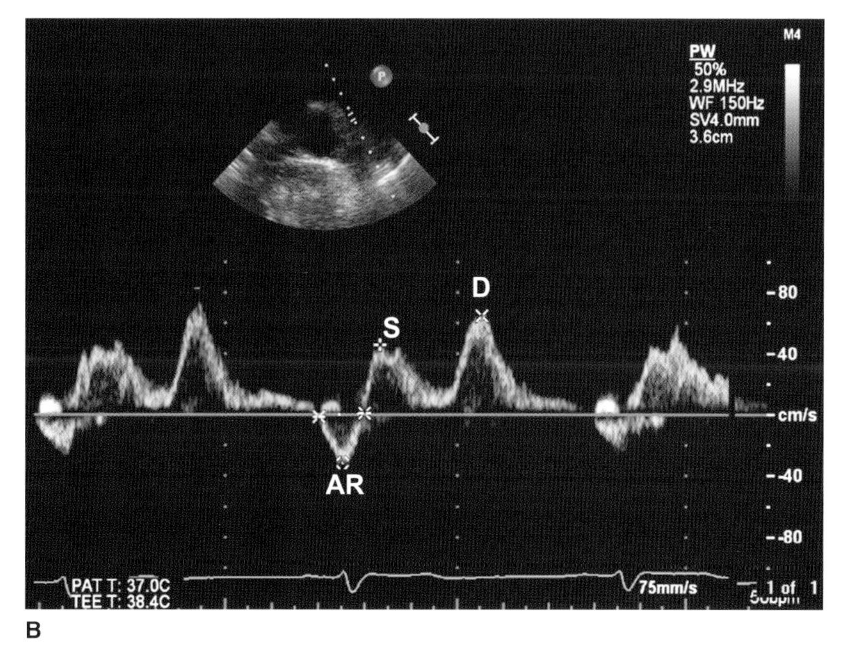

FIGURE 12–11. **A:** Abnormal pulmonary venous flow pattern with a prominent systolic component in a patient with grade I (impaired relaxation) diastolic dysfunction **B:** Abnormal pulmonary venous flow pattern with a blunted systolic component in a patient with diastolic dysfunction and elevated filling pressures. (S, peak systolic flow velocity; D, peak diastolic flow velocity; AR, atrial reversal flow.)

the time difference between the duration of PV AR wave and the mitral A wave (ARdur-Adur) are not affected by age and can provide an age-independent assessment of late diastolic LV pressures.[48]

Changes in the PV flow profile observed during spontaneous respirations include an increase in global flow and a relative increase of diastolic components during the expiratory period. Therefore, PV flow should be recorded during apnea or during the end-expiratory period in mechanically ventilated patients. Heart rate can also alter the PV flow profile. Tachycardia reduces the duration of the diastolic phase; thus, at rates greater than 100 beats per minute, the diastolic component of PV flow is reduced with an increase in systolic fraction and PV AR may be absent[40] Atrial fibrillation also produces an absent PV AR wave; decreased systolic filling fraction, probably caused by the loss of the atrial relaxation as well as by the reduced amplitude of the downward displacement of mitral leaflets; and at times, late systolic reversal of flow in the absence of significant mitral regurgitation.[49] Loading conditions can affect the PV flow profile even when diastolic properties remain constant. Fluid loading affects the PV flow profile by decreasing systolic components and the systolic fraction, with little effect on early diastolic flow. Major changes are observed during the late diastolic phase, with an increase of peak velocity and duration of PV AR.

Mitral stenosis induces an enlargement of the LA and increases LA wall stiffness. Impaired atrial relaxation and reduced mitral annulus displacement result in a decrease in the systolic filling fraction, which is a predictor of increased LA pressure. However, because of impaired LV filling, there is no relation between LV filling pressure and PV flow profile in mitral stenosis.[50] Elevation of LAP as a result of mitral regurgitation also produces a decrease in the systolic fraction; in cases of severe mitral regurgitation, reversal of systolic flow is observed.[51]

MITRAL ANNULUS TISSUE DOPPLER IMAGING

The physical principles of tissue Doppler imaging (TDI) are analogous to those of conventional PW Doppler. Doppler shift is typically measured either from blood cell movement (with a normal velocity of up to 150 cm/s) or solid tissues movement (with usual velocities rarely > 15 cm/s). In conventional PW Doppler studies, the low-velocity, high-amplitude signals of tissue motion are filtered out, leaving only Doppler signals from blood flow. With TDI, the opposite is true, and red blood cell Doppler shifts are filtered, leaving only tissue velocity data. Advantages of TDI over conventional ultrasound techniques include the fact that high-energy signals generated by wall motion are minimally affected by tissue interfaces, thus a high-quality two-dimensional image is not always necessary in order to obtain adequate tissue Doppler data. Furthermore, the high temporal resolution of pulsed TDI allows for quantifying systolic and diastolic events during isovolumic periods. Finally, intramyocardial velocities can easily be analyzed over the cardiac cycle, thus changes with physiologic or pathologic conditions can be readily observed. TDI velocities can be displayed as a spectral PW Doppler signal, a color velocity-encoded M mode, or a two-dimensional color map.

Left ventricular diastolic function assessment using the TDI technique evaluates the mitral annular motion. The movement of the mitral annulus can be easily recorded by placing the PW Doppler sample gate at the level of the lateral or septal mitral annulus in the ME4C view (Figure 12–12A). Although the myocardial fibers have both translational and rotational components, in the ME4C view, axial motion of the LV is parallel to the Doppler beam, and therefore the recorded velocities are primarily related to LV contraction and relaxation.

Normal Pattern and Basic Variables

A typical spectral display of TDI consists of a negative (below the baseline) systolic component (S′) and two positive signals (above the baseline), one occurring during early diastole (E′) and the other one during atrial contraction (A′) (Figure 12–12B). S′ is caused by the descent of the mitral annulus toward the apex in LV systole. E′ represents myocardial elongation during early diastole and relates to the velocity of relaxation, and A′ represents the passive myocardial distension caused by atrial contraction, either by retraction of the annular ring or due to the subsequent late ventricular filling.[34] These TDI diastolic velocities are simultaneous to the transmitral flow components. However, in healthy subjects the peak of E′ occurs before the peak of the transmitral flow E velocity, suggesting that E′ represents the active relaxation of the myocardium that precedes filling of the LV. E′ is strongly correlated to cardiac catheterization indices of LV relaxation.[52,53] In subjects with normal diastolic function, the ratio of E′ to A′ is always greater than one. E′ and E′/A′ ratio decline with age and with pathologic conditions such as dilated cardiomyopathy, myocardial ischemia, or LV hypertrophy. Some studies have suggested that the threshold values of E′ used to identify diastolic dysfunction should be approximately 12.5 cm/s in young adults and 8.5 cm/s for older subjects.[54]

Technical Recommendations

With the TDI function of the TEE machine activated, in the ME4C view, a PW Doppler sample volume of 2.5 to 5.0 mm is placed in the myocardial wall of interest (lateral or septal mitral annulus). The Doppler beam should be aligned as parallel as possible with the longitudinal axial motion of the LV. Some investigators recommend the lateral mitral annulus as the location of choice since the velocities tend to be higher, are less influenced by the velocities of the blood flow, and tend to be more reproducible than the septal annulus.[42,55] As the mitral annular velocities are usually less than 20 cm/s, the velocity scales should be lowered. Doppler gain and wall filters should be minimized in order to display the lower myocardial velocities. Sweep speed is commonly set at 100 or 200 mm/s.[21]

Abnormal Patterns

An E′ value less than 8 cm/s is consistent with diastolic dysfunction (Figure 12–12C).[42] Similar to transmitral flow velocity profiles, patients with impaired ventricular relaxation often have an E′/A′ ratio less than one, but unlike transmitral flow, this ratio does not pseudonormalize with increased LA pressures.[56] Therefore, in patients with diastolic dysfunction and increased filling pressures, a reduced E′ can be used to identify patients with pseudonormal LV filling pattern.[57] While some clinical studies have suggested that early diastolic myocardial velocity E′ is less preload dependent than mitral flow velocity, this may not be true in healthy subjects with normal or enhanced LV relaxation or in patients with normal LV systolic function and volume overload owing to mitral or aortic regurgitation.[21,56,57]

As mitral E velocity is dependent on LV relaxation and filling pressure and E′ relates mostly to LV relaxation, the E/E′ ratio relates well to LV filling pressures

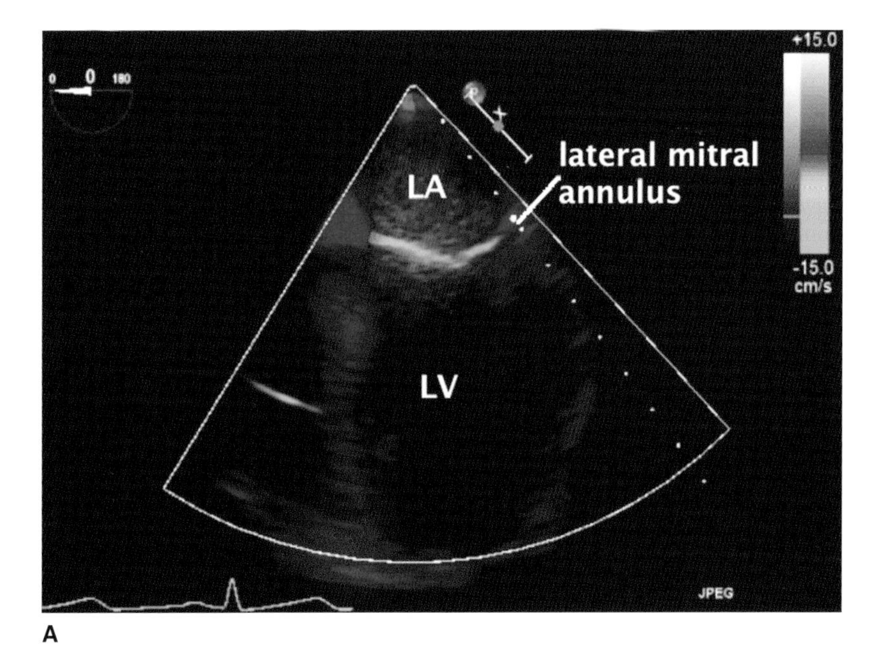

A

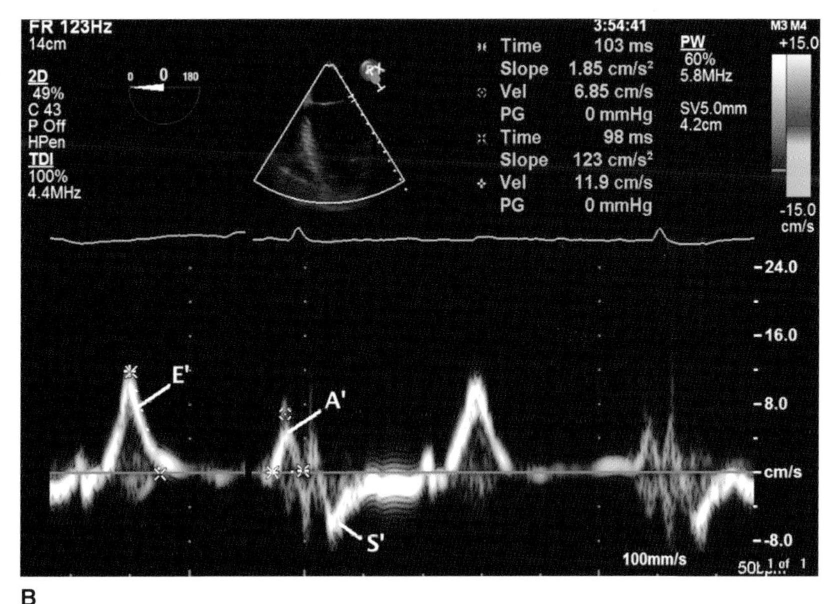

B

FIGURE 12–12. **A:** Midesophageal four-chamber view with color map of tissue velocities. The sample gate of the pulsed-wave Doppler beam is placed at the lateral mitral annulus. (LA, left atrium; LV, left ventricle.) **B:** Normal pattern of spectral Doppler displays tissue velocities recorded at the lateral mitral annulus. There is a negative systolic signal (S′) and two positive signals in early (E′) and late diastole (A′). **C:** Tissue Doppler imaging recorded with pulsed-wave Doppler at the lateral annulus of the mitral valve in diastolic dysfunction. Note the decreased E′ velocity and the inverted E′/A′ ratio.

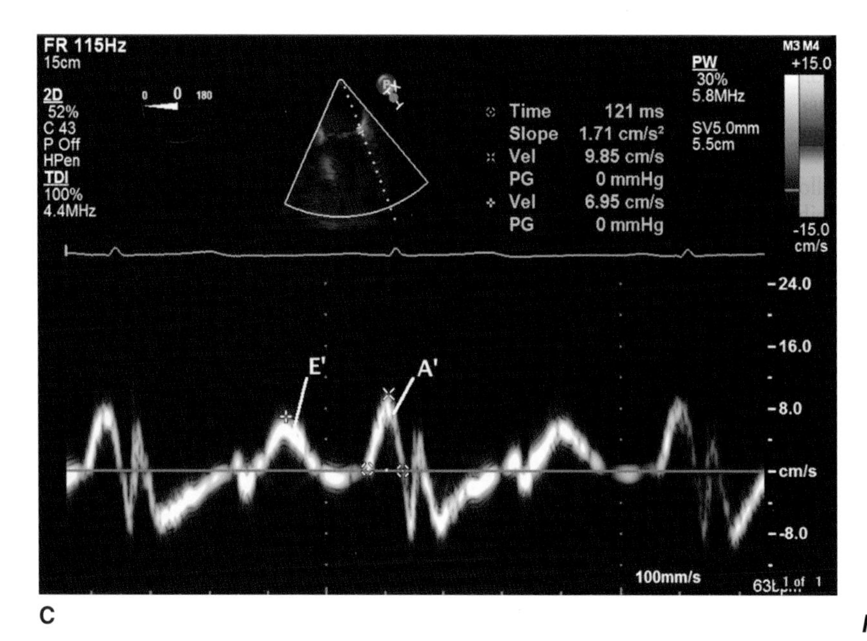

C

FIGURE 12–12. *(Continued)*

irrespective of the LV ejection fraction.[58] Nagueh et al showed that an E/E′ ratio greater than 10 detected a mean pulmonary capillary wedge pressure greater than 15 mm Hg with a sensitivity of 97% and a specificity of 78%.[57] Other investigators have shown that an E/E′ ratio greater than 15 was highly specific for LA pressures higher than 15 mm Hg, and a ratio of less than 8 is highly specific for normal LA pressures, while a wide variability is present in patients with an E/E′ ratio between 8 and 15.[59] This difference might result from the fact that while the former study used the lateral mitral annulus velocities, the latter used the septal mitral annulus for measurements. In patients with a normal EF, lateral E/E′ seems to have the highest correlation with LV filling pressures with the caveat that in these patients E′ may not be preload independent.[58] The ability of the E/E′ ratio to estimate LV filling pressures has been described in patients with sinus tachycardia, atrial fibrillation, and hypertrophic cardiomyopathy. In patients after cardiac transplant the increase in E/E′ ratio can detect early rejection.[33,60-62] TDI is also helpful in differentiating constrictive pericarditis from restrictive cardiomyopathies. Both entities are characterized by elevated transmitral flow peak E wave, but patients with constriction and normal LV relaxation have normal E′ velocities, while patients with restriction have lower than normal E′ velocities.[63]

Limitations

E′ may not be a true indicator of LV relaxation and filling pressures in the setting of wall motion abnormalities and myocardial tethering. An average of lateral and septal E′ velocities may offer a better estimate of global LV diastolic properties when wall motion abnormalities are present in the basal segments.[34] Patients with severe mitral annular calcification have lower mitral annular velocities caused by decreased mitral annular motion.[64] Mitral annular velocities are also inaccurate after MV annulopasty and MV replacement.

Other TDI Measurements and Technological Advancements

In patients with abnormal myocardial relaxation there is a delay in the onset of E′ velocity, irrespective of the LA pressure. In patients with increased LV filling pressures, the MV opens prematurely due to the increased LA pressure, which decreases the time to the onset of the transmitral flow E velocity and results in the E′ velocity occurring later than mitral E velocity. Therefore, the time difference between the onset of mitral inflow E velocity and the onset of mitral annulus E′ velocity (TE-E′) is used to infer characteristics of both LV relaxation and LV filling pressure. This time difference is prolonged in diastolic dysfunction,[26,65] and an IVRT/TE-E′ less than 2 has high accuracy in identifying patients with a pulmonary capillary wedge pressure greater than 15 mm Hg.[65]

A novel application of TDI is the noninvasive measurement of myocardial deformation by using strain and strain rate (see Chapter 24). Myocardial strain (S) is defined as the change in segment length (L) relative to the resting length of muscle (L0): S = (L – L0)/L0. The rate at which the length of the segment changes is the strain rate (SR = dS/dt). The strain rate is defined as the rate of change of tissue velocity over distances within the myocardium. It is therefore theoretically less susceptible than tissue velocity to cardiac translational motion and myocardial tethering.[66] During ventricular contraction, the myocardium shortens in the longitudinal and circumferential dimensions (negative strain) and thickens or lengthens in the radial direction (positive strain). Although most of the investigational studies on strain rate have focused on systolic function, strain and strain rate can be used to assess regional and global diastolic function.

One of the most important limitations of TDI-based strain and strain rate measurements is the angle dependency of the ultrasound beam with respect to tissue motion. A recently introduced angle-independent method of measuring myocardial deformation is two-dimensional (2D) speckle tracking. Speckle tracking is based on tracking, frame-to-frame throughout the cardiac cycle, the unique speckle patterns created by scattering, reflection, and interference of the ultrasound beams within the myocardial tissue.[67] By tracking different speckles in the same myocardial segments, the distance between the speckles can be measured and segmental shortening or strain can be calculated.[68] In addition, the measurement of rotation with speckle tracking has enabled assessment of LV twist and untwist around its long axis, which plays a pivotal role in the assessment of LV systolic and diastolic function. LV untwisting velocity has emerged as a novel index of LV diastolic function. It has a powerful correlation with the intraventricular pressure gradients, which are responsible for the LV diastolic suction effect. In addition, delayed timing of untwisting seems to be related to LV relaxation and is considered an early sign of diastolic dysfunction.[69-71] Two-dimensional speckle tracking is not affected by the Doppler angle, but is highly dependent on the quality of 2D images.

COLOR M-MODE DOPPLER: PROPAGATION VELOCITY

Another echocardiographic diastolic index is flow propagation velocity in early diastole (Vp), which represents the spatiotemporal velocity distribution along a scan line that extends from the mitral annulus to the apex. Unlike the traditional measure of mitral inflow velocities, Vp provides information equivalent to multiple simultaneous pulsed-wave Doppler echocardiographic measurements from the mitral orifice to the LV apex.[47] Two mechanisms have been proposed as determinants of Vp: the presence of intracavitary pressure gradients and the formation of flow vortices. In patients with normal diastolic function, LV relaxation and untwisting around its axis generate an intraventricular pressure gradient and suction effect, which results in the flow of blood from the base towards the apex in early diastole.

Technical Recommendations

Vp is measured in the ME4C view by applying color-flow Doppler with a narrow color sector that includes the LA, MV, and LV apex. Attention should be paid to eliminating any foreshortening of the LV. The M-mode cursor is placed through the center of the mitral inflow blood column (as identified by color Doppler), from the LA through the MV and towards the LV apex. The color velocity map should be adjusted to alias at 75% of the peak E mitral inflow velocity and the sweep rate should be maximized. In subjects in sinus rhythm, color M-mode Doppler generates two waves, corresponding to the mitral inflow E and A waves. In order to measure Vp, a slope should be drawn from the mitral valve at the first aliasing velocity during early filling to 4 cm distally towards the LV apex (Figure 12–13A).

Interpretation of Propagation Velocity

A Vp greater than 55 cm/s (normal values are 80 ± 25 cm/s) is associated with normal diastolic function in young, healthy subjects (Figure 12–13A).[72] In patients with abnormal diastolic function the diminished intraventricular pressure gradient and increased vortex formation lead to slower propagation of early LV filling flow and a reduced Vp.[47] Impaired diastolic function has been reported to generally reduce Vp to less than 45 cm/s (Figure 12–13B). In contrast to transmitral flow velocities, Vp appears less preload sensitive.[73] In a large group of patients with normal, impaired relaxation and pseudonormal pulsed Doppler patterns of LV filling, Takatsuji et al showed that while transmitral flow Doppler indices did not distinguish between patients with normal and pseudonormal filling patterns, color M-mode Doppler Vp did not "pseudonormalize," being equally low in patients with impaired relaxation and in patients with a pseudonormal pattern.[74] Recent reports, however, have questioned this preload independence, both in patients with normal or depressed ejection fraction.[75,76]

Garcia et al have shown that the pulmonary wedge pressure can be inferred noninvasively from the peak transmitral flow E velocity and Vp.[77] While mitral peak E velocity is dependent on relaxation and preload, Vp is related to LV relaxation; therefore, the ratio E/Vp, which corrects for the influence of LV relaxation on

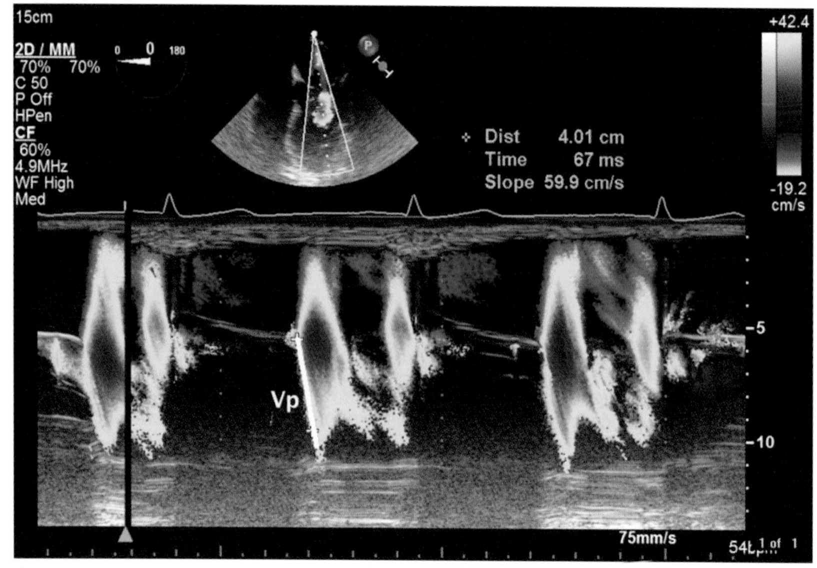

A

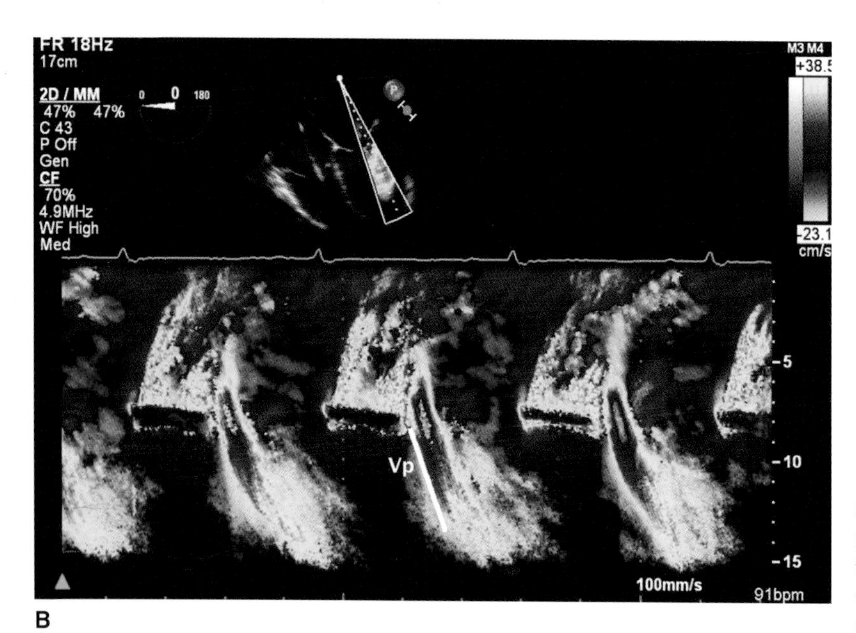

B

FIGURE 12–13. **A:** Normal propagation velocity (Vp) profile. **B:** Reduced propagation velocity (Vp) in a patient with diastolic dysfunction.

transmitral flow, should reflect the LV filling pressures. It is considered that a ratio of E/Vp greater than 1.5 is associated with increased LA pressure.[77] This ratio has also been validated in patients with atrial fibrillation.[33] Similar to the mitral annulus TDI, Vp may be useful in distinguishing restrictive cardiomyopathy from constrictive pericarditis in patients with preserved LV systolic function. Although these patients may have similar PW Doppler transmitral flow velocity patterns, patients with constrictive pericarditis often have a rapid Vp (steeper slope), whereas patients with restrictive cardiomyopathy have a slower Vp.[63]

Limitations

Flow propagation velocity is influenced by age. These age-related variations are present in healthy individuals, in the absence of any apparent cardiovascular disease, and can differ by as much as 44% from the youngest to the oldest individuals.[78] Rivas-Gotz et al have concluded that Vp is inversely related to end-systolic volume and directly related to EF, stroke volume, and cardiac output.[58] Therefore, it is possible for the Vp to fall in the normal range in patients with normal EF despite the presence of diastolic dysfunction, making E/Vp ratio a less optimal index for estimating filling pressures in this population of patients. In patients with moderate or severe aortic insufficiency color M-mode propagation velocity can be difficult to obtain if the regurgitant jet crosses the path of mitral inflow.[35]

GRADING OF DIASTOLIC FUNCTION

Assessment of LV diastolic function should be an integral part of a standard echocardiographic examination. Diastolic function assessment should begin with 2D anatomical imaging and evaluation of LA diameter and volume, LV size and wall thickness, LV systolic function, and valvular and pericardial disease. Accurate evaluation of diastolic function should include transmitral flow PW Doppler evaluation, PW Doppler analysis of PV flow, and TDI of the mitral annulus motion. Mitral flow velocities under a Valsalva maneuver and color M-mode Vp of the mitral inflow can be useful adjuncts.

Assessment of cardiac chamber size and thickness is an essential part of the echocardiographic evaluation of diastolic function. LA enlargement can be present in the absence of diastolic dysfunction in patients with atrial flutter or fibrillation, significant valvular disease, severe bradycardia, or normal athlete's heart. However, in the absence of primary atrial pathology or valvular disease, LA enlargement can be a marker of the chronicity and severity of diastolic dysfunction and a sign of chronic elevation of atrial pressure. LA volume can be evaluated by several methods, among which are the biplane Simpson's method and three-dimensional (3D) echocardiography. LA size is best measured at end-systole when the chamber is at its greatest dimension, with care to exclude the LA appendage and the pulmonary veins. When using transesophageal echocardiography (TEE), however, especially in situations of LA enlargement, the LA does not always entirely fit in the imaging sector. Therefore, the dimensions can be estimated by performing measurements in different imaging planes.[79] Increased LA size has been found to be an independent predictor of adverse cardiovascular outcomes, especially atrial fibrillation, heart failure, stroke, and death.[38,80] Calculation of LV thickness in relation to mass is necessary to diagnose cardiac hypertrophy, a major cause of diastolic dysfunction. LV dilation is another indication of diastolic dysfunction. Diastolic heart failure with normal systolic function is frequent, so parameters of systolic function have to be integrated into the final diagnosis. However, contraction and relaxation are coupled, and impaired myocardial contractility is always associated with relaxation abnormalities. Therefore, a normal mitral flow profile in patients with LV systolic dysfunction should be interpreted as a pseudonormal pattern.

According to the American Society of Echocardiography (ASE) recommendations for evaluation of LV diastolic function, grade I diastolic dysfunction (impaired relaxation) is characterized by E/A ratio less than 0.8, DT greater than 200 milliseconds, IVRT greater than 100 milliseconds, predominant systolic flow in PVF (S>D), mitral annulus velocity E′ less than 8 cm/s and E/E′ ratio less than 8 (septal and lateral) (Figure 12–14).[38] Patients with grade I diastolic dysfunction may become symptomatic if the contribution from atrial contraction is lost, as occurs with development of atrial fibrillation or with exercise because of shortening of the diastolic filling period. In grade II diastolic dysfunction (pseudonormal) mitral E/A ratio is between 0.8 and 1.5 and decreases more than 50% during a Valsalva maneuver, E/E′ ratio is between 9 and 12 and E′ is less than 8 cm/s. Also, PV flow provides supporting data for elevated LV filling pressures (S<D, AR velocity >30 cm/s, AR-A duration >30 milliseconds) (Figure 12–15). Grade III diastolic dysfunction (restrictive filling) is characterized by E/A ratio greater than 2, DT less than 160 milliseconds, IVRT less than 60 milliseconds, systolic filling fraction less than 40%, and average E/E′ ratio greater than 13 (septal E/E′ greater than 15, lateral E/E′ greater than 12) (Figure 12–16). Treatment in these patients may produce changes in the mitral flow velocity curve with improvement to grade II or even grade I diastolic dysfunction, in which case they are considered to be grade IIIa (reversible) diastolic dysfunction. Patients who exhibit severe abnormalities of ventricular compliance and end-stage heart disease maintain a severe restrictive pattern even after aggressive treatment. These patients have grade IIIb (irreversible) diastolic dysfunction and carry the worst prognosis.[38] Values of the parameters discussed above in various stages of diastolic dysfunction are presented in Table 12–3.

When evaluating diastolic function, one should take into consideration the previously-mentioned limitations of each parameter, the age of the patient, the presence or absence of cardiac disease, and the loading conditions. The various diastolic parameters should be interconnected with each other and interpreted in the context of the given clinical setting.

A practical approach to grading diastolic dysfunction, as suggested by the ASE recommendations for evaluation of LV diastolic function, is shown in Figure 12–17.[38]

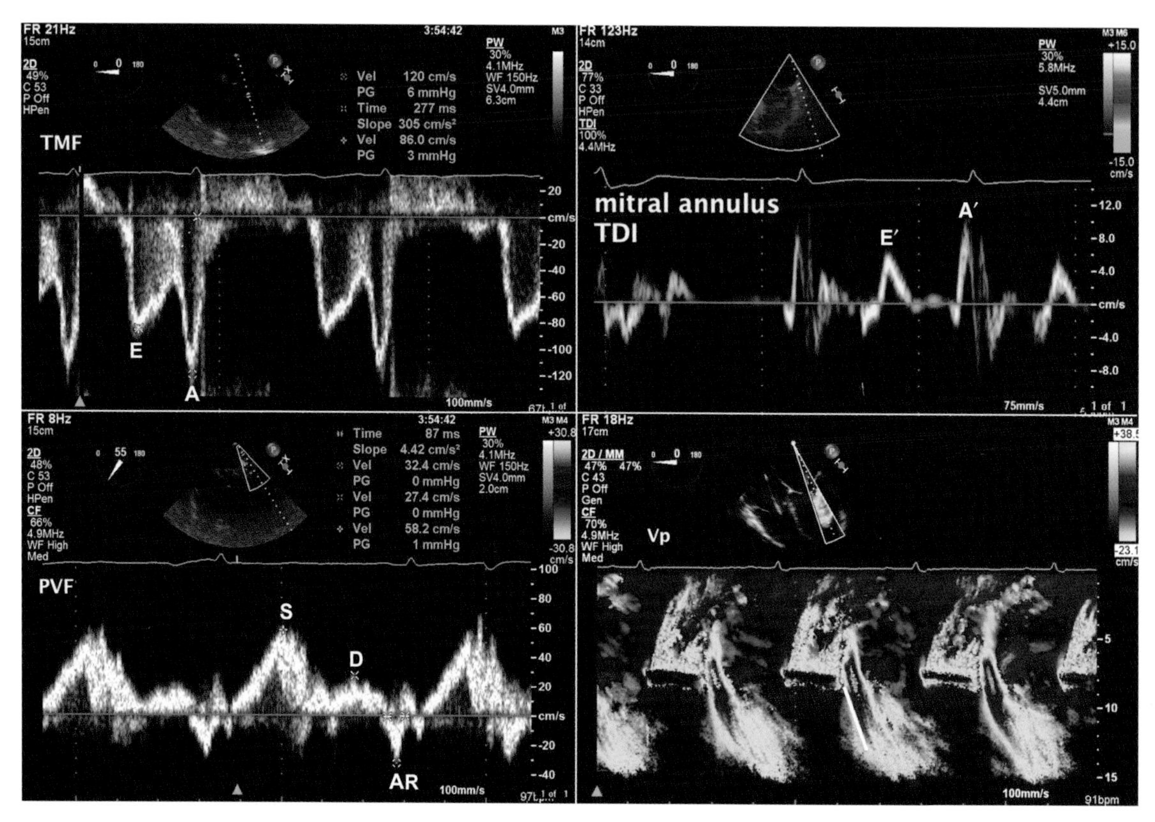

FIGURE 12–14. Patterns of Doppler echocardiographic indices of diastolic function in grade I diastolic dysfunction. (TMF, transmitral flow; TDI, tissue Doppler imaging; PVF, pulmonary venous flow; Vp, color M-mode propagation velocity.)

RIGHT VENTRICULAR DIASTOLIC FUNCTION

Right ventricle (RV) filling differs from LV filling in that the diastolic filling period is slightly shorter and maximal velocities are lower as a result of the larger tricuspid annulus.[81] Tricuspid flow recordings are accomplished with the same methods and adjustments as for mitral flow and may be best visualized in the midesophageal RV inflow-outflow view. Just as with the transmitral velocity profile, the transtricuspid profile is affected by loading conditions, heart rate, aging, and respiration. Respiratory variations are accentuated as compared with mitral flow, and it is common to observe an inversion of the E/A ratio during the inspiratory phase of positive pressure ventilation.

Assessment of RV diastolic function also includes PW Doppler interrogation of hepatic venous flow (HVF). The hepatic veins join the intrahepatic inferior vena cava (IVC) tangentially and can be visualized by advancing and turning the TEE probe rightward from a midesophageal bicaval view. The wave pattern of normal HVF velocity consists of two forward flows and two reverse flows (Figure 12–18). During ventricular systole there is an antegrade systolic flow during atrial filling (S wave), which is influenced by tricuspid valve annular motion, right atrial (RA) relaxation, and tricuspid regurgitation. This is followed by a small flow reversal at the end of systole (V wave), which is influenced by RV and RA compliance and possibly by the recoil of the tricuspid annulus at the end of ventricular contraction. During diastole there is a second phase of forward flow when the RA functions as a conduit during RV filling (D wave). At the end of diastole there is a small reversal of flow during atrial contraction (AR wave).[81]

Abnormal relaxation patterns characterized by a decreased E velocity, a decreased E/A ratio, and an

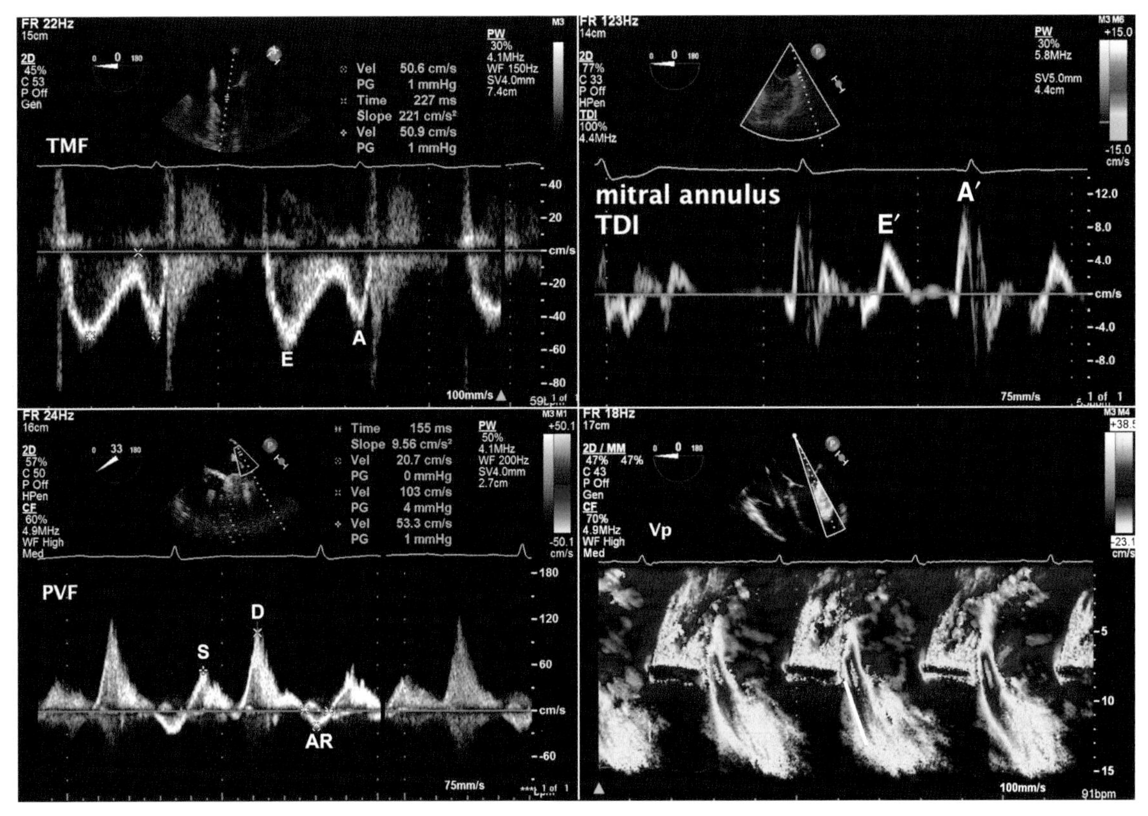

FIGURE 12–15. Patterns of Doppler echocardiographic indices of diastolic function in grade II diastolic dysfunction. (TMF, transmitral flow; TDI, tissue Doppler imaging; PVF, pulmonary venous flow; Vp, color M-mode propagation velocity.)

increased DT of the E wave have been described in association with heart failure or chronic obstructive pulmonary disease with pulmonary hypertension, but detailed descriptions of the time course and patterns of RV dysfunction are lacking.[82,83] The ratio of the total hepatic reverse flow integral to total forward flow integral calculated by measuring the time-velocity integral (TVI) for the S, V, D, and A waves ($TVI_A + TVI_V/TVI_S + TVI_D$) increases with RV diastolic dysfunction or significant tricuspid regurgitation. A marked shortening of the DT and diastolic predominance of hepatic vein flow with prominent V- and A-wave reversals during spontaneous inspiration indicate significant decreases in RV compliance and restrictive physiology.[84] Also, in restrictive right ventricular conditions and in the presence of normal pulmonary vascular resistance and intact pulmonary valve, the pulmonary valve leaflets will reopen in late diastole and laminar flow will be detectable by Doppler ultrasound, usually with a velocity of greater than 20 cm/s.[85]

MEASURING DIASTOLIC FUNCTION IN THE PERIOPERATIVE SETTING

The perioperative setting is characterized by fluctuation in hemodynamics and changes in loading conditions, as well as potential changes in intrathoracic pressures (institution of positive pressure ventilation, Trendelenburg position, or pneumoperitoneum), all of which can adversely impact the diastolic performance of the heart. Therefore, such instances may unmask diastolic dysfunction in patients with subclinical forms of disease[86] or may promote acute decompensation of diastolic heart failure in patients carrying such a diagnosis.[87] Various studies have shown that the presence of diastolic dysfunction in the perioperative period represents a prognostic factor. In a prospective study, Liu et al demonstrated that pseudonormal or restrictive transmitral flow filling patterns in the postoperative period after coronary artery bypass graft surgery (CABG) are strong predictors of adverse cardiac events.[88] In a

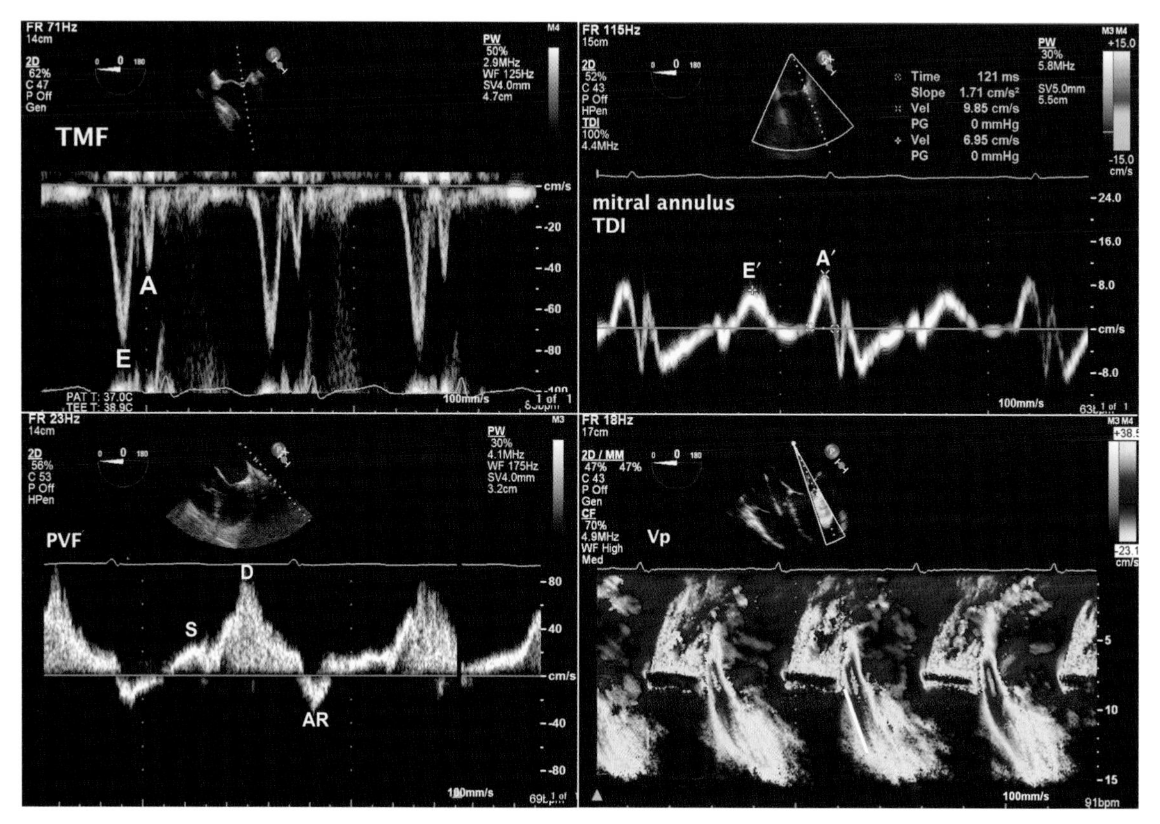

FIGURE 12–16. Patterns of Doppler echocardiographic indices of diastolic function in grade III diastolic dysfunction. (TMF, transmitral flow; TDI, tissue Doppler imaging; PVF, pulmonary venous flow; Vp, color M-mode propagation velocity.)

Table 12–3. Classification of Different Stages of Diastolic Dysfunction With Mitral Flow, Pulmonary Venous Flow, Propagation Velocity, and Mitral Annular VelocityAge Groups

	Normal	Impaired Relaxation	Pseudonormal	Restrictive Filling
TMF				
E/A	1-2	<0.8	0.8-1.5	≥2
DT (ms)	150-220	>200	150-220	<160
IVRT (ms)	60-100	>100	>100	<60
PVF				
PV-S/PV-D	>1	>1	<1	<1
PV-AR (cm/s)	<35	<35	>35	>35
ARdur-Adur	<30	<30	>30	>30
Vp	>55	<45	<45	<45
E′	>8 (septal) >10 (lateral)	>8 (septal) >10 (lateral)	<8 (septal) <10 (lateral)	<8 (septal) <10 (lateral)
E/E′	<8 (septal) <8 (lateral)	≤8 (septal) ≤8 (lateral)	9-12 (average)[a]	>15 (septal) >12 (lateral)

[a] Average of septal and lateral velocities.

TMF, transmitral flow; E, early filling peak velocity; A, late filling peak velocity; DT, deceleration time of E wave; IVRT, isovolumic relaxation time; PV-S, peak velocity of systolic component; PV-D, peak velocity of diastolic component; PV-AR, peak velocity of atrial reversal flow; PV-ARdur, duration of atrial reversal flow; Adur, duration of A wave; PVF, pulmonary venous flow; E′, peak tissue velocity in early diastole; Vp, velocity of propagation.

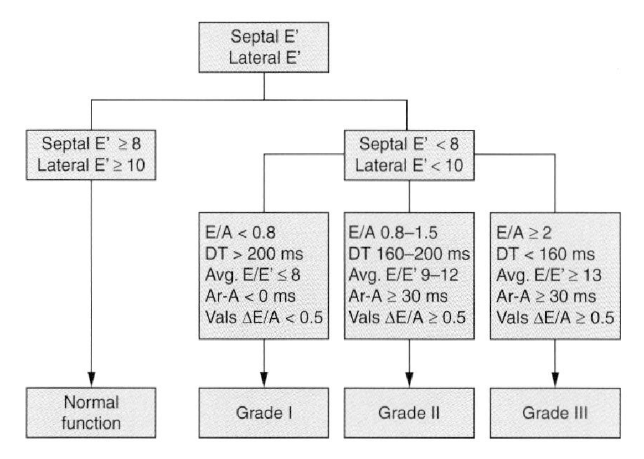

FIGURE 12–17. A practical algorithm for grading diastolic dysfunction as suggested by the American Society of Echocardiography recommendations for evaluation of left ventricular diastolic function. (Avg, average; Val, Valsalva; E′, peak tissue velocity in early diastole; E, transmitral early filling peak velocity; A, transmitral late filling peak velocity; DT, deceleration time of E wave; AR-A, duration of pulmonary vein atrial reversal flow minus duration of transmitral A wave.) *(Reproduced with permission from Nagueh, et al. Recommendations for the evaluation of left ventricular diastolic function by echocardiography. JASE. 2009;22(2):127.)*

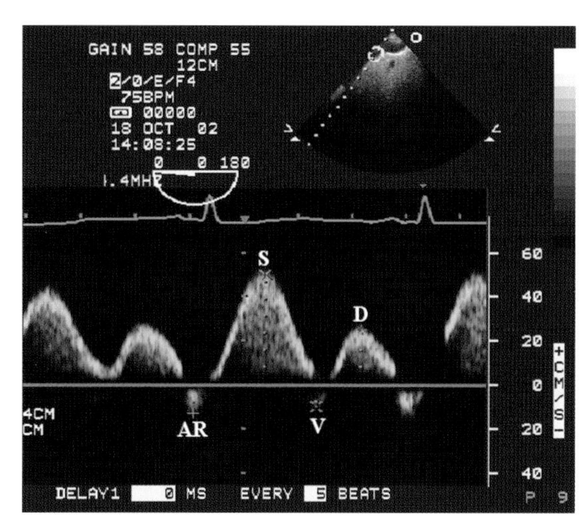

FIGURE 12–18. Normal hepatic venous profile recorded by pulsed-wave Doppler. There are two forward flows (S wave and D wave) and two reverse flows (V wave and AR wave).

retrospective study of diastolic function in patients undergoing on-pump CABG surgery, Nicoara et al observed that although diastolic function did not change in most patients, it worsened in a smaller proportion of cases and was associated with a higher incidence of heart failure and postoperative inotropic use.[89]

Intraoperative assessment of diastolic function and filling pressures is of paramount clinical importance, guiding the clinician in developing a perioperative management plan and potentially improving the outcome of patients. Transesophageal echocardiography represents an excellent noninvasive tool in the operating room, used to diagnose and grade diastolic dysfunction. Due to significant load changes during this period, diastolic indices such as mitral annulus TDI and Vp render themselves more suitable for intraoperative assessment of diastolic function as compared to the conventional Doppler indices (transmitral flow and PV flow velocities). However, mitral annular TDI and Vp lack linearity, thus these indices can accurately diagnose the presence or absence of diastolic dysfunction but cannot grade its severity.[89,90] In the near future, the availability of less load-dependent echocardiographic applications, such as strain, strain rate, and 2D speckle tracking, may improve our capacity to grade diastolic dysfunction and monitor therapeutic interventions.

CONCLUSION

Assessment of LV diastolic function should be an integral part of the routine echocardiographic examination.[38] Although frequently underestimated, diastolic dysfunction is common and can be a cause of hemodynamic instability in patients undergoing surgery or in patients in the intensive care unit. A systematic, stepwise Doppler evaluation of diastolic function complements 2D imaging and provides clinically relevant information in a noninvasive and prompt fashion.

ACKNOWLEDGMENTS

The authors would like to acknowledge the contributions of Drs. Jean Pierre Goarin and Ghassan Abiad from the previous edition.

REFERENCES

1. Bernard F, Denault A, Babin D, et al. Diastolic dysfunction is predictive of difficult weaning from cardiopulmonary bypass. *Anesth Analg.* 2001;92(2):291-298.
2. Priebe HJ. The aged cardiovascular risk patient. *Br J Anaesth.* 2000;85(5):763-778.
3. Dar O, Cowie MR. Acute heart failure in the intensive care unit: epidemiology. *Crit Care Med.* 2008;36(1 Suppl):S3-8.

4. Bhatia RS, Tu JV, Lee DS, et al. Outcome of heart failure with preserved ejection fraction in a population-based study. *N Engl J Med.* 2006;355(3):260-269.
5. Zile MR, Brutsaert DL. New concepts in diastolic dysfunction and diastolic heart failure. Part I: diagnosis, prognosis, and measurements of diastolic function. *Circulation.* 2002;105(11): 1387-1393.
6. Sabbah HN, Stein PD. Pressure-diameter relations during early diastole in dogs. Incompatibility with the concept of passive left ventricular filling. *Circ Res.* 1981;48(3):357-365.
7. Suga H, Goto Y, Igarashi Y, Yamada O, Nozawa T, Yasumura Y. Ventricular suction under zero source pressure for filling. *Am J Physiol.* 1986;251(1 Pt 2):H47-55.
8. Nishimura RA, Housmans PR, Hatle LK, Tajik AJ. Assessment of diastolic function of the heart: background and current applications of Doppler echocardiography. Part I. Physiologic and pathophysiologic features. *Mayo Clin Proc.* 1989;64(1):71-81.
9. Brutsaert DL, Housmans PR, Goethals MA. Dual control of relaxation. Its role in the ventricular function in the mammalian heart. *Circ Res.* 1980;47(5):637-652.
10. Grossman W. Diastolic dysfunction in congestive heart failure. *N Engl J Med.* 1991;325(22):1557-1564.
11. Schunkert H, Dzau VJ, Tang SS, Hirsch AT, Apstein CS, Lorell BH. Increased rat cardiac angiotensin converting enzyme activity and mRNA expression in pressure overload left ventricular hypertrophy. Effects on coronary resistance, contractility, and relaxation. *J Clin Invest.* 1990;86(6): 1913-1920.
12. Little WC, Badke FR, O'Rourke RA. Effect of right ventricular pressure on the end-diastolic left ventricular pressure-volume relationship before and after chronic right ventricular pressure overload in dogs without pericardia. *Circ Res.* 1984;54(6): 719-730.
13. Brutsaert DL, Sys SU, Gillebert TC. Diastolic failure: pathophysiology and therapeutic implications. *J Am Coll Cardiol.* 1993;22(1):318-325.
14. Pagel PS, Grossman W, Haering JM, Warltier DC. Left ventricular diastolic function in the normal and diseased heart. Perspectives for the anesthesiologist (2). *Anesthesiology.* 1993;79(5):1104-1120.
15. Chen W, Gibson D. Relation of isovolumic relaxation to left ventricular wall movement in man. *Br Heart J.* 1979;42(1): 51-56.
16. Lew WY. Evaluation of left ventricular diastolic function. *Circulation.* 1989;79(6):1393-1397.
17. Samuelsson S, Brodin LA, Broman M, Owall A, Settergren G. Comparison between transesophageal Doppler echocardiography and nuclear cardioangiography for the evaluation of left ventricular filling during coronary artery bypass grafting. *Anesth Analg.* 1995;80(1):41-46.
18. Nishimura RA, Tajik AJ. Evaluation of diastolic filling of left ventricle in health and disease: Doppler echocardiography is the clinician's Rosetta Stone. *J Am Coll Cardiol.* 1997;30(1):8-18.
19. Little WC, Ohno M, Kitzman DW, Thomas JD, Cheng CP. Determination of left ventricular chamber stiffness from the time for deceleration of early left ventricular filling. *Circulation.* 1995;92(7):1933-1939.
20. Oh JK, Appleton CP, Hatle LK, Nishimura RA, Seward JB, Tajik AJ. The noninvasive assessment of left ventricular diastolic function with two-dimensional and Doppler echocardiography. *J Am Soc Echocardiogr.* 1997;10(3):246-270.
21. Appleton CP, Firstenberg MS, Garcia MJ, Thomas JD. The echo-Doppler evaluation of left ventricular diastolic function. A current perspective. *Cardiol Clin.* 2000;18(3):513-546, ix.
22. Appleton CP, Jensen JL, Hatle LK, Oh JK. Doppler evaluation of left and right ventricular diastolic function: a technical guide for obtaining optimal flow velocity recordings. *J Am Soc Echocardiogr.* 1997;10(3):271-292.
23. Rossi A, Cicoira M, Golia G, Anselmi M, Zardini P. Mitral regurgitation and left ventricular diastolic dysfunction similarly affect mitral and pulmonary vein flow Doppler parameters: the advantage of end-diastolic markers. *J Am Soc Echocardiogr.* 2001;14(6):562-568.
24. Giannuzzi P, Imparato A, Temporelli PL, et al. Doppler-derived mitral deceleration time of early filling as a strong predictor of pulmonary capillary wedge pressure in postinfarction patients with left ventricular systolic dysfunction. *J Am Coll Cardiol.* 1994;23(7):1630-1637.
25. Nishimura RA, Appleton CP, Redfield MM, Ilstrup DM, Holmes DR Jr, Tajik AJ. Noninvasive doppler echocardiographic evaluation of left ventricular filling pressures in patients with cardiomyopathies: a simultaneous Doppler echocardiographic and cardiac catheterization study. *J Am Coll Cardiol.* 1996;28(5):1226-1233.
26. Wang J, Nagueh SF. Echocardiographic assessment of left ventricular filling pressures. *Heart Fail Clin.* 2008;4(1):57-70.
27. Hoffmann R, Lambertz H, Jutten H, Flachskampf FA, Hanrath P. Mitral and pulmonary venous flow under influence of positive end-expiratory pressure ventilation analyzed by transesophageal pulsed Doppler echocardiography. *Am J Cardiol.* 1991;68(6):697-701.
28. Firstenberg MS, Levine BD, Garcia MJ, et al. Relationship of echocardiographic indices to pulmonary capillary wedge pressures in healthy volunteers. *J Am Coll Cardiol.* 2000;36(5): 1664-1669.
29. Nishimura RA, Abel MD, Housmans PR, Warnes CA, Tajik AJ. Mitral flow velocity curves as a function of different loading conditions: evaluation by intraoperative transesophageal Doppler echocardiography. *J Am Soc Echocardiogr.* 1989;2(2): 79-87.
30. Choong CY, Abascal VM, Thomas JD, Guerrero JL, McGlew S, Weyman AE. Combined influence of ventricular loading and relaxation on the transmitral flow velocity profile in dogs measured by Doppler echocardiography. *Circulation.* 1988;78(3): 672-683.
31. Hurrell DG, Oh JK, Mahoney DW, Miller FA Jr, Seward JB. Short deceleration time of mitral inflow E velocity: prognostic implication with atrial fibrillation versus sinus rhythm. *J Am Soc Echocardiogr.* 1998;11(5):450-457.
32. Matsukida K, Kisanuki A, Toyonaga K, et al. Comparison of transthoracic Doppler echocardiography and natriuretic peptides in predicting mean pulmonary capillary wedge pressure in patients with chronic atrial fibrillation. *J Am Soc Echocardiogr.* 2001;14(11):1080-1087.
33. Nagueh SF, Kopelen HA, Quinones MA. Assessment of left ventricular filling pressures by Doppler in the presence of atrial fibrillation. *Circulation.* 1996;94(9):2138-2145.
34. Groban L, Dolinski SY. Transesophageal echocardiographic evaluation of diastolic function. *Chest.* 2005;128(5):3652-3663.
35. Frogel J, Soranno L, Humphrey T. Aortic insufficiency confounding transesophageal echocardiograph assessment of left ventricular diastolic function. *Anesth Analg.* 2008;106(2):409-411.

36. Oh JK, Hatle LK, Sinak LJ, Seward JB, Tajik AJ. Characteristic Doppler echocardiographic pattern of mitral inflow velocity in severe aortic regurgitation. *J Am Coll Cardiol.* 1989;14(7): 1712-1717.
37. Castini D, Gentile F, Siffredi M, et al. Does aortic regurgitation affect transmitral flow? An echo-Doppler study. *Acta Cardiol.* 1993;48(4):345-353.
38. Nagueh SF, Appleton CP, Gillebert TC, et al. Recommendations for the evaluation of left ventricular diastolic function by echocardiography. *J Am Soc Echocardiogr.* 2009;22(2):107-133.
39. Bartzokis T, Lee R, Yeoh TK, Grogin H, Schnittger I. Transesophageal echo-Doppler echocardiographic assessment of pulmonary venous flow patterns. *J Am Soc Echocardiogr.* 1991;4(5): 457-464.
40. Appleton CP. Hemodynamic determinants of Doppler pulmonary venous flow velocity components: new insights from studies in lightly sedated normal dogs. *J Am Coll Cardiol.* 1997;30(6):1562-1574.
41. Nishimura RA, Abel MD, Hatle LK, Tajik AJ. Relation of pulmonary vein to mitral flow velocities by transesophageal Doppler echocardiography. Effect of different loading conditions. *Circulation.* 1990;81(5):1488-1497.
42. Khouri SJ, Maly GT, Suh DD, Walsh TE. A practical approach to the echocardiographic evaluation of diastolic function. *J Am Soc Echocardiogr.* 2004;17(3):290-297.
43. Lester SJ, Tajik AJ, Nishimura RA, Oh JK, Khandheria BK, Seward JB. Unlocking the mysteries of diastolic function: deciphering the Rosetta Stone 10 years later. *J Am Coll Cardiol.* 2008;51(7):679-689.
44. Rossvoll O, Hatle LK. Pulmonary venous flow velocities recorded by transthoracic Doppler ultrasound: relation to left ventricular diastolic pressures. *J Am Coll Cardiol.* 1993;21(7): 1687-1696.
45. Yamamuro A, Yoshida K, Hozumi T, et al. Noninvasive evaluation of pulmonary capillary wedge pressure in patients with acute myocardial infarction by deceleration time of pulmonary venous flow velocity in diastole. *J Am Coll Cardiol.* 1999;34(1): 90-94.
46. Klein AL, Tajik AJ. Doppler assessment of pulmonary venous flow in healthy subjects and in patients with heart disease. *J Am Soc Echocardiogr.* 1991;4(4):379-392.
47. Garcia MJ, Thomas JD, Klein AL. New Doppler echocardiographic applications for the study of diastolic function. *J Am Coll Cardiol.* 1998;32(4):865-875.
48. Klein AL, Abdalla I, Murray RD, et al. Age independence of the difference in duration of pulmonary venous atrial reversal flow and transmitral A-wave flow in normal subjects. *J Am Soc Echocardiogr.* 1998;11(5):458-465.
49. Chao TH, Tsai LM, Tsai WC, Li YH, Lin LJ, Chen JH. Effect of atrial fibrillation on pulmonary venous flow patterns assessed by Doppler transesophageal echocardiography. *Chest.* 2000;117(6):1546-1550.
50. Klein AL, Bailey AS, Cohen GI, et al. Effects of mitral stenosis on pulmonary venous flow as measured by Doppler transesophageal echocardiography. *Am J Cardiol.* 1993;72(1):66-72.
51. Klein AL, Stewart WJ, Bartlett J, et al. Effects of mitral regurgitation on pulmonary venous flow and left atrial pressure: an intraoperative transesophageal echocardiographic study. *J Am Coll Cardiol.* 1992;20(6):1345-1352.
52. Nagueh SF, Sun H, Kopelen HA, Middleton KJ, Khoury DS. Hemodynamic determinants of the mitral annulus diastolic velocities by tissue Doppler. *J Am Coll Cardiol.* 2001;37(1): 278-285.
53. Ohte N, Narita H, Hashimoto T, Akita S, Kurokawa K, Fujinami T. Evaluation of left ventricular early diastolic performance by color tissue Doppler imaging of the mitral annulus. *Am J Cardiol.* 1998;82(11):1414-1417.
54. Dumesnil JG, Paulin C, Pibarot P, Coulombe D, Arsenault M. Mitral annulus velocities by Doppler tissue imaging: practical implications with regard to preload alterations, sample position, and normal values. *J Am Soc Echocardiogr.* 2002;15(10 Pt 2): 1226-1231.
55. Garcia MJ, Thomas JD. Tissue Doppler to assess diastolic left ventricular function. *Echocardiography.* 1999;16(5):501-508.
56. Sohn DW, Chai IH, Lee DJ, et al. Assessment of mitral annulus velocity by Doppler tissue imaging in the evaluation of left ventricular diastolic function. *J Am Coll Cardiol.* 1997;30(2): 474-480.
57. Nagueh SF, Middleton KJ, Kopelen HA, Zoghbi WA, Quinones MA. Doppler tissue imaging: a noninvasive technique for evaluation of left ventricular relaxation and estimation of filling pressures. *J Am Coll Cardiol.* 1997;30(6):1527-1533.
58. Rivas-Gotz C, Manolios M, Thohan V, Nagueh SF. Impact of left ventricular ejection fraction on estimation of left ventricular filling pressures using tissue Doppler and flow propagation velocity. *Am J Cardiol.* 2003;91(6):780-784.
59. Ommen SR, Nishimura RA, Appleton CP, et al. Clinical utility of Doppler echocardiography and tissue Doppler imaging in the estimation of left ventricular filling pressures: a comparative simultaneous Doppler-catheterization study. *Circulation.* 2000;102(15):1788-1794.
60. Mankad S, Murali S, Kormos RL, Mandarino WA, Gorcsan J 3rd. Evaluation of the potential role of color-coded tissue Doppler echocardiography in the detection of allograft rejection in heart transplant recipients. *Am Heart J.* 1999;138(4 Pt 1):721-730.
61. Nagueh SF, Bachinski LL, Meyer D, et al. Tissue Doppler imaging consistently detects myocardial abnormalities in patients with hypertrophic cardiomyopathy and provides a novel means for an early diagnosis before and independently of hypertrophy. *Circulation.* 2001;104(2):128-130.
62. Nagueh SF, Mikati I, Kopelen HA, Middleton KJ, Quinones MA, Zoghbi WA. Doppler estimation of left ventricular filling pressure in sinus tachycardia. A new application of tissue doppler imaging. *Circulation.* 1998;98(16):1644-1650.
63. Garcia MJ, Rodriguez L, Ares M, Griffin BP, Thomas JD, Klein AL. Differentiation of constrictive pericarditis from restrictive cardiomyopathy: assessment of left ventricular diastolic velocities in longitudinal axis by Doppler tissue imaging. *J Am Coll Cardiol.* 1996;27(1):108-114.
64. Soeki T, Fukuda N, Shinohara H, et al. Mitral inflow and mitral annular motion velocities in patients with mitral annular calcification: evaluation by pulsed Doppler echocardiography and pulsed Doppler tissue imaging. *Eur J Echocardiogr.* 2002;3(2):128-134.
65. Rivas-Gotz C, Khoury DS, Manolios M, Rao L, Kopelen HA, Nagueh SF. Time interval between onset of mitral inflow and onset of early diastolic velocity by tissue Doppler: a novel index of left ventricular relaxation: experimental studies and clinical application. *J Am Coll Cardiol.* 2003;42(8):1463-1470.
66. Castro PL, Greenberg NL, Drinko J, Garcia MJ, Thomas JD. Potential pitfalls of strain rate imaging: angle dependency. *Biomed Sci Instrum.* 2000;36:197-202.

67. Leitman M, Lysyansky P, Sidenko S, et al. Two-dimensional strain-a novel software for real-time quantitative echocardiographic assessment of myocardial function. *J Am Soc Echocardiogr.* 2004;17(10):1021-1029.
68. Marcucci C, Lauer R, Mahajan A. New echocardiographic techniques for evaluating left ventricular myocardial function. *Semin Cardiothorac Vasc Anesth.* 2008;12(4):228-247.
69. Notomi Y, Lysyansky P, Setser RM, et al. Measurement of ventricular torsion by two-dimensional ultrasound speckle tracking imaging. *J Am Coll Cardiol.* 2005;45(12):2034-2041.
70. Saito M, Okayama H, Nishimura K, et al. Determinants of left ventricular untwisting behaviour in patients with dilated cardiomyopathy: analysis by two-dimensional speckle tracking. *Heart.* 2009;95(4):290-296.
71. Takeuchi M, Borden WB, Nakai H, et al. Reduced and delayed untwisting of the left ventricle in patients with hypertension and left ventricular hypertrophy: a study using two-dimensional speckle tracking imaging. *Eur Heart J.* 2007;28(22): 2756-2762.
72. Brun P, Tribouilloy C, Duval AM, et al. Left ventricular flow propagation during early filling is related to wall relaxation: a color M-mode Doppler analysis. *J Am Coll Cardiol.* 1992;20(2): 420-432.
73. Garcia MJ, Smedira NG, Greenberg NL, et al. Color M-mode Doppler flow propagation velocity is a preload insensitive index of left ventricular relaxation: animal and human validation. *J Am Coll Cardiol.* 2000;35(1):201-208.
74. Takatsuji H, Mikami T, Urasawa K, et al. A new approach for evaluation of left ventricular diastolic function: spatial and temporal analysis of left ventricular filling flow propagation by color M-mode Doppler echocardiography. *J Am Coll Cardiol.* 1996;27(2):365-371.
75. Graham RJ, Gelman JS, Donelan L, Mottram PM, Peverill RE. Effect of preload reduction by haemodialysis on new indices of diastolic function. *Clin Sci (Lond).* 2003;105(4): 499-506.
76. Troughton RW, Prior DL, Frampton CM, et al. Usefulness of tissue doppler and color M-mode indexes of left ventricular diastolic function in predicting outcomes in systolic left ventricular heart failure (from the ADEPT study). *Am J Cardiol.* 2005;96(2):257-262.
77. Garcia MJ, Ares MA, Asher C, Rodriguez L, Vandervoort P, Thomas JD. An index of early left ventricular filling that combined with pulsed Doppler peak E velocity may estimate capillary wedge pressure. *J Am Coll Cardiol.* 1997;29(2):448-454.
78. Mego DM, DeGeare VS, Nottestad SY, et al. Variation of flow propagation velocity with age. *J Am Soc Echocardiogr.* 1998;11(1): 20-25.
79. Lang RM, Bierig M, Devereux RB, et al. Recommendations for chamber quantification: a report from the American Society of Echocardiography's Guidelines and Standards Committee and the Chamber Quantification Writing Group, developed in conjunction with the European Association of Echocardiography, a branch of the European Society of Cardiology. *J Am Soc Echocardiogr.* 2005;18(12):1440-1463.
80. Abhayaratna WP, Seward JB, Appleton CP, et al. Left atrial size: physiologic determinants and clinical applications. *J Am Coll Cardiol.* 2006;47(12):2357-2363.
81. Otto CM. Echocardiographic evaluation of ventricular diastolic filling and function. In: Otto CM, ed. *Textbook of Clinical Echocardiography.* 2nd ed. Philadelphia: Saunders; 2000:132.
82. Ozer N, Tokgozoglu L, Coplu L, Kes S. Echocardiographic evaluation of left and right ventricular diastolic function in patients with chronic obstructive pulmonary disease. *J Am Soc Echocardiogr.* 2001;14(6):557-561.
83. Yu CM, Sanderson JE, Chan S, Yeung L, Hung YT, Woo KS. Right ventricular diastolic dysfunction in heart failure. *Circulation.* 1996;93(8):1509-1514.
84. Djaiani GN, Shernan SK. Intraoperative assessment of diastolic function: utility of echocardiography. *Curr Opin Anaesthesiol.* 2003;16(1):11-19.
85. Redington AN. Right ventricular function. *Cardiol Clin.* 2002;20(3):341-349.
86. Popescu WM, Bell R, Duffy A, Perrino AC. Morbidly obese patients undergoing laparscopic surgery: evidence for impaired cardiac performance. *Anesthesiology.* 2007;107:A1232.
87. Pirracchio R, Cholley B, De Hert S, Solal AC, Mebazaa A. Diastolic heart failure in anaesthesia and critical care. *Br J Anaesth.* 2007;98(6):707-721.
88. Liu J, Tanaka N, Murata K, et al. Prognostic value of pseudonormal and restrictive filling patterns on left ventricular remodeling and cardiac events after coronary artery bypass grafting. *Am J Cardiol.* 2003;91(5):550-554.
89. Nicoara A, Phillips-Bute B, Gorrin-Rivas M, Nikolov N, Swaminathan M. Determinants of change in diastolic function after CABG surgery. *Anesthesiology.* 2007;107:A1230.
90. Mahmood F, Matyal R. Assessment of perioperative diastolic function and dysfunction. *Int Anesthesiol Clin.* 2008;46(2):51-62

REVIEW QUESTIONS

Select the *one* best answer for each of the following questions.

1. In patients with LV systolic dysfunction, elevation of PCWP is likely to occur when E-wave DT is:
   a. <220 milliseconds
   b. >300 milliseconds
   c. <150 milliseconds
   d. <300 milliseconds
   e. >150 milliseconds

2. Which of following statements concerning IVRT is ***INCORRECT***?
   a. IVRT is the interval between aortic valve closure and onset of mitral inflow.
   b. IVRT represents the interval between LV relaxation and LV pressure decline.
   c. IVRT is influenced by the velocity of active relaxation.
   d. IVRT is influenced by the aortic pressure and the atrial pressure.
   e. IVRT is best acquired from a deep transgastric long-axis view.

3. Transmitral Doppler flow in patients with isolated relaxation abnormality and normal LV filling pressure is characterized by:

a. Decreased IVRT
b. Decreased early diastolic peak velocity
c. Decreased DT of the E wave
d. Increased E/A ratio
e. Increased early diastolic peak velocity

4. Transmitral Doppler flow peak E velocity is dependent on all of the following ***EXCEPT***:
   a. Active left ventricular relaxation
   b. Myocardial elastic properties
   c. Left atrial pressure
   d. Left atrial contraction
   e. Heart rate

5. E-wave deceleration time of the transmitral Doppler flow is increased by all of the following ***EXCEPT***:
   a. Hypovolemia
   b. Relaxation abnormality
   c. Hypertension
   d. Decreased LV compliance
   e. Mitral stenosis

6. Which of the following statements is ***FALSE***?
   a. Mitral regurgitation results in an increase in E-wave velocity.
   b. Mitral stenosis results in a decrease in E-wave deceleration time.
   c. Severe acute aortic regurgitation results in a restrictive pattern of the transmitral flow.
   d. Mitral stenosis results in increased E-wave velocity.
   e. Mitral regurgitation results in a restrictive pattern of the transmitral flow.

7. A normal transmitral Doppler flow pattern can be considered pseudonormal if:
   a. A systolic fraction of PVF defined as the ratio of the systolic velocity integral to the sum of systolic and diastolic components is equal to 60%.
   b. LV filling Vp <80 cm/s.
   c. LV filling Vp >50 cm/s.
   d. E′ velocity is more than 8 cm/s.
   e. E′ velocity is less than 8 cm/s.

8. Changes in transmitral Doppler flow parameters induced by severely increased LV stiffness are:
   a. Increased E-wave DT
   b. Increased IVRT
   c. Decreased E/A ratio
   d. Increased early diastolic flow velocity
   e. Increased late diastolic flow velocity

9. A Doppler mitral recording shows the following: E = 83 cm/s, DT = 180 milliseconds, and A = 72 cm/s. The septal E′ velocity recorded with TDI is 7.2 cm/s. Which of the following statements best describes this Doppler examination?
   a. Healthy adult
   b. Ischemic cardiomyopathy with pseudonormal filling pattern
   c. Hypertrophic cardiomyopathy with normal filling pressures
   d. Restrictive filling pattern related to fibrosis cardiomyopathy

10. RV failure may alter LV diastolic function by all these mechanisms ***EXCEPT***:
    a. Septal wall ischemia
    b. Direct compression of the left cardiac chamber in intact pericardium
    c. Paradoxical septal wall motion
    d. Tricuspid regurgitation

11. The systolic component of the pulmonary venous flow is decreased by all of the following ***EXCEPT***:
    a. Impairment of LA relaxation
    b. Impairment of LV systolic function
    c. Elevation of LA pressure
    d. LV hypertrophy
    e. Atrial fibrillation

12. Which of the following statements is true regarding atrial systole?
    a. It contributes 30% of the LV filling in young healthy subjects.
    b. It contributes 35% to 40% of the LV filling in elderly subjects.
    c. It contributes less to LV filling in grade I (impaired relaxation) diastolic dysfunction.
    d. It contributes more to LV filling in grade III (restrictive filling) diastolic dysfunction.
    e. It occurs in diastole before diastasis.

13. An LV end-diastolic pressure higher than 15 mm Hg is more likely if:
    a. E/E′ ratio is higher than 15.
    b. E/Vp is less than 1.5.
    c. Pulmonary venous flow AR velocity is less than 35 cm/s.
    d. Pulmonary venous flow AR duration exceeds transmitral flow A duration by 20 milliseconds.
    e. E/A ratio is less than 0.8.

14. In a healthy 20-year-old patient with an E/A ratio greater than 1.5, which is more likely to be true?
    a. Increased IVRT
    b. Decreased IVRT
    c. E′ less than 8 cm/s
    d. Vp more than 55 cm/s
    e. Vp less than 45 cm/s

15. In a 70-year-old with uncontrolled hypertension and normal E/A ratio, which is more likely to occur?
    a. E′ more than 10 cm/s
    b. Increased IVRT
    c. E/E′ less than 10
    d. Pulmonary venous flow with systolic predominance
    e. Pulmonary venous flow with diastolic predominance

16. Which of the following statements is more likely to be true?
    a. A 40-year-old patient with severe acute aortic insufficiency has an E/A ratio less than 1.
    b. A 60-year-old patient with restrictive cardiomyopathy has an E/A ratio less than 0.8.
    c. A 20-year-old marathon runner has an E/A ratio more than 1.5.
    d. A 70-year-old patient with severe mitral regurgitation has an E/A ratio less than 1.
    e. A 60-year-old patient with chronic aortic regurgitation has an E/A ratio more than 1.5.

17. Mitral annulus tissue Doppler imaging:
    a. Measures low-amplitude high-velocity signals
    b. Measures low-amplitude low-velocity signals
    c. Displays velocities higher than 15 cm/s
    d. Displays septal velocities higher than lateral velocities
    e. Can be displayed as both spectral Doppler and color map

18. Which of the following distinguishes constrictive pericarditis with normal systolic function from restrictive cardiomyopathy?
    a. Increased E-wave DT in constrictive pericarditis
    b. Increased E-wave velocity in restrictive cardiomyopathy
    c. Decreased E/A ratio in restrictive cardiomyopathy
    d. Normal E′ velocity in constrictive pericarditis
    e. Decreased Vp in constrictive pericarditis

19. Which of the following parameters measured during Doppler examination suggests an elevation of LV filling pressure in patients with chronic atrial fibrillation?
    a. Transmitral E-wave velocity more than 80 cm/s
    b. Transmitral E-wave DT more than 200 milliseconds
    c. Mitral E/A ratio more than 2
    d. E/E′ ratio more than 15
    e. E/Vp ratio less than 1.5

20. A reverse systolic flow can be observed in the pulmonary vein flow in:
    a. Moderate mitral regurgitation
    b. Impaired LV relaxation
    c. Severe mitral stenosis
    d. Tachycardia
    e. Atrial fibrillation

21. Constrictive pericarditis is suspected in a 60-year-old patient. Which of the following parameters is consistent with this diagnosis?
    a. Transmitral E-wave DT = 200 milliseconds
    b. Color M-mode Vp = 60 cm/s
    c. Mitral annulus E′ velocity = 6.2 cm/s
    d. E/A ratio = 0.8
    e. Color M-mode Vp = 32 cm/s

22. Which of the following statements is ***TRUE***?
    a. Strain rate measured by TDI is dependent on myocardial tethering.
    b. Strain rate measured by TDI is independent on the angle of the Doppler beam.
    c. Speckle tracking is dependent on the angle of the Doppler beam.
    d. Negative strain measures lengthening of the myocardium.
    e. Speckle tracking measures myocardial deformation.

23. Performing a Valsalva maneuver will result in:
    a. Decreased E/A ratio in a healthy adult
    b. Increased E and A velocities in a healthy adult
    c. Increased E/A ratio in a patient with pseudonormal filling pattern
    d. Increased E/A ratio in a patient with grade IIIa diastolic dysfunction
    e. Unchanged E/A ratio in a healthy adult

24. Which of the following statements regarding the effects of mitral stenosis is ***TRUE***?
    a. Transmitral flow velocities are decreased.
    b. E/E′ ratio accurately estimates left ventricular end-diastolic pressure.
    d. Transmitral E and A waves are fused.
    e. Systolic predominance is seen on the pulmonary vein flow.

25. Which of the following statements is true regarding tissue Doppler imaging (TDI)?
    a. Usually radially oriented fibers are interrogated by Doppler.
    b. Longitudinally oriented fibers cannot be interrogated by Doppler.
    c. Fibrotic myocardium may sometimes have a normal velocity.

d. Doppler interrogation of the velocities is independent of the angle of the Doppler beam.
e. TDI is highly dependent on a high-quality 2D image.

26. The administration of diuretics in a healthy subject:
a. May mimic a relaxation abnormality
b. May increase the E-wave velocity
c. May decrease the E-wave DT
d. May decrease the IVRT
e. Does not change the E and A velocities

27. Which is of the following statements is true regarding pulmonary venous flow variables?
a. The S_1 wave depends on LV relaxation.
b. The S_2 wave depends on LA relaxation.
c. The S_2 wave depends on RV function.
d. The D wave depends on LA relaxation.
e. The AR wave depends on LV relaxation.

28. Which of the following statements regarding the transmitral flow is ***TRUE***?
a. The transmitral E/A ratio can be more than 2 in a healthy 18-year-old.
b. The transmitral E-wave DT decreases with age.
c. The isovolumic relaxation time decreases with age.
d. The transmitral E/A ratio increases with age.
e. Age has no effect on the E and A velocities.

29. The initial abnormality of diastolic dysfunction is:
a. Increased ventricular compliance
b. Ventricular interdependence
c. Decreased ventricular compliance
d. Increased ventricular stiffness
e. Impaired ventricular relaxation

30. A 38-year-old patient has a previous history of stroke. He presents to the OR for closure of a patent foramen ovale. After induction of anesthesia, the assessment of diastolic function via transmitral flow Doppler reveals the following: E = 75 cm/s, A = 51 cm/s, DT = 190 milliseconds. Pulmonary vein flow Doppler reveals S/D ratio less than 1. During sternotomy the lung is injured and 700 cc of blood loss occurs. A new assessment of the diastolic function will most likely reveal:
a. E = 75 cm/s, A = 51 cm/s, DT = 190 milliseconds
b. E = 50 cm/s, A = 68 cm/s, DT = 250 milliseconds
c. E = 75 cm/s, A = 51 cm/s, DT = 190 milliseconds
d. E = 90 cm/s, A = 34 cm/s, DT = 150 milliseconds
e. E = 85 cm/s, A = 35 cm/s, DT = 140 milliseconds

31. A 70-year-old patient presents to the OR for coronary artery bypass graft surgery. After induction of anesthesia 1-mm ST segment depression is present. The assessment of diastolic function via transmitral flow Doppler reveals the following: E = 71 cm/s, A = 69 cm/s, DT = 200 milliseconds. Tissue Doppler imaging of the lateral mitral annulus reveals E′ = 5 cm/s. After 30 minutes of nitroglycerine infusion, assessment of the diastolic pattern will most likely be consistent with:
a. Normal pattern
b. Reversible restrictive pattern
c. Pseudonormal pattern
d. Impaired relaxation pattern
e. Irreversible restrictive pattern

32. The isovolumic relaxation time:
a. Shortens with increasing age
b. Shortens in patients with a restrictive filling pattern
c. Lengthens with increases in heart rate
d. Is defined as the time between mitral valve closure and aortic valve opening
e. Shortens with increases in afterload

33. On the transmitral flow velocity profile, the deceleration time of the E wave:
a. Shortens in patients with acute aortic regurgitation
b. Shortens in patients with mitral stenosis
c. Lengthens in patients with a restrictive filling pattern
d. Shortens in patients with impaired relaxation pattern
e. Shortens with increasing age

34. Tissue Doppler imaging of the mitral annulus:
a. Uses the continuous-wave Doppler technique
b. Has a low temporal resolution
c. Measures intramyocardial velocities
d. Evaluates the translational and rotational movement of the left ventricle
e. Measures red blood cell velocities

35. In a patient with atrial fibrillation, the echocardiographic measurement associated with increased filling pressures is:
a. Transmitral E/A velocity ratio greater than 2
b. Decreased pulmonary venous systolic flow
c. Less beat-to-beat variability on mitral inflow parameters
d. Increased transmitral E-wave velocity
e. Decreased propagation velocity

36. A 65-year-old patient with aortic stenosis presents to the OR for an aortic valve replacement. The initial assessment of diastolic function reveals a normal transmitral flow Doppler pattern. Which of the following statements is ***TRUE***?
    a. Nitroglycerine infusion will decrease both E-wave and A-wave velocities.
    b. A Valsalva maneuver will decrease only E-wave velocity.
    c. Administration of metoprolol will decrease both E-wave and A-wave velocities.
    d. Placement in Trendelenburg position will decrease only E-wave velocity.
    e. A 500-cc blood loss will not change the E/A ratio.

37. Which of the following statements pertaining to the pulmonary venous flow pattern is ***TRUE***?
    a. In grade II diastolic dysfunction the diastolic filling fraction is more than 55%.
    b. In grade I diastolic dysfunction PVS velocity declines.
    c. Impaired relaxation is associated with an increased PVD velocity.
    d. In healthy subjects AR duration is equal or more than transmitral A duration.
    e. In young, healthy subjects the systolic component can be blunted.

38. The compensatory mechanism responsible for pseudonormalization of the transmitral flow pattern is:
    a. Increased ventricular compliance
    b. Decreased pericardial restraint
    c. Decreased ventricular stiffness
    d. Decreased intracavitary diastolic pressures
    e. Increased left atrial pressures

39. In which of the following clinical situations is the E/E′ ratio ***NOT*** accurate for estimating LV filling pressures?
    a. Atrial fibrillation
    b. Hypertrophic obstructive cardiomyopathy
    c. After heart transplant
    d. Sinus tachycardia
    e. Severe mitral regurgitation with normal ejection fraction

40. Which of the following is ***TRUE*** regarding estimating LV filling pressures?
    a. E/E′ ratio accurately estimates LV filling pressures in constrictive pericarditis.
    b. E/Vp ratio accurately estimates filling pressures in atrial fibrillation.
    c. E/E′ ratio less than 10 is highly sensitive for increased LV filling pressures.
    d. E/E′ ratio accurately estimates LV filling pressures in patients with mitral stenosis.
    e. E/A ratio less than 0.8 is highly sensitive of increased LV filling pressures.

41. Which of the following statements is ***TRUE***?
    a. Impaired relaxation results in a prolongation in peak –dP/dt.
    b. Impaired relaxation results in a reduction of the time constant of relaxation.
    c. Impaired relaxation results in a prolongation of the time constant of relaxation.
    d. Isovolumic relaxation time depends on the time of mitral valve opening.
    e. Impaired relaxation results in a decreased isovolumic relaxation time.

42. Which of the following statements is ***TRUE*** regarding myocardial compliance and relaxation?
    a. Compliance is the ratio of change in pressure to unit change in volume.
    b. Stiffness is the ratio of change in volume to unit change in pressure.
    c. Compliance affects mostly early diastole.
    d. An increase in afterload delays myocardial relaxation.
    e. Active relaxation starts at the closure of the aortic valve.

43. Which of the following statements is ***TRUE*** regarding tissue Doppler imaging?
    a. TE-E′ is decreased is diastolic dysfunction.
    b. Lateral E′ is less than septal E′ in constrictive pericarditis.
    c. E′ velocity is preload independent in healthy individuals.
    d. Lateral E′ is more accurate than septal E′ after mitral annuloplasty.
    e. E′ occurs after transmitral E in healthy subjects.

44. Which of the following statements is ***TRUE*** regarding hepatic venous flow?
    a. Retrograde systolic flow S wave depends on right atrium relaxation.
    b. Retrograde systolic flow V wave depends on right atrium compliance.
    c. Retrograde flow in the hepatic veins occurs only in late diastole.
    d. Decreased RV compliance is associated with systolic predominance of the hepatic venous flow.

45. The following clinical situations can result in diastolic dysfunction ***EXCEPT***:
    a. Tachycardia
    b. Acute hypertension

c. Elevated right atrial pressure
d. Administration of diuretics
e. Renin-angiotensin-aldosterone activation

46. Which of the following statements is ***TRUE*** regarding the compliance of the left ventricle?
    a. The modulus of chamber stiffness is inversely related to the chamber stiffness.
    b. The modulus of chamber stiffness is proportional to the myocardial stiffness.
    c. The modulus of myocardial stiffness reflects the relation between stiffness and pressure.
    d. Chamber stiffness is constant throughout ventricular filling.
    e. The modulus of chamber stiffness is independent of chamber geometry.

47. In a patient with constrictive pericarditis, which of the following changes will happen with spontaneous inspiration?
    a. Increased E′ velocity
    b. Decreased E′ velocity
    c. Increased mitral A-wave velocity
    d. Increased mitral E-wave velocity
    e. Increased tricuspid E-wave velocity

48. All the following changes could be expected with tachycardia ***EXCEPT***:
    a. Fused E and A waves
    b. Increased A-wave velocity
    c. Decreased pulmonary venous D wave
    d. Decreased E′ velocity
    e. Positive pulmonary venous AR wave

49. All the following changes could be expected with aging ***EXCEPT***:
    a. Decrease in E-wave velocity
    b. Increase in A-wave velocity
    c. Unchanged pulmonary venous AR wave
    d. Blunting of the pulmonary venous S wave
    e. Increase in E-wave deceleration time

50. After induction of general anesthesia, a patient with grade I diastolic dysfunction (impaired relaxation pattern) is placed in steep Trendelenburg position. Which of the following changes would you expect?
    a. Increase in IVRT
    b. Decrease in E′ velocity
    c. Increase in A-wave velocity
    d. Increase in E-wave DT
    e. Increase in E-wave velocity

Evaluation of Right Heart Function 13

Rebecca A. Schroeder, Shahar Bar-Yosef, and Jonathan B. Mark

STRUCTURE AND FUNCTION

As the role of the right ventricle (RV) in overall cardiac function has been more fully appreciated, greater efforts have been made to describe and quantify RV function using TEE in ways useful to clinicians. These efforts have been frustrated by the non-geometric, asymmetric shape of the chamber, its sequential contraction pattern, and the obscuring effect of epicardial fat on RV wall motion and thickness. In addition, the RV is exquisitely sensitive to loading conditions, overall pulmonary function, and the interdependence of the two ventricles.

The RV is anatomically divided into its inflow and outflow portions reflecting its dual embryonic origin. The inflow portion begins at the tricuspid valve and extends towards the apex to include the trabeculated, posteroinferior segments, while the outflow portion is usually free of trabeculations and includes the infundibulum (anterosuperior segments) and pulmonic valve. A series of muscular bands divide the two portions, the most important to the echocardiographer being the moderator band. This structure extends from the base of the anterior papillary muscle to the ventricular septum and should not be mistaken for a thrombus or intracavitary mass (see Chapter 3).[1,2]

Ventricular systolic ejection of the RV has a different pattern than that of the left ventricle. The ejection phase begins earlier and lasts longer, while the velocity profile is characterized by a lower and delayed peak.[3] Right ventricular ejection is largely due to a bellows-like motion of the free wall and longitudinal shortening of the ventricle (apex to annulus) rather than the twisting and rotational motions that predominate on the left side.[2,4] Finally, contraction of the RV is sequential, beginning with the free wall and moving towards the infundibulum.[5]

TOMOGRAPHIC VIEWS OF THE RIGHT VENTRICLE

Although the vast majority of information about the RV can be obtained from a small number of images, the chamber's complexity defies standardized description or definition. The RV is a paradoxical structure, appearing triangular in one view but of an elongated, crescent shape in another. Likewise, while it usually appears smaller than the left ventricle (LV), its end-diastolic volume is actually greater.[2]

As the RV cannot be completely seen in any single image, multiple scan planes are required to adequately assess RV structure and function. The RV has approximately one-sixth the mass of the LV, and performs about one-quarter of its partner's stroke work.[6] It consists of a free wall, an inferior or diaphragmatic wall, a septal wall, and an outflow tract (RVOT) region, although there is no formal segmental scheme for classifying wall motion as exists for the LV.

Despite this, a series of guidelines have been developed that attempt to establish standards for measurement of global RV size and function. Most important of these are the Recommendations for Chamber Quantification, developed jointly by the American Society of Echocardiography and the European Association of Echocardiography.[7] These standards were developed by a combination of methods, including statistical calculation of standard deviation, expert opinion, and assessment of associated outcome. It is recommended that the same values be used to assess RV size for both transesophageal (TEE) and transthoracic echocardiography (TTE), even though the actual images obtained may be markedly different.[7] Quantification with TEE is frequently very challenging due to the increased difficulty in achieving standard image planes and views.

Midesophageal Views

Probably the most useful view for RV assessment is the midesophageal four-chamber (ME-4C) view. To image the right ventricle, the standard ME-4C view is obtained and the probe is then turned slightly to the right to bring the tricuspid valve into the middle of the screen (Figure 13–1). The basilar RV free wall will be to the left of the screen while the apical portion of the free wall will be in the far field or slightly to the right, depending on the orientation of the heart. It may be useful to increase the multiplane angle to 10° to 20° to optimize the view of the RV cavity. A normal RV will

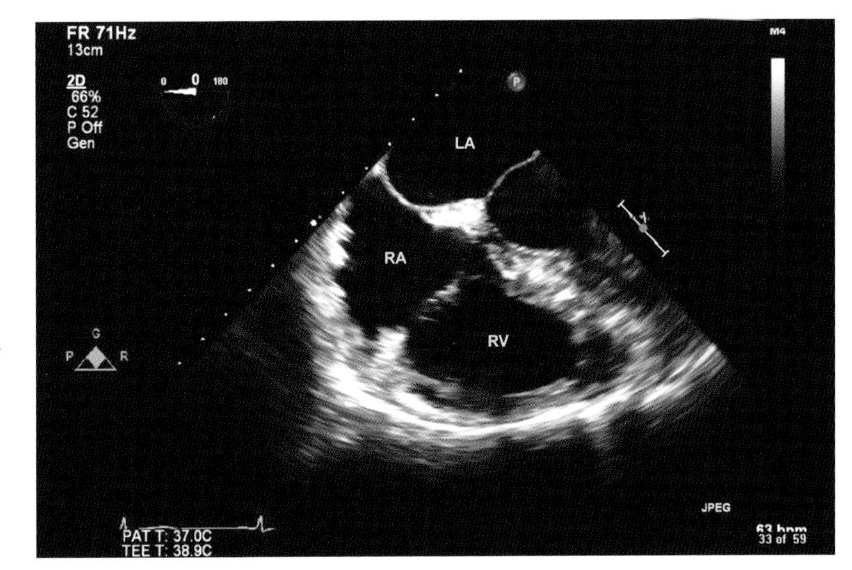

FIGURE 13–1. Midesophageal four-chamber view, with the probe turned to the patient's right side, the RA and RV come into view. Note the right ventricular hypertrophy in this image. (RA, right atrium; LA, left atrium; RV, right ventricle.)

be no more than two-thirds the longitudinal extent of the LV with the LV comprising the apex of the heart. From this imaging plane, the mid-cavity and longitudinal diameters of the RV may be measured and systolic motion qualitatively assessed (Figure 13–2). In addition, color-flow (CFD) and spectral Doppler analysis of trans-tricuspid flow as well as tissue Doppler examination of the tricuspid annulus may be performed from this image to evaluate possible valvular pathology and diastolic dysfunction. The ME-4C view is also an excellent view in which to quantify the right atrium (RA) by measuring its major and minor axes and comparing it to its partner to the left. As opposed to the left atrium (LA), normal ranges for RA size are not different for men and women. Normal reference limits for RV and RA size as well as partition values for mild, moderate, and severe enlargement are listed in Table 13–1.[7]

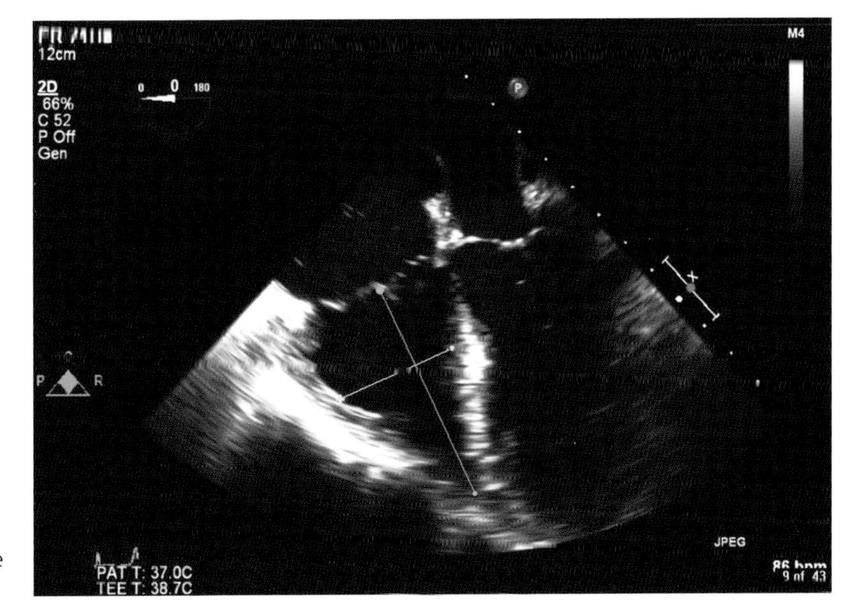

FIGURE 13–2. Midesophageal four-chamber view with long- and short-axis dimensions marked. Normal and abnormal dimensions are noted in Table 13–1.

Table 13–1. Reference Values for Right Atrium, Right Ventricle, and Pulmonic Valve (all measurements are in centimeters)

		Enlargement		
	Normal	**Mild**	**Moderate**	**Severe**
RA	2.9-4.5	4.6-4.9	5.0-5.4	≥5.5
RV				
Mid-cavity	2.7-3.3	3.4-3.7	3.8-4.1	≥4.2
Longitudinal	7.1-7.9	8.0-8.5	8.6-9.1	≥9.2
RVOT	2.5-2.9	3.0-3.2	3.3-3.5	≥3.6
PV	1.7-2.3	2.4-2.7	2.8-3.1	≥3.2

RA, right atrium; RV, right ventricle; RVOT, right ventricular outflow tract; PV, pulmonic valve annulus.
From Lang RM, Bierig M, Devereux RB, et al. Recommendations for chamber quantification: a report from the American Society of Echocardiography's Guidelines and Standards Committee and the Chamber Quantification Writing Group, developed in conjunction with the European Association of Echocardiography, a branch of the European Society of Cardiology. J Am Soc Echocardiogr. 2005;18(12):1440-1463; and Foale R, Nihoyannopoulos P, McKenna W, et al. Echocardiographic measurement of the normal adult right ventricle. Br Heart J. 1986;56(1):33-44.

Rotation of the TEE multiplane angle to approximately 30° to 60° and slight rotation of the probe to the right will bring the inflow-outflow or wrap-around view onto the screen (Figure 13–3). In this view, the RA, tricuspid valve (TV), RV, pulmonic valve (PV), and proximal pulmonary artery (PA) appear in order from the left side of the screen in an arc sweeping counter-clockwise in the far field around the aortic valve to the right. The RV inferior or diaphragmatic free wall is visible in the far field and the infundibular portion of the RV is particularly well seen closer to the right side of the screen. This is also an excellent view in which to use CFD to interrogate the TV and PV and to measure the dimensions of the PV annulus as well as the RV outflow tract (RVOT) or the immediate subpulmonary regions (Figure 13–4; see Table 13–1).

Further rotation of the multiplane angle to 90° to 120° while keeping the RA in view will bring the bicaval view onto the screen with the left atrium in the near field, the superior vena cava to the right, and

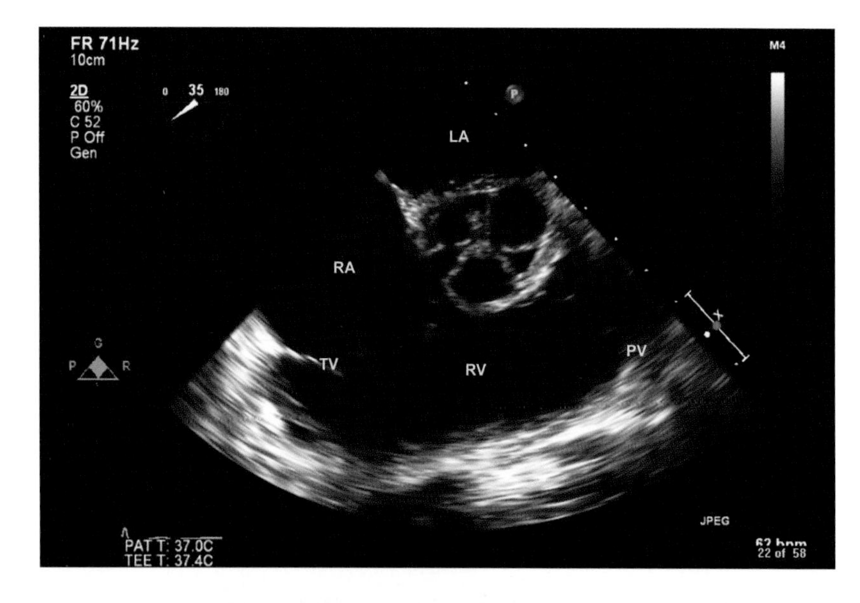

FIGURE 13–3. Midesophageal inflow-outflow view. Note the aortic valve in short axis in the mid-field, the right atrium (RA) to the left, the right ventricle (RV) in the far field, and the pulmonic valve (PV) to the right. (LA, left atrium; TV, tricuspid valve.)

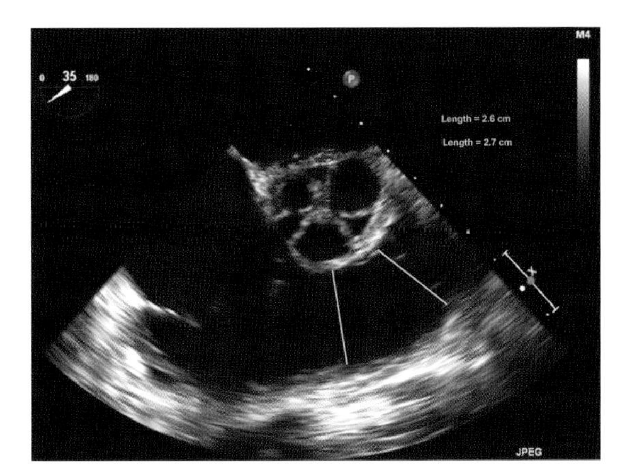

FIGURE 13–4. Midesophageal inflow-outflow view with right-ventricular outflow tract and pulmonic valve dimensions marked.

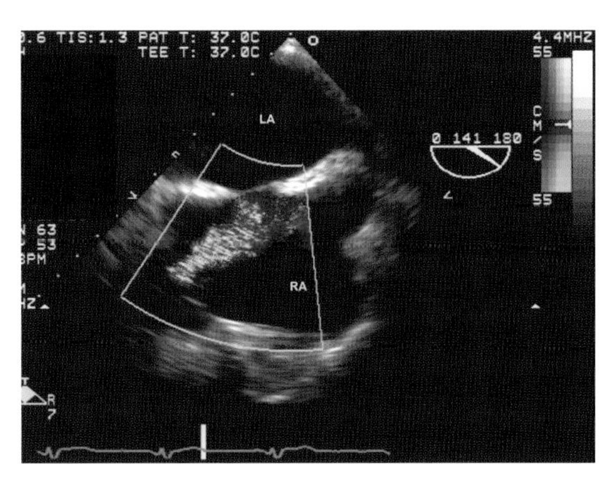

FIGURE 13–6. Midesophageal view of modified bicaval view with color Doppler. Note that the regurgitant jet and the ultrasound beam are closely aligned in this view. (RA, right atrium; LA, left atrium.)

the inferior vena cava (IVC) to the left (Figure 13–5). Frequently, the eustachian valve is seen emanating from the junction of the RA with the IVC at the lower end of the crista terminalis. This fetal remnant may have a mobile, filamentous structure associated with it that is known as a Chiari network, and is considered a normal variant (see Chapter 3). The interatrial septum is visible in the center of the screen and may be easily examined for a patent foramen ovale or other abnormalities. The tricuspid valve may be brought into this image at the far left field by further multiplane transducer angle rotation. This modified bicaval view is ideal for spectral Doppler analysis of a tricuspid regurgitation jet as the direction of the jet is usually closely aligned with the direction of the ultrasound beam (Figure 13–6). The coronary sinus is often seen just underneath the IVC to the left side of the screen and may prove useful in placement of a coronary sinus catheter during cardiac surgery (see Chapter 5).

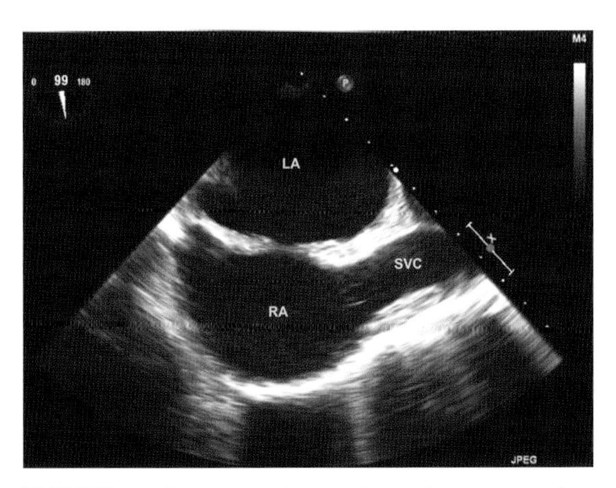

FIGURE 13–5. Midesophageal bicaval view. Note the left atrium (LA) in the near field, the interatrial septum and right atrium (RA) in the mid-field, and the superior vena cava (SVC) to the right of the display.

Transgastric Images

Transgastric images of the RV should be carefully examined as it is not uncommon that some of the best images of the RV are obtained from this position. A transgastric short-axis (TG-SAX) view of the RV is obtained by advancing the TEE probe into the stomach (35 to 45 cm from the incisors), flexing the probe, identifying the LV, and turning the probe to the patient's right. The RV will appear crescent shaped and wrapped around the LV. The tricuspid leaflets are often seen in short axis with extreme flexion (Figure 13–7). A long-axis or inflow RV view may be obtained one of two ways. From the LV short-axis view, the probe is turned to the right to bring the RV short-axis view into the center of the screen and the multiplane angle is rotated to 90° to 140°, yielding a view with the RV to the left of the screen, the TV in the middle, and the RA to the right (Figure 13–8A). The inferior free wall will appear in the near field and the anterior free wall in the far field. Alternatively, from the LV short-axis view, the transducer angle is advanced to 100° to 120°, identifying the LV long-axis view, and the probe is then turned to the right to reveal the RV inflow or long-axis view. Spectral Doppler analysis is not optimal from this position given the divergence between the

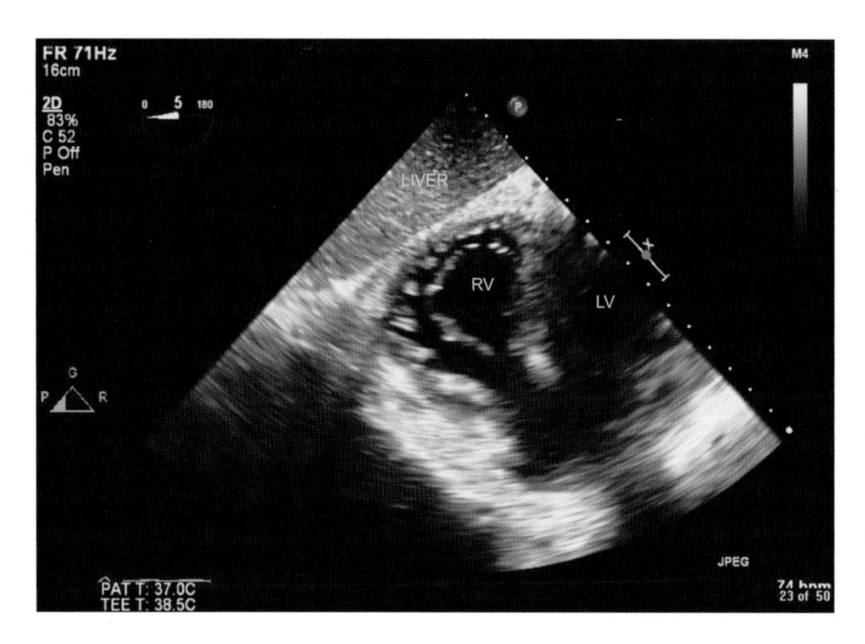

FIGURE 13–7. Transgastric short-axis view of the right ventricle (RV), note the triangular shape of the ventricular cavity and the leaflets of the tricuspid valve. (LV, left ventricle.)

angle of the ultrasound beam and the direction of blood flow (Figure 13–8B).

An RV outflow view may occasionally be developed from the RV short-axis view by rotating the multiplane angle slowly towards 100° to 130°, but also turning the probe slightly towards the patient's left (Figure 13–9A). The RVOT and PV will appear in the mid–far field, parallel to the beam, often in optimal position for color and spectral Doppler analysis, should that be desired (Figure 13–9B).

The deep transgastric image of right-sided structures is sometimes optimal for assessment of tricuspid annular motion with tissue Doppler methods.[8] This image is obtained by advancing the probe to the deep transgastric position, flexing the tip to identify the deep transgastric images of the LV, and turning

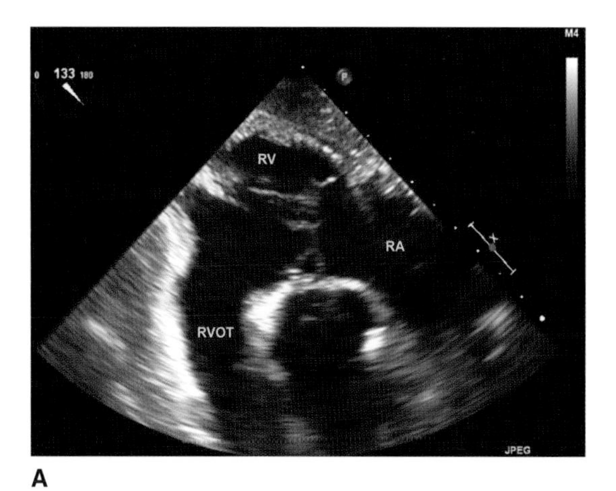

A

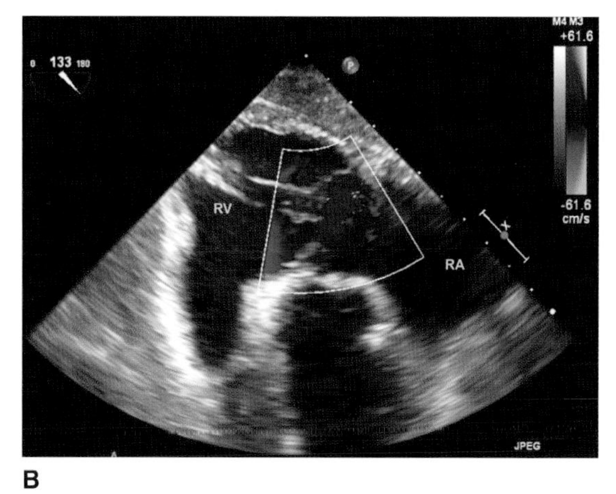

B

FIGURE 13–8. Transgastric RV inflow two-dimensional **(A)** and color-flow Doppler **(B)** views. Note that the direction of any regurgitant jet may not be appropriate for spectral Doppler analysis. The right ventricular outflow tract (RVOT) is partially visible in the mid–far field. (RV, right ventricle; RA, right atrium.)

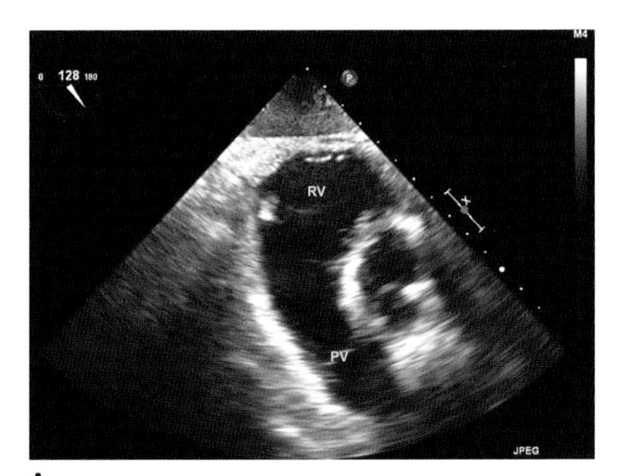

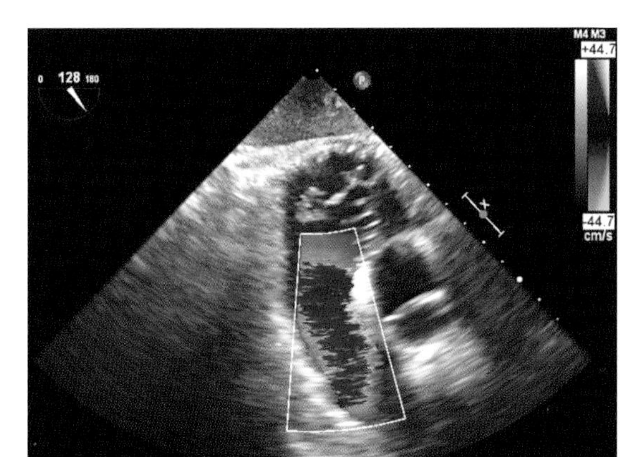

FIGURE 13–9. Transgastric RV outflow two-dimensional **(A)** and color-flow Doppler **(B)** views. Note that the direction of flow through the pulmonic valve (PV) does allow for spectral Doppler analysis of flow. (RV, right ventricle.)

the probe slightly towards the patient's right side (Figure 13–10). The result often resembles an apical four-chamber image obtained with transthoracic echocardiography.

The transgastric position is also the appropriate position from which to examine hepatic vein flow (Figure 13–11). From the transgastric position, the probe is turned to the patient's right side until the liver is seen. An appropriately sized and positioned vein is chosen and the multiplane angle is rotated such that the vein is as linear and as parallel with the ultrasound beam as possible. Spectral Doppler analysis of flow is then performed to examine flow patterns, in a manner analogous to that of pulmonary venous flow.

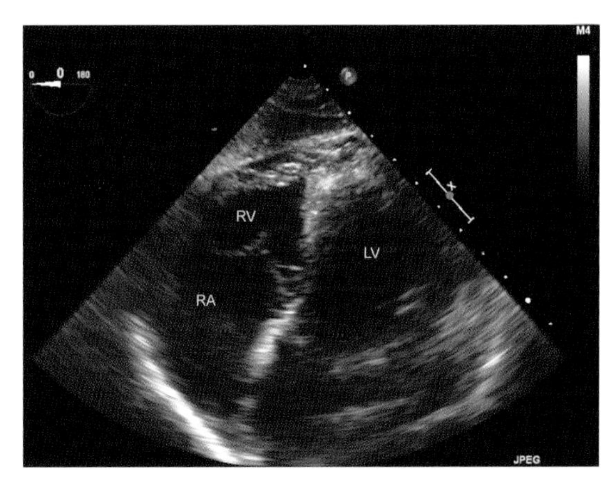

FIGURE 13–10. Deep transgastric view of the right atrium (RA) and right ventricle (RV) with both chambers marked. This view closely resembles a transthoracic apical four-chamber view. (LV, left ventricle.)

MECHANICAL ADAPTATIONS OF THE RIGHT VENTRICLE

Exposure to chronic conditions of excessively high preload or afterload will eventually result in fundamental changes to the structure of the RV. However, the mechanisms by which the RV copes with pathologic changes depends on whether it is facing increases in pressure work or increases in volume work.

Normal RV free-wall thickness is less than half that of the LV due to low pressures characteristic of the right-side system. However, elevated pressures in the

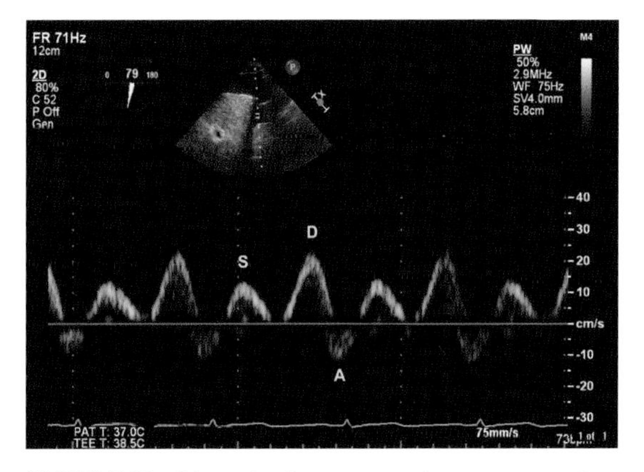

FIGURE 13–11. Pulsed-wave Doppler spectrum of hepatic vein flow includes two antegrade waves (systolic [S] and diastolic [D]) and a retrograde A wave.

right ventricular cavity, be they a result of pulmonary hypertension, pulmonic valvular pathology, or intrinsic myocardial disease, will cause patterns of ventricular hypertrophy that are indistinguishable from those of the left. Furthermore, the diagnosis of RV hypertrophy may be confounded by the appearance of trabeculations, which often become extremely dense and prominent in cases of pulmonary hypertension, especially near the apex. Right ventricular wall thickness is best measured using the inferior or lateral wall rather than the anterior wall, and measures 5 mm or less in a normal heart but may exceed 10 mm in cases of *cor pulmonale*.[9,10] Increased RV wall thickness may also be caused by primary myocardial infiltrative diseases such as amyloidosis or endocardial fibroelastosis.[11]

Under normal conditions, the center of mass in the heart is in the LV, and the ventricular septum maintains its concave curvature towards the LV throughout the cardiac cycle. As such, the LV maintains its circular shape in the transgastric midpapillary view. However, as the RV hypertrophies, the center of mass shifts rightward, towards the septum itself (Figure 13–12). The septum begins to flatten, and the LV thus begins to assume a D shape. Furthermore, this septal deformation results in the loss of the normal triangular or crescent shape of the RV in the transgastric view and the RV assumes a more spherical shape. Indeed, from the transgastric, midpapillary view, the two ventricles may begin to appear as two similar cavities with a flat wall dividing them. However, because the deformity in septal configuration is due to elevations in pressure within the ventricular cavities, this flattening is greatest when the intracavitary pressures are greatest, that is, at end-systole.[12-14]

In cases of myocardial failure, the RV will begin to dilate as a compensatory mechanism to maintain its stroke volume regardless of whether the failure is primary, secondary to volume overload, or following a long period of hypertrophy. This is detectable in a variety of echocardiographic views but the midesophageal four-chamber view adjusted to maximize the tricuspid annulus is the most useful. As noted, the LV should constitute the apex of the heart and the RV should extend no farther than two-thirds the length of the LV. A moderately dilated RV will reach to more than two-thirds the longitudinal extent of the LV, and a severely dilated RV will actually form the apex of the heart, displacing the LV completely (Figure 13–13).[7] In addition, the RV will transform from a triangular to a circular shape as it dilates.[9] More quantitative measurements have been established and are obtained from the midesophageal four-chamber as well as from the inflow-outflow view (see Table 13–1).

Septal motion is also abnormal in conditions of RV dilatation when the exaggerated motion of the septum occurs without any real shift in the center of mass, as is seen with RV hypertrophy. The septum appears to flatten, resulting in a D-shaped LV, but this occurs during the period of maximal filling, that is, during end-diastole.[12,14] Then, as the ventricles

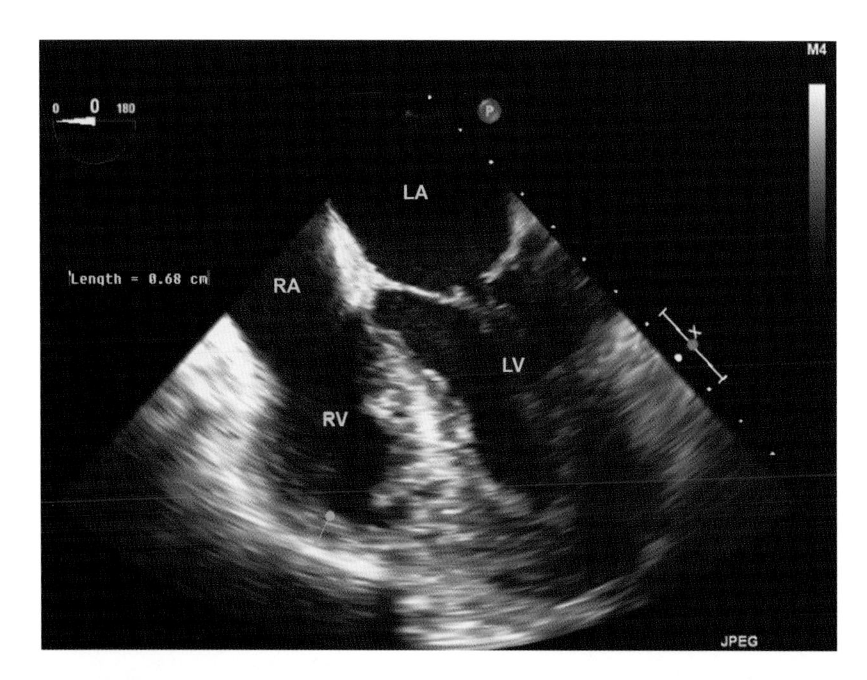

FIGURE 13–12. Midesophageal four-chamber view demonstrating moderate right ventricular hypertrophy (wall thickness measuring 6.8 mm). (RA, right atrium; RV, right ventricle; LA, left atrium; LV, left ventricle.)

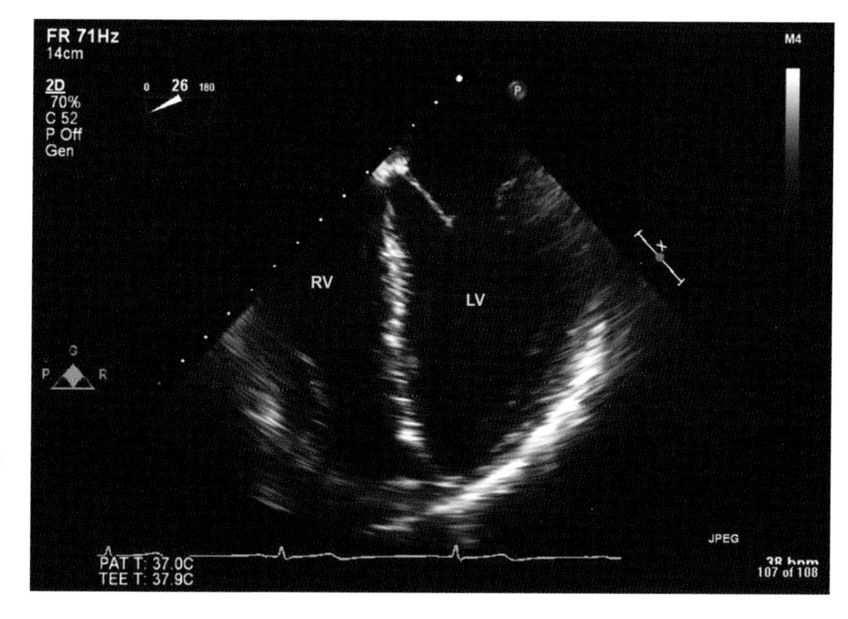

FIGURE 13–13. Midesophageal four-chamber view demonstrating RV dilatation. Note the equal dimensions of the right and left ventricle indicating moderate dilatation of the right ventricle (RV). (LV, left ventricle.)

empty, the septum is free to assume a more normal curvature. It is important, though, not to confuse this motion with the septal "bounce" that is commonly seen with ventricular pacing using epicardial leads following cardiac surgery and attributed to an abnormal pattern of contraction.[15]

ASSESSMENT OF REGIONAL SYSTOLIC FUNCTION

Any assessment of RV function is complicated by the combined interplay of factors that distinguish it from the LV. As discussed above, its geometry is complex and difficult to image due to its distance from the probe as well as its structure. Because the wall is thinner and less muscular, systolic inward excursion is less than that of the LV, and it is affected by LV function by way of sharing a common wall. Furthermore, its size varies significantly during the respiratory cycle in opposing directions, depending on whether the patient is breathing spontaneously or is being mechanically ventilated.

Due in part to these difficulties, the ASE-SCA guidelines for intraoperative TEE examination concluded that mild degrees of RV hypocontractility are hard to define accurately, and have recommended that RV dysfunction would only be diagnosed when a wall segment is either akinetic or dyskinetic.[16] In the ME-4C view (see Figure 13–1) one can evaluate the function of the free anterolateral RV wall. The midesophageal inflow-outflow view (see Figure 13–3) allows assessment of the RV diaphragmatic wall (in the far field and to the left) and of the infundibular portion of the RV (at the right side of the view). Last, the transgastric RV inflow view (see Figure 13–8) also allows evaluation of the RV diaphragmatic wall.

Similar to the LV, regional RV dysfunction can coexist with preserved global function, for example, when one of the acute marginal branches of the right coronary artery is occluded. A small portion of the anterior RV free wall is supplied by the left anterior descending artery through its conal branch, and this can lead to regional RV dysfunction with left coronary artery disease.[17] During cardiac surgery, cardioplegia delivery may be inadequate for RV protection, especially with retrograde techniques.[18] Also, the right coronary artery arises from the anterior aspect of the ascending aorta, serving as a common site for coronary air embolism during separation from cardiopulmonary bypass.

Hypercontractility of the infundibular RV outflow tract leading to obstruction of blood flow has been described in approximately 5% of patients after cardiac surgery.[19] The end-systolic obliteration of RV outflow can be associated with significant pressure gradient across the RV outflow tract (>25 mm Hg). Several risk factors for this condition have been described, including RV hypertrophy, hypovolemia, and increased adrenergic tone. Clinically, it is associated with tricuspid regurgitation and hemodynamic instability.

ASSESSMENT OF GLOBAL SYSTOLIC FUNCTION

The technical difficulties that hamper accurate assessment of regional RV function also confound assessment of global function, leading to a diverse array of quantitative indices (Table 13–2).

Ejection phase indices are especially affected by the non-geometric shape of the RV. In addition, tricuspid regurgitation is very common and the decreased afterload might compensate for decreased contractility. The unidimensional index *shortening fraction* can be calculated along either the short or long axis of the RV from the ME-4C view or the TG-SAX (with the probe rotated rightward to show the RV), but is rarely adequately reflective of RV contraction.[20] A variant of shortening fraction that has been found more useful is *tricuspid annular plane systolic excursion (TAPSE).* It has been shown that the main contribution to RV systole is the contraction of longitudinal muscle fibers that cause the tricuspid annulus to move toward the RV apex. The majority of this movement occurs in the lateral aspect of the ventricular free wall, as the medial septal attachment of the tricuspid annulus is relatively fixed. Hence the tricuspid annulus moves like a hinge during systole, resulting in a measurable long-axis excursion of the lateral aspect of the tricuspid annulus. In TTE, TAPSE is usually measured in the apical four-chamber view. However, for TEE imaging, the transgastric RV inflow view (see Figure 13–8A) more accurately aligns the axis of annular movement with the direction of the ultrasound beam, allowing more accurate measurement of annular motion using M-mode (Figure 13–14).[21] In one study, TAPSE had a better correlation with radionuclide-measured RV ejection fraction compared to RV fractional area change.[22] Other studies have shown that decreased TAPSE is associated with a worse prognosis in patients with acute myocardial infarction and in patients after mitral valve repair surgery.[23,24] It should be mentioned, though, that TAPSE can also be affected by LV function independent of RV function.[25]

Table 13–2. Indices of right ventricular systolic function

Index	Normal Values
Tricuspid annular plane systolic excursion	15-20 mm
Fractional area change	32%-60%
Ejection fraction	45%-65%
dP/dT	>1000 mm Hg/s
Myocardial performance index	0.3-0.4

Data are from Haddad F, Couture P, Tousignant C, Denault AY. The right ventricle in cardiac surgery, a perioperative perspective: I. Anatomy, physiology, and assessment. Anesth Analg. 2009;108(2):407-421; and Lang RM, Bierig M, Devereux RB, et al. Recommendations for chamber quantification: a report from the American Society of Echocardiography's Guidelines and Standards Committee and the Chamber Quantification Writing Group, developed in conjunction with the European Association of Echocardiography, a branch of the European Society of Cardiology. J Am Soc Echocardiogr. 2005;18(12):1440-1463.

A two-dimensional ejection phase index is the *fractional area change (FAC),* calculated as follows:

$$\text{FAC} = \left(\frac{\text{End-Diastolic Area} - \text{End-Systolic Area}}{\text{End-Diastolic Area}}\right) \times 100$$

Similar to shortening fraction, it can be measured by planimetry in either the ME-4C or the TG-SAX views. The degree of RV dysfunction can be classified as mild (FAC 25% to 31%), moderate (FAC 18% to 24%), or severe dysfunction (FAC <18%).[7] In patients undergoing coronary artery bypass surgery, RV FAC values less than 35% were associated with a worse early and late postoperative outcome.[26]

A three-dimensional *ejection fraction* can be calculated using a summation of smaller geometric volumes (ellipsoid, prism, or pyramid) to model the RV.[27,28] Similar to the LV, a modified Simpson's method can also be used to calculate RV ejection fraction.[29] In the future, three-dimensional echocardiography might be employed to obtain more accurate measurements of RV size (see Chapter 24).[30]

Several non-geometric indices of RV function have been suggested. In patients with tricuspid regurgitation, the acceleration of the regurgitant jet into the right atrium (*dP/dt*) reflects the rate of increase in RV pressure during systole, and is determined by RV contractility. To calculate dP/dt, the tricuspid regurgitation jet is identified at the transesophageal RV inflow-outflow view with color-flow Doppler. The omniplane angle is adjusted to align the tricuspid regurgitation jet with the ultrasound beam, and the continous-wave spectral Doppler trace of the regurgitation jet is examined (Figure 13–15). dt is defined as the time interval between jet velocities of 1 m/s (corresponding to a ventriculo-atrial pressure gradient of 4 mm Hg) and 2 m/s (corresponding to a pressure gradient of 16 mm Hg). The dP/dt is then calculated by dividing the pressure difference (16 – 4 = 12 mm Hg) by the time interval (in seconds). Calculation of RV dP/dt using echocardiography has a good correlation with values derived from invasive cardiac catheterization.[31] Compared to ejection phase indices, dP/dt is more sensitive to preload changes but less sensitive to afterload.[32]

Another ventricular function index free of any geometrical assumptions is the *myocardial performance*

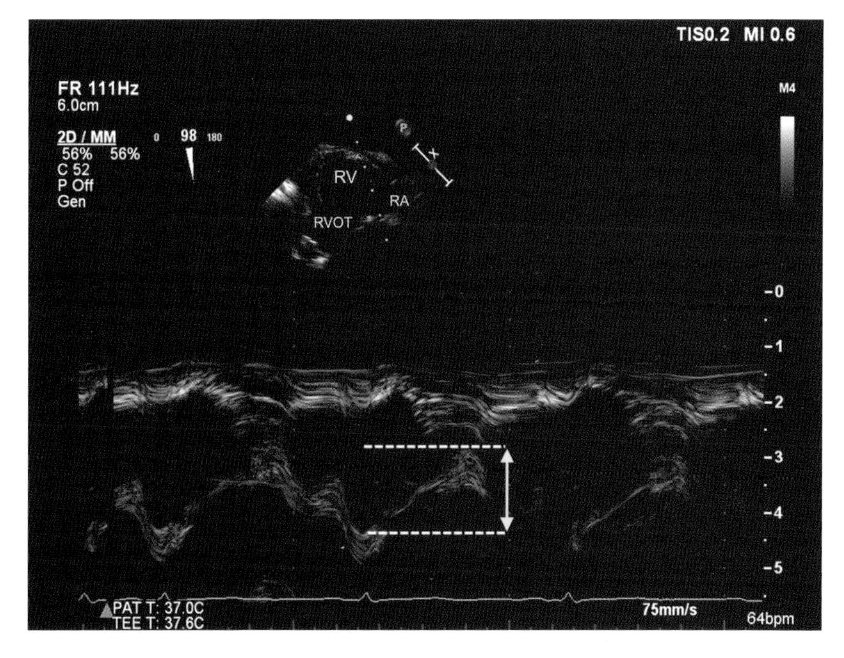

FIGURE 13–14. Measurement of tricuspid annular plane systolic excursion (TAPSE) from the transgastric RV inflow view. Using M-mode, the movement of the leading edge of the lateral tricuspid annulus attachment is tracked during systole, and its excursion is measured; here, it is 15 mm. (RA, right atrium; RV, right ventricle; RVOT, right ventricular outflow tract.)

index (MPI), originally defined for the left ventricle as the sum of the two isovolumic intervals (isovolumic contraction and isovolumic relaxation) divided by ejection time (Figure 13–16).[33] For the RV, a spectral pulsed-wave Doppler trace of pulmonary artery flow provides the ejection time and is recorded either from the upper esophageal aortic arch short-axis or the transgastric RV outflow view. Total systolic time can be measured as the duration of a tricuspid regurgitation jet if it exists, or as the interval between the end of the A and the start of the E wave on a tricuspid inflow spectral Doppler trace (Figure 13–17). The isovolumic period is calculated by subtracting the ejection time from the total systolic time. MPI is affected by both systolic and diastolic function, and is relatively independent of heart rate, afterload, and preload.[33] MPI value above 0.5 was found to predict hemodynamic instability and mortality after cardiac valvular surgery.[34]

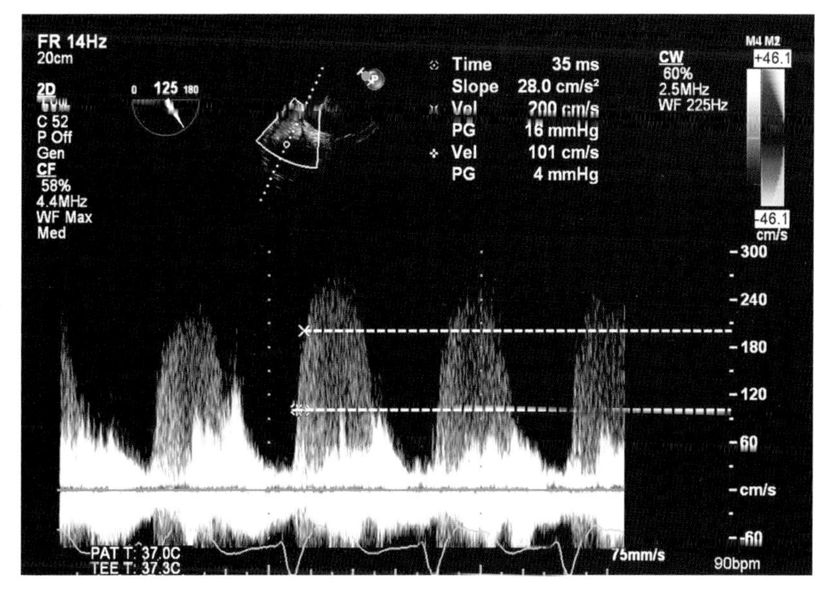

FIGURE 13–15. Spectral Doppler analysis of the tricuspid regurgitation jet showing calculation of dP/dt. Flow velocities of 1 m/s and 2 m/s are marked and the time interval between them is measured (35 milliseconds or 0.035 seconds). The change in pressure in this case is 16 − 4 = 12 mm Hg. dP/dt is calculated as 12 mm Hg/0.035 seconds = 343 mm Hg/s, suggesting significant right ventricular dysfunction.

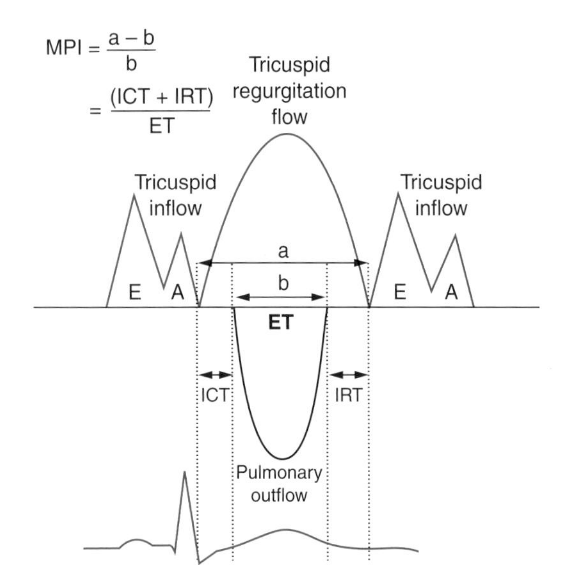

FIGURE 13–16. Schematic demonstrating calculation of myocardial performance index (MPI) as the sum of the isovolumic contraction time (ICT) and relaxation time (IRT), divided by the right ventricular ejection time (ET).

Several important hemodynamic values can be derived from spectral Doppler interrogation of right-side flows. *Cardiac output* can be calculated by placing the pulsed-wave Doppler sample volume just proximal to the pulmonary valve either in the transgastric RV outflow view or the upper esophageal aortic arch view to measure the velocity-time integral (Figure 13–18A and B). The RVOT diameter is measured in the same view or in the midesophageal RV inflow-outflow view (see Figure 13–4). Stroke volume is then calculated as follows:

$$SV = RVOT_{Area} \times RVOT_{VTI}$$

In patients without significant tricuspid valve regurgitation, this measurement correlates well with cardiac output measured by thermodilution.[35]

In the presence of tricuspid regurgitation and in the absence of RV outflow obstruction, continuous-wave Doppler can be used to estimate *pulmonary artery (PA) systolic pressure* because the peak velocity of the tricuspid regurgitant jet reflects the pressure gradient between the RV and RA (Figure 13–19A and B). Most patients with pulmonary hypertension have some degree of tricuspid regurgitation, making quantitative estimation possible. It is important to align the ultrasound beam to within 20° of parallel to the regurgitant jet to avoid significant underestimation of the pressure gradient.

Estimation of *RA pressure* is based on the absolute measurement and respiratory variation of IVC size using the TG-SAX view with the probe rotated to the right (Figure 13–20). A maximal diameter less than 20 mm quite accurately differentiates patients with RA pressures less than 10 mm Hg from those with greater than 10 mm Hg.[36] While the decrease in diameter in response to a forced sniffing maneuver (normal decrease

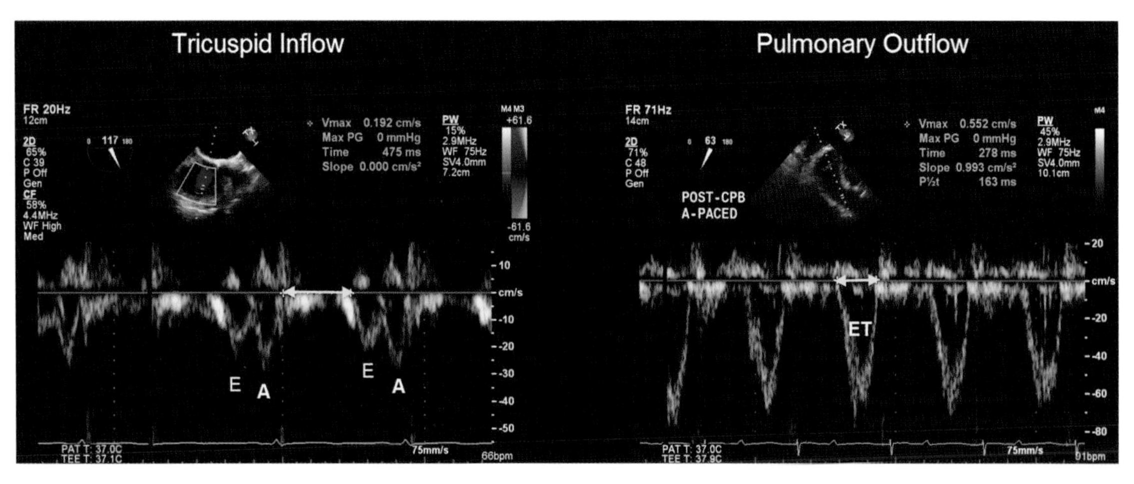

FIGURE 13–17. Spectral Doppler trace of the tricuspid inflow *(left)* with the systolic time measured between the end of the A wave to the beginning of the next E wave, and of the pulmonary outflow *(right)* with measurement of the ejection time (ET). Here, systolic duration is 475 milliseconds and ET is 278 milliseconds. Therefore, the MPI = (475 – 278)/278 = 0.71.

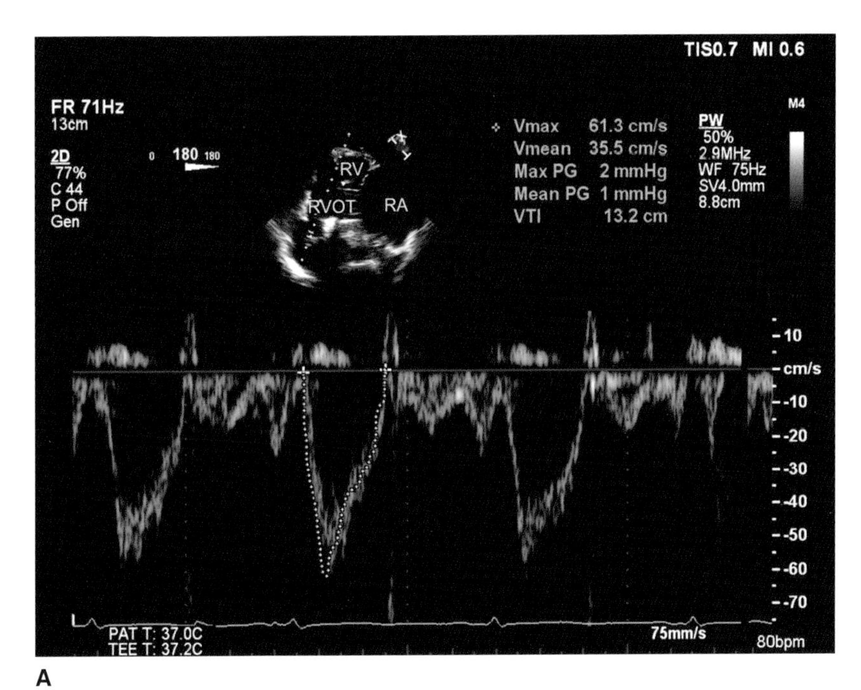

A

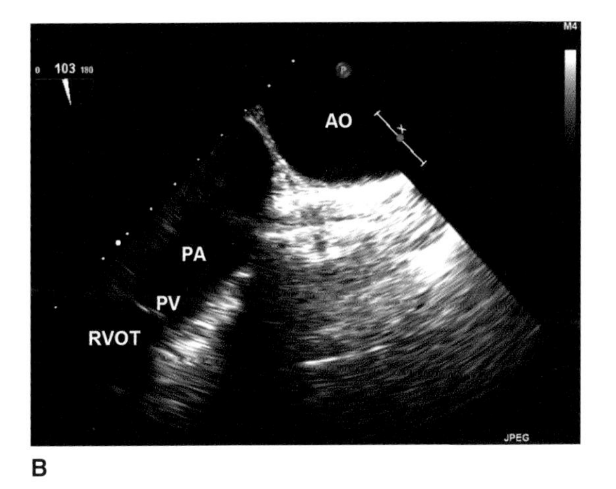

B

FIGURE 13–18. **A:** Spectral Doppler tracing of pulmonary outflow at the transgastric RV inflow-outflow view, showing the calculation of the velocity-time integral (VTI), in this case 13.2 cm. Right ventricular stroke volume = $RVOT_{VTI} \times RVOT_{area}$. **B:** Pulmonary outflow can be aligned with the ultrasound beam with the probe at the upper esophageal level rotated rightward and the multiplane angle at ~100°. (RA, right atrium; RV, right ventricle; RVOT, right ventricular outflow tract; AO, aorta; PA, pulmonary artery; PV, pulmonic valve.)

is 35% to 55%) can add some information about RA pressure within 5 mm Hg gradations, it is significantly less reliable.[36] In spontaneously breathing patients, IVC diameter decreases during inspiration, while in mechanically ventilated patients the opposite is usually true depending on intravascular volume status. An increase of more than 12% during inspiration predicts an increase in cardiac output in response to volume loading.[37]

RIGHT VENTRICULAR DIASTOLIC FUNCTION

Right ventricular diastolic function can be evaluated in a manner analogous to the left ventricle, although it has been less studied and its clinical significance is still largely unknown. Compared to the mitral annulus, the tricuspid annulus diameter is larger, resulting in lower inflow velocities.[38] Also, tricuspid inflow is more subject

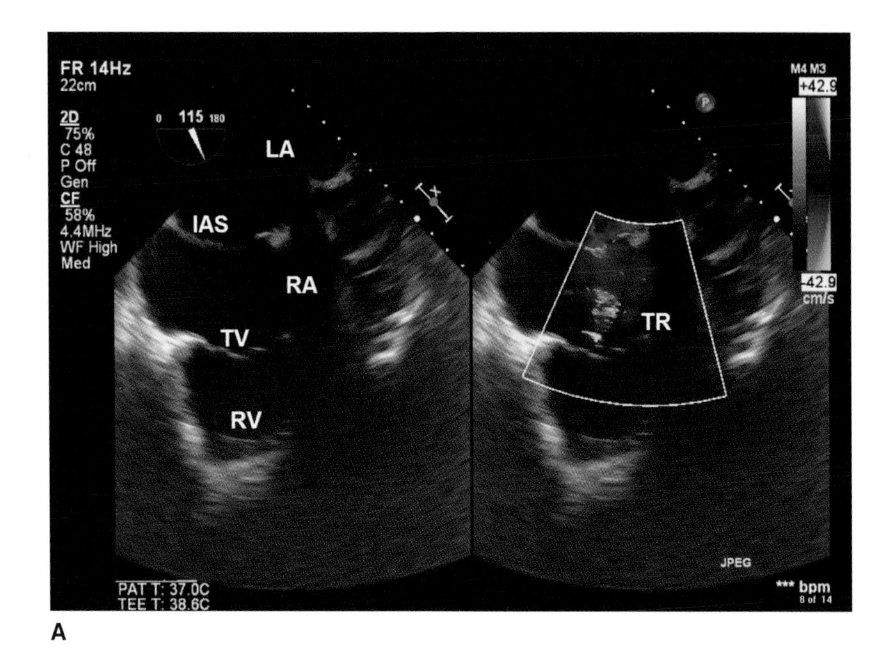

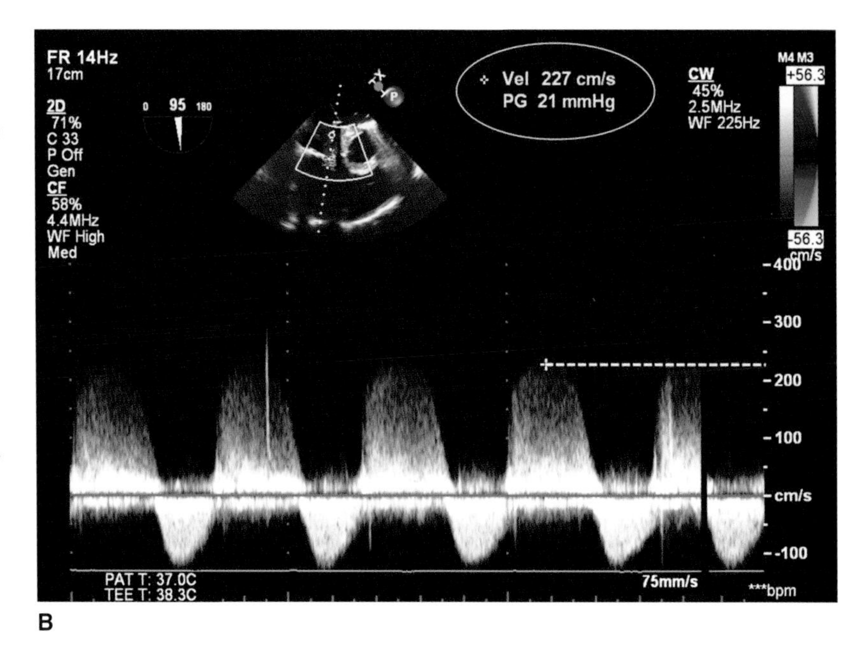

FIGURE 13–19. **A:** Aligning the tricuspid regurgitation (TR) jet in parallel with the ultrasound beam is often possible with the probe at the midesophageal level, rotated to the right and with the multiplane angle around 100° to 120°. This view shows the left (LA) and right atria (RA), the interatrial septum (IAS), the tricuspid valve (TV), and a small portion of the right ventricle (RV). **B:** Spectral Doppler trace of the tricuspid regurgitation jet reflecting a RV-to-RA pressure gradient of 21 mm Hg.

to respiratory variations, with inflow velocities increasing during spontaneous inspiration.[39] When evaluating diastolic function, it is important to ensure that the respiratory variation measured is not an artifact resulting from respiratory-induced translocation and rotation movements of the heart itself, which might lead to situations in which the interrogated flow is not parallel to the ultrasound beam.

Right ventricular filling is evaluated by measuring tricuspid inflow velocities, and can usually be measured from the midesophageal, modified bicaval view with the probe turned to the right and the transducer

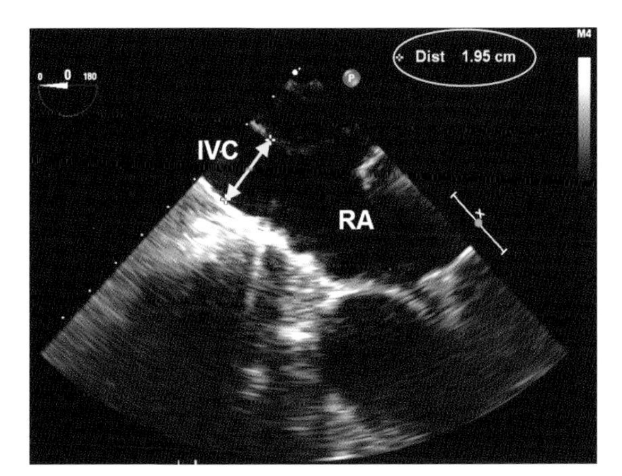

FIGURE 13–20. Inferior vena cava (IVC) diameter where it enters the right atrium (RA). This is a deep transgastric view with the probe rotated rightward.

angle rotated to somewhere between 90° and 120°. The ideal position of the transducer angle is determined by attempting to align the direction of blood flow with the direction of the ultrasound beam, and is highly dependent on how the heart is positioned in the chest with respect to the esophagus. Normal tricuspid inflow consists of an early diastolic E wave corresponding to right atrial emptying upon opening of the tricuspid valve, and a late diastolic A wave corresponding to atrial contraction (Figure 13–21). Right atrial filling is usually evaluated using TEE by interrogating hepatic vein flow or IVC flow. From the transgastric position, the probe is rotated to the right, and adjusted such that a hepatic vein branch is as parallel as possible with the ultrasound beam. The hepatic vein inflow usually includes two antegrade flows—S during systole and D during early diastole—and a retrograde end-diastolic A wave corresponding to atrial contraction (see Figure 13–11). A second retrograde end-systolic V wave is variably present. Normal values for these flow velocities are summarized in Table 13–3.

A third modality used to assess RV diastolic function is tricuspid annular tissue Doppler analysis. The normal spectral curve includes one negative systolic wave (S′) and two positive diastolic waves—an early (E′) wave and a late (A′) wave. Normally, the E′ wave is higher than the A′ wave. In a pattern similar to the LV, the first stage of diastolic dysfunction is related to impaired ventricular relaxation, and is denoted by decreased E- and E′-wave velocities, E/A and E′/A′ ratios of less than 1, and increased deceleration times on trans-tricuspid flow assessment. More severe diastolic dysfunction resulting from decreased ventricular compliance and restricted filling is characterized by a high E/A ratio (usually >1.5), normal or short trans-tricuspid deceleration times, and an S-wave peak velocity that is lower than the D wave on the hepatic

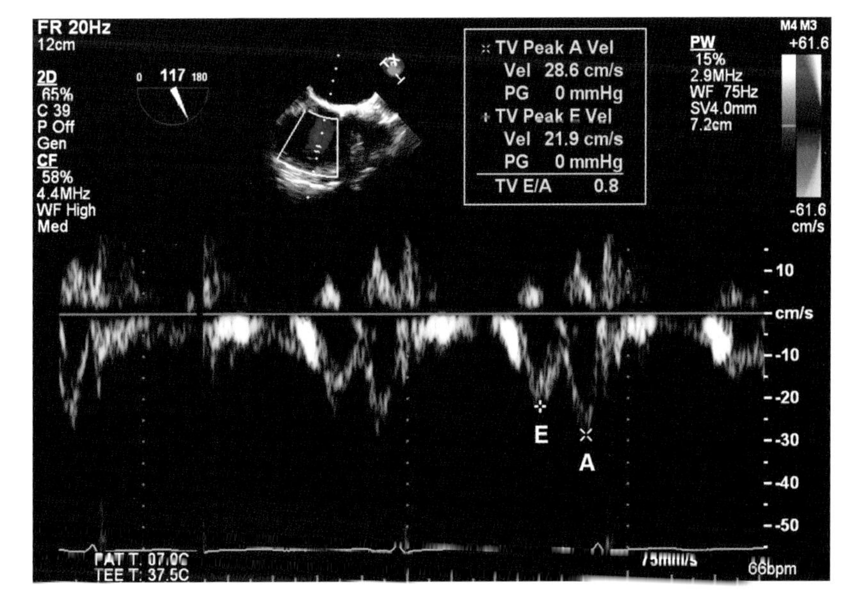

FIGURE 13–21. Pulsed-wave Doppler interrogation of tricuspid inflow at the midesophageal level. The E/A ratio of 0.8 indicates impaired RV relaxation.

Table 13–3. Flow velocities in the right heart

	Wave	Normal Values
Tricuspid inflow	E wave	41 ± 8 cm/s
	A wave	33 ± 8 cm/s
	E/A ratio	1.3 ± 0.4
	Deceleration time	198 ± 23 s
Hepatic vein flow	S wave	41 ± 15 cm/s
	D wave	24 ± 10 cm/s
	A wave	17 ± 5 cm/s
Tricuspid annulus tissue Doppler	E′	13-17 cm/s
	A′	12-18 cm/s
	E′/A′ ratio	0.8-1.2

Data are for normal subjects older than 50 years, taken from Klein AL, Leung DY, Murray RD, Urban LH, Bailey KR, Tajik AJ. Effects of age and physiologic variables on right ventricular filling dynamics in normal subjects. Am J Cardiol. 1999;84(4):440-448; and Alam M, Wardell J, Andersson E, Samad BA, Nordlander R. Characteristics of mitral and tricuspid annular velocities determined by pulsed wave Doppler tissue imaging in healthy subjects. J Am Soc Echocardiogr. 1999;12(8):618-628.

vein flow. In contrast to the E/A ratio on the tricuspid inflow trace, the E′/A′ ratio on the tricuspid annulus tissue Doppler tracing remains less than 1 and continues to diminish with worsening function.

REFERENCES

1. Netter F. Heart. In: Yonkman F, ed. *The CIBA Collection of Medical Illustrations.* New York: CIBA Pharmaceuticals Co; 1978:9.
2. Dell'Italia LJ. The right ventricle: anatomy, physiology, and clinical importance. *Curr Probl Cardiol.* 1991;16(10): 653-720.
3. Jiang L, Wiegers SE, Weyman AE. Right ventricle. In: Weyman AE, ed. *Principles and Practice of Echocardiography.* 2nd ed. Philadelphia: Lea & Febiger; 1994:901-921.
4. Petitjean C, Rougon N, Cluzel P. Assessment of myocardial function: a review of quantification methods and results using tagged MRI. *J Cardiovasc Magn Reson.* 2005;7(2): 501-516.
5. Lee FA. Hemodynamics of the right ventricle in normal and disease states. *Cardiol Clin.* 1992;10(1):59-67.
6. Lorenz CH, Walker ES, Morgan VL, Klein SS, Graham TP Jr. Normal human right and left ventricular mass, systolic function, and gender differences by cine magnetic resonance imaging. *J Cardiovasc Magn Reson.* 1999;1(1):7-21.
7. Lang RM, Bierig M, Devereux RB, et al. Recommendations for chamber quantification: a report from the American Society of Echocardiography's Guidelines and Standards Committee and the Chamber Quantification Writing Group, developed in conjunction with the European Association of Echocardiography, a branch of the European Society of Cardiology. *J Am Soc Echocardiogr.* 2005;18(12):1440-1463.
8. Haddad F, Couture P, Tousignant C, Denault AY. The right ventricle in cardiac surgery, a perioperative perspective: I. Anatomy, physiology, and assessment. *Anesth Analg.* 2009;108(2): 407-421.
9. Otto C. Echocardiographic evaluation of left and right ventricular systolic function. In: Otto CM, ed. *Textbook of Clinical Echocardiography.* 2nd ed. Philadelphia: Saunders; 2000: 100-131.
10. Cacho A, Prakash R, Sarma R, Kaushik VS. Usefulness of two-dimensional echocardiography in diagnosing right ventricular hypertrophy. *Chest.* 1983;84(2):154-157.
11. Child JS, Krivokapich J, Abbasi AS. Increased right ventricular wall thickness on echocardiography in amyloid infiltrative cardiomyopathy. *Am J Cardiol.* 1979;44(7):1391-1395.
12. Louie EK, Rich S, Levitsky S, Brundage BH. Doppler echocardiographic demonstration of the differential effects of right ventricular pressure and volume overload on left ventricular geometry and filling. *J Am Coll Cardiol.* 1992;19(1):84-90.
13. Jardin F, Dubourg O, Bourdarias JP. Echocardiographic pattern of acute cor pulmonale. *Chest.* 1997;111(1):209-217.
14. Davlouros PA, Niwa K, Webb G, Gatzoulis MA. The right ventricle in congenital heart disease. *Heart.* 2006;92 Suppl 1: i27-38.
15. Little WC, Reeves RC, Arciniegas J, Katholi RE, Rogers EW. Mechanism of abnormal interventricular septal motion during delayed left ventricular activation. *Circulation.* 1982;65(7): 1486-1491.
16. Shanewise JS, Cheung AT, Aronson S, et al. ASE/SCA guidelines for performing a comprehensive intraoperative multiplane transesophageal echocardiography examination: recommendations of the American Society of Echocardiography Council for Intraoperative Echocardiography and the Society of Cardiovascular Anesthesiologists Task Force for Certification in Perioperative Transesophageal Echocardiography. *Anesth Analg.* 1999;89(4): 870-884.
17. Wilson BC, Cohn JN. Right ventricular infarction: clinical and pathophysiologic considerations. *Adv Intern Med.* 1988;33: 295-309.
18. Christakis GT, Fremes SE, Weisel RD, et al. Right ventricular dysfunction following cold potassium cardioplegia. *J Thorac Cardiovasc Surg.* 1985;90(2):243-250.
19. Denault AY, Chaput M, Couture P, Hebert Y, Haddad F, Tardif JC. Dynamic right ventricular outflow tract obstruction in cardiac surgery. *J Thorac Cardiovasc Surg.* 2006;132(1): 43-49.
20. Bommer W, Weinert L, Neumann A, Neef J, Mason DT, DeMaria A. Determination of right atrial and right ventricular size by two-dimensional echocardiography. *Circulation.* 1979;60(1):91-100.
21. David JS, Tousignant CP, Bowry R. Tricuspid annular velocity in patients undergoing cardiac operation using transesophageal echocardiography. *J Am Soc Echocardiogr.* 2006;19(3):329-334.
22. Mishra M, Swaminathan M, Malhotra R, Mishra A, Trehan N. Evaluation of right ventricular function during CABG: transesophageal echocardiographic assessment of hepatic venous flow versus conventional right ventricular performance indices. *Echocardiography.* 1998;15(1):51-58.
23. Samad BA, Alam M, Jensen-Urstad K. Prognostic impact of right ventricular involvement as assessed by tricuspid annular motion in patients with acute myocardial infarction. *Am J Cardiol.* 2002;90(7):778-781.

24. Di Mauro M, Calafiore AM, Penco M, Romano S, Di Giammarco G, Gallina S. Mitral valve repair for dilated cardiomyopathy: predictive role of right ventricular dysfunction. *Eur Heart J.* 2007;28(20):2510-2516.
25. Lopez-Candales A, Rajagopalan N, Saxena N, Gulyasy B, Edelman K, Bazaz R. Right ventricular systolic function is not the sole determinant of tricuspid annular motion. *Am J Cardiol.* 2006;98(7):973-977.
26. Maslow AD, Regan MM, Panzica P, Heindel S, Mashikian J, Comunale ME. Precardiopulmonary bypass right ventricular function is associated with poor outcome after coronary artery bypass grafting in patients with severe left ventricular systolic dysfunction. *Anesth Analg.* 2002;95(6):1507-1518, table of contents.
27. Benchimol A, Desser KB, Hastreiter AR. Right ventricular volume in congenital heart disease. *Am J Cardiol.* 1975;36(1):67-75.
28. Ferlinz J, Gorlin R, Cohn PF, Herman MV. Right ventricular performance in patients with coronary artery disease. *Circulation.* 1975;52(4):608-615.
29. Panidis IP, Ren JF, Kotler MN, et al. Two-dimensional echocardiographic estimation of right ventricular ejection fraction in patients with coronary artery disease. *J Am Coll Cardiol.* 1983;2(5):911-918.
30. Ota T, Fleishman CE, Strub M, et al. Real-time, three-dimensional echocardiography: feasibility of dynamic right ventricular volume measurement with saline contrast. *Am Heart J.* 1999;137(5):958-966.
31. Imanishi T, Nakatani S, Yamada S, et al. Validation of continuous wave Doppler-determined right ventricular peak positive and negative dP/dt: effect of right atrial pressure on measurement. *J Am Coll Cardiol.* 1994;23(7):1638-1643.
32. Kass DA, Maughan WL, Guo ZM, Kono A, Sunagawa K, Sagawa K. Comparative influence of load versus inotropic states on indexes of ventricular contractility: experimental and theoretical analysis based on pressure-volume relationships. *Circulation.* 1987;76(6):1422-1436.
33. Tei C, Ling LH, Hodge DO, et al. New index of combined systolic and diastolic myocardial performance: a simple and reproducible measure of cardiac function—a study in normals and dilated cardiomyopathy. *J Cardiol.* 1995;26(6):357-366.
34. Haddad F, Denault AY, Couture P, et al. Right ventricular myocardial performance index predicts perioperative mortality or circulatory failure in high-risk valvular surgery. *J Am Soc Echocardiogr.* 2007;20(9):1065-1072.
35. Maslow A, Comunale ME, Haering JM, Watkins J. Pulsed wave Doppler measurement of cardiac output from the right ventricular outflow tract. *Anesth Analg.* 1996;83(3):466-471.
36. Brennan JM, Blair JE, Goonewardena S, et al. Reappraisal of the use of inferior vena cava for estimating right atrial pressure. *J Am Soc Echocardiogr.* 2007;20(7):857-861.
37. Feissel M, Michard F, Faller JP, Teboul JL. The respiratory variation in inferior vena cava diameter as a guide to fluid therapy. *Intensive Care Med.* 2004;30(9):1834-1837.
38. Otto CM. *Textbook of Clinical Echocardiography.* 3rd ed. Philadelphia, PA: Elsevier Saunders; 2004.
39. Klein AL, Leung DY, Murray RD, Urban LH, Bailey KR, Tajik AJ. Effects of age and physiologic variables on right ventricular filling dynamics in normal subjects. *Am J Cardiol.* 1999;84(4):440-448.

REVIEW QUESTIONS

Select the *one* best answer for each of the following questions.

1. Which of the following TEE scan planes displays both the right atrium and right ventricle?
   a. Midesophageal bicaval
   b. Midesophageal long axis
   c. Midesophageal RV inflow-outflow
   d. Midesophageal two chamber

2. Which of the following structures is attached to the moderator band?
   a. Crista terminalis
   b. Right ventricular apex
   c. Tricuspid valve
   d. Ventricular septum

3. All of the following confound assessment of right ventricular wall thickness EXCEPT:
   a. Epicardial fat
   b. Far field location
   c. Prominent trabeculations
   d. Pericardial effusion

4. Compared to left ventricular ejection, right ventricular ejection:
   a. Begins later
   b. Has a shorter duration
   c. Has a shorter pre-ejection period
   d. Involves more twisting

5. Compared to the left ventricle, which of the following structural features distinguishes the right ventricle?
   a. Larger mass
   b. Smaller volume
   c. Smooth inflow region
   d. Trabeculated apex

6. In this figure, the arrow identifies the:

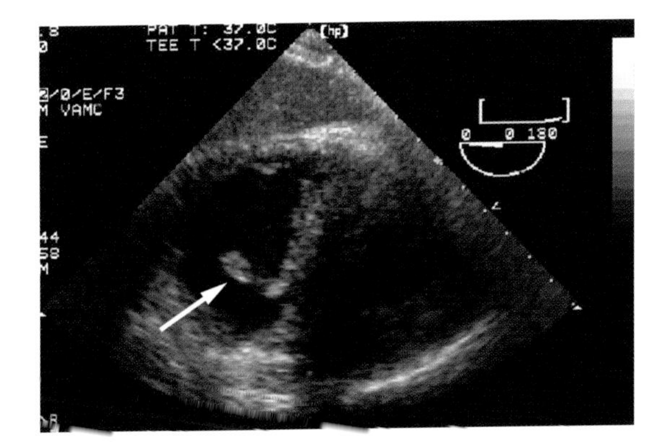

a. Crista supraventricularis
b. Eustachian valve
c. Moderator band
d. Tricuspid valve

7. The right ventricular anterior wall is seen in which of the following scan planes?
   a. Deep transgastric
   b. Midesophageal bicaval
   c. Midesophageal four-chamber
   d. Transgastric RV inflow

8. The modified midesophageal bicaval view provides good spectral Doppler alignment for assessment of:
   a. Hepatic vein flow velocity
   b. Pulmonary artery diastolic pressure
   c. Pulmonic stenosis
   d. Tricuspid regurgitation

9. Which of the following is demonstrated in the figure?

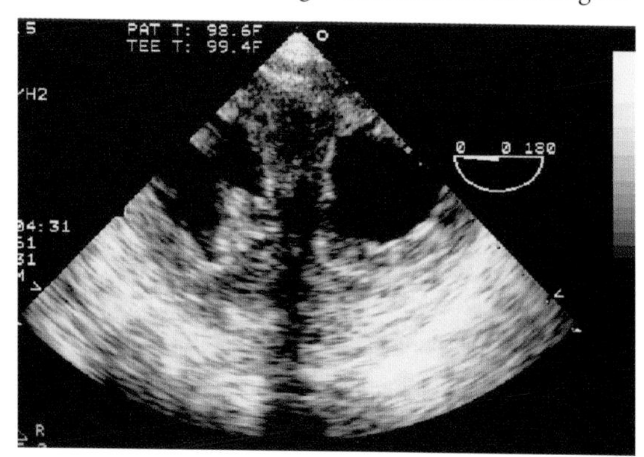

   a. Hypovolemia
   b. Pericardial effusion
   c. Right ventricular dilatation
   d. Right ventricular hypertrophy

10. Which of the following is demonstrated in the figure?

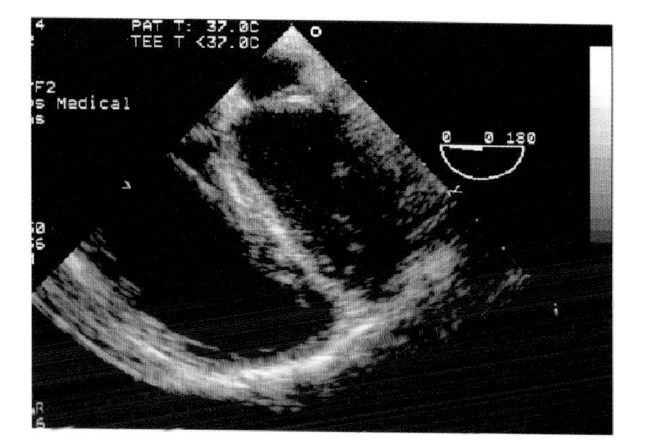

   a. Pericardial effusion
   b. Pleural effusion
   c. Right ventricular enlargement
   d. Right ventricular infarction

11. Which of the following TEE scan planes allows calculation of cardiac output from the right ventricular outflow tract?
    a. Midesophageal four-chamber
    b. Midesophageal long axis
    c. Transgastric long axis
    d. Transgastric RV outflow

12. Which of the following structures is shown in the figure?

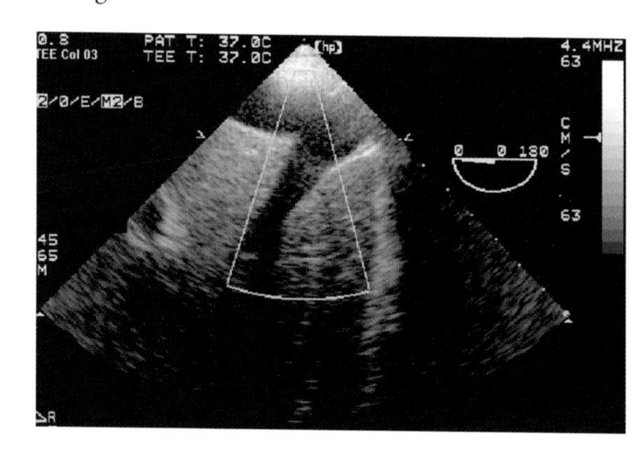

    a. Descending aorta
    b. Hepatic vein
    c. Pulmonary artery
    d. Superior vena cava

13. Which of the following contributes to infundibular RV outflow tract obstruction?
    a. Hypovolemia
    b. Inotropic therapy
    c. Myocardial ischemia
    d. Ventricular pacing

14. Tricuspid annular plane systolic excursion is:
    a. An indicator of RV contractility
    b. Greater medially than laterally
    c. Normally less than 15 mm
    d. Negatively correlated with RV ejection fraction

15. Normal RV ejection fraction:
    a. Is greater than left ventricular ejection fraction
    b. Is less than RV fractional area change
    c. Is directly related to pulmonary artery systolic pressure
    d. Is directly related to tricuspid annular plane systolic excursion

16. The RV myocardial performance index:
    a. Is dependent on systolic and diastolic function
    b. Is independent of isovolumic phase duration
    c. Is normally greater than 0.6
    d. Requires measurement of tricuspid regurgitation velocity

17. Right atrial pressure:
    a. Increases during spontaneous inspiration
    b. Is directly related to inferior vena caval diameter
    c. Is increased when inferior vena caval diameter is 15 mm
    d. Is inversely related to the severity of tricuspid regurgitation

Echocardiographic Evaluation of Cardiomyopathies

14

Andrew Maslow and Stanton K. Shernan

INTRODUCTION

Cardiomyopathy is generally defined as a "disease of the myocardium associated with cardiac dysfunction."[1] *Primary cardiomyopathies* are divided into four major classifications: (a) dilated cardiomyopathy (DCM), (b) hypertrophic cardiomyopathy (HCM), (c) restrictive (or infiltrative) cardiomyopathy (RICM), and (d) miscellaneous group including left ventricular non-compaction (LVNC), arrhythmogenic right ventricular dysplasia (AVRD), and Tako-tsubo cardiomyopathy. Each of the primary cardiomyopathies has distinctive morphological and functional characteristics even though they may present clinically in a similar fashion. The etiology of primary or idiopathic cardiomyopathies is not attributable to another systemic disease process. Alternatively, primary cardiomyopathies refer to primary diseases of the heart muscle (Table 14–1).

The incidence of cardiomyopathy is less than 1% in the general population, with DCM representing the vast majority of cases.[2] Hypertrophic cardiomyopathy is less prevalent, while RICM, LVNC, and AVRD are the least common. The incidence of cardiomyopathy varies depending on a number of factors including diagnostic testing, the type of institution reporting the data, and the referral patterns. When all cardiomyopathies are considered, the incidence varies depending on the prevalence of cardiac pathology associated with coronary artery disease, valvular pathology, systemic hypertension, and a host of other systemic pathophysiologic conditions. Accurate diagnostic assessment of patients suspected of having a cardiomyopathy is important to establish prognosis and to institute appropriate treatment. This chapter focuses on salient echocardiographic features of primary cardiomyopathies, but also includes discussion and description of non-primary cardiomyopathies for completeness.

DILATED CARDIOMYOPATHY

Etiology and Clinical Presentation

Dilated cardiomyopathy (DCM) accounts for 60% of all cardiomyopathies and is defined as an intrinsic myocardial disease process characterized by progressive myocyte hypertrophy, dilation, and contractile dysfunction of one or both ventricles.[1,3,4] Although ventricular wall thickness can be increased, the degree of hypertrophy is proportionally less compared to the amount of dilatation.[5] The development of left ventricular (LV) hypertrophy is initially beneficial in reducing systolic wall stress, a major determinant of myocardial oxygen consumption. However, wall stress is never fully normalized and eventually stimulates LV remodeling, resulting in a reduced ejection fraction (EF) as the ventricle continues to dilate and assume a spherical shape.[6] The combination of apoptotic and necrotic cell death, myocardial fibrosis, and cytoskeletal uncoupling contributes to eventual myocardial mechanical failure. In contrast to hypertrophic and restrictive cardiomyopathies, which often present with normal end-diastolic volumes and preserved or increased EF, DCM is defined by increased end-systolic and end-diastolic volumes and a reduced LV EF (<45%).[7] Furthermore, mitral (MV) and tricuspid valve (TV) regurgitation may be present in association with increased ventricular volume and/or pressure load. Cardiac mural thrombi may also develop in the presence of stasis associated with reduced cardiac function and blood flow velocity, and are most commonly found in the LV apex or left atrial appendage (LAA).

A variety of distinctive pathological processes including viral myocarditis, autoimmune-mediated inflammation, cytoskeletal/contractile protein abnormalities, metabolic derangements, growth factor/cytokine signaling pathways, and cardiovascular disease may be responsible for initiating the myocyte injury, ventricular dilatation, and myocardial dysfunction associated with DCM.[5,8] In addition, genetic factors, peripartum cardiomyopathy, and cytotoxic insults (alcohol, chemotherapeutic agents) have been implicated. Interestingly, many affected patients are classified as having idiopathic DCM since a specific etiology cannot be determined.

DCM may occur at any age including childhood; however, it most commonly affects those 18 to 50 years old. The incidence of DCM is reported to be five to eight cases per 100,000 per year, and is more prevalent

Table 14–1. Etiology of Cardiomyopathy

Etiologies	Congestive (Dilated)	Restrictive	Hypertrophic
Idiopathic	Idiopathic Peripartum	Endocardial fibrosis Hypereosinophilia Idiopathic hypereosinophilia	Obstructive Nonobstructive
Toxic	Ethyl alcohol Heavy metals (cobalt, arsenic, lead) Chemotheraphy (ie, Doxorubicin)		
Inflammatory	Myocarditis:		
Infectious	Viral, bacterial, fungal, parasite		
Noninfectious	Transplant rejection Autoimmune Hypersensitivity reaction	Scleroderma Neoplasm	
Metabolic	Nutritional deficiency: Thiamine Selenium Carnitine Protein Endocrine: Acromegaly Hyperthyroidism Hypothyroidism Electrolyte abnormalities	Amyloidosis Iron (hemochromatosis) Glycogen storage disease	
Neuromuscular	Muscular dystrophy Friedreich ataxia		
Other	Coronary artery disease Valve disease		

in blacks and males than in Caucasians and females.[5] Many patients with DCM may be asymptomatic. The typical presentation of patients with progressive deteriorating DCM include clinical signs (third and/or fourth heart sounds, systolic murmurs consistent with atrial-ventricular valve regurgitation, pulmonary congestion, atrial fibrillation, consequences of systemic embolization from intracardiac thrombi) and symptoms (fatigue, exertional intolerance, and angina often in the absence of coronary artery disease [CAD]), all of which are consistent with LV heart failure.[9] The right ventricle (RV) may be independently involved in rare cases of a familial form of DCM; however, RV failure is usually a later and more ominous consequence of primary LV failure, and is usually associated with a particularly poor prognosis.[10]

Mortality associated with DCM can be significant. As much as 50% of patients die within 2 years. Five-year survival following the initial diagnosis has been reported in the 50% to 75% range depending upon the initiation of therapy,[11] extent of cardiac remodeling and dysfunction, and advanced age.[12,13] About 25% of patients with recent-onset DCM improve spontaneously.[14] Patients with DCM and advanced CHF with LV end-diastolic diameters greater than 4 cm/m^2 body surface area have twice the 1-year mortality rate compared to those patients with less significant ventricular dilatation.[13]

Echocardiographic Evaluation

DCM can be identified using a number of diagnostic modalities including electrocardiography (sinus tachycardia, ventricular dysrhythmias, poor R-wave progression, intraventricular conduction delays, anterior Q waves even without evidence of CAD), radionucleotide ventriculography (biventricular dilatation, reduced EF, regional wall motion abnormalities [RWMA]), and cardiac catheterization (elevated LV filling pressures, ventricular dilatation, reduced EF, RWMA, mitral regurgitation [MR] and occasional mural thrombi).[10] Two-dimensional (2D) and Doppler echocardiography are important noninvasive techniques for defining the degree of ventricular impairment, assessing valve function, and diagnosing intracardiac thrombi. In addition, echocardiography is essential for monitoring the response to pharmacological therapy and, when necessary, to assist in the optimal timing and planning of valve surgery, remodeling procedures, or cardiac transplantation.

Two-Dimensional Echocardiographic Evaluation of Anatomic Features

Classic 2D echocardiographic features of DCM include the presence of increased systolic and diastolic LV dimensions. The diameter of the LV in the transgastric midpapillary short-axis view is often larger than the diameter measured at the base because of the spherical configuration that develops with progressive remodeling. End-diastolic diameters may exceed 8 cm in severe DCM, and volumes can double.[9] The LV wall can vary from normal to increased thickness; however, relative wall thickness (ie, the ratio of end-diastolic wall thickness to end-diastolic cavity radius) is severely diminished. In addition to increased cardiac mass and diminished contractile function, left atrial (LA) and right heart dilatation are common (Figure 14–1). RV dilatation may result from primary myocardial failure or can develop secondary to pulmonary hypertension associated with increased LV end-diastolic pressure (LVEDP). Although not pathognomonic, LV and/or RV wall motion tends to be *symmetrically and globally* reduced in patients with DCM compared to the typical *segmental and focal* wall motion abnormalities more commonly associated with ischemic heart disease and coronary artery narrowing.

Dobutamine stress echocardiography may be helpful in demonstrating provocable differences in RWMA in patients with LV dysfunction associated with CAD, and thus differentiating them from those patients with idiopathic DCM.[10,15] It is important to make this distinction since patients with ischemic cardiomyopathy may experience significant improvement in functional capacity with coronary revascularization. A central caveat of coronary revascularization is the recovery of myocardial function after resumption of flow to a chronically underperfused heart in a region known as 'viable' myocardium. The term *hibernating myocardium* refers to myocardium that is viable but exists in a state of contractile dysfunction due to hypoperfusion. Restoration of perfusion can reverse the hibernation and result in contractile recovery. *Stunned myocardium* is also viable and demonstrates decreased contractility, but has normal perfusion.

Evaluation of myocardial viability is based on the contractile response to inotropic stimulation, identification

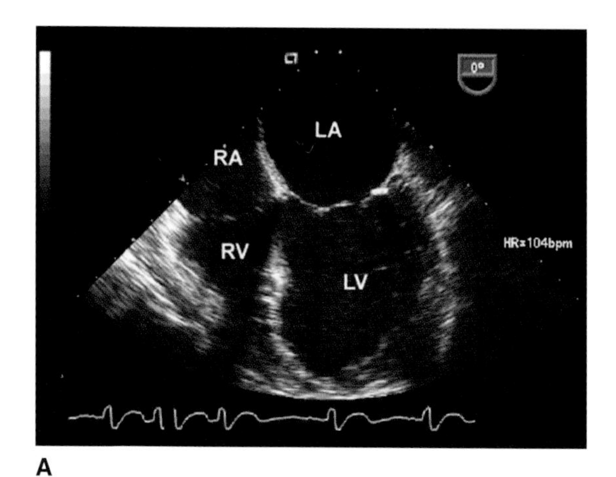

A

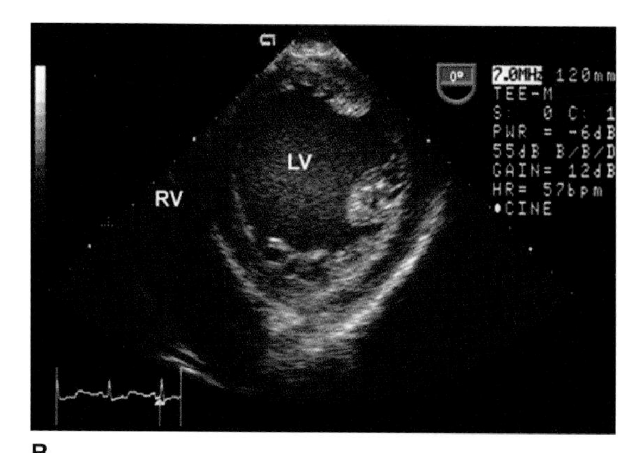

B

FIGURE 14–1. Transesophageal echocardiographic views demonstrating two-dimensional anatomic features of idiopathic dilated cardiomyopathy. **A:** Severe dilatation and sphericity of the left ventricle (LV) is noted in this midesophageal four-chamber view. **B:** Midtransgastric short-axis view of the LV demonstrating severe dilatation (LV diameter = 6.5 cm). (RA, right atrium; LA, left atrium; RV, right ventricle.)

of perfusion, or assessment of myocardial cellular and metabolic integrity. All these techniques involve administration of an 'uptake' agent and an imaging modality. Contractility can be enhanced by an inotrope such as dobutamine, while imaging can be performed with echocardiography (dobutamine stress echocardiography, or DSE). Over the last 20 years, DSE has emerged as a popular, safe and cost-efficient technique for assessment of myocardial viability. While low dose dobutamine (5-10 mcg/kg/min) allows contractile reserve to be assessed, higher doses of dobutamine (up to 40 mcg/kg/min) are used to assess ischemia. At low dose, viable myocardium demonstrates an improvement in contractility. A higher dobutamine dose increases myocardial oxygen demand and if coronary flow is unable to meet the demand for increased perfusion, contractile function may worsen, indicating ischemia. Thus, low-dose dobutamine will improve function in hibernating myocardium but function will worsen with high-dose dobutamine. Both low-dose and high-dose dobutamine will improve function in stunned myocardium.

Four different patterns of response to high dose DSE are recognized: (1) *monophasic* (initial improvement and no deterioration) suggesting viable myocardium with no coronary stenoses; (2) *biphasic* (initial improvement with subsequent deterioration) indicating viability with ischemia; (3) *ischemic* (deterioration without initial improvement) indicating severe ischemia with critical coronary stenosis; and (4) *no change* throughout study, representing a transmural scar. When DSE indicates viable myocardium as well as ischemia, functional response to revascularization is more likely.

The presence of intra-atrial and intraventricular spontaneous echocardiographic contrast associated with a low cardiac output should raise concern for the presence of an intracavitary thrombus in patients with DCM and the potential need for anticoagulation to prevent systemic embolism (Figure 14–2). Thrombi tend to develop more commonly in the LV compared to the LA,[16] perhaps due to the "protective" effect of blood flow turbulence associated with concurrent MR. Thrombi may be flat, laminated, and immobile, or protuberant and very mobile thus increasing the risk for systemic embolization (Figure 14–3). Echocardiography is the gold standard for diagnosing LV thrombus. Two-dimensional echocardiography combined with color-flow Doppler has a reported sensitivity of 100% and a specificity of 97% for diagnosing LV thrombus compared to angiography, which has only a 20% to 50% sensitivity and a 75% specificity.[17] Diagnostic echocardiographic criteria for identifying an LV thrombus include a usual location adjacent to, but distinct from, abnormally contracting myocardium, visualization in at least two planes, demarcation by a clear thrombus-blood interface, and an abnormal LV Doppler flow pattern.[18] Transesophageal echocardiography (TEE) may be superior to transthoracic echocardiography (TTE) for visualizing LV apical thrombi.[19] However, the differential diagnosis of apical thrombi may be complicated by the presence of thickened false tendinae or trabeculae in the apical region. In addition, a smooth, laminated mural thrombus may be more difficult to visualize in the LV apex than a pedunculated, mobile thrombus. Further echocardiographic interrogation using contrast enhancement or an epicardial-placed transducer may be helpful in delineating the presence of a LV apical thrombus.[20]

EVALUATION OF VENTRICULAR SYSTOLIC FUNCTION

Reduced ventricular contractile function (EF <45%) is fundamental to the diagnosis of DCM. Global echocardiographic evaluation of myocardial contraction can be obtained by using 2D-echocardiography to measure the percentage of fractional shortening, EF-area, or ejection fraction using Simpson method of disks (see Chapter 6). Doppler findings may include a reduced aortic ejection

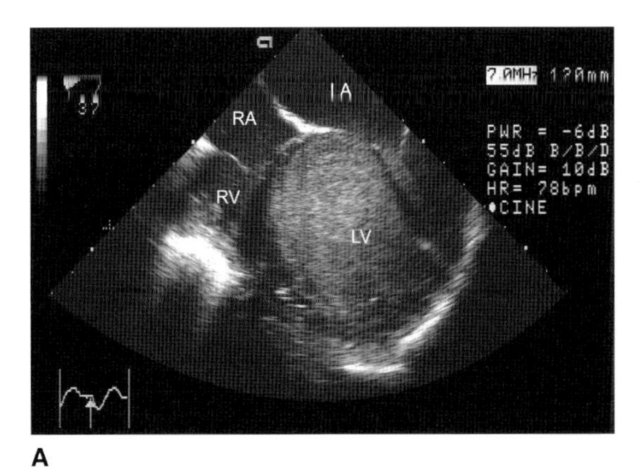

A

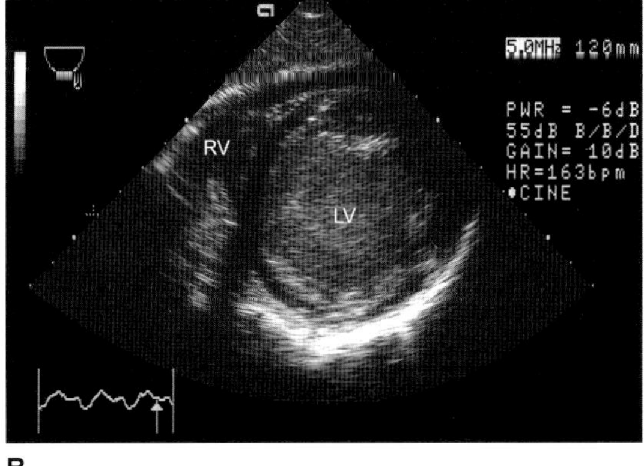

B

FIGURE 14–2. Transesophageal echocardiographic midesophageal four-chamber **(A)** and midtransgastric short-axis **(B)** views demonstrating spontaneous contrast within the left ventricle (LV) of a patient with severe idiopathic dilated cardiomyopathy. (RA, right atrium; LA, left atrium; RV, right ventricle.)

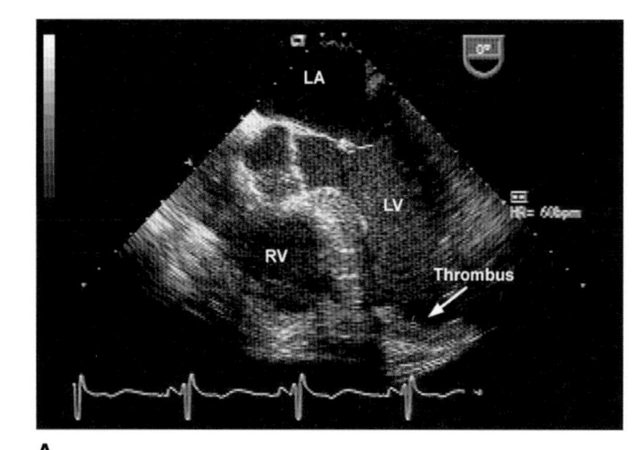

A

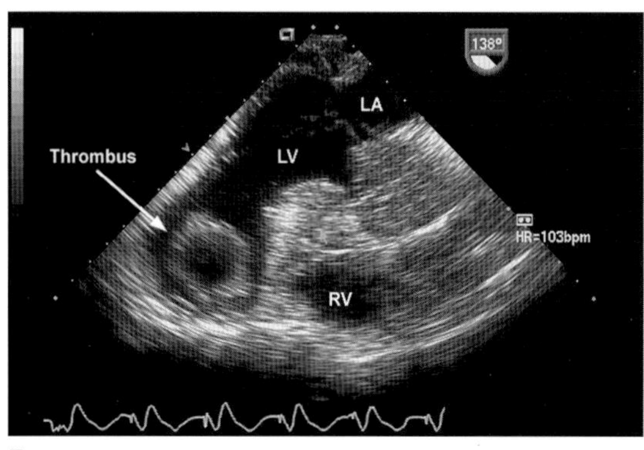

B

FIGURE 14–3. Transesophageal echocardiographic views of left ventricular (LV) apical thrombus associated with dilated cardiomyopathy. **A:** Midesophageal four-chamber view of a laminated, LV apical thrombus *(arrow)*. **B:** Midesophageal two-chamber view of a mobile, protuberant, LV apical thrombus *(arrow)*. (LA, left atrium; RV, right ventricle.)

velocity and time-velocity integral reflecting a diminished stroke volume. Indices of ventricular systolic function related to isovolumic contraction such as dP/dt are less influenced by loading conditions compared to ejection phase indices, and can be estimated from MR jet velocities using continuous-wave Doppler (CWD) echocardiography.[21] All echocardiographic measurements of systolic performance are typically reduced in patients with DCM.

Evaluation of Ventricular Diastolic Function

Left Ventricle. Although DCM is defined by the presence of significant systolic dysfunction, concurrent diastolic dysfunction is common and may manifest anywhere within the full spectrum of severity from impaired relaxation to restriction. Symptoms of congestive heart failure (CHF) in patients with DCM appear to be related to the severity of diastolic dysfunction.[22-25] Normal LV diastolic performance can be defined as sufficient LV filling to produce an adequate cardiac output at a pulmonary venous pressure of less than 12 mm Hg. In patients with DCM, elevation of pulmonary venous pressures compensates for decreased diastolic function.

The main determinants of LV diastolic filling include myocardial relaxation, passive filling characteristics (LV compliance), LA contractility and pressure, heart rate, and MV integrity. Doppler echocardiographic evaluation of the transmitral (TMDF) and pulmonary venous (PVDF) Doppler flow velocity profiles can provide information pertaining to LV diastolic function.[26] In early diastolic dysfunction associated with DCM, the ratio of the early-to-late TMDF velocities (E/A ratio), which is normally greater than 1, decreases to less than 1 in response to *impaired LV relaxation* (E-to-A reversal) (Figure 14–4 and Table 14–2). In addition, the deceleration time (DT: time between the peak transmitral E wave and the return of the velocity to baseline) and isovolumic relaxation time (IVRT: time between the cessation of LV outflow and the beginning of LV inflow) are prolonged. Similarly, in the presence of impaired LV relaxation, the diastolic component of the PVDF becomes significantly diminished compared to the systolic component. In more severe cases of DCM, increased LV stiffness due to myocardial fibrosis contributes to progressive diastolic dysfunction and reduced LV compliance, resulting in an increased LVEDP and LA pressure (LAP). When the elevated LAP becomes the driving force for transmitral flow, a *restrictive* pattern develops characterized by a supranormal TMDF E/A ratio, and decreased DT and IVRT. Diminished LV compliance is also associated with a significantly blunted PVDF systolic velocity compared to the diastolic velocity. The PVDF atrial-reversal velocity (PV_{AR}) and duration may be increased in the presence of an elevated LAP and preserved contractility, or decreased in later stages of diastolic dysfunction because of excessive afterload associated with an elevated LVEDP (see Figure 14–4).[26] The transitional, *pseudo-normal* phase of diastolic dysfunction that develops in between impaired relaxation and restriction, is characterized by a TMDF profile that appears identical to the normal profile since the gradual increasing LAP compensates for impaired LV relaxation to maintain the transmitral pressure gradient (see Figure 14–4). However, the systolic component of the PVDF profile tends to remain blunted relative to the diastolic component as long as the LAP is abnormally elevated.

Conventional measures of diastolic function including TMDF and PVDF velocity profiles can be influenced

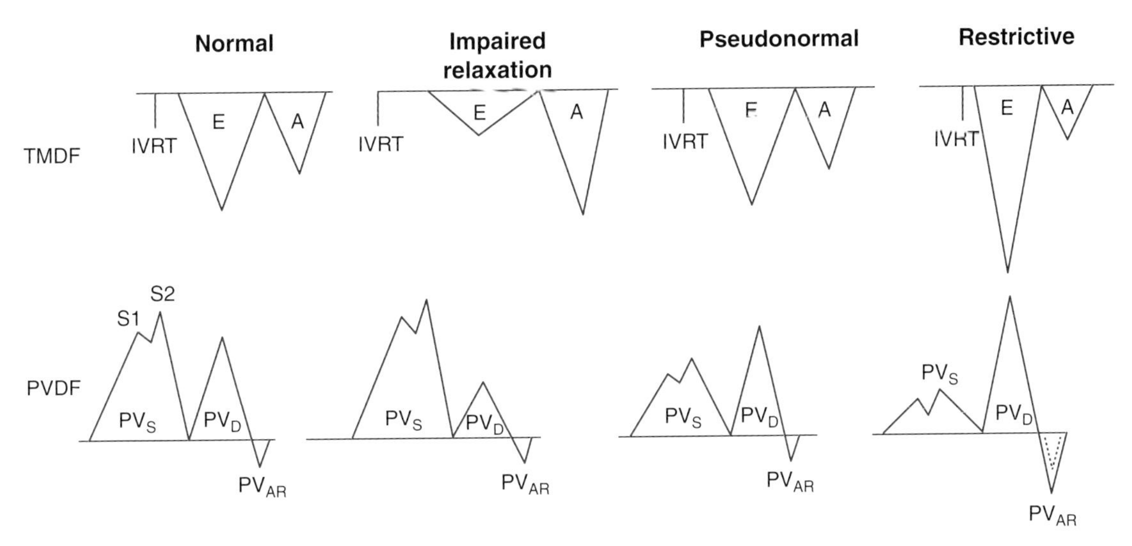

FIGURE 14–4. The impact of progressive left ventricular (LV) diastolic dysfunction on transmitral (TMDF, *top*) and pulmonary venous (PVDF, *bottom*) Doppler flow velocity profiles. Note the change in TMDF early/late (E/A) ratio, which decreases when impaired relaxation develops, and gradually becomes supernormal as LV compliance is reduced with restriction. Changes in the PVDF compliment those in the TMDF profile over the spectrum of diastolic dysfunction. Progressive increases in LV stiffness is associated with blunting of the systolic (PV_{S1} and PV_{S2}) component of the PVDF profile and increased early diastolic (PV_D) velocities, while the left atrium serves as an open conduit between the pulmonary veins and left ventricle (see text for details). (PV_{AR}, late diastolic, atrial reversal component of the PVDF profile.)

by acute changes in loading conditions, tachycardia, dysrhythmias, tethering, stunning, and pacing. Recently, newer echocardiographic techniques for assessing LV diastolic function have been described including Doppler tissue imaging, color kinesis, color M-mode transmitral flow propagation velocity, myocardial strain, and strain rate.[27] These echocardiographic modalities are reportedly less vulnerable to the effects of acute changes in loading conditions, and may therefore complement the use of conventional echocardiographic

Table 14–2. Doppler Assessment of Left Ventricular Diastolic Function by Transmitral and Pulmonary Venous Doppler Flow Velocities

	Normal	Impaired Relaxation	Pseudonormal	Restrictive
TMDF:				
E/A	0.7-1.7	<0.7	>0.7	>1.7
IVRT (ms)	90-110	>110	<110	<90
DT (ms)	140-240	>240	<240	<140
PVDF				
S/D	1.0-1.5	>1.5	<1.2	<0.8
AR (ms)	<35	<35	>35	>35
$PVDF_{AR}/TMDF_A$	<0.8	<0.8	≤ or > 0.8	> 0.8

TMDF, transmitral Doppler flow velocity; PVDF, pulmonary venous Doppler flow velocity; E, early transmitral filling; A, late transmitral filling (atrial contraction), IVRT, isovolumic relaxation time; DT, deceleration time; S, atrial filling during ventricular systole; D, atrial filling during ventricular diastole; AR, pulmonary venous flow reversal wave during atrial contraction; $PVDF_{AR}/TMDF_A$, ratio of the respective AR and A wave durations.

techniques for evaluating diastolic dysfunction in patients with DCM. It is also important to appreciate that MR, which is common among patients with DCM, can have a considerable impact on the LV diastolic filling pattern. Significant MR is often associated with an elevated LAP, which produces an increased TMDF E/A ratio and systolic blunting of the PVDF velocity profile, making the assessment of concurrent diastolic dysfunction even more challenging. Rossi et al have identified that the relationship between the increased duration of PVDF atrial-reversal relative to the TMDF A wave in patients with diminished LV compliance is preserved even in the presence of MR, and thus can be used to identify diastolic dysfunction while other measurements fail.[28]

Right Ventricle. Indirect evidence of RV diastolic function in patients with DCM can also be obtained from a comprehensive 2D echocardiographic examination by examining RV mass or volume. A thorough assessment of RV diastolic function, however, requires a Doppler echocardiographic evaluation of transtricuspid Doppler flow (TTDF) velocities.[26] Transtricuspid Doppler flow velocities tend to be lower due to the larger TV annular size, but they are affected by the same physiologic variables that affect LV filling. Direct comparisons of RV and LV inflow velocities also reveal differences in timing and reciprocal respiratory variation. During spontaneous inspiration, negative intrapleural pressure results in an increase in right atrial (RA) volume and subsequent greater RV diastolic filling velocities up to 20% compared to end-expiratory values.[29] LA and LV filling are actually reduced during spontaneous inspiration relative to end-expiration. These reciprocal patterns of respiratory variation become exaggerated in patients with diastolic dysfunction. Although not thoroughly investigated, positive pressure ventilation would presumably have an opposite effect on TTDF velocity patterns in comparison to spontaneous ventilation.

Echocardiographic evaluation of RV diastolic function in patients with DCM also includes an assessment of RA inflow velocities including the hepatic venous (HV), inferior vena cava (IVC), and superior vena cava (SVC) Doppler profiles, all of which have similar contours and components. The HVs join the intrahepatic IVC tangentially, and can be visualized by advancing and turning the TEE probe rightward from a midesophageal, bicaval acoustic window. The normal HV Doppler profile is characterized by (1) a small reversal of flow following atrial contraction (AR wave); (2) an antegrade systolic phase during atrial filling from the SVC and IVC (S wave) that is influenced by TV annular motion, RA relaxation, and tricuspid regurgitation (TR); (3) a second small flow reversal at end-systole (V wave) that is influenced by RV and RA compliance; and (4) a second antegrade filling phase while the RA acts as a passive conduit during RV filling (D wave).[29]

Diastolic RV dysfunction can manifest with the same relative changes in TTDF peak E- and A-wave velocities, E/A-wave ratios, and DT that occur with TMDF profiles associated with alterations in LV relaxation and compliance.[30] The ratio of the total hepatic reverse flow integral/total forward flow integral (TVI_A + TVI_V/TVI_S + TVI_D) increases with either RV diastolic dysfunction or significant TR, but appears to be more affected by the former.[31] In addition, a marked shortening of the TTDF DT and diastolic predominance of HV flow with prominent V- and A-wave reversals during spontaneous inspiration indicates significant decreases in RV compliance and increased diastolic filling pressures. Changes in IVC diameter during spontaneous inspiration also reflect RA pressure (RAP). In general, low RAP (0 to 5 mm Hg) is associated with a small IVC (<1.5 cm diameter) and a spontaneous inspiratory collapse greater than 50% of the original diameter. In contrast, significant increases in RAP (>20 mm Hg) are associated with dilated IVC (>2.5 cm) and HVs with little respiratory variation (<50%). Diastolic RV dysfunction (lower TTDF peak E-wave velocity, lower E/A ratios, and prolonged RV IVRT) has also been demonstrated in patients with pulmonary hypertension (PHT) and in those with symptomatic CHF even in the absence of PHT, suggesting a potential role for ventricular interdependence in impaired RV filling.[32]

EVALUATION OF MITRAL AND TRICUSPID VALVE LESIONS

Ventricular dilatation associated with DCM may produce functional atrioventricular valve incompetence. Incomplete closure of the MV and TV may develop due to annular dilatation; however, an independent role of mitral annular dilatation in the development of MR in patients with DCM remains controversial.[33,34] Abnormal alignment of the papillary muscles related to the development of ventricular sphericity is more consistently responsible for atrioventricular valve incompetence due to apical displacement of the coaptation point, which increases tension on the leaflets (ie, "apical tenting"; Figure 14–5).[35] Aikawa et al utilized three-dimensional (3D) echocardiography to demonstrate that functional MR associated with nonischemic DCM is related to annular dilatation.[36] Furthermore, dilation of the anterior and anterolateral LV walls results in displacement of the anterior papillary muscle, narrowing of the angle of the anterior chordae to the mitral annulus, and widening of the central angle between the anterior and posterior chordae. Kwan et al also used 3D echocardiography to demonstrate that MV deformation from the medial to lateral side is asymmetrical in

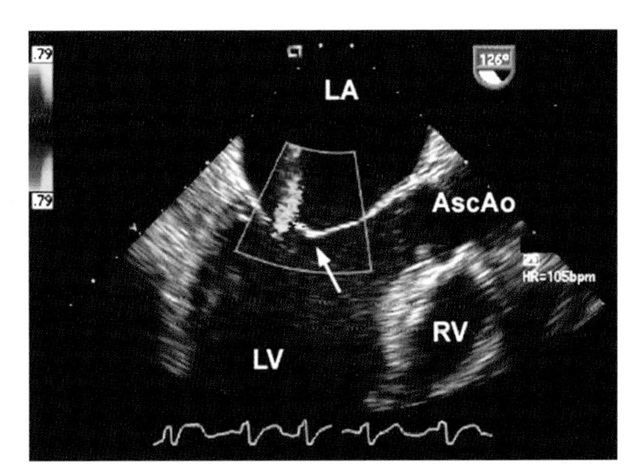

FIGURE 14–5. Transesophageal echocardiographic midesophageal four-chamber views demonstrating a color-flow Doppler signal of significant mitral regurgitation associated with dilated cardiomyopathy. The mechanism of functional mitral regurgitation in dilated cardiomyopathy is related to annular dilatation and/or abnormal alignment of the papillary muscles causing apical tenting *(arrow)* of the anterior MV leaflet. (LA, left atrium; LV, left ventricle; RV, right ventricle; AscAO, acsending aorta.)

patients with ischemic cardiomyopathy, whereas it is symmetrical in those with DCM.[37]

Mitral and tricuspid regurgitation should be semi-quantified using color-flow, pulsed-wave, and continuous-wave Doppler to measure regurgitant jet length, jet area, vena contracta, proximal isovelocity surface area, effective regurgitant surface area, and regurgitant fraction, which may be helpful when corrective valve surgery is anticipated. Reductive annuloplasty of both MV and TV orifices in patients with DCM significantly changes LV morphology, reverses ventricular remodeling, decreases LV sphericity, and slows the progression of heart failure.[38]

Utility of Echocardiography in Determining Prognosis

A number of 2D echocardiographic findings have prognostic value in patients with DCM.[22] In particular, marked chamber dilatation (LV, LA, RV)[39] and depressed ventricular function (LV, RV)[40] are associated with poor survival. In addition, decreased end-systolic and end-diastolic LV volumes following low-dose dobutamine infusion also indicate a more favorable prognosis. Furthermore, Doppler echocardiographic measurements including MR severity,[41] significant pulmonary hypertension assessed from the TR Doppler flow velocity,[42] and a restrictive TMDF velocity profile that does not respond to pharmacological intervention have been correlated with a worse outcome.[43,44]

HYPERTROPHIC CARDIOMYOPATHY

Etiology and Pathophysiology

Hypertrophic cardiomyopathy has been described with a variety of terms including "idiopathic hypertrophic subaortic stenosis" (IHSS) and "asymmetric septal hypertrophy," reflecting a narrowed LV outflow tract (LVOT) due to a focal pattern of hypertrophy. More recently, the classification has been simplified to reflect the pathophysiology and to accommodate the varied patterns of hypertrophy. While diastolic dysfunction occurs in almost all individuals with HCM, only 25% experience a dynamic, intermittent, or episodic obstruction to ventricular systolic outflow.[45,46] Patients are therefore subdivided into two related but distinct groups: (1) hypertrophic cardiomyopathy (HCM) and (2) hypertrophic obstructive cardiomyopathy (HOCM), which includes those with obstruction to ventricular systolic outflow.

Hypertrophic cardiomyopathy (HCM/HOCM) is defined as an abnormal thickening of the myocardium without chamber dilation, in the absence of a demonstrable cause (eg, aortic stenosis [AS], systemic hypertension). The incidence is approximately 0.2% in the general population, but reporting may vary depending on the referral patterns of the institution, and the diagnostic criteria.[45,46] Diagnosis may be based on presentation, family history, hemodynamic evaluation, and echocardiographic examination. A more definitive diagnosis may require myocardial biopsy and/or genetic testing.

Hypertrophic cardiomyopathy is inherited as an autosomal dominant trait with variable expression.[45] Gene mutations involving the regulatory proteins of the sarcomere as well as the myofilaments have been reported. Defects of at least nine genes contributing to more than 130 mutations help to explain the heterogeneity of the disease. An anticipated increase in the frequency of genetic testing may have an impact on the currently reported incidence. In addition, improvement in the quality of genetic testing will help to pave the way for preventative and more targeted therapeutic intervention.

The histology of HCM/HOCM displays a range of abnormalities from simple hypertrophy of organized, longitudinally directed muscle fibers to a disarray of abnormal-appearing fibers.[47] Over time, myocardial fibrosis may replace normal muscle, resulting in a less compliant ventricle. Abnormal concentric thickening can also be seen in the coronary arteries. These changes, when coupled with ventricular hypertrophy and elevated intracavitary pressures, increase the risk of myocardial ischemia.

The age of onset, morphology, and pathophysiology of HCM/HOCM vary greatly. More commonly, HCM/HOCM presents in young adulthood from the second to fifth decades, and is characterized by a diffuse or asymmetric ventricular hypertrophy. Presentation of HCM/HOCM in older patients (≥65 years old) is becoming increasingly recognized.[48,49] Whether elderly patients have previously asymptomatic hypertrophy or develop hypertrophy later in life is not known. Although commonly ascribed to HCM/HOCM, asymmetric hypertrophy has also been reported as an adaptive response to AS, systemic hypertension, and in certain congenital cardiac anomalies.

Hypertrophic cardiomyopathy is classically defined by the presence of LV hypertrophy (>11mm thickness), which occurs disproportionately in the ventricular septum by a ratio of greater than 1.3:1.0 relative to the measured free-wall thickness (Figure 14–6).[46] The inferolateral basal wall is infrequently involved. However, different patterns of hypertrophy have been reported including isolated proximal basal septal hypertrophy ("septal bulge"),[48-50] inferlolateral wall hypertrophy,[51] concentric or diffuse hypertrophy,[52] and RV hypertrophy in a small number of cases. Four types of hypertrophic cardiomyopathy have been described: type I—hypertrophy limited to the anterior septum; type II—hypertrophy of anterior and posterior septum; type III—diffuse hypertrophy sparing only the basal inferlolateral wall; type IV—apical hypertrophy.[53]

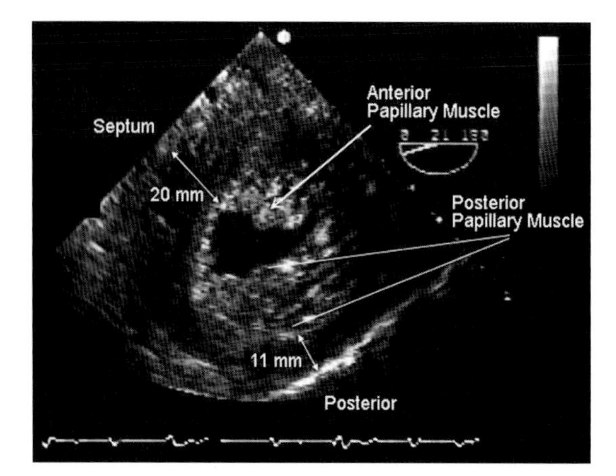

FIGURE 14–6. Asymmetric septal hypertrophy. Transthoracic echocardiographic short-axis view of the left ventricle. The septal (20 mm) to posterior wall (11 mm) thickness ratio is greater than 1.3 and consistent with asymmetric hypertrophy.

The mechanism of LVOT obstruction (LVOTO) is complex, involving ventricular hypertrophy and abnormalities of the MV apparatus.[54-56] The common pathway is represented by a narrower ventricular cavity with or without distortion of MV leaflet coaptation and subsequent MR. Scenarios more likely to result in LVOTO include asymmetric hypertrophy, a prominent basal septum, a narrowed outflow cavity (<25 mm), and structural abnormalities of the MV apparatus. The latter includes anteriorly positioned papillary muscles,[57] abnormal insertion of the papillary muscles into the mitral leaflet,[58] elongated mitral leaflets,[59-61] and disturbances in MV annular function (eg, posterior annular calcification). LVOTO has also been reported with concentric hypertrophy. Delineation of the mechanism of LVOTO is important for planning therapeutic interventions, especially in regard to the requirement for and timing of surgery.

Presentation, Signs, and Symptoms

The annual mortality of patients with HCM/HOCM ranges from 2.5% to 4%. The 4-year mortality rate of asymptomatic patients is extremely low compared to severely compromised patients with New York Heart Association class III/IV symptoms. Patients with HCM/HOCM may be severely symptomatic early in life or remain asymptomatic for decades. Symptoms including decreased exercise capacity, angina, dyspnea, dizziness, syncope, and/or sudden death are due to ventricular diastolic dysfunction, myocardial ischemia, arrhythmias, LVOTO, and MR. Physical examination may be normal at rest. The cardiac apex may be displaced, reflecting the hypertrophy and overall increase in cardiac mass. Third or fourth cardiac sounds (S_3 or S_4) indicate decreased ventricular compliance and congestive heart failure (CHF). A harsh crescendo-decrescendo systolic murmur suggests LVOTO. Electrocardiography demonstrates a ventricular strain pattern including nonspecific ST- and T-wave changes. Prominent T waves have been noted in patients with apical hypertrophy.

Coronary ischemia may occur in the absence of coronary artery narrowing due to poor perfusion through the thickened myocardium and increased intracavitary pressures and/or a reduction in coronary artery vasodilatory reserve.[62,63] Concentric hypertrophy of the coronary arteries increases the risk of myocardial ischemia. Dyspnea or CHF often occur despite normal or even supranormal systolic function. Myocardial ischemia, abnormal diastolic function, and/or systolic outflow obstruction with or without MR all contribute to development of CHF. These processes are dynamic and may not be present at rest, but may require provocative maneuvers such as a Valsalva or the administration of a systemic vasodilator such as amyl nitrate. Such interventions reduce ventricular preload resulting in a smaller or narrower cavity and LVOTO.

Atrial and ventricular arrhythmias are a primary cause of syncope, stroke, and sudden death. The electrical abnormalities of the hypertrophic heart are related to atrial chamber pressures and size, and abnormal myocardial architecture. Atrial fibrillation is the most common rhythm disturbance, while sudden death is the most significant cause of mortality. The risk of sudden death is highest for younger patients with severe LV hypertrophy (>20- to 30-mm thickness), LVOT gradient greater than 50 mm Hg, LA dilatation (>45 mm), a reduction in blood pressure during exercise, a history of syncope, and/or a family history of syncope. Interestingly, LVOTO has not been directly related to morbidity or sudden death.[45,46] Risk assessment is important since placement of an implantable cardiac defibrillator is the recommended prophylaxis or treatment to prevent sudden death.

Echocardiographic Examination

Echocardiography is essential to assess and diagnose the etiology of hypertrophy as well as to assess ventricular function, diagnose LVOTO, and to quantify the severity of valve dysfunction. It is an important tool in formulating a prognosis and for initiating and planning treatment. For patients having surgery, intraoperative echocardiographic examination is important to re-evaluate cardiac function, help determine the surgical plan, and assess results immediately after cardiopulmonary bypass (CPB).[64-66]

Two-dimensional and M-mode echocardiography permit assessment of cardiac function, myocardial thickness, chamber size, valve function, and to locate the level of ventricular cavity narrowing. Two-dimensional imaging is complemented by Doppler evaluation. Color-flow Doppler examination permits the assessment of valve function and areas of high flows, and directs the pulsed-wave (PWD) and CWD Doppler exams, which are used to measure velocities and gradients within the ventricular cavity.

Ventricular Function and Morphology

In patients with HCM/HOCM, systolic function is usually preserved (LVEF ≥55%) or hyperdynamic (LVEF ≥65%) and the ventricular cavity is normal or reduced in size. A smaller percentage (<5% to 10%) of patients may have reductions in systolic function with or without chamber dilation, suggestive of late- or end-stage cardiomyopathy. Focal and global systolic dysfunction is due to disarray of the myocardial fibers with or without fibrosis. In addition, decreases in myocardial performance may be due to atheromatous CAD, hypertrophic involvement of the coronary arteries, reduction of coronary perfusion in a hypertrophied ventricle, or decreased coronary artery vasodilatory reserve.[62,63]

Echocardiographic assessment of ventricular wall thickness and intracavitary dimensions should be performed at the base, mid, and apical segments to delineate the pattern of hypertrophy and identify where systolic outflow obstruction may occur. Wall thickness in HCM/HOCM ranges from normal (≤11 mm) to greater than 30 mm. The absence of hypertrophy does not rule out HCM/HOCM since development of myocardial thickening may be delayed until the second or third decade, emphasizing the need for routine follow-up of patients with a family history of HCM/HCOM.

A number of patterns of myocardial hypertrophy have been reported including diffuse, asymmetric, concentric, or even isolated focal hypertrophy. While asymmetric septal hypertrophy is classically described, hypertrophy may be diffuse or concentrated elsewhere including the mid-, apical, or inferolateral ventricular segments (Figure 14–7). Narrowing of the ventricular cavity (<25 mm during systole) may be associated with abnormal systolic outflow velocities (>1.4 m/s). A variant of hypertrophy is isolated to the basal septum (septal bulge). The risk of LVOTO for these patients may be determined by the angle between LVOT outflow and ventricular (transmitral) inflow (Figure 14–8).[49,50] A greater intrusion of septal tissue into the LVOT yields a larger angle and greater disturbance to outflow. Angles greater than 35° are predictive of LVOTO with provocation.[50] Angles greater than 80° are associated with high velocity flows at rest.

Diastolic Function

Diastolic dysfunction associated with ventricular hypertrophy, myocardial disarray, fibrosis, and/or coronary artery insufficiency occurs in almost all patients. Reduced ventricular filling can also be due to inadequate systolic emptying caused by dynamic outflow obstruction. Relief of LVOTO and subsequent reduction in LV pressures also improves coronary blood flow, myocardial oxygen balance, and ventricular filling. The assessment of diastolic function can be achieved with a number of echocardiographic techniques including TMDF and PVDF velocity profiles (see Table 14–2). Doppler profiles of LV diastolic function in patients with HCM/HOCM range from normal to restrictive filling patterns, the latter reflecting greater degrees of hypertrophy and fibrosis. More commonly, abnormal ventricular relaxation is present. The severity of diastolic function correlates with reductions in exercise tolerance and CHF.

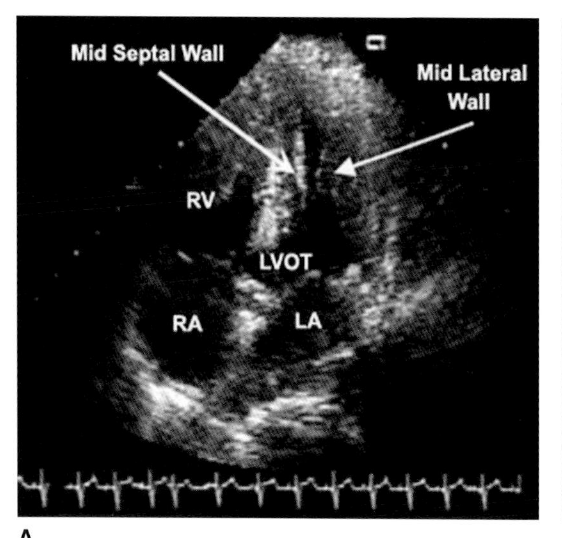

A

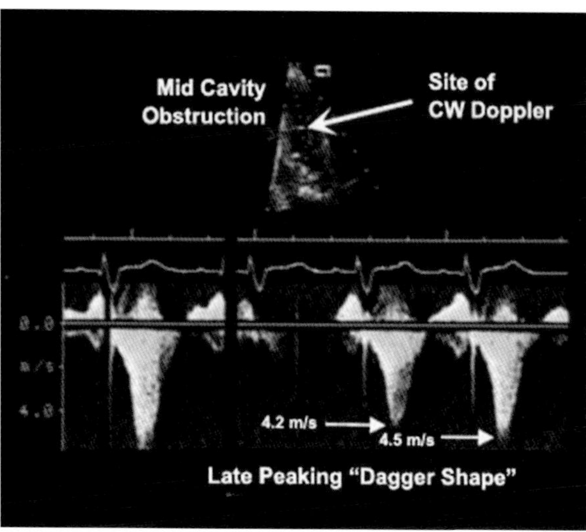

B

FIGURE 14–7. Mid–left ventricular cavity obstruction. **A:** Transthoracic echocardiographic apical five-chamber view of the right (RV) and left ventricles, right (RA) and left (LA) atria, and the left ventricular outflow tract (LVOT). **B:** Continuous-wave Doppler (CW) analysis through the LV. Peak velocities are greater than 4 m/s (ie, intracavitary gradient >64 mm Hg). The Doppler profile is characteristically late peaking or "dagger shaped," which is consistent with a dynamic LVOT obstruction occurring in mid-systole.

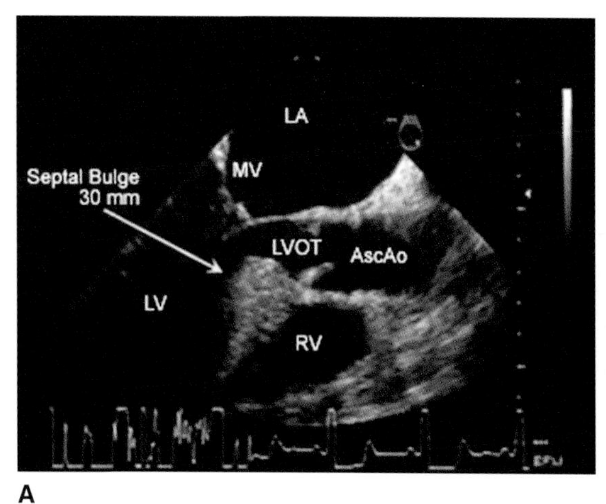

A

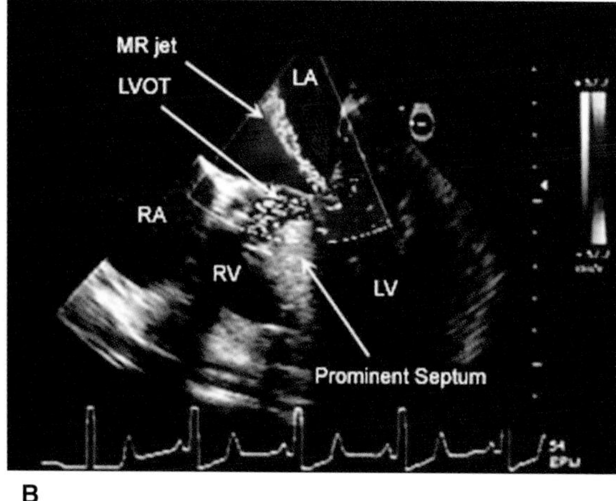

B

FIGURE 14–8. Left ventricular (LV) septal bulge. **A:** Transesophageal echocardiographic (TEE) midesophageal long-axis view of the left ventricular outflow tract (LVOT) demonstrating a prominent septum of approximately 30-mm thickness. The angle between mitral inflow and LVOT outflow is approximately 70° to 90°. **B:** Color-flow Doppler imaging in the TEE midesophageal five-chamber view in which turbulence (consistent with high velocity) is seen in the LVOT (obstruction to outflow) and left atrium, which is consistent with mitral regurgitation (MR). (LA, left atrium; MV, mitral valve; RA, right atrium; RV, right ventricle; Asc Ao, ascending aorta.)

MITRAL VALVE REGURGITATION AND SYSTOLIC OUTFLOW OBSTRUCTION

Mitral regurgitation and systolic outflow obstruction are not uniformly found in patients with HCM and may require provocation to identify. Both medical and/or surgical therapy may be indicated to treat MR and systolic outflow obstruction. Systolic outflow obstruction whether at the level of the LVOT or at the middle portion of the ventricular cavity results in high systolic flow velocities, incomplete systolic emptying, and increased ventricular cavity pressures. PWD sampling of the ventricular cavity from the apex to the subaortic valve (AV) area can be utilized to identify the location of abnormal systolic outflow. The Doppler profile is described as late peaking (>1.4 m/s) and "dagger shaped" in appearance (see Figure 14–7B; Figure 14–9). CWD may be necessary to quantify the outflow velocity when aliasing occurs during PWD examination. Although transesophageal windows allow Doppler sampling from the ventricular apex to the middle of the cavity, transgastric views allow better assessment of the LVOT and AV flows. LVOTO can also be demonstrated by using M-mode to interrogate the AV leaflets from the short- or long-axis AV views (see Figure 14–9). The AV leaflets will open normally but close prematurely in mid-systole due to dynamic obstruction of systolic outflow.

Two-dimensional echocardiographic assessment may display systolic anterior motion (SAM) of the mitral leaflets and chordae (Figure 14–10). Esophageal imaging demonstrates SAM more easily and clearly. A number of investigations describe how a narrowed LVOT creates a high-velocity flow, which subsequently creates a Venturi or vacuum effect on the MV leaflets causing them to move anteriorly, further narrowing the LVOT resulting in LVOTO.[50,56] In these patients, SAM distorts MV leaflet coaptation causing MR. The Venturi effect, however, does not fully explain LVOTO and SAM, which may or may not occur with high-velocity systolic flows. Specific features of the MV associated with SAM and LVOTO include redundant or elongated mitral leaflets, lax chordae, abnormally positioned papillary muscles, and mitral annular dysfunction.

Color Doppler analysis of the LVOT and MV from the midesophageal three- or five-chamber and long-axis windows demonstrates aliasing of the CFD jet in LVOT at the level of narrowing consistent with high-velocity flow, and across the MV indicating significant MR. This "Y"-shaped CFD is consistent with LVOTO/SAM and MR (Figure 14–11). Quantitation of MR is discussed in detail in Chapter 7.

Clinical and experimental evidence suggests that manipulation of the MV annulus and/or subvalvular apparatus can either prevent or precipitate SAM and LVOTO.[48,54,58,59] Normally, the MV annulus is dynamic in that it enlarges and contracts during the cardiac cycle.[67] During systole,, all of the posterior and much of the anterior annular segments contract and move posteriorly. A small portion of the anterior annulus that abuts the LVOT lengthens in an anterior and superior direction. These movements result in a wider

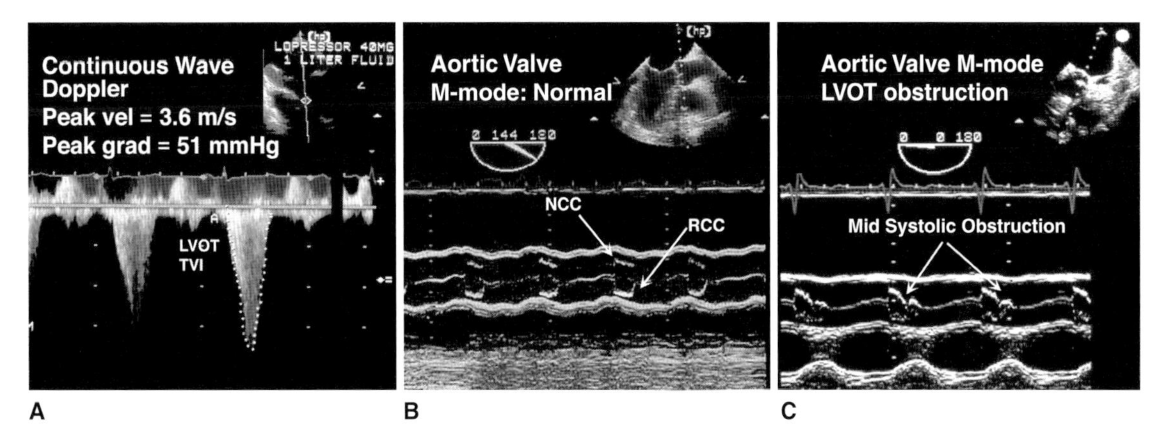

FIGURE 14–9. Doppler and M-mode assessment of left ventricular systolic outflow. **A:** Continuous-wave Doppler assessment of systolic blood flow across the left ventricular outflow tract (LVOT) and aortic valve (AV). The time-velocity integral (TVI) is late peaking and "dagger shaped." **B:** Normal M-mode of the AV demonstrating the opening of the non- (NCC) and right (RCC) coronary cusps. Note that the AV leaflets open and remain open throughout systole. **C:** M-mode of the AV demonstrating dynamic outflow tract obstruction. Although the leaflets open initially, they close in mid-systole as demonstrated by the arrow.

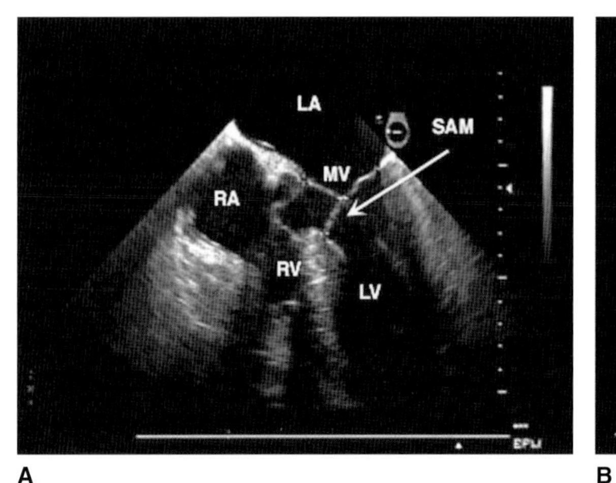

A

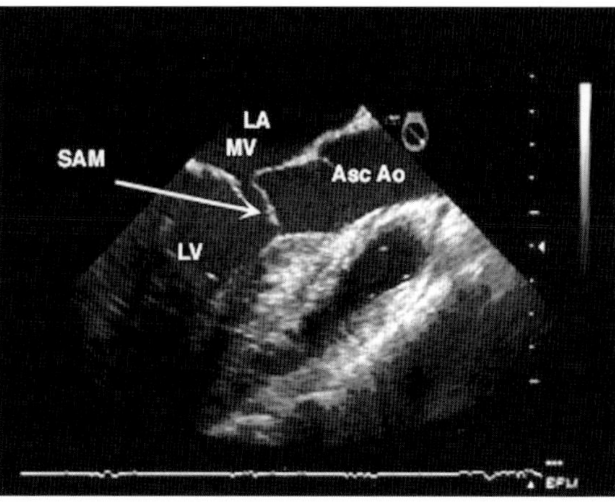

B

FIGURE 14–10. Systolic anterior motion (SAM) of the mitral valve (MV) leaflets associated with anterior leaflet (AL) displacement anteriorly toward the left ventricular (LV) septum causing obstruction to ventricular systolic outflow, and distortion of the MV leaflet coaptation point. **A:** Imaging from the transesophageal echocardiographic (TEE) midesophageal five-chamber view demonstrates MV SAM. The LV septal thickness in diastole is approximately 11 mm. **B:** Imaging from the TEE midesophageal long-axis window showing MV SAM and clear disruption of leaflet coaptation. During diastole the LV septal thickness is 15 mm. In these two cases, the MV leaflets are significantly redundant. (LA, left atrium; RA, right atrium; RV, right ventricle; Asc Ao, ascending aorta.)

LVOT. Annular movement also moves the MV leaflets and coaptation more posteriorly during ventricular systole, resulting in a wider LVOT and making SAM/LVOTO less likely. Abnormalities of the MV annulus including calcification along the posterior annulus distorts normal annular posterior motion and increases the risk of SAM/LVOTO. Mitral annular calcification (MAC) alone does not contribute significantly to SAM/LVOTO as few patients with this single abnormality have this problem, and conversely, not all patients with SAM/LVOTO have MAC. However, posterior annular calcification hinders the

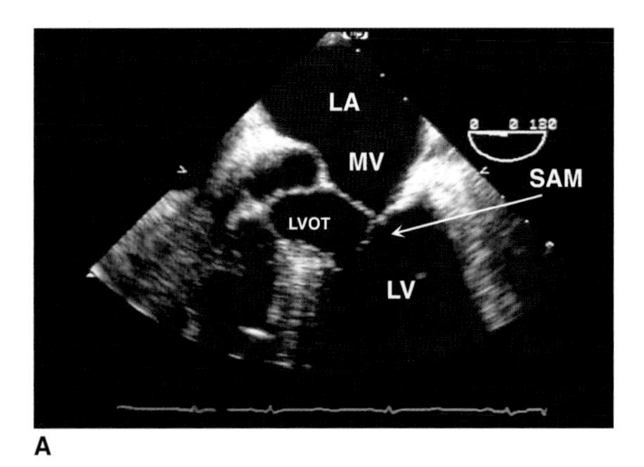

A

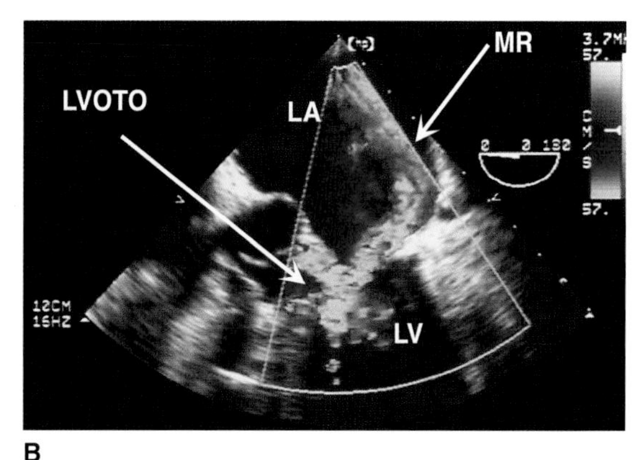

B

FIGURE 14–11. Color-flow Doppler (CFD) aliasing seen simultaneously in the left ventricular outflow tract (LVOT) and across the mitral valve (MV) consistent with left ventricular outflow tract obstruction (LVOTO), and mitral regurgitation (MR). **A:** Two-dimensional transesophageal echocardiographic (TEE) imaging of the midesophageal five-chamber view demonstrating systolic anterior motion (SAM, *arrow*) of the MV leaflets. **B:** CFD analysis showing turbulence *(arrows)* in the LVOT and across the MV. (LA, left atrium; LV, left ventricle.)

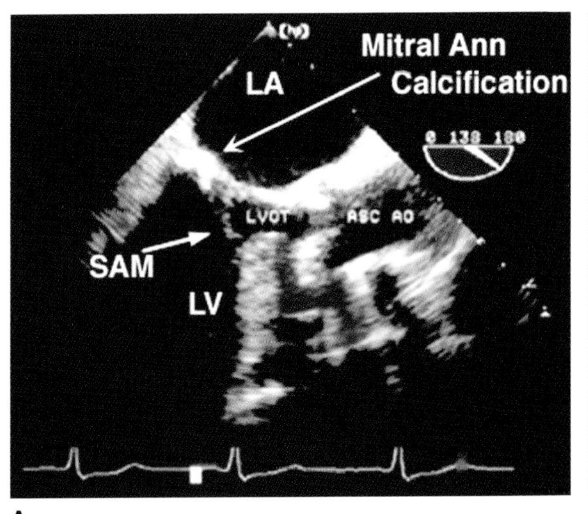

A

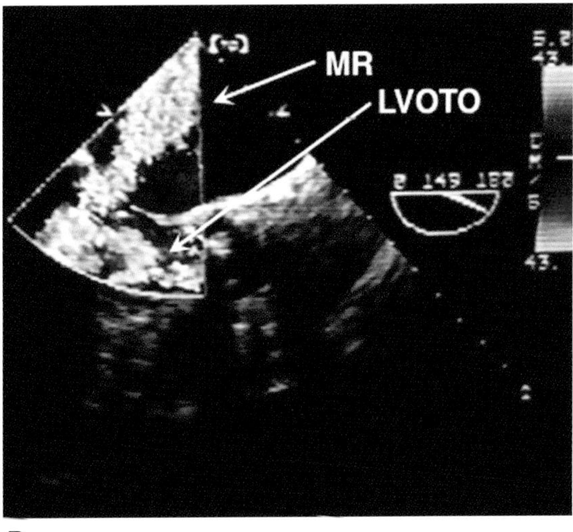

B

FIGURE 14–12. Mitral annular (Ann) calcification contributing to systolic anterior motion (SAM). **A:** Calcification of the posterior annulus hinders the normal posterior movement of the mitral valve (MV) apparatus and places the leaflets closer to the outflow tract during systole increasing the risk of SAM *(short arrow)*. **B:** When combined with a prominent left ventricular (LV) septum with or without MV leaflet redundancy, SAM, mitral regurgitation (MR), and left ventricular outflow tract obstruction (LVOTO) develop as demonstrated by color-flow Doppler aliasing. (LVOT, left ventricular outflow tract; Asc Ao, ascending aorta.)

normal posterior movement of the mitral apparatus, and the mitral leaflets are positioned closer to the outflow tract during systole thus increasing the risk of SAM (Figure 14–12). Conversely, normal posterior motion of the mitral apparatus decreases the likelihood of SAM/LVOTO as demonstrated after MV repair.

A large anterior mitral leaflet (AL >2.0 cm in length), measured in end-diastole from the midesophageal 5 chamber view, contributes to LVOTO.[55,59-61] During ventricular systole, a relatively greater posterior leaflet (PL) contribution to MV coaptation also contributes to the development of SAM/LVOTO (Figure 14–13).[55,60,61,68] More specifically, when the heights of the posterior leaflet (posterior annulus to coaptation point) and anterior leaflet (anterior annulus to coaptation point) are similar (AL:PL ≤1.3), the risk of SAM/LVOTO is increased.[68] The larger PL coapts with the AL closer to its base, resulting in increased residual or "slack" leaflet portions that lie closer to the LVOT and are thus more susceptible to ventricular outflow exposure. The distance between the coaptation point and the ventricular septum (C-Sept) measured from the TEE midesophageal three- or five-chamber window reflects the position of the coaptation point and the thickness of the ventricular septum. A C-Sept distance of 2.5 cm or less is sufficiently narrowed to increase LVOT velocities for patients with HCM/HOCM, and also increase the risk of SAM/LVOTO/MR after MV repair.[50,68,69]

In vitro flow models demonstrate that anterior and inward displacement of the papillary muscle alters chordal tension resulting in excess leaflet mobility. Anterior displacement of the papillary muscles also shifts the mitral coaptation point toward the base of the leaflets and more anterior toward the LVOT.[54,55] These alterations result in excess and lax mitral tissue in the LVOT, increasing the risk of SAM/LVOTO with or without LV hypertrophy (Figure 14–14). In contrast, when the papillary muscle(s) are positioned posteriorly along with the coaptation point, no SAM was seen despite severe septal hypertrophy and flow velocities of 3.3 m/s.

The angle at which the mitral leaflets open affects the direction of blood flow into the LV during diastole and subsequently the direction of ventricular systolic outflow (Figure 14–15).[57] Normally, ventricular inflow is directed along the posterior wall, and outflow is directed along the septum exerting minimal forces on the mitral leaflets. However, anterior displacement of the papillary muscle(s) results in movement of the mitral coaptation point toward the LVOT,

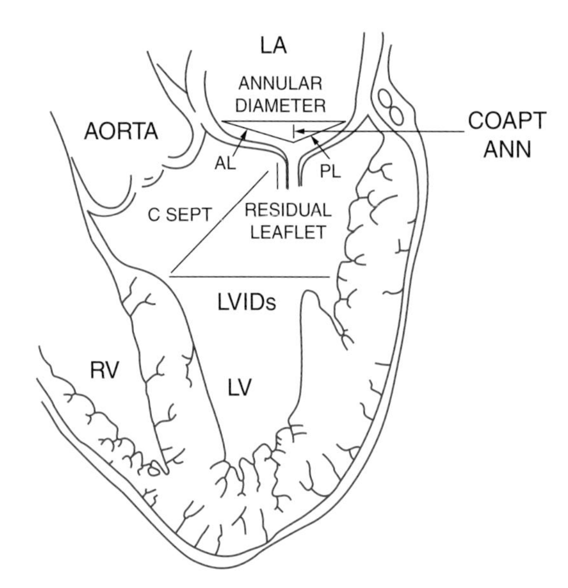

FIGURE 14–13. Schematic representation of measurements performed to assess risk of systolic anterior motion (SAM) of the anterior (AL) and posterior (PL) mitral (MV) leaflets. The relative heights of the two MV leaflets (distance from annulus to the AL and PL coaptation point) and the distance from the coaptation point to the nearest point of the septum (C-Sept) may predict SAM and left ventricular outflow tract obstruction (LVOTO) for patients with hypertrophic cardiomyopathy (HCM) and/or hypertrophic obstructive cardiomyopathy (HOCM) or those undergoing MV repair. In addition, the angle between the LVOT and trans-MV inflow predicts the occurrence of high-velocity blood flow in the LVOT. An AL/PL ratio of less than 1.3 and/or C-Sept distance less than 2.5 cm is demonstrated with SAM/LVOTO after MV repair. These measurements also differentiate patients with HCM from those with HOCM. (LA, left atrium; LV, left ventricle; RV, right ventricle; LVID, left ventricular internal diameter; COAPT ANN, coaptation point to the mitral annulus.) *(Reprinted with permission from Maslow AD, Regan MM, Haering JM, Johnson RG, Levine RA. Echocardiographic predictors of left ventricular outflow tract obstruction and systolic anterior motion of the mitral valve after mitral valve reconstruction for myxomatous valve disease. J Am Coll Cardiol 1999;34:2096-2104.)*

directing ventricular inflow toward the ventricular septum. Blood then moves from the septum toward the posterior wall during diastole, and during systole is subsequently directed toward the LVOT, thus pushing the MV leaflets toward the LVOT and causing SAM. Redirecting ventricular inflow toward the posterior wall will minimize mitral leaflet distortion during ventricular systolic outflow.

The mechanism of SAM/LVOTO and MR is likely to involve some combination of the Venturi effect and abnormalities of the mitral apparatus. These variables may contribute differently from one patient to another. Nevertheless, delineating the mechanisms of SAM/LVOTO/MR provides useful information when considering the best mode of therapy for patients who are symptomatic from outflow tract obstruction and MR. Reassessment of heart function after treatment is necessary to determine the need for adjustments and/or additional interventions. Nonsurgical goals and treatments include the use of β-receptor and calcium channel blockers, maintenance of preload and afterload (Figure 14–16), and avoidance of arrhythmias. Other treatments include ventricular pacing (to induce a left bundle branch block) and alcohol ablation of the ventricular septum. The goal of these therapies is to maintain ventricular function and enlarge the LVOT in order to reduce ventricular outflow gradients. Patients who remain refractory to these noninvasive therapies may be referred for surgical intervention.

Surgical procedures for SAM/LVOTO vary depending upon the mechanism of outflow obstruction and the presence and etiology of MR. The preoperative echocardiographic exam is particularly important to assess myocardial performance and valve integrity, and delineate the mechanisms of dysfunction. Routine intraoperative echocardiographic evaluation prior to and immediately after cardiopulmonary bypass (CPB) is performed to help guide surgical decisions and assess results. Surgical options include myomectomy/myotomy, which involves resecting a significant portion of the ventricular septum at the level of obstruction. In addition, MV surgery may be considered, especially if native valve abnormalities exist including prolapse, ruptured cordae, and redundant/elongated leaflets. Mitral valve replacement with a low-profile bileaflet mechanical valve should reliably eliminate MR and reduce LVOTO involving the mitral apparatus. Mitral valve repair has also been reported for patients with HOCM and MR[70] and avoids complications associated with prosthetic valves. The feasibility of repair can be determined and guided by echocardiographic assessment. The primary goal of MV repair is to move the coaptation point posteriorly in order to (1) produce a posteriorly directed ventricular inflow while maintaining systolic flow along the septum, and (2) to keep the MV leaflets posterior and away from the LVOT, thereby minimizing or eliminating the effects of systolic "drag" forces on the leaflets. If the AL is considered

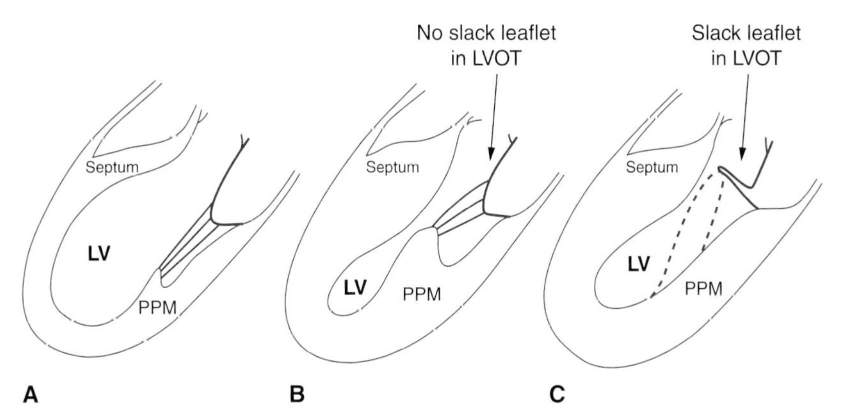

FIGURE 14–14. Schematic representation of the effects of anterior displacement of the left ventricular (LV) papillary muscles on chordal tension and mitral valve (MV) leaflet position. **A:** Normal position of the papillary muscle (PPM) and normal LV septal thickness result in a wide left ventricular outflow tract (LVOT). **B:** Thickened LV septum with mild anteriorly positioned PPM. Normal chordal tension prevents any slack MV leaflet tissue from obstructing the LVOT. **C:** Thickened LV septum with significantly anterior displacement of the PPM results in increased chordal laxity and subsequent slack MV leaflets which rest in the LVOT and obstruct flow. *(Reprinted with permission from Levine RA, Vlahakes GJ, Lefebvre X, Guerrero JL, Cape EG, Yoganathan AP, Weyman AE. Papillary muscle displacement causes systolic anterior motion of the mitral valve. Experimental validation and insights into the mechanism of subaortic obstruction. Circulation. 1995;91:1189-95.)*

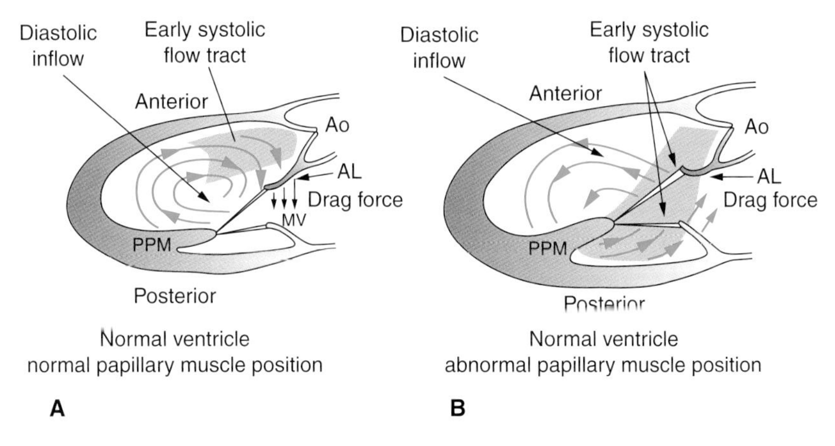

FIGURE 14–15. Schematic of transmitral left ventricular (LV) inflow and LV outflow for normal posterior papillary muscle (PPM) position and anterior displacement of the PPM. **A:** Normal PPM position places the mitral valve (MV) apparatus more posteriorly and directs LV inflow more posteriorly, while systolic outflow is directed along the septum. While blood exits the LV it also forces the MV leaflets to a posterior position and away from the LV outflow tract (LVOT). **B:** Anterior displacement of the PPM positions the MV apparatus more anteriorly. Left ventricular inflow is directed along the septum, while ventricular systolic outflow moves from the posterior wall toward the LVOT pushing the MV leaflets anteriorly toward the LVOT, thereby increasing the risk of systolic anterior motion and outflow tract obstruction. (AL, anterior mitral valve leaflet; Ao, aorta.) *(Reprinted with permission from Lefebvre XP, He S, Levine RA, Yoganathan AP. Systolic anterior motion of the mitral valve in hypertrophic cardiomyopathy: an in vitro pulsatile flow study. J Heart Valve Dis 1995;4:422-438.)*

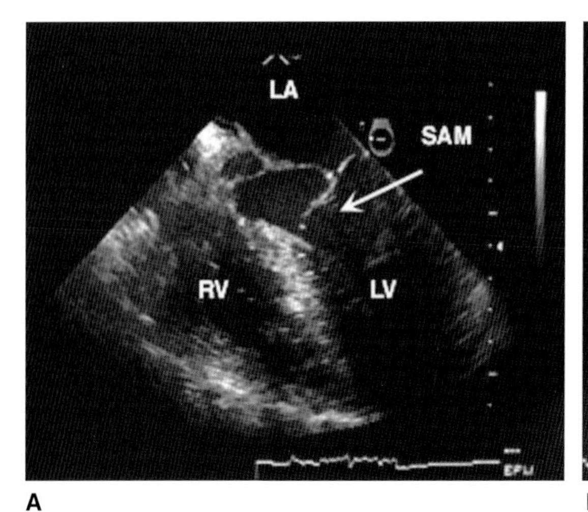

A

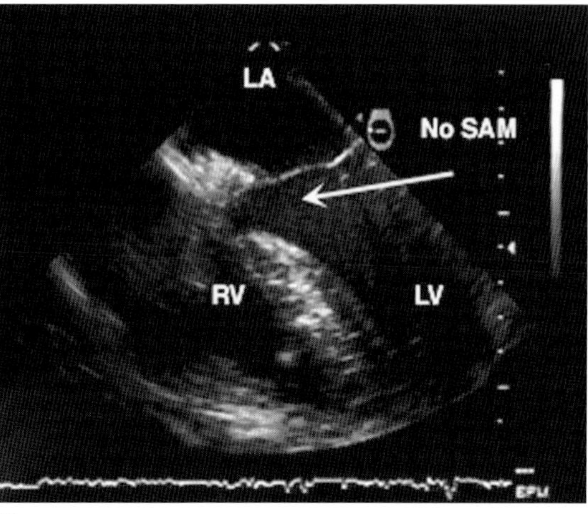

B

FIGURE 14–16. Resolution of mitral leaflet systolic anterior motion (SAM) after increasing afterload by administering vasopressin. **A:** Transesophageal echocardiographic midesophageal four-chamber view demonstrating SAM associated with left ventricular outflow tract obstruction. **B:** Resolution of SAM after the administration of 40 units of vasopressin. (LA, left atrium; RV, right ventricle; LV, left ventricle.)

excessively redundant, a triangular resection may also be necessary. Although MV repair eliminates complications of prosthetic valves, it is a more complex surgery.

The range of overall surgical mortality is 2% to 5%, and is higher for elderly patients (8% to 27%). Surgical resection of the myocardium can be complicated by a severed septal perforator artery,the creation of an iatrogenic ventricular septal defect and varying degrees of heart block.[71] Furthermore, injury to the MV has been reported during myotomy-myectomy procedures.[66] The importance of intraoperative echocardiography in diagnosing complications following surgical procedures for SAM/LVOTO/MR therefore cannot be overemphasized.

Systolic Outflow Tract Obstruction After Cardiac Procedures

LVOTO with SAM and MR may develop after cardiac surgical procedures including, but not limited to, AV replacement, especially for AS, and MV repair. Dynamic outflow tract obstruction or its potential has been recognized prior to and as long as 2 to 3 years after AVR.[72] While it is not clear whether or not these patients have variants of HCM/HOCM, the mechanisms of LVOTO/SAM/MR are similar and may include asymmetric hypertrophy of the ventricular septum, a prominent septal bulge, smaller ventricular cavity, hyperdynamic systolic function, excess or redundant MV leaflets, an increased incidence of posterior MAC, and/or a shorter C-Sept distance (ie, narrower LVOT). Recognition for the potential for SAM/LVOTO/MR allows for the opportunity to initiate medical therapy and/or surgical intervention.

Predictors of LVOTO/SAM/MR after MV surgery include a relatively greater contribution of the PL to mitral coaptation (AL [coaptation point to anterior annulus]:PL <1.3), and a shorter C-Sept distance (<2.5 cm).[68,69] Resolution of LVOTO/SAM/MR was seen with a relative increase in AL contribution to coaptation (AL:PL >2.0) and an increase in C-Sept distance, both of which result in posterior movement of the mitral coaptation point. LVOTO has also been reported after MV replacement with a bioprosthetic valve. While imaging from esophageal windows may suggest LVOT narrowing due to the location of the bioprosthetic valve struts, assessment of the LVOT from TEE transgastric windows is necessary for confirmation. Three-dimensional TEE may also permit confirmation of MV bioprosthetic strut location within the vicinity of the LVOT, yet without obstructing blood flow, when 2D TEE imaging planes are not definitive (Figure 14–17). Aortic valve M-mode may also be useful in detecting early valve closure.

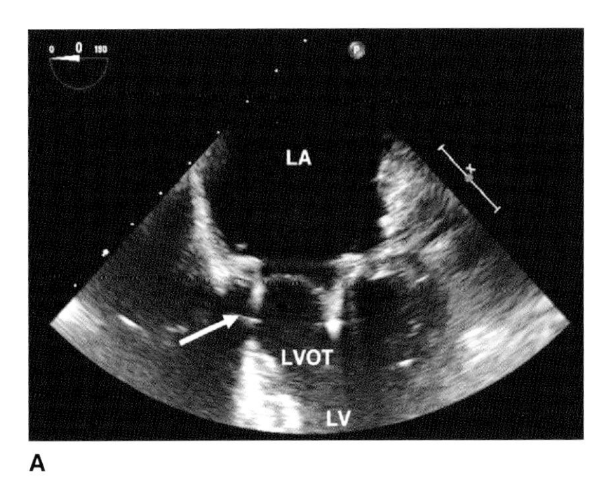

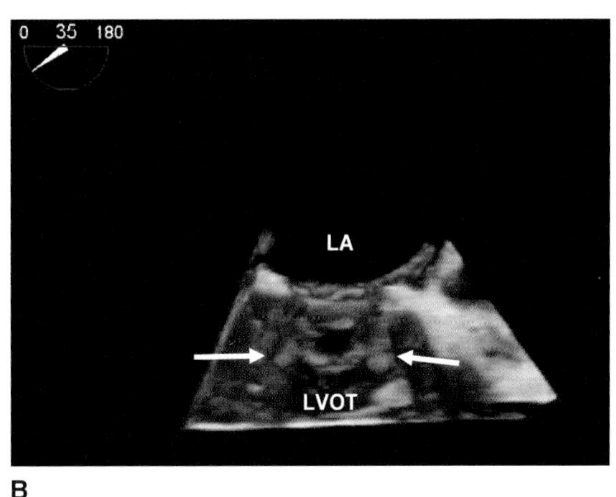

A B

FIGURE 14–17. Transesophageal echocardiographic (TEE) two-dimensional (2D) and real time, full-volume three-dimensional (RT-3D) imaging using a matrix array (Philips Healthcare, Inc, Andover, MA) in a patient following bioprosthetic mitral valve replacement (MVR). **A:** Midesophageal five-chamber view demonstrating the appearance of a bioprosthetic MVR strut *(arrow)* in the vicinity of the left ventricular outflow tract (LVOT) appearing to potentially obstruct outflow. **B:** Full-volume RT-3D TEE image rotated to view the LVOT in short axis from the left ventricular (LV) perspective in the same patient. Two of the three bioprosthetic MVR struts *(arrows)* can be seen straddling the LVOT in a nonobstructive orientation. (LA, left atrium.)

RESTRICTIVE AND INFILTRATIVE CARDIOMYOPATHY (RICM)

Etiology and Pathophysiology

Restrictive cardiomyopathy (RCM) is a pathologic process in which diastolic function of one or both ventricles is severely impaired in the absence of a definitive systemic disease. Although restrictive pathophysiology is implied, a range in severity of diastolic dysfunction occurs in relation to the extent of disease. While several diseases are associated with restrictive filling, only Loeffler hypereosinophilic endocarditis, endomyocardial fibrosis, and idiopathic restrictive cardiomyopathy qualify as primary restrictive cardiomyopathies.[1,73] Secondary causes of RICM include infiltrative diseases such as amyloidosis, sarcoidosis, and storage diseases (eg, glycogen storage disease, hemochromatosis), certain drugs (anthracyclines, ergotamine, methysergide, serotonin), and a number of miscellaneous causes (transplant rejection, radiation, cancers, toxins). Collectively, these diseases have significant overlap and have been categorized as restrictive/constrictive, infiltrative, congestive, or obliterative cardiomyopathies reflecting the range of clinical and morphological presentations. Congestive cardiomyopathy more accurately reflects this group of disorders due to the presence of either pulmonary venous or vena caval congestion, which results in signs of left and right heart failure, respectively. However, since this term is vague and could include all cardiomyopathies, the diseases in this section will be referred to as "restrictive/infiltrative cardiomyopathies" [RICM]; Table 14–3).

RICM should be suspected when a patient presents with CHF, nondilated ventricles, dilated atria, diastolic dysfunction, and poor response to medical therapy. While chest x-ray reveals cardiomegaly and a thickened heart, electrocardiogram (ECG) demonstrates low QRS voltage consistent with replacement of the normal myocardium with non- or poorly conducting tissue. Tissue biopsy frequently confirms the diagnosis; however, it may also show nonspecific and nondiagnostic fibrotic changes of the endomyocardium and myocardium.[74]

Two-Dimensional Echocardiographic Evaluation

Establishing the diagnosis and determining the severity of ventricular dysfunction is important for treatment and prognosis. Differentiation from more treatable causes of heart dysfunction (eg, CAD, valvular heart disease, pericardial disease) is necessary to allow prompt performance of therapeutic procedures (eg, pericardiectomy for pericarditis) when indicated. There are a number of clinical and echocardiographic findings that are unique for each disease in this group of cardiomyopathies.

Table 14–3. Etiologies of Primary and Secondary Restrictive and Infiltrative Cardiomyopathy

Myocardial
Ischemic cardiomyopathy
Non-infiltrative:
Idiopathic cardiomyopathy
Familial cardiomyopathy:
Hypertrophic cardiomyopathy
Scleroderma
Pseudoxanthoma elasticum
Diabetic cardiomyopathy
Infiltrative:
Amyloidosis
Sarcoidosis
Gaucher disease
Hurler disease
Fatty infiltration
Storage diseases:
Hemochromatosis
Fabry disease
Glycogen storage disease
Endomyocardial:
Endomyocardial fibrosis
Hypereosinophilic syndrome
Carcinoid heart
Metastatic cancer
Radiation
Toxic effects of anthracycline
Drug-related fibrosis (serotonin, methysergide, ergotamine, mercury, bisulfan)

Amyloidosis is the most commonly reported etiology of RICM and is caused by an abnormal layering of protein within the myocardial tissues including all cardiac chambers as well as the coronary arteries, cardiac conduction system, and heart valves. Four types of amyloidosis have been described: (a) primary, (b) secondary, (c) familial, and (d) senile. The protein that is present in *primary amyloidosis* comes from plasma cells, possibly associated with multiple myeloma. *Secondary amyloidosis* is associated with chronic inflammatory diseases such as rheumatoid arthritis, and tuberculosis. Of the four types, primary and senile amyloidosis involve cardiac tissues, with the former involving other systemic organs and the latter occurring in older patients. Mortality for patients with cardiac amyloidosis is high, and survival beyond 2 to 3 years for patients presenting with CHF is less than 50%.[75] Prognosis is related to the extent of infiltration, thickness of the ventricular walls, severity of diastolic dysfunction, presence of systolic dysfunction, and RV involvement.[76,77]

An autopsy study of 54 patients who died of cardiac amyloidosis highlights the extensive amyloid infiltration of the cardiac tissues.[78] Amyloid deposition was found within the interstitium (53 of 54), endocardium, valves (46 of 54; 86%), and intramurally within the coronary arteries (54 of 54). No disease was found in the epicardial coronary arteries, distinguishing it from atheromatous disease. Forty-four of 54 (85%) patients with amyloidosis who died from cardiac causes had a history of CHF. Of the eight patients without CHF, three had sudden death, two had familial amyloidosis, two had multiple myeloma, and one had cirrhosis due to amyloid infiltration. Forty-five percent had varying degrees of heart block, and 18% had complete heart block. During autopsy, the heart was described as "rubbery" and noncompliant. Although all patients in this study had bi-atrial enlargement, only 20% had ventricular dilation, which was associated with other pathologies (eg, CAD, primary pulmonary disease). Intracardiac thrombi were found in 26% of patients, with a greater incidence in the atria. In 50 of 54 patients, the ventricular septum and free wall had equal or near equal thickness. Four (7%) of patients had asymmetric thickening with a septal/free-wall ratio greater than 1.3:1.

A number of echocardiographic features differentiate the amyloid heart from other causes of hypertrophy and/or diastolic dysfunction.[77,79] The echocardiographic appearance of the amyloid heart is classically described as "speckled," granular, or "starry skied" (Figure 14–18). Speckling may be due to the acoustic interface created by myocytes and amyloid protein. All cardiac tissues may be symmetrically or, infrequently, asymmetrically thickened and "speckled." Similar to other etiologies of RICM, the atria are enlarged, while the ventricular cavity size is often normal or reduced. However, infiltration of the atrial walls, especially the interatrial septum, differentiates amyloidosis from other causes of CHF. In addition, RV thickening and speckling are more common with amyloidosis than other diseases. While speckling has been found in other diseases (eg, uremia), its presence is highly sensitive and specific for cardiac amyloidosis. Systolic dysfunction, when it occurs, is rarely associated with chamber enlargement or RWMA except in those patients with coronary artery involvement. Prognosis in patients with amyloidosis is based on myocardial wall thickness, severity of diastolic dysfunction, and systolic function.[73,75] For patients with wall thickness 12 mm or less the median survival is about 2.5 years, while survival is reduced for those with wall thickness between 12 and 15 mm (1.3 years), and least for those with wall thickness 15 mm or greater (0.4 years). The incidence of systolic dysfunction is 0%, 35%, and 70% in these three groups, respectively. In patients with systolic dysfunction, only 5% have LV

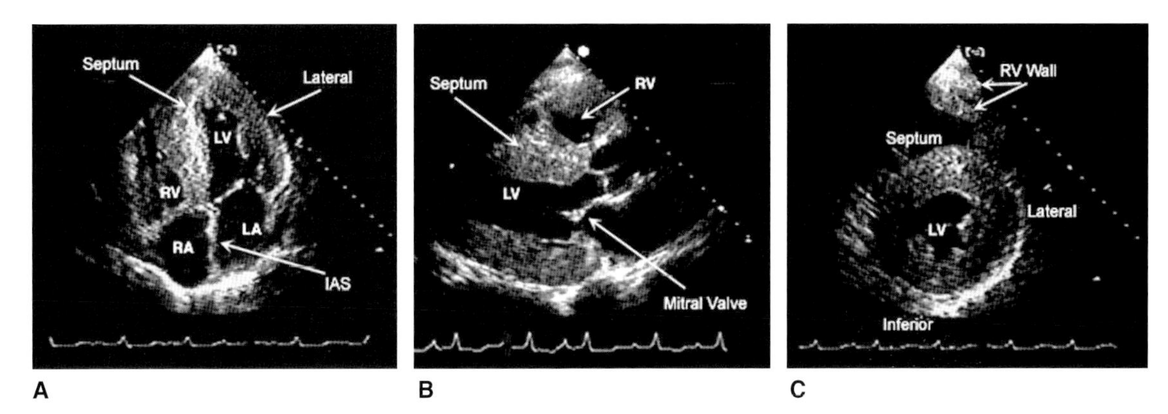

FIGURE 14–18. Transthoracic echocardiographic (TTE) two-dimensional imaging in a patient with cardiac amyloidosis. **A:** TTE apical four-chamber view demonstrating thickened walls involving both the left (LV) and right (RV) ventricles. The echocardiographic appearance of the walls is "speckled," or "starry skied," suggesting amyloid infiltration. Amyloid infiltration is also apparent in the interatrial septum. (LA, left atrium, IAS, interatrial septum.) **B:** TTE parasternal view of the LV, RV, left ventricular outflow tract and aortic valve, mitral valve (MV), and left atrium. In addition to involvement of both ventricles, the MV leaflets appear thickened and infiltrated. **C:** TTE parasternal short-axis view of the LV and RV free wall. Both chambers appeared to be thickened and infiltrated with amyloid. (RA, right atrium.)

dilation and/or focal RWMA. These patients have significant amyloid involvement of the coronary arteries. Prognosis is also related to the severity of diastolic dysfunction, which in turn is correlated with ventricular wall thickening. For patients with milder cardiac involvement, wall thickness is less than 15 mm, and Doppler profiles suggest a pattern consistent with abnormal relaxation. In contrast, patients with wall thickness 15 mm or greater have flow profiles suggestive of a restrictive filling defect. Comparable profiles are found when assessing filling of the right heart of patients with amyloidosis.[80] The TTDF, caval, or hepatic vein flow profiles for patients with RV free wall thickness less than 7 mm are usually consistent with abnormal relaxation. For patients with RV wall thickness 7 mm or greater the patterns suggest a restrictive filling defect.

Idiopathic restrictive cardiomyopathy is an autosomal dominant disease associated with heart block and skeletal myopathy, which presents in the third and fourth decades.[73,75,81] Histologic examination reveals variable degrees of interstitial fibrosis throughout the heart, which cannot be explained by a specific etiology. For children under 10 years of age, the survival is less than 2 years, while more than 60% of adults survive beyond 4 years. Echocardiographic evaluation reveals diastolic dysfunction, relatively normal systolic function, variable myocardial thickening, atrial enlargement with or without thrombi, and pulmonary hypertension.

Endocardial fibroelastosis is found in children and characterized by a thick endocardium.[35] Histology demonstrates infiltration of the endocardium with collagen and elastic tissue causing LV endocardial thickening with or without MV involvement. While the primary form is not associated with other congenital cardiac abnormalities, a secondary form may be found with LVOTO, aortic coarctation, coronary artery abnormalities, or hypoplastic left heart.

Hypereosinophilic syndrome (*Loffler endocarditis*) and *endomyocardial fibrosis* are a continuum of the same disease differing only by their presenting pathology.[82] Although these diseases are uncommon, their occurrence is greater in parts of Africa and Asia, accounting for as much as 25% of cardiac deaths. While both are the result of cardiac eosinophilia, Loffler endocarditis presents with significant cardiac hypereosinophilia, while endomyocardial fibrosis represents a later stage characterized mainly by fibrosis. As both diseases progress, endocardial thickening and fibrosis develop with greater involvement of the MV and TV subvalvular apparatus producing valve insufficiency and/or stenosis. Involvement of the ventricular apex results in obliteration of the cavity, which may be further complicated by thrombus formation. Echocardiography demonstrates bi-atrial enlargement, endocardial thickening, or deposits along the MV and TV associated papillary muscles, and along the apices of both ventricles (Figure 14–19). The involved tissues appear

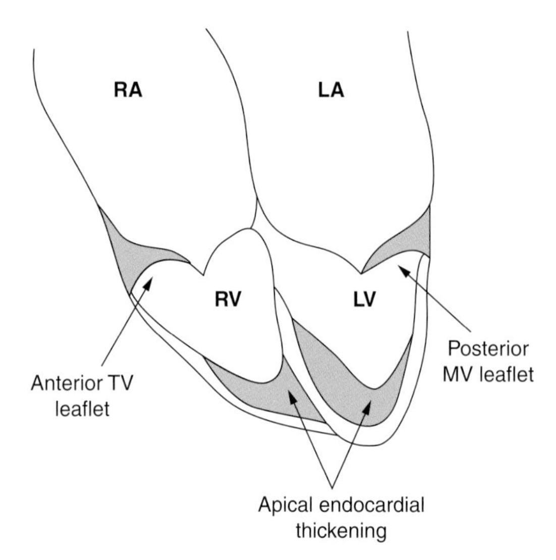

FIGURE 14–19. Schematic representation of hypereosinophilic syndrome or endomyocardial fibrosis. The right (RA) and left (LA) atria are enlarged. There is thickening noted *(arrows)* along the posterior mitral valve (MV) annulus and leaflet as well as the anterior tricuspid valve (TV) annulus and leaflet. Ventricular apical obliteration reduces the ventricular cavity size. (LV, left ventricle; RV, right ventricle.)

bright and echo-dense, consistent with calcium deposition. While impairment to ventricular filling is present, systolic motion of the ventricular walls is usually preserved.

Hemochromatosis is an infiltrative process due to abnormal deposition of iron in a number of organs including the liver, heart, kidneys, pancreas, skin, and pituitary gland. Iron deposits within the cells cause degeneration and subsequent fibrosis. Cardiac involvement is the leading cause of death in these patients, occurring in as many as 40% of patients with primary hemochromatosis.[83] Cardiac pathology is rarely seen without other organ system involvement. Echocardiographic features that are typical of this infiltrative disease include primary involvement of the LV associated with chamber enlargement and significant systolic dysfunction. In sharp contrast to primary RCM, a restrictive filling defect is rare. Wall thickening and RWMA are also uncommon; however, the latter may be present in infrequent cases of coronary artery involvement and microcirculatory insufficiency. Echocardiographic evaluation may be useful to monitor the beneficial effects of chelation.

Sarcoidosis is a systemic disease in which organs are infiltrated with non-caseating granulomas. Cardiac involvement is found in approximately 20% to 25% of cases, and is rarely seen without involvement of other organ systems.[84] The LV free wall and papillary muscles are more commonly affected, causing ventricular dysfunction, conduction system abnormalities, and an increased risk of sudden death. Initially, patients have diastolic dysfunction, which gradually progresses to include systolic dysfunction. Echocardiographic features are less specific and include RWMA and chamber enlargement with ventricular thinning that may lead to aneurysm formation. Other less commonly found features include pericardial effusions, LV thrombi, and diastolic dysfunction. RV thickness and dysfunction usually develop from sarcoid involvement of the lung parenchyma producing pulmonary hypertension.

A number of miscellaneous etiologies of RICM have also been described. *Carcinoid* infiltration of the heart is associated with fibrous plaques within the TV, MV, and along the RV free wall. *Radiation therapy* results in both myocardial and endocardial fibrosis, especially of the RV, causing a restrictive pathophysiology. A number of pharmacologic agents also cause restrictive cardiac disease including anthracyclines (Doxorubicin), which are also known to cause a dilated cardiomyopathy and can aggravate the effects of radiation therapy on the heart. *Glycogen, lipid, and mucopolysaccharide storage diseases* are uncommon diseases, and therefore echocardiographic descriptions are not well established. These disorders share commonalties with both HCM/HOCM as well as with other RCM. For example, echocardiographic evaluation of Pompe disease (type II glycogen storage disease) may include asymmetric LV hypertrophy with SAM. Fabry disease (X-linked recessive, lysosomal storage disorder resulting from α-galactosidase deficiency) may share similar features with amyloidosis including biventricular abnormalities and reduced diastolic and systolic dysfunction.

Doppler Assessment of Diastolic Function: Restrictive Physiology

The demonstration of restrictive TMDF and PVDF profiles in patients with RICM is an inherent component of the diagnosis and has been shown to correlate with outcome. While distinct differences have been drawn between abnormal relaxation and restrictive physiology, it is likely that they are part of a continuum of diastolic dysfunction. For example, patients with cardiac amyloidosis progress over time from normal diastolic function to impaired relaxation, through pseudonormal pathophysiology, and then to a restrictive pattern (Figure 14–20; see Table 14–2). The Doppler flow profiles seen with mild diastolic dysfunction are primarily the result of reduced ventricular relaxation while atrial pressures and function are relatively normal.

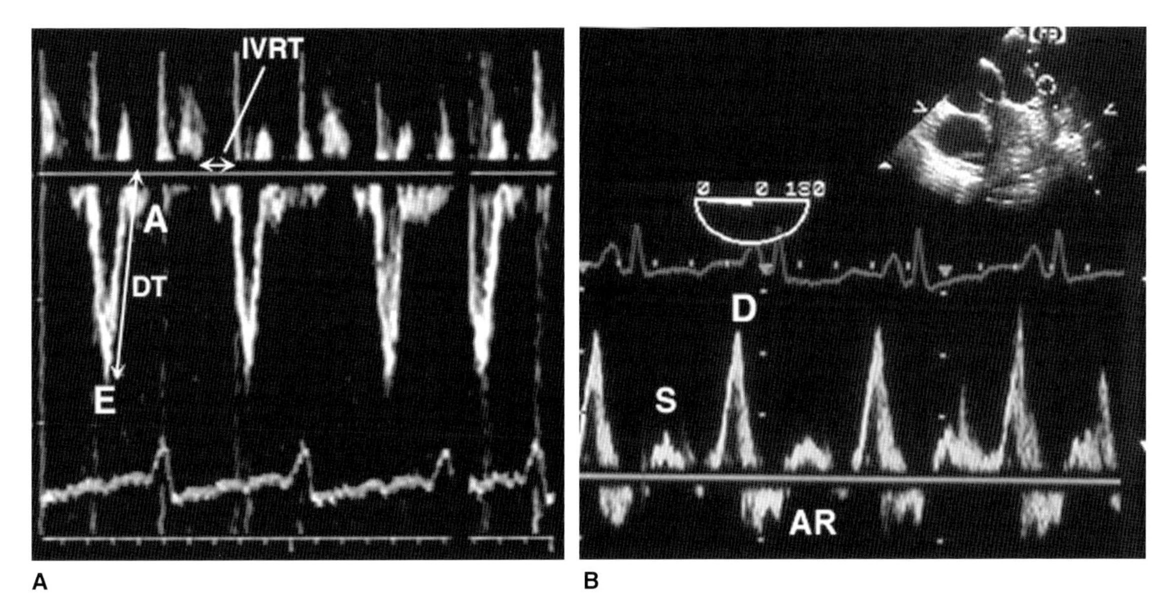

FIGURE 14–20. Transmitral (TMDF) and pulmonary venous Doppler flow (PVDF) velocity profiles consistent with restrictive left ventricular filling. **A:** TMDF profile demonstrating an early (E) to late (A) ratio much greater than 2.0. The deceleration time (DT = 100 milliseconds) and isovolumic relaxation time (IVRT = 60 milliseconds) are decreased. **B:** PVDF profile from the left pulmonary vein demonstrating a systolic (S) to diastolic (D) ratio S/D much less than 0.5 consistent with an elevated left atrial pressure. The peak velocity of the late diastolic flow reversal during atrial contraction (AR) is 40 cm/s.

As diastolic function deteriorates, ventricular stiffness increases along with ventricular and atrial pressures. Atrial contractility and compliance subsequently decrease with further reductions in ventricular compliance.

Flow profiles suggesting a restrictive filling include an E/A ratio greater than 2.0, DT less than 150 milliseconds, IVRT less than 80 milliseconds, PV_D less than 30 cm/s, a $PV_{S/D}$ much less than 1.0, an PV_{AR} greater than 35 milliseconds, and a $PV_{AR}/TMDF_A$ duration or peak velocity ratio of greater than 0.6 (see Figures 14–4 and 14–20).[77] These filling patterns result from elevated LAP forcing early transmitral flow (decreased IVRT) into a stiff LV (decreased propagation velocity and DT), which subsequently limits transmitral flow during a diminished atrial contraction (ie, increased E/A ratio). A relatively larger LA volume is ejected backwards toward the pulmonary veins during atrial contraction, thus producing an increased $PV_{AR}/TMDF_A$ ratio. Incomplete LA emptying during atrial contraction subsequently limits pulmonary venous inflow during ventricular systole, resulting in a decreased PV_S/PV_D. RV failure is associated with similar Doppler flow velocity profiles into the RA and across the tricuspid valve.

Restrictive filling patterns are associated with poor exercise tolerance, CHF, and mortality across a number of different populations including patients with RICM.[43,77,85-87]

Differential Diagnosis

Differentiation between RICM and from other causes of CHF is important to establish both prognosis and a treatment plan. While treatment for RICM is largely supportive and prognosis is comparatively poor, treatment for other causes of heart failure have greater success. The differential diagnosis includes CAD, hypertension, HCM/HOCM, DCM, valvular pathology, and pericardial disease. These etiologies are usually known or suspected based on the patient's history and examination, or are diagnosed with echocardiography and/or coronary angiography. The echocardiographic appearance of the myocardium is normal in these disease processes unless scarring is present (thin and bright echoes). Hypertrophic cardiomyopathies have been discussed in detail above. Although myocardial thickening is present with HCM/HOCM, hypertension, or aortic stenosis, the echocardiographic appearance does not typically appeared "speckled." In addition, atrial infiltration and thickening are not likely. Furthermore, a restrictive pattern is less commonly reported with other causes of myocardial thickening. Valvular dysfunction may also occur with RICM; however, a pattern of valve apparatus infiltration is usually noted during 2D echocardiography. Valve surgery may improve functional capacity of patients with RICM.

Pericardial diseases including effusion/tamponade, tumor, and constrictive pericarditis are often included in the differential diagnosis of CHF. Differentiation from RICM is important since pericardial diseases can be treated with resection of the constrictive pericardium or pericardiocentesis.[77,85] An accurate diagnosis of cardiomyopathy may prevent an unnecessary surgical procedure.

Since a range in the severity of diastolic dysfunction may be present in patients with RICM, similarities with constrictive pericarditis may be demonstrated in the resting TMDF and PVDF profiles. However, other differences allow distinction between the two pathological processes (Table 14–4). In patients with constrictive pericarditis, RAP and LAP waveforms demonstrate normal or reduced "a" and "v" waves along with a deep "y" descent. The "x" descent may also be normal or deep. RV pressure waveforms classically reveal a "dip" and "plateau" or "square root" appearance. There is equalization (within 5 mm Hg) of diastolic pressures in all four cardiac chambers, and pulmonary vascular pressures may be mildly elevated. In contrast, pressure waveforms in RICM reveal elevated RA and LA "a" and "v" waves along with a prominent "y" descent. Although a similar RV waveform may occur with RICM, equalization of diastolic pressures is unusual, and more severe pulmonary hypertension is often present.

A number of echocardiographic findings also help differentiate constrictive pericarditis from RICM (see Chapter 15). In constrictive pericarditis, 2D and M-mode echocardiography reveal a thickened and/or calcified (echo-dense) pericardium without apparent abnormalities elsewhere in the ventricular myocardium, valve tissues, or atrial walls (Figure 14–21). The inferolateral ventricular wall may be flat due to the adherent pericardium, limiting its mobility. In addition, the ventricular septum may appear to "bounce" during diastole due to the near equal pressures in both ventricles, and limitation of filling during diastole.[85] A dilated IVC is consistent with an elevated RAP or impaired filling.

Doppler echocardiography is also useful to distinguish constrictive pericarditis from RICM. By surrounding the heart, the abnormal pericardium attenuates the affects of intrathoracic pressure changes on the heart, while changes in intrathoracic pressures are transmitted

Table 14–4. Differentiation between Constrictive Pericarditis and Restrictive Cardiomyopathy

Indices	Pericardial Constriction	Myocardial Restriction
Peripheral signs	Ascites, edema	Ascites, edema
RA wave	Prominent "x" and "y" descent	Prominent "y" descent
RA pressure	Elevated	Elevated
RV wave	Dip and plateau; square root sign	Dip and plateau; square root sign
RVEDP	One-third RVSP; equal to LVEDP	Less than one-third RVSP; <LVEDP
LVEDP	Normal or increased	Increased
PASP	<40-50 mm Hg	>40-50 mm Hg
PCWP	Equal to RAP	>RAP
CO	Normal or decreased	Decreased
Systolic function	Normal	Normal or decreased
Auscultation	Pericardial rub	S_3 heart sound, MR, TR
CXR	Pericardial calcification	Bi-atrial enlargement
ECG	Nonspecific ST changes	Decreased voltage
Echocardiography	Pericardial thickening and calcification Restriction to inflow Normal muscle appearance >10% changes in transmitral and tricuspid flows	Myocardial thickening Restriction to inflow Infiltration <10% changes in transmitral and tricuspid flows
Biopsy	Abnormal pericardium; normal myocardium	Abnormal myocardium

RA, right atrium; RV, right ventricle; RVEDP, right ventricular end-diastolic pressure; RVSP, right ventricular systolic pressure; LVEDP, left ventricular end-diastolic pressure; PASP, pulmonary artery systolic pressure; PCWP, pulmonary capillary wedge pressure; RAP, right atrial pressure; CO, cardiac output; MR, mitral regurgitation; TR, tricuspid regurgitation; ECG, electrocardiogram.

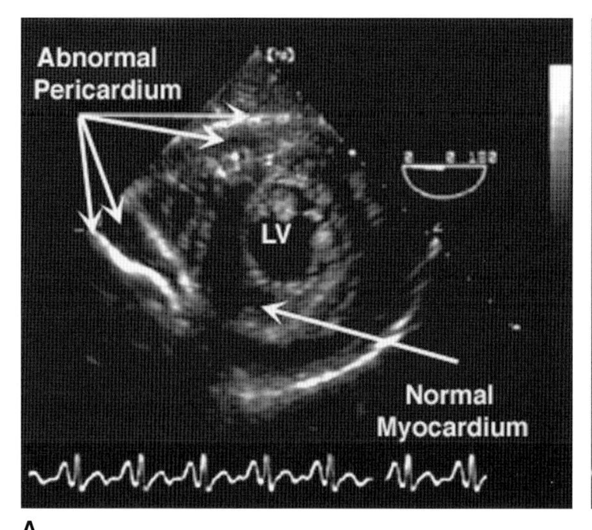

A

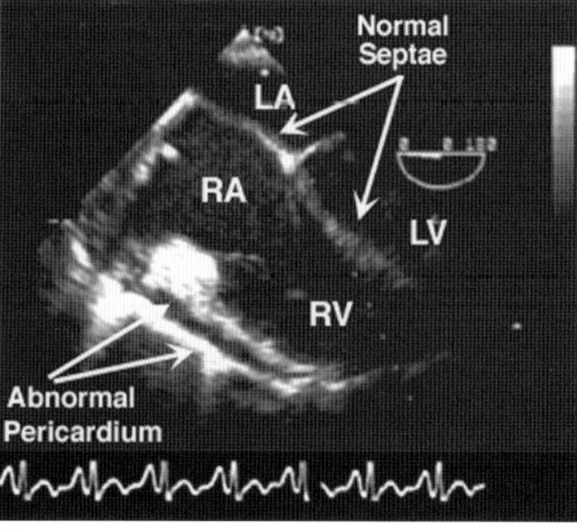

B

FIGURE 14–21. Transesophageal echocardiographic (TEE) two-dimensional images of patient with constrictive pericarditis. **A:** TEE transgastric mid–short-axis view of the left (LV) and right ventricle . The pericardium appears unusually bright (calcified) and thickened, while the pericardial space is echolucent. The myocardium appears normal. In this particular case, opening the pericardium revealed an empyema. **B:** TEE midesophageal four-chamber view demonstrating abnormal pericardium along the right atrium (RA) and RV. The pericardium appears bright and thickened. In this image the atrial and ventricular septae appear normal. (LA, left atrium.)

to the central vessels (cavae and pulmonary veins that are not encased by the constricting pericardium). During spontaneous ventilation, inspiration lowers intrathoracic and also pulmonary venous pressures. This leads to reduction in LAP, which is reflected by reductions in TMDF peak velocities (E and A waves), an increase in IVRT, and a reduction in PVDF velocities into the LA. The opposite changes are seen during expiration. The corresponding right heart flows and velocities are opposite to the left side of the heart. Changes in right and left heart flows are opposite during positive pressure ventilation. Peak velocities change more than 15% from one respiratory phase to another. In contrast, for patients with RICM, there is little change (<15%) in Doppler measured flows across the TV and MV, since changes in intrathoracic pressure are transmitted to the heart and central venous tissues equally.

MISCELLANEOUS CARDIOMYOPATHIES

Left Ventricular Non-Compaction

Left ventricular non-compaction (LVNC) or hypertrabeculation results from an arrest of the normal fetal development of the myocardium. During its initial developmental stages, the heart muscle has a spongy texture and appearance, ie, non-compacted. At this time and through the 17th week of gestation, the developing myocardium receives its nutrition via diffusion across cell membranes, since the coronary arteries are not yet developed. This loose network of muscle trabeculations and bands maximizes the amount of surface area, thereby facilitating the diffusion of blood into the tissue beds. The coronary arteries develop around the 18th week of gestation as the spongy trabeculated myocardium becomes more compacted in preparation for contraction required for normal ventricular function. Beyond the 18th week, the prominent trabeculations further reduce in size and appear even closer to the surface, while the spongy myocardium becomes increasingly more compacted.

Approximately 0.015% to 0.05% of echocardiograms display images consistent with LVNC, although the actual incidence is difficult to ascertain.[88] Among patients presenting with heart failure, this incidence may be greater.[89] The timing of arrested development dictates the degree of myocardial dysfunction. In its most severe form, the pumping function of the myocardium is severely impaired. The genetic inheritance varies significantly, and mutations generally include genes coding for the myocardial filaments, cytoskeleton, and possibly coronary vasculature. Sponge-like interlacing smaller muscle bundles have been described during autopsy, along with non-compacted broad and coarse trabeculae; however, well-developed papillary muscles are usually absent.[90]

The clinical presentation of LVNC varies from asymptomatic to severe heart failure, the latter being characterized by a number of nonspecific signs and symptoms including peripheral edema, dyspnea, fatigue, and reduced functional capacity. A variety of atrial and ventricular arrhythmias, conduction delays, and blocks may develop; however, tachycardias are generally not well tolerated. There is also an increased incidence of intra-cavitary thrombi located within the trabecular mesh; however, they are not likely to develop in the absence of systolic dysfunction.

The diagnosis of LVNC is usually based on echocardiography and cardiac magnetic resonance imaging (CMRI). Jenni et al proposed the following echocardiographic criteria for the diagnosis of LVNC:

1. Thickened LV wall consisting of two layers: a thin, compacted epicardial layer and a markedly thickened endocardial layer with numerous prominent trabeculations and deep recesses with a maximum ratio of non-compacted to compacted myocardium greater than 2:1 at end-systole in a TTE parasternal short-axis view.[91,92]
2. Color Doppler highlighted flow within the recesses created by the deep trabeculations.
3. Involvement of the mid to apical inferior and lateral wall segments.

All three of these findings are required to make the diagnosis of LVNC. Apical and midventricular inferior and lateral walls may be affected most often. Hypokinesis of the affected walls, diastolic dysfunction, and thrombi may be observed; however, these are not required to establish the diagnosis.

Chin et al have also suggested that echocardiographic criteria for LVNC include a ratio of the distance from the epicardial surface to the trough of the trabecular recess and the distance from the epicardial surface to the peak of the trabeculations of 0.5 or less as viewed in a TTE apical four-chamber or sub-xiphoid view at end-diastole.[93] Although both of these criteria highlight the presence of prominent trabeculations, the Jenni criteria have been shown to be more sensitive.[94]

Cardiac magnetic resonance imaging displays a maximum ratio during diastole, of non-compacted to compacted myocardial thickness of greater than 2.3 as assessed in three long-axis views (sensitivity 86%, specificity 99%). This finding distinguishes LVNC from other cardiovascular etiologies of prominent trabeculations including HCM associated with aortic stenosis and systemic hypertension.[95]

Treatment of LVNC is generally supportive, including standard therapies for heart failure and arrhythmia prevention. Oechslin et al described the outcome for 34 adults with LVNC over 44 ± 40 months.[88] The mean age at diagnosis was 42 ± 17 years with 12 patients experiencing significant heart failure at the time of diagnosis. The mean LV end-diastolic diameter was 65 ± 12 mm and an LV ejection fraction of 33 ± 13%. Apical and midventricular segments of the inferior and lateral walls were involved in more than 80% of cases. Complications included heart failure (n = 18; 53%), thromboembolic events (n = 8; 24%), and ventricular tachycardias (n = 14; 41%). Sudden death occurred in 12 individuals, which was associated with heart failure in four patients, while two others died of noncardiac causes. Four patients underwent heart transplantation and four received automatic implantable cardioverter/defibrillators. Presentation in the neonatal period carries a 14% mortality at 3 years. For unclear reasons, there may be a period of recovery followed by significant deterioration.[96]

Arrhythmogenic Right Ventricular Cardiomyopathy

Arrhythmogenic right ventricular cardiomyopathy (ARVC) or arrhythmogenic right ventricular dysplasia (ARVD) is characterized histologically by fatty and/or fibrous infiltrate of the right ventricle. The severity varies from a functionally normal patient with mild structural changes to complete involvement of the RV myocardium with severe ventricular dysfunction and arrhythmias. The ventricular septum is typically spared. The left ventricle is also less commonly involved.

Patients with ARVC present between the ages of 10 and 50 years (mean age of 30 years). It is rarely diagnosed in infancy and uncommonly before age 10. The incidence is regionally different, although rare in the United States, with a maximum occurrence of approximately 1 in 1000. However, ARVC may account for 11% of sudden cardiac death in younger patients, and in 22% of athletes.[97,98] The diagnosis is suspected for sudden cardiac death brought on by exercise.

The presentation of patients with ARVC varies depending on the extent of infiltration. Symptoms include palpitations, syncope, atypical chest pain, and dyspnea.[99] Symptomatic atrial fibrillation and ventricular arrhythmias, the latter ranging from frequent premature ventricular contractions to ventricular tachycardia/fibrillation, are typical.[100] High-risk patients include those with symptoms including syncope, hemodynamic instability, and/or ventricular dysrhythmias, evidence of right ventricular failure, evidence of left ventricular involvement, and an increase in QRS duration of greater than 40 milliseconds.[101]

The diagnosis of ARVC is suspected for young patients with ventricular tachycardia and a left bundle branch block (LBBB) configuration or multiple morphologies. The QRS morphology usually resembles a LBBB configuration since the arrhythmia is more likely to originate from the right ventricle. The diagnosis, however, depends on histologic demonstration of fibrofatty replacement of the right ventricle. Nevertheless, since the sensitivity of tissue biopsy may be as low as 67%, other criteria have been established to determine the diagnosis of ARVC[102]:

1. Global and/or regional dysfunction and structural alterations
2. Repolarization or depolarization and conduction abnormalities on the ECG
3. Arrhythmias
4. Family history of ARVC

The evaluation of suspected patients includes ECG, echocardiography, radionucleotide ventriculography, and magnetic resonance imaging (MRI) studies. Forty to fifty percent of patients with ARVC have normal ECG at presentation; however, within 6 years, almost all patients present with of one of the following ECG findings[103]:

1. Prolonged QRS
2. Incomplete or complete bundle branch block
3. Epsilon wave (30%)
4. T-wave inversion that correlates with degree of RV enlargement
5. QT dispersion
6. Prolonged S-wave upstroke

Electrophysiologic testing often demonstrates inducible ventricular arrhythmias and typically localizes the foci to the right ventricle.

Echocardiographic evidence of ARVC includes right ventricular enlargement ± regional wall motion abnormalities.[104] Right heart enlargement characteristically involves the right ventricular outflow tract (>30-mm diameter).[105] Although right ventricular enlargement and dysfunction is common, RV failure is present in only 6% of patients. At a later stage, however, the right ventricle becomes increasing dilated and dysfunctional.

Disease severity can be classified echocardiographically as[104]:

1. Mild: Right ventricular end-diastolic volume (RVEDV) less than 75 mL/m^2 with localized hypokinesis or akinesis
2. Moderate: RVEDV 75 to 120 mL/m^2 with localized hypokinesis or akinesis
3. Severe: RVEDV 120 mL/m^2 or greater with widespread akinesis/dyskinesis and diastolic bulging

Qualitative echocardiographic findings include trabecular derangement and a hyper-reflective moderator band.[105]

Treatment of ARVC is directed toward preventing sudden cardiac death. Although not well defined, placement of an implantable cardiac defibrillator may be indicated for both primary and secondary therapies.[106] Sotalol may be the best pharmacologic therapy especially when an "electrical storm" occurs with an implantable cardiac defibrillator.[106] Amiodarone can also be effective.[106] Treatment of atrial fibrillation also follows similar protocols as for the general population including cardioversion, rate control, and anticoagulation. Since exercise is known to precipitate tachyarrhythmias, avoidance of exercise may be advised. More invasive therapies include radiofrequency ablation of a documented arrhythmogenic foci and surgical resection of the right ventricular free wall to decrease the ventricular mass responsible for initiating ventricular tachycardias, and to prevent the spread of ventricular arrhythmias to the left ventricle.

Tako-tsubo Cardiomyopathy

Tako-Tsubo cardiomyopathy or Tako-Tsubo syndrome (TTS), also known as "stress cardiomyopathy" or "broken-heart syndrome" mimics an acute coronary syndrome and is accompanied by reversible left ventricular apical ballooning in the absence of angiographically significant coronary artery stenosis. In Japanese, "takotsubo" means "fishing pot for trapping octopus," and the left ventricle of a patient diagnosed with this condition resembles that shape. About 70-80% of cases of TTS occur in post-menopausal women under some form of extreme, exceptional and prolonged mental stress. In the remaining 20%, the stress is physical such as massive trauma, surgery or severe pain. In very rare cases, no "cause" can be found.[107,108]

The etiology of TTS is not fully understood, but several mechanisms have been proposed. Dote and associates[109] suggested coronary vasospasm as the pathogenic mechanism; however, induction of coronary vasospasm by acetylcholine or ergonovine has yielded mixed results. The possibility of myocardial injury due to microvascular spasm has also been suggested. Ako and coworkers,[110] by using of an intracoronary Doppler wire technique, demonstrated microcirculation impairments in instances of transient LV hypocontraction. Another putative mechanism is neurogenic stunned myocardium. This condition is also observed during acute cerebrovascular accidents and during the catecholamine-induced cardiomyopathy in patients with pheochromocytoma. Enhanced sympathetic activity appears to play a very important role in the pathophysiology of TTS.

The electrocardiogram in patients with TTS often demonstrates non-specific ST-T abnormalities, ST elevation, and/or QT prolongation with large negative T waves while cardiac biomarkers (troponin, creatine kinase) are only very slightly elevated. Echocardiography typically shows significantly decreased left ventricular wall motion with hypokinesis or akinesis of the anterior wall and anterior septum from the mid-papillary level to the apex. A hallmark of this syndrome is apical ballooning with sparing of the base of the heart. The apex is thought to be structurally vulnerable because it does not have a 3-layered myocardial configuration, has a limited elasticity reserve, can easily become ischemic as a consequence of its relatively limited coronary circulation, and is more responsive to adrenergic stimulation. [111,1126]

An inverted Tako-Tsubo syndrome has also been recently described in patients with severe intracranial processes or with pheochromocytoma crisis. In those rare cases, instead of the tip of the left ventricle becoming stunned and "paralyzed", the tip of the left ventricle is hyperdynamic while the base of the heart appears stunned and "paralyzed".[113,114]

Treatment of TTS relies largely on support measures as short-term outcomes are excellent, with complete resolution in a few weeks in most but not all patients. Data on long-term outcome is limited but TTS recurs in approximately 5% and appears to be a marker for increased noncardiac mortality. [115]

REFERENCES

1. Richardson P, McKenna W, Bristow M, et al. Report of the 1995 World Health Organization/International Society and Federation of Cardiology Task Force on the Definition and Classification of Cardiomyopathies. *Circulation.* 1996;93(5): 841-842.
2. Abelmann WH. Classification and natural history of primary myocardial disease. *Prog Cardiovasc Dis.* 1984;27(2): 73-94.
3. Bachinski LL, Roberts R. New theories. Causes of dilated cardiomyopathy. *Cardiol Clin.* 1998;16(4):603-610, vii.
4. Stevenson LW, Perloff JK. The dilated cardiomyopathies: clinical aspects. *Cardiol Clin.* 1988;6(2):187-218.
5. Dec GW, Fuster V. Idiopathic dilated cardiomyopathy. *N Engl J Med.* 1994;331(23):1564-1575.
6. Hirota Y, Shimizu G, Kaku K, Saito T, Kino M, Kawamura K. Mechanisms of compensation and decompensation in dilated cardiomyopathy. *Am J Cardiol.* 1984;54(8):1033-1038.
7. Davies MJ. The cardiomyopathies: an overview. *Heart.* 2000;83(4):469-474.
8. Colucci WS. Molecular and cellular mechanisms of myocardial failure. *Am J Cardiol.* 1997;80(11A):15L-25L.
9. Fonarow GC. Pathogenesis and treatment of cardiomyopathy. *Adv Intern Med.* 2001;47:1-45.
10. Wynne J, Braunwald E. The cardiomyopathies and myocardities. In: Braunwald E ZD, Libby P, ed. *Heart Disease.* 6th ed. Philadelphia: W.B. Saunders Company; 2001:1751-1799.
11. Felker GM, Thompson RE, Hare JM, et al. Underlying causes and long-term survival in patients with initially unexplained cardiomyopathy. *N Engl J Med.* 2000;342(15):1077-1084.
12. Lauer MS, Evans JC, Levy D. Prognostic implications of subclinical left ventricular dilatation and systolic dysfunction in men free of overt cardiovascular disease (the Framingham Heart Study). *Am J Cardiol.* 1992;70(13):1180-1184.
13. Lee TH, Hamilton MA, Stevenson LW, et al. Impact of left ventricular cavity size on survival in advanced heart failure. *Am J Cardiol.* 1993;72(9):672-676.
14. Semigran MJ, Thaik CM, Fifer MA, Boucher CA, Palacios IF, Dec GW. Exercise capacity and systolic and diastolic ventricular function after recovery from acute dilated cardiomyopathy. *J Am Coll Cardiol.* 1994;24(2):462-470.
15. Vigna C, Russo A, De Rito V, et al. Regional wall motion analysis by dobutamine stess echocardiography to distinguish between ischemic and nonischemic dilated cardiomyopathy. *Am Heart J.* 1996;131(3):537-543.
16. Khan IA. Left atrial thrombus in dilated cardiomyopathy. *Am J Geriatr Cardiol.* 2002;11(2):130.
17. Maze SS, Kotler MN, Parry WR. The contribution of color Doppler flow imaging to the assessment of a left ventricular thrombus. *Am Heart J.* 1988;115(2):479-482.
18. Delemarre BJ, Visser CA, Bot H, Dunning AJ. Prediction of apical thrombus formation in acute myocardial infarction based on left ventricular spatial flow pattern. *J Am Coll Cardiol.* 1990;15(2):355-360.
19. Chen C, Koschyk D, Hamm C, Sievers B, Kupper W, Bleifeld W. Usefulness of transesophageal echocardiography in identifying small left ventricular apical thrombus. *J Am Coll Cardiol.* 1993;21(1):208-215.
20. Thanigaraj S, Schechtman KB, Perez JE. Improved echocardiographic delineation of left ventricular thrombus with the use of intravenous second-generation contrast image enhancement. *J Am Soc Echocardiogr.* 1999;12(12):1022-1026.
21. Chen C, Rodriguez L, Guerrero JL, et al. Noninvasive estimation of the instantaneous first derivative of left ventricular pressure using continuous-wave Doppler echocardiography. *Circulation.* 1991;83(6):2101-2110.
22. Pinamonti B, Di Lenarda A, Sinagra G, Camerini F. Restrictive left ventricular filling pattern in dilated cardiomyopathy assessed by Doppler echocardiography: clinical, echocardiographic and hemodynamic correlations and prognostic implications. Heart Muscle Disease Study Group. *J Am Coll Cardiol.* 1993;22(3):808-815.
23. Nishimura RA, Appleton CP, Redfield MM, Ilstrup DM, Holmes DR Jr, Tajik AJ. Noninvasive Doppler echocardiographic evaluation of left ventricular filling pressures in patients with cardiomyopathies: a simultaneous Doppler echocardiographic and cardiac catheterization study. *J Am Coll Cardiol.* 1996;28(5):1226-1233.
24. Rihal CS, Nishimura RA, Hatle LK, Bailey KR, Tajik AJ. Systolic and diastolic dysfunction in patients with clinical diagnosis of dilated cardiomyopathy. Relation to symptoms and prognosis. *Circulation.* 1994;90(6):2772-2779.

25. Richartz BM, Werner GS, Ferrari M, Figulla HR. Comparison of left ventricular systolic and diastolic function in patients with idiopathic dilated cardiomyopathy and mild heart failure versus those with severe heart failure. *Am J Cardiol.* 2002;90(4): 390-394.
26. Shernan S, Zile M. A practical approach to the echocardiographic evaluation diastolic function. In: Perrino A, Reeves, S, eds. *A Practical Approach to Transesophageal Echocardiography.* Baltimore: Lippincott, Williams & Wilkins; 2003:110-130.
27. Djaiani GN, Shernan SK. Intraoperative assessment of diastolic function: utility of echocardiography. *Curr Opin Anaesthesiol.* 2003;16(1):11-19.
28. Rossi A, Cicoira M, Golia G, Anselmi M, Zardini P. Mitral regurgitation and left ventricular diastolic dysfunction similarly affect mitral and pulmonary vein flow Doppler parameters: the advantage of end-diastolic markers. *J Am Soc Echocardiogr.* 2001;14(6):562-568.
29. Otto CM. Echocardiographic evaluation of ventricular diastolic filling and function. In: Otto CM, ed. *Textbook of Clinical Echocardiography.* Philadelphia: W.B. Saunders; 2000:132-152.
30. Klein AL, Hatle LK, Burstow DJ, et al. Comprehensive Doppler assessment of right ventricular diastolic function in cardiac amyloidosis. *J Am Coll Cardiol.* 1990;15(1):99-108.
31. Nomura T, Lebowitz L, Koide Y, Keehn L, Oka Y. Evaluation of hepatic venous flow using transesophageal echocardiography in coronary artery bypass surgery: an index of right ventricular function. *J Cardiothorac Vasc Anesth.* 1995;9(1):9-17.
32. Yu CM, Sanderson JE, Chan S, Yeung L, Hung YT, Woo KS. Right ventricular diastolic dysfunction in heart failure. *Circulation.* 1996;93(8):1509-1514.
33. Boltwood CM, Tei C, Wong M, Shah PM. Quantitative echocardiography of the mitral complex in dilated cardiomyopathy: the mechanism of functional mitral regurgitation. *Circulation.* 1983;68(3):498-508.
34. Kono T, Sabbah HN, Stein PD, Brymer JF, Khaja F. Left ventricular shape as a determinant of functional mitral regurgitation in patients with severe heart failure secondary to either coronary artery disease or idiopathic dilated cardiomyopathy. *Am J Cardiol.* 1991;68(4):355-359.
35. Levine RA. Echocardiographic assessment of the cardiomyopathies. In: Weyman AE, ed. *Principles and Practice of Echocardiography.* Phildelphia: Lea & Febiger; 1994:781-823.
36. Aikawa K, Sheehan FH, Otto CM, Coady K, Bashein G, Bolson EL. The severity of functional mitral regurgitation depends on the shape of the mitral apparatus: a three-dimensional echo analysis. *J Heart Valve Dis.* 2002;11(5):627-636.
37. Kwan J, Shiota T, Agler DA, et al. Geometric differences of the mitral apparatus between ischemic and dilated cardiomyopathy with significant mitral regurgitation: real-time three-dimensional echocardiography study. *Circulation.* 2003;107(8): 1135-1140.
38. Radovanovic N, Petrovic LJ, Zorc M, et al. Changes in left ventricular morphology and function in end-stage dilated cardiomyopathy after reductive annuloplasty of double mitral and tricuspid orifices. *J Card Surg.* 2002;17(3):201-204.
39. Dini FL, Cortigiani L, Baldini U, et al. Prognostic value of left atrial enlargement in patients with idiopathic dilated cardiomyopathy and ischemic cardiomyopathy. *Am J Cardiol.* 2002;89(5):518-523.
40. Ghio S, Recusani F, Klersy C, et al. Prognostic usefulness of the tricuspid annular plane systolic excursion in patients with congestive heart failure secondary to idiopathic or ischemic dilated cardiomyopathy. *Am J Cardiol.* 2000;85(7):837-842.
41. Junker A, Thayssen P, Nielsen B, Andersen PE. The hemodynamic and prognostic significance of echo-Doppler-proven mitral regurgitation in patients with dilated cardiomyopathy. *Cardiology.* 1993;83(1-2):14-20.
42. Abramson SV, Burke JF, Kelly JJ Jr, et al. Pulmonary hypertension predicts mortality and morbidity in patients with dilated cardiomyopathy. *Ann Intern Med.* 1992;116(11):888-895.
43. Werner GS, Schaefer C, Dirks R, Figulla HR, Kreuzer H. Prognostic value of Doppler echocardiographic assessment of left ventricular filling in idiopathic dilated cardiomyopathy. *Am J Cardiol.* 1994;73(11):792-798.
44. Faris R, Coats AJ, Henein MY. Echocardiography-derived variables predict outcome in patients with nonischemic dilated cardiomyopathy with or without a restrictive filling pattern. *Am Heart J.* 2002;144(2):343-350.
45. Wigle ED, Rakowski H, Kimball BP, Williams WG. Hypertrophic cardiomyopathy. Clinical spectrum and treatment. *Circulation.* 1995;92(7):1680-1692.
46. Wigle ED. Cardiomyopathy: The diagnosis of hypertrophic cardiomyopathy. *Heart.* 2001;86(6):709-714.
47. Rezkalla SH, Kloner RA. Cardiomyopathy. *Cardiovasc Rev Rep.* 1991;12:53-66.
48. Lewis JF, Maron BJ. Clinical and morphologic expression of hypertrophic cardiomyopathy in patients > or = 65 years of age. *Am J Cardiol.* 1994;73(15):1105-1111.
49. Krasnow N. Subaortic septal bulge simulates hypertrophic cardiomyopathy by angulation of the septum with age, independent of focal hypertrophy. An echocardiographic study. *J Am Soc Echocardiogr.* 1997;10(5):545-555.
50. Nakatani S, Marwick TH, Lever HM, Thomas JD. Resting echocardiographic features of latent left ventricular outflow obstruction in hypertrophic cardiomyopathy. *Am J Cardiol.* 1996;78(6):662-667.
51. Lewis JF, Maron BJ. Hypertrophic cardiomyopathy characterized by marked hypertrophy of the posterior left ventricular free wall: significance and clinical implications. *J Am Coll Cardiol.* 1991;18(2):421-428.
52. Maron BJ, Clark CE, Henry WL, et al. Prevalence and characteristics of disproportionate ventricular septal thickening in patients with acquired or congenital heart diseases: echocardiographic and morphologic findings. *Circulation.* 1977;55(3); 489-496.
53. Otto CM. The cardiomyopathies, hypertensice heart disease, post-cardiac-tranplant patient, and pulmonary heart disease. In: Otto CM, ed. *Textbook of Clinical Echocardiography.* Philadelphia: W.B. Saunders; 2000:183-212.
54. Levine RA, Vlahakes GJ, Lefebvre X, et al. Papillary muscle displacement causes systolic anterior motion of the mitral valve. Experimental validation and insights into the mechanism of subaortic obstruction. *Circulation.* 1995;91(4): 1189-1195.
55. Jiang L, Levine RA, King ME, Weyman AE. An integrated mechanism for systolic anterior motion of the mitral valve in hypertrophic cardiomyopathy based on echocardiographic observations. *Am Heart J.* 1987;113(3):633-644.
56. Levine RA, Lefebvre X, Guerrero JL, et al. Unifying concepts of mitral valve function and disease: SAM, prolapse and ischemic mitral regurgitation. *J Cardiol.* 1994;24(38 Suppl): S157-169.

57. Lefebvre XP, He S, Levine RA, Yoganathan AP. Systolic anterior motion of the mitral valve in hypertrophic cardiomyopathy: an in vitro pulsatile flow study. *J Heart Valve Dis.* 1995;4(4):422-438.
58. Klues HG, Roberts WC, Maron BJ. Anomalous insertion of papillary muscle directly into anterior mitral leaflet in hypertrophic cardiomyopathy. Significance in producing left ventricular outflow obstruction. *Circulation.* 1991;84(3):1188-1197.
59. Pai RG, Jintapakorn W, Tanimoto M, Shah PM. Role of papillary muscle position and mitral valve structure in systolic anterior motion of the mitral leaflets in hyperdynamic left ventricular function. *Am J Cardiol.* 1995;76(8):623-628.
60. Schwammenthal E, Nakatani S, He S, et al. Mechanism of mitral regurgitation in hypertrophic cardiomyopathy: mismatch of posterior to anterior leaflet length and mobility. *Circulation.* 1998;98(9):856-865.
61. Klues HG, Roberts WC, Maron BJ. Morphological determinants of echocardiographic patterns of mitral valve systolic anterior motion in obstructive hypertrophic cardiomyopathy. *Circulation.* 1993;87(5):1570-1579.
62. Dellsperger KC, Marcus ML. Effects of left ventricular hypertrophy on the coronary circulation. *Am J Cardiol.* 1990;65(22):1504-1510.
63. Cannon RO 3rd, Dilsizian V, O'Gara PT, et al. Impact of surgical relief of outflow obstruction on thallium perfusion abnormalities in hypertrophic cardiomyopathy. *Circulation.* 1992;85(3):1039-1045.
64. Marwick TH, Stewart WJ, Lever HM, et al. Benefits of intraoperative echocardiography in the surgical management of hypertrophic cardiomyopathy. *J Am Coll Cardiol.* 1992;20(5):1066-1072.
65. Grigg LE, Wigle ED, Williams WG, Daniel LB, Rakowski H. Transesophageal Doppler echocardiography in obstructive hypertrophic cardiomyopathy: clarification of pathophysiology and importance in intraoperative decision making. *J Am Coll Cardiol.* 1992;20(1):42-52.
66. Roberts CS, Gertz SD, Klues HG, et al. Appearance of or persistence of severe mitral regurgitation without left ventricular outflow obstruction after partial ventricular septal myotomy-myectomy in hypertrophic cardiomyopathy. *Am J Cardiol.* 1991;68(17):1726-1728.
67. Glasson JR, Komeda MK, Daughters GT, et al. Three-dimensional regional dynamics of the normal mitral anulus during left ventricular ejection. *J Thorac Cardiovasc Surg.* 1996;111(3): 574-585.
68. Maslow AD, Regan MM, Haering JM, Johnson RG, Levine RA. Echocardiographic predictors of left ventricular outflow tract obstruction and systolic anterior motion of the mitral valve after mitral valve reconstruction for myxomatous valve disease. *J Am Coll Cardiol.* 1999;34(7):2096-2104.
69. Lee KS, Stewart WJ, Lever HM, Underwood PL, Cosgrove DM. Mechanism of outflow tract obstruction causing failed mitral valve repair. Anterior displacement of leaflet coaptation. *Circulation.* 1993;88(5 Pt 2):II24-29.
70. Matsui Y, Shiiya N, Murashita T, Sasaki S, Yasuda K. Mitral valve repair and septal myectomy for hypertrophic obstructive cardiomyopathy. *J Cardiovasc Surg (Torino).* 2000;41(1):53-56.
71. Swaminathan M, Debruijn NP, Glower DD, Mathew JP. Unexpected transesophageal echocardiographic finding after septal myectomy. *J Cardiothorac Vasc Anesth.* 2002;16(3):384-385.
72. Bartunek J, Sys SU, Rodrigues AC, van Schuerbeeck E, Mortier L, de Bruyne B. Abnormal systolic intraventricular flow velocities after valve replacement for aortic stenosis. Mechanisms, predictive factors, and prognostic significance. *Circulation.* 1996;93(4):712-719.
73. Kushwaha SS, Fallon JT, Fuster V. Restrictive cardiomyopathy. *N Engl J Med.* 1997;336(4):267-276.
74. Edwards WD. Endomyocardial biopsy and cardiomyopathy. *Cardiovasc Rev Rep.* 1990;11:26-43.
75. Katritsis D, Wilmshurst PT, Wendon JA, Davies MJ, Webb-Peploe MM. Primary restrictive cardiomyopathy: clinical and pathologic characteristics. *J Am Coll Cardiol.* 1991;18(5):1230-1235.
76. Patel AR, Dubrey SW, Mendes LA, et al. Right ventricular dilation in primary amyloidosis: an independent predictor of survival. *Am J Cardiol.* 1997;80(4):486-492.
77. Klein AL, Cohen GI. Doppler echocardiographic assessment of constrictive pericarditis, cardiac amyloidosis, and cardiac tamponade. *Cleve Clin J Med.* 1992;59(3):278-290.
78. Roberts WC, Waller BF. Cardiac amyloidosis causing cardiac dysfunction: analysis of 54 necropsy patients. *Am J Cardiol.* 1983;52(1):137-146.
79. Nishikawa H, Nishiyama S, Nishimura S, et al. Echocardiographic findings in nine patients with cardiac amyloidosis: their correlation with necropsy findings. *J Cardiol.* 1988;18(1):121-133.
80. Klein AL, Hatle LK, Taliercio CP, et al. Prognostic significance of Doppler measures of diastolic function in cardiac amyloidosis. A Doppler echocardiography study. *Circulation.* 1991;83(3): 808-816.
81. Siegel RJ, Shah PK, Fishbein MC. Idiopathic restrictive cardiomyopathy. *Circulation.* 1984;70(2):165-169.
82. Fauci AS, Harley JB, Roberts WC, Ferrans VJ, Gralnick HR, Bjornson BH. NIH conference. The idiopathic hypereosinophilic syndrome. Clinical, pathophysiologic, and therapeutic considerations. *Ann Intern Med.* 1982;97(1):78-92.
83. Furth PA, Futterweit W, Gorlin R. Refractory biventricular heart failure in secondary hemochromatosis. *Am J Med Sci.* 1985;290(5):209-213.
84. Valantine H, McKenna WJ, Nihoyannopoulos P, et al. Sarcoidosis: a pattern of clinical and morphological presentation. *Br Heart J.* 1987;57(3):256-263.
85. Klein AL, Cohen GI, Pietrolungo JF, et al. Differentiation of constrictive pericarditis from restrictive cardiomyopathy by Doppler transesophageal echocardiographic measurements of respiratory variations in pulmonary venous flow. *J Am Coll Cardiol.* 1993;22(7):1935-1943.
86. Poulsen SH, Jensen SE, Egstrup K. Longitudinal changes and prognostic implications of left ventricular diastolic function in first acute myocardial infarction. *Am Heart J.* 1999;137(5):910-918.
87. Poulsen SH, Jensen SE, Gotzsche O, Egstrup K. Evaluation and prognostic significance of left ventricular diastolic function assessed by Doppler echocardiography in the early phase of a first acute myocardial infarction. *Eur Heart J.* 1997;18(12):1882-1889.
88. Oechslin EN, Attenhofer Jost CH, Rojas JR, Kaufmann PA, Jenni R. Long-term follow-up of 34 adults with isolated left ventricular noncompaction: a distinct cardiomyopathy with poor prognosis. *J Am Coll Cardiol.* 2000;36(2):493-500.

89. Kovacevic-Preradovic T, Jenni R, Oechslin EN, Noll G, Seifert B, Attenhofer Jost CH. Isolated left ventricular noncompaction as a cause for heart failure and heart transplantation: a single center experience. *Cardiology.* 2009;112(2):158-164.
90. Burke A, Mont E, Kutys R, Virmani R. Left ventricular noncompaction: a pathological study of 14 cases. *Hum Pathol.* 2005;36(4):403-411.
91. Jenni R, Oechslin E, Schneider J, Attenhofer Jost C, Kaufmann PA. Echocardiographic and pathoanatomical characteristics of isolated left ventricular non-compaction: a step towards classification as a distinct cardiomyopathy. *Heart.* 2001;86(6):666-671.
92. Frischknecht BS, Attenhofer Jost CH, Oechslin EN, et al. Validation of noncompaction criteria in dilated cardiomyopathy, and valvular and hypertensive heart disease. *J Am Soc Echocardiogr.* 2005;18(8):865-872.
93. Chin TK, Perloff JK, Williams RG, Jue K, Mohrmann R. Isolated noncompaction of left ventricular myocardium. A study of eight cases. *Circulation.* 1990;82(2):507-513.
94. Murphy RT, Thaman R, Blanes JG, et al. Natural history and familial characteristics of isolated left ventricular noncompaction. *Eur Heart J.* 2005;26(2):187-192.
95. Petersen SE, Selvanayagam JB, Wiesmann F, et al. Left ventricular non-compaction: insights from cardiovascular magnetic resonance imaging. *J Am Coll Cardiol.* 2005;46(1):101-105.
96. Lofiego C, Biagini E, Pasquale F, et al. Wide spectrum of presentation and variable outcomes of isolated left ventricular non-compaction. *Heart.* 2007;93(1):65-71.
97. Corrado D, Fontaine G, Marcus FI, et al. Arrhythmogenic right ventricular dysplasia/cardiomyopathy: need for an international registry. Study Group on Arrhythmogenic Right Ventricular Dysplasia/Cardiomyopathy of the Working Groups on Myocardial and Pericardial Disease and Arrhythmias of the European Society of Cardiology and of the Scientific Council on Cardiomyopathies of the World Heart Federation. *Circulation.* 2000;101(11):E101-106.
98. Corrado D, Basso C, Schiavon M, Thiene G. Screening for hypertrophic cardiomyopathy in young athletes. *N Engl J Med.* 1998;339(6):364-369.
99. Hulot JS, Jouven X, Empana JP, Frank R, Fontaine G. Natural history and risk stratification of arrhythmogenic right ventricular dysplasia/cardiomyopathy. *Circulation.* 2004;110(14):1879-1884.
100. Dalal D, Nasir K, Bomma C, et al. Arrhythmogenic right ventricular dysplasia: a United States experience. *Circulation.* 2005;112(25):3823-3832.
101. Corrado D, Leoni L, Link MS, et al. Implantable cardioverter-defibrillator therapy for prevention of sudden death in patients with arrhythmogenic right ventricular cardiomyopathy/dysplasia. *Circulation.* 2003;108(25):3084-3091.
102. McKenna WJ, Thiene G, Nava A, et al. Diagnosis of arrhythmogenic right ventricular dysplasia/cardiomyopathy. Task Force of the Working Group Myocardial and Pericardial Disease of the European Society of Cardiology and of the Scientific Council on Cardiomyopathies of the International Society and Federation of Cardiology. *Br Heart J.* 1994;71(3):215-218.
103. Jaoude SA, Leclercq JF, Coumel P. Progressive ECG changes in arrhythmogenic right ventricular disease. Evidence for an evolving disease. *Eur Heart J.* 1996;17(11):1717-1722.
104. Nava A, Bauce B, Basso C, et al. Clinical profile and long-term follow-up of 37 families with arrhythmogenic right ventricular cardiomyopathy. *J Am Coll Cardiol.* 2000;36(7):2226-2233.
105. Yoerger DM, Marcus F, Sherrill D, et al. Echocardiographic findings in patients meeting task force criteria for arrhythmogenic right ventricular dysplasia: new insights from the multidisciplinary study of right ventricular dysplasia. *J Am Coll Cardiol.* 2005;45(6):860-865.
106. Zipes DP, Camm AJ, Borggrefe M, et al. ACC/AHA/ESC 2006 guidelines for management of patients with ventricular arrhythmias and the prevention of sudden cardiac death: a report of the American College of Cardiology/American Heart Association Task Force and the European Society of Cardiology Committee for Practice Guidelines (Writing Committee to Develop Guidelines for Management of Patients With Ventricular Arrhythmias and the Prevention of Sudden Cardiac Death). *J Am Coll Cardiol.* 2006;48(5):e247-346.
107. Virani SS, Khan AN, Mendoza CE, Ferreira AC, de Marchena E. Takotsubo cardiomyopathy, or broken-heart syndrome. Tex Heart Inst J. 2007;34(1):76-9.
108. Seth PS, Aurigemma GP, Krasnow JM, Tighe DA, Untereker WJ, Meyer TE. A Syndrome of Transient Left Ventricular Apical Wall Motion Abnormality in the Absence of Coronary Disease: A Perspective from the United States. Cardiology, 2003;100:61-66
109. Dote K, Sato H, Tateishi H, Uchida T, Ishihara MJ. Myocardial stunning due to simultaneous multivessel coronary spasms: a review of 5 cases J Cardiol. 1991;21(2):203-14.
110. Ako J, Takenaka K, Uno K, Nakamura F, Shoji T, Iijima K, Ohike Y, Kim S, Watanabe T, Yoshizumi M, Ouchi Y. Reversible left ventricular systolic dysfunction--reversibility of coronary microvascular abnormality. Jpn Heart J. 2001 May;42(3):355-63.
111. Tsuchihashi K, Ueshima K, Uchida T, Oh-mura N, Kimura K, Owa M, Yoshiyama M, Miyazaki S, Haze K, Ogawa H, Honda T, Hase M, Kai R, Morii I; Transient left ventricular apical ballooning without coronary artery stenosis: a novel heart syndrome mimicking acute myocardial infarction. Angina Pectoris-Myocardial Infarction Investigations in Japan. J Am Coll Cardiol. 2001 Jul;38(1):11-8.
112. Mori H, Ishikawa S, Kojima S, Hayashi J, Watanabe Y, Hoffman JI, Okino H. Increased responsiveness of left ventricular apical myocardium to adrenergic stimuli. Cardiovasc Res. 1993 Feb;27(2):192-8.
113. Ennezat PV, Pesenti-Rossi D, Aubert JM, Rachenne V, Bauchart JJ, Auffray JL, Logeart D, Cohen-Solal A, Asseman P. Transient left ventricular basal dysfunction without coronary stenosis in acute cerebral disorders: a novel heart syndrome (inverted Takotsubo). Echocardiography. 2005 Aug;22(7):599-602.
114. Sanchez-Recalde A, Costero O, Oliver JM, Iborra C, Ruiz E, Sobrino JA. Images in cardiovascular medicine. Pheochromocytoma-related cardiomyopathy: inverted Takotsubo contractile pattern. Circulation. 2006 May 2;113(17):738-9.
115. Sharkey SW, Windenburg DC, Lesser JR, Maron MS, Hauser RG, Lesser JN, Haas TS, Hodges JS, Maron BJ. Natural history and expansive clinical profile of stress (tako-tsubo) cardiomyopathy. J Am Coll Cardiol 2010 Jan 26;55(4):333-41

REVIEW QUESTIONS

Select the ONE BEST answer for each item.

1. Which one of the following primary cardiomyopathies is most common?
   a. Dilated
   b. Hypertrophic
   c. Infiltrative
   d. Restrictive

2. Dilated cardiomyopathy can typically be distinguished from other primary cardiomyopathies by the presence of which one of the following?
   a. Decreased ejection fraction
   b. Impaired left ventricular relaxation
   c. Decreased end-diastolic volume
   d. Mitral regurgitation

3. Which one of the following locations is the most common site for the development of thrombi in patients with dilated cardiomyopathy?
   a. Main pulmonary artery
   b. Left atrium
   c. Left ventricular apex
   d. Right atrial appendage

4. All of the following factors are associated with decreased 5-year survival following the initial diagnosis of dilated cardiomyopathy *except*:
   a. Biventricular dysfunction
   b. Childhood onset
   c. Delayed initiation of therapy
   d. Increased extent of cardiac remodeling

5. What percentage of patients with dilated cardiomyopathy will die within 2 years?
   a. 20% to 25%
   b. 45% to 50%
   c. 70% to 75%
   d. 90% to 95%

6. What percentage of patients with dilated cardiomyopathy improve spontaneously?
   a. 20% to 25%
   b. 45% to 50%
   c. 70% to 75%
   d. 90% to 95%

7. Idiopathic dilated cardiomyopathy can most commonly be distinguished from ischemic cardiomyopathy by which one of the following characteristics?
   a. Absence of coronary artery disease
   b. Angina
   c. Improvement in regional ventricular wall motion following dobutamine
   d. Symmetric and globally reduced ventricular wall motion

8. Which one of the following echocardiographic findings pertaining to left ventricular dilatation in patients with dilated cardiomyopathy is correct?
   a. Basal diameter exceeds midventricular diameter.
   b. Decreased end-systolic diameter.
   c. Diminished relative wall thickness.
   d. Left ventricular dilatation is usually less than right ventricular dilatation.

9. Which of the following echocardiographic findings is most consistent with a diagnosis of right ventricular dilatation?
   a. Apex-forming right ventricle
   b. Hepatic vein Doppler flow velocity reversal during systole
   c. Right ventricular free wall akinesis
   d. Tricuspid regurgitation

10. Which of one the following echocardiographic findings is fundamental to the diagnosis of dilated cardiomyopathy?
    a. Left ventricular end-systolic diameter less than 4 cm^2
    b. Left ventricular ejection fraction less than 45%
    c. Right ventricular dilatation
    d. Severe mitral regurgitation

11. Which one of the following echocardiographic findings is consistent with the greatest risk for systemic embolization of thrombus?
    a. Dilated left atrium
    b. Left atrial appendage laminated thrombus
    c. Protuberant left ventricular apical thrombus
    d. Spontaneous contrast in the left ventricle

12. Diagnostic echocardiographic criteria for identifying a left ventricular thrombus in a patient with dilated cardiomyopathy include all of the following, *except*:
    a. Demarcation by a clear thrombus-blood interface
    b. Normal transmitral Doppler flow velocity profile
    c. Usual location adjacent to but distinct from abnormally contracting myocardium
    d. Visualization in at least two planes

13. In patients with dilated cardiomyopathy, impaired left ventricular relaxation is indicated by which one of the following characteristics of the transmitral Doppler flow velocity profile?
    a. Decreased A-wave velocity
    b. Decreased isovolumic relaxation time
    c. Increased deceleration time
    d. Increased E-wave velocity

14. In patients with dilated cardiomyopathy, impaired left ventricular relaxation is indicated by which one of the following characteristics of the pulmonary venous Doppler flow velocity profile?
    a. Atrial reversal component duration exceeding the transmitral A-wave duration
    b. Atrial reversal velocity greater than 35 cm/s
    c. Peak diastolic velocity less than peak systolic velocity
    d. Systolic flow reversal

15. In patients with dilated cardiomyopathy, mitral regurgitation is most commonly due to which one of the following mechanisms?
    a. Apical displacement of the coaptation point
    b. Mitral annular calcification
    c. Posterior leaflet prolapse
    d. Systolic anterior motion

16. All of the following echocardiographic findings have been correlated with a worse outcome in patients with dilated cardiomyopathy, *except*:
    a. Decreased left ventricular end-systolic volumes following dobutamine
    b. Increased tricuspid regurgitation peak Doppler flow velocity
    c. Restrictive transmitral Doppler flow velocity profile
    d. Severe mitral regurgitation

17. In patients with dilated cardiomyopathy, decreased right ventricular compliance is indicated by which one of the following echocardiographic findings?
    a. Increased transtricuspid E-wave deceleration time
    b. Inferior vena cava diameter less than 1.5 cm^2
    c. Decreased transtricuspid peak E-wave velocity
    d. Predominant hepatic vein V- and A-wave reversals during spontaneous inspiration

18. In patients with dilated cardiomyopathy, which one of the following most likely accounts for the relative increased incidence of thrombi found in the left ventricle compared to the left atrium?
    a. Atrial fibrillation
    b. Concurrent left ventricular apical myocardial infarction
    c. Decreased left atrial compliance
    d. Protective effect of mitral regurgitation

19. All of the following echocardiographic findings are commonly associated with dilated cardiomyopathy, *except*:
    a. Dilated left atrium
    b. Impaired left ventricular relaxation
    c. Focal regional wall motion abnormalities
    d. Mitral regurgitation

20. Etiologies for the development of dilated cardiomyopathy include all of the following, *except*:
    a. Familial linkage
    b. Autoimmunity
    c. Systemic hypertension
    d. Viral myocarditis

21. Primary cardiomyopathies:
    a. Can be associated with coronary artery narrowing
    b. Are associated with systemic disease
    c. Are commonly found in the general population
    d. Always involve all four chambers
    e. Are always associated with diastolic dysfunction

22. True statements regarding primary cardiomyopathies include all of the following, *except*:
    a. They overlap with each other with respect to clinical symptoms.
    b. All may have diastolic dysfunction.
    c. All may have systolic dysfunction.
    d. They are associated with a systemic disease.
    e. The incidence in the general population is less than 1%.

23. All patients with hypertrophic cardiomyopathy have a globally hypertrophied ventricle.
    a. True
    b. False

24. Approximately 25% of patients with hypertrophic cardiomyopathy have left ventricular outflow tract obstruction.
    a. True
    b. False

25. All of the following contribute to systolic anterior motion and left ventricular outflow tract obstruction, *except*:
    a. Posterior mitral annular calcification
    b. Septal hypertrophy
    c. Elongated mitral leaflets
    d. Direction of ventricular inflow
    e. Posterior shift of papillary muscle

26. The incidence of HCM/HOCM in the general population is:
    a. Less than 1%
    b. Less than restrictive/infiltrative cardiomyopathy
    c. Greater than 10%
    d. Between 1% and 10%
    e. Greater than for dilated cardiomyopathy

27. Genetic testing for patients with HCM/HOCM:
    a. Has found abnormalities on only one gene
    b. Is performed in all patients
    c. Has found mutations on at least nine genes
    d. Has not revealed any genetic abnormalities
    e. Is routinely performed in all family members of patients with HCM/HOCM

28. All patients with ventricular hypertrophy:
    a. Have a primary cardiomyopathy
    b. Have an asymmetric pattern of hypertrophy
    c. Have aortic stenosis and/or systemic hypertension
    d. Have involvement of the interatrial septum
    e. Are more likely to have echocardiographic evidence of diastolic dysfunction

29. All of the following are true *except*:
    a. Hypertrophic cardiomyopathy may be symptomatic or asymptomatic.
    b. Diastolic dysfunction is found in the majority of patients with ventricular hypertrophy.
    c. Systolic outflow obstruction can be dynamic and episodic.
    d. Restrictive filling is found only in restrictive cardiomyopathy.
    e. Varying degrees of diastolic dysfunction are found in patients with hypertrophy.

30. Hypertrophic cardiomyopathy:
    a. Incidence is greatest in the elderly patient
    b. Incidence is greatest in patients under 10 years old
    c. Can occur only after the second decade
    d. Is more commonly discovered between the 2nd and 5th decades
    e. Does not predict risk of complications

31. Risk factors for sudden death in hypertrophic cardiomyopathy include all of the following, *except*:
    a. Personal or family history of syncope
    b. Presence of left ventricular outflow tract obstruction
    c. Young patients
    d. Severe left ventricular hypertrophy (>20-mm thickness)
    e. A reduction in blood pressure with exercise

32. Relationships between the mitral coaptation point and the left ventricular outflow tract that predispose to outflow tract obstruction include:
    a. Distance between the mitral coaptation point and the ventricular septum 25 mm or less
    b. Mitral inflow/aortic outflow angle of less than 30°
    c. Relative lengths of the anterior and posterior leaflets of greater than 2.0:1.0
    d. Distance between the mitral annulus and septum less than 25 mm
    e. Posterior displacement of the coaptation point

33. For hypertrophic cardiomyopathies, coronary ischemia may be due to all of the following, *except*:
    a. Hypertrophy of the coronary arteries
    b. Elevated intraventricular pressures
    c. Coronary artery aneurysm and thrombosis
    d. Coronary atheromatous disease
    e. Reduced coronary vasodilatory reserve

34. Which of the following is least likely to be performed as a primary treatment in patients with hypertrophic cardiomyopathy?
    a. Mitral valve replacement with a bioprosthetic valve
    b. Placement of an internal cardiac defibrillator
    c. Mitral valve repair
    d. Surgical resection of the hypertrophic ventricular septum
    e. Administration of antibiotic prophylaxis

35. True statements regarding hypereosinophilic syndrome include all of the following, *except*:
    a. It is also known as Loffler endocarditis.
    b. It is continuous with endomyocardial fibrosis (ie, same disease).
    c. It is known to cause endocardial thickening of the mitral and tricuspid annuli.
    d. It is associated with significant systolic dysfunction.
    e. Endocardial thickening is associated with obliteration of the ventricular apex.

36. Differential diagnosis of restrictive filling defect include all of the following, *except*:
    a. Myocardial ischemia/infarct
    b. Cardiac amyloidosis
    c. Mitral regurgitation
    d. Hypereosinophilic syndrome
    e. End-stage aortic stenosis

37. Histologic examination of hypertrophic cardiomyopathy may include all of the following, *except*:
    a. Myocardial disarray
    b. Myocardial fibrosis

c. Myocardial hypertrophy
d. Amyloid infiltration
e. Asymmetric distribution of hypertrophy

38. Doppler data suggestive of restrictive filling pattern include all except:
a. Transmitral deceleration time less than 150 milliseconds
b. Isovolumic relaxation time less than 80 milliseconds
c. Transmitral early to late filling fraction ratio (E/A) less than 0.70
d. Pulmonary venous systolic to diastolic inflow ratio (E/A) of less than 0.5
e. Pulmonary venous atrial reversal (A_{rev}) velocity greater than 35 cm/s

39. Which of the following statements is true regarding patients with hypertrophic cardiomyopathy?
a. Hypertrophy is frequently found in the right ventricle.
b. Hypertrophy is not found in the inferolateral wall.
c. Hypertrophy is typically asymmetric with greater involvement of the septum.
d. Hypertrophy typically involves the interatrial septum.

40. Which of the following statements is true regarding patients with hypertrophic cardiomyopathy?
a. Coronary arteries may exhibit abnormal concentric thickening.
b. Always coexists with pulmonary hypertension.
c. It is inherited as an autosomal recessive trait with variable expression.
d. Diastolic dysfunction occurs in 25% of patients.

41. In patients with hypertrophic cardiomyopathy, ventricular hypertrophy can involve:
a. Basilar septum
b. Inferolateral wall
c. Mid-cavity
d. Apex
e. All of the above

42. Which of the following echocardiogarphic findings is most likely associated with hypertrophic cardiomyopathy?
a. Increased intracavitary dimensions
b. Decreased systolic function
c. Symmetric ventricular hypertrophy
d. Systolic anterior motion of the mitral valve

43. Which of the following statements is true regarding echocardiographic evidence of left ventricular out flow tract obstruction?
a. M-mode demonstrates late closure of the aortic valve.
b. M-mode demonstrates premature opening of the aortic valve.
c. M-mode demonstrates late opening of the aortic valve.
d. M-mode demonstrates premature closure of the aortic valve.

44. Which of the following statement is true regarding patients with hypertrophic cardiomyopathy?
a. Ventricular dysrhythmias are the main cause of death.
b. Left ventricular outflow obstruction has been directly related the sudden death.
c. Left ventricular outflow obstruction is directly related to arrhythmias.
d. The annual mortality rate ranges from 0.5% to 1%.

45. Which of the following increases the risk of sudden death in patients with hypertrophic cardiomyopathy?
a. LVOT gradient of 35 mm Hg
b. Reduction in blood pressure during exercise
c. LV hypertrophy of 20 mm
d. Old age

46. With regard to systolic anterior motion of the mitral valve and outflow tract obstruction:
a. It is found in approximately 70% of patients with hypertrophic cardiomyopathy.
b. It has different mechanisms across different populations.
c. It is related, in part, to abnormalities of the mitral apparatus.
d. The Bernoulli effect is responsible for outflow tract obstruction.

47. M-mode echocardiography is useful for the evaluation of hypertrophic cardiomyopathy by detecting or measuring:
a. Ventricular diastolic function
b. Ventricular wall thickness
c. Mitral insufficiency when combined with color Doppler
d. Aortic insufficiency when combined with color Doppler evaluation of the left ventricular outflow tract

48. True statements regarding diastolic dysfunction include:
a. It occurs in all patients with hypertrophic cardiomyopathy.
b. Doppler assessment is often affected by changes in loading conditions.

c. It is always associated with systolic dysfunction.
d. It occurs in 25% of patients with restrictive cardiomyopathy.

49. Which of the following is associated with a restrictive cardiomyopathy?
a. Myocarditis
b. Friedreich ataxia
c. Lead poisoning
d. Cardiac hemochromatosis

50. Typical echocardiographic features in patients with restrictive cardiomyopathy include:
a. Left ventricular free-wall thickening
b. Right ventricular free-wall thickening
c. Decreased LV systolic function
d. Normal right and left atrial size

51. The typical mitral inflow velocity in patients with restrictive cardiomyopathy includes:
a. Short IVRT, tall E wave, short DT
b. Short IVRT, short E wave, short DT
c. Short IVRT, tall E wave, long DT
d. Short IVRT, short E wave, long DT

52. The prognosis for patients with cardiac amyloidosis is:
a. Poor for patients with a pulmonary venous systolic/diastolic inflow ratio less than 0.5
b. Poor for patients with LV wall thickness in diastole greater than 15 mm
c. Poor for patients with a transmitral deceleration time less than 140 milliseconds
d. All of the above

53. When differentiating cardiac amyloidosis from other causes of restrictive patterns:
a. Speckling or a "starry-skied" appearance of the myocardium is found only in patients with amyloidosis.
b. Left ventricular systolic dysfunction is more likely to be present in amyloidosis.
c. Involvement of the interatrial septum is strongly suggestive of amyloid infiltration.
d. Dilation of the atria is diagnostic of amyloidosis.

54. In patients with amyloid infiltration of the heart:
a. The incidence of left ventricular systolic dysfunction is not related to wall thickness.
b. Left ventricular systolic dysfunction is present in 70% of cases.
c. Left ventricular dilation is present in less than 10% of cases with systolic dysfunction.
d. Biventricular dilation is an end-stage event.

55. Cardiac involvement in hemochromatosis:
a. Commonly presents with restrictive pathophysiology
b. Is commonly seen without other organ system involvement
c. Uncommonly contributes to mortality
d. Is associated with systolic dysfunction and chamber enlargement

56. Which of the following statements is correct regarding constrictive pericarditis and restrictive cardiomyopathy?
a. Both have a similar clinical presentation.
b. Both have decreased LV systolic function.
c. Both have the same pattern of impaired diastolic filling.
d. Both are associated with pulmonary hypertension.

57. Echocardiographic data that differentiate constrictive pericarditis from restrictive cardiomyopathy include:
a. Respiratory variation of transmitral and pulmonary venous flows
b. Presence of a thickened and/or calcified pericardium
c. Normal-appearing interatrial septum
d. All of the above

58. Intracardiac thrombi may occur:
a. With all three categories of cardiomyopathy
b. With abnormalities of the endocardium due to infiltrative diseases
c. In the dilated and dysfunctional atrium
d. In areas of low flow velocity (<25 cm/s)
e. All of the above

Pericardial Diseases

15

Nikolaos J. Skubas and Manuel L. Fontes

Pericardial diseases constitute pathologic processes that involve the pericardium, the pericardial sac and its contents, and the thoracic structures surrounding the heart. Cardiovascular perturbations associated with pericardial disease range from the asymptomatic electrocardiographic findings in uremic pericarditis to catastrophic circulatory collapse observed in the setting of acute hemorrhagic pericardial tamponade. The clinical features of pericardial diseases may resemble right-side failure, notably right ventricular (RV) failure and tricuspid insufficiency, but can also present as left-side failure manifesting as shortness of breath, reduced exercise tolerance, and multiorgan hypoperfusion. However, clinical management of pericardial pathology may differ significantly from that of ventricular dysfunction or valvular heart disease. As a consequence, timely diagnosis and initiation of appropriate medical or surgical therapy is imperative. This chapter deals specifically with the clinical utility of transesophageal echocardiography (TEE) in the evaluation, diagnosis, and characterization of pericardial disease including constrictive pericarditis and cardiac tamponade.

PERICARDIAL ANATOMY AND PHYSIOLOGY

The pericardium consists of three layers: a fibrous layer that blends with the adventitia of the great vessels and systemic and pulmonary venous inflows, a parietal layer lining the inner surface of the fibrous pericardium, and a visceral layer lining the epicardium.[1] The visceral component is made up of a single layer of mesothelial cells, is attached to the surface of the heart and epicardial fat, and regulates the production of pericardial fluid (normally 5 to 30 mL may be seen in the pericardial space).[2] This layer also reflects back on itself to line the outer fibrous layer forming the parietal pericardium.[1] The latter is composed of collagen fibers meshed with elastic fibers that allow considerable flexibility of the pericardium during childhood and early adult years, although this elasticity is lost with advancing age. The pericardial space conforms to the shape of the heart, and extends superiorly for a short distance along the great vessels to form a small pocket posteriorly, known as the *transverse sinus*. Similarly, the *oblique sinus* is formed by an extension of the pericardium posterior to the left atrium between the pulmonary veins. The function of the pericardium includes protection of the heart from the spread of infection or malignancy from surrounding structures, reduction of friction between the heart and the adjacent tissues, control of hydrostatic forces on the heart, prevention of acute chamber dilatation, and maintenance of diastolic coupling between the ventricles.[2]

PERICARDITIS

Despite its ability to isolate the heart from direct extension of infectious and noninfectious pathogens, pericardial inflammation occurs in nearly 5% of the population according to autopsy findings, but is clinically detected in fewer than 0.1% of hospital admissions.[3] The causes of pericarditis are numerous: idiopathic, infectious (viral, tuberculosis, acute bacterial, fungal, toxoplasmosis, or amebiasis), acute myocardial infarction, uremia, neoplastic disease, radiation, autoimmune (acute rheumatic fever, systemic lupus erythematosus, or rheumatoid arthritis), sarcoidosis, amyloidosis, drugs (hydralazine, procainamide, phenytoin, or penicillin), trauma, postcardiotomy for cardiac surgery, dissecting aortic aneurysm, myxedema, and chylopericardium.[4] Most cases tend to be idiopathic or viral in origin and produce pathologic findings consistent with acute inflammation. These findings include infiltration with lymphocytes, polymorphonuclear neutrophils, and macrophages; alterations in pericardial vascularity; deposition of fibrin; and increase in pericardial fluid content that, depending on the rate of accumulation and the amount of exudate fluid within the pericardial sac, can result in clinical features of cardiac tamponade.[5] Following the acute inflammatory phase, fibrous adhesions may be present between the pericardium and the epicardium, pleura, sternum, and any other tissues contiguous with the pericardium.[6] In constrictive pericarditis the two pericardial layers are not necessarily thickened, but they are always fused together. As the pericardial compliance decreases, increases in tissue oxygen demand can be met only by increases in heart rate because stroke volume is fixed or progressively declining.

CONSTRICTIVE PERICARDITIS

The symptomatology associated with constrictive pericarditis is dependent on the cause and severity of acute pericarditis, the degree of progression to chronic constrictive pericarditis, and the limitation to chamber filling. Most often, patients complain of retrosternal chest pain that is extremely variable in intensity and quality and may be suggestive of acute abdomen or myocardial ischemia. Frequently, patients find relief by sitting up and bending forward. In contrast, lying supine, coughing, or deep breathing exacerbates the pain. Notable findings on physical examination include a pericardial rub, distant heart sounds, increased jugular venous pressure, edema, ascites, and Kussmaul's sign (increased right atrial pressure with inspiration resulting in a paradoxical elevation in jugular venous distention). The physical findings often are indistinguishable from those of severe RV dysfunction and tricuspid insufficiency: liver congestion, abdominal ascites, and lower extremity edema. The electrocardiogram typically demonstrates diffuse ST-segment concave elevation (without reciprocal ST-segment depression as seen in myocardial ischemia). However, these ST changes are detected primarily during the early stages of pericarditis. In addition, the electrocardiogram may have a low-voltage pattern. In chronic pericarditis, the chest radiographs may show calcification of the pericardium principally on lateral views with a normal cardiac silhouette, or there may be evidence of cardiomegaly (Figure 15–1). In addition, large pleural effusions may be seen.

In constrictive pericarditis, the diastolic filling is impaired, and the total cardiac volume is decreased. Ventricular and atrial volume changes are governed by the noncompliant pericardium, not by the compliance of the chambers. Because of the pericardial constriction, ventricular filling is characterized by an early rapid increase in diastolic pressure such that the pressure gradient between atrium and ventricle dissipates abruptly and filling terminates (plateaus) in early diastole. On a ventricular pressure waveform, this characteristic finding of constrictive pericarditis is referred to as the *dip and plateau* or *square-root sign* (Figure 15–2).[7-11] Similarly, recording of the central venous tracing exhibits the classic "M" or "W" pattern in which the V wave is enhanced secondary to noncompliance of the atrium arising from pericardial constraint.[7,8] Increased right atrial (RA) pressures also lead to a rapid *y* descent, reflecting abrupt emptying of the atrium with tricuspid valve opening. In all, the prominent features of constrictive pericarditis include a fused pericardium, a relatively fixed intracardiac volume, and equalization of diastolic chamber pressures. That is, the central venous pressure (CVP) equalizes with the RA pressure, the RV end-diastolic pressure, the left atrial (LA) pressure, and the left ventricular (LV) end-diastolic pressure,

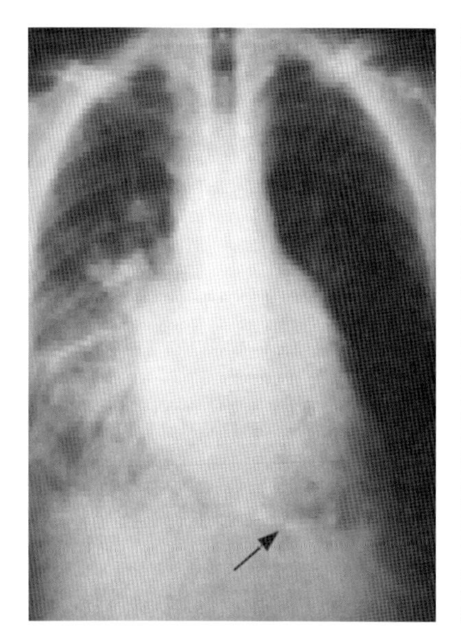

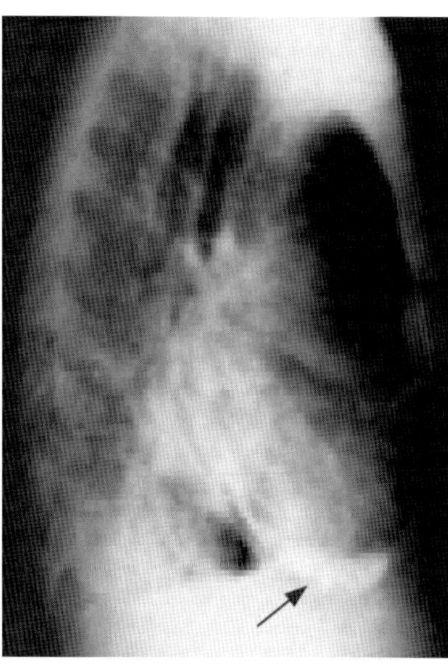

FIGURE 15–1. Chest radiograph (*left*, anterior-posterior; *right*, lateral) showing calcified pericardium *(arrows)*.

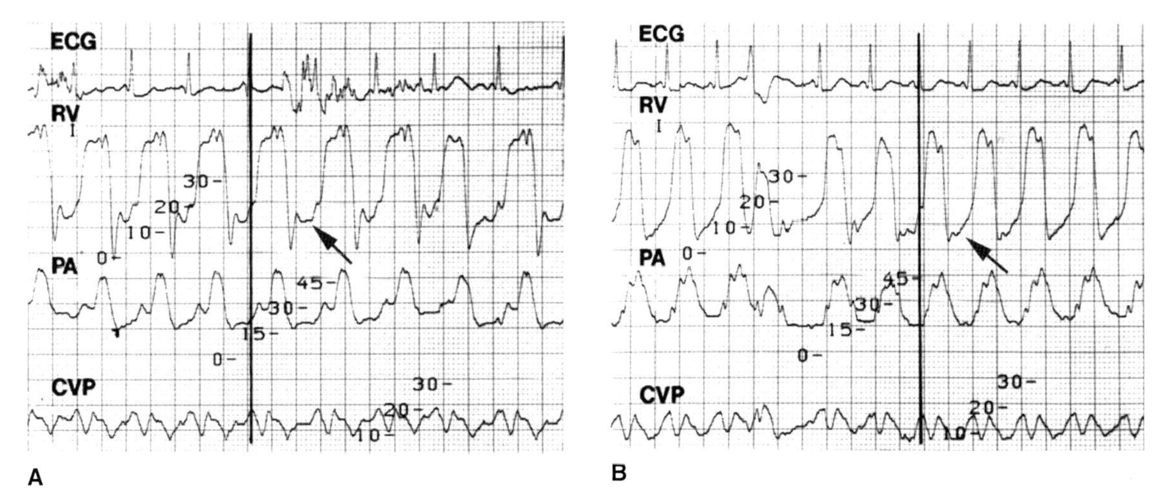

FIGURE 15–2. Hemodynamic tracings in a patient with constrictive pericarditis. **A:** Before pericardiectomy. **B:** After pericardiectomy. Before pericardiectomy, the diastolic right ventricular tracing shows a characteristic abrupt rise in diastolic pressure followed by a plateau (square-root sign) demonstrating equalization of right ventricular and atrial pressures *(arrow)*, which disappeared after pericardiectomy. (CVP, central venous pressure; ECG, electrocardiogram; PA, pulmonary artery pressure; RV, right ventricular pressure.) *(Reproduced with permission from Skubas NJ, Beardslee M, Barzilai B, Pasque M, Kattapuram M, Lappas DG. Constrictive pericarditis: intraoperative hemodynamic and echocardiographic evaluation of cardiac filling dynamics. Anesthesia and Analgesia 2001;92:1424.)*

or its surrogate, the pulmonary artery occlusion pressure (PAOP).

Two-Dimensional Echocardiography

The echocardiographic assessment of thickened pericardium by the transthoracic approach is often limited and is diagnostic in less than one third of cases of constrictive pericarditis. In contrast, two-dimensional TEE examination can identify pericardial thickening in constrictive pericarditis in nearly 90% of cases.[12] A comprehensive TEE approach has the advantage of better image resolution and enhanced definition of the pericardial interface with fat, fluid, and surrounding tissue that is comparable to ultrafast computer tomography and magnetic resonance imaging techniques (Figure 15–3).[13,14] Normally, the pericardium is an echo-dense line, 1 to 2 mm in thickness, separated from the myocardium by an area of lucency (fluid or pericardial fat). Pericardial thickening appears as increased echogenicity on two-dimensional echo and as multiple parallel reflections at the surface of the LV on M-mode.

Midesophageal (ME) four-chamber, ME two-chamber, ME long-axis (LAX), deep transgastric, and transgastric short-axis views allow for imaging of LV and RV walls and surrounding pericardium. The pericardium should be examined for echo-density, homogeneity, and thickening. Thickness of the pericardium is measured from the outer border of the myocardium to the outer edge of the pericardium, avoiding areas of echolucent space between the two borders, with a pericardium

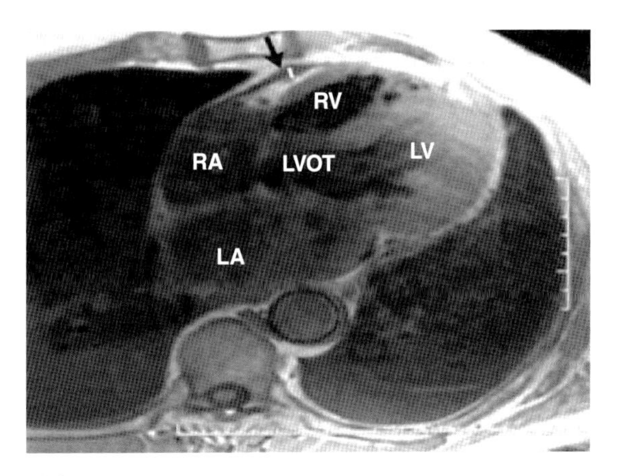

FIGURE 15–3. Constrictive pericarditis by magnetic resonance imaging. Segmental pericardial thickening is seen anteriorly, just above the right ventricle *(arrow)*. (RA, right atrium; RV, right ventricle; LA, left atrium; LV, left ventricle; LVOT, left ventricular outflow tract)

thicker than 3 mm considered abnormal.[15,16] Multiple measurements should be performed to obtain an average thickness, and multiple views of the pericardium should be imaged because pericardial thickening may be asymmetric in distribution. This heterogeneity of pericardial involvement accounts for some of the limitations in diagnosing and detecting pericardial disease when using TTE. Additional features of the echocardiographic examination that assist in the diagnosis of constrictive pericarditis include abnormal interventricular septal motion (see below) and atrial compression by the thickened pericardium.

Examination of the venous inflow to the right and left heart (vena cava and pulmonary veins) also may assist in the diagnosis of pericardial disease. As previously described, by advancing the probe to the ME depth and optimizing the view of LA and RA separated by the interatrial septum, the bicaval view can be imaged by rotating the multiplane angle forward to 90°. The inferior vena cava (IVC) will appear on the top left of the screen as it enters the atrium. Maintaining this view while advancing the probe more distally into the esophagus will demonstrate the entire length of the IVC and the intrahepatic veins as they enter the IVC. A dilated and nonpulsatile IVC is a nonspecific indicator of constrictive pericarditis.[7] Moreover, a decrease with spontaneous inspiration in IVC diameter of less than 50% at the junction of the RA is a marker of elevated RA pressure. Similarly, variations in pulmonary vein flow velocities with respiration (see below) aid in the diagnosis of constriction.

M-mode

On TTE M-mode echocardiography, diagnostic features in constrictive pericarditis, include pericardial thickening, flattening of the LV inferolateral wall during mid- to late diastole, LA enlargement, abnormal diastolic and systolic motions of the interventricular septum, atrial systolic notch (a posterior rather than the normal anterior interventricular septal motion occurring after the onset of electrocardiographic P wave that terminates before the QRS complex), and premature pulmonic valve closure.[17] Diastolic septal motion is related primarily to the trans-septal pressure gradient, which in constrictive pericarditis is derived from the abrupt filling of the ventricles. Therefore, during the early phase of diastole, the interventricular septum can exhibit a sudden posterior deflection followed by a more gradual posterior septal motion occurring later in diastole (atrial systolic notch). Whereas these findings may be apparent in constrictive pericarditis, Engel and associates reported a low sensitivity in the diagnosis of constrictive pericarditis with the use of M-mode.[17] In a series of 40 patients with a diagnosis of constrictive pericarditis confirmed by hemodynamic criteria, surgical examination, or necropsy, the most common findings by M-mode were abnormal septal motion and flattening of the LV inferolateral wall motion in diastole.[17] However, posterior septal motion abnormality is seen in other pathologic states including RV volume overload, ischemic heart disease, and in the setting of cardiac surgery. Although the use of M-mode may have limitations in the assessment of constrictive pericarditis, in general, all patients with this pathology will display abnormal findings on M-mode. Thus, M-mode should be considered an adjunct to other modalities of echocardiographic diagnosis of constrictive pericarditis.

Pulsed-Wave Doppler

Doppler examination of flow dynamics is often diagnostic of constrictive pericarditis and is an important adjunct in differentiating pericardial processes from myocardial pathology associated with diastolic dysfunction. The Doppler findings characterize the flow dynamics due to the rigid, noncompliant pericardium encompassing both ventricles, minimizing their diastolic volume, exaggerating their interdependence, and isolating them from intrathoracic respiratory changes. RV and LV diastolic inflow velocities show high early inflow velocities (E wave) consistent with rapid early filling and rapid equalization of pressures. This is a reflection of the restraining effect of the thickened pericardium and of the decreased filling of the ventricles in mid- to late diastole. The mitral and tricuspid late inflow velocities (A wave) are extremely low or virtually absent, as in a restrictive filling pattern, with the atrial contraction contributing little to LV filling. In addition, the deceleration time of the E velocity is short.

In constrictive pericarditis, pulmonary vein flow dynamics should correlate with the expected findings of pericardial impediment of atrial filling during ventricular systole (blunting of the S wave), followed by relatively larger diastolic flow (D wave). Although the D wave is greater in magnitude than the S, it also becomes limited by poor chamber compliance during the latter part of diastole as ventricular pressure rapidly equilibrates with atrial pressure. Consequently, atrial contraction will have little to no contribution to ventricular filling, resulting in redirection of blood flow from the atrium to the pulmonary vein depicted as a larger A wave.[18] However, the clinical validity of Doppler findings is highly dependent on the ultrasonographer's technical expertise, the clinical setting at the time of the examination (ie, loading conditions), and, more importantly, its confirmation or support of other clinical or echocardiographic correlates of the underlying pathophysiology.

The aforementioned findings are highly influenced by respiratory variations and by ventricular interaction (please refer to the Cardiac Tamponade section for additional details). Normally, decreases in intrathoracic pressure with spontaneous inhalation are transmitted to the heart and the pulmonary veins. In healthy, spontaneously ventilating subjects, this decreased intrathoracic pressure results in *minor* decreases in pulmonary vein to LA pressure gradient, resulting in mild decrease in LV filling (<10% to 15% fluctuation of the mitral inflow E wave).[19] In constrictive pericarditis, the thickened pericardium isolates the intrapericardial cardiac chambers (but not the extrapericardially located pulmonary veins) from changes in intrathoracic pressure during the respiratory cycle. As a result, mitral inflow E and pulmonary vein D velocities decrease during inspiration. This decrease in diastolic flow is due to a significant decrease in the pressure gradient between the pulmonary vein and the LA. During spontaneous exhalation, mitral inflow E and pulmonary vein D velocities increase (>25% compared with the inspiratory values) as intrathoracic pressure rises and the flow of blood previously pooled in the lungs during inspiration increases.[20,21] Reciprocal changes are seen on the right side of the heart such that RV filling increases with spontaneous inspiration and decreases with exhalation. A variation greater than 25% between inspiratory and expiratory velocities on the right side is also indicative of constrictive pericarditis. In addition, prominent hepatic vein diastolic flow reversal may be noticed as a result of increased RA pressure.

As compared with spontaneous breathing, positive pressure ventilation reverses the respiratory variation of mitral inflow and pulmonary vein inflow velocities in subjects with constrictive pericarditis.[22] Relative to exhalation, a mechanical breath increases the intrathoracic pressure, leading to greater mitral inflow E and pulmonary vein D velocities during Doppler examination.

Increased respiratory variation in mitral inflow E velocities in conjunction with pulmonary vein inflow velocity variation is virtually pathognomonic for constrictive pericarditis (Figure 15–4).[7] This is an important finding that helps to distinguish constrictive pericarditis from restrictive cardiomyopathy in which there is no respiratory variation in velocities, as well as no pericardial thickening. Of note, there is a subset of patients with constrictive pericarditis who do not exhibit respiratory variation, namely those with atrial fibrillation or severely elevated LA pressures.

Tissue Doppler

Doppler tissue imaging of the lateral mitral annulus in the ME four-chamber view allows the measurement of myocardial wall velocities. The diastolic E′ and

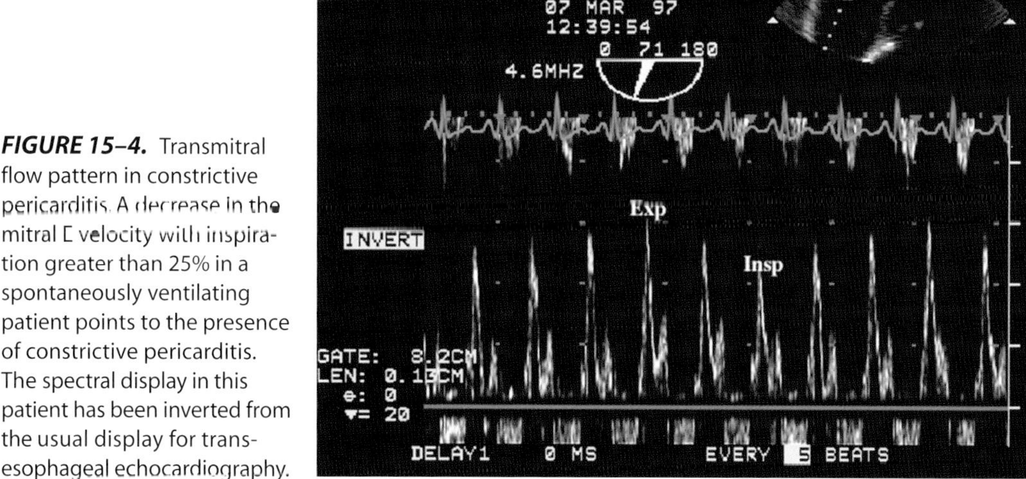

FIGURE 15–4. Transmitral flow pattern in constrictive pericarditis. A decrease in the mitral E velocity with inspiration greater than 25% in a spontaneously ventilating patient points to the presence of constrictive pericarditis. The spectral display in this patient has been inverted from the usual display for transesophageal echocardiography.

A′ velocities of Doppler tissue parallel transmitral E and A velocities, but are relatively independent of preload (see Chapter 12). Doppler tissue velocities reflect LV expansion and contraction and therefore aid in differentiating constrictive pericarditis from restrictive cardiomyopathy. In constrictive pericarditis, E′ tends to be preserved (>8 cm/s) despite increased LV filling pressure, whereas a significantly decreased E′ (<8 cm/s) is evident in restrictive cardiomyopathy.[18,23] To offset the decreased lateral expansion imposed by the thickened pericardium, the preserved E′ in constrictive pericarditis represents a greater longitudinal expansion of the myocardium.

CARDIAC TAMPONADE

The syndrome of acute cardiac compression was first described in 1935 as Beck's triad: hypotension, increased jugular venous pressure, and muffled heart sounds. Cardiac tamponade is defined as significant compression of the heart by accumulating pericardial contents. These contents include blood and clots (postcardiotomy, chamber perforation, dissecting aortic aneurysm, trauma, or anticoagulant therapy), exudative effusions (malignant states, infective pericarditis, or idiopathic pericarditis), nonexudative effusions (uremia, systemic lupus erythematosus, rheumatoid arthritis, idiopathic, or radiation), and air. Any pericardial effusion or collection can advance to cardiac tamponade; pericardial collection is a pathophysiologic continuum that, at one extreme, may be clinically insignificant or, at the other extreme, may present as a life-threatening condition requiring emergent surgical attention, irrespective of the amount of pericardial contents. Any pericardial content that exceeds the ability of the pericardium to expand will result in positive transmural pressure, which overcomes the distending pressure of the cardiac chambers and impairs diastolic filling.

Normally, about 5 to 30 mL of pericardial fluid is found inside the pericardial space—an amount sufficient for detection by echocardiography. The physiologic effect of fluid in the pericardial space depends not only on the volume but also on the rate of accumulation. Slowly expanding effusions can become quite large (>1000 mL) with very little increase in pericardial pressure and no symptomatology. Conversely, rapid accumulations of very small volumes (50 to 100 mL) or a strategically located mass can lead to marked elevations in pericardial pressure and clinical decompensation.[24]

Once pericardial collection exceeds the ability of pericardium to expand, the total intrapericardial volume (fluid/content and cardiac structures and volume) becomes constant throughout the cardiac cycle. Because the intracardiac pressures vary during the cardiac cycle, the compressive effects of a pericardial fluid collection are seen first on low-pressure chambers, ie, atria during atrial relaxation (ie, ventricular systole) and ventricles during diastole. Therefore, systolic atrial inversion will be noticed before diastolic RV outflow tract compression. An increasing pericardial pressure also will equilibrate more rapidly with the pressures of the thinner-walled right heart than with the pressures of the left heart.[25,26] Coronary blood flow is reduced in cardiac tamponade, but this reduction is not sufficient to add an ischemic injury to the myocardium. In the absence of coronary artery disease there is a proportionate decrease in both ventricular preload (decreased chamber filling) and afterload. As a consequence, myocardial work and oxygen consumption are reduced. However, patients with preexistent coronary artery disease may be at increased risk for myocardial ischemia and/or infarction.

Under normal conditions, ventricular interaction is extremely important for maintenance of adequate cardiac performance. The average stroke volume of the RV equals the stroke volume of the LV; however, respiration causes cyclical differences in LV and RV stroke volumes. During spontaneous inspiration, negative intrapleural pressure facilitates venous return to the right heart. At the same time venous return to the left heart is diminished because (1) lung expansion increases the pulmonary venous blood volume and (2) increase in RV filling causes the interventricular septum to "bulge" leftward, thereby reducing LV dimension and altering its compliance and filling (ventricular interaction/interdependence). During spontaneous exhalation, the reverse process occurs. This ventricular interdependence is exaggerated in cardiac tamponade, because the total cardiac volume is limited by the pressurized pericardial content. As the intrapericardial content increases, it reaches a point at which the parietal pericardium cannot stretch commensurate with the rising pressure. Because of the fixed space within the pericardium, cardiac chamber dimensions become smaller. Thus, the normal effects of respiration will be pronounced: the increased extra-intrathoracic pressure gradient during spontaneous inspiration favors filling of RV at the expense of LV filling, while there is more LV filling during spontaneous exhalation (when there is less RV filling).

Echocardiographic studies of patients with cardiac tamponade have described phasic respiratory changes in which LV filling (and mitral valve excursions) decreased during inspiration.[25] In contrast, RV dimensions increased in association with a shifting of the interventricular septum toward the LV. In the case of cardiac tamponade, ventricular interaction involves not only the interventricular septum but also other cardiac chambers, depending on the etiology of the tamponade (fluid vs clot; regional vs global tamponade). Therefore, the magnitude of diastolic changes is related to the severity of pericardial fluid collection, chamber pressure and volume, and transpulmonary pressures during inspiration and exhalation. Overall, the physiology of ventricular interaction in clinical cardiac tamponade becomes more complex as the pressure-volume relation of mediastinal and chest structures is altered with each heartbeat and by respiratory and neuroendocrine influences.

Normally, there is an inspiratory decrease of less than 10 mm Hg in the arterial systolic pressure and an accompanying inspiratory decrease in the venous pressure. However, in patients with tamponade, there is *pulsus paradoxus*: an inspiratory decrease of arterial pressure greater than 10 mm Hg with venous pressure that remains steady or increases.[27] The magnitude of paradoxical pulse is directly proportional to the inspiratory (spontaneous breathing) decrease of LV dimension, diastolic volume, and stroke volume. Of importance, pulsus paradoxus and the phasic respiratory changes in ventricular dimensions are not unique to cardiac tamponade. These changes can be present in constrictive pericarditis and in a variety of clinical conditions in which intrapleural pressure is significantly diminished, such as respiratory distress, airway obstruction, chronic obstructive pulmonary disease, and pulmonary embolism. Of note, this clinical feature of cardiac tamponade may be absent in patients with chest wall trauma, neuromuscular disease, and pneumothorax because they cannot produce sufficient negative intrapleural pressure during inspiration to produce changes in chamber dimension and decrease in LV stroke volume. Similarly, those under positive pressure mechanical ventilation or with severe aortic regurgitation may or may not exhibit hemodynamic findings suggestive of pulsus paradoxus.

In the setting of cardiac surgery, cardiac tamponade can occur acutely over minutes or hours or after a few days postoperatively. The reported incidence of acute cardiac tamponade is 0.5% to 5.8%.[28,29] The typical patient has significant chest tube drainage (>200 mL/h) in the immediate postoperative period with or without hemodynamic signs of inadequate cardiac output. Alternatively, the chest tubes may become obstructed by blood clots, thus impeding mediastinal drainage. Delayed tamponade has been defined arbitrarily as cardiac tamponade occurring more than 5 to 7 days after pericardiotomy.[25,28,29] The incidence is 0.3% to 2.6% and is often misdiagnosed because of a low index of suspicion or because the clinical signs and symptoms are similar to those of congestive heart failure, pulmonary embolism, and generalized fatigue (ie, failure to thrive postoperatively).

Thus, diagnosis of cardiac tamponade after cardiac surgery is often difficult and requires a high degree of clinical suspicion, proficient knowledge of pulmonary artery catheter derived hemodynamics, physical examination, and use of diagnostic tools such as echocardiography, chest roentgenography, and magnetic resonance imaging (Figure 15–5). Relying on a single diagnostic modality can lead to inaccurate management and increased patient morbidity. The classic teaching of equalization of diastolic blood pressures in cardiac tamponade (CVP = PA diastolic pressure = PAOP) is infrequently observed postoperatively because the pericardium is left open. As such, blood and clot do not distribute around the heart homogeneously to produce equalization of pericardial diastolic pressures. In general, CVP is elevated, but PA diastolic pressure and the PAOP can be normal, elevated, or, in some cases, decreased.

Regional cardiac tamponade occurs when one or more cardiac chambers are compressed. Postoperative RA hematomas often become localized to the anterior and lateral walls, whereas LA clots are found more commonly behind the left atrium in the oblique sinus.[30] After cardiotomy, diastolic regional collapse of RA or RV is the most common echocardiographic finding in "early" cardiac tamponade.[29-31] However, Russo and

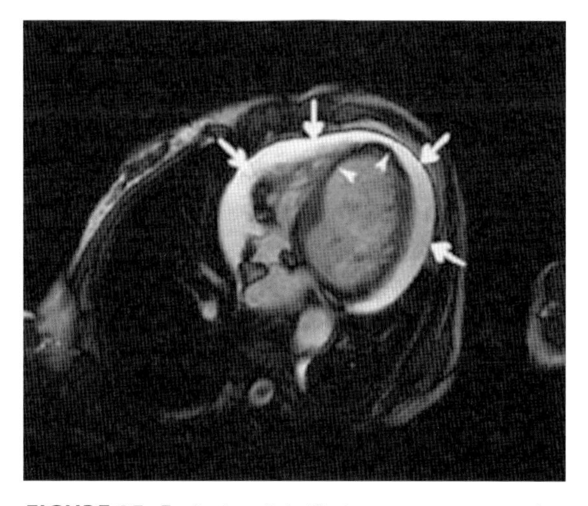

FIGURE 15–5. Pericardial effusion seen on magnetic resonance imaging. The pericardium is distended *(large white arrows)* and separated from the surface of the heart *(small arrows)* by a fluid collection.

colleagues found that only 33% of patients with the diagnosis of cardiac tamponade had right heart catheterization findings that reflected equalization of diastolic blood pressures.[32] Overall, 90% of patients with postcardiotomy cardiac tamponade had atypical clinical, hemodynamic, or echocardiographic findings. Therefore, the diagnosis of postoperative cardiac tamponade should be considered whenever hemodynamic deterioration is encountered, particularly when reduction in cardiac output and blood pressure are not readily responsive to conventional management. Selective compression of the right heart by hematoma becomes less prominent in "delayed" tamponade as the right heart becomes adherent or tethered to the anterior chest wall. The clinical presentation in such a case may be mistaken for congestive heart failure, acute LV or RV infarction, septic shock, or pulmonary embolism. In delayed tamponade, the complaints tend to be vague, and fewer hemodynamic data are available (ie, pulmonary artery catheter) to allow prompt diagnosis of tamponade.

Although transthoracic echocardiography (TTE) is generally less invasive than TEE, imaging constraints in the post–cardiac surgical patient often leads to inconclusive diagnosis (see below). In contrast, TEE can be very helpful in diagnosis and clinical management of tamponade. Electrocardiography and chest roentgenography are adjunct diagnostic techniques. Electrocardiographic changes seen with cardiac tamponade include nonspecific ST- and T-wave abnormalities, low-voltage QRS complex, signs of myocardial ischemia and pericarditis, and *electrical alternans*.[33] The latter is seen in patients with large effusions and is characterized by beat-to-beat shifts in the electrical axis. This beat-to-beat alteration may be due to the increased distance between the heart and the chest wall, resulting in a "pendulum"-like motion of the heart.[25,33] However, it has been shown that minimal amount of pericardial fluid removal abolishes electrical alternans despite an enlarged pericardial space. Thus, the electrocardiographic changes of electrical alternans may reflect a hemodynamic pathology rather than an anatomic abnormality. This finding, although sensitive for cardiac tamponade, is not very specific (very few patients with tamponade present with electrical alternans).

On standard anterior-posterior chest roentgenography, the cardiac silhouette may appear normal in size or extremely enlarged depending on the acuity of the tamponade process. With large effusions, the cardiac silhouette will appear "widened" with or without features such as obscuring of the pulmonary vessels at the hilum and a globular or "water bottle" configuration of the heart.

Two-Dimensional Echocardiography

Several echocardiographic features of cardiac tamponade may be detected by TTE and TEE: (1) diminished LV dimension (and mitral valve excursion) during inspiration, (2) shift of the interventricular septum toward the LV, (3) changes in transvalvular (mitral and aortic) flow characteristics seen by Doppler techniques (see below), (4) diastolic posterior motion of the RV wall, and (5) in some cases, a systolic notch on the RV epicardium. Although many of the signs on a roentgenogram or echocardiogram can be suggestive of cardiac tamponade, it should be remembered that no finding by itself is 100% sensitive and specific.

TTE can be compromised by postoperative factors: the surgical site may preclude use of an optimal transthoracic window, chest tubes affect imaging and proper positioning of the patient, compression of the chest wall with the TTE probe may worsen incisional pain, and some loculated effusions may not be amenable to TTE imaging. TEE can overcome many of these imaging constraints. Pericardial effusions can be readily seen and graded, and pericardial blood clots can be visualized to compress the atria and the ventricle.

Detection of pericardial effusion with two-dimensional imaging may commence by advancing the TEE probe to obtain a transgastric midpapillary short-axis (SAX) view at 0° and assess for the presence of an echolucent fluid-filled space surrounding one or both ventricles (Figure 15–6). Hemorrhagic or purulent fluid is more echogenic than serous collections. Often, fibrin strands are visible. Of note, the absence of pericardial contents around the LV should not necessarily exclude the absence of pericardial collection around other heart structures such as the RV. RV and LV function should be assessed in this view. When the effusion is significant, ventricular function can be depressed if the pericardial pressure overwhelms ventricular diastolic pressures to the point that myocardial blood flow is reduced. Next, the transgastric two-chamber and long-axis (LAX) views are obtained by rotating the probe to about 90° to 110°. In these views, the anterior and inferior walls of the LV are visualized and, if present, a pericardial collection appears as an echolucent space separating the aforementioned LV walls from the parietal pericardium. In all transgastric views, in the absence of previous surgery or pericardial disease, any pericardial effusion will be diffuse, with clear separation between the parietal and visceral pericardia. Diffuse collections are visualized first posterior to the heart, as the patient is usually supine during examination, and when small they are seen in systole only. Pericardial effusions are

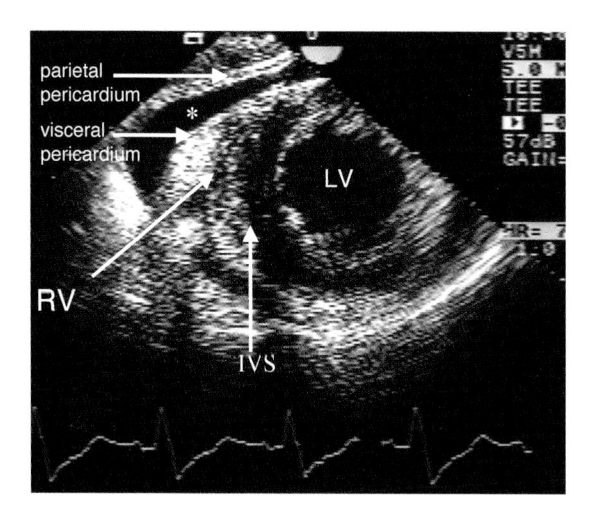

FIGURE 15–6. Pericardial effusion detected on the midpapillary short-axis view. The right ventricle is almost obliterated and its cavity is barely visible. Around both ventricles, there is an echolucent space filled with fluid *(asterisk)*. The visceral pericardium is indistinguishable from the epicardial surface of the two ventricles. The parietal pericardium is the outer border of the pericardial effusion. The distance between the two pericardial layers is 1.3 cm, so the pericardial fluid collection is graded as moderate. Notice the absence of electrical alternans in the electrocardiographic tracing at the bottom of the picture. (IVS, interventricular septum; RV, right ventricle; LV, left ventricle.)

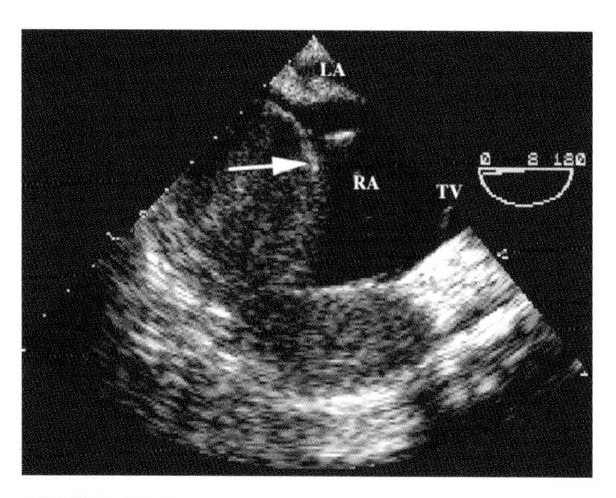

FIGURE 15–7. Right atrial compression by a large localized thrombus in a modified midesophageal four-chamber view. The arrow points to the invagination in the right atrium wall created by the thrombus. Particularly in the post–cardiac surgical setting, loculated pericardial collections can form around the right or left atrium, restrict ventricular filling, and cause hemodynamic collapse. (LA, left atrium; RA, right atrium; TV, tricuspid valve.)

graded as minimal (50 to 100 mL) if the visceral and parietal pericardial layers are separated by less than 0.5 cm in *diastole*, small (100 to 250 mL) if separated by 0.5 to 1.0 cm, moderate (250 to 500 mL) if separated by 1.0 to 2 cm, and large (>500 mL) when greater than 2 cm.[34] The absence of pericardial effusion in the transgastric views should not limit further echocardiographic examination because loculated pericardial collections (Figure 15–7) can exist around the RA or the LA (seen in the ME four-chamber view or the ME bicaval view). In the latter view, one can perform an M-mode examination through the RA free wall, to identify systolic RA free wall inversion or collapse. The same can be done in the ME LAX view to diagnose RV outflow tract diastolic collapse. Significant pericardial effusion may also dilate potential spaces formed by the pericardial folds, such as the transverse sinus (Figure 15–8), found between the posterior ascending aorta and the anterior LA wall (visualized in the ME LAX view, where one can see that the left atrium and ascending aorta are not next to each other but are separated by the dilated transverse sinus).

RA Collapse

The RA is a thin and flexible structure and, under normal conditions, brief wall inversion can occur. As a consequence, the specificity of RA systolic collapse for tamponade increases when systolic compression persists for one-third or longer of the duration of the cardiac cycle.[28] Atrial compression has a 95% sensitivity, 100% specificity, and positive predictive value of 90%.[30] It is best visualized by TTE on parasternal LAX and apical four-chamber views; on TEE, the ME four-chamber view (Figure 15–9) or the ME bicaval views are recommended. RA systolic collapse is a sensitive sign in the diagnosis of tamponade and is best evaluated by using M-mode through the RA (Figure 15–10).

RV Collapse

RV collapse may occur when the pericardial pressure exceeds RV pressure. This typically occurs during diastole, when the RV pressure is at its lowest. Diastolic RV collapse is more specific than RA collapse for confirming tamponade[35] and can be identified by an abnormal posterior inward motion of the anterior RV wall during diastole (Figure 15–11).[30,36] Timing of collapse may be

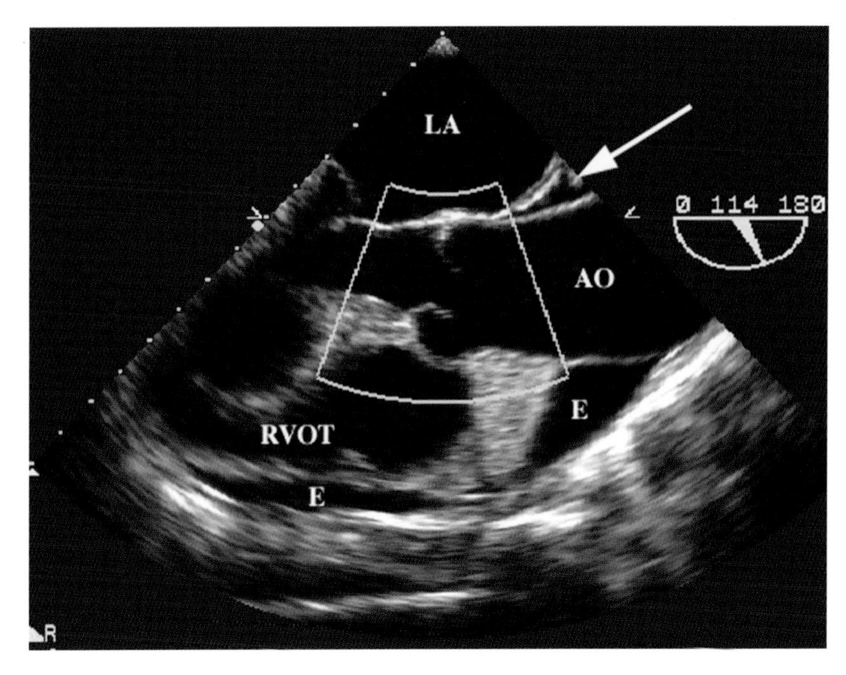

FIGURE 15–8. In this midesophageal long-axis view, pericardial effusion compresses the free wall of the right ventricle and the right ventricular outflow tract. The transverse sinus *(arrow)*, a potential space created by the pericardial folds between the left atrium and the ascending aorta, is also filled with pericardial fluid. In large pericardial effusions, this space can be markedly dilated and serve as a helpful diagnostic finding. (AO, ascending aorta; E, effusion; LA, left atrium; RVOT, right ventricular outflow tract.)

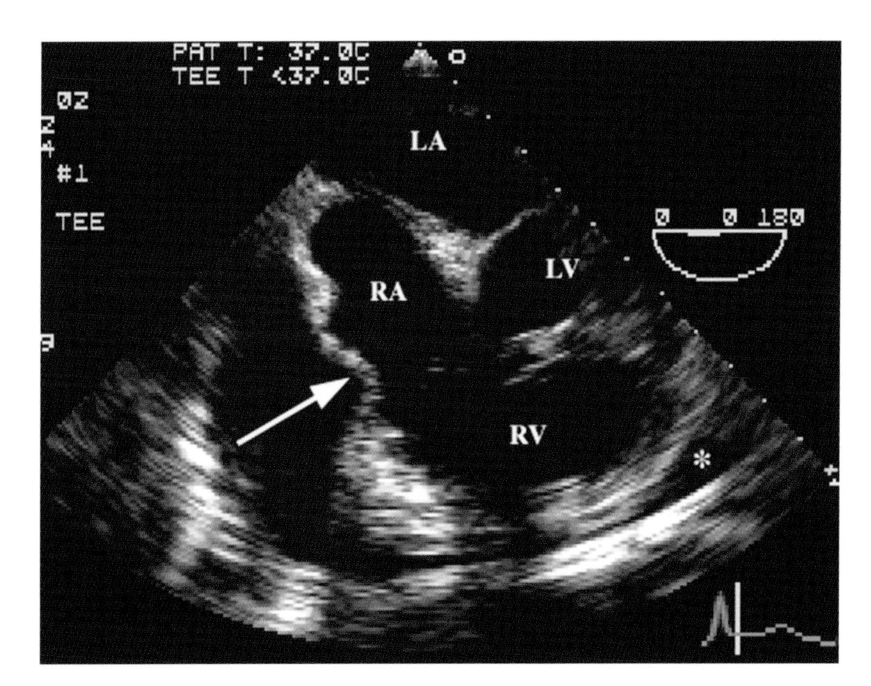

FIGURE 15–9. Right atrial collapse. The left atrium, right atrium, right ventricle, and left ventricle are seen in a midesophageal four-chamber view with the probe rotated toward the right atrium. There is pericardial effusion around the heart (*asterisk*, outside the free wall of the right ventricle). The picture is significant because the free wall of the right atrium is inverted *(white arrow)* during systole *(white mark on the electrocardiograph at the bottom of the echo display)*. Systolic right atrial collapse should always raise the suspicion of hemodynamically significant pericardial fluid collection. (LA, left atrium; LV, left ventricle; RA, right atrium; RV, right ventricle.)

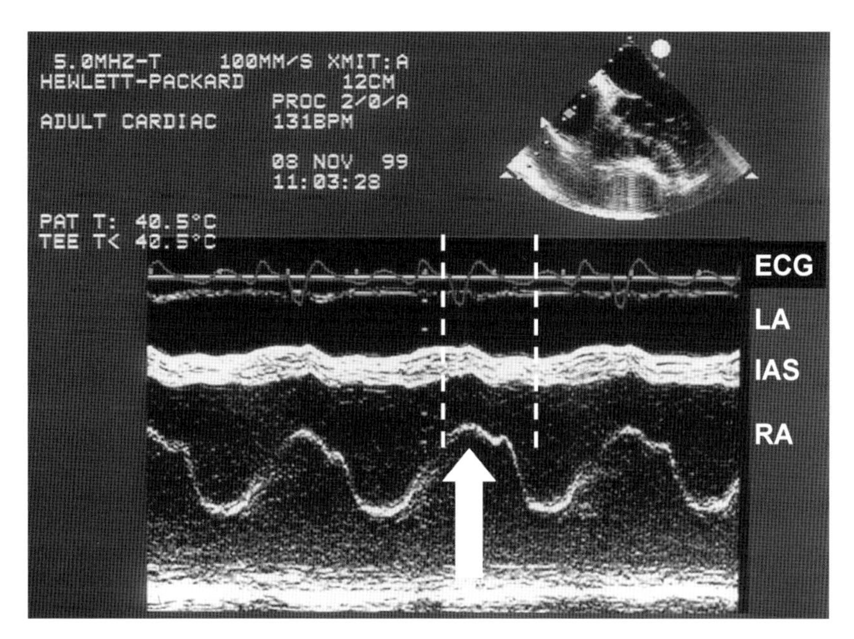

FIGURE 15–10. M-mode image of right atrial free wall compression in cardiac tamponade. While in the transesophageal echocardiographic midesophageal four-chamber view, the cursor line is positioned so that it transects the left atrium, interatrial septum, and the free wall of the right atrium. Dashed lines coincide with the systolic interval on the electrocardiographic tracing. The inward motion of the right atrial free wall during systole is apparent. Although this may be normal if short lived, it is indicative of cardiac tamponade if the duration of the inward motion lasts longer than one-third of the systolic period *(white arrow)*. (IAS, interatrial septum; LA, left atrium; RA, right atrium.)

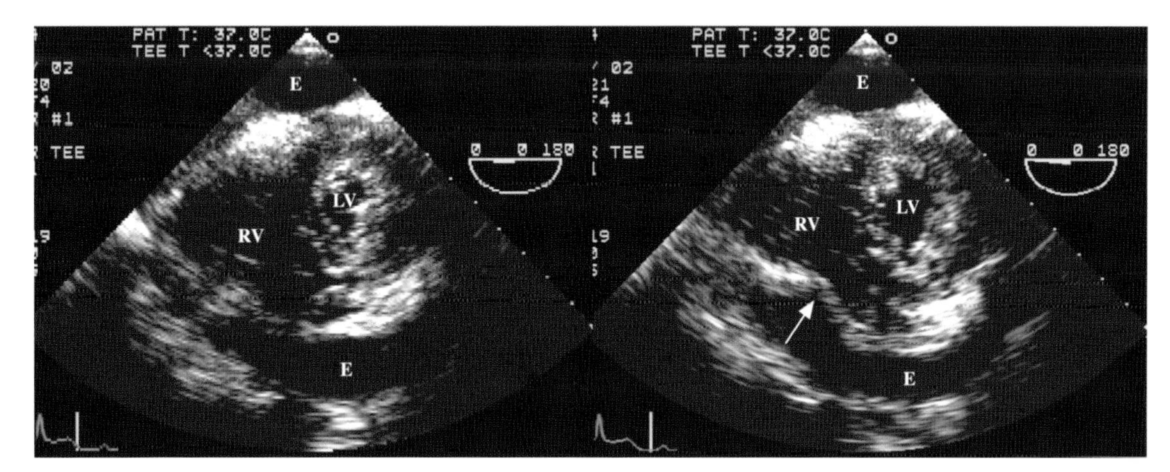

FIGURE 15–11 Right ventricular diastolic collapse. The left and right ventricles are seen in a transgastric short-axis view with a large pericardial effusion detected anteriorly and posteriorly. In the left panel, the right ventricle is seen at end-systole; in the right panel, the right ventricle is inverted during diastole *(arrow)*. (E, effusion; LV, left ventricle; RV, right ventricle.)

Table 15–1. Echocardiographic Findings in Cardiac Tamponade, Constrictive Pericarditis, and Restrictive Cardiomyopathy

	Cardiac Tamponade	Constrictive Pericarditis	Restrictive Cardiomyopathy
2D	Moderate to large pericardial effusion	Pericardial thickening, sometimes (20%-30%) with calcification	Normal pericardium, thickened LV
	RA, LA, and RV free wall inversion (collapse)	Small RA and LA	Major enlargement of RA and LA
	IVC plethora	IVS moves toward the LV during spontaneous inspiration	Relatively little IVS movement in most cases
Doppler			
LV Inflow	Respiratory variation present: spontaneous exhalation E > inspiration E	E variation: spontaneous exhalation > inspiration by ≥25%	Little respiratory variation, E:A ≥2.0, DT <160 ms
PV Flow	Respiratory variation present: spontaneous exhalation D > inspiration D	D variation: exhalation > inspiration by ≥25%, S:D >1.0	Little respiratory variation, S:D <1.0
MV Annulus Tissue Velocities		E′ >8.0 cm/s	E′ <8.0 cm/s

2D, two-dimensional; A, late diastolic wave of mitral inflow; D, diastolic wave of pulmonary vein flow; DT, deceleration time; E, early diastolic wave of mitral inflow; E′, early diastolic myocardial tissue velocity; IVC, inferior vena cava; IVS, interventricular septum; LA, left atrium; LV, left ventricle; MV, mitral valve; PV, pulmonary vein; RA, right atrium; RV, right ventricle; S, systolic wave of pulmonary vein flow.

more apparent on the M-mode recording, provided the M-mode cursor line can intersect the RV free wall. RV collapse lasting more than one-third of diastole is a specific sign for cardiac tamponade.[5]

It is important to note that RV collapse may not occur in the presence of RV hypertrophy or with significantly elevated RV end-diastolic pressures (as is the case in pulmonary hypertension, where significant elevation of pericardial pressure is required before RV collapses). Further, cardiac tamponade may exist without evidence of chamber collapse if the mechanical compression arises from a regional process such as blood clot. Such a scenario is common postoperatively or may develop from recurrent episodes of pericarditis complicated by loculated pericardial effusions.

Pulsed-Wave Doppler

Cardiac tamponade reduces compliance of the various cardiac chambers affecting filling and their systolic and diastolic function. As such, transvalvular and transpulmonary vein filling patterns can be interrogated with Doppler echocardiography to allow diagnosis and differentiation between cardiac tamponade and restrictive and constrictive lesions (Table 15–1). As with constrictive pericarditis, during spontaneous inspiration RV early inflow velocity (E wave) is augmented with tamponade while LV filling (mitral inflow E wave) diminishes. Reciprocal changes are seen with spontaneous exhalation, and a variation between inspiratory and expiratory velocities greater than 25% is used to diagnose tamponade (Figures 15–12 through 15–14). The decreased LV early filling can also be detected as delayed mitral valve opening and prolonged isovolumic relaxation time.[37] Respiratory variations in mitral inflow velocities may or may not be detected in the setting of positive pressure ventilation. Faehnrich and colleagues reported that the LV filling gradient changes minimally under mechanical ventilation, with only a modest increase in mitral inflow during delivery of a mechanical breath, followed by a reduction in flow in relation to exhalation.[38] This suggests that the operative force affecting cardiac output is the increased pericardial pressure from the effusion so that changes in transthoracic pressures have minimal effects on ventricular filling.

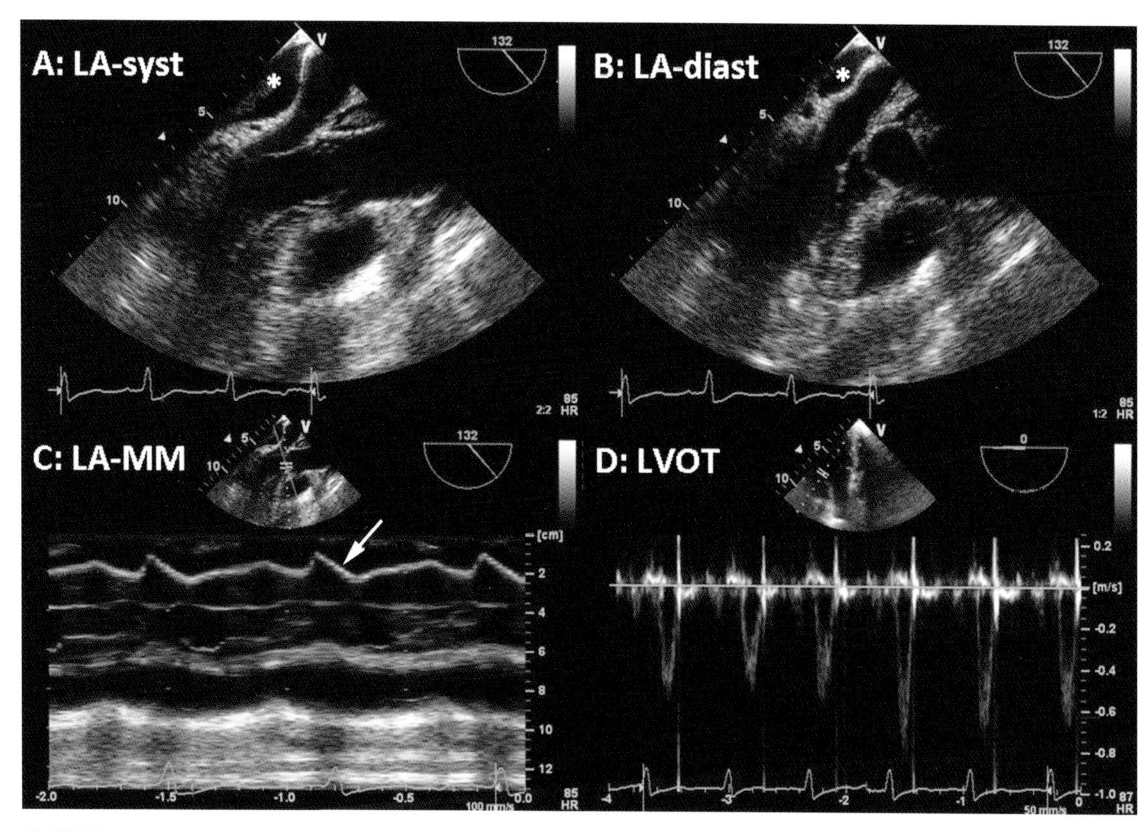

FIGURE 15–12. Localized pericardial collection (*) around the left atrium (LA) as imaged in the midesophageal long-axis view. LA inversion is seen in **(A)** systole (syst) but not in **(B)** diastole (diast) and can be better appreciated with **(C)** M-mode imaging (*arrow*). **D:** Low velocity and fluctuation of left ventricular outflow tract (LVOT) blood flow.

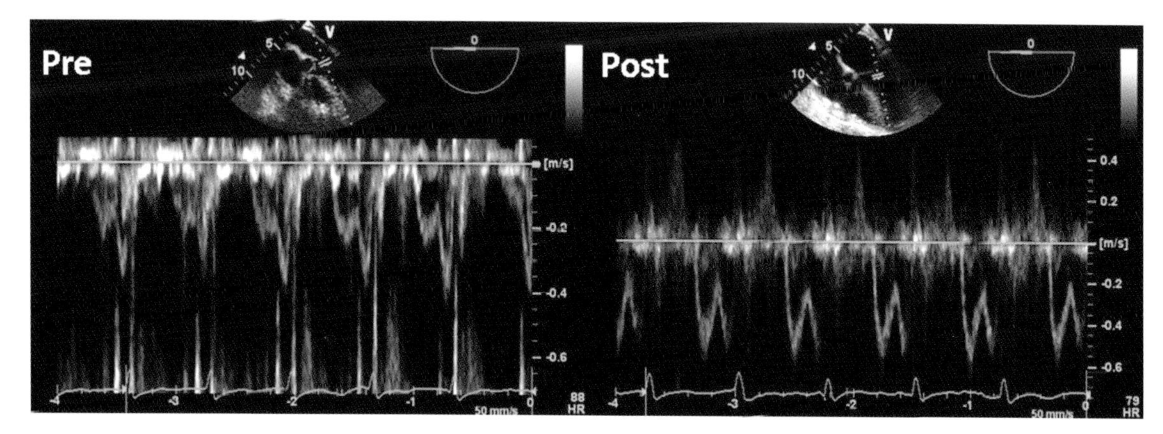

FIGURE 15–13. Mitral inflow velocities recorded with a pulsed-wave sample volume between the mitral leaflet tips in pericardial tamponade. The early diastolic velocities are reduced in the presence of tamponade (pre) and recover after evacuation of the pericardial collection (post).

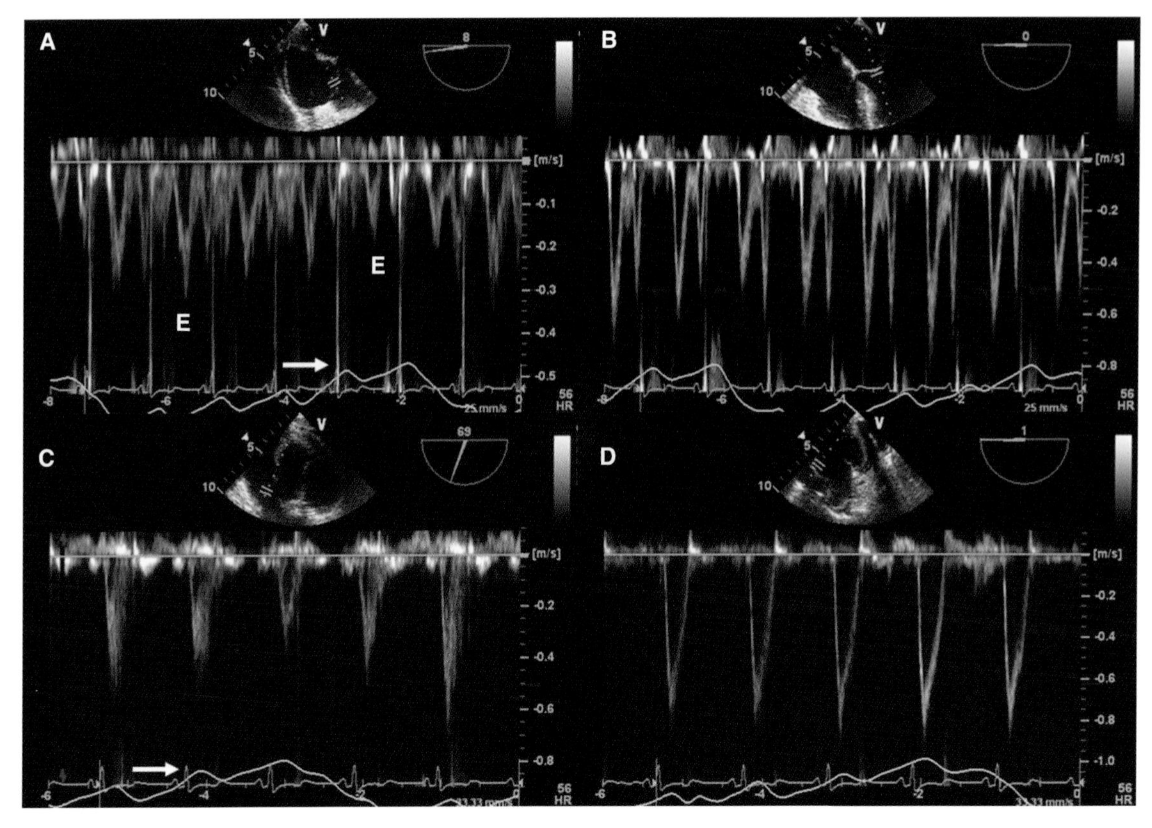

FIGURE 15–14. Regional cardiac tamponade. **A:** Right ventricular inflow velocities recorded with a pulsed-wave Doppler sample volume between the tips of tricuspid valve demonstrate a 47% decrease in early (E) velocity with mechanical inspiration. **B:** Left ventricular inflow velocities recorded in a similar manner at the tips of mitral valve show lack of significant respiratory variation. **C:** Right ventricular outflow velocities decrease with mechanical inspiration, while left ventricular outflow velocities **(D)** are unaffected.

REFERENCES

1. Holt JP. The normal pericardium. *Am J Cardiol.* 1970;26(5):455-465.
2. Watkins MW, LeWinter MM. Physiologic role of the normal pericardium. *Annu Rev Med.* 1993;44:171-180.
3. Song H, Choi YW, Jang IS, et al. Pericardium: anatomy and spectrum of disease on computed tomography. *Curr Probl Diagn Radiol.* 2002;31(5):198-209.
4. Manner J, Perez-Pomares JM, Macias D, Munoz-Chapuli R. The origin, formation and developmental significance of the epicardium: a review. *Cells Tissues Organs.* 2001;169(2):89-103.
5. Little WC, Freeman GL. Pericardial disease. *Circulation.* 2006;113(12):1622-1632.
6. Spodick DH. Macrophysiology, microphysiology, and anatomy of the pericardium: a synopsis. *Am Heart J.* 1992;124(4):1046-1051.
7. Skubas NJ, Beardslee M, Barzilai B, Pasque M, Kattapuram M, Lappas DG. Constrictive pericarditis: intraoperative hemodynamic and echocardiographic evaluation of cardiac filling dynamics. *Anesth Analg.* 2001;92(6):1424-1426.
8. Aikat S, Ghaffari S. A review of pericardial diseases: clinical, ECG and hemodynamic features and management. *Cleve Clin J Med.* 2000;67(12):903-914.
9. Talreja DR, Nishimura RA, Oh JK, Holmes DR. Constrictive pericarditis in the modern era: novel criteria for diagnosis in the cardiac catheterization laboratory. *J Am Coll Cardiol.* 2008;51(3):315-319.
10. Goldstein JA. Cardiac tamponade, constrictive pericarditis, and restrictive cardiomyopathy. *Curr Probl Cardiol.* 2004;29(9):503-567.
11. Higano ST, Azrak E, Tahirkheli NK, Kern MJ. Hemodynamic rounds series II: hemodynamics of constrictive physiology: influence of respiratory dynamics on ventricular pressures. *Catheter Cardiovasc Interv.* 1999;46(4):473-486.

12. Hutchison SJ, Smalling RG, Albornoz M, Colletti P, Tak T, Chandraratna PA. Comparison of transthoracic and transesophageal echocardiography in clinically overt or suspected pericardial heart disease. *Am J Cardiol.* 1994;74(9):962-965.
13. Giorgi B, Mollet NR, Dymarkowski S, Rademakers FE, Bogaert J. Clinically suspected constrictive pericarditis: MR imaging assessment of ventricular septal motion and configuration in patients and healthy subjects. *Radiology.* 2003;228(2): 417-424.
14. Kim JS, Kim HH, Yoon Y. Imaging of pericardial diseases. *Clin Radiol.* 2007;62(7):626-631.
15. Izumi C, Iga K, Sekiguchi K, Takahashi S, Konishi T. Usefulness of the transgastric view by transesophageal echocardiography in evaluating thickened pericardium in patients with constrictive pericarditis. *J Am Soc Echocardiogr.* 2002;15(9): 1004-1008.
16. Myers RB, Spodick DH. Constrictive pericarditis: clinical and pathophysiologic characteristics. *Am Heart J.* 1999;138(2 Pt 1): 219-232.
17. Engel PJ, Fowler NO, Tei CW, et al. M-mode echocardiography in constrictive pericarditis. *J Am Coll Cardiol.* 1985;6(2): 471-474.
18. Yazdani K, Maraj S, Amanullah AM. Differentiating constrictive pericarditis from restrictive cardiomyopathy. *Rev Cardiovasc Med.* 2005;6(2):61-71.
19. Sun JP, Abdalla IA, Yang XS, et al. Respiratory variation of mitral and pulmonary venous Doppler flow velocities in constrictive pericarditis before and after pericardiectomy. *J Am Soc Echocardiogr.* 2001;14(11):1119-1126.
20. Oh JK, Hatle LK, Seward JB, et al. Diagnostic role of Doppler echocardiography in constrictive pericarditis. *J Am Coll Cardiol.* 1994;23(1):154-162.
21. Dal-Bianco JP, Sengupta PP, Mookadam F, Chandrasekaran K, Tajik AJ, Khandheria BK. Role of echocardiography in the diagnosis of constrictive pericarditis. *J Am Soc Echocardiogr.* 2009;22(1):24-33; quiz 103-104.
22. Abdalla IA, Murray RD, Awad HE, Stewart WJ, Thomas JD, Klein AL. Reversal of the pattern of respiratory variation of Doppler inflow velocities in constrictive pericarditis during mechanical ventilation. *J Am Soc Echocardiogr.* 2000;13(9): 827-831.
23. Ha JW, Oh JK, Ling LH, Nishimura RA, Seward JB, Tajik AJ. Annulus paradoxus: transmitral flow velocity to mitral annular velocity ratio is inversely proportional to pulmonary capillary wedge pressure in patients with constrictive pericarditis. *Circulation.* 2001;104(9):976-978.
24. Weitzman LB, Tinker WP, Kronzon I, Cohen ML, Glassman E, Spencer FC. The incidence and natural history of pericardial effusion after cardiac surgery—an echocardiographic study. *Circulation.* 1984;69(3):506-511.
25. Hoit BD. Pericardial disease and pericardial tamponade. *Crit Care Med.* 2007;35(8 Suppl):S355-364.
26. Spodick DH. Threshold of pericardial constraint: the pericardial reserve volume and auxiliary pericardial functions. *J Am Coll Cardiol.* 1985;6(2):296-297.
27. Barash P. Pulsus paradoxus. *Hosp Phys.* 2000;36(1):49-50.
28. Feigenbaum H, Armstrong WF, Ryan T. Pericardial diseases. In: Feigenbaum H, Armstrong WF, Ryan T, eds. *Feigenbaum's Echocardiography.* 6th ed. Philadelphia: Lippincott Williams & Wilkins; 2005:247.
29. Tsang TS, Barnes ME, Hayes SN, et al. Clinical and echocardiographic characteristics of significant pericardial effusions following cardiothoracic surgery and outcomes of echo-guided pericardiocentesis for management: Mayo Clinic experience, 1979-1998. *Chest.* 1999;116(2):322-331.
30. Kronzon I, Cohen ML, Winer HE. Diastolic atrial compression: a sensitive echocardiographic sign of cardiac tamponade. *J Am Coll Cardiol.* 1983;2(4):770-775.
31. Kuvin JT, Harati NA, Pandian NG, Bojar RM, Khabbaz KR. Postoperative cardiac tamponade in the modern surgical era. *Ann Thorac Surg.* 2002;74(4):1148-1153.
32. Russo AM, O'Connor WH, Waxman HL. Atypical presentations and echocardiographic findings in patients with cardiac tamponade occurring early and late after cardiac surgery. *Chest.* 1993;104(1):71-78.
33. Longo MJ, Jaffe CC. Images in clinical medicine. Electrical alternans. *N Engl J Med.* 1999;341(27):2060.
34. Munt B, Moss R, Thompson C. Pericardial disease. In: Otto CM, ed. *The Practice of Clinical Echocardiography.* 3rd ed. Philadelphia, PA: WB Saunders; 2007:726.
35. Cheitlin MD, Alpert JS, Armstrong WF, et al. ACC/AHA Guidelines for the Clinical Application of Echocardiography. A report of the American College of Cardiology/American Heart Association Task Force on Practice Guidelines (Committee on Clinical Application of Echocardiography). Developed in collaboration with the American Society of Echocardiography. *Circulation.* 1997;95(6): 1686-1744.
36. Kronzon I, Cohen ML, Winer HE. Contribution of echocardiography to the understanding of the pathophysiology of cardiac tamponade. *J Am Coll Cardiol.* 1983;1(4): 1180-1182.
37. Wann S, Passen E. Echocardiography in pericardial disease. *J Am Soc Echocardiogr.* 2008;21(1):7-13.
38. Faehnrich JA, Noone RB Jr, White WD, et al. Effects of positive-pressure ventilation, pericardial effusion, and cardiac tamponade on respiratory variation in transmitral flow velocities. *J Cardiothorac Vasc Anesth.* 2003;17(1):45-50.

REVIEW QUESTIONS

Choose the *one* best answer for the following questions.

1. Cardiac tamponade is:
   a. A collection of fluid around the heart causing compression of heart chambers
   b. An augmentation of ventricular ejection
   c. Equalization of atrial and ventricular systolic pressures
   d. Compression of cardiac chambers due to excessive pulmonary pressures

2. The best method to diagnose cardiac tamponade is:
   a. Echocardiography
   b. Clinical impression
   c. Electrocardiography
   d. Capnography

3. The amount of fluid in the pericardial space determines the physiologic effects of cardiac tamponade.
   a. True
   b. False

4. The rate of accumulation of fluid in the pericardial space determines the physiologic effects of tamponade.
   a. True
   b. False

5. Cardiac tamponade manifests clinically as:
   a. Hypotension
   b. Tachycardia
   c. Increased jugular venous distention
   d. Low cardiac output
   e. All of the above

6. Pulsus paradoxus is:
   a. A systolic blood pressure increase greater than 10 mm Hg during spontaneous breathing
   b. A systolic blood pressure decrease greater than 10 mm Hg during spontaneous inspiration
   c. A systolic blood pressure increase greater than 10 mm Hg during controlled ventilation
   d. A systolic blood pressure decrease greater than 10 mm Hg during controlled ventilation
   e. None of the above

7. Pulsus paradoxus is diagnostic for cardiac tamponade.
   a. True
   b. False

8. Spontaneous inspiration augments RV filling.
   a. True
   b. False

9. Electrical alternans is exclusively dependent on the amount of fluid contained in the pericardial sac.
   a. True
   b. False

10. TEE is the most useful technique for diagnosing cardiac tamponade.
    a. True
    b. False

11. The cardiac chamber most commonly compressed in cardiac tamponade is:
    a. Right atrium
    b. Right ventricle
    c. Left atrium
    d. Left ventricle

12. Patients with long-standing pulmonary hypertension exhibit the typical findings of tamponade.
    a. True
    b. False

13. All of the following are causes for pulsus paradoxus *except*:
    a. Asthma
    b. Emphysema
    c. Cardiac tamponade
    d. Pericarditis
    e. Myocardial infarction

14. The following statement about the pathophysiology of pulsus paradoxus is true:
    a. Changes in intrathoracic pressure associated with breathing lead to changes in the pressure gradients along which blood exits or enters the thorax.
    b. Pulsus paradoxus results from the intimate association between the left ventricle and the systemic circulation (ie, distension of the arterial system affects filling of the left ventricle).
    c. The decrease of pleural pressures causes a concomitant decrease in the gradient from the venous system to the right ventricle.
    d. The small increase in venous return causes an increase in preload of the right ventricle and an increase in LV inflow.

15. All of the following are features of pericardial tamponade *except*:
    a. Electrical alternans on electrocardiography
    b. Pulsus paradoxus
    c. Pulsus alternans
    d. Equalization of diastolic pressures
    e. Blunted *y* descent seen on central venous pressure waveform

16. Cardiac tamponade occurring after cardiac surgery generally causes pericardial pressures to be distributed evenly around the heart chambers.
    a. True
    b. False

17. Doppler echocardiography is helpful in differentiating restrictive from constrictive pericardial processes by examining:
    a. Tricuspid flow patterns *only*
    b. Transmitral and transtricuspid flow patterns
    c. Transmitral and pulmonary venous flows
    d. Pulmonary venous flow *only*

18. In cardiac tamponade, transmitral flow velocities show the following patterns:
    a. E/A = 1
    b. E/A >3
    c. Prolonged E-wave deceleration time
    d. Absent E wave
    e. Rapid E-wave deceleration time

19. Positive pressure ventilation minimally affects transmitral flow profile in patients with cardiac tamponade.
    a. True
    b. False

20. Normal pericardial thickness is:
    a. 1 to 2 mm
    b. 3 to 4 mm
    c. Less than 1 mm
    d. 4 to 6 mm

21. Transmitral Doppler in constrictive pericarditis demonstrates an early, rapid diastolic (E wave) downslope.
    a. True
    b. False

22. Two-dimensional echocardiography of the pericardium includes assessment of the following parameters *except*:
    a. Echogenicity
    b. Calcification
    c. Thickness
    d. Motion

23. Posterior septal motion is a common finding on M-mode in patients with constrictive pericarditis and is related mostly to abnormal motion of the interatrial septum during systole.
    a. True
    b. False

24. The transmitral and the tricuspid late filling velocities in constrictive pericardial disease are:
    a. Increased as a result of higher atrial pressures
    b. Nearly absent due to rapid equalization of transvalvular pressures
    c. Decreased because of inadequate preload
    d. Normal
    e. None of the above

25. The pericardium is composed of the following structures *except*:
    a. Visceral pericardium
    b. Parietal pericardium
    c. Epicardial fat
    d. Lymphatics

26. Bacterial infections are the most common cause of pericarditis.
    a. True
    b. False

27. The pericardial pressure-volume relation is best described by which of the following statements?
    a. Acute increase in pericardial fluid causes a sudden rise in pericardial pressure followed by minimal changes in pressure with additional accumulation of fluid.
    b. For a large change in volume there is minimal change in pressure.
    c. The pericardial compliance is unaffected by preload.
    d. Ventricular interaction provides compensation for increases in pericardial fluid.
    e. None of the above.

28. The clinical features of pericardial diseases may resemble:
    a. Right-side failure, notably RV failure
    b. Tricuspid insufficiency
    c. Left-side failure manifesting as shortness of breath, reduced exercise tolerance, and multiorgan hypoperfusion
    d. All of the above

29. The visceral component of the pericardium is made up of a single layer of mesothelial cells that is attached to the surface of the heart and epicardial fat, and it regulates the production of pericardial fluid lubricating the heart.
    a. True
    b. False

30. The function of the pericardium includes protection of the heart from:
    a. Spread of infection and malignancy from surrounding structures
    b. Reduction of friction between the heart and the adjacent tissues
    c. Control of hydrostatic forces on the heart
    d. Prevention of acute chamber dilatation and maintenance of diastolic coupling of the ventricles
    e. All of the above

31. The causes of pericarditis are numerous and include all of the following *except*:
    a. Idiopathic
    b. Infectious
    c. Acute myocardial infarction
    d. Amiodarone
    e. Autoimmune

32. After the acute inflammatory phase, fibrous adhesions may be present only between the pericardium and the myocardium.
    a. True
    b. False

33. Most patients with constrictive pericarditis complain of:
    a. Retrosternal chest pain that is extremely variable in intensity and quality
    b. Nausea and vomiting
    c. Headache
    d. Productive cough

34. Notable findings on physical examination of patients with pericarditis include all of the following *except*:
    a. A pericardial rub
    b. Distant heart sounds
    c. Increased jugular venous pressure
    d. Kussmaul sign
    e. Electrical alternans

35. The electrocardiogram in a patient with pericarditis typically will demonstrate diffuse ST-segment elevation that concaves upwardly with reciprocal ST-segment depression as seen in myocardial ischemia.
    a. True
    b. False

36. The classic *dip and plateau* or *square-root sign* is:
    a. A waveform of ventricular pressures demonstrating a truncation of ventricular filling in early diastole as atrial and ventricular pressures equalize
    b. A mathematical formula that is used to derive cardiac output from Doppler studies of the mitral inflow in mitral stenosis
    c. A ventricular pressure waveform seen in hypertrophic cardiomyopathy
    d. A classic sign of pericarditis denoting rapid equalization of ventricular pressure in mid- to late diastole

37. The echocardiographic assessment of thickened pericardium by the transthoracic approach is often limited by:
    a. A high sensitivity and a low specificity
    b. Poor image quality
    c. Positioning of the transducer
    d. Transducer frequency, gain, and gray-scale settings
    e. None of the above

38. Two-dimensional TEE examination can identify pericardial thickening in constrictive pericarditis in nearly 90% of cases, whereas TTE has a detection rate as low as 30%.
    a. True
    b. False

39. A comprehensive TEE approach for assessing pericardial constriction has the advantage over the TTE approach by having:
    a. Better image resolution and enhanced definition of the pericardial interface with fat, fluid, and surrounding tissue
    b. Larger imaging windows than TTE
    c. Better penetration through lung tissue
    d. None of the above

40. The best views for assessing pericardial constriction include all of the following *except*:
    a. ME four-chamber
    b. ME two-chamber
    c. ME LAX
    d. Transgastric short axis
    e. ME short axis

41. All of the following are key features of the echocardiographic examination that assist in the diagnosis of constrictive pericarditis *except*:
    a. Interventricular septal motion.
    b. Delayed closure of the aortic valve due to increased pericardial pressure.
    c. Atrial compression by the thickened pericardium.
    d. The deep transgastric view is especially helpful in defining myocardial borders and it may be the best view to determine pericardial properties.

42. Examination of the vena cava (inferior and superior) and the pulmonary veins provide important information for diagnosing pericardial disease in spontaneous and mechanically ventilated patients.
    a. True
    b. False

43. An increase in IVC diameter at the junction of the right atrium of greater than 50% with inspiration is a marker of RA hypertension.
    a. True
    b. False

44. Thickness of the pericardium is measured from the outer border of the myocardium to the inner edge of the pericardium, avoiding areas of echolucent space between the two borders.
    a. True
    b. False

45. Properties of the parietal pericardium include:
    a. Collagen fibers meshed with elastic fibers
    b. Flexibility
    c. Rigidity in older patients
    d. Lining of the fibrous pericardium
    e. All of the above

46. The inflammatory phase of pericarditis is marked by all of the following *except*:
    a. Infiltration with leukocytes such as lymphocytes, polymorphonuclear leukocytes, and macrophages
    b. Alterations in pericardial vascularity
    c. Deposition of fibrin
    d. Decrease in pericardial fluid content

47. In patients over 60 years of age, the D wave of pulmonary vein flow Doppler examination is generally greater in magnitude than the S wave.
    a. True
    b. False

48. In constrictive pericarditis, the thickened pericardium isolates the intrapericardial cardiac chambers (but not the extrapericardially located pulmonary veins) from changes in intrathoracic pressure during the respiratory cycle.
    a. True
    b. False

49. Prominent hepatic vein diastolic flow reversal may be noticed as a result of increased RA pressure only in patients with significant tricuspid regurgitation and sinus tachycardia.
    a. True
    b. False

Echocardiography for Aortic Surgery

16

Christopher Hudson, Jose Coddens, and Madhav Swaminathan

INTRODUCTION

Diseases involving the aorta can present a challenge to both surgeons and anesthesiologists. Aortic dissection and rupture are life threatening, require rapid and accurate diagnosis, and need definitive medical and/or surgical management due to their high risk of morbidity and mortality.[1,2] A key ingredient in the efficient management of these patients is imaging of the thoracic aorta. Transesophageal echocardiography (TEE) has become an essential noninvasive diagnostic modality for acute thoracic aortic pathologies, and is a standard part of the echocardiographer's armamentarium in the operating room.[3-6] It is important for the echocardiographer to quickly and accurately verify the diagnosis, distinguish true pathology from the many common confounding artifacts, and clearly communicate precise echocardiographic findings of the aorta and related cardiac anatomy to the surgeon in order to guide intervention. The following text reviews aortic anatomy and pathology and associated echocardiographic features that assist with imaging during aortic surgery.

ANATOMY OF THE AORTA

In order to truly appreciate the invaluable role that TEE plays in the assessment for diseases of the aorta, a detailed understanding of the aorta and surrounding anatomic structures is crucial. The thoracic aorta can be divided into three anatomic segments: ascending thoracic aorta, aortic arch, and descending thoracic aorta (Figure 16–1). The ascending thoracic aorta originates at the level of the aortic valve annulus. As previously described in Chapter 9, the aortic valve comprises three crescent-shaped leaflets that coapt to form three commissures. Immediately distal to the aortic valve apparatus is a short and dilated aortic segment—the sinus of Valsalva—which is subdivided into the noncoronary, left coronary, and right coronary sinuses. As the nomenclature suggests, the left and right coronary arteries each originate from their respectively named sinus. Distal to the sinus of Valsalva, the aorta slightly narrows, forming the sinotubular junction (STJ). From this point, the ascending aorta crosses beneath the main pulmonary artery, then courses in an anterior, cranial, and rightward direction over the origin of the right pulmonary artery.

The ascending aorta terminates and continues as the aortic arch at the origin of the brachiocephalic (innominate) artery. The aortic arch then proceeds to curve in a posterior and leftward direction with cranial convexity. Three arteries arise from the aortic arch: the brachiocephalic, left common carotid, and left subclavian arteries. It is often difficult to visualize the distal ascending thoracic aorta and proximal aortic arch with TEE because the trachea is positioned between the esophagus and aorta, effectively preventing ultrasound transmission. Immediately beyond the origin of the left subclavian artery, at the point of attachment of ligamentum arteriosum (remnant of the fetal ductus arteriosus), is a second narrowing called the aortic isthmus. Unlike the heart and proximal part of the aorta, the aortic isthmus and descending thoracic aorta are relatively fixed. Consequently, deceleration injury secondary to trauma is most often confined to this level. Distal to the aortic isthmus, the descending aorta follows a caudal, slightly anterior, and rightward trajectory towards the aortic diaphragmatic hiatus. Along its intrathoracic course, the descending thoracic aorta and the esophagus are in close proximity. While the esophagus courses almost straight downward, anterior to the midline of the vertebral bodies, the aorta travels in a smooth, curved direction from the anterolateral side of the 4th thoracic vertebral body to the anterior side of the 11th vertebral body.

During its thoracic descent, multiple intercostal arteries branch off the aorta and may occasionally be imaged with TEE using color-flow Doppler (CFD). Spinal branches of these intercostal arteries supply blood to the spinal cord through radicular arteries. The radicular artery anatomy in this area is quite variable, with 4 to 10 radicular branches typically contributing to the thoracic spinal cord. The anterior spinal cord blood supply is tenuous in the thoracic region, thus it is

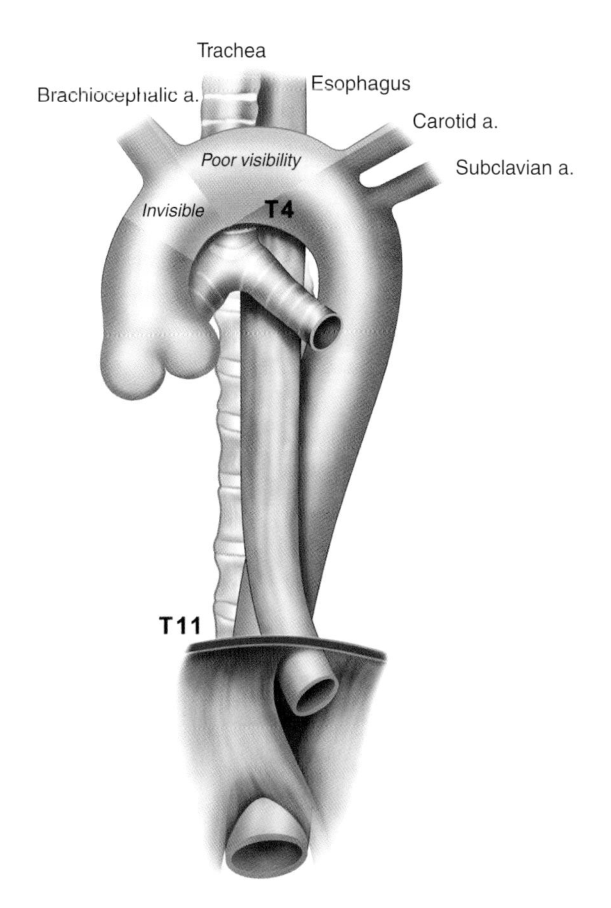

FIGURE 16–1. Anatomic course of the thoracic aorta. The relationship with the esophagus is particularly important with regard to orientation of the probe and the aorta in each of its thoracic sections: the ascending aorta, aortic arch, and descending aorta. The interposition of the trachea makes portions of the ascending aorta and arch either completely invisible or partially visible.

at great risk for cord ischemia. Frequently, one radicular artery—the *arteria radicularis magna*, or the artery of Adamkiewicz—is very developed and is responsible for the majority of anterior spinal cord blood supply, and it is typically found between T9 and T12.

Below the diaphragm, the abdominal aorta lies posterior to the stomach. Because the stomach is a large cavity that is highly deformable, the position of the abdominal aorta in relation to the intragastric TEE probe is somewhat variable. The celiac artery and mesenteric arteries originate from the anterior side of the abdominal aorta. The renal arteries arise from the left and right sides of the aorta, slightly below the mesenteric vessels.

The wall of the aorta is composed of three tunicae: the intima, media, and adventia. The inner layer, the intima, consists of simple squamous epithelium and underlying connective tissue. The tunica media consists of circularly arranged smooth muscle and elastic tissue. The outer adventitial layer is mainly a loose layer of connective tissue, lymphatics, and vasa vasorum (ie, "vessels of the vessels"). TEE provides the ability to assess the aortic wall for many pathologies including thickening of the tunica intima due to arteriosclerosis and/or atherosclerosis, intimal tears/dissections, and aneurysmal dilatation.

ECHOCARDIOGRAPHIC EVALUATION OF THE THORACIC AORTA

As described in Chapter 5, insertion of the TEE probe must be performed gently and should never be forced through areas of resistance. This is especially important in patients with suspicion of major aortic pathology. First, intubation of the esophagus with the TEE probe can be very stimulating and may result in hypertensive episodes, increasing the risk of further tearing or rupture of a dissection or aneurysm. Second, resistance encountered during advancement of the probe may represent esophageal compression by a large aneurysm, and if so, consideration should be given to abandon the examination. Finally, in aortic dissection, because the adventitia is the sole layer of the wall of the false lumen, aortic rupture may occur if the TEE probe is not manipulated cautiously.

As with any TEE examination, a systematic approach is required to thoroughly evaluate the thoracic aorta. As per the SCA/ASE guidelines, there are six short-axis and two long-axis imaging planes that enable imaging of most of the thoracic aorta.[7] Although many sequences are possible, the authors recommend the following order: Begin with the midesophageal (ME) aortic valve (AV) short-axis (SAX), "Mercedes-Benz" view, which is obtained at the midesophageal level with the scan angle rotated forward to 30° to 60° (see Figure 5–19B). From here, the angle can be rotated by another 90° to about 120° to 150° to identify the ME AV long-axis (LAX) view (see Figure 5–20D). The long-axis view is particularly important because it allows evaluation of the aortic valve and proximal ascending aorta. Measurements can be made of the left ventricular outflow tract (LVOT), aortic valve annulus, sinuses of Valsalva, STJ, and ascending aorta if aortic valve repair and/or root reconstruction are planned (Figure 16–2). In order to visualize the ascending aorta in short axis, rotate back to a scan angle of 0° and slowly withdraw from the level of the aortic valve (ie, ME ascending aorta SAX view; see Figure 5–30B). By rotating forward to a 120° scan angle, a ME ascending

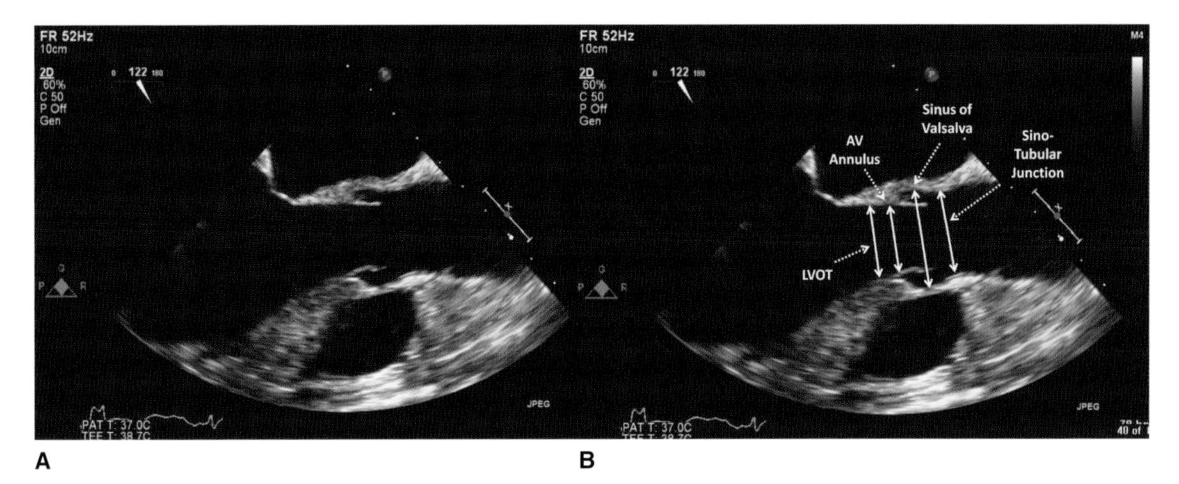

FIGURE 16–2. Midesophageal aortic valve long-axis view shown as a mid-systolic frame (panel **A**) and with relevant measurements (panel **B**). See text for details. (AV, aortic valve; LVOT, left ventricular outflow tract)

aorta LAX view is obtained (see Figure 5–32B). It is crucial in these two views to carefully examine the aorta for dissections. Artifacts are frequently encountered within the ascending aorta, and it is important to distinguish artifacts from true pathology as discussed in Chapter 3.

Following examination of the ascending aorta, the TEE probe should be advanced to the level of the ME four-chamber view and rotated towards the patient's left. This should result in the descending aorta SAX view in which the aorta appears as a circular image at the top of the screen (Figure 16–3). As the descending aorta is about 3 to 4 cm in diameter at this level, reducing the scan depth to 6 to 8 cm and selecting a high transducer frequency improves both the spatial and temporal resolutions of the image. Almost the entire descending thoracic aorta may be visualized in short axis by advancing and withdrawing the TEE probe. By rotating the scan angle forward to 90°, the descending aorta can be seen longitudinally (see Figure 16–3).

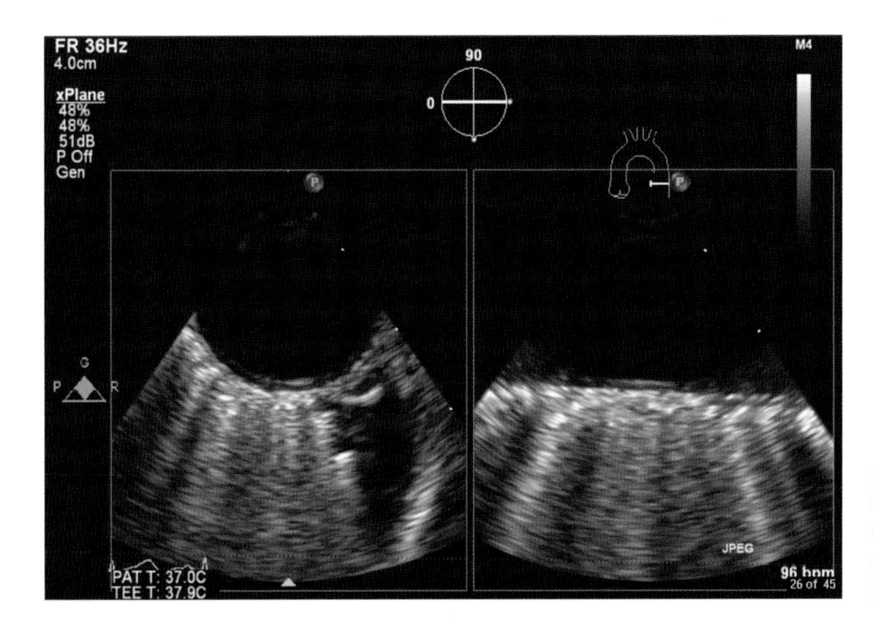

FIGURE 16–3. Short- *(left)* and long-axis *(right)* views of the descending aorta shown simultaneously with x-plane imaging.

Alternating between short- and long-axis views may help demonstrate aortic pathology more comprehensively. While withdrawing the TEE probe and maintaining the descending aorta in the short-axis view (at 0°), the aorta will change in appearance from circular to longitudinal at the level of the aortic arch (upper esophageal [UE] aortic arch LAX; see Figure 5–34). Frequently, the origins of the left subclavian and carotid arteries can be seen. Adding CFD with the Nyquist limit set at 50 cm/s may aid in visualizing these vessels. Finally, by rotating forward to 90°, the UE aortic arch SAX will be obtained (see Figure 5–31B). Most aortic pathologies can be identified by adding pulsed-wave Doppler (PWD) and continuous-wave Doppler (CWD), as well as gray-scale and color M-mode to the two-dimensional (2D) examination above.

AORTIC ANEURYSMS

An aortic aneurysm is a localized or diffuse dilation of the aorta to twice its diameter involving all three layers of the vessel wall. The estimated annual incidence is six cases per 100,000 persons.[8] TEE is useful for the diagnosis and classification of thoracic and upper abdominal aortic aneurysms. Thoracoadominal aneurysms (TAAs) are categorized into four types based on the Crawford classification system (Figure 16–4).[9] Type I involves the entire descending thoracic aorta to the abdominal aorta above the renal arteries. Type II originates in the proximal descending thoracic aorta and terminates distal to the renal arteries. Type III affects the distal half of the thoracic aorta and the abdominal aorta to the bifurcation. Type IV is limited to the distal portion of the descending thoracic aorta and the abdominal aorta to the bifurcation.

Aneurysms are generally thought to be a disease of aging and a consequence of degeneration and atherosclerosis. Aging results in a pathological process that involves the development of eccentric fibrous intimal thickening, lipid deposition, and calcification, leading to weakening of the aortic wall and dilation.[10] According to Laplace law (Tension = Pressure × Radius), as the diameter of the lumen increases, the wall tension increases resulting in progressive dilation. Other causes of TAAs include connective tissue diseases (ie, Marfan's, type IV Ehlers-Danlos and Loeys-Dietz syndromes), infections (ie, bacteria, mycotic, or syphilitic), trauma, and increased wall tension secondary to hypertension or a high-velocity jet originating from aortic stenosis.

The decision to surgically repair a TAA is based upon the size and etiology of the aneurysm. According to recommendations by the Society of Thoracic Surgeons, a thoracic fusiform aneurysm should be surgically repaired if it is greater than 5.5 cm in diameter or twice the diameter of the normal contiguous aorta.[11] Indications for saccular aneurysm have not been determined, but it is considered reasonable to intervene if the width is greater than 2 cm. Patients with connective tissue diseases, such as Marfan's syndrome, may be considered for early operative repair because of their increased risk of dissection or rupture. A strong family history of aortic aneuryms may also prompt early intervention. Finally, symptomatic patients should be considered for operative treatment regardless of the size of the aneurysm. Symptoms include persistent pain, malperfusion, and compression of nearby structures leading to dysphagia, cough, hoarseness, or Horner's syndrome. Descending TAAs can also be treated by endovascular stent grafting. There are no established guidelines regarding which patients should be managed

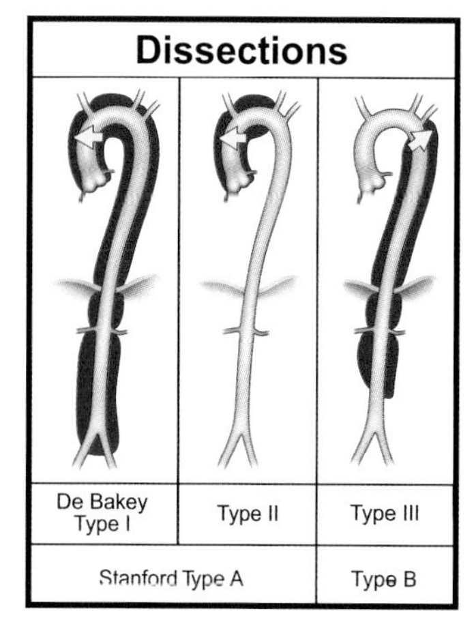

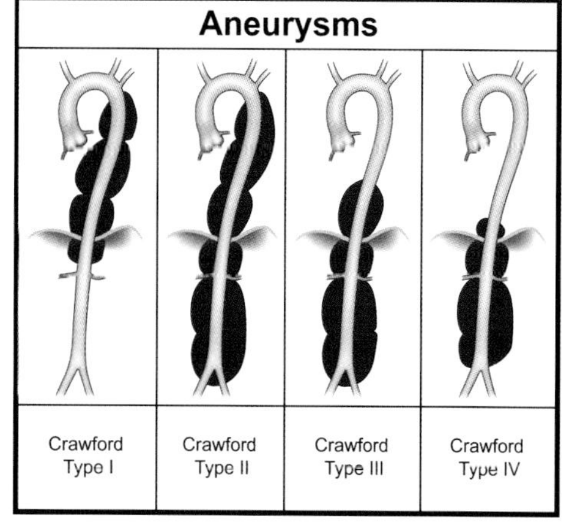

FIGURE 16–4. Classification of aortic dissection and aneurysms.

with endovascular aortic repair (EVAR). In general, patients at high risk for complications from either conventional open repair or medical management may benefit from this relatively less invasive approach. Another emerging alternative for complex aortic pathology is the "hybrid" approach in which an open surgical technique is combined with an EVAR. This approach is thought to maximize the benefit of complete repair of complex lesions while minimizing the risk of a total open technique.

TEE may be used to detect the patency of aortic side branches and to evaluate for the presence of organ malperfusion. In the thoracic region, the identification of the left subclavian artery and its patency may be particularly important in EVAR and hybrid approaches. Intraoperative TEE is also an excellent monitoring tool, especially if aortic cross-clamping is performed, and may be helpful during cannulation if total or partial extracorporeal circulatory support is required. Monitoring of cardiac function is an added benefit of TEE during aortic aneurysm surgery. While the aorta remains the focus of intraoperative imaging, the effects of aortic manipulation on cardiac function can also be evaluated. This enables clinicians to make informed decisions on pharmacological support, should it be required.

AORTIC DISSECTION

An aortic dissection is a separation in the aortic wall that allows blood flow within the tunica media. Currently, there are two proposed etiologies for aortic dissections.[12] In the first hypothesis, the intima is ruptured along the edge of an atheromatous plaque or at a penetrating ulcer. The high pressure in the aorta forces blood through the intimal tear into the tunica media, creating a false lumen. The intimal layer that separates the false lumen from the true lumen (normal conduit of blood in the aorta) is termed the intimal flap. While intimal injury per se does not lead to dissection, it is a common precipitating factor, especially when the aortic medial layer is diseased. In the second hypothesis, the dissection is attributed to spontaneous rupture of the vasa vasorum or degeneration of the collagen and elastin that make up the tunica media. This medial layer can be affected by poor structural integrity as seen in old age or with primary connective tissue diseases such as Marfan's syndrome. Apart from medial integrity, the time required for extension of an intimal tear and development of a dissection depends on the rate of rise of systolic pressure, pulsatile pressure, diastolic recoil, and mean arterial pressure.

Aortic dissection is the most common cause of death among all conditions involving the aorta. The incidence of thoracic aortic dissection in North America is about 5 to 10 cases per million people per year.[13] The mortality associated with acute aortic dissection is extremely high, with 21% of patients dying before hospital admission.[14] The mortality rate from acute aortic dissection has been shown to be 1% to 3% per hour for the first 24 to 48 hours, and as high as 80% by 2 weeks.[15] Due to this high mortality, early diagnosis is considered crucial for appropriate management to be initiated.

Magnetic resonance imaging (MRI) is currently the gold standard test for the detection and assessment of aortic dissections with a sensitivity and specificity of 98% and 98%, respectively.[16] However, there are many contraindications to MRI examination including implanted medical devices (ie, pacemaker, orthopedic hardware, etc) and hemodynamic instability. Consequently, TEE is increasingly becoming an important and convenient modality for diagnosis of acute aortic dissection. TEE, similar to MRI, is highly sensitive and specific for the diagnosis of aortic dissection, with a sensitivity of 97% and specificity of 100%.[17] TEE is an attractive first-choice diagnostic procedure because of its accuracy, speed, relatively low cost, portability, and noninvasiveness.[18] However, a major limitation of TEE in the diagnosis of aortic dissection is the inability to reliably visualize the distal ascending aorta and proximal aortic arch. The frequent presence of artifacts such as mirror images in aortic imaging makes TEE prone to important false-positive diagnoses of dissection (Figure 16–5).

There are two main classification systems utilized for thoracic aortic dissections (see Figure 16–4).[19] The DeBakey classification system recognizes three types of aortic dissections.[19,20] In type I, the entire aorta is dissected; in type II, only the ascending aorta is involved; and in type III, the ascending aorta and arch are spared, while the descending aorta is dissected. Type III is further subclassified into type IIIA, involving the descending thoracic aorta alone, and type IIIB, extending into the abdominal aorta. The Stanford system classifies dissections into two types.[20] In Type A the ascending aorta is affected, while in Type B the ascending aorta is spared. A classification system from Europe has also been proposed to replace the DeBakey and Stanford classification systems.[21,22] This classification groups dissection into five types based on etiology (Table 16–1).

These classification systems have important prognostic and therapeutic consequences.[11,23] Type A aortic dissection is a formal indication for surgical intervention because the reported mortality rate with medical therapy far exceeds that reported for surgical treatment.[24-26] Unlike Type A aortic dissections, the correct management for Type B aortic dissections remains controversial.[27-29] Medical management is advocated for most Type B dissections as most studies show no clear survival advantage with surgical management. Some indications for surgery in Type B dissection include organ malperfusion, persistent pain, hemodynamic instability, or

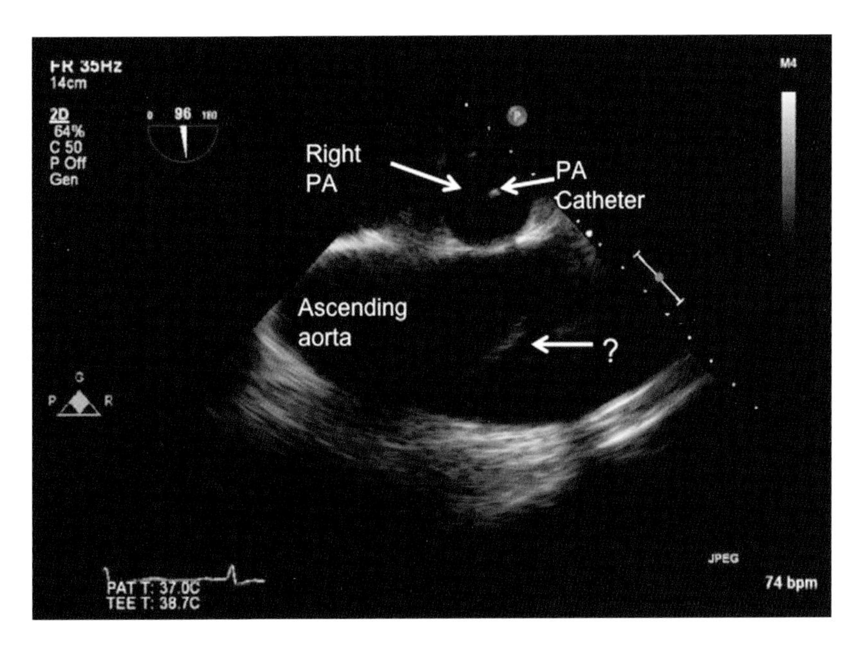

FIGURE 16–5. Midesophageal ascending aortic long-axis view with a suspicious shadow (?) in the aortic lumen. The pulmonary artery (PA) catheter may cast a mirror image artifact in the ascending aorta that displays a similar "bounce" to that of an intimal flap, creating an impression of a dissection. Similarly, an actual dissection flap may be erroneously mistaken for an artifact.

any signs of impending or ongoing rupture, notably the accumulation of pleural, pericardial, periaortic, or mediastinal fluid; propagation of the dissection; increasing size of hematoma; and development of a saccular aneurysm. In addition, echocardiographic evidence of a wide-open false lumen with communication to the true lumen increases the risk of progression of the dissection, and therefore is considered an indication for surgery.

Though an intimal tear is the classic finding for aortic dissection, it is not always present. The presence of an intimal flap is therefore considered a classical sign of dissection, but not a mandatory one. The TEE examination of a patient with aortic dissection involves several components including characterization of the dissection, assessment of flow in aortic branches, and determination of cardiac complications. The dissection flap is a thin, mobile echogenic membrane found within

Table 16–1. European Society of Cardiology Classification of Aortic Dissections.

Class	Description
I	Classic aortic dissection (DeBakey and Stanford)
II	Intramural hematoma/hemorrhage
III	Discrete/subtle dissection without hematoma
IV	Plaque rupture leading to aortic ulceration
V	Traumatic or iatrogenic

the aortic lumen; however, to avoid a false-positive diagnosis, the intimal flap must be identified in multiple image planes.[18,30,31] Although identification of the site of the intimal tear can be challenging, CFD imaging is useful in the assessment of entry and exit sites. It can sometimes be very difficult to distinguish the true lumen from the false lumen. In contrast to the false lumen, the true lumen tends to be smaller, round in appearance, shows enlargement during systole, and often has normal PWD and CFD profiles. In addition, M-mode imaging can help determine the direction of movement of the flap in systole, and thereby identify the location of the true lumen (Figure 16–6). The false lumen is usually larger and crescent shaped, and often demonstrates spontaneous echo contrast suggesting sluggish blood flow.

Closure of the tear to prevent further spread of the dissection is an essential part of the surgical repair.[32] Ascending aortic dissection usually requires a formal sternotomy, while descending aortic dissections can be managed by open (thoracotomy), EVAR, or hybrid techniques. The two most common sites of intimal tear are 1 to 3 cm above the sinuses of Valsalva (70%) and the ligamentum arteriosum (30%).[33-35]

Other variants of aortic dissection include intramural hematoma (IMH) and aortic ulcers. Intramural hematoma (ie, European Heart Society class II dissection) is a common finding with a prevalence of up to 30%.[36,37] The false lumen is believed to be due to rupture of vasa vasorum in the tunica media resulting

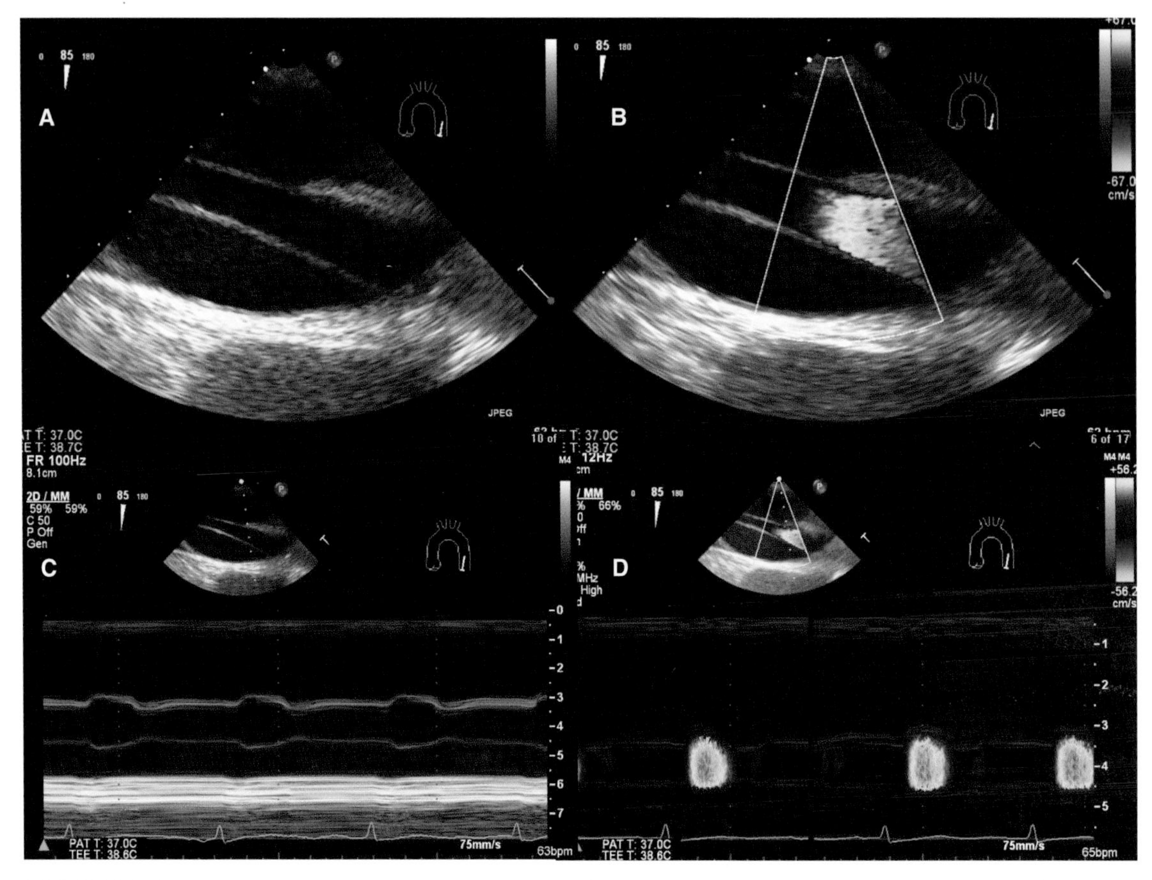

FIGURE 16–6. Techniques of determining flow in the true lumen. Panel **(A)** is a two-dimensional midesophageal long-axis view of the descending aorta showing two possible lumens. The application of color-flow Doppler (panel **B**) demonstrates higher velocity flow in the true lumen. M-mode imaging across the long axis of the aorta (panel **C**) demonstrates the two sides of the true lumen expanding in systole as the intraluminal pressure increases. Color M-mode imaging (panel **D**) shows color-flow signals within the true lumen in systole corresponding with the expanding lumen in panel **(C)**.

in hematoma formation.[12] There are two distinctive types of IMH.[38] Type I IMH has a smooth intraluminal surface, a diameter less than 3.5 cm, and a wall thickness greater than 0.5 cm, while type II IMH has a rough intraluminal surface, a diameter greater than 3.5 cm, and a wall thickness greater than 0.6 cm. Both types have a longitudinal extension of at least 11 cm.

Atherosclerotic aortic plaques can also ulcerate (ie, European Heart Society class IV dissection) leading to the formation of aneuryms, aortic rupture, or dissections.[39] The ulcers predominantly affect the descending thoracic aorta and are not usually associated with longitudinal extension. On TEE, these lesions are characterized by a discrete ulcer penetrating the aortic wall with or without intramural hematoma.

While identification and characterization of the dissection remains extremely important, there are several other crucial aspects of the echocardiographic examination for a patient with aortic dissection. Functional aortic insufficiency (AI) occurs frequently in patients with acute Type A aortic dissection, with approximately 44% being severe AI.[5] The mechanisms of the AI include incomplete leaflet closure due to leaflet tethering in a dilated aorta, aortic leaflet prolapse due to disruption of leaflet attachments, and dissection flap prolapse through the aortic valve orifice. The management of AI associated with aortic dissection is controversial. If the aortic valve leaflets are otherwise normal, preservation of the native valve can be achieved in up to 86% of Type A dissections.[40]

The aorta has several side branches, including the coronary arteries, cerebral vessels, celiac and mesenteric vessels, renal arteries, and spinal cord vessels, which can be compromised as a consequence of dissection. The incidence of coronary artery involvement in aortic dissection can be as high as 10% to 20%.[41] The left main and right coronary arteries can often be reliably visualized in the ME AV SAX view.[17] Direct evidence of coronary involvement is the presence of a dissection flap extending into the ostium of the coronary vessel. Indirect evidence includes electrocardiographic (ECG) changes, cardiovascular instability, and echocardiographic findings of regional wall motion abnormalities. Although branch arteries of the aortic arch can be reliably visualized with TEE,[42,43] the use of additional modalities including epiaortic scanning and surface Doppler directly over the carotid arteries to assess dissection extent into the arch vessels is highly recommended.[44] The remaining side branches including the renal, intestinal, and spinal cord vessels are more difficult to examine with TEE.

Other important echocardiographic findings include the presence of pericardial and left pleural effusions. Although pericardial effusions can result from the rupture of the dissection through the wall of the aortic root, the most common cause is from the transudation of fluid across the false lumen.[4,45] The development of left pleural effusion is similar except for the fact that the rupture occurs in the descending thoracic aorta.[46,47] A pericardial effusion appears as an echolucent space between the parietal and visceral pericardium on TEE. Echocardiographic signs suggesting tamponade include early diastolic collapse of the right ventricle, late diastolic/early systolic collapse of the right or left atrium, decreased size of the cardiac chambers, and abnormal ventricular septal wall motion with inspiration. A left pleural effusion is best seen in the descending aorta SAX view as an echolucent space that resembles a "claw" (Figure 16–7).

Intraoperatively, TEE is a valuable tool to monitor volume status and global and regional left ventricular function. It can also assist with cannulation and discern whether the malperfused side branches originate from the false or the true lumen—information that is essential in the surgical decision to reimplant these vessels. Finally, TEE can be used to evaluate the success of the surgical repair (ie, absence of blood flow in the false lumen) and assess for the presence of residual AI and resolution of wall motion abnormalities or pericardial and pleural effusions.

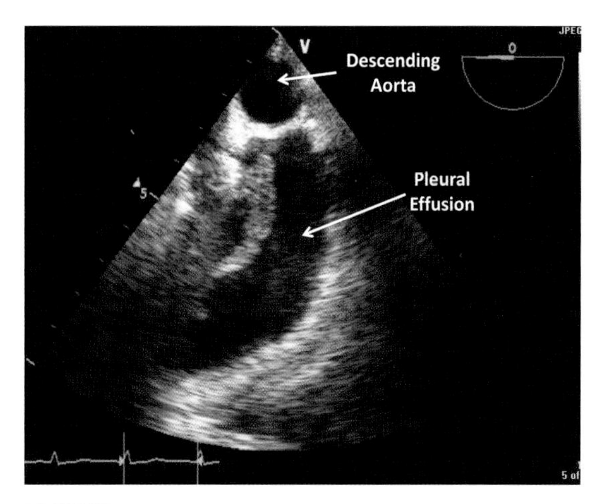

FIGURE 16–7. Midesophageal short-axis view of the descending aorta demonstrating a crescent-shaped echolucent space that suggests a significant left pleural effusion.

AORTIC ATHEROSCLEROSIS

Stroke continues to be a significant cause of morbidity and mortality after cardiac surgery. Strokes occur in approximately 1% to 6% of patients following cardiac surgery and account for nearly 20% of deaths.[48-50] The association between aortic atheromatous disease and stroke has been clearly defined.[51-53] Techniques for detecting the presence of aortic atheromas include manual palpation, x-ray, magnetic resonance and tomographic scans, and cardiac catheterization. However, TEE and epiaortic ultrasound are generally considered to be superior imaging modalities.[54,55]

Several classification systems for grading the severity of aortic atheromas have been proposed. A commonly used system is that of Katz and colleagues who divided the severity of atherosclerosis into five grades (Table 16–2).[52] It should be noted, however, that these measurement and categorization schemes are limited because they

Table 16–2. Classification of thoracic aortic atheroma.

Grade	Description
1	Normal aorta
2	Severe intimal thickening
3	Atheroma protruding <5 mm into aortic lumen
4	Atheroma protruding >5 mm into aortic lumen
5	Mobile atheroma

measure only maximal thickness and do not account for total plaque area (ie, "atheroma burden") within any given segment of aorta. Furthermore, the thickness measurement is just a one-dimensional estimate of a three-dimensional atherosclerotic lesion. Another limitation of grading systems is that gray-scale density, calcification, surface texture, and ulceration are highly subjective atheroma characteristics and prone to interobserver variability. Irrespective of the specific classification system used, patients with advanced aortic atherosclerosis are at high risk for adverse outcomes—patients with grade 5 lesions have a 1-year mortality rate of 25%.[52,56]

Although TEE has been useful in diagnosing aortic atheromatous disease, it is not without limitations. The usual site for aortic cannulation and cross-clamping during cardiopulmonary bypass is the distal ascending aorta and proximal arch, which are difficult areas to visualize with TEE.[57,58] It is also believed that aortic manipulation may result in plaque embolism and subsequent neurological injury.[59] It is therefore possible to miss the presence of severe aortic disease with TEE alone. Konstadt et al found that severe atherosclerosis in the ascending aorta was not detected in 19% of cases.[57] Epiaortic ultrasound has been shown to overcome this limitation and has emerged as the gold standard for detecting the extent and distribution of ascending aortic atherosclerosis.[44,60] It is important to note that although it is possible to accurately detect atheromatous disease with a combination of TEE and epiaortic scanning, any subsequent alteration in surgical management has not been conclusively shown to reduce the incidence of neurological sequelae.[61,62] There are numerous surgical techniques that focus on reducing the manipulation of the ascending aorta in an effort to decrease embolic events. These include using alternate atheroma-free sites for cannulation, cross-clamping, and placement of proximal anastomoses; deep hypothermic circulatory arrest for improved neurologic protection; off-pump approaches; and avoidance of cross-clamping altogether.[60,63-66]

AORTIC TRAUMA

Traumatic aortic disease is associated with an exceptionally high mortality.[67,68] The reported mortality rate of patients who present to the hospital with a traumatic aortic injury is about 30%. Severe deceleration is the most common etiology, with the injury most commonly occurring at the aortic isthmus (approximately 54% to 67% of the time).[67] Other sites of injury, in order of decreasing frequency, are the descending thoracic aorta, the aortic arch, and the abdominal aorta. Computed tomography (CT) scan and aortography remain the diagnostic imaging modalities of choice.[69] However, these modalities can be time consuming, require transport of a potentially unstable patient, and necessitate administration of nephrotoxic contrast agents. In contrast, TEE, with a reported 91% sensitivity and 100% specificity, is noninvasive, can be performed at the bedside, and avoids the use of contrast agents, but may also be limited by availability of suitably trained personnel.[6]

Three types of lesions may be encountered: a subadventitial traumatic aortic rupture, a traumatic aortic intimal tear, or a mediastinal hematoma.[6] The subadventitial traumatic aortic rupture may be partial, subtotal, or complete, and is characterized by the presence of blood flow on both sides of the disruption. A flap consisting of intima and media can also be found. There may be a disrupted aortic wall and a deformed aortic contour, although the aortic diameter is usually preserved. It can sometimes be very difficult to differentiate subadventitial traumatic aortic rupture from aortic dissection. Echocardiographic findings supporting subadventitial traumatic aortic rupture include asymmetrical contour at the level of aortic isthmus, thick and highly mobile medial flap, absence of tear, presence of mediastinal hematoma, similar blood flow velocities on both sides of the flap, and mosaic color Doppler flow surrounding the disruption. In contrast, TEE findings supporting aortic dissection include symmetrical enlargement of the aortic contour, thin and less mobile intimal flap, entry and exit tears, no mediastinal hematoma, thrombus formation in the false lumen, different blood flow velocities in both the true and false lumens, and finally, absence of mosaic color Doppler flow mapping on both sides of the intimal flap.

Traumatic aortic intimal tears appear echocardiographically as thin, mobile intraluminal appendages of aortic wall that are located in the region of the aortic isthmus. Since these lesions are small and superficial, the contour and diameter are unaffected, and color-flow mapping does not demonstrate turbulence. Mediastinal hematomas have three characteristic TEE findings: increasing space between the probe and the wall of the aorta, double contour aortic wall, and a distinct echogenic space between the bright aortic wall and the visceral pleura. This space is typically seen in the far field adjacent to the posterolateral aortic wall.

Associated lesions with traumatic aortic injury have been reported by Goarin and colleagues.[70] These consist of pulmonary contusion, left pleural effusion, rib fractures, diaphragmatic rupture, mediastinal hematoma, hemopericardium, myocardial contusion, valvular lesions, and hypovolemia. Some of these lesions become apparent much later after the initial injury; hence, a follow-up TEE examination is mandatory.

ENDOVASCULAR STENTING

In the early 1990s, the use of endovascular stents to treat aortic pathologies was introduced. Since then, stents have become an increasingly utilized alternative to conventional aortic surgery.[71,72] There was initial skepticism for their use in the thoracic aorta due to concerns about their durability in this region with higher hemodynamic stress. However, as experience grew with their use in the thoracic aorta, endovascular stenting became a widely adopted practice and has been routinely used since the early 2000s for the treatment of complex aortic diseases.

On March 23, 2005, the U.S. Food and Drug Administration (FDA) approved the Gore TAG thoracic endoprosthesis. Since then, two other thoracic stent graft systems have received approval: the Medtronic Talent (Medtronic Vascular, Santa Rosa, CA, USA) and the Zenith TX-2 (Cook Medical Inc, Bloomington, IN, USA). Currently, the only FDA-approved indication for the use of these devices is for the treatment of thoracic aortic aneurysmal disease. However, endovascular stents are now being successfully used for other aortic pathology such as acute and chronic dissection, transection, and aorto-bronchial fistulae. The early results have been very promising, and long-term data on durability are awaited.[73] In aneurysmal disease, the goal of the stent is to exclude the aneurysmal sac so that further dilation and disease progression can be prevented. In aortic dissection, the goal of the sent is to exclude the intimal tear, thus preventing its evolution. During an EVAR procedure, TEE is extremely valuable and can be used to verify pathology such as the site of the intimal tear, to identify the true and false lumen, to guide stent placement, to detect endoleaks, and to assess cardiac performance.[74] It can also be used to take measurements of the aorta and the aortic lesion, document side branch patency, and detect static or dynamic obstruction. An added benefit of TEE is the noninvasive visualization and direction of guidewires and catheters on short- and long-axis views of the aorta, thus reducing the need for nephrotoxic contrast agents. A guidewire appears as a linear echo dense intraluminal structure. TEE is also an excellent hemodynamic monitor, especially during inflation of the balloon to unfold the stent. Similar to cross-clamping of the aorta, inflation of the balloon can cause significant aortic occlusion and subsequent strain on the heart, and result in regional or global myocardial ischemia. Newer endoaortic balloons, however, incorporate a nonocclusive design that permits partial flow, thereby reducing the extent of myocardial strain. However, TEE use is limited by the poor visualization of the distal ascending aorta and proximal arch, and by the need for general anesthesia. There is also the potential interference of the TEE probe with fluoroscopy during procedures in the aortic arch.

Although an off-label indication, the use of EVAR for dissection deserves special consideration. First, sizing of the endograft is based solely on the diameter of the aorta at the proximal landing zone, since the distal zone will include both the true and false lumens. This is in contrast to aneurysms where both proximal and distal aortic diameters must be considered. Second, it is critical for the guidewire of the endograft delivery system to be within the true lumen. This can be easily facilitated with TEE, which is superior to angiography in this regard. Finally, TEE can be useful in identifying distal fenestrations between the true and false lumens, which may determine the number of endografts to be used.

Another emerging indication for EVAR is traumatic aortic transections. These patients are typically young, have multiple injuries, and are critically ill. They are also hyperdynamic, which makes endograft deployment challenging. TEE imaging can also be difficult in a setting where there may be multiple surgical specialties involved, and facial or spinal injuries may limit the opportunities for esophageal imaging. A distinct feature from an echocardiographic perspective is that the left subclavian artery is almost always covered, and loss of flow on CFD imaging should be expected.

An endoleak is a common complication following endovascular repair of the aorta. It is characterized by persistent blood flow within the aneurysmal sac or adjacent vascular segment being treated by the stent, and may occur in 20% of patients.[75] Endoleaks are characterized into four types based on location (Table 16–3)[76] and can also be classified on the basis of time of occurrence: primary endoleaks are detected within the first 30 days postoperatively while secondary endoleaks occur after 30 days. Endoleaks can also be detected by TEE, which has been demonstrated to be more sensitive than angiography (Figure 16–8).[77,78] A limitation of

Table 16–3. Classification of endoleaks.

Type	Description
I	Attachment site leak **A** Proximal leak **B** Distal leak **C** Iliac occluder
II	Branch leaks **A** To and fro simple flow from branch vessel into aneurysmal sac **B** Complex flow through two or more branch vessels into the aneurysmal sac
III	Graft defect **A** Midgraft hole **B** Junctional leak or graft disconnection **C** Other mechanisms, eg, failure from suture holes
IV	Graft wall porosity

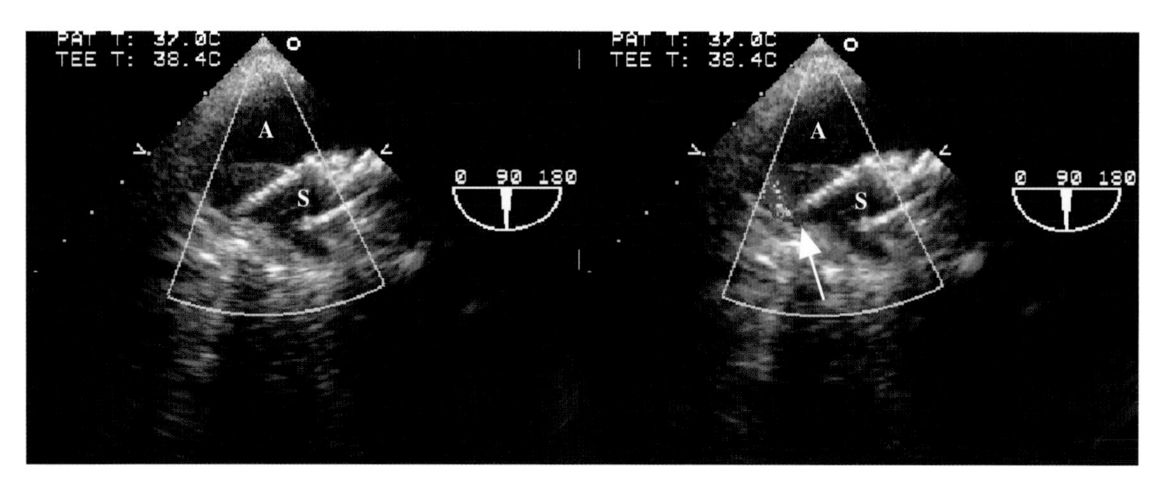

FIGURE 16–8. Type IB (distal) endoleak. The stent (S) and aneurysmal sac (A) are shown in two-dimensional *(left panel)* and color-flow *(right panel)* imaging. A small jet *(arrow)* is seen entering the aneurysmal sac from the distal portion of the stent.

angiography is that it relies on a fixed volume of contrast to circulate within the endoleak. Therefore, smaller leaks may be overlooked because the volume of contrast within the leak may not be detectable by fluoroscopy, or the imaging angle may not be aligned to detect the endoleak. Most endoleaks can be detected using CFD in the region of the aneurysmal sac. However, endoleaks that are in the far field may be obscured by echo-dense endograft material. Additionally, the color scale for CFD may need to be reduced in order to visualize low-flow leaks. Another echocardiographic sign of an endoleak is the development of spontaneous echo contrast (SEC, or "smoke") within the aneurysmal sac following the deployment of the stent.[79] The sudden development of SEC in a previously quiescent aneurysmal sac should alert the echocardiographer to the potential presence of an endoleak. Contrast that swirls or moves around the sac may indicate an endoleak, while static contrast indicates no movement or flow within the sac, suggesting the absence of any endoleak. Detecting endoleaks intraoperatively also provides the opportunity for immediate corrective interventions.

AORTIC COARCTATION

Coarctation of the aorta is a congenital narrowing of the aorta at the level of the aortic isthmus. Described more completely in Chapter 18, a coarctation can be preductal, ductal, or postductal, and can vary in length. It is commonly associated with other cardiac abnormalities including bicuspid aortic valve and patent ductus arteriosus. The classical presentation is arterial hypertension in the right arm with normal to low blood pressure in the lower extremities. TEE findings include narrowing of the aorta distal to the subclavian artery and turbulent blood flow on CFD. The anatomical position of this lesion makes transthoracic echocardiography the imaging modality of choice. The coarctation is best visualized with the transducer at the suprasternal notch.

SUMMARY

Transesophageal echocardiography is invaluable for perioperative imaging of the aorta. The anatomical juxtaposition of the aorta and esophagus makes TEE an ideal imaging tool, especially for thoracic aortic pathology. From complex lesions in the ascending aorta to endovascular stenting, TEE can provide valuable information to the intraoperative echocardiographer, including lesion identification, measurement of aortic dimensions, quantification of associated abnormalities like aortic incompetence, and detection of complications such as endoleaks.

REFERENCES

1. Miller DC, Mitchell RS, Oyer PE, Stinson EB, Jamieson SW, Shumway NE. Independent determinants of operative mortality for patients with aortic dissections. *Circulation.* 1984;70(3 Pt 2):I153-164.
2. Olsson C, Thelin S, Stahle E, Ekbom A, Granath F. Thoracic aortic aneurysm and dissection: increasing prevalence and improved outcomes reported in a nationwide population-based study of more than 14,000 cases from 1987 to 2002. *Circulation.* 2006;114(24):2611-2618.

3. Blanchard DG, Kimura BJ, Dittrich HC, DeMaria AN. Transesophageal echocardiography of the aorta. *JAMA.* 1994;272(7):546-551.
4. Armstrong WF, Bach DS, Carey L, et al. Spectrum of acute dissection of the ascending aorta: a transesophageal echocardiographic study. *J Am Soc Echocardiogr.* 1996;9(5):646-656.
5. Movsowitz HD, Levine RA, Hilgenberg AD, Isselbacher EM. Transesophageal echocardiographic description of the mechanisms of aortic regurgitation in acute type A aortic dissection: implications for aortic valve repair. *J Am Coll Cardiol.* 2000;36(3):884-890.
6. Vignon P, Gueret P, Vedrinne JM, et al. Role of transesophageal echocardiography in the diagnosis and management of traumatic aortic disruption. *Circulation.* 1995;92(10):2959-2968.
7. Shanewise JS, Cheung AT, Aronson S, et al. ASE/SCA guidelines for performing a comprehensive intraoperative multiplane transesophageal echocardiography examination: recommendations of the American Society of Echocardiography Council for Intraoperative Echocardiography and the Society of Cardiovascular Anesthesiologists Task Force for Certification in Perioperative Transesophageal Echocardiography. *Anesth Analg.* 1999;89(4):870-884.
8. Bickerstaff LK, Pairolero PC, Hollier LH, et al. Thoracic aortic aneurysms: a population-based study. *Surgery.* 1982;92(6):1103-1108.
9. Crawford ES, Crawford JL, Safi HJ, et al. Thoracoabdominal aortic aneurysms: preoperative and intraoperative factors determining immediate and long-term results of operations in 605 patients. *J Vasc Surg.* 1986;3(3):389-404.
10. Richards JM, Moores C, Nimmo A, Chalmers RT. Thoracoabdominal aneurysm disease. *Scott Med J.* 2008;53(4):38-42.
11. Svensson LG, Kouchoukos NT, Miller DC, et al. Expert consensus document on the treatment of descending thoracic aortic disease using endovascular stent-grafts. *Ann Thorac Surg.* 2008;85(1 Suppl):S1-41.
12. Wilson SK, Hutchins GM. Aortic dissecting aneurysms: causative factors in 204 subjects. *Arch Pathol Lab Med.* 1982;106(4):175-180.
13. Chen K, Varon J, Wenker OC, Judge DK, Fromm RE Jr, Sternbach GL. Acute thoracic aortic dissection: the basics. *J Emerg Med.* 1997;15(6):859-867.
14. Meszaros I, Morocz J, Szlavi J, et al. Epidemiology and clinicopathology of aortic dissection. *Chest.* 2000;117(5):1271-1278.
15. Pitt MP, Bonser RS. The natural history of thoracic aortic aneurysm disease: an overview. *J Card Surg.* 1997;12(2 Suppl):270-278.
16. Cigarroa JF, Isselbacher EM, DeSanctis RW, Eagle KA. Diagnostic imaging in the evaluation of suspected aortic dissection. Old standards and new directions. *N Engl J Med.* 1993;328(1):35-43.
17. Ballal RS, Nanda NC, Gatewood R, et al. Usefulness of transesophageal echocardiography in assessment of aortic dissection. *Circulation.* 1991;84(5):1903-1914.
18. Nienaber CA, Spielmann RP, von Kodolitsch Y, et al. Diagnosis of thoracic aortic dissection. Magnetic resonance imaging versus transesophageal echocardiography. *Circulation.* 1992;85(2):434-447.
19. Debakey ME, Henly WS, Cooley DA, Morris GC Jr, Crawford ES, Beall AC Jr. Surgical management of dissecting aneurysms of the aorta. *J Thorac Cardiovasc Surg.* 1965;49:130-149.
20. Daily PO, Trueblood HW, Stinson EB, Wuerflein RD, Shumway NE. Management of acute aortic dissections. *Ann Thorac Surg.* 1970;10(3):237-247.
21. Svensson LG, Labib SB, Eisenhauer AC, Butterly JR. Intimal tear without hematoma: an important variant of aortic dissection that can elude current imaging techniques. *Circulation.* 1999;99(10):1331-1336.
22. Erbel R, Alfonso F, Boileau C, et al. Diagnosis and management of aortic dissection. *Eur Heart J.* 2001;22(18):1642-1681.
23. Nienaber CA, Eagle KA. Aortic dissection: new frontiers in diagnosis and management: Part I: from etiology to diagnostic strategies. *Circulation.* 2003;108(5):628-635.
24. David TE, Armstrong S, Ivanov J, Barnard S. Surgery for acute type A aortic dissection. *Ann Thorac Surg.* 1999;67(6):1999-2001; discussion 2014-1999.
25. DeBakey ME, McCollum CH, Crawford ES, et al. Dissection and dissecting aneurysms of the aorta: twenty-year follow-up of five hundred twenty-seven patients treated surgically. *Surgery.* 1982;92(6):1118-1134.
26. Laas J, Jurmann MJ, Heinemann M, Borst HG. Advances in aortic arch surgery. *Ann Thorac Surg.* 1992;53(2):227-232.
27. Glower DD, Fann JI, Speier RH, et al. Comparison of medical and surgical therapy for uncomplicated descending aortic dissection. *Circulation.* 1990;82(5 Suppl):IV39-46.
28. Lansman SL, Hagl C, Fink D, et al. Acute type B aortic dissection: surgical therapy. *Ann Thorac Surg.* 2002;74(5):S1833-1835; discussion S1857-1863.
29. Wheat MW Jr. Current status of medical therapy of acute dissecting aneurysms of the aorta. *World J Surg.* 1980;4(5):563-569.
30. Erbel R, Engberding R, Daniel W, Roelandt J, Visser C, Rennollet H. Echocardiography in diagnosis of aortic dissection. *Lancet.* 1989;1(8636):457-461.
31. Marx GR, Bierman FZ, Matthews E, Williams R. Two-dimensional echocardiographic diagnosis of intracardiac masses in infancy. *J Am Coll Cardiol.* 1984;3(3):827-832.
32. Cooley DA. Surgical management of aortic dissection. *Tex Heart Inst J.* 1990;17(4):289-301.
33. Khalil A, Helmy T, Porembka DT. Aortic pathology: aortic trauma, debris, dissection, and aneurysm. *Crit Care Med.* 2007;35(8 Suppl):S392-400.
34. Hagan PG, Nienaber CA, Isselbacher EM, et al. The International Registry of Acute Aortic Dissection (IRAD): new insights into an old disease. *JAMA.* 2000;283(7):897-903.
35. Sorensen HR, Olsen H. Ruptured and dissecting aneurysms of the aorta. Incidence and prospects of surgery. *Acta Chir Scand.* 1964;128:644-650.
36. Alfonso F, Goicolea J, Aragoncillo P, Hernandez R, Macaya C. Diagnosis of aortic intramural hematoma by intravascular ultrasound imaging. *Am J Cardiol.* 1995;76(10):735-738.
37. Nienaber CA, von Kodolitsch Y, Petersen B, et al. Intramural hemorrhage of the thoracic aorta. Diagnostic and therapeutic implications. *Circulation.* 1995;92(6):1465-1472.
38. Mohr-Kahaly S, Erbel R, Kearney P, Puth M, Meyer J. Aortic intramural hemorrhage visualized by transesophageal echocardiography: findings and prognostic implications. *J Am Coll Cardiol.* 1994;23(3):658-664.

39. Movsowitz HD, Lampert C, Jacobs LE, Kotler MN. Penetrating atherosclerotic aortic ulcers. *Am Heart J.* 1994;128(6 Pt 1): 1210-1217.
40. Mazzucotelli JP, Deleuze PH, Baufreton C, et al. Preservation of the aortic valve in acute aortic dissection: long-term echocardiographic assessment and clinical outcome. *Ann Thorac Surg.* 1993;55(6):1513-1517.
41. Hirst AE Jr, Johns VJ Jr, Kime SW Jr. Dissecting aneurysm of the aorta: a review of 505 cases. *Medicine (Baltimore).* 1958;37(3): 217-279.
42. Katz ES, Konecky N, Tunick PA, Rosenzweig BP, Freedberg RS, Kronzon I. Visualization and identification of the left common carotid and left subclavian arteries: a transesophageal echocardiographic approach. *J Am Soc Echocardiogr.* 1996;9(1): 58-61.
43. Orihashi K, Matsuura Y, Sueda T, et al. Aortic arch branches are no longer a blind zone for transesophageal echocardiography: a new eye for aortic surgeons. *J Thorac Cardiovasc Surg.* 2000;120(3):466-472.
44. Glas KE, Swaminathan M, Reeves ST, et al. Guidelines for the performance of a comprehensive intraoperative epiaortic ultrasonographic examination: recommendations of the American Society of Echocardiography and the Society of Cardiovascular Anesthesiologists; endorsed by the Society of Thoracic Surgeons. *J Am Soc Echocardiogr.* 2007;20(11): 1227-1235.
45. Patel YD. Rupture of an aortic dissection into the pericardium. *Cardiovasc Intervent Radiol.* 1986;9(4):222-224.
46. Gandelman G, Barzilay N, Krupsky M, Resnitzky P. Left pleural hemorrhagic effusion. A presenting sign of thoracic aortic dissecting aneurysm. *Chest.* 1994;106(2):636-638.
47. Little S, Johnson J, Moon BY, Mehta S. Painless left hemorrhagic pleural effusion: an unusual presentation of dissecting ascending aortic aneurysm. *Chest.* 1999;116(5):1478-1480.
48. Bucerius J, Gummert JF, Borger MA, et al. Stroke after cardiac surgery: a risk factor analysis of 16,184 consecutive adult patients. *Ann Thorac Surg.* 2003;75(2):472-478.
49. Roach GW, Kanchuger M, Mangano CM, et al. Adverse cerebral outcomes after coronary bypass surgery. Multicenter Study of Perioperative Ischemia Research Group and the Ischemia Research and Education Foundation Investigators. *N Engl J Med.* 1996;335(25):1857-1863.
50. Peterson ED, Cowper PA, Jollis JG, et al. Outcomes of coronary artery bypass graft surgery in 24,461 patients aged 80 years or older. *Circulation.* 1995;92(9 Suppl):II85-91.
51. Davila-Roman VG, Barzilai B, Wareing TH, Murphy SF, Schechtman KB, Kouchoukos NT. Atherosclerosis of the ascending aorta. Prevalence and role as an independent predictor of cerebrovascular events in cardiac patients. *Stroke.* 1994;25(10): 2010-2016.
52. Katz ES, Tunick PA, Rusinek H, Ribakove G, Spencer FC, Kronzon I. Protruding aortic atheromas predict stroke in elderly patients undergoing cardiopulmonary bypass: experience with intraoperative transesophageal echocardiography. *J Am Coll Cardiol.* 1992;20(1):70-77.
53. Tunick PA, Perez JL, Kronzon I. Protruding atheromas in the thoracic aorta and systemic embolization. *Ann Intern Med.* 1991;115(6):423-427.
54. Hartman GS, Yao FS, Bruefach M, 3rd, et al. Severity of aortic atheromatous disease diagnosed by transesophageal echocardiography predicts stroke and other outcomes associated with coronary artery surgery: a prospective study. *Anesth Analg.* 1996;83(4):701-708.
55. Marschall K, Kanchuger M, Kessler K, et al. Superiority of transesophageal echocardiography in detecting aortic arch atheromatous disease: identification of patients at increased risk of stroke during cardiac surgery. *J Cardiothorac Vasc Anesth.* 1994;8(1):5-13.
56. Montgomery DH, Ververis JJ, McGorisk G, Frohwein S, Martin RP, Taylor WR. Natural history of severe atheromatous disease of the thoracic aorta: a transesophageal echocardiographic study. *J Am Coll Cardiol.* 1996;27(1):95-101.
57. Konstadt SN, Reich DL, Quintana C, Levy M. The ascending aorta: how much does transesophageal echocardiography see? *Anesth Analg.* 1994;78(2):240-244.
58. Royse C, Royse A, Blake D, Grigg L. Screening the thoracic aorta for atheroma: a comparison of manual palpation, transesophageal and epiaortic ultrasonography. *Ann Thorac Cardiovasc Surg.* 1998;4(6):347-350.
59. Tenenbaum A, Fisman EZ, Schneiderman J, et al. Disrupted mobile aortic plaques are a major risk factor for systemic embolism in the elderly. *Cardiology.* 1998;89(4):246-251.
60. Ribakove GH, Katz ES, Galloway AC, et al. Surgical implications of transesophageal echocardiography to grade the atheromatous aortic arch. *Ann Thorac Surg.* 1992;53(5):758-761; discussion 762-753.
61. Grigore AM, Grocott HP. Pro: epiaortic scanning is routinely necessary for cardiac surgery. *J Cardiothorac Vasc Anesth.* 2000;14(1):87-90.
62. Ostrowski JW, Kanchuger MS. Con: epiaortic scanning is not routinely necessary for cardiac surgery. *J Cardiothorac Vasc Anesth.* 2000;14(1):91-94.
63. Byrne JG, Aranki SF, Cohn LH. Aortic valve operations under deep hypothermic circulatory arrest for the porcelain aorta: "no-touch" technique. *Ann Thorac Surg.* 1998;65(5):1313-1315.
64. Cheng DC, Bainbridge D, Martin JE, Novick RJ. Does off-pump coronary artery bypass reduce mortality, morbidity, and resource utilization when compared with conventional coronary artery bypass? A meta-analysis of randomized trials. *Anesthesiology.* 2005;102(1):188-203.
65. Gaspar M, Laufer G, Bonatti J, Muller L, Mair P. Epiaortic ultrasound and intraoperative transesophageal ecocardiography for the thoracic aorta atherosclerosis assessment in patient undergoing CABG. Surgical technique modification to avoid cerebral stroke. *Chirurgia (Bucur).* 2002;97(6): 529-535.
66. Kouchoukos NT, Wareing TH, Daily BB, Murphy SF. Management of the severely atherosclerotic aorta during cardiac operations. *J Card Surg.* 1994;9(5):490-494.
67. Wall MJ, Jr., Hirshberg A, LeMaire SA, Holcomb J, Mattox K. Thoracic aortic and thoracic vascular injuries. *Surg Clin North Am.* 2001;81(6):1375-1393.
68. Fabian TC, Richardson JD, Croce MA, et al. Prospective study of blunt aortic injury: Multicenter Trial of the American Association for the Surgery of Trauma. *J Trauma.* 1997;42(3):374-380; discussion 380-373.
69. Brasel KJ, Weigelt JA. Blunt thoracic aortic trauma. A cost-utility approach for injury detection. *Arch Surg.* 1996;131(6): 619-625; discussion 625-616.
70. Goarin JP, Catoire P, Jacquens Y, et al. Use of transesophageal echocardiography for diagnosis of traumatic aortic injury. *Chest.* 1997;112(1):71-80.

71. Dake MD, Miller DC, Semba CP, Mitchell RS, Walker PJ, Liddell RP. Transluminal placement of endovascular stent-grafts for the treatment of descending thoracic aortic aneurysms. *N Engl J Med.* 1994;331(26):1729-1734.
72. Parodi JC, Palmaz JC, Barone HD. Transfemoral intraluminal graft implantation for abdominal aortic aneurysms. *Ann Vasc Surg.* 1991;5(6):491-499.
73. Verhoye JP, de Latour B, Heautot JF, et al. Mid-term results of endovascular treatment for descending thoracic aorta diseases in high-surgical risk patients. *Ann Vasc Surg.* 2006;20(6):714-722.
74. Swaminathan M, Lineberger CK, McCann RL, Mathew JP. The importance of intraoperative transesophageal echocardiography in endovascular repair of thoracic aortic aneurysms. *Anesth Analg.* 2003;97(6):1566-1572.
75. van Marrewijk C, Buth J, Harris PL, Norgren L, Nevelsteen A, Wyatt MG. Significance of endoleaks after endovascular repair of abdominal aortic aneurysms: The EUROSTAR experience. *J Vasc Surg.* 2002;35(3):461-473.
76. Veith FJ, Baum RA, Ohki T, et al. Nature and significance of endoleaks and endotension: summary of opinions expressed at an international conference. *J Vasc Surg.* 2002;35(5):1029-1035.
77. Fattori R, Caldarera I, Rapezzi C, et al. Primary endoleakage in endovascular treatment of the thoracic aorta: importance of intraoperative transesophageal echocardiography. *J Thorac Cardiovasc Surg.* 2000;120(3):490-495
78. Rapezzi C, Rocchi G, Fattori R, et al. Usefulness of transesophageal echocardiographic monitoring to improve the outcome of stent-graft treatment of thoracic aortic aneurysms. *Am J Cardiol.* 2001;87(3):315-319.
79. Swaminathan M, Mackensen GB, Podgoreanu MV, McCann RL, Mathew JP, Hughes GC. Spontaneous echocardiographic contrast indicating successful endoleak management. *Anesth Analg.* 2007;104(5):1037-1039.

REVIEW QUESTIONS

Select the *one* best answer for each of the following questions.

1. Which of the following is TRUE regarding the anatomy of the ascending thoracic aorta?
   a. It travels anterior to the main pulmonary artery.
   b. It travels in a posterior, cranial, and rightward direction over the right pulmonary artery.
   c. It travels in an anterior, cranial, and rightward direction over the right pulmonary artery.
   d. It travels in a posterior, cranial, and rightward direction over the left pulmonary artery.

2. Which of the following anatomical segments of the aorta includes the aortic isthmus?
   a. Ascending thoracic aorta
   b. Aortic arch
   c. Mid–descending thoracic aorta
   d. Distal descending thoracic aorta

3. Which of the following is TRUE regarding the descending thoracic aorta?
   a. It starts distal to the right side of the body of T4.
   b. It runs downward from the side of T4 to the anterior side of T11.
   c. It runs vertically along the vertebral column towards the esophageal hiatus.
   d. It starts anterior to the esophagus.

4. The artery of Adamkiewicz most commonly originates from which of the following thoracic levels?
   a. T2 to T8
   b. T4 to T9
   c. T6 to T10
   d. T9 to T12

5. Which of the following techniques is most likely to result in optimal visualization of a normal descending thoracic aorta?
   a. Using an imaging depth of 12 cm to optimize measurements
   b. The use of a low transducer frequency to improve spatial resolution
   c. Concurrent use of color-flow Doppler to improve temporal resolution
   d. Leftward rotation of the probe at the level of the left atrium

6. Which of the following is the optimal technique for evaluating the anatomy of the ascending aorta?
   a. The ME aortic valve short-axis view at 30° to 60°
   b. Using tissue Doppler with high frame rates
   c. Epiaortic imaging with a high-frequency transducer
   d. Using color M-mode to improve temporal resolution

7. Which of the following are ideal for imaging the proximal aortic arch?
   a. The upper esophageal short-axis view using high frequencies.
   b. The midesophageal short-axis view at the level of the main pulmonary trunk.
   c. An upper esophageal long-axis view.
   d. Scanning the arch in a short-axis plane with rotation of the shaft from left to right may display the arch vessels.

8. A 54-year-old male is admitted with chest pain and suspected Type A dissection. He was imaged in an outside hospital emergency room but the imaging details are unavailable. He remains symptomatic with ST changes on his ECG in the LAD territory, and is scheduled for emergent surgery. The surgeon requests a TEE examination immediately after induction of anesthesia. Which of the following

views is likely to confirm the diagnosis of Type A dissection AND associated wall motion abnormalities?
a. Midesophageal RV inflow-outflow
b. Transgastric mid–short axis
c. Midesophageal long axis
d. Upper esophageal arch short axis

9. In the patient in question 8, the echocardiographer suspects a possible intimal flap in the descending aorta. Which of the following techniques will most likely help establish the presence of a dissection in the descending aorta?
a. Use of color-flow Doppler to determine differential flow velocities in true and false lumens
b. Use of tissue Doppler to image aortic tissue velocity throughout the cardiac cycle
c. Use of M-mode to determine differential flow in the true and false lumens
d. Use of pulsed-wave Doppler to determine holodiastolic flow in the true lumen

10. Which of the following classifications accurately describes an aortic dissection involving only the ascending aorta?
a. DeBakey type I
b. Stanford type B
c. European System class IV
d. DeBakey type II

11. The development of the Stanford and European classification systems for aortic dissections was primarily based on which of the following clinical needs?
a. Different lesions have distinct management strategies.
b. Different imaging modalities have distinct diagnostic sensitivities for different lesions.
c. The identification of true and false lumens will impact management.
d. Complications of different types need to be managed appropriately.

12. Which of the following accurately describes the appropriate type of thoracoabdominal aortic aneurysm that involves the distal half or less of the descending thoracic aorta and substantial segments of the abdominal aorta according to Crawford's classification system?
a. Type I
b. Type II
c. Type III
d. Type IV

13. Which of the following factors is most likely involved in the etiology of aortic dissections?
a. Connective tissue diseases
b. Cystic medial necrosis
c. Syphilitic infections
d. Trauma

14. Which of the following best describes the pathology of an aortic dissection?
a. Formation of an intimal tear is frequently a late phenomenon.
b. Blood flow between the tunica media and tunica adventia.
c. Intramural hematoma cannot progress to dissection or rupture.
d. Intramural hematoma may account for up to 30% of early aortic dissections.

15. A 62-year-old female presents with a saccular aneurysm in the descending thoracic aorta 4 cm below the aortic origin of the subclavian artery. An endovascular repair is planned. Standard monitoring is employed, including left radial arterial pressure. Immediately after graft deployment and endo-balloon inflation, severe systemic hypotension is observed. Which of the following is most likely to explain this clinical finding?
a. Inadvertent stent coverage of the left subclavian artery
b. Myocardial strain due to balloon occlusion of the aorta
c. Coronary ischemia following balloon deflation
d. Bleeding due to possible rupture from balloon overinflation

16. A 48-year-old male is admitted with chest pain and suspected aortic dissection. He is scheduled for emergent surgery since his CT scan revealed a Type A dissection. However, in the operating room, the echocardiographer does not observe a dissection flap in the ascending aorta with TEE. Although a sternotomy has been performed, the aorta has not yet been manipulated. Which of the following is the approach most likely to establish the diagnosis of a Type A dissection?
a. Angiography in the operating room with contrast.
b. Color-flow Doppler with TEE in the ascending aorta.
c. Comprehensive epiaortic scan with a high-frequency tranducer.
d. Defer surgery pending repeat magnetic resonance imaging.

17. In aortic dissection, which of the following aortic side branches can be reliably assessed for malperfusion defects using TEE?
a. Coronary arteries
b. Spinal cord arteries
c. Renal arteries
d. Mesenteric arteries

18. A patient presents to the operating room for an emergent repair of a Type A dissection. History is significant for gradually worsening delirium and confusion in addition to chest and back pain, and shortness of breath. Prior to induction, the systemic arterial pressure is 92/66 mm Hg, central venous pressure is 21 mm Hg, and the heart rate is 110/min. Which of the following are most likely to be seen during intraoperative imaging?
    a. Pericardial effusion, wall motion abnormalities, and ascending aortic atheroma
    b. Pleural effusion, wall motion abnormalities, and ascending aortic atheroma
    c. Pericardial effusion, wall motion abnormalities, and carotid dissection
    d. Pleural effusion, ascending aortic atheroma, and carotid dissection

19. Which of the following imaging modalities may reliably be used to distinguish between the true and false lumen in aortic dissections?
    a. Tissue velocity and strain of aortic walls on either side of an intimal flap
    b. Flow velocity aliasing seen in the false lumen on color-flow Doppler
    c. Movement of the intimal flap towards the true lumen in systole on 2D imaging
    d. Higher-velocity flow in the true lumen on color M-mode imaging

20. During intraoperative TEE imaging in a patient undergoing repair of a Type A dissection with extension into the descending aorta up to the celiac vessels, the echocardiographer notes fluttering of the anterior mitral leaflet in diastole. Which of the following is most likely to suggest severe aortic regurgitation in this patient?
    a. Diastolic mitral regurgitation on color-flow Doppler (CFD)
    b. Systolic turbulence on CFD in the LV outflow tract
    c. Holodiastolic flow in one lumen in the descending aorta
    d. Dissection flap in the ascending aortic short-axis view

21. An intimal flap of a Type A aortic dissection is most likely to be mistaken for a mirror image artifact of which of the following structures?
    a. Pulmonary artery catheter
    b. Intra-aortic balloon pump catheter
    c. Pacing catheters in the superior vena cava
    d. Pericardial reflection of the oblique sinus

22. Which of the following is the most common location for an intimal tear?
    a. Sinuses of Valsalva
    b. Distal ascending aorta
    c. Ligamentum arteriosum
    d. Sinotubular junction

23. Which of the following attributes of an aortic atheroma are particularly significant for adverse outcome and should be reported during intraoperative imaging?
    a. Irregularities on the plaque surface
    b. Gray-scale density of the atheroma
    c. Mobility of the atheromatous plaque
    d. On which wall the lesion is located

24. While several grading systems have been advocated and used in practice, they use variable measures of atheroma severity. Which of the following attributes is common to all atheroma classification systems?
    a. Thickness or height of the atheroma
    b. Gray-scale density or calcification
    c. Ulceration of plaque surface
    d. Plaque area as a measure of burden

25. Intraoperative TEE is particularly suited for detecting atheromatous lesions in which of the following areas of the aorta?
    a. Distal ascending
    b. Proximal arch
    c. Mid ascending
    d. Proximal descending

26. Epiaortic scanning is particularly suited for detecting atheromatous lesions in which of the following areas of the aorta?
    a. Mid descending
    b. Proximal ascending
    c. Distal arch
    d. Proximal descending

27. According to the European Society, an aortic dissection caused by an intramural hematoma is what class of aortic lesion?
    a. Class I
    b. Class II
    c. Class III
    d. Class IV

28. Pleural effusions are commonly the result of transudation of fluid in which of the following aortic lesions?
    a. Type II dissection
    b. Intramural hematoma
    c. Penetrating ulcer
    d. Type B dissection

29. During endovascular repair, measurement of the aortic diameter is more important in the proximal landing zone than the distal landing zone in which of the following conditions?
    a. Saccular aneurysm
    b. Penetrating ulcer
    c. Aortic transaction
    d. Type B dissection

30. Which of the following is the optimal view to assess for the presence of a left pleural effusion?
    a. Midesophageal long-axis view
    b. Deep transgastric long-axis view
    c. Midesophageal descending aortic short-axis view
    d. Midesophageal ascending aorta short-axis view

31. Which of the following is an indication for surgical therapy of an aortic aneurysm?
    a. Symptomatic patient
    b. A fusiform aneurysm of 5.0 cm
    c. Saccular aneurysm less than 1.5 cm
    d. A thoracic aortic diameter of 3.5 cm

32. During endovascular repair, TEE is most likely to be useful for which of the following?
    a. Measurement of distal ascending aortic diameter
    b. Flow in the innominate artery branch of the aorta
    c. Type 1 endoleak in the proximal descending aorta
    d. Graft sizing in the distal landing zone for dissections

33. A 74-year-old man presents for endovascular repair of an aortic aneurysm that extends from 1 cm below the origin of the left subclavian artery to the level of the diaphragm. The surgeon plans to cover the subclavian artery due to a narrow landing zone. After endograft employment, the anesthesiologist notes that the cerebral oxygen saturation is low on the left side and the bi-spectral index is below that expected. Which of the following is the most likely explanation for the sudden developments of these neuromonitoring values?
    a. Expected coverage of the left subclavian
    b. Dissection of the left carotid from endografting
    c. Inadvertent coverage of the left common carotid
    d. Air embolism from endoballoon rupture

34. A patient undergoes endografting for repair of a thoracoabdominal aortic aneurysm. During his endograft deployment, the surgeon suspected that the patient may develop a future type II endoleak. Which of the following imaging modalities is ideal for detecting this type of endoleak?
    a. Transesophageal echo
    b. Cine-angiography
    c. Intravascular ultrasound
    d. Spiral CT scan

35. Which of the following is most likely to be mistaken for a Type B dissection on intraoperative imaging with TEE?
    a. Left pleural effusion
    b. Mobile atheroma
    c. Mirror image artifact
    d. Pulmonary artery catheter

36. Which of the following echocardiographic findings is considered a classic sign of an aortic dissection?
    a. Penetrating ulcer
    b. Intramural hematoma
    c. An intimal flap
    d. Entry and exit tear

37. Which of the following echocardiographic findings indicates an endoleak on TEE?
    a. Static echo contrast in the aneurysmal sac
    b. Turbulent flow in the sac on color Doppler
    c. Flow within the dissection true lumen
    d. Pulsatile movement of the endograft

38. Which of the following lesions is most often present in the descending aorta, does not extend longitudinally, is associated with atherosclerotic disease, and may lead to aortic rupture?
    a. Fusiform aneurysm
    b. Type B dissection
    c. Ulcerating plaque
    d. Intramural hematoma

39. Which of the following lesions is most often associated with subadventitial traumatic aortic disruption?
    a. Esophageal rupture
    b. Right pleural effusion
    c. Clavicular fracture
    d. Mediastinal hematoma

40. Which of the following echocardiographic findings is most likely in a patient admitted to the emergency room following a motor vehicle accident with multiple injuries?
    a. Thick intimal tear in the aortic arch
    b. Wall motion abnormalities
    c. Sinotubular calcification
    d. Aortic root aneurysm

Transesophageal Echocardiography for Heart Failure Surgery

17

Susan M. Martinelli, Joseph G. Rogers, and Carmelo A. Milano

The epidemic of heart failure is a worldwide problem that is anticipated to increase with both an aging population and the improved survival from cardiac complications producing left ventricular systolic dysfunction (e.g. myocardial infarction). Increasingly, these patients who survive a serious cardiac injury but have persistent ventricular dysfunction precluding normal end-organ function experience a poor quality of life and high rates of morbidity and mortality. At the age of 40, the lifetime risk of developing heart failure is 20%, and the 1-year heart failure mortality rate is 20%.[1] The number of hospitalizations for heart failure has tripled between the 1970s and 2004, and contemporary data indicate that heart failure was the primary or secondary cause of 3.8 million annual admissions in the United States.[2] It is estimated that the direct and indirect costs of heart failure in the United States will exceed $37 billion in 2009, highlighting the economic importance of this disease.[1]

While most heart failure patients are managed medically, surgical options for refractory heart failure include orthotopic heart transplantation and mechanical circulatory support. Advances in donor and recipient selection, organ procurement, and immunosuppressant therapy have led to an increase in the survival of grafted organs. Transplant surgery is currently considered the treatment of choice for end-stage heart, lung, and liver diseases, but the predominant limiting factor is a shortage of donors. Mechanical circulatory support has therefore emerged as a valuable and viable adjunct to transplantation in the management of heart failure patients.

Echocardiography plays an essential role in the donor organ selection process and preoperative screening, perioperative management, and post-transplant follow-up of recipients. Similarly, perioperative transesophageal echocardiography (TEE) provides invaluable anatomic and functional information in patients receiving circulatory support devices, which influence not only anesthetic management but also surgical decision making. The following text will first describe the role of TEE in heart transplantation, followed by a discussion of its value in the implantation of mechanical circulatory support devices.

HEART TRANSPLANTATION

The application of TEE as a diagnostic and monitoring modality in heart transplant surgery can be divided into five categories:

1. Cardiac donor screening
2. Intraoperative monitoring in the pretransplant period
3. Intraoperative evaluation of cardiac allograft function and surgical anastomoses in the immediate posttransplantation period
4. Management of early postoperative hemodynamic abnormalities in the intensive care unit
5. Postoperative follow-up studies of cardiac allograft function

Role of TEE in Cardiac Donor Screening

As a result of the shortage of available donor hearts, many institutions are now liberalizing their acceptance criteria to include higher-risk (marginal) donor hearts.[3] Table 17–1 presents the conventional cardiac contraindications to the use of a donor heart. Despite the potential risk for transmitting atherosclerotic, hypertensive, and valvular heart diseases, organs from older donors are increasingly being used. This aggressive approach has proved particularly successful when matching for higher-risk recipients (alternate recipient list) with a greater short-term mortality risk or with significant comorbid factors.[4]

Echocardiography plays an important role in the effort to improve the yield of donor evaluation.[5] By ruling out donors with structural abnormalities, severe ventricular dysfunction, or significant wall motion abnormalities (WMAs), the need for costly and time-consuming cardiac catheterization can be circumvented. In potential donors on ventilatory support, TEE has been shown to be particularly useful in providing

Table 17–1. Contraindications to the Use of a Potential Donor Heart.

Donor hearts with preexisting heart disease: coronary artery disease, valvular heart disease, or significant congenital anomalies
Hemodynamic instability requiring excessive inotropic support
Cardiac contusion
Severe wall motion abnormalities on echocardiogram
Persistent left ventricular dysfunction (ejection fraction <0.4) despite optimization of preload, afterload, and inotropic support
Severe left ventricular hypertrophy on inspection of the heart
Intractable ventricular or supraventricular arrhythmias
Brain death as a result of cardiac arrest
Prolonged or repeated episodes of cardiopulmonary resuscitation

consistent high-quality imaging when transthoracic echocardiography (TTE) has proved inadequate.

An initial echocardiogram should *not* be obtained before adequate hemodynamic and metabolic resuscitation. In particular, volume status, acidosis, hypoxemia, hypercarbia, and anemia should be corrected, and inotropic support should be weaned to a minimum compatible with adequate blood pressure and cardiac output (CO). The goals of the echocardiogram are to rule out structural abnormalities and assess regional and global functions. It is unclear if donor hearts with left ventricular (LV) hypertrophy, defined as a wall thicker than 11 mm in the absence of underfilling of the ventricle (pseudohypertrophy), can safely be used for transplantation. One study shows that LV hypertrophy (LVH) may increase the incidence of early graft failure,[6] but a more recent study demonstrated that hearts with mild (12 to 13 mm) or moderate (13 to 17 mm) LVH do not increase morbidity.[3] Most valvular and congenital abnormalities preclude transplantation, with the possible exception of mild lesions such as mitral valve prolapse in the absence of significant regurgitation, a normal functioning bicuspid aortic valve, or an easily repairable secundum-type atrial septal defect.

Segmental WMAs in donor hearts may be the result of coronary artery disease, myocardial contusion, or ventricular dysfunction after brain injury. Contused myocardial tissue resembles infarcted myocardial tissue histologically and functionally.[7] The pattern of ventricular dysfunction after spontaneous intracranial hemorrhage is usually segmental and often spares the apex of the left ventricle.[8] This pattern correlates with the sympathetic innervation of the ventricle. In contrast, ventricular dysfunction after traumatic brain injury may be global or regional. For both types of brain injury, there is a poor correlation between the distribution of echocardiographic dysfunction and actual histologic evidence of myocardial injury. Some studies have suggested that WMA and global function improve shortly after heart transplantation, but a recent multi-institutional study identified WMA on the donor echocardiogram as a powerful independent predictor of early graft failure.[9] WMA on the donor echocardiogram may be particularly important when associated with a donor age older than 40 years and an ischemic time longer than 4 hours.

The lowest fractional area change in a donor heart permitting safe transplantation is unknown, but it has been suggested that a fractional area change greater than 35%, in the absence of other cardiac abnormalities, could be used as a guide.[8]

Intraoperative Monitoring in the Pretransplant Period

Idiopathic and ischemic cardiomyopathies are the two most common causes of cardiac failure in the transplant recipient. Regardless of the cause of failure, global cardiac dilatation is a common feature and the term *dilated cardiomyopathy* has been applied to this end-stage condition. These patients have fixed, low stroke volumes and are very dependent on an adequate preload. Further, even mild increases in afterload may result in a marked reduction in stroke volume. Patients in cardiac failure compensate for their low CO by an increase in sympathetic activity, which leads to generalized vasoconstriction and to sodium and water retention. This delicate balance among preload, contractility, and afterload can be dramatically disturbed after the induction of general anesthesia. TEE is therefore ideally suited to rapidly evaluate and guide intraoperative management in these patients. Several factors commonly seen in recipients, including diastolic dysfunction, regurgitant valvular lesions, and positive pressure ventilation, result in a poor correlation between measured filling pressures and LV volumes. Thus, optimization of LV filling and inotropic support can be more readily and rapidly achieved under TEE guidance. Right ventricular (RV) size and function also should be assessed in these patients. The presence of RV hypertrophy is suggestive of long-standing pulmonary hypertension, which may lead to acute RV dysfunction in the transplanted heart.

TEE is similarly sensitive in detecting intracardiac thrombi, with the possible exception of an apical thrombus. Prethrombotic sluggish blood flow is characterized echocardiographically as spontaneous contrast or "smoke." Patients with dilated cardiomyopathy, especially in the presence of spontaneous echo contrast, have a high incidence of thrombus formation in the apex of the left ventricle. The left atrial (LA) appendage also should be inspected for possible thrombi, particularly in patients with atrial fibrillation. When thrombi are present in the left heart, manipulation of the heart before cardiopulmonary bypass (CPB) should proceed with great caution in an effort to avoid systemic thromboembolism. Other sources of embolism during the pretransplant period include atheromatous plaque from the ascending aorta during aortic cannulation or air entrainment during the explantation of ventricular assist devices. As in all CPB cases, the aorta (ascending aorta, arch, and descending aorta) should be examined for atherosclerotic plaque before aortic cannulation. TEE is extremely sensitive in the detection of intravascular air and early detection and intervention may potentially limit this complication.

It is common practice to place a pulmonary artery (PA) catheter into the PA only after CPB because it is often difficult to pass these catheters through large dilated ventricles, incompetent tricuspid valves, and in low CO states. PA catheter placement is also more prone to induce arrhythmias. TEE therefore can be used to determine CO and PA pressures during the pre-CPB period (see Chapter 4).

Intraoperative Monitoring in the Posttransplantation Period

TEE imaging of the heart during and after weaning from CPB provides invaluable information with important diagnostic and prognostic implications. Before weaning from CPB, TEE is used to detect retained air and to assist venting and de-airing maneuvers. The most common sites of air retention are the right and left upper pulmonary veins, the LV apex, the left atrium, and the coronary sinus. The right coronary artery is commonly affected by air embolism because of its more superior location in the ascending aorta, resulting in a hypocontractile dilated right ventricle and ST-segment changes in the inferior electrocardiographic leads. After separation from CPB, a detailed examination of the transplanted heart should include the elements listed in Table 17–2.

The function of the newly transplanted heart depends on many factors: baseline function before brain death, degree of myocyte damage before and during harvesting, amount of donor inotropic support, ischemic time, myocardial protection during the ischemic interval, reperfusion injury, cardiac denervation, donor-recipient size mismatch, and degree of pulmonary hypertension in the recipient. To accurately assess cardiac allograft anatomy and physiology, the echocardiographer needs to understand the surgical procedure and appreciate the changes that normally occur in the transplanted heart.

Table 17–2. Intraoperative Examination of the Transplanted Heart.

Assessment of:
Left ventricular regional and global systolic function
Left ventricular diastolic function
Right ventricular function
Atrioventricular valves
Atria and atrial anastomoses
Pulmonary arterial anastomosis
Pulmonary venous anastomoses

The standard or biatrial technique, originally described by Lower and Shumway, was the primary method for nearly 30 years.[10] However, more transplantation centers are now using the bicaval anastomotic technique as the method of choice, except in infants and small children. The advantages of the bicaval technique include preserved geometry and function of the atria, improved CO, and less disruption in the geometry of the atrioventricular valves, resulting in reduced valvular regurgitation, fewer conduction abnormalities, less thrombus formation in the left atrium, and decreased perioperative mortality.[11] In the standard technique, most of the native atrial walls and the interatrial septum are left in situ, leaving the inferior vena cava (IVC), superior vena cava, and pulmonary venous inflow tracts undisturbed. In the donor heart, an LA cuff is created by incising through the pulmonary vein orifices, whereas the right atrial (RA) cuff is created by incising through the inferior vena caval orifice and extending the incision up toward the base of the RA appendage. When the bicaval technique is performed, most of the native atrial tissue is excised, thereby creating superior vena cava and IVC cuffs for end-to-end anastomoses with the donor vena cavae. Divisions and end-to-end anastomoses of the great vessels are the same for both techniques.

Intraoperative TEE assessment of allograft LV systolic function early after separation from CPB has been shown to better predict early requirements for inotropic and mechanical support than routinely measured hemodynamic variables, particularly when ischemic times are prolonged.[12] In general, allograft LV systolic function after CPB is expected to be normal, and impaired LV systolic function at this stage, usually the result of ischemic injury or early acute rejection, is often transient. It is important to document any intraoperative regional WMAs because coronary atherosclerosis and myocardial infarction, often silent, are major

Table 17–3. Characteristic Two-Dimensional Echocardiographic Changes in the Left Ventricle After Heart Transplant.

Increased wall thickness, especially inferolateral and septal walls
Paradoxical or flat interventricular septal motion and decreased septal systolic thickening
Clockwise rotation and medial shift of the left ventricle within the mediastinum, necessitating nonstandard transesophageal echocardiographic transducer positions and angles
Small postoperative pericardial effusions

causes of morbidity and mortality after heart transplant surgery.

There are several echocardiographic findings that could be considered abnormal in the general population but are characteristic in the allograft left ventricle. These are listed in Table 17–3. Increases in LV wall thickness and LV mass are thought to represent myocardial edema resulting from manipulation and transport of the heart. Because the donor heart is typically smaller than the original dilated failing heart, it tends to be positioned more medially in the mediastinum and tends to be rotated clockwise. This could result in difficulties in obtaining the standard tomographic planes, and nonstandard TEE probe positions and angles may have to be used.

Diastolic compliance is often decreased in the first few days or weeks after cardiac transplant, but typically improves in the first year.[4] This is most likely the result of ischemia or reperfusion injury, a smaller donor heart in a larger recipient, or a larger heart implanted into a restricted pericardial space. Unfortunately, Doppler echocardiographic assessment of LV diastolic function is complicated by a variety of factors, outlined in Table 17–4. When remnant atrial tissues retain mechanical activity, atrial contractions become asynchronous, resulting in beat-to-beat variations in transmitral inflow velocities. Atrial dysfunction can also result in abnormal transmitral and pulmonary venous flow patterns.[13] LV diastolic dysfunction therefore is not the sole cause of altered transmitral flow patterns, and atrial dysfunction has to be ruled out. The echocardiographic indicators of atrial dysfunction include a decreased ratio of systolic to diastolic maximum pulmonary venous flow velocity in the presence of normal pulmonary capillary wedge pressures, reduced LA area change, and reduced mitral annulus motion.[13]

Table 17–4. Factors Complicating Doppler Echocardiographic Left Ventricular Diastolic Function Assessment After Heart Transplantation.

Asynchronous atrial contractions may result in beat-to-beat variations in transmitral flow
Left atrial dysfunction also may result in abnormal transmitral and pulmonary venous flow patterns
Recipient P waves and various pacing modes complicate measurements

The thin-wall right ventricle is particularly susceptible to injury during the period of ischemia and reperfusion and also compensates poorly for any increase in pulmonary vascular resistance, which often is elevated in patients with end-stage heart failure. Therefore, it is not surprising that acute RV failure is more common than LV failure and accounts for 50% of all cardiac complications and 19% of all early deaths after heart transplantation.[14] Once the diagnosis of RV dysfunction is established, stenosis at the PA anastomosis or kinking of the PA should first be ruled out. A systolic gradient higher than 10 mm Hg may indicate the need for surgical revision. TEE should then be used to optimize RV filling to avoid overdistention of the ventricle and to assess the response to inotropic support. In the setting of maximum inotropic support and pulmonary vasodilator therapy, the presence of a small hyperdynamic left ventricle with a dilated right ventricle (Figure 17–1), especially when accompanied by marginal urine output, arrhythmias, or coagulopathy, should prompt the consideration of the implantation of an RV assist device.

The size and geometry of the atria and the atrial anastomoses depend entirely on the transplantation technique employed. In the standard biatrial technique, different-sized portions of the native atria are left in situ (Figure 17–2), resulting in biatrial enlargement, asynchronous contraction, and intraluminal protrusion of the atrial anastomoses. This method also often gives the atria a multichamber configuration on the TEE (Figure 17–3). The anastomotic protrusions appear echo-dense and should not be confused with thrombi, although thrombi may form along the suture line. These protrusions may also occasionally contact the posterior mitral leaflet in systole, or even result in a mild constriction with a step-up of intraatrial Doppler flow velocities. Severe cases of supra-mitral valve obstruction, or acquired cor triatriatum, have been described after heart transplantation and should be suspected intraoperatively when the LA remnant is markedly enlarged and LV volume is reduced. Turbulent flow by color-flow Doppler (CFD), fluttering of the mitral valve leaflets, and elevated blood flow velocities by pulsed-wave Doppler also may aid in the confirmation of the diagnosis.

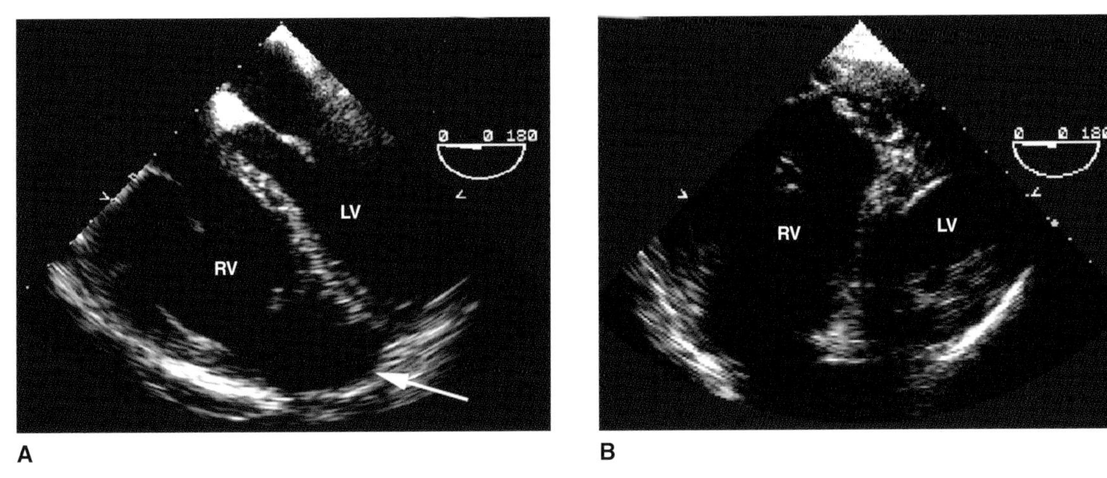

FIGURE 17–1. Right ventricular dilation. **A:** In the long-axis view, the right ventricle appears to be greater than two-thirds the size of the left ventricle, and the apex of the heart includes the right ventricle *(arrow)*. **B:** In the short-axis view, a small, usually hyperdynamic left ventricle is seen with a dilated right ventricle. (LV, left ventricle; RV, right ventricle.)

The integrity of the interatrial septum should be assessed intraoperatively by using color-flow Doppler and contrast echocardiography (agitated saline or saline microcavitation). Shunts can occur at the atrial anastomotic site or through a patent foramen ovale (PFO). Although uncommon, shunting through a PFO that is not apparent preoperatively may become hemodynamically significant postoperatively. As the relative pressure difference between the left and right atria changes as a result of pulmonary hypertension, RV dysfunction, or tricuspid regurgitation (TR), right-to-left shunting can occur and present as refractory postoperative hypoxemia.[15] Identification of a left-to-right shunt across the interatrial anastomoses also should prompt surgical repair because it can contribute to progressive RV volume overload and TR.

Spontaneous echo contrast can be detected in up to 55% of heart transplant recipients. This is usually

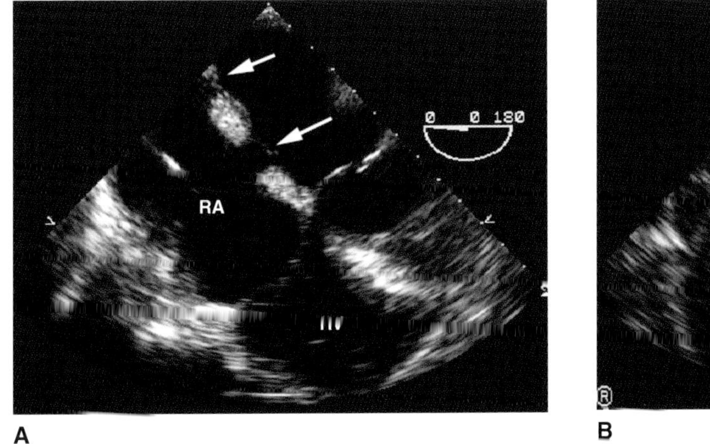

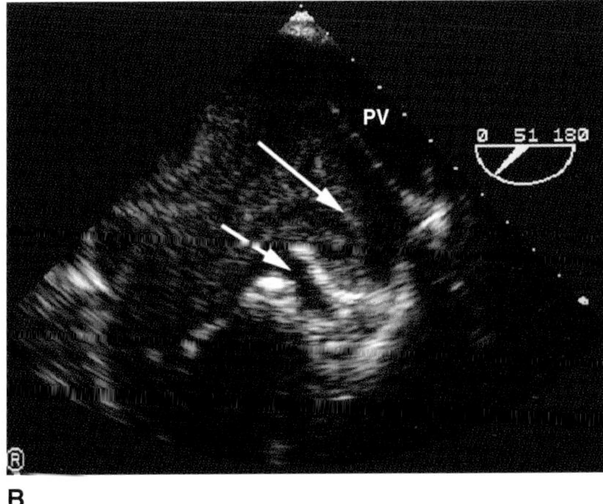

FIGURE 17–2. Posttransplantation transesophageal echocardiography demonstrating consequences of the different-sized portions of the native atria left in situ. **A:** Two fossa ovale *(arrows)*. **B:** Two atrial appendages *(arrows)*. (PV, pulmonary vein; RA, right atrium; RV, right ventricle.)

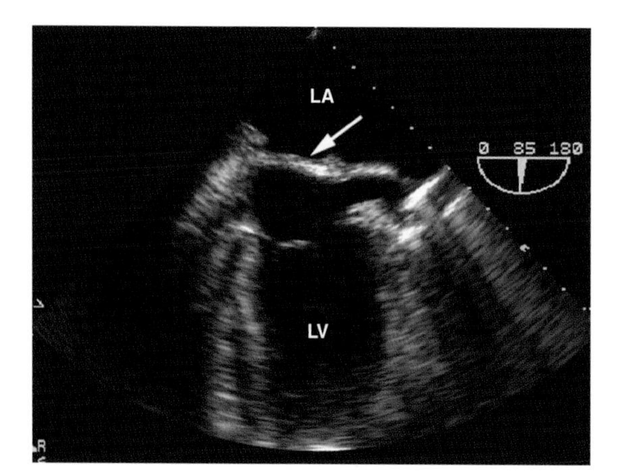

FIGURE 17–3. Anastomotic protrusions *(arrow)* creating the impression of a multi-chamber left atrium. (LA, left atrium; LV, left ventricle.)

confined to the donor atrial component and is associated with thrombi, usually attached to the LA free wall underneath the protruding suture line. The incidence of thrombus formation in the left atrium is reduced with the bicaval anastomosis technique.

The PA anastomosis should be examined for possible stenosis, and, although rare, kinking or torsion of the donor or recipient pulmonary artery should be ruled out, especially in the setting of RV dysfunction.[16] Color-flow Doppler may detect turbulent flow, and the pressure gradient should be measured with continuous-flow Doppler. Pulmonary venous inflow also should be assessed with color-flow and pulsed-wave Doppler.

Mild to moderate degrees of TR and mitral regurgitation (MR) are common after heart transplantation. MR is usually mild, produces an eccentric jet toward the LA free wall, and has a reported incidence of 48% to 87%.[16,17] TR, the most common valvular abnormality after heart transplantation with a reported incidence of 85%, is usually mild with an eccentric jet directed toward the interatrial septum.[18] TR after heart transplantation is best quantified by using the ratio of the maximum area of the regurgitant jet to the RA area.[19] The etiology of atrioventricular valve regurgitation in the transplanted heart is thought to be related to distortion of annular geometry. Annular distortion after the standard biatrial anastomotic technique is predominantly the result of disturbed atrial geometry and function, whereas donor heart and recipient pericardial cavity size mismatch is thought to play an important role after the bicaval anastomotic technique. This hypothesis is supported by the fact that the incidence and severity of TR and MR are reduced after the bicaval technique as compared with the standard biatrial technique.

The natural history of these regurgitant lesions varies, but the incidence of severe TR appears to increase with time, and some patients may require tricuspid valve repair or replacement for refractory symptoms. However, in many of these patients, the subvalvular apparatus was damaged during subsequent endomyocardial biopsy.[19] When patients were examined 1 year after transplantation, those with significant TR were more symptomatic and had poorer right-side heart function and greater mortality than those with mild or no TR.[20,21]

Management of Early Postoperative Hemodynamic Abnormalities in the Intensive Care Unit

TEE has become an invaluable tool in the management of seriously ill intensive care patients in whom transthoracic acoustic images may be poor. Particular uses in these circumstances include assessment of biventricular function, anastomotic problems (kinks, torsion, or stenosis), valvular abnormalities, sources of systemic emboli, and the detection of pericardial tamponade.

Postoperative Follow-Up Studies of Cardiac Allograft Function

Echocardiography, a noninvasive means of diagnosing transplant rejection, plays a significant role in the follow-up of recipients after heart transplantation. Proposed echocardiographic indicators of rejection in heart transplant patients are listed in Table 17–5. In addition, two- or three-dimensional echocardiography may be used to guide transvenous endomyocardial biopsies to prevent inadvertent damage to the tricuspid valve and its supporting apparatus. Dobutamine stress echocardiography, used in the detection of allograft vasculopathy, also has been shown to have a high negative predictive value for

Table 17–5. Echocardiographic Indicators of Rejection.

Increasing left ventricular mass and left ventricular wall thickness
Increased myocardial echogenicity
New or increasing pericardial effusion
Greater than 10% decrease in left ventricular ejection fraction
Restrictive left ventricular filling pattern (>20% decrease in mitral valve pressure half-time and 20% decrease in isovolumic relaxation time)
New-onset mitral regurgitation

determining future cardiac events and death in heart transplant recipients.[22]

MECHANICAL CIRCULATORY SUPPORT

Mechanical circulatory support devices include intra-aortic balloon pumps and ventricular assist devices (VADs) that may be inserted for supporting the failing left and/or right ventricle.

Intra-aortic Balloon Pumps

Intra-aortic balloon pumps (IABPs) are placed perioperatively in 2% to 12% of cardiac surgical patients, with the majority being placed intraoperatively.[5] When IABPs are placed, TEE can be useful in determining the need for the IABP, assessing for contraindications such as aortic insufficiency or severe aortic atherosclerosis, and guiding its placement into the descending aorta. TEE can also rapidly assess the effects of counterpulsation upon LV function and determine if there were any complications such as aortic dissection or aortic valve perforation. Inappropriate placement is the most common complication, and inadvertent passage of the IABP into the aortic arch, left ventricle, subclavian artery, renal artery, contralateral femoral artery, and right atrium have all been reported.[23,24]

Assessment of IABP placement begins with visualization of the guidewire within the lumen of the descending aorta. This is particularly important in the setting of aortic dissection, when identification of the true aortic lumen may be challenging. Optimal placement of the IABP tip is 3 to 4 cm distal to the origin of the left subclavian artery, or when the tip is seen at the inferior border of the transverse aortic arch.[25] To confirm proper placement, the balloon is first identified in the descending aorta short-axis view. Proper placement has been defined by the disappearance of the tip of the IABP from the aortic arch in the upper esophageal aortic arch long-axis view. Placement below the subclavian artery can also be visualized in a descending aorta long-axis view by slowly withdrawing the probe until the subclavian artery is seen at the level of the aortic arch (which is now seen in cross-section). The common carotid artery is sometimes mistaken for the subclavian artery but can be differentiated by its larger diameter and by turning the probe to the left (to visualize subclavian) and then to the right (to visualize the common carotid). The balloon itself typically appears as an echodense image when deflated (Figure 17–4) and a scattered echo image when inflated. A side lobe artifact is commonly seen when the tip of the IABP is visualized in the short-axis view.

Left Ventricular Assist Devices

Transesophageal echocardiography plays a critical role in each step of the management of patients with left ventricular assist devices (LVADs), including the preplacement evaluation of cardiac structure and function,

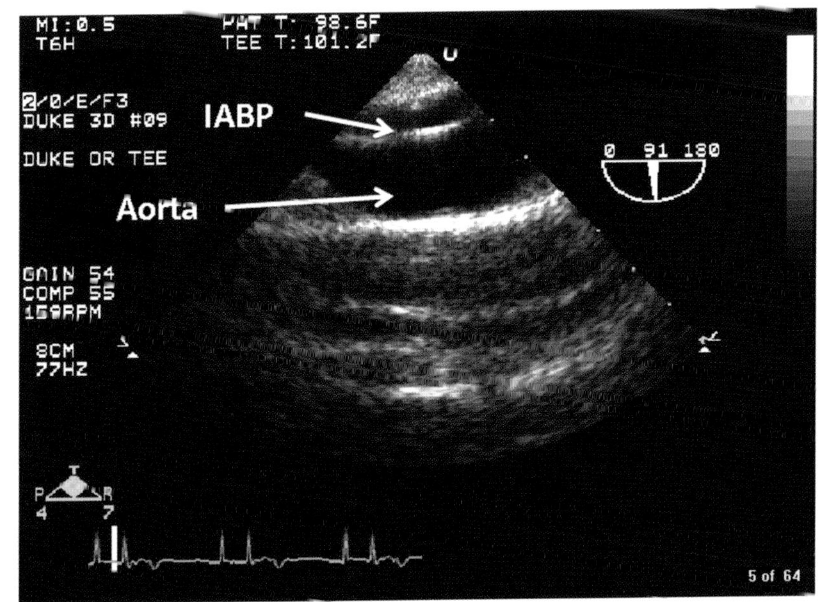

FIGURE 17–4. A midesophageal descending aorta long-axis view demonstrates the aortic lumen and an echodense intra-aortic balloon pump (IABP) within the aortic lumen.

detection of interatrial shunts, determination of aortic and tricuspid valve pathology, separation from CPB, and assessment of device function in the postoperative period.

PRE-PROCEDURE ASSESSMENT

A pre-procedure TEE is typically performed in the operating room following induction of general anesthetic and prior to institution of CPB. Determination of the patency of the foramen ovale, aortic valve insufficiency, mitral valve stenosis, tricuspid regurgitation, left heart thrombus, and assessment of right ventricular function are critical to intraoperative planning and management.

Patent Foramen Ovale. While it is important to recognize an atrial or ventricular septal defect, the more common cause of an intracardiac shunt is a patent foramen ovale (PFO). Intracardiac shunts are important to diagnose and repair to reduce the risk of paradoxical embolism or hypoxemia following LVAD placement. An appropriately functioning LVAD will significantly reduce LV diastolic pressures (often to <5 to 10 mm Hg) but right heart filling pressures can remain abnormally elevated, resulting in a right-to-left shunt and hypoxemia. Even small PFOs should be surgically repaired because of the significant incidence of shunting seen in patients with LVADs.

The normal foramen ovale is best seen in a midesophageal (ME) bicaval view; it appears as a thin slice of tissue bound by thicker ridges of tissue, one of which appears as a "flap." TEE evaluation of the foramen ovale should include two-dimensional (2D) assessment for flap movement and color-flow Doppler assessment, optimized for measurement of lower-velocity flow. Injection of agitated saline (a "bubble study") along with a Valsalva maneuver is typically used to provoke right-to-left shunting.[26] In such a study, the bubbles should be injected after the Valsalva maneuver produces a decrease in RA volume, and the Valsalva should be released (so as to transiently increase RA pressure over LA pressure) when the microbubbles are first seen to enter the RA. Bowing of the septum to the left upon release of Valsalva confirms the transient increase in right atrial pressures. Admixture of agitated saline with small quantities of blood has been reported to improve the acoustic signal of the microbubbles. The bubble study is positive if bubbles appear in the left atrium within five cardiac cycles (Figure 17–5). In patients with severe LV failure, it may be difficult to sufficiently decrease left atrial pressure. In such cases, an alternative method involves partial obstruction of the pulmonary artery by the surgeon after the aortic cannula is placed.[27]

Aortic Pathology. The LVAD outflow cannula is typically placed in the ascending aorta (except for the Jarvik 2000, which may be attached to the descending aorta). Thus, a thorough examination of the ascending aorta is an essential component of the intraoperative TEE evaluation. The ascending aorta is optimally viewed in the midesophageal ascending aortic short- and long-axis

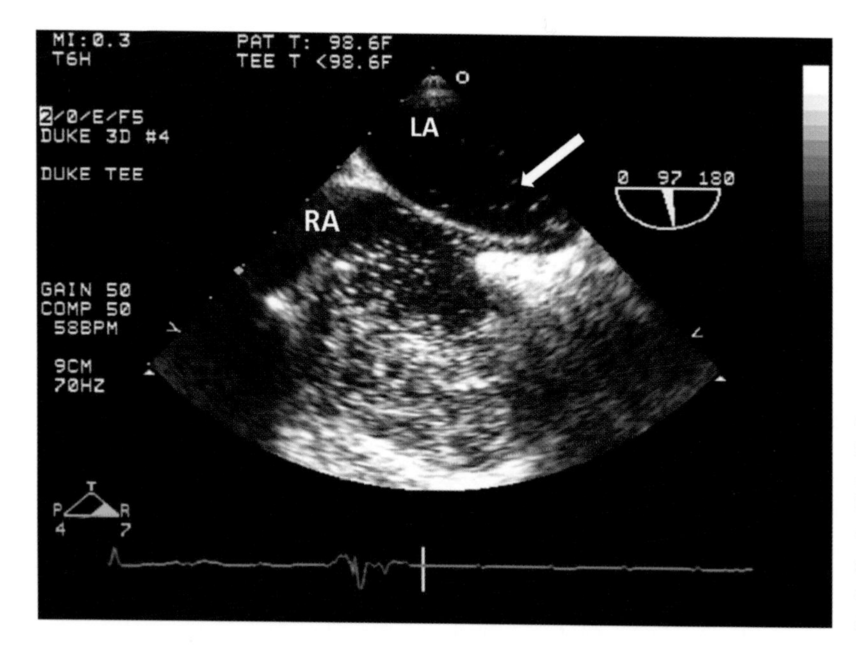

FIGURE 17–5. Mid-esophageal bicaval view with agitated saline contrast injected into the right atrium (RA). A few bubbles are seen simultaneously in the left atrium *(arrow)*. (LA, left atrium.)

views. An ascending aortic aneurysm may require repair prior to LVAD placement.[26] Protruding atheroma or mobile atheroma increase stroke risk, and their presence must be communicated to the surgeon. These plaques can be difficult to palpate; therefore, an epiaortic image at the site of cannulation for CBP and for the outflow cannula may assist the surgeon with precise placement.[28]

Aortic Valve Insufficiency. Significant aortic valve regurgitation (AR) results in chronic volume overload of the LV with consequent ventricular dilation and dysfunction. Reduction of the transaortic (valve) pressure gradient secondary to elevated LV end-diastolic pressure and reduced aortic diastolic pressure may confound determination of AR severity and lead to underestimation in a heart failure population.[26,29] In LVAD patients with AR, LV volume loading may be more pronounced as blood being returned from the LVAD is delivered to the aorta just above the aortic valve and regurgitant volume is increased because the LV end-diastolic pressure is low relative to the aortic pressure. If the resultant regurgitant volume exceeds 1 to 2 L/min, patients may remain in clinical heart failure despite the LVAD, since this volume is not delivered systemically but remains within a circuit formed by the LV, LVAD, and the ascending aorta. Older, volume displacement LVADs typically eject blood each time the device is full; therefore, AR in these patients increases the pump rate.[29]

Aortic insufficiency is best assessed in the midesophageal aortic valve short- and long-axis views as discussed in Chapter 9. It has been suggested that patients with worse than mild AR should undergo a concomitant aortic valve repair or replacement.[30,31] However, the decision to correct AR is complex since the addition of a valve procedure significantly increases procedural mortality.[32] Important considerations include the degree of aortic valve calcification and the characteristics of the regurgitant jet. An eccentric regurgitant jet in a heavily calcified valve may be more likely to worsen with VAD support and usually warrants surgical correction. Another consideration relates to the planned duration of LVAD support. If the LVAD is being used to bridge the patient to transplant and a relatively short period of support is anticipated, then moderate AR may be tolerated, anticipating that LVAD speeds/rates may be higher than normal. On the other hand, if the device is being used as a permanent or "destination" treatment, such aortic regurgitation is likely to progress and may impact the durability of the device.

There are several methods of surgically addressing AR. One option is replacement of the aortic valve. Mechanical valves are not typically used because of the potential for thrombus formation on the valve as a consequence of the immobility of the leaflets during most LVAD cycles. Furthermore, intermittent opening of the aortic valve renders the patient at risk for embolization.[29,30] Thus, if the valve requires replacement, most surgeons recommended the use of a bioprosthesis.[32] Another alternative to managing AR in the LVAD patient is partial or complete surgical ligation of the aortic valve cusps. This should not be performed if there is a chance of ventricular recovery with subsequent removal of the device.[29,30] A third option in patients without the possibility for native heart recovery is placement of an occlusive LV outflow tract patch graft. In this situation, all blood must be delivered from the LV to the LVAD, and pump failure may result in severe hemodynamic instability as the native heart would be required to eject through the LVAD.[30,32]

Mitral Valve Stenosis. A significant mitral gradient will lead to impairment of LVAD filling, persistent elevation of pulmonary venous pressure, and symptoms of heart failure. While rheumatic mitral stenosis (MS) is rare in this group of patients, previous procedures such as mitral valve repair or replacement are common. TEE should evaluate for the presence of severe MS across repaired mitral valves or prosthetic valves. It is recommended that severe MS be surgically repaired, with a commissurotomy or concomitant replacement of the mitral valve.[26,29] Mitral valve stenosis is optimally assessed by TEE in the midesophageal four-chamber view using CFD and spectral Doppler to determine peak and mean transvalvular gradients as described in Chapter 7.

Tricuspid Regurgitation. Careful evaluation of tricuspid regurgitation (TR) is also warranted. Severe TR with hepatic vein flow reversal usually warrants concomitant tricuspid repair, as elimination of severe TR may improve right ventricular function and device filling following LVAD placement. The tricuspid valve is optimally viewed in the midesophageal four-chamber and the midesophageal right ventricular inflow-outflow views (see Chapter 10).

Left Heart Thrombus. Abnormal blood flow patterns in the left atrium and ventricle predispose to thrombus formation. Common sites of left heart thrombus include the left atrial appendage (Figure 17–6) and the left ventricular apex.[31,33] In an attempt to reduce the risk for embolization, TEE should be utilized to rule out the presence of LV apical thrombus prior to the ventriculotomy for placement of the LVAD inflow cannula. Epicardial scanning may be helpful when the apex cannot be visualized with TEE.

Right Ventricular Dysfunction. An LVAD only supports the left heart and is dependent on a functional right ventricle (RV) to provide adequate preload. While

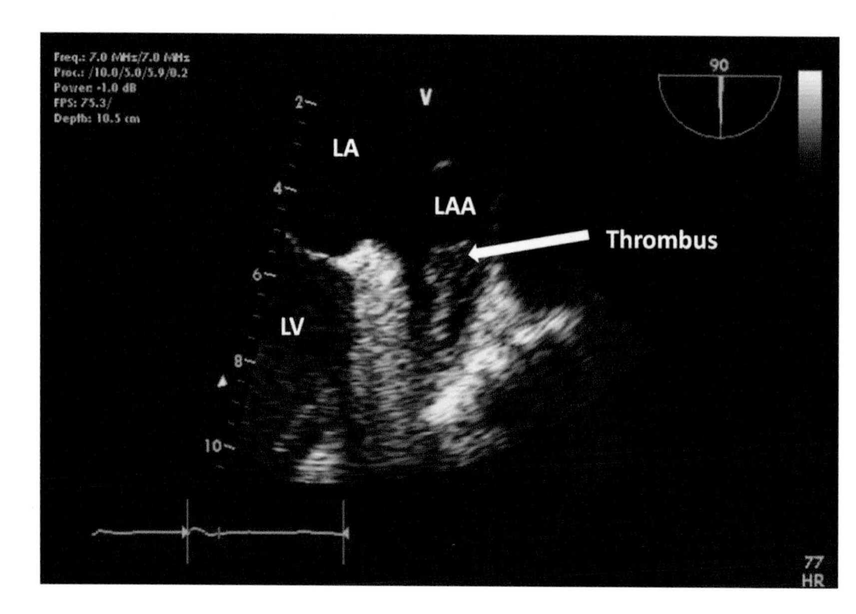

FIGURE 17–6. A midesophageal two-chamber "zoom" view of the left atrial appendage (LAA) demonstrating a thrombus within its cavity. (LA, left atrium; LV, left ventricle.)

the LVAD may enhance RV performance by decreasing its afterload, it may also worsen RV function by increasing its preload.[26] When evaluating the RV, it may be helpful to determine the RV fractional area change (RVFAC), defined as:

$$\frac{\text{End Diastolic Area} - \text{End Systolic Area}}{\text{End Diastolic Area}} \times 100$$

A normal RVFAC is greater than 40%, while most patients receiving an LVAD have an RVFAC of 20% to 30%.[31] An RVFAC less than 20% predicts a high risk for RV failure following LVAD placement.[31] Right ventricular dysfunction remains one of the important clinical challenges in left-side mechanical circulatory support. Combinations of inotropic agents, systemic and inhaled vasodilators, and mechanical RV support may be needed to ensure proper function of the LVAD.

SEPARATION FROM CARDIOPULMONARY BYPASS

The TEE exam must be repeated during separation from CPB initially to assist in the de-airing process. As the pressure gradients within the heart change dramatically with a functional LVAD, it is also important to repeat the assessment for a PFO, AR, and RV dysfunction. Aortic valve opening, placement and orientation of the inflow cannula, flow in the inflow cannula and outflow graft, and assessment of LV size and ventricular septal position are critical in the intraoperative management of these patients.

De-airing. Following open heart surgery, ambient air (Figure 17–7) can be retained in multiple locations of the heart including the right and left upper pulmonary veins, the LV apex, the left atrial appendage, the right coronary sinus of Valsalva, and the pulmonary artery.[26,34] In addition, air can be retained in the VAD cannulas and the pump itself.[26] The de-airing process is more complicated for this procedure compared to valvular heart procedures. Most LVAD designs are able to generate negative intraventricular pressure or suction, which can lead to entrainment of extracardiac air. This is most commonly seen when device rate or speed is inappropriately increased during a time when the delivery of blood into the LV is reduced. Thus, the complex de-airing process for LVADs includes removal of intracardiac air as well as vigilance to avoid entrainment and reintroduction. A potential negative impact is when entrained air is delivered into the right coronary artery with subsequent RV dysfunction, reduced LV filling, and further entrainment of air by the pump. In this scenario, the TEE will demonstrate a distended RV, a collapsed LV, and significant air in the aorta. Preserving RV function while weaning from CPB so as to maintain LV preload during the period of reduced LVAD flows and until protamine reversal is therefore highly desirable. TEE examination for air should be conducted continually from before initiation of CPB weaning until after protamine reversal.

Patent Foramen Ovale. Although it is optimal to diagnose a PFO prior to CPB, LVAD-induced reductions in LV end-diastolic pressure and left atrial pressure

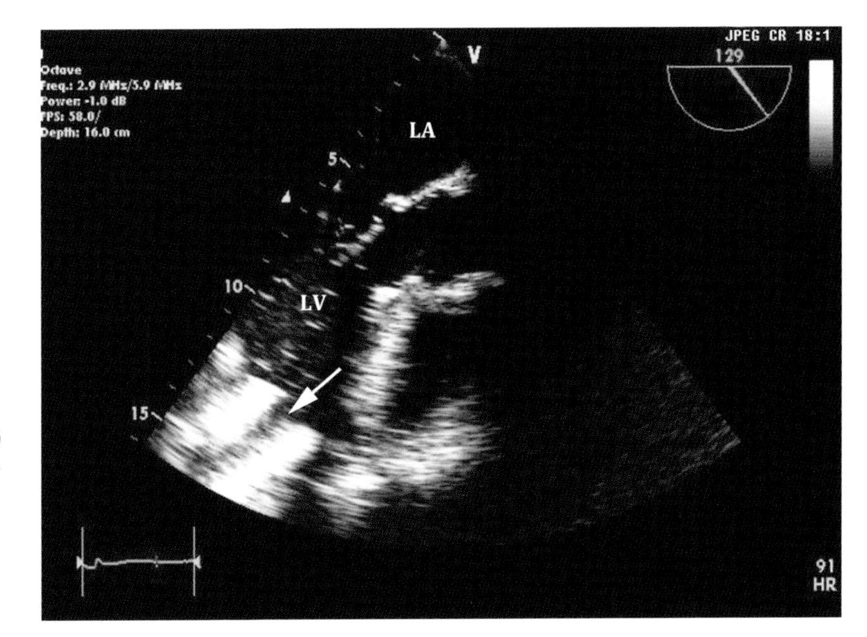

FIGURE 17–7. Midesophageal long-axis view showing a left ventricular assist device cannula (*arrow*) at the apex of the left ventricle (LV). Air bubbles can be seen as echo-dense spots within the LV cavity, moving with blood flow. (LA, left atrium.)

increase the likelihood of right-to-left shunting. Discovery of a previously unrecognized PFO following CPB has been described and may require reinstitution of CPB for repair if there is significant shunt flow.[35,36]

Aortic Valve. Ideally the severity of AR should be determined preoperatively to allow for correction during LVAD placement. However, the increased transaortic (valve) gradient associated with reduction of the LV end-diastolic pressure and increased flow into the ascending aorta through the outflow graft after CPB is discontinued may worsen preexistent AR. If worse than mild AR is identified, the aortic valve may need to be surgically corrected.[37]

In addition to examining the aortic valve for severity of AR, the frequency of aortic valve opening should be determined. A functioning LVAD is capable of reducing LV end-diastolic pressure to a level at which the aortic valve does not open during a normal cardiac cycle. However, if the LVAD is only providing partial or variable support, the aortic valve will open intermittently.[26]

Right Ventricular Dysfunction. As the LVAD provides a normal cardiac output, a commensurate amount of blood is returning to the right heart as preload. Patients with RV dysfunction may be unable to accommodate for this change, and signs of right heart failure may develop including RV distension, acute severe tricuspid regurgitation, increase in pulmonary pressures, and LV failure secondary to a low preload.[31] Another cause of RV dysfunction after LVAD placement is based on the concept of ventricular interdependence. Rapid reductions in LV end-diastolic pressure may result in movement of the ventricular septum toward the LV free wall. Functionally this causes abrupt alternations in RV size and geometry and can influence the severity of tricuspid regurgitation. If identified, the most effective short-term treatment is to reduce the LVAD flow, which subsequently increases the LV end-diastolic pressure and returns the septum to a more normal anatomic position.

Inflow Cannula. The inflow cannula is usually placed in the LV apex and is often directed anteroseptally and toward the mitral valve opening but away from the interventricular septum and lateral wall. It should not abut any of the LV walls in order to avoid obstruction of blood flow into the cannula.[31] If the cannula is misdirected, withdrawal and inferior displacement by the surgeon generally rectifies the situation. Proper inflow cannula placement should be evaluated in at least two views: the midesophageal four-chamber view and the midesophageal long-axis view. A CFD sector should be placed across the opening of the inflow cannula and should demonstrate low-velocity, unidirectional, laminar (nonturbulent) flow (Figure 17–8). In addition, unobstructed flow should be demonstrated using continuous-wave Doppler from the inflow cannula with peak velocities less than 2.5 m/s (Figure 17–9).[31] The cannula position should be assessed again after chest closure to ensure that it remains correctly positioned.

Outflow Cannula. The outflow cannula of most devices is placed in the ascending aorta. This cannula may be seen in the midesophageal ascending aorta short-axis

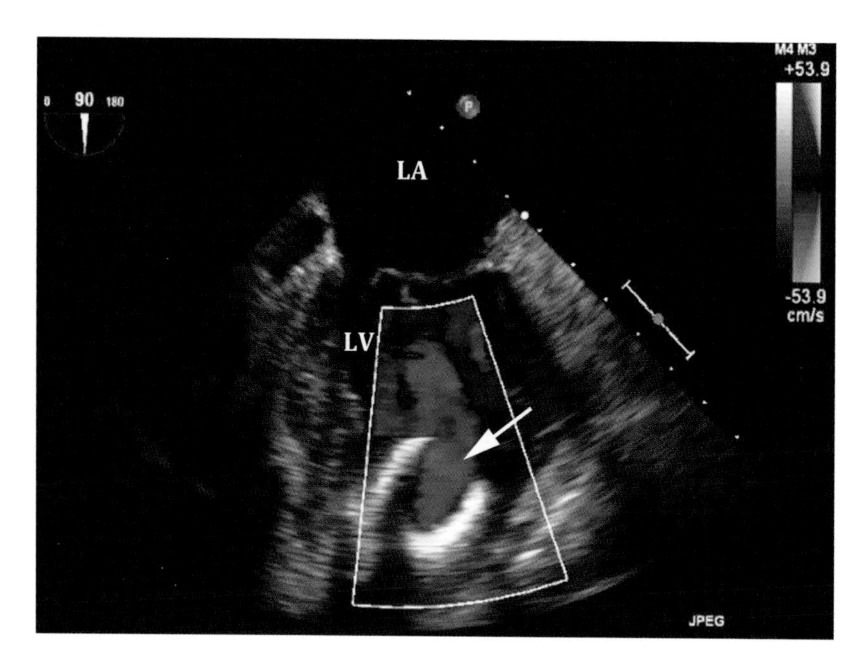

FIGURE 17–8. Midesophageal two-chamber view of the left ventricle (LV) demonstrating laminar flow with color-flow Doppler across the left ventricular assist device inflow cannula (*arrow*) positioned at the LV apex. (LA, left atrium)

(Figure 17–10) or long-axis views. In order to assess the blood flow at the cannula anastomotic site, pulsed- or continuous-wave Doppler can be used. The peak velocity should be 1.0 to 2.0 m/s for an axial device and around 2 m/s for a pulsatile device.[26]

Left Ventricle. After protamine administration, the LVAD speed can be safely increased and TEE should confirm LV unloading. A properly functioning LVAD should reduce the LV diameter, and the interventricular septum should remain in a neutral position. Persistent deviation of the septum to the right suggests inadequate reduction of left ventricular pressure, and an increased pump speed is warranted. Septal displacement towards the LV cavity is indicative of excessive LV unloading and may have adverse implications for RV function as discussed above. Detection of specific wall motion abnormalities and determination of ejection fraction are unreliable with a functional LVAD as preload reduction precludes normal contractility.[26]

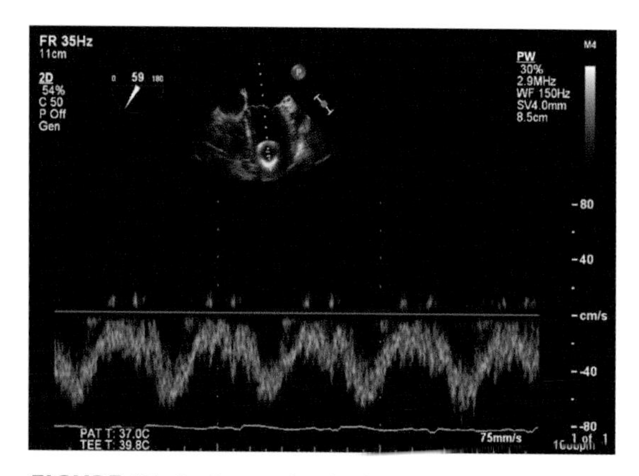

FIGURE 17–9. Spectral pulsed-wave Doppler flow velocity across a left ventricular device inflow cannula in the midesophageal four-chamber view demonstrating low-velocity laminar flow.

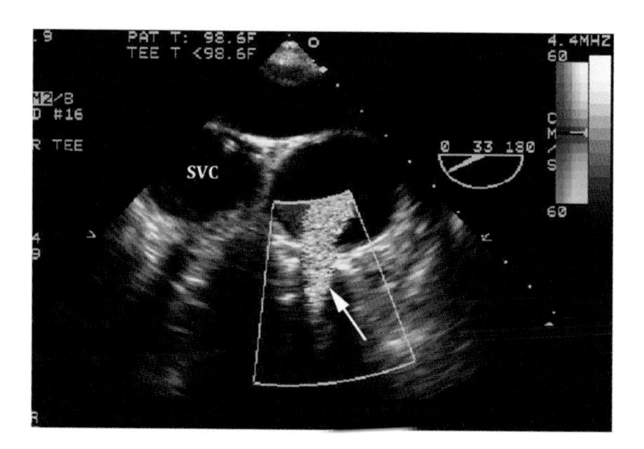

FIGURE 17–10. Midesophageal ascending aortic short-axis view demonstrating a left ventricular assist device outflow cannula *(arrow)* with color-flow Doppler showing flow across the cannula into the ascending aorta. (SVC, superior vena cava.)

POSTOPERATIVE PERIOD

TEE can be used to assess patients with reduced LVAD flows or function. The differential diagnosis includes right ventricular failure, pulmonary embolus, cardiac tamponade, hypovolemia, cannula obstruction or malposition, and device failure.[31,38]

Right Ventricular Failure or Pulmonary Embolus. RV failure and pulmonary embolus present with a similar echocardiographic picture. As mentioned previously, RV failure limits the preload for the LVAD, causing a low output state. The typical findings on TEE include a dilated and dysfunctional RV, severe tricuspid regurgitation, and an underfilled left ventricle. Patients with a pulmonary embolus tend to have elevated pulmonary artery pressures, whereas those with isolated RV failure may actually have low pulmonary artery pressures. If there is concern of a pulmonary embolus, the pulmonary arteries should also be examined.[31]

Cardiac Tamponade. Tamponade can be difficult to diagnose after LVAD placement, as fluid collections may be loculated, making them difficult to identify. For example, the typical findings of right heart compression may be absent if the fluid collection is located posteriorly and compresses the left atrium. Normal LVAD physiology, which reduces left heart filling pressures, also confounds this assessment.[31]

Hypovolemia. Clinically, hypovolemia will present with systemic hypotension, reduced jugular venous pressure or central venous pressure, and reduced LVAD output. Although this diagnosis does not typically require imaging, TEE may be a useful adjunct, demonstrating small RV and LV dimensions and ruling out other possible etiologies for the clinical picture, including RV failure and tamponade.

Inflow Cannula. Inflow cannula obstruction has a severely detrimental impact on VAD function and can be caused by a variety of pathological processes (Table 17–6).[26,39] The cannula should again be examined in at least two views, typically the midesophageal four-chamber view and the midesophageal long-axis view.[31] Color-flow Doppler across the cannula inlet demonstrating turbulent flow during LVAD diastole, and continuous-wave Doppler demonstrating a peak velocity greater than 2.5 m/s are suggestive of obstruction.[26,39-41] Three dimensional (3D) TEE images have also been used to visualize thrombus in the inflow cannula (Figure 17–11).

The pulsatile LVADs contain valved conduits that direct flow through the device and prevent regurgitation in a manner similar to the native heart. Inflow valve regurgitation (IVR) is a common cause of LVAD mechanical dysfunction and is usually due to a torn cusp or commissural dehiscence of the prosthetic valve secondary to high pressures.[37,41] The patient with significant IVR presents with clinical evidence of heart failure and elevated pump rates that result from increased device filling. Echocardiography will demonstrate ineffective LV unloading characterized by increased LV dimensions and aortic valve opening in addition to decreased outflow graft velocity and a decreased stroke volume.[37,41]

Table 17–6. Potential Causes of Inflow Cannula Obstruction.

Hypovolemia
Thrombus
Compression of the ventricular septum
Compression of the papillary muscles
Compression of the left atrial wall (if the cannula is placed in the left atrium)
Migration of thrombus from an intracardiac site

Outflow Cannula. Documented complications of the outflow cannulae include perforation and malposition. Air bubbles in the aorta near the outflow cannula anastamosis may suggest cannula perforation.[26] An extreme case of cannula misplacement was reported in a hemodynamically unstable patient in whom the LV was dilated and the AV was opening with LVAD systole. The outflow cannula was not visualized on TEE and upon surgical exploration, was found in the right superior pulmonary vein.[40]

RIGHT VENTICULAR ASSIST DEVICE

Mechanical assist devices can be used for right ventricular support either in isolation or in combination with a left-sided device. The etiology of right heart failure after cardiac surgery includes prolonged cardiopulmonary bypass time, inadequate myocardial protection, or right coronary occlusion from vasospasm, air embolus, or thrombus.[42] Isolated right heart failure is rare, occurring in only about 0.3% of cardiac surgical patients.[43] However, it is associated with a very poor prognosis.[42,43]

Most right ventricular assist devices (RVADs) are placed after a failed attempt to separate from CPB or within the same day as LVAD placement.[44] The RVAD inflow cannula is typically placed in the right atrium (but can occasionally be placed in the right ventricle).[26] This cannula should be visualized using either the midesophageal four-chamber view or the midesophageal bicaval view. The RVAD outflow cannula is attached to the main pulmonary artery. This cannula can be difficult to image by TEE, but may be seen in the midesophageal right ventricle inflow-outflow view (Figure 17–12). As with the LVAD cannula, flow should be laminar and of low velocity when examined with CFD.

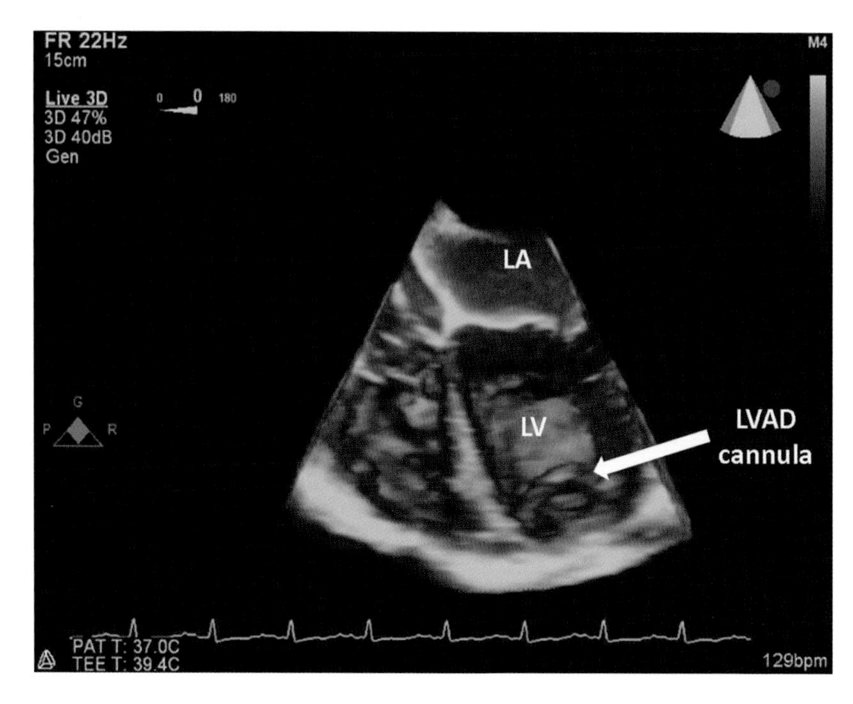

FIGURE 17–11. A three-dimensional transesophageal echocardiographic view demonstrating a left ventricular assist device (LVAD) inflow cannula *(arrow)* in the apical region. A thrombus could be seen within the lumen of the cannula. (LV, left ventricle; LA, left atrium.)

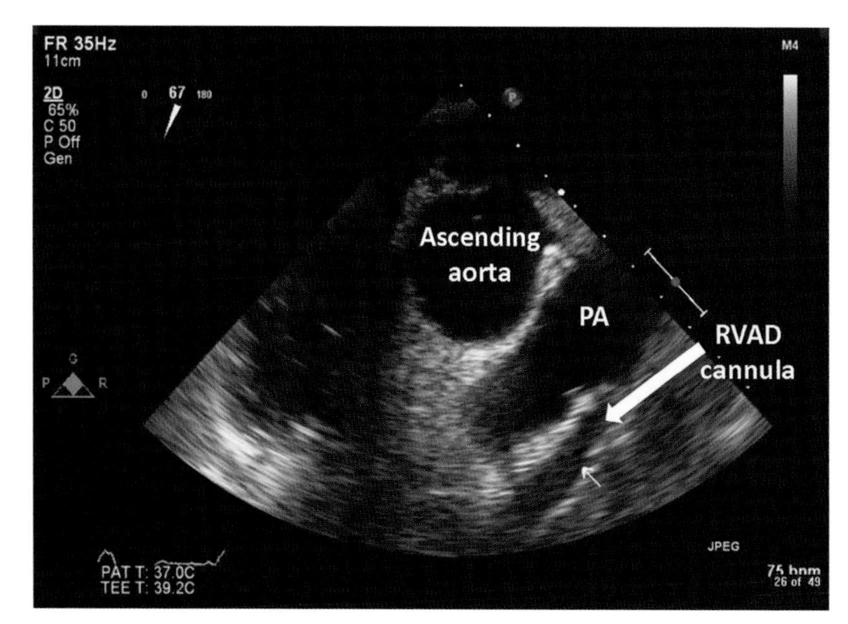

FIGURE 17–12. Midesophageal right ventricle inflow-outflow view demonstrating a right ventricular assist device (RVAD) outflow cannula *(arrow)* adjacent to the RV outflow tract just before it enters the main pulmonary artery (PA).

SUMMARY

The current surge in the heart failure patient population will produce a concomitant increase in the number of VAD insertions and heart transplants performed worldwide. The option of VAD support is particularly attractive in the face of a shortage of donor organs. As a consequence of the significant technological advances in mechanical cardiac support devices seen in the last decade, patients will benefit from a reduced complication rate and improved survival. Intraoperative TEE imaging is a critical part of successful device placement and cardiac transplantation.

REFERENCES

1. Lloyd-Jones D, Adams R, Carnethon M, et al. Heart disease and stroke statistics—2009 update. a report from the American Heart Association Statistics Committee and Stroke Statistics Subcommittee. *Circulation.* 2009;119(3):e21-181.
2. Butler J, Kalogeropoulos A. Worsening heart failure hospitalization epidemic we do not know how to prevent and we do not know how to treat! *J Am Coll Cardiol.* 2008;52(6):435-437.
3. Goland S, Czer LS, Kass RM, et al. Use of cardiac allografts with mild and moderate left ventricular hypertrophy can be safely used in heart transplantation to expand the donor pool. *J Am Coll Cardiol.* 2008;51(12):1214-1220.
4. Tallaj JA, Kirklin JK, Brown RN, et al. Post-heart transplant diastolic dysfunction is a risk factor for mortality. *J Am Coll Cardiol.* 2007;50(11):1064-1069.
5. Naunheim KS, Swartz MT, Pennington DG, et al. Intraaortic balloon pumping in patients requiring cardiac operations. Risk analysis and long-term follow-up. *J Thorac Cardiovasc Surg.* 1992;104(6):1654-1660; discussion 1660-1651.
6. Aziz S, Soine LA, Lewis SL, et al. Donor left ventricular hypertrophy increases risk for early graft failure. *Transpl Int.* 1997;10(6):446-450.
7. Tenzer ML. The spectrum of myocardial contusion: a review. *J Trauma.* 1985;25(7):620-627.
8. Vedrinne JM, Vedrinne C, Coronel B, Mercatello A, Estanove S, Moskovtchenko JF. Transesophageal echocardiographic assessment of left ventricular function in brain-dead patients: are marginally acceptable hearts suitable for transplantation? *J Cardiothorac Vasc Anesth.* 1996;10(6):708-712.
9. Young JB, Hauptman PJ, Naftel DC, et al. Determinants of early graft failure following cardiac transplantation, a 10-year, multi-institutional, multivariable analysis. *J Heart Lung Transplant.* 2001;20(2):212.
10. Shumway NE, Lower RR, Stofer RC. Transplantation of the heart. *Adv Surg.* 1966;2:265-284.
11. Schnoor M, Schafer T, Luhmann D, Sievers HH. Bicaval versus standard technique in orthotopic heart transplantation: a systematic review and meta-analysis. *J Thorac Cardiovasc Surg.* 2007;134(5):1322-1331.
12. Kaye DM, Bergin P, Buckland M, Esmore D. Value of postoperative assessment of cardiac allograft function by transesophageal echocardiography. *J Heart Lung Transplant.* 1994;13(2):165-172.
13. Spes CH, Tammen AR, Fraser AG, Uberfuhr P, Theisen K, Angermann CE. Doppler analysis of pulmonary venous flow profiles in orthotopic heart transplant recipients: a comparison with mitral flow profiles and atrial function. *Z Kardiol.* 1996;85(10):753-760.
14. Hosenpud JD, Bennett LE, Keck BM, Boucek MM, Novick RJ. The Registry of the International Society for Heart and Lung Transplantation: eighteenth official report—2001. *J Heart Lung Transplant.* 2001;20(8):805-815.
15. Ouseph R, Stoddard MF, Lederer ED. Patent foramen ovale presenting as refractory hypoxemia after heart transplantation. *J Am Soc Echocardiogr.* 1997;10(9):973-976.
16. de Marchena E, Futterman L, Wozniak P, et al. Pulmonary artery torsion: a potentially lethal complication after orthotopic heart transplantation. *J Heart Transplant.* 1989;8(6):499-502.
17. De Simone R, Lange R, Sack RU, Mehmanesh H, Hagl S. Atrioventricular valve insufficiency and atrial geometry after orthotopic heart transplantation. *Ann Thorac Surg.* 1995;60(6):1686-1693.
18. Angermann CE, Spes CH, Tammen A, et al. Anatomic characteristics and valvular function of the transplanted heart: transthoracic versus transesophageal echocardiographic findings. *J Heart Transplant.* 1990;9(4):331-338.
19. Chan MC, Giannetti N, Kato T, et al. Severe tricuspid regurgitation after heart transplantation. *J Heart Lung Transplant.* 2001;20(7):709-717.
20. Aziz TM, Saad RA, Burgess MI, Campbell CS, Yonan NA. Clinical significance of tricuspid valve dysfunction after orthotopic heart transplantation. *J Heart Lung Transplant.* 2002;21(10):1101-1108.
21. Marelli D, Esmailian F, Wong SY, et al. Tricuspid valve regurgitation after heart transplantation. *J Thorac Cardiovasc Surg.* 2009;137(6):1557-1559.
22. Akosah KO, Olsovsky M, Kirchberg D, Salter D, Mohanty PK. Dobutamine stress echocardiography predicts cardiac events in heart transplant patients. *Circulation.* 1996;94(9 Suppl):II283-288.
23. Coffin SA. The misplaced intraaortic balloon pump. *Anesth Analg.* 1994;78(6):1182-1183.
24. Varadarajan B, Karski J, Vegas A, Heinrich L. A rare complication of intra-aortic balloon pump placement. *J Cardiothorac Vasc Anesth.* 2005;19(2):259-260.
25. Shanewise JS, Sadel SM. Intraoperative transesophageal echocardiography to assist the insertion and positioning of the intraaortic balloon pump. *Anesth Analg.* 1994;79(3):577-580.
26. Chumnanvej S, Wood MJ, MacGillivray TE, Melo MF. Perioperative echocardiographic examination for ventricular assist device implantation. *Anesth Analg.* 2007;105(3):583-601.
27. Majd RE, Kavarana MN, Bouvette M, Dowling RD. Improved technique to diagnose a patent foramen ovale during left ventricular assist device insertion. *Ann Thorac Surg.* 2006;82(5):1917-1918.
28. Katz ES, Tunick PA, Rusinek H, Ribakove G, Spencer FC, Kronzon I. Protruding aortic atheromas predict stroke in elderly patients undergoing cardiopulmonary bypass: experience with intraoperative transesophageal echocardiography. *J Am Coll Cardiol.* 1992;20(1):70-77.
29. Rao V, Slater JP, Edwards NM, Naka Y, Oz MC. Surgical management of valvular disease in patients requiring left ventricular assist device support. *Ann Thorac Surg.* 2001;71(5):1448-1453.
30. Bryant AS, Holman WL, Nanda NC, et al. Native aortic valve insufficiency in patients with left ventricular assist devices. *Ann Thorac Surg.* 2006;81(2):e6-8.
31. Scalia GM, McCarthy PM, Savage RM, Smedira NG, Thomas JD. Clinical utility of echocardiography in the management of implantable ventricular assist devices. *J Am Soc Echocardiogr.* 2000;13(8):754-763.
32. Savage EB, d'Amato TA, Magovern JA. Aortic valve patch closure: an alternative to replacement with HeartMate LVAS insertion. *Eur J Cardiothorac Surg.* 1999;16(3):359-361.
33. Miyake Y, Sugioka K, Bussey CD, Di Tullio M, Homma S. Left ventricular mobile thrombus associated with ventricular assist device: diagnosis by transesophageal echocardiography. *Circ J.* 2004;68(4):383-384.
34. Orihashi K, Matsuura Y, Hamanaka Y, et al. Retained intracardiac air in open heart operations examined by transesophageal echocardiography. *Ann Thorac Surg.* 1993;55(6):1467-1471.

35. Loyalka P, Idelchik GM, Kar B. Percutaneous left ventricular assist device complicated by a patent foramen ovale: importance of identification and management. *Catheter Cardiovasc Interv.* 2007;70(3):383-386.
36. Liao KK, Miller L, Toher C, et al. Timing of transesophageal echocardiography in diagnosing patent foramen ovale in patients supported with left ventricular assist device. *Ann Thorac Surg.* 2003;75(5):1624-1626.
37. Horton SC, Khodaverdian R, Powers A, et al. Left ventricular assist device malfunction: a systematic approach to diagnosis. *J Am Coll Cardiol.* 2004;43(9):1574-1583.
38. Nicoara A, Mackensen GB, Podgoreanu MV, Milano CA, Mathew JP, Swaminathan M. Malpositioned left ventricular assist device cannula: diagnosis and management with transesophageal echocardiography guidance. *Anesth Analg.* 2007;105(6):1574-1576.
39. Szymanski P, Religa G, Klisiewicz A, Baranska K, Hoffman P. Diagnosis of biventricular assist device inflow cannula obstruction. *Echocardiography.* 2007;24(4):420-424.
40. Pu M, Stephenson ER Jr, Davidson WR Jr, Sun BC. An unexpected surgical complication of ventricular assist device implantation identified by transesophageal echocardiography: a case report. *J Am Soc Echocardiogr.* 2003;16(11):1194-1197.
41. Horton SC, Khodaverdian R, Chatelain P, et al. Left ventricular assist device malfunction: an approach to diagnosis by echocardiography. *J Am Coll Cardiol.* 2005;45(9):1435-1440.
42. Osaki S, Edwards NM, Johnson MR, Kohmoto T. A novel use of the implantable ventricular assist device for isolated right heart failure. *Interact Cardiovasc Thorac Surg.* 2008;7(4): 651-653.
43. Moazami N, Pasque MK, Moon MR, et al. Mechanical support for isolated right ventricular failure in patients after cardiotomy. *J Heart Lung Transplant.* 2004;23(12):1371-1375.
44. Ochiai Y, McCarthy PM, Smedira NG, et al. Predictors of severe right ventricular failure after implantable left ventricular assist device insertion: analysis of 245 patients. *Circulation.* 2002;106(12 Suppl 1):I198-202.

REVIEW QUESTIONS

Select the *one* best answer for each of the following questions.

1. Which of the following is a relative contraindication to inserting an intra-aortic balloon pump?
   a. Severe mitral regurgitation
   b. Patent foramen ovale
   c. Severe aortic regurgitation
   d. Endovascular stent in aortic arch

2. Which of the following correctly describes the final location of the tip of an intra-aortic balloon pump?
   a. 3 to 4 cm distal to the aortic valve
   b. 7 to 10 cm distal to the origin of the left subclavian artery
   c. Anywhere in the descending aorta
   d. 3 to 4 cm below the takeoff of the left subclavian artery

3. A patent foramen ovale is best seen in which of the following TEE views?
   a. ME two chamber
   b. ME long axis
   c. ME bicaval
   d. Deep transgastric long axis

4. Which of the following are true with regard to a patent foramen ovale (PFO)?
   a. During a Valsalva maneuver, the interatrial septum should bow towards the right atrium.
   b. It is unnecessary to reevaluate for a PFO after cardiopulmonary bypass.
   c. A PFO can lead to right-to-left shunt.
   d. An interatrial septal aneurysm rules out a PFO.

5. The severity of aortic stenosis is often underestimated in heart failure patients because of which of the following reasons?
   a. Transmitral flow velocity is higher than normal.
   b. Left ventricular end-diastolic pressure is high.
   c. Left atrial pressure is greater than right atrial pressure.
   d. Transaortic flow velocity is lower than expected.

6. In a patient with a left ventricular assist device, aortic regurgitation that is moderate or worse should be fixed by all of the following *except*:
   a. Mechanical valve replacement
   b. Bioprosthetic valve replacement
   c. Suturing the valve closed
   d. Left ventricular outflow graft patch

7. In which of the following indications for left ventricular assist device implantation is it acceptable to permanently close the aortic valve for severe incompetence?
   a. Temporary cardiac support.
   b. Bridge to recovery.
   c. Destination therapy.
   d. It is never appropriate.

8. Mitral stenosis in a patient with a left ventricular assist device will most likely lead to which of the following conditions?
   a. A high output state
   b. Increased device filling
   c. Improved right heart function
   d. Increased pulmonary pressures

9. Patients presenting for LVAD placement are most likely to have thrombi in which of the following locations?
   a. Mitral valve
   b. Proximal ascending aorta

c. Left atrial appendage
d. Right ventricular apex

10. Pulmonary vasodilators should be strongly considered in patients undergoing left ventricular assist device implantation, especially in which of the following preexisting conditions?
a. Mitral stenosis
b. Aortic regurgitation
c. Patent foramen ovale
d. Right ventricular dysfunction

11. Following placement of a left ventricular assist device, intracardiac air is most commonly seen by TEE in which of the following structures?
a. Right atrial appendage
b. Left pulmonary artery
c. The assist device itself
d. Left ventricle

12. In a patient with an LVAD, which of the following describes the appropriate management of a patent foramen ovale?
a. It need not be repaired if there is left-to-right shunting.
b. It should be repaired during placement of the device.
c. It should be repaired only if there is hypoxia.
d. It may be ignored unless there is a history of stroke.

13. Following placement of a left ventricular assist device, a TEE reveals that the aortic valve does not open during systole. Which of the following best describes the reason for this phenomenon?
a. Left ventricular pressure is higher than aortic pressure.
b. The aortic valve is severely stenosed.
c. The left ventricular preload is high.
d. The device is working normally.

14. Which of the following best describes the effect of aortic valve insufficiency AFTER left ventricular device (LVAD) placement?
a. It limits effective output from the LVAD.
b. It indicates that pump speed should be increased.
c. It suggests severe left ventricular dysfunction.
d. It is normal and will eventually resolve.

15. Which of the following suggests right ventricular failure after placement of a left ventricular assist device?
a. Systolic reversal of hepatic vein flow
b. Severe mitral regurgitation
c. Central venous pressure of 8 mm Hg
d. Systemic hypertension

16. Which of the following best describes the correct orientation of an LVAD inflow cannula?
a. In the left ventricle pointing towards the interventricular septum
b. In the ascending aorta directed towards the posterior aortic wall
c. In the descending aorta below the subclavian artery origin
d. In the left ventricle directed towards the mitral valve

17. Which of the following views are most likely to enable assessment of an LVAD inflow cannula?
a. ME ascending aorta short axis
b. ME long-axis view
c. ME RV inflow-outflow view
d. ME ascending aorta long-axis view

18. Which of the following best describes the character of Doppler-assessed flow into the LVAD inflow cannula under normal operating conditions?
a. Turbulent flow pattern
b. Bidirectional flow pattern
c. Laminar flow pattern
d. High velocity flow pattern

19. Which of the following best describes the correct orientation of an LVAD outflow cannula?
a. In the left ventricle pointing towards the interventricular septum
b. In the ascending aorta directed towards the posterior aortic wall
c. In the descending aorta below the subclavian artery origin
d. In the left ventricle directed towards the mitral valve

20. On TEE examination, the interventricular septum is seen bowing towards the left ventricle. Which of the following best describes the subsequent LVAD management plan?
a. The device output should be increased.
b. Diuresis should be instituted.
c. Left ventricle preload may be increased.
d. The device is working normally.

21. Which of the following best describes the effect of a regurgitant inflow valve in an LVAD cannula?
a. The left ventricle will be collapsed.
b. LVAD stroke volume will increase.

c. Increased aortic regurgitation.
d. Aortic valve will open more frequently.

22. Which of the following is most likely to result in right ventricular failure following cardiopulmonary bypass?
    a. Short cardiopulmonary bypass time
    b. Inadequate de-airing of the heart
    c. Vasospasm of the left circumflex
    d. Undiagnosed aortic stenosis

23. The ideal location of an outflow cannula for a right ventricular assist device is:
    a. In the ascending aorta
    b. In the descending aorta
    c. In the main pulmonary artery
    d. In the superior vena cava

24. Which of the following best describes a common echocardiographic finding in the immediate postoperative period in heart transplant recipients?
    a. Restrictive left ventricular filling pattern
    b. Frequent pericardial effusions
    c. Shadow of atrial tissue in the right atrial cavity
    d. Moderate mitral regurgitation

25. Which of the following is the most likely explanation for severe right heart dysfunction in a heart transplant recipient?
    a. Preexisting pulmonary hypertension in the recipient
    b. Pericardial thrombus causing extrinsic obstruction
    c. Undiagnosed tricuspid regurgitation in the donor heart
    d. New mitral regurgitation in the donor heart

26. Which of the following echocardiographic findings best supports an indication for right ventricular assist device (RVAD) implantation in a transplanted heart?
    a. An under-filled, hypocontractile right ventricle
    b. A dilated, hypocontractile RV after administration of protamine
    c. A hyperdynamic left ventricle, dilated RV, and paradoxical interventricular septal shift
    d. A dilated, hypocontractile RV after inadequate de-airing of the left heart

27. Which of the following is the most likely reason for a finding of spontaneous echo contrast (SEC) in the transplanted heart left atrium?
    a. Atrial enlargement and dyssynchronous contraction
    b. Atrial fibrillation or flutter
    c. Severe pulmonary hypertension
    d. Undetected patent foramen ovale

28. Which of the following statements best describes the reason for tricuspid regurgitation in a transplant recipient?
    a. The use of a bicaval anastomotic technique
    b. Patent foramen ovale in the donor heart
    c. Significant pulmonary hypertension in the recipient
    d. Atrial fibrillation or flutter after cardiopulmonary bypass

29. Upon separation from cardiopulmonary bypass, the right ventricle appears hypocontractile and dilated, the pulmonary artery pressure is 16/8 mm Hg, and the ST-segments in leads II, III, and aVF are depressed. Which of the following is the most likely explanation for this finding?
    a. Reperfusion injury
    b. Aortic dissection
    c. Coronary air embolism
    d. Acute rejection
    e. Pulmonary embolism

Questions 30 through 33 involve the following case: A 72-year-old patient is undergoing coronary artery bypass graft surgery and possible mitral valve repair for ischemic mitral regurgitation. Preoperative TEE demonstrates a left ventricular ejection fraction of 40% and a normal right ventricle. Immediately after discontinuation of cardiopulmonary bypass, the left ventricle has new wall motion abnormalities in the mid-inferior and mid-inferoseptal segments. The mitral repair appears adequate. The right ventricle is hypokinetic and dilated.

30. Which of the following is the most likely explanation for the echo findings?
    a. Inadequate right heart protection
    b. Severe tricuspid regurgitation
    c. High transmitral flow velocity
    d. Coronary air embolism
    e. Trans-septal mitral approach

31. Which of the following TEE views is most likely to show the described abnormalities?
    a. Midesophageal two chamber
    b. Midesophageal RV inflow-outflow
    c. Midesophageal long axis
    d. Transgastric mid–short axis
    e. Transgastric two chamber

32. The surgeon requests quantification of right ventricular dysfunction (RVD). Which of the following echocardiographic parameters are most likely to indicate severe RVD?
    a. Systolic reversal in hepatic vein flow
    b. Increased tricuspid annular systolic excursion

c. RV diastolic internal diameter of 28 mm
d. Tricuspid regurgitation vena contracta of 7 mm

33. Which of the following echocardiographic parameters is most likely to demonstrate diastolic heart disease in this patient?
    a. Early transmitral flow velocity of 120 cm/s
    b. Transmitral early-to-late (E/A) ratio of 2.0
    c. Early diastolic myocardial tissue velocity of 4 cm/s
    d. Respiratory variation in diastolic tissue velocity

34. A 66-year-old female patient presents for coronary surgery but also has an ejection fraction of 30% and what appears to be severe aortic stenosis with a calculated valve area of 0.7 cm^2, but with a mean gradient of only 28 mm Hg. Which of the following responses to a dobutamine infusion will confirm true aortic stenosis rather than low gradient due to severe LV dysfunction?
    a. A mean gradient of 28 mm Hg that does not increase
    b. A valve area of 0.8 cm^2 that increases to 1.3 cm^2
    c. Stroke volume of 56 mL that increases to 78 mL
    d. Calculated valve area of 0.8 cm^2 that does not change

35. Which of the following is the most likely mechanism for mitral regurgitation in a patient with heart failure?
    a. Restriction of the posterior leaflet
    b. Prolapse of the P2 scallop
    c. Flail of the anterior leaflet
    d. Increase in left atrial pressure

Transesophageal Echocardiography for Congenital Heart Disease

18

Stephanie S. F. Fischer and Mathew V. Patteril

The incidence of congenital heart disease (CHD) is 0.5% to 1%, and common malformations are less frequent (0.15%).[1] An increasing percentage of these infants survive to adulthood largely due to advances in cardiology, cardiac surgery, and perioperative anesthetic and critical care management.[2] At present, adults with congenital heart disease constitute a significant and growing cardiac population of 5%.

In patients with CHD, transesophageal echocardiography (TEE) allows for the real-time acquisition of both anatomic and hemodynamic information, thereby helping in clinical decision making. During interventional cardiac catheterization procedures, TEE is instrumental in the monitoring and guidance of valvuloplasties, angioplasties, closure of intracardiac shunts, trans-septal atrial puncture, and electrophysiological ablation. During palliative and corrective surgical procedures, TEE is fundamental in confirming diagnosis; detection of unanticipated findings; modification of surgical procedures; assessment of the adequacy of the procedure; guidance of revision; monitoring of intracardiac air, ventricular volume, and myocardial performance; and formulation of anesthetic and postoperative management. The primary objectives of TEE in patients with CHD are to define important anatomic and hemodynamic information when data provided by other modalities are inadequate, establish a complete evaluation of complex congenital heart disease, and confirm or exclude a diagnosis of clinical relevance.

Congenital heart disease has been classified based on the level of complexity, presence or absence of cyanosis, and primary physiologic alterations. TEE image interpretation is therefore best performed using a segmental approach,[3] where the heart is considered in terms of three segments (atria, ventricles, and arterial trunks), and these are connected via two junctions (atrioventricular and ventriculoarterial).[4] The use of a segmental approach provides a systematic guide for verification that all significant chambers and valves and their relationships have been recorded. Important determinants in this segmental analysis include:

- Visceral situs
- Venoatrial connections (systemic and pulmonary veins)
- Atrial situs (normal, inversus, right isomerism, or left isomerism)
- Ventricular morphology (right versus left)
- Atrioventricular septae
- Atrioventricular valves
- Semilunar valves
- Ventricular outflows
- Great arteries
- Atrioventricular connections (concordant, discordant, double inlet, straddling, absent)
- Ventriculoarterial connections (concordant, discordant, double outlet, single outlet)

VISCERAL SITUS

The usual orientation of the organs with the liver on the right and the spleen on the left is referred to as *situs solitus. Situs inversus* refers to a situation where given organs, or even all bodily organs, are reversed (eg, liver on the left and spleen on the right). Asplenia is associated with bilateral right-sidedness (right isomerism—liver on both sides), while polysplenia is associated with bilateral left-sidedness (left isomerism—spleen on both sides).

ANOMALIES OF VENOATRIAL CONNECTIONS

Persistent Left Superior Vena Cava

A persistent left superior vena cava (PLSVC) is the most common thoracic venous anomaly and occurs in 0.4% of the general population and in 4% to 11% of patients with congenital heart disease.[5] The etiology of this defect is thought to be the failure of regression of left anterior and common cardinal veins and left sinus horn. In 90% of cases, the PLSVC connects to the right atrium through the coronary sinus (Figure 18–1). In

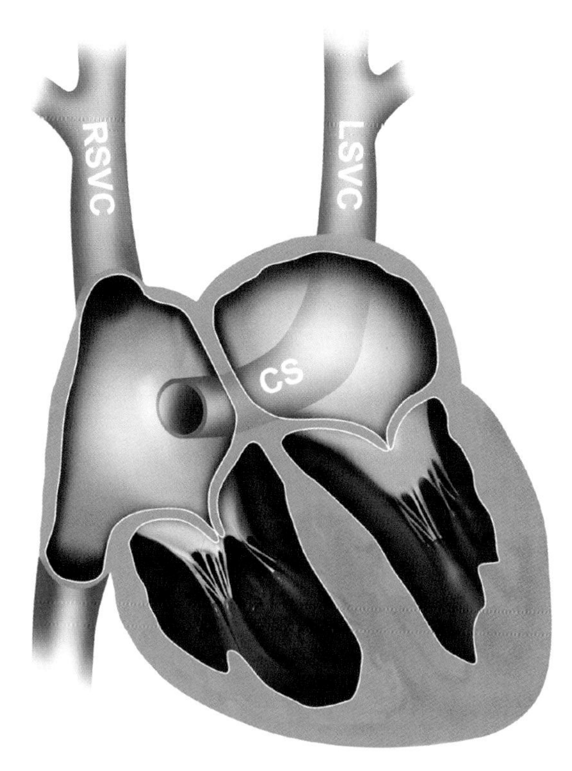

FIGURE 18–1. Persistent left superior vena cava (LSVC). In its most common form, the LSVC drains into the coronary sinus (CS). (RSVC, right superior vena cava.)

the remainder, the PLSVC connects to the left atrium. A PLSVC is associated with atrioventricular canal defects, tetralogy of Fallot, and anomalies of the inferior vena cava. The clinical presentation and physiologic consequence of a PSLVC depend on its association with other anomalies. If the PSLVC is isolated, patients may remain asymptomatic.

The diagnosis of this defect in patients undergoing cardiac surgery raises several issues. First, the passage of a pulmonary artery catheter into the right ventricle via puncture of the *left* internal jugular vein may be difficult because the catheter may traverse the coronary sinus. Similarly, a PSLVC can complicate placement of permanent pacemakers and automatic implantable cardioverter defibrillators. Second, placement of a separate cannula in the coronary sinus may be necessary for complete venous drainage into the cardiopulmonary bypass machine. Third, retrograde cardioplegia in these patients will be ineffectively delivered to the myocardium. Finally, if patients with PLSVC undergo a heart transplant, the coronary sinus would have to be carefully dissected so that the PLSVC can be re-anastomosed to the right atrium

Echocardiographic Assessment

The bicaval view, midesophageal (ME) four-chamber view, and ME two-chamber view are the most useful in assessing this lesion. On two-dimensional examination, an enlarged coronary sinus (normal coronary sinus size is 1 cm) is most often the first clue to the presence of a PLSVC (Figure 18–2). The diagnosis can be confirmed

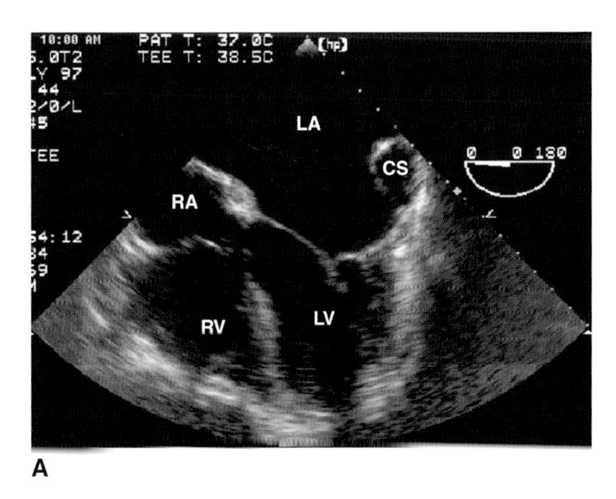

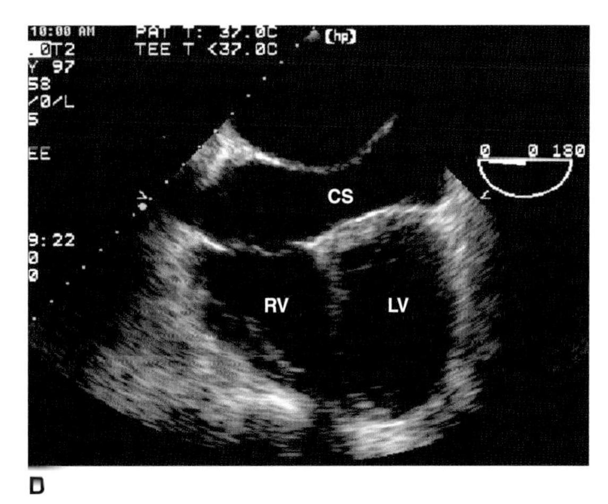

FIGURE 18–2. **A:** In the four-chamber view, a large coronary sinus is seen to the right of the image and often is the first clue to the presence of a persistent left superior vena cava. **B:** Advancing the probe from the four-chamber view shows a dramatically enlarged coronary sinus. **C:** Injection of agitated saline solution into the left arm demonstrating near opacification of the coronary sinus *(arrow)* before bubble entry into the right atrium confirms the presence of the persistent left superior vena cava. (CS, coronary sinus; LA, left atrium; LV, left ventricle; RA, right atrium; RV, right ventricle.)

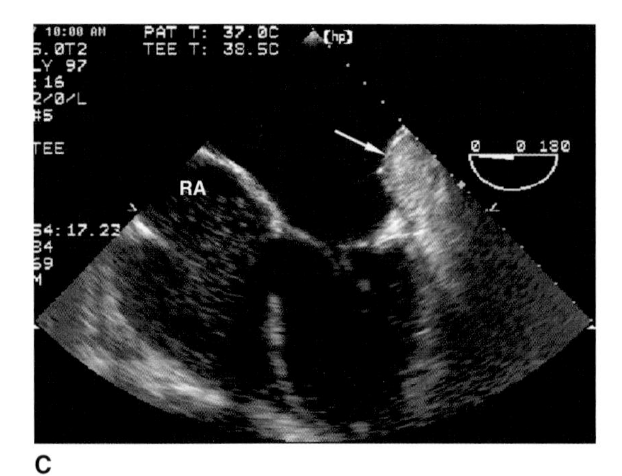

C

FIGURE 18–2. *(Continued)*

by injecting agitated saline solution into a vein in the left arm. In patients with a PLSVC, the "contrast" will be seen first in the coronary sinus before arriving into the right atrium (see Figure 18–2C).

Anomalous Pulmonary Venous Return

Anomalous drainage of the pulmonary veins results from in utero failure of the pulmonary veins to fuse with the left atrium. Two types have been identified. In patients with *total* anomalous pulmonary venous drainage, all pulmonary venous return is directed into a systemic venous system, creating a large left-to-right shunt. The site of pulmonary venous drainage may be supracardiac (into the innominate vein or left- or right-sided superior vena cava), cardiac (into an enlarged coronary sinus), or infracardiac (into the portal vein, ductus venosus, hepatic vein, or inferior vena cava) (Figure 18–3). Some degree of interatrial mixing (usually atrial septal defect [ASD] or patent foramen ovale [PFO]) is mandatory and provides the only access for pulmonary venous blood to the left heart. Survival beyond infancy without surgical intervention is unlikely; hence, this entity is not encountered in the adult population.

Partial anomalous pulmonary venous drainage is characterized by failure of one or two of the pulmonary veins to connect with the left atrium. Most commonly, the right upper and/or right lower pulmonary veins drain into the superior vena cava or the junction of the right atrium and superior vena cava. A sinus venosus ASD often accompanies this lesion. In the scimitar syndrome, the right lower pulmonary vein anomalously joins the inferior vena cava.

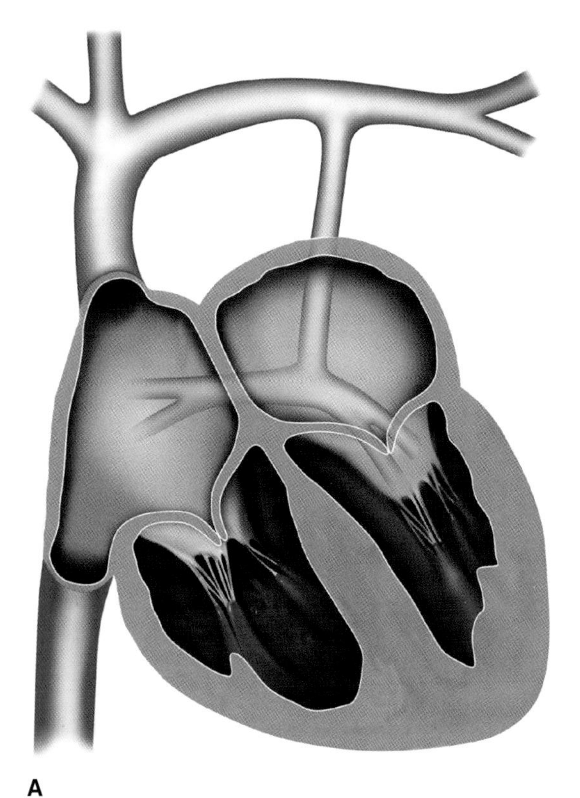

A

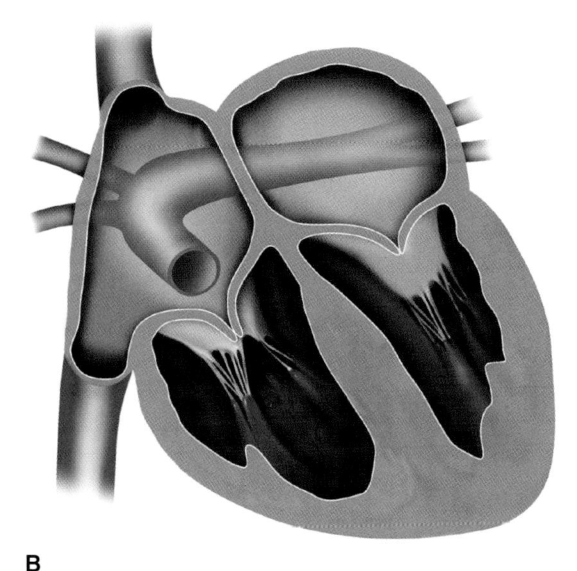

B

FIGURE 18–3. **(A)** Supracardiac (innominate vein), **(B)** cardiac (coronary sinus), and **(C)** infracardiac (inferior vena cava) drainage sites for anomalous pulmonary venous return.

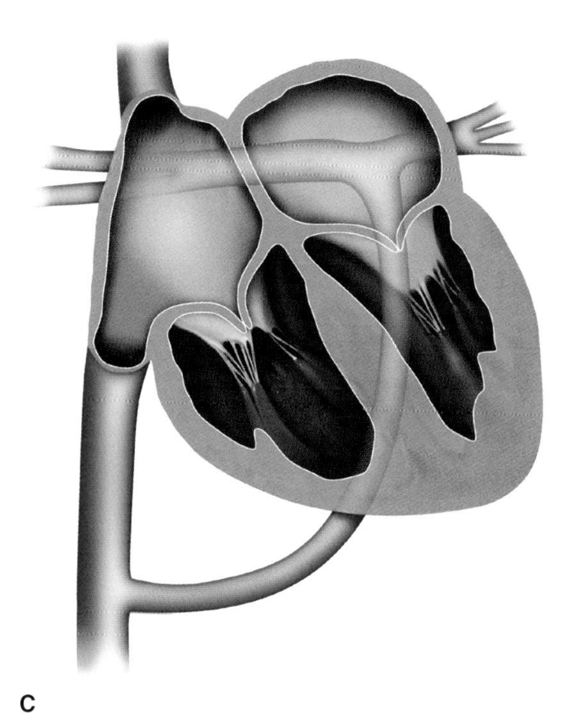

C

FIGURE 18–3. *(Continued)*

The physiologic consequences of partial anomalous pulmonary venous drainage may be minor. If more of the pulmonary venous drainage is diverted to the right atrium, evidence of right-side volume overload will be present. Associated anomalies include sinus venosus ASD, patent ductus arteriosus, transposition of the great arteries, and pulmonic valve atresia.

ECHOCARDIOGRAPHIC ASSESSMENT

A dilated coronary sinus, evidence of right ventricular (RV) and right atrial dilatation, and an ASD are sometimes the only initial abnormal echocardiographic findings and should prompt a careful search for all four pulmonary veins. The diagnosis of total anomalous pulmonary venous drainage relies on visualization of the termination of all four pulmonary veins and defining a venous confluence connecting to the right atrium, coronary sinus, or vena cava. Partial anomalous pulmonary venous drainage most often is an anomaly involving the right pulmonary vein, and the abnormal connection is usually near the right side of the atrial septum or the base of the superior vena cava and is best viewed in the bicaval view. Agitated saline injection proximal to the anomalous connection with the superior vena cava may be useful in delineating the anomalous pulmonary vein from the superior vena cava (Figure 18–4). Color Doppler aids in the detection of individual veins, the direction of flow, and the presence of turbulence. Spectral Doppler confirms or excludes pulmonary venous obstruction. Surgically corrected lesions may require reinvestigation with color and pulsed-wave Doppler to determine the patency of the venous connection. Normal pulmonary vein flow should have a biphasic systolic–diastolic pattern with a maximal velocity of less than 1 m/s. A continuous nonphasic pattern and a peak velocity of greater than 2 m/s signifies restrictive pulmonary venous flow.[4]

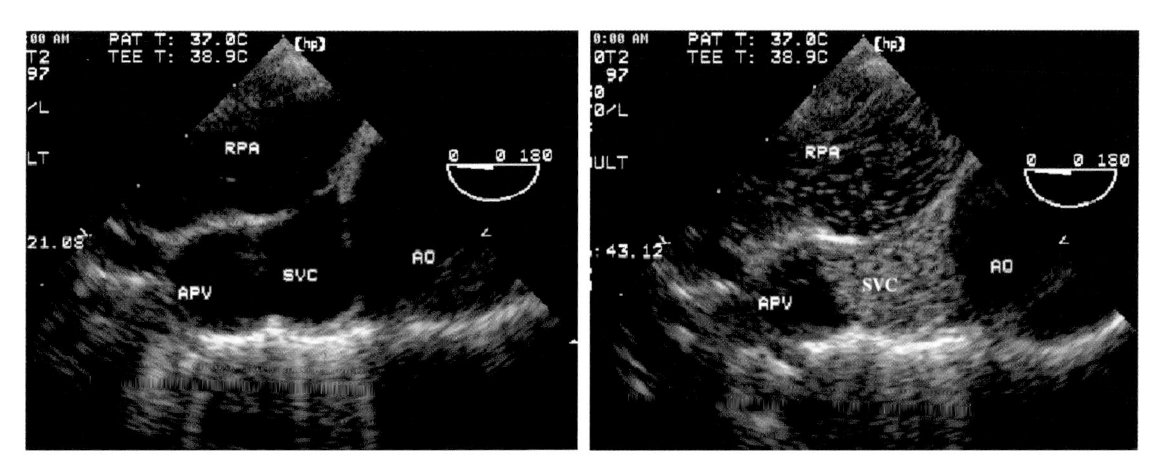

FIGURE 18–4. Anomalous pulmonary venous drainage into the superior vena cava *(left)*. Injection of agitated saline solution proximal to the anomalous connection with the superior vena cava shows no contrast *(right)* within the anomalous pulmonary vein, indicating that it is a vessel distinct from the superior vena cava. (AO, ascending aorta; APV, anomalous pulmonary vein; RPA, right pulmonary artery; SVC, superior vena cava.)

ATRIAL SITUS

Four possible atrial arrangements can be encountered: (1) *situs solitus*—normal arrangement of right and left atrium; (2) *situs inversus*—right atrium is on the left and the left atrium is on the right; (3) *right atrial isomerism*—bilateral right atria; and (4) *left atrial isomerism*—bilateral left atria. The morphological right atrium and left atrium can be differentiated by the anatomy of the atrial appendages. The right atrial appendage is broad, whereas the left atrial appendage is narrow and pointed.

VENTRICULAR MORPHOLOGY

Complex CHD lesions may demonstrate one or two ventricular chambers, ventricular inversion with the RV on the left and LV on the right (atrioventricular discordance), or abnormal arterial connections to the ventricles (ventriculoarterial discordance). Hence, the ventricles need to be identified by their structure and not by their positions or connections.[6] The morphologically right and left ventricles have distinctive features, which are summarized in Table 18–1. Atrioventricular valves are always associated with their respective ventricles; therefore a tricuspid valve will identify the right ventricle and a mitral valve the left ventricle.

ANOMALIES OF ATRIOVENTRICULAR SEPTAE

Atrial Septal Defect (ASD)

ASD is the second most common congenital heart defect, occurring in women two to three times as often as in men. ASDs include the following types: ostium secundum (70%), ostium primum (20%), sinus venosus (10%), and coronary sinus (rare).

Table 18–1. Morphological features that distinguish the right and left ventricles.

Right Ventricle	Left Ventricle
Heavily trabeculated	Smooth walls
Three papillary muscles	Two papillary muscles
Moderator band	No moderator band
Tricuspid valve has chordal attachments to ventricular septum	Mitral valve has no chordal attachment to ventricular septum
Tricuspid valve has three leaflets	Mitral valve has two leaflets
Tricuspid valve has a more apical septal insertion point	Mitral valve has a higher septal insertion point

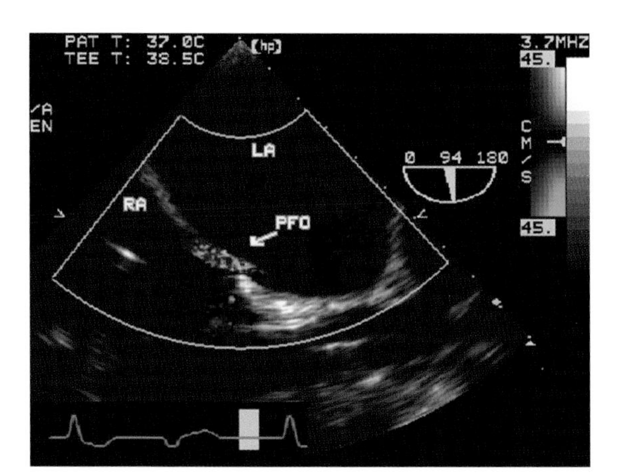

FIGURE 18–5. Color-flow Doppler imaging across a patent foramen ovale (PFO) showing left-to-right shunting. (LA, left atrium; RA, right atrium.)

Although not a "true" ASD, a patent foramen ovale (PFO) persists secondary to failure of fusion of the septum primum and secundum (Figure 18–5). The prevalence of probe patent PFO is as high as 26% in autopsy series. Clinical problems attributed to PFO include paradoxical embolism leading to cerebrovascular accidents, decompression illness in divers, and migraine headaches. In a meta-analysis, the presence of a PFO alone increased the risk of recurrent cerebrovascular events fivefold, with an even higher risk in the presence of an atrial septal aneurysm.[7] Other identified risk factors are the size of the PFO, the number of microbubbles in the left atrium during the first seconds after release of a Valsalva maneuver, and the presence of a eustachian valve directed toward the PFO,[8] hence the rationale of PFO closure to protect against recurrent strokes. Elective surgical closure of a PFO diagnosed as an incidental finding during routine intraoperative TEE is not currently thought to be of benefit unless the patient has experienced a prior stroke of uncertain etiology or as a result of known paradoxical embolism. Some surgeons choose to repair a PFO if the atrium is to be opened as part of the scheduled surgical procedure. However, it should be noted that, even when the PFO is surgically repaired, the risk of recurrent neurologic events is not completely eliminated. Catheter-based PFO closure can be performed as an outpatient procedure, is associated with minimal risk, and has superseded surgical closure.[9]

Ostium secundum defects are located in the midportion of the interatrial septum in the region of the fossa ovalis and are associated with mitral valve prolapse and mitral regurgitation. *Ostium primum* defects are located at the inferior portion of the interatrial septum and are associated with a cleft mitral valve with variable degrees

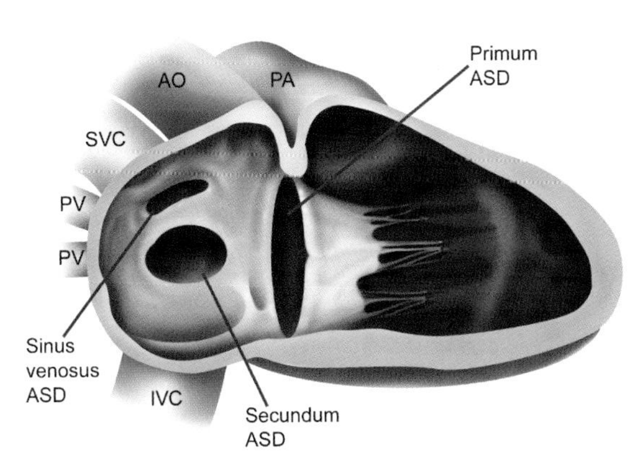

FIGURE 18–6. Schematic showing the anatomic locations of the three most common atrial septal defects. (ASD, atrial septal defect; IVC, inferior vena cava; SVC, superior vena cava; PA, pulmonary artery; AO, aorta; PV, pulmonary vein.)

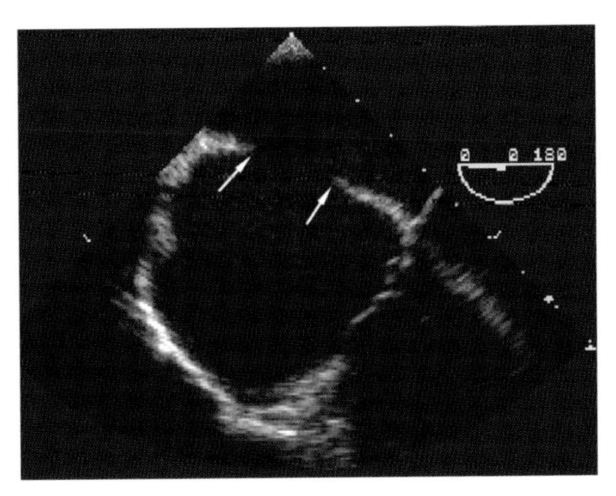

FIGURE 18–7. An ostium secundum atrial septal defect located in the midportion of the interatrial septum in the region of the fossa ovale. Arrows point to the margins of the defect.

of mitral regurgitation. *Sinus venosus* defects may be of the superior or inferior vena caval type. Most defects in this category are located near the entrance of the superior vena cava and right pulmonary veins high in the atrial septum (superior vena caval type) and are associated with anomalous return of the right upper and lower pulmonary veins (Figure 18–6). The relatively uncommon defects in the inferior vena caval–atrial junction are characterized by a deficiency of the inferior limbic septum. *Coronary sinus* defects occur from a partial or complete absence of the roof of the coronary sinus, creating a left-to-right shunt from the left atrium to the coronary sinus and then into the right atrium. These lesions are associated with a persistent left superior vena cava. The fundamental physiology of all these lesions is a transatrial shunt, and the direction and magnitude of shunting is determined by the size of the defect and the relative compliance of the ventricles.

ECHOCARDIOGRAPHIC ASSESSMENT

TEE provides excellent interrogation of the interatrial septum, with a sensitivity exceeding that of transthoracic echocardiography for the detection of ASDs. Two-dimensional interrogation of the entire atrial septum should be performed in transverse and longitudinal planes to ensure that small defects at the margins of the septum are not missed. The dimension of and the relative size of the defect to the entire interatrial septum should be determined. The best views are midesophageal four chamber, two chamber, and bicaval.

Secundum defects are located in the midportion of the interatrial septum in the region of the fossa ovalis (Figure 18–7), and ostium primum defects are located at the inferior portion of the interatrial septum (Figure 18–8). The bicaval view is particularly useful in detecting inferior and superior sinus venosus ASDs (Figure 18–9). The least common type of atrial septal defect, the coronary sinus communication, is defined by an enlarged coronary sinus with a deficient roof (unroofed coronary sinus), and is found in association with a persistent left superior vena cava. In the transverse axis, this is seen as an echo-free space wedge between the left upper pulmonary vein and left atrial appendage, and in the longitudinal plane, it can be identified as it enters the coronary sinus.

Color-flow Doppler allows for evaluation of flow across the defect and the detection of mitral or tricuspid regurgitation. Saline contrast injection may be useful in confirming right-to-left shunting and aid in detection of small lesions, but it must be used cautiously in light of the potential for cerebral embolism. Spectral Doppler is used to assess the hemodynamic consequences of the lesion. Measurement of the tricuspid regurgitant jet velocity can estimate systolic pulmonary artery pressures and diagnose pulmonary hypertension. In the absence of significant valvular disease, the shunt magnitude can be determined by measuring the velocity time integrals (VTIs) across the RV and LV outflow tracts. A ratio of pulmonary to systemic flow (Q_p/Q_s) of greater than 1.5 is considered significant. Further intraoperative evaluation includes detection of associated lesions, assessment of adequacy of surgical repair and postoperative atrioventricular valve competency, and evaluation of ventricular function.

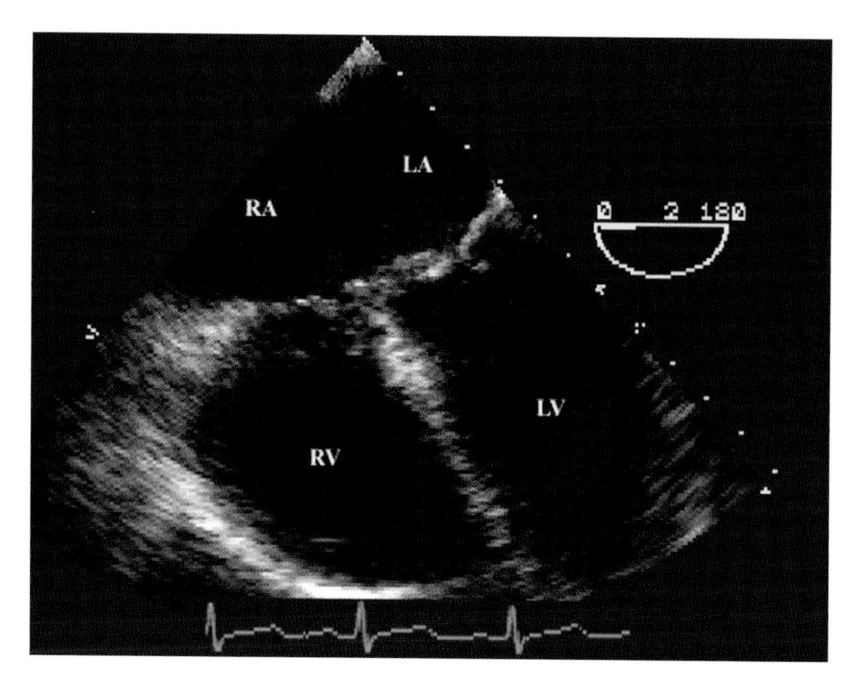

FIGURE 18–8. An ostium primum defect located at the inferior portion of the interatrial septum often is best seen on the midesophageal four-chamber view. (LA, left atrium; LV, left ventricle; RA, right atrium; RV, right ventricle.)

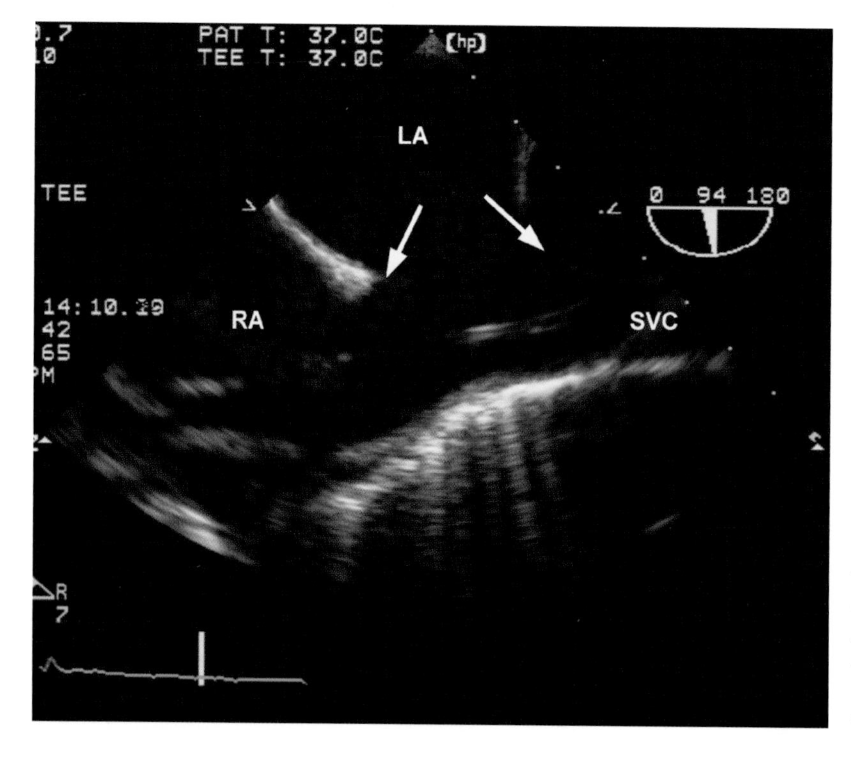

FIGURE 18–9. A sinus venosus defect in the posterior portion of the interatrial septum near the entrance of the superior vena cava is often best visualized with the bicaval view. A central venous catheter is seen passing through the superior vena cava into the right atrium. Arrows point to the margins of the defect. (LA, left atrium; RA, right atrium; SVC, superior vena cava.)

Ventricular Septal Defect (VSD)

Even though VSDs are the most common congenital anomaly recognized at birth, they account for only 10% to 15% of defects observed in adults with CHD.[10] VSDs can occur in isolation or as part of complex lesions, and are classified by location into four major groups: (1) supracristal (also known as subarterial, outlet, subpulmonic, doubly committed, and infundibular); (2) infracristal (perimembranous); (3) muscular; and (4) atrioventricular canal (inlet) types (Figure 18–10).

The *perimembranous* type (Figure 18–11) accounts for 70% of all VSDs and involves the membranous septum. The defect is adjacent to the aortic valve and the annulus of the tricuspid valve contributes to the rim of the defect. When the VSD is primarily adjacent to the tricuspid valve, it is called a *perimembranous inlet* defect but when the defect extends primarily toward the aortic valve, it is referred to as a *perimembranous outlet* defect. In an *inlet* defect, shunting of blood occurs from the LV outflow tract to the right ventricle just beneath the septal leaflet of the tricuspid valve. There may be an associated tricuspid valve aneurysm or redundant tricuspid septal leaflet tissue that may plug the defect. In 10% of cases, a perimembranous defect can undermine the right aortic cusp, causing herniation of the cusp and aortic insufficiency. Rarely, a perimembranous VSD may lead to the formation of a communication between the LV outflow tract and the right atrium known as Gerbode defect. Small membranous VSDs may close spontaneously during childhood by approximation of the tricuspid valve septal leaflet across the defect. This defect closure may be undetectable in adulthood, or a residual anatomic abnormality, a "ventricular septal aneurysm," may be visualized at the closure site.

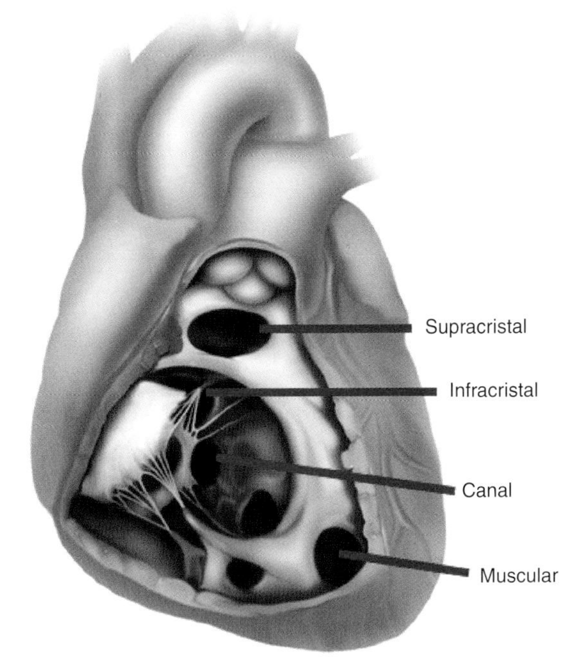

FIGURE 18–10. Schematic showing the anatomic locations of ventricular septal defects.

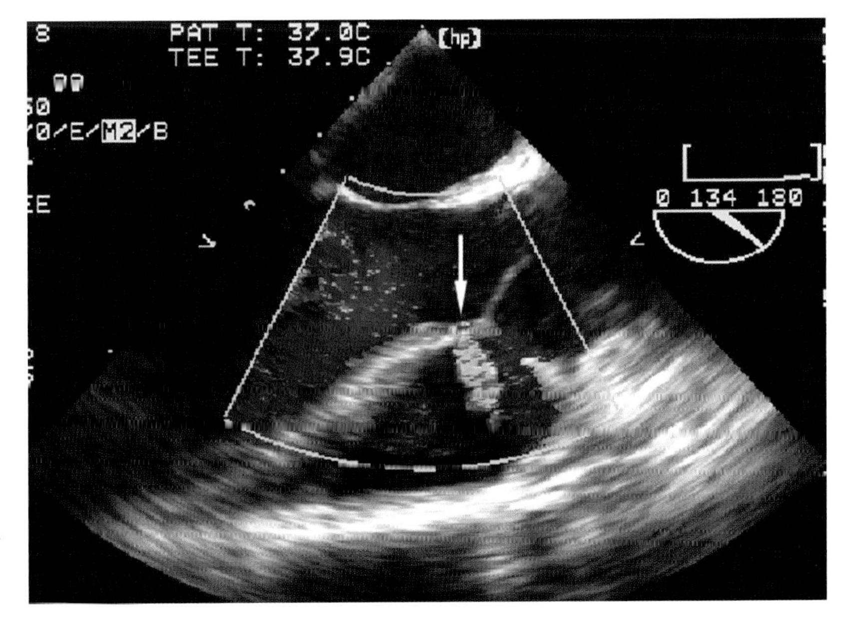

FIGURE 18–11. Small perimembranous outlet ventricular septal defect *(arrow)* with left-to-right shunting.

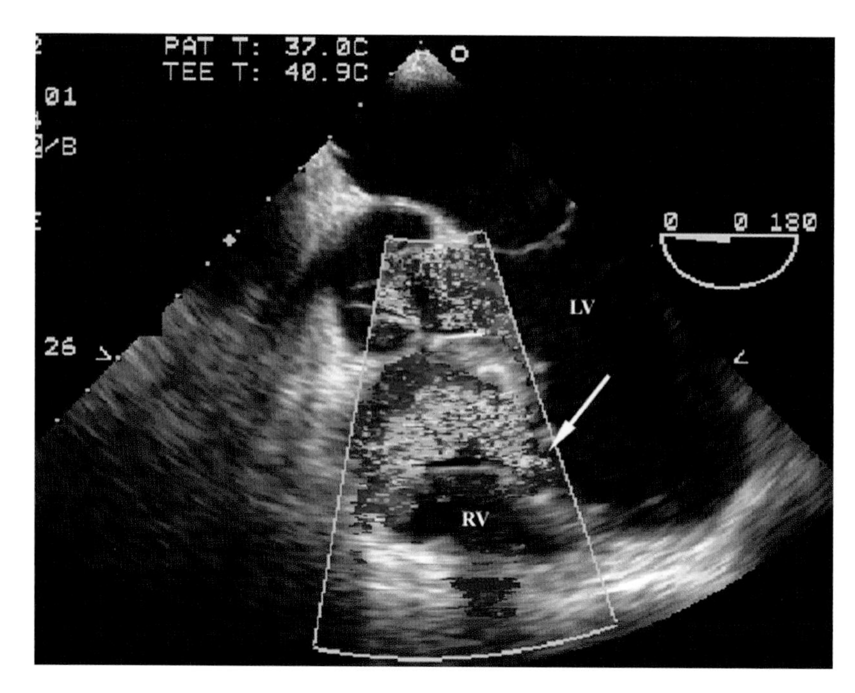

FIGURE 18–12. Large muscular-type ventricular septal defect *(arrow)*, in this case occurring as a complication of myocardial infarction. (LV, left ventricle; RV, right ventricle.)

Muscular-type VSDs (20%) are located in the central (Figure 18–12) or apical trabecular portion of the septum. They are often quite large, isolated, or multiple, and can be associated with pulmonary vascular disease. In some cases, RV outflow tract hypertrophy occurs in association with the VSD and serves to limit the severity of pulmonary hypertension (known as Gasul phenomenon).

The crista supraventricularis can be considered synonymous with the infundibular septum—the muscle separating the outflow tracts of the left and the right ventricles. The *supracristal* defects (5%) are usually circular and are located within the infundibular portion of the right ventricular outflow tract. The superior edge of the VSD is the conjoined annulus of the aortic and pulmonary valves; both the outlet septum and septal component of subpulmonary infundibulum are absent. Thus, the superior rim may have a direct relationship with the right coronary cusp of the aortic valve such that the right aortic leaflet may prolapse into the VSD, resulting in functional restriction of the size of the VSD but worsening aortic regurgitation. Even in the presence of only mild aortic regurgitation and a small VSD, this defect should be surgically closed to prevent rapid progression of aortic valve regurgitation.[11]

The *atrioventricular* canal or inlet type defects (5%) are seen close to the atrioventricular valves in the posterior or inlet portion of the septum and usually are caused by a defect in the formation of the atrioventricular septum. As such, they can be a part of a complex defect (see below), and are associated with a cleft in the mitral or tricuspid valve, common atrioventricular valve, and fibrous aneurysms.

The physiologic consequences of these lesions are determined by the size of the defect and the relative vascular resistance in the pulmonary bed. Patients are also at a higher risk for infective endocarditis.

ECHOCARDIOGRAPHIC ASSESSMENT

Two-dimensional echocardiographic assessment is focused on defining the anatomic abnormality, whereas color-flow Doppler enhances the sensitivity of detection of all forms of VSD and helps to determine the magnitude and direction of the shunt. The ventricular septum is best interrogated in the ME four-chamber view, ME long-axis (LAX) view, ME RV inflow-outflow view, and the transgastric short-axis (TG SAX) view.[4] The ME RV inflow-outflow view is especially helpful in differentiating a perimembranous VSD from a supracristal VSD (Figure 18–13). Unlike the more common perimembranous type of VSD, a supracristal VSD does not lie near the tricuspid valve, and the tricuspid valve is not involved in partial closure of the defect. Color Doppler of a supracristal defect in this view shows left-to-right shunting with turbulent flow directed into the pulmonary outflow tract. It is important to remember that this defect may be missed in the ME four-chamber view. Distortion of the right aortic leaflet and aortic

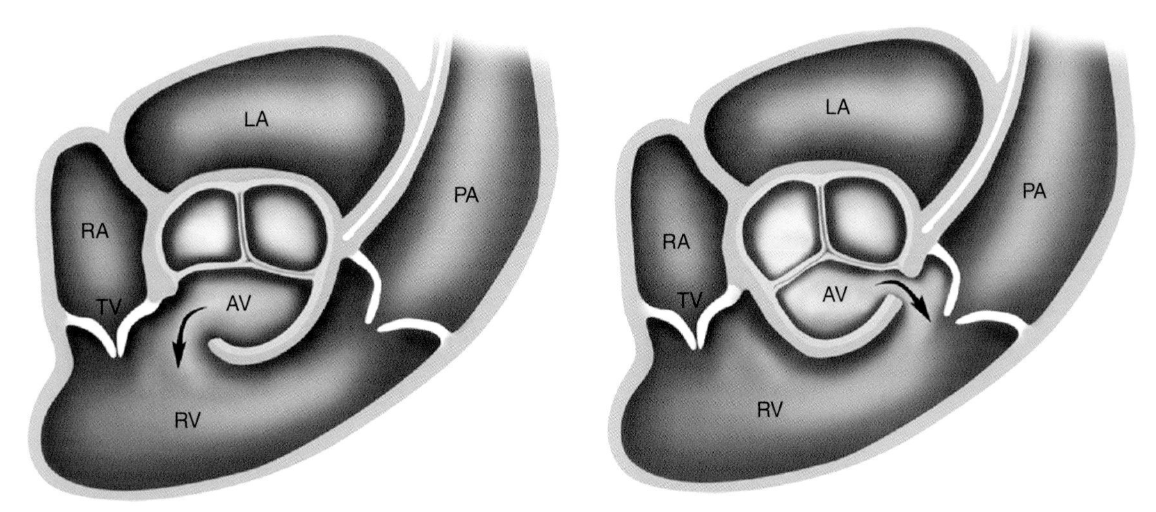

FIGURE 18–13. Schematic of the right ventricular inflow-outflow view showing the locations of a perimembranous *(left)* and supracristal *(right)* ventricular septal defect. (LA, left atrium; PA, pulmonary artery; RA, right atrium; TV, tricuspid valve; AV, aortic valve; RV, right ventricle.)

regurgitation may be the only clue to the presence of a significant supracristal defect.

"Ventricular septal aneurysms" are characterized on M-mode echocardiography by a pattern of multiple linear echoes moving into the right ventricle during systole. Two-dimensional imaging reveals a saccular protuberance with a rapid flicking motion extending into the right ventricle during systole and realigning with the ventricular septum during diastole.

For all types of VSDs, continuous-wave Doppler helps in measuring the peak jet velocity, and hence estimating RV systolic pressures and pulmonary artery systolic pressures. The pressure gradient between the right and left ventricle can be calculated by using the simplified Bernoulli equation as follows:

$$P_{LV} - P_{RV} = 4 \times (V_{VSD\ Peak\ Velocity})^2$$

$$P_{RV} = P_{LV} - 4 \times (V_{VSD\ Peak\ Velocity})^2$$

where P_{LV} is the LV systolic pressure, which equals the aortic systolic blood pressure in the absence of LV outflow obstruction, and P_{RV} is the RV systolic pressure, which equals the pulmonary artery systolic blood pressure in the absence of RV outflow obstruction.

The intracardiac shunt can be quantified by calculating the stroke volume across the pulmonic and aortic valves to develop the Q_p/Q_s ratio. The location for determining the stroke volume depends on the location of the shunt. Q_p is typically measured at the level of the RV outflow tract, whereas Q_s is measured at the level of the LV outflow tract. A Q_p/Q_s of 1.5 or greater is considered significant. The shunt volume (different from the shunt fraction) is the product of the cross-sectional area of the color-flow jet at the defect and the flow-velocity integral of the continuous-wave Doppler systolic flow signal.[12]

$$\text{VSD Shunt Volume} = \pi \left(\frac{\text{Diameter}_{VSD}}{2} \right)^2 \times \text{VTI}_{VSD}$$

Postoperatively, residual shunting across the patch has to be excluded. A large dehiscence of the patch ($>$3 mm) is an indication for immediate surgical revision. The tricuspid valve also needs to be investigated carefully as surgical repair of a VSD through the right atrium may involve detachment of the septal tricuspid leaflet and reconstruction of the leaflet once the VSD is repair is completed. Also, both the right coronary cusp and the septal tricuspid leaflet can be tethered during repair of a perimembranous VSD.[4]

Atrioventricular Canal Defects

Also known as atrioventricular septal defects (AVSDs) or endocardial cushion defects, these lesions are produced by anomalies of the atrial and ventricular septa and the adjacent parts of the atrioventricular (AV) valve. Three types are described: (1) partial AVSDs, consisting of two separate atrioventricular valves, an ostium primum ASD as well as a cleft mitral valve, (2) transitional AVSDs made up of an ostium primum ASD, a small ventricular

Table 18–2. Rastelli Classification.

Rastelli type A	Superior bridging leaflet is divided in two portions at the septum, one mitral portion and one tricuspid portion, both attached firmly to the left and right side of the interventricular septum (IVS), respectively, with long chordae.
Rastelli type B	Superior bridging leaflet is divided but not attached to IVS. Mitral and tricuspid components are attached to anomalous papillary muscle arising in right ventricle.
Rastelli type C	Superior bridging leaflet is not divided and is not attached to the IVS (free-floating leaflet).

septal defect, and two distinct atrioventricular valves; and (3) complete AVSDs, the most common defect, made up of an ostium primum ASD, inlet-type VSD, and a common atrioventricular valve that bridges both the right and the left sides of the heart, creating superior (anterior) and inferior (posterior) bridging leaflets. The Rastelli classification describes three types of complete AV canal defects based on the morphology of the anterior (superior) bridging leaflet, its degree of bridging, and its chordal attachments (Table 18–2).[13] These bridging leaflets may have chordal insertions into both ventricles. In such cases it must be surgically divided into left and right portions and resuspended from a central patch to create separate atrioventricular orifices.

Down syndrome occurs in 35% of patients with atrioventricular septal defect. Other associated cardiac lesions include tetralogy of Fallot, double-outlet right ventricle (DORV), total anomalous pulmonary venous connection, and pulmonary atresia. Subaortic stenosis also may occur from a discrete fibromuscular narrowing or from abnormal chordal insertions traversing the outflow tract. Subaortic obstruction can also develop postoperatively as a consequence of the reduction of LV outflow tract size after repair of the mitral valve cleft. Based on the size of the ventricular septal communication and the competence of the atrioventricular valves, patients may become symptomatic early in life or remain relatively asymptomatic until young adulthood. Surgical repair consists of patch closure of ASDs and/or VSDs and repair of the atrioventricular valves.

Echocardiographic Assessment

TEE defines the precise anatomy and allows detection of intracardiac shunts, chordal attachments, subaortic stenosis, and the presence and severity of left and right atrioventricular valve regurgitation. Shunting may occur left to right across the atria, left to right across the ventricles, or left ventricle to right atrium. Atrioventricular canal defects are readily visualized in the ME views. A four-chamber view shows that both atrioventricular valves are inserted at the same level and defines the presence and size of ASDs and VSDs (Figure 18–14).

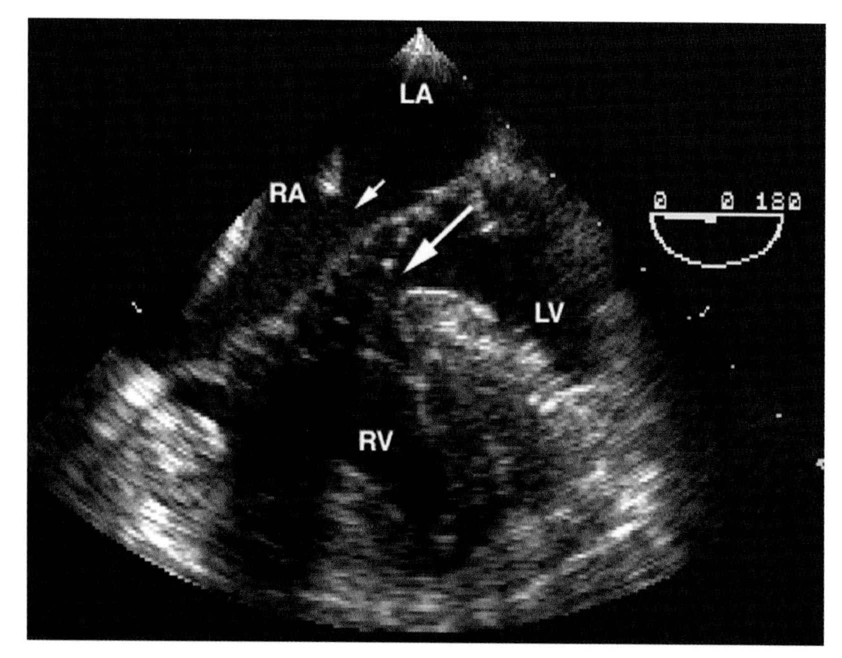

FIGURE 18–14. Complete atrioventricular canal defect with a primum atrial septal defect *(small arrow)*, inlet-type ventricular septal defect *(large arrow)*, and a common atrioventricular valve. (LA, left atrium; LV, left ventricle; RA, right atrium; RV, right ventricle.)

Chordal and papillary muscle arrangements of both atrioventricular valves also should be defined. The mitral valve is well visualized in a basal transgastric view at 0° and 90° and with three-dimensional imaging for number of leaflets and presence of a cleft. Color Doppler is useful to determine the presence and severity of atrioventricular valve regurgitation and to determine the location and size of shunts. Careful inspection of the right ventricle for signs of volume overload, inspection of the LV outflow tract for signs of obstruction, and exclusion of associated cardiac lesions completes the examination. Postoperative assessment includes detection of residual shunting, evaluation of atrioventricular valve regurgitation, iatrogenic atrioventricular valve stenosis, and subaortic stenosis.

ANOMALIES OF ATRIOVENTRICULAR VALVES

Mitral Valve Anomalies

Most patients with congenital anomalies of the mitral valve present in adulthood with clinical findings of mitral insufficiency. A cleft in the anterior leaflet of the mitral valve presents by itself or as a part of a complex involving the atrioventricular septum. A double-orifice mitral valve occurs due to the abnormal fusion of the embryonic endocardial cushions and may present functionally as a stenotic or regurgitant lesion. The leaflets of a parachute mitral valve typically are attached to a single, central papillary muscle. The abnormal pattern of flow associated with these lesions predisposes these patients to infective endocarditis.

ECHOCARDIOGRAPHIC ASSESSMENT

The four ME and two transgastric views define the number of leaflets, a single or double orifice, the presence of a cleft, the number and location of the papillary muscles, and chordal attachments (see Chapters 5 and 7). Color, continuous-wave, and pulsed-wave Doppler are important in assessing the functional significance of these anomalies. The possibility of endocarditis in these patients should not be overlooked. For quantification of the severity of the stenotic or regurgitant lesions, please refer to Chapter 7.

Ebstein's Anomaly of the Tricuspid Valve

Ebstein's anomaly is a rare defect, accounting for less than 1% of all congenital heart defects, but constitutes 40% of the congenital malformations of the tricuspid valve. The principal aberration occurring with Ebstein's anomaly is a malformation of the tricuspid valve. Two of the three leaflets of the valve, the septal and the posterior, are displaced downward into the right ventricle. The anterior leaflet is typically large and redundant and is often described as "sail-like." It is abnormally attached to the RV free wall but is not displaced. The portion of the right ventricle between the atrioventricular junction and the displaced tricuspid leaflets is usually referred to as *atrialized*. The remaining right ventricle is hypoplastic and functionally impaired. Most commonly, the tricuspid valve is regurgitant, often with multiple eccentric jets. Eighty percent of patients with Ebstein's anomaly have an interatrial communication such as an ASD or a patent foramen ovale. With severe tricuspid regurgitation and elevated right atrial pressures, right-to-left shunting of blood may occur. The clinical presentation varies widely, depending on the degree of displacement of the tricuspid leaflets, and ranges from severe cyanosis and heart failure in the newborn to mild tricuspid insufficiency or absence of symptoms in the adult. Arrhythmias also may be the only clinical symptom occurring as a result of marked right atrial enlargement or because of Wolff-Parkinson-White syndrome, found in 10% to 15% of patients with Ebstein's anomaly.[14] Arrhythmias, cyanosis, dyspnea, and exercise intolerance are the frequently seen symptoms in older patients.

ECHOCARDIOGRAPHIC ASSESSMENT

The echocardiography views include midesophageal four-chamber, RV inflow and outflow, transgastric RV inflow, and short-axis views. The four-chamber view shows the extent of apical displacement of the tricuspid valve (Figure 18–15). Ebstein's anomaly is diagnosed when the distance from the mitral valve annulus to the displaced tricuspid septal leaflet measures more than 20 mm. In addition, the four-chamber plane is optimal for defining the degree of adherence of the anterior leaflet to the RV free wall, the size of the right atrium, and the size of the true right ventricle. Attention should be directed to the relative sizes and contractility of the atrialized and the true right ventricle. An atrialized-to-functional right ventricle ratio of greater than 0.5 indicates poor RV systolic function. The long-axis view of the RV inflow tract (RV inflow-outflow) allows evaluation of posterior leaflet displacement and demonstrates the sail-like anterior leaflet arising normally from the tricuspid annulus (see Figure 18–15B). M-mode may show increased excursion with a rounded off appearance of the anterior tricuspid valve leaflet, decreased E-F slope of the anterior leaflet, and premature opening of the pulmonic valve. Color-flow Doppler is used to determine the presence and severity of tricuspid regurgitation. Detailed Doppler and two-dimensional examination of the interatrial septum for associated defects and assessment of direction of flow across these defects should be performed.

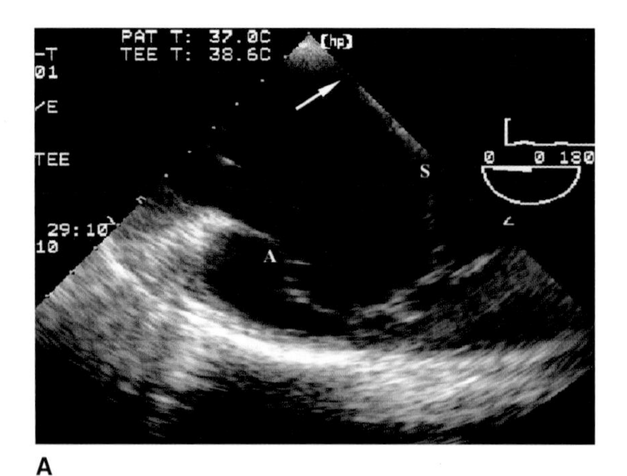

A

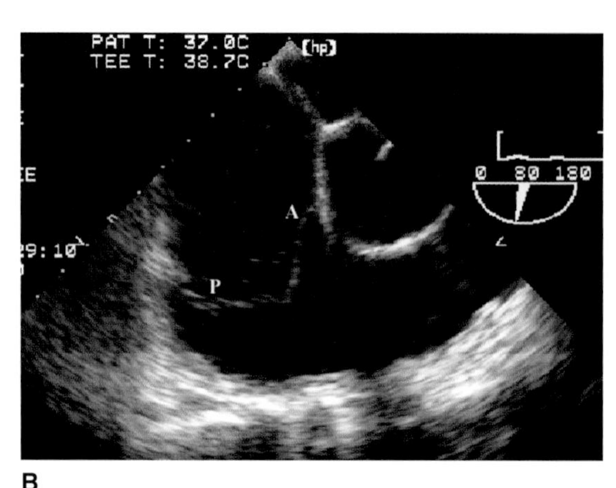

B

FIGURE 18–15. Ebstein's malformation. **A:** In a low four-chamber view with the probe rotated toward the right ventricle, the large anterior leaflet is seen with clear apical displacement of the septal leaflet. In Ebstein's malformation, the anterior leaflet usually is not displaced. The arrow points to the coronary sinus. **B:** In the right ventricular inflow-outflow view, the anterior and apically displaced posterior leaflets are seen. (A, anterior leaflet; P, posterior leaflet; S, septal leaflet.)

Echocardiography is also useful in separating patients who would require valve replacement from those in whom valve repair might be successful. Information with potential implications for surgical repair includes anterior leaflet size, valve mobility and excursion, presence or absence of restriction or tethering of the anterior leaflet, size of the right ventricle, and associated defects.[15] Postoperatively, TEE is used to determine the mobility and functionality of the repaired or replaced tricuspid valve.

ANOMALIES OF THE SEMILUNAR VALVES

Bicuspid Aortic Valve

The most commonly encountered congenital heart defect, bicuspid aortic valve may be present in up to 2% to 3% of the general population, with a male-to-female ratio of 4:1 or greater.[10] Anatomically, the bicuspid valve is composed of two leaflets or cusps, usually of unequal size, with an eccentric commissure or "raphe," or the cusps may be equal in size with a single central commissure. The disparity in the cusp size leads to redundancy and inappropriate valve coaptation resulting in regurgitation. Patients may be completely asymptomatic or develop aortic regurgitation at an early age secondary to redundancy or prolapse of cusp tissue. The mechanism of progressive valvular dysfunction appears to be related to abnormal hemodynamic stress leading to fibrosis and calcification of the leaflets. Symptomatic aortic stenosis usually occurs before the age of 65 years. Twenty percent of patients with bicuspid aortic valve have an associated cardiovascular abnormality,[10] such as patent ductus arteriosus, or abnormalities of the aorta including aortic coarctation, dissection (due to decreased connective tissue), and poststenotic dilatation. The Shone complex, a left-side obstructive lesion, includes a biscuspid aortic valve, supravalvular mitral ring, parachute mitral valve, discrete subaortic membrane, and coarctation of aorta. Infective endocarditis is a significant problem for these patients, with a 35-times higher incidence than the general population.

ECHOCARDIOGRAPHIC ASSESSMENT

TEE should be used to assess valve morphology (commissure and position of raphe), lateral mobility and separation, and annular size (see Chapter 9). Distinctive echo features include systolic doming in the long-axis view and the demonstration of a single commissural line with two functional valve cusps in the short-axis view (Figure 18–16). In patients with asymmetric leaflets and a prominent raphe, the valve may appear tricuspid in diastole; however, the elliptical "football" (sometimes referred to as "fishmouth" or "clamshell") shape of the systolic orifice indicates that the raphe is not a functional commissure. When extensive calcification occurs, doming may no longer be noted and the morphology of the cusps in the short-axis views may be difficult to distinguish from the calcific stenosis of a tricuspid aortic valve.[14]

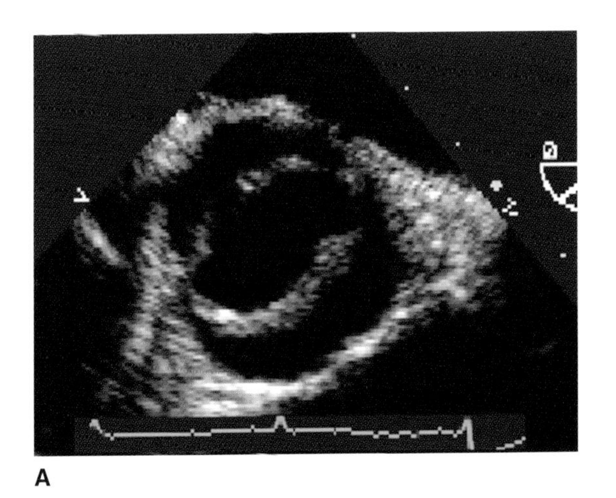

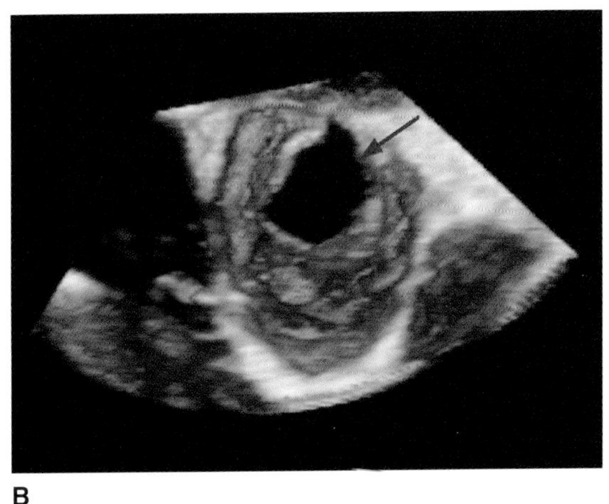

A B

FIGURE 18–16. Bicuspid aortic valve with the "fishmouth" or "clamshell" shape of the systolic orifice seen with two-dimensional **(A)** and three-dimensional (**B**; *arrow*) imaging.

Using a transgastric approach, a quantitative evaluation of the degree of outflow obstruction can be obtained by Doppler echocardiography. Complete evaluation includes detection of left ventricular (LV) hypertrophy or dilation, identification of poststenotic aortic root dilatation and other associated cardiovascular anomalies (aortic coarctation or dissection), and an evaluation of the number of sinuses of Valsalva present (there may only be two instead of three). Planimetry of the bicuspid aortic valve, however, is unreliable as an estimation of aortic valve area. Pre- and intraoperative aortic valve annulus dimensions can be measured if a Ross procedure is planned or to guide the sizing of a mechanical valve. Severity of aortic regurgitation or stenosis and residual defects on completion of the surgical intervention are assessed as for the tricuspid aortic valve described earlier (see Chapter 9). As the Ross procedure involves reimplantation of the coronary arteries, the pre- and postoperative assessment of segmental and global left ventricular function is important.

Pulmonic Stenosis

Pulmonic stenosis constitutes 8% of all congenital heart defects. The stenosis can be valvular, subvalvular, or supravalvular. In general, pulmonic stenosis follows a benign course; with mild pulmonic stenosis (peak gradient <30 mm Hg), there is only a 5% chance of requiring valvotomy; while a moderate degree of stenosis, there is a 20% likelihood of requiring intervention.[16] Pulmonic valve morphology usually involves a supple but thickened valve with commissural fusion or a bicuspid valve. Pulmonic stenosis is usually isolated but can be associated with other anomalies including congenital rubella, atrial septal defects, Noonan syndrome (small stature, shield chest, and web neck), Williams syndrome, and trisomy 13 to 15 and 18.

Echocardiographic Assessment

The best views to assess the pulmonic valve are the ME RV inflow-outflow and upper esophageal aortic arch short-axis views (see Chapter 10). Echocardiographic findings may include thickened pulmonic valve leaflets (bicuspid, tricuspid, quadricuspid, or dysplastic), systolic doming of the pulmonary leaflets, diastolic doming (pulmonary valve prolapse), and a D-shaped left ventricle in systole (if RV pressures are elevated). Measuring the pulmonic valve thickness and annulus dimensions is useful in the assessment for percutaneous balloon valvuloplasty. Variable degrees of poststenotic dilatation of the main and left pulmonary arteries may be present. Right ventricular hypertrophy develops secondary to long-standing pulmonary valve stenosis, and the hypertrophied muscle may cause significant right ventricular infundibular obstruction. Pulsed-wave Doppler sampling of the entire RV outflow is required to exclude infundibular, subinfundibular, and main or pulmonary branch stenoses. Continuous-wave Doppler is the most useful in determining the transvalvular pressure gradient and pulmonic valve area. A dagger-shaped, late-peaking systolic gradient characterizes dynamic infundibular obstruction. Color-flow Doppler aids in determining the location of the stenotic jet and quantifying the severity of pulmonary regurgitation. Pulmonary regurgitation is especially common post pulmonary valvotomy. Detection of associated lesions such as ASD or VSD is essential

ANOMALIES OF VENTRICULAR OUTFLOW

Tetralogy of Fallot

Tetralogy of Fallot (TOF) is the most common cyanotic heart disease. It is typically characterized by four anomalies: a VSD, an overriding aorta, pulmonary valve stenosis, and RV hypertrophy. The hallmark of TOF is an anterocephalic deviation of the infundibular septum causing subpulmonary obstruction in the right ventricular outflow tract.[17] The aorta is committed to both ventricles to a variable degree, but by definition is committed to the left ventricle by at least 50%. Other anomalies can be present with tetralogy of Fallot, including ASD in 10% to 15% (so-called pentalogy of Fallot), right aortic arch in 25%, anomalous origin of the left anterior descending coronary artery in 10%,[18] absence of the pulmonary valve, aortopulmonary collaterals, and systemic venous anomalies (in patients with pulmonary atresia and VSD). The physiologic consequences of tetralogy of Fallot are related mainly to the RV outflow tract obstruction and the large, nonrestrictive perimembranous VSD. The severity of cyanosis depends on the degree of the ventricular right-to-left shunting and the degree of obstruction in the RV outflow tract. Clinical presentation can vary from cyanotic spells, dyspnea, and limited exercise tolerance to erythrocytosis, hyperviscosity, cerebral abscess, stroke, and endocarditis. Survival beyond childhood is unlikely in the majority of patients who have not been surgically treated. Complete correction is performed in early infancy. However, these adult patients may yet have significant problems after successful repair with the most common being residual right ventricular outflow tract obstruction and pulmonary regurgitation leading to right ventricular failure. A subset of patients may present with ongoing aortic root dilatation and aortic regurgitation.

ECHOCARDIOGRAPHIC ASSESSMENT

Because it is a complex anomaly, a combination of scanning planes (ME, transgastric, and deep transgastric views) is required to define all the defects (Figure 18–17).

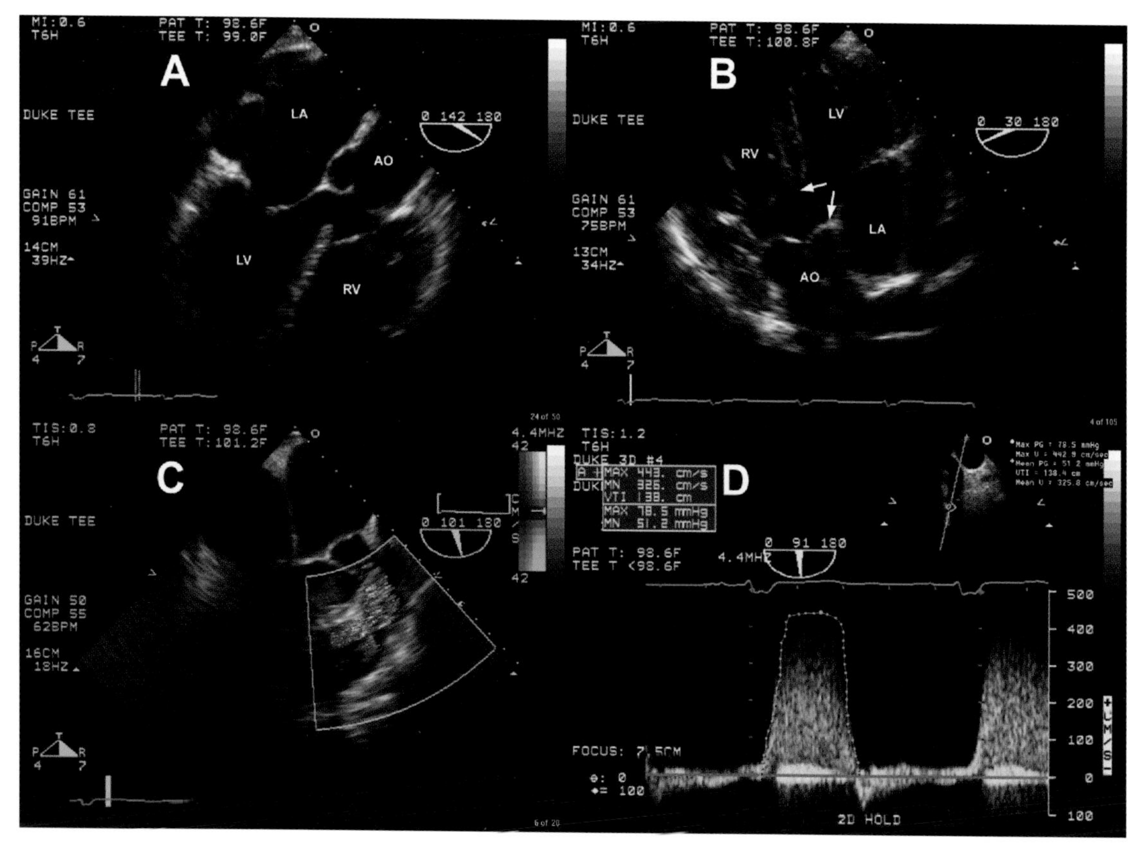

FIGURE 18–17. Tetralogy of Fallot with an overriding aorta (**A** and **B**), VSD (*arrows* in **B**), and pulmonic stenosis seen with color-flow **(C)** and continuous-wave Doppler **(D)**. (LA, left atrium; AO, aorta; LV, left ventricle; RV, right ventricle.)

The two-dimensional examination should identify RV hypertrophy, overriding aorta, VSDs, small pulmonic annulus, RV outflow obstruction, size of the main pulmonary artery, and ventricular dimensions and function. The perimembranous VSD is seen as a large subaortic defect on the ME aortic short- and long-axis views. An overriding aorta is best appreciated in the ME aortic valve long-axis view; evaluation of the descending thoracic aorta is helpful in detecting aortic to pulmonary artery collaterals. Color and pulsed Doppler help in assessing the direction and velocity of the ventricular shunt. Continuous-wave Doppler measures the systolic gradient across the stenotic outflow tract in the upper esophageal aortic arch short-axis view. Associated pulmonary valve anomalies such as pulmonary artery stenosis and hypoplasia are best seen as the TEE probe is withdrawn from the ME RV inflow-outflow view and by using a transgastric approach to visualize the right ventricular outflow tract (RVOT). Surgical correction involves closing the VSD and relieving the right ventricular outflow obstruction. This may be achieved with resection of infundibular muscle, an RVOT patch, a transannular patch (a patch extended across the pulmonary valve annulus), or a valved conduit placed between the RV and the pulmonary artery. After surgical intervention, TEE is helpful in evaluating residual shunt or RVOT obstruction (a peak gradient up to 20 mm Hg is considered normal; gradients above 40 mm Hg indicate significant stenosis), pulmonary valvular regurgitation after transannular repair, and ventricular function.

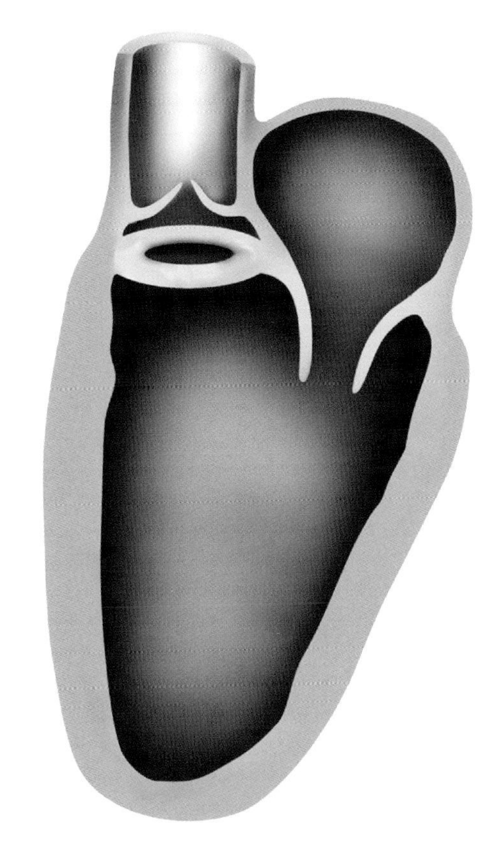

FIGURE 18–18. Membranous subaortic stenosis produced by a connective tissue ring obstructing the outflow tract of the left ventricle.

Subaortic Stenosis

The most common type of congenital aortic subvalvular stenosis is an abnormal fibromuscular ridge that may encircle the LV outflow tract (LVOT; Figure 18–18). A less common type is caused by a diaphragm-like membrane adherent to the base of the aortic leaflets, the junction of muscular and membranous septum, or the anterior leaflet of the mitral valve itself. In patients with hypertrophic obstructive cardiomyopathy, obstruction of the LVOT is due to septal hypertrophy plus systolic anterior motion of the mitral valve leaflets.

Subaortic stenosis obstructs LV outflow, producing effects similar to valvular aortic stenosis: LV hypertrophy, myocardial ischemia, heart failure, and sudden death. In addition, a subaortic membrane may alter LV outflow dynamics and injure the aortic valve without any significant obstructive component. Abnormal flow patterns can produce structural damage to the aortic valve and cause aortic insufficiency. There may be other effects from a subaortic membrane, including structural injury to the mitral valve and direct damage to the aortic valve if the membrane invades the aortic valve. Surgical repair involves excision of the membrane or ridge, septal myomectomy, and aortic valve replacement if severe aortic regurgitation is present. The abnormal flow characteristics that initiated the growth of a subaortic membrane may allow the regrowth of the membrane, even after complete resection. Associated anomalies include supramitral rings, bicuspid aortic valve and aortic coarctation, and a complex that includes a perimembranous VSD and an obstructive muscle bundle in the right ventricle. In the adult population, subaortic stenosis may occur following surgical repair of congenital heart lesions including AVSD, TOF, DORV, and transposition of the great arteries

ECHOCARDIOGRAPHIC EVALUATION

The subaortic membrane is visualized most easily in the ME long-axis view, where a linear structure extends from the left surface of the interventricular septum and the base of the anterior mitral leaflet, causing narrowing of the LV outflow tract.

Unexplained turbulence on color-flow Doppler examination in the ME long-axis, five-chamber, and transgastric or deep transgastric long-axis views is often the first indication of the presence of an obstruction (Figure 18–19A). Measurement of increased subvalvular velocities and estimation of pressure gradients by spectral Doppler help to confirm the diagnosis (Figure 18–19B). Aortic insufficiency often is found as a result of the long-standing flow disturbance. A preoperative search for associated congenital anomalies and postoperative assessment of adequacy of resection, aortic and mitral valve injuries during the repair, and the presence of iatrogenic interventricular communications occurring as a consequence of the myomectomy concludes the TEE study.

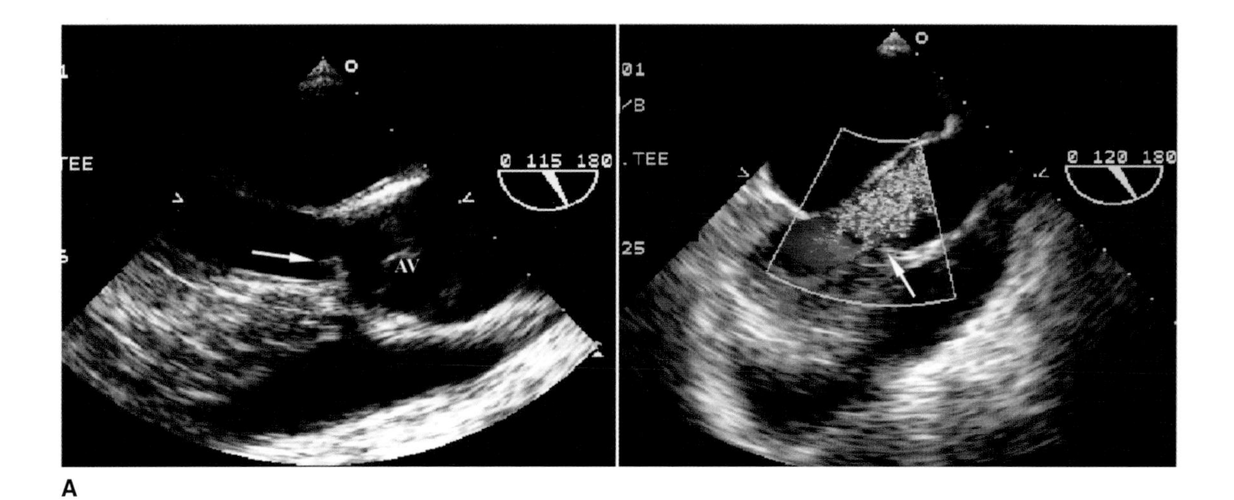

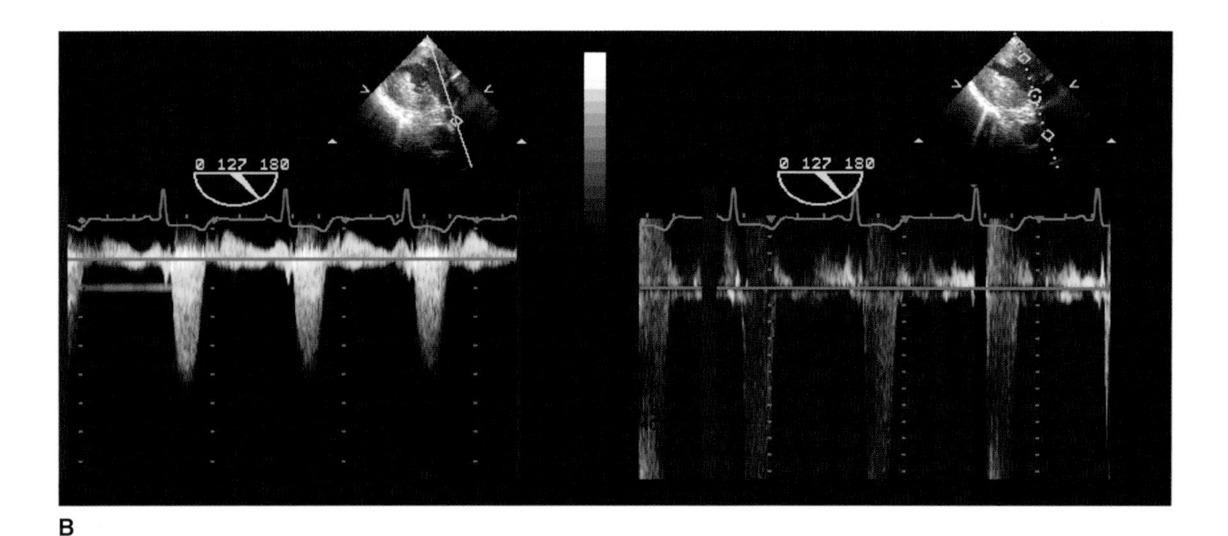

FIGURE 18–19. **A:** The subaortic membrane *(arrow)* is clearly visible on the two-dimensional examination *(left)* and as outflow tract turbulence on the color-flow examination *(right)*. **B:** Continuous-wave Doppler interrogation through the left ventricular outflow tract and aortic valve shows a velocity of almost 4 m/s, whereas pulsed-wave Doppler interrogation in the left ventricular outflow tract results in aliasing, thus indicating elevated subvalvular velocities. (AV, aortic valve.)

ANOMALIES OF THE GREAT ARTERIES

Coronary Artery Anomalies

Coronary artery anomalies are seen in a wide range of congenital abnormalities and involve the origin, course, and structure of epicardial coronary arteries. The incidence is about 0.3% to 1.3% in the general population and in 4% to 15% of young people who experience sudden death. Presence of coronary artery anomalies may, at times, create challenges during coronary angiography, percutaneous coronary interventions, and coronary artery surgery.

Clinically they remain quiescent and do not influence the quality of life or lifespan. Certain types of coronary anomalies, such as the origin of the left main coronary artery from the pulmonary trunk, the aberrant course of the arteries between the great vessels in association with anomalous and slit-like ostium, and large coronary artery fistulas, may be associated with sudden death, myocardial ischemia, congestive heart failure, or endocarditis. Hypoplastic coronary arteries and high takeoff of coronary ostia have also been occasionally reported to have been associated with sudden death. Congenital heart diseases found to have strong association with coronary artery anomalies include truncus arteriosus, transposition of great vessels, pulmonary valve atresia, double-outlet right ventricle, bicuspid aortic valve, and tetralogy of Fallot.

In general, the coronary anomalies can be classified into normal variations, abnormal number, anomalous origin, anomalous course, anomalous termination, and abnormal coronary structure. Normal variations include (1) absence of the left main coronary artery with separate origin of the left anterior descending (LAD) and left circumflex coronary (LCX) arteries from the left coronary sinus of the aorta (described in roughly 1% of patients undergoing angiography); (2) minor variations in the position of the ostia within the coronary sinus; and (3) separate origin of conal branches. Duplication of the LAD and right coronary artery (RCA), and anomalous origin of the coronary arteries from the pulmonary artery, left/right ventricle, internal mammary, subclavian, right carotid, or higher up on the aorta (>1 cm from the sinotubular junction) have all been reported. Similarly, the left main may give rise to LAD, LCX, and RCA. An anomalous artery may course along one of four pathways: A (Anterior to the right ventricular outflow tract), B (Between the aorta and the pulmonary trunk), C (through the Crista supraventricularis), and D (Dorsal to aorta). The coronaries can also take an intramyocardial course (myocardial bridging). From a structural point of view, the coronary arteries may be stenotic, hypoplastic, or atretic.

ECHOCARDIOGRAPHIC ASSESSMENT

A careful assessment is fundamental to viewing these anomalies. Upper esophageal and midesophageal (aortic short-axis and long-axis) views are very useful in examining the origin and course of the vessels. Special attention needs to be paid to assess for other congenital associations, segmental wall motion abnormalities, and ventricular function.

Coronary Fistula

A coronary fistula is any abnormal communication between the coronary artery and a cardiac chamber, great vessel, or vascular structure. Fistulas result from persistence of embryonic channels between the chambers and coronary arteries, and can involve the right coronary (most common), the left coronary, or both. They tend to terminate more toward the low-pressure right-side chambers (pulmonary artery, coronary sinus, or superior vena cava). Very rarely, a fistula will drain into the left heart.[19] The overall incidence of coronary fistulas is 2.1%. The clinical presentation and physiologic consequence of this lesion depend on the degree of shunting, location of the fistula, and termination site. Long-standing left-to-right shunting can produce ventricular volume overload and congestive heart failure. When the fistula diverts coronary flow, angina and, rarely, myocardial infarction can occur. Coronary fistula should not be confused with the *Thebesian veins*, or *venae cordis minimae* which are tiny cardiac venous tributaries that normally drain directly into the cardiac chambers.

ECHOCARDIOGRAPHIC ASSESSMENT

The primary objective of the echocardiographic examination is to ascertain the site and dimensions of the fistula, and the receiving chamber and the degree of the shunt. Evaluation of the coronary artery fistula involves upper esophageal aortic arch, ME aortic valve short-axis, and ME long-axis views. Two-dimensional echocardiography may detect an enlarged proximal coronary artery. RV enlargement denotes the presence of left-to-right shunting. Color-flow Doppler detects a continuous flow pattern within the enlarged and tortuous coronary artery or turbulent flow patterns within the receiving chamber. Contrast echocardiography (using agitated saline solution to visualize an area of negative contrast) also can be used to detect the termination of the fistula into the right heart.

Sinus of Valsalva Aneurysm

A higher incidence of sinus of Valsalva aneurysms has been reported in Far Eastern countries than in Western countries, with a 4:1 male predominance. A weakness in the aortic media at its junction with the annulus fibrosis is thought to be the cause of the congenital aneurysm of the aortic sinuses of Valsalva. These aneurysms are associated with other lesions such as

VSD (40%), bicuspid aortic valve, ASD, pulmonary stenosis, and patent ductus arteriosus. They occur most commonly in the right (69%) and noncoronary sinus (26%), but can be seen in the left coronary sinus (5%). They also may extend into other regions of the heart, most frequently the right ventricle and right atrium.[20] An enlarged aneurysm can present with RV outflow tract obstruction, LV outflow tract obstruction, and compression of the main coronary arteries or tricuspid valve. It also can cause atrioventricular conduction abnormalities or VSDs by burrowing into the septum. Mild aortic regurgitation occurs due to aortic root enlargement. Clinically, symptoms typically occur when the aneurysm ruptures into the receiving chamber, which is usually the right atrium or ventricle. Patients often present with retrosternal chest pain, epigastric pain, congestive heart failure, or evidence of outflow tract obstruction.

ECHOCARDIOGRAPHIC ASSESSMENT

The aortic root, sinuses of Valsalva, LV outflow tract, and the ascending aorta can be examined in detail by using the following views: ME aortic valve short axis, ME aortic valve long axis, transgastric long axis, deep transgastric long axis, upper esophageal aortic arch short and long axis, and epiaortic scanning. Two-dimensional echocardiographic findings include abnormal dilatation of one or more of the sinuses, an extended aneurysmal channel typically seen as a finger-like projection ("windsock" appearance) with echo dropout at the tip of the aneurysm (Figure 18–20), diastolic expansion of the aneurysm, aortic valve prolapse, RV volume overload (in rupture of the noncoronary or right coronary type), or LV volume overload (in rupture of the left coronary type). Doppler findings include a swirling flow pattern in an intact aneurysm and a high-velocity systolic and diastolic turbulent flow pattern into the receiving chamber, if the aneurysm has ruptured. Doppler also helps in determining the presence and severity of associated VSDs and aortic or tricuspid regurgitation. Lesions that should be differentiated from a sinus of Valsalva aneurysm include membranous ventricular septum aneurysms (originates below the plane of the aortic valve), acquired aortic fistulas (do not show the extended aneurysmal channel), and coronary artery fistulas (coronary artery origin and abnormal coronary lumen size).

Supravalvular Obstruction

Supravalvular aortic obstruction is a narrowing of the ascending aorta. This type of stenosis is uncommon and often associated with Williams syndrome or congenital rubella, or it may be familial. The three major types of obstruction are the *hourglass* type (an infolding of the aorta at the sinotubular junction producing an hourglass deformity), *membranous* type (a membranous web-like obstruction), and *tubular* type (diffuse tubular hypoplasia of the ascending aorta). Supravalvular obstruction is usually progressive and aortic regurgitation is common. The origins of the coronary arteries become dilated and tortuous secondary to exposure to high pressures from the more distal aortic obstruction. With Williams syndrome, there often are associated peripheral pulmonary or systemic arterial stenoses. Patients with supravalvular aortic obstruction are at an increased risk for sudden death.

ECHOCARDIOGRAPHIC ASSESSMENT

Echocardiographic detection of supravalvular stenosis relies on careful inspection of the sinotubular junction and the proximal ascending aorta in the ME long-axis view of the aorta. In a normal aorta, the diameter at the sinotubular junction equals or slightly exceeds that of the aortic annulus, and the tubular portion of the ascending aorta should never be smaller than the aortic annulus. Imaging of the proximal branch pulmonary arteries also should be attempted in patients with Williams syndrome.

Coarctation of the Aorta

Coarctation of the aorta accounts for 8% of all cases of congenital heart disease (CHD). The anatomic lesion most commonly found is a discrete ridge or diaphragm comprised of localized medial thickening, infolding of the media, and superimposed neointimal tissue that narrows the aortic segment just below the left subclavian artery and opposite the ductus arteriosus or ligamentum arteriosum. Coarctation of the aorta can be one of the causes of left ventricular outflow obstruction in the very young. In the older age group, coarctation is most often diagnosed after the identification of incidental hypertension during a routine physical examination or after the detection of diminished or absent pulses in the lower extremities. Coarctation is categorized as *preductal*, *juxtaductal*, or *postductal* depending on the position relative to the ligamentum arteriosum, and may be discrete or involve a long segment of the aorta. The lesion may also occur at the level of the abdominal aorta. Associated defects include bicuspid aortic valve (80% to 85%), patent ductus arteriosus (50%), VSDs, valvular aortic stenosis, subaortic stenosis, and Turner syndrome. It also can occur as a part of Shone complex (supravalvular mitral valve ring, parachute mitral valve, subaortic stenosis, and coarctation). Clinically, patients with coarctation present with a history of systemic hypertension (33%), headache, epistaxis, and congestive heart failure. Physical

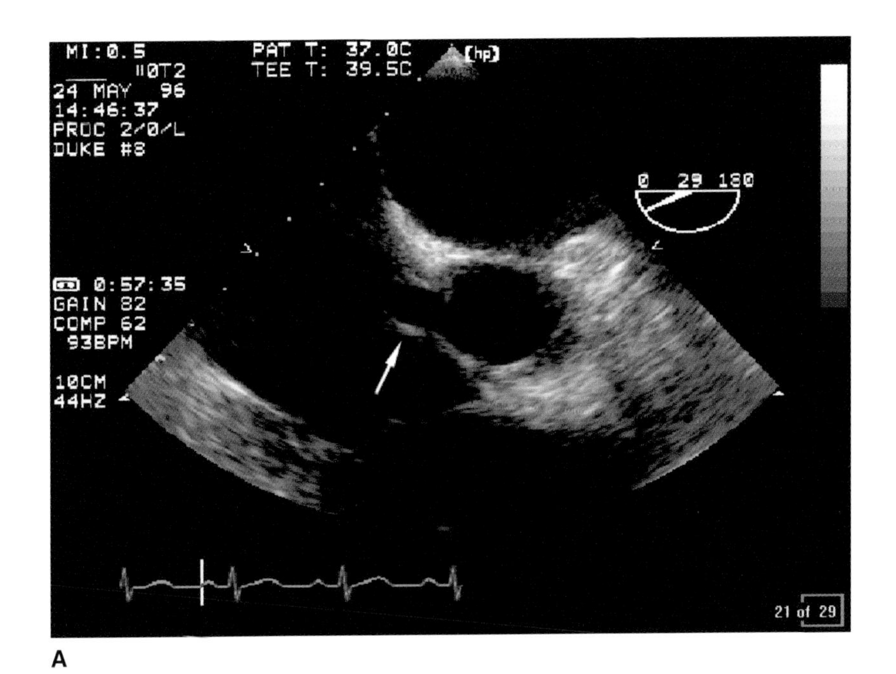

A

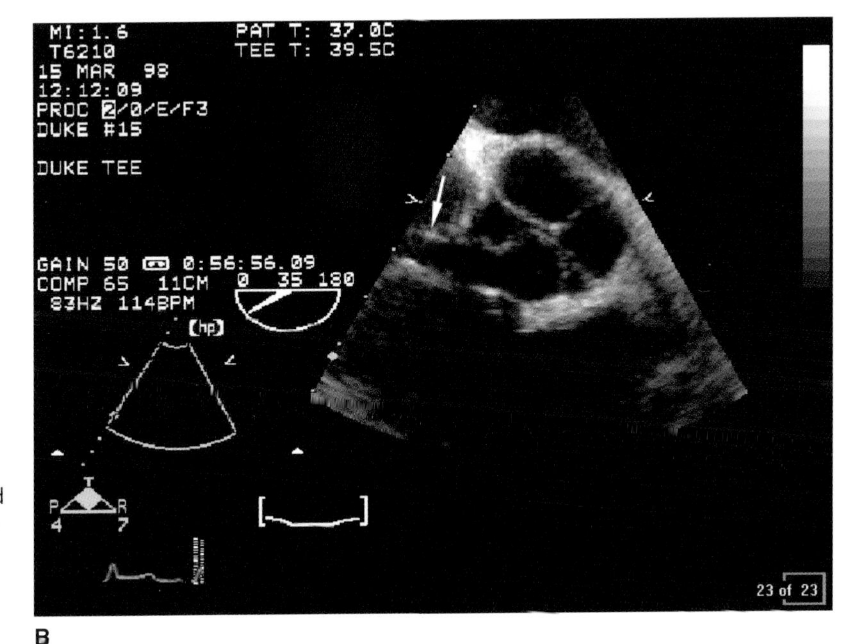

B

FIGURE 18–20. **A** and **B:** Two-dimensional imaging in two patients with a ruptured sinus of Valsalva aneurysm shows an extended aneurysmal channel typically seen as a finger-like projection or "windsock" *(arrow)* with echo dropout at the tip of aneurysm.

examination findings include elevated systolic blood pressure in the upper extremity when compared with the lower extremity (systolic blood pressure differential in arm vs leg of 20 mm Hg or more), radial to femoral pulse delay, diminished femoral pulses, and cyanosis with exercise (in preductal). The primary physiologic consequence of this defect is an increased LV afterload.

Echocardiographic Assessment

A detailed examination can be conducted by using the short- and long-axis views of the aortic arch and descending aorta. Two-dimensional findings include a long, tubular narrowing of the descending thoracic aorta usually distal to the left subclavian artery, increased systolic pulsation of the aorta proximal to the lesion, decreased systolic pulsation of abdominal aorta, poststenotic dilatation of the aorta, enlarged intercostal arteries distal to coarctation, and increased diameter of the left subclavian artery. Evaluation of the associated defects is also important. The severity of coarctation is assessed by measuring the narrowest diameter of the coarctation and comparing it with the descending thoracic aorta diameter (a ratio of 0.4 or less indicates severe coarctation). Pulsed-wave Doppler may detect increased velocity and turbulent flow at the site of obstruction. Continuous-wave Doppler through the coarctation demonstrates the characteristic flow pattern of increased systolic flow velocity and continuous flow in diastole. The profile of the abdominal aortic flow is typically damped and has a delay in the systolic upstroke, turbulence in systole, and variable degrees of diastolic antegrade flow.[21] Color-flow Doppler demonstrates flow acceleration proximal to and turbulent flow through the site of obstruction (Figure 18–21).

Patent Ductus Arteriosus

An inevitable part of fetal life, the ductus arteriosus usually closes within the first 24 to 48 hours of life. Patent ductus accounts for about 2% to 10% of cases of CHD. The ductus arises from the pulmonary artery bifurcation near the left pulmonary artery and connects to the descending aorta just opposite the left subclavian artery (Figure 18–22). It can occur as an isolated anomaly or in association with other defects such as VSDs and coarctation. In later life, the ductus can become calcified, friable, or even aneurysmal. Patients may present with symptoms of infective endocarditis, chest pain, palpitations, congestive heart failure, or pulmonary hypertension. The nature and severity of symptoms is dependent on the size of the ductus and the difference between the systemic and pulmonary vascular resistances.

Echocardiographic Assessment

The main goals in the evaluation include morphologic portrayal of the ductus and surrounding structures, appraisal of the shunt magnitude, estimation of pulmonary artery pressures, and exclusion of associated anomalies. The ductus is best viewed where the left pulmonary artery crosses the descending thoracic aorta. A full evaluation of this lesion often requires a combination of the upper esophageal aortic arch, descending aorta long- and short-axis views, and the deep transgastric long-axis views. Two-dimensional findings include left atrial and ventricular dilatation, LV volume overload, dilated pulmonary artery, and signs of pulmonary hypertension. The length and diameter of the ductus also should be measured. Color-flow Doppler is probably

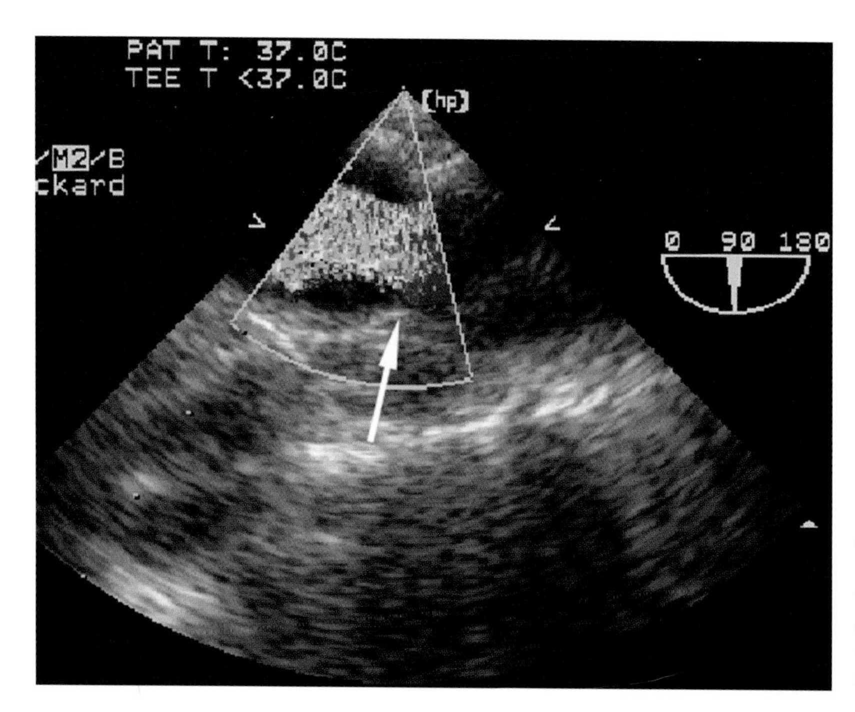

FIGURE 18–21. Color-flow Doppler imaging in a patient with aortic coarctation demonstrating turbulent flow through the site of obstruction *(arrow).*

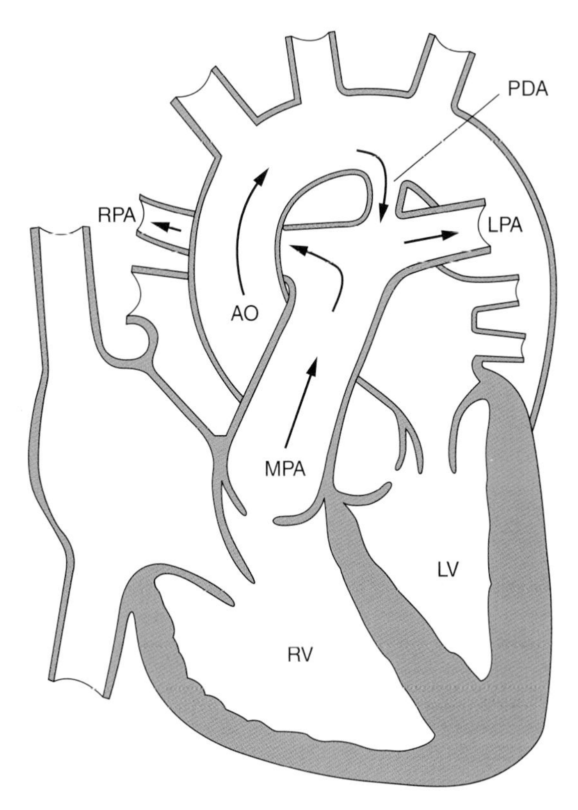

FIGURE 18–22. Schematic diagram demonstrating the origin of the patent ductus arteriosus (PDA) from the pulmonary artery bifurcation near the left pulmonary artery and its termination in the descending aorta opposite the left subclavian artery. (AO, aorta; LPA, left pulmonary artery; LV, left ventricle; MPA, main pulmonary artery; RPA, right pulmonary artery; RV, right ventricle.)

the best aid in diagnosing the ductus. The continuous ductal flow presents as a jet entering the main pulmonary artery near the origin of the left pulmonary during diastole, but the systolic component of the shunt flow usually is eclipsed by the systolic flow in the main pulmonary artery. As pulmonary artery pressures rise, the shunt velocity and flow decrease, making visualization of even the diastolic component more difficult. In a similar fashion, pulsed Doppler with an accurate recording of the electrocardiogram helps to differentiate shunt flow from normal pulmonary artery flow. Continuous-wave Doppler measurement of the peak systolic velocity of the shunt jet can be used to calculate the systolic gradient between the aorta and the pulmonary artery (by using the simplified Bernoulli equation). Subtracting this gradient from the systemic systolic blood pressure yields the systolic pulmonary artery pressure. In patients with a patent ductus arteriosus, the shunt occurs after the pulmonary valve, so Q_p is measured at the level of the left ventricular outflow tract and Q_s is measured at the level of the right ventricular outflow tract.

ANOMALIES OF ATRIOVENTRICULAR CONNECTIONS

The Univentricular Heart

The definition of univentricular heart encompasses a broad group of congenital cardiac malformations. Specifically, it includes double-inlet left ventricle or double-inlet right ventricle, mitral atresia, tricuspid atresia, and unbalanced atrioventricular canal defects. All are characterized by both atria being related entirely to one functional ventricle. In most univentricular hearts there are two ventricular chambers—one well-developed ventricle (the functional ventricle) and a second rudimentary ventricle. The well-developed ventricle may be designated left, right, or indeterminate.[22] The dominant ventricle has a left ventricular morphology in 80% of cases. Ventricular morphology can be established by the unique features of each ventricle as listed in Table 18–1. The univentricular circulation is inherently inefficient because of the recirculation of the pulmonary and systemic venous return; therefore, the palliative plan for patients with single ventricle physiology is diversion of all the systemic venous blood directly into the pulmonary arteries. Adult patients with single ventricle physiology would have undergone a systemic to pulmonary artery shunt, followed by a Glenn shunt, and finally a Fontan procedure.

ECHOCARDIOGRAPHIC ASSESSMENT

TEE should delineate details of the atrioventricular connection, the ventriculoarterial connection, and ventricular morphology. When more than 50% of both AV valves open into a single ventricle, it is considered an echocardiographic hallmark of a double-inlet ventricle. Similarly, the hallmark of an unbalanced atrioventricular canal defect is more than 75% of a common AV valve opening into one ventricular chamber.[22] Tricuspid atresia is characterized by the lack of a direct connection between the right atrium and ventricle, and mitral atresia by the lack of direct connection between left atrium and ventricle. AV valve insufficiency is common in these hearts and also a marker for adverse prognosis. Abnormalities of the ventriculoarterial connection form an integral part of univentricular hearts.[17] Most often, the ventriculoarterial connection is discordant, with the pulmonary artery arising from the main left ventricle and the aorta arising from a rudimentary right ventricle. TEE definition of the ventricular morphology may be difficult, but as a rule, anterior rudimentary chambers are of right ventricular morphology and posterior rudimentary chambers are usually of left ventricular morphology.[17] The evaluation on an adult post–Fontan-type operation is discussed in the section below on surgical procedures.

ANOMALIES OF VENTRICULOARTERIAL CONNECTIONS

Truncus Arteriosus

Truncus arteriosus is a rare anomaly characterized by a single arterial trunk arising from the normally formed ventricles by means of a single semilunar valve (ie, truncal valve) and accounts for 1% to 2% of the congenital heart disease. This anomaly is thought to result from incomplete or failed septation of the distal conus, truncus arteriosus, and the aortic sac. A large VSD usually coexists with the truncus defect, essentially making the right and left ventricles into a single chamber. The pulmonary arteries originate from the common arterial trunk distal to the coronary arteries and proximal to the first brachiocephalic branch of the aortic arch. Pulmonary arteries may arise from the common trunk in one of several patterns, which often are used to classify subtypes of truncus arteriosus. In type I (most common), an aortopulmonary septum is recognized and a single main pulmonary artery is identified to originate from the posterior wall of the truncus. In type II the aortopulmonary septum is absent and separate right and left pulmonary arteries arise from the posterior truncal wall. Type III has only one pulmonary artery arising from the lateral wall of the truncal vessel and the blood supply to the other lung is from either the base of the aortic arch or the systemic arteries. In type IV (rare), the pulmonary arteries arise from the descending aorta, and this type often is called a *pseudotruncus* (probably a severe tetralogy of Fallot with pulmonary atresia and large bronchial collaterals). A variety of abnormalities may be associated with truncus arteriosus such as structural abnormalities of the truncal valve, including dysplastic and supernumerary leaflets,[23] significant regurgitation (moderate or severe) through the truncal valve, abnormal proximal coronary arteries, interruption of the aortic arch (which almost always occurs between the left common carotid and subclavian arteries), right aortic arch, left superior caval vein, aberrant subclavian artery, ASD, atrioventricular septal defect, double aortic arch, and various forms of functionally univentricular heart. The physiologic sequelae of this anomaly depend on the degree of cyanosis and ventricular volume overload. The single most important issue in the description of truncus arteriosus is whether a right ventricular to pulmonary artery conduit can be performed as a primary repair. The surgical management of this condition involves removal of the pulmonary arteries from the truncal root, closure of the root defect, patch closure of the ventricular septal defect, and reconstruction of the right ventricular outflow.

Echocardiographic Assessment

A full set of echocardiographic views is necessary to guarantee complete and precise definition of the anatomy and associated anomalies. The primary objectives are to identify and confirm the conotruncal abnormalities, the number of VSDs, the morphology of the truncal valve, anomalies of the coronary arteries, size of the aortic arch, and location of the pulmonary artery orifices. The most characteristic finding is the identification of the truncal root, which overrides a ventricular septal defect and deficiency of the infundibular septum. The midesophageal and aortic arch views demonstrate the single arterial trunk arising from the ventricles, with variable override of the ventricular septum. The single trunk is also seen to be in continuity with the mitral valve. The left atrium is large due to increased pulmonary blood flow. These views also demonstrate the thickness and mobility of the truncal valve leaflets, and origins and course of the proximal coronary arteries. The aortic arch view allows delineation of the pulmonary arterial origin(s) from the common trunk, although additional views are helpful to more completely characterize the pulmonary arterial anatomy. Demonstration of pulmonary arteries arising from the truncus is necessary to distinguish this anomaly from pulmonary atresia with VSD.

Transposition of the Great Arteries (TGA)

Also known as D-transposition, with this lesion there is atrioventricular concordance and ventriculoarterial discordance. The aorta arises in an anterior position from the right ventricle, and the pulmonary artery arises from the anatomic left ventricle (Figure 18–23). Systemic venous blood returns to the right atrium, from where it goes to the morphologic right ventricle and then to the aorta. Pulmonary venous blood returns to the left atrium, from where it goes to the morphologic left ventricle and then to the pulmonary artery. Therefore, there is complete separation of the pulmonary and systemic circulation and survival depends on a communication such as ASD, VSD, or patent ductus arteriosus between the two circuits, allowing for intracardiac mixing. Other associated cardiac anomalies include obstruction to pulmonary outflow, atrioventricular valve abnormalities, anomalous origin and course of the coronary arteries, and aortic arch anomalies.

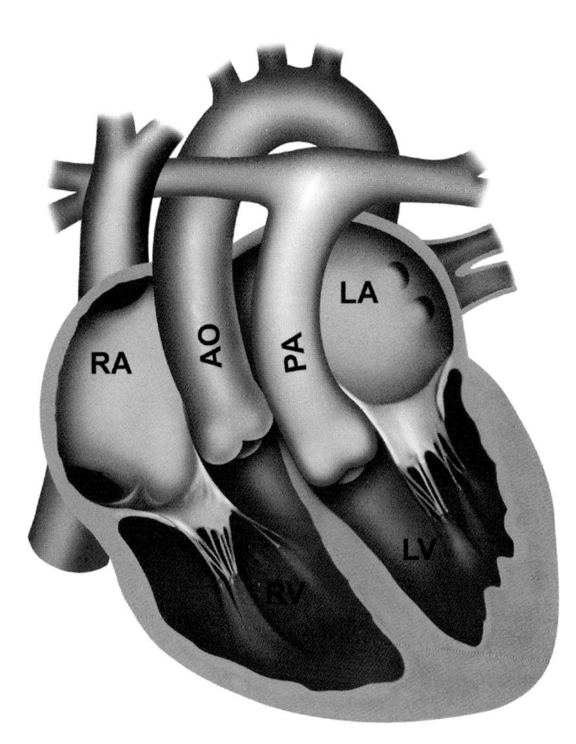

FIGURE 18–23. Transposition of the great arteries. (RA, right atrium; LA, left atrium; RV, right ventricle; LV, left ventricle; PA, pulmonary artery; AO, aorta.)

Most patients who are currently adults with D transposition have undergone surgery to redirect blood at an atrial level by using a baffle (Mustard procedure) or atrial flaps (Senning procedure). These so-called physiologic procedures correct cyanosis, but the right ventricle continues to function as the systemic ventricle and late dysfunction and dilatation are not uncommon. The Jatene procedure, also described as anatomic repair, has supplanted the atrial switch procedures and involves transection of the pulmonary artery and ascending aorta and switching of the arteries, so that the left ventricle supports the systemic circulation. The coronary arteries are also translocated to the neo-aorta, formerly the pulmonary artery.

ECHOCARDIOGRAPHIC ASSESSMENT

TEE is valuable in the assessment of these patients in the perioperative period. Preoperatively, a variety of transesophageal planes including long- and short-axis views are used to view the anomalies. The aortic long-axis view can be used to visualize the parallel relationship of the outflow tracts and great vessels with a posterior course of the pulmonary artery. The pulmonary artery (LVOT in this anomaly) should be viewed for the presence of obstruction or valve regurgitation in the long-axis, apical, and transgastric views. The deep transgastric view demonstrates the discordant ventriculoarterial connections. Evaluation of the tricuspid valve (systemic atrioventricular valve) for regurgitation is fundamental because the severity of ventricular dysfunction and the extent of tricuspid regurgitation may have long-term and short-term prognostic implications.

Echocardiographic evaluation after the arterial switch procedure should focus on detection of RV outflow tract obstruction (the most common problem), neo-pulmonary stenosis, neo-aortic root dilatation, neo-aortic valve regurgitation, and assessment of RV function and coronary ostial patency.

Congenitally Corrected Transposition of the Great Arteries (ccTGA)

Also known as L-transposition, congenitally corrected transposition of the great arteries is characterized by inversion of the ventricles and transposition of the great arteries (discordant atrioventricular connections plus discordant ventriculoarterial connections). Systemic venous blood returns to the right atrium, and flows across the mitral valve and into the morphologic left ventricle, which is connected to the pulmonary artery. Pulmonary venous blood returns to the left atrium, and flows across the tricuspid valve and into the morphologic right ventricle, which is connected to the aorta. Therefore, the systemic and pulmonary circulations are in series and physiologically corrected, but the morphologic right ventricle supports the systemic circulation.

This lesion is a rare form of CHD. Associated abnormalities occur in most cases and consist of VSD, pulmonary or subpulmonary stenosis, and tricuspid valve anomalies. Patients with no associated abnormalities may have undetected L-transposition until problems arise in the sixth or seventh decade. Surgery is complex but may be feasible in certain patients and involves an atrial baffle procedure plus an arterial switch operation—the so-called double switch operation.

ECHOCARDIOGRAPHIC ASSESSMENT

The ME four-chamber view confirms the diagnosis by demonstrating the abnormal inferiorly placed atrioventricular valve (tricuspid valve) in the left-side morphologic right ventricle (Figure 18–24). The tricuspid valve is often Ebsteinoid in character in this form of CHD. The aortic valve is located leftward, anterior, and superior to the pulmonic valve. The great vessels connection can be appreciated from a variety of views as previously described. With advancing age, RV dilatation is common and is accompanied by decreased systolic function

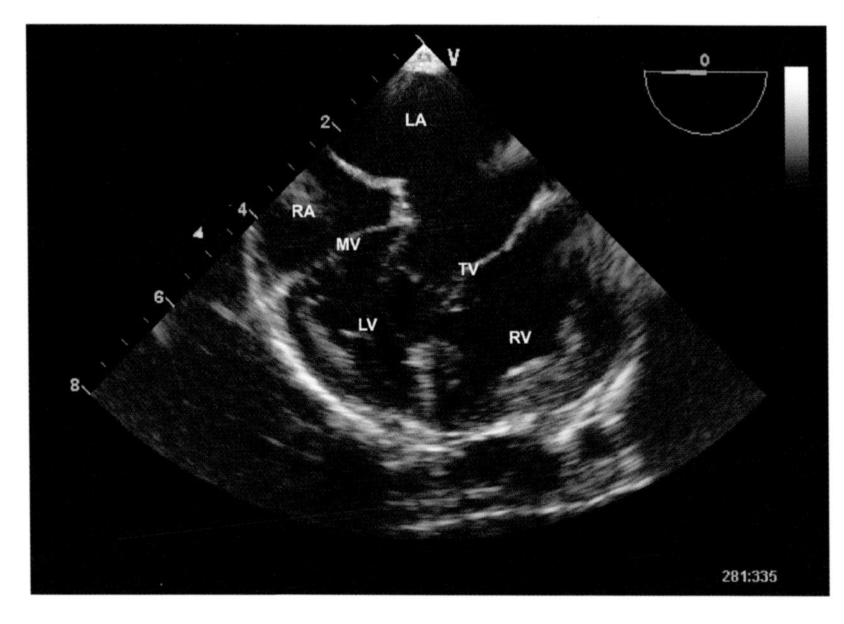

FIGURE 18–24. Congenitally corrected transposition of the great arteries. Characteristic features help to differentiate the morphologic right ventricle located on the left-hand side from the morphologic left ventricle on the right-hand side. The right ventricle displays heavy trabeculations, septal chordal attachment of the tricuspid valve, and lower septal insertion of the tricuspid valve. The tricuspid valve is also characterized as ebsteinoid. (LA, left atrium; RA, right atrium; MV, mitral valve; LV, left ventricle; TV, tricuspid valve; RV, right ventricle.)

The TEE examination should include a search for associated abnormalities of the left-side tricuspid valve (present in 90%), VSD (70%), LV outflow obstruction (40%, usually subvalvular), RV outflow tract obstruction, and subaortic stenosis.

Double-Outlet Right Ventricle

DORV represents a continuum of congenital heart disease that ranges from VSD with significant override of the aorta, to both great arteries arising from the right ventricle, to transposition of the great arteries with pulmonary override of the VSD. DORV lesions are classified according to the anatomic relation of the VSD to the great vessels. The VSD is usually large and may be *subaortic*, which is most common, or *subpulmonary* (Taussig-Bing form), *noncommitted* (VSD is remote from the great vessels), or *doubly committed* (VSD is shared equally by the aorta and pulmonary artery). Pulmonary or aortic stenosis, valvular or subvalvular, is present in up to 50% of patients. Coarctation of the aorta is a common associated lesion, and interrupted aortic arch also may be present. The location of the VSD determines the physiologic picture, and the presence of pulmonary stenosis or increased pulmonary vascular resistance restricting flow across the VSD determines outcome in these patients. A subaortic VSD with pulmonary stenosis resembles the hemodynamic picture of tetralogy of Fallot, whereas a subpulmonary VSD resembles complete transposition with blood from the LV flowing through the VSD to the pulmonary artery and blood from the RV flowing mainly to the aorta. Surgical approach varies according to the type of DORV.

Echocardiographic Assessment

The principal diagnostic feature is the appearance of both great arteries primarily committed to the right ventricle (Figure 18–25). Deep TG views and ME LAX views are helpful in delineating the spatial relationship between the great arteries, the outflow tract of each artery, and the type of VSD and its location relative to the great arteries. Associated cardiac lesions also need to be excluded.

Adult patients who have had a Rastelli repair for DORV with subaortic VSD and pulmonary stenosis require careful TEE evaluation to exclude kinking or obstruction along these conduits. Patients with DORV of a tetralogy of Fallot type usually have had the VSD closed with a septal patch and primary repair of the pulmonic stenosis site. Residual defects in the ventricular septum or around the patch may frequently occur. Color-flow imaging confirms the residual shunt.

COMMON SURGICAL PROCEDURES

Cavopulmonary Connections

Glenn Shunt

A Glenn shunt is typically used as the initial palliative procedure for single ventricle physiology. It consists of an anastomosis between the end of the superior vena cava to the side of the right pulmonary artery, which is divided from the main pulmonary artery in the classic form; alternatively, superior vena cava flow is directed

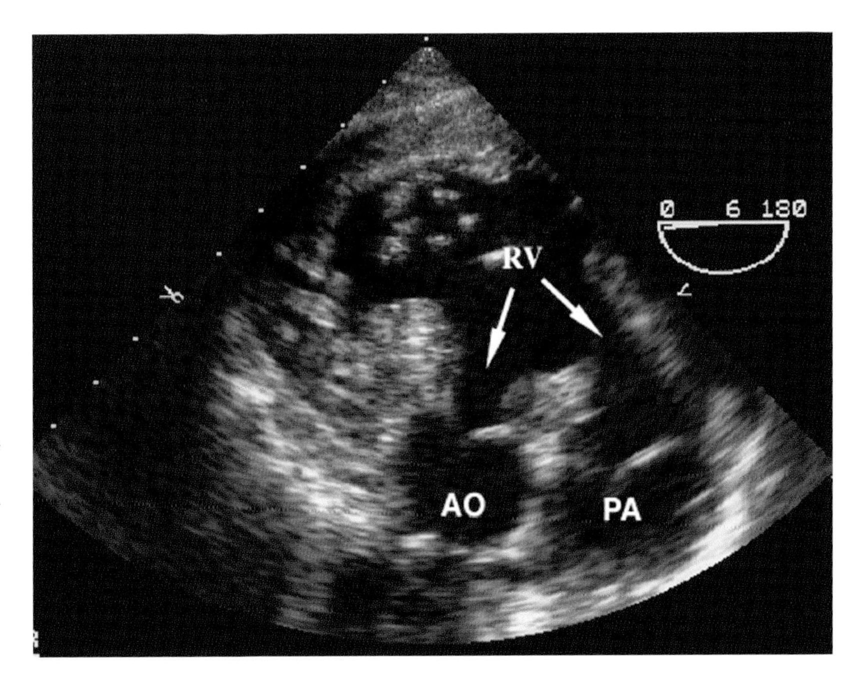

FIGURE 18–25. Deep transgastric long-axis view showing a double-outlet right ventricle with two great arteries originating from a hypertrophied right ventricle. (AO, aorta; RV, right ventricle; PA, pulmonary artery.)

to both (undivided) pulmonary arteries in the bidirectional form (Figure 18–26). The shunt improves arterial saturation, although cyanosis remains because blood draining from the inferior vena cava still mixes with pulmonary venous return at the atrial level. The Glenn

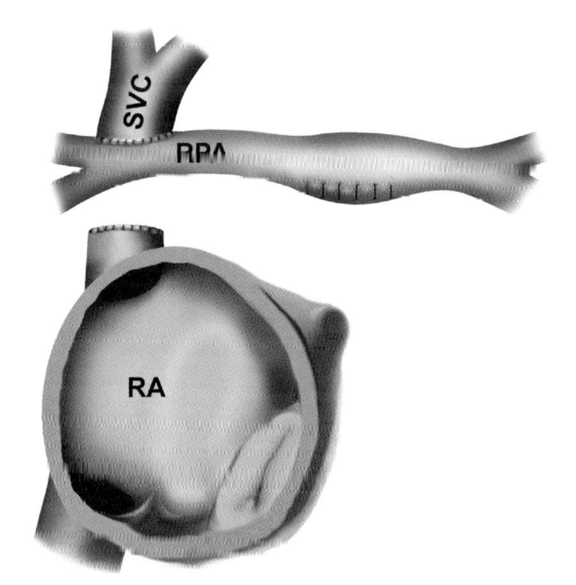

FIGURE 18–26. Bidirectional Glenn shunt. (SVC, superior vena cava; RPA, right pulmonary artery; RA, right atrium.)

shunt is performed at about 6 months of age followed by the Fontan procedure between 18 months and 4 years of age.

Echocardiographic Assessment. TEE imaging in a vertical plane alignment at the level of the right atrium identifies the upper part of the superior vena cava, and then, with rotation of the probe rightward, the upper to middle superior anastomosis to the right pulmonary artery can be visualized. Combined color-flow and pulsed Doppler imaging rules out stenosis or thrombus at the level of anastomosis. Agitated saline solution injected peripherally may be used to exclude pulmonary arteriovenous fistula. Doppler findings of low-velocity, biphasic, and laminar flow with an inspiratory increase (spontaneous ventilation) in the velocity of flow within the shunt are normal. Turbulent flow, on the other hand, may indicate obstruction at the superior vena cava to pulmonary artery anatomosis.

FONTAN PROCEDURE

The Fontan procedure has evolved over many years. The objective of this procedure is to direct inferior venal caval flow into the pulmonary arteries, bypassing the right ventricular chamber. Previously this was achieved by a direct right atrial to pulmonary artery connection, whereas more recently a total cavopulmonary connection is performed as a staged procedure. Stage I is a bidirectional Glenn shunt (as discussed above), and stage II is a technique in which inferior vena cava blood is directed through a lateral tunnel within the right atrium or a tube

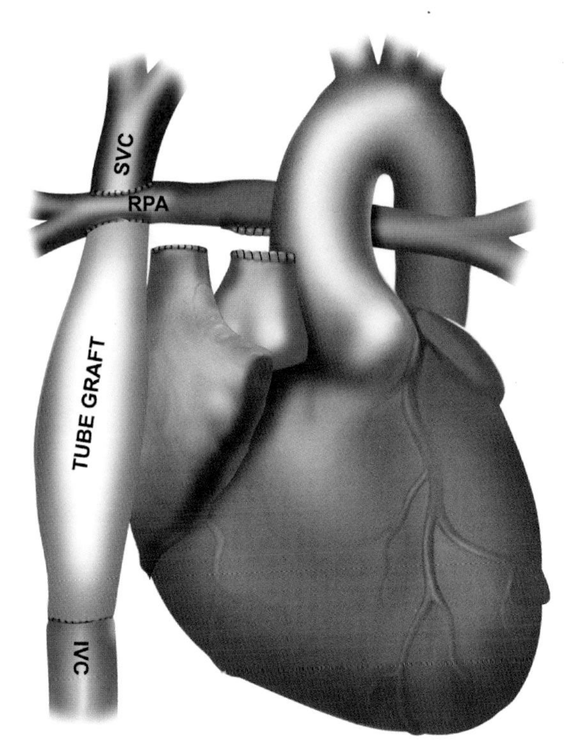

FIGURE 18–27. Extracardiac Fontan procedure. (SVC, superior vena cava; RPA, right pulmonary artery; IVC, inferior vena cava.)

graft external to the right atrium into the pulmonary artery (extracardiac Fontan; Figure 18–27). Once complete, all of the systemic venous return is diverted directly into the pulmonary arteries. Pulmonary blood flow is passive without an intervening ventricular chamber to propel it across the lungs. The transpulmonary gradient (systemic venous pressure–left atrial pressure) becomes the driving pressure across the pulmonary bed. Consideration of pulmonary vascular resistance, systemic atrioventricular valve competency, and systemic ventricular function determine whether the procedure can be performed. Outcome in these patients is determined by systemic ventricular function and atrioventricular valve competency.

Echocardiographic Assessment. Complications of the Fontan circulation such as cavoatrial shunting, thrombus formation, and obstruction within the systemic venous pathways must be excluded. The inferior venous pathway may be best visualized with a transgastric view. A normal flow profile through the venopulmonary anastomosis or in the conduit has a biphasic forward pattern of moderate velocity (0.2 to 0.5 m/s). A flow profile with a velocity of greater than 1.5 m/s is suggestive of obstruction.[4] Pulsed-wave Doppler in the pulmonary artery should show increase in flow with inspiration during spontaneous ventilation.

Ross Procedure

The Ross procedure is used in patients who require aortic valve replacement. It consists of excision of the aortic valve and placement of the native pulmonary valve and trunk into the aortic position with reimplantation of the coronary arteries. On the pulmonary side, a homograft conduit is placed between the right ventricle and the pulmonary artery.

Preoperatively, comparison of aortic annulus and pulmonic annulus diameters, and detection of presence and severity of pulmonary regurgitation determines the feasibility of the procedure. Postoperative and follow-up evaluations should focus on visualization of the pulmonary autograft for aneurysmal dilatation and presence of regurgitation.

Atrial Switch Operations

Several decades ago the atrial switch operation was the standard surgical approach for transposition of the great arteries. Intra-atrial baffles that redirect blood at an atrial level were fashioned from pericardial tissue in the Mustard procedure and from right atrial flaps in the Senning procedure. Systemic venous blood from the caval veins is then directed through the baffle across the mitral valve into the left ventricle and out the pulmonary artery (Figure 18–28). Pulmonary venous

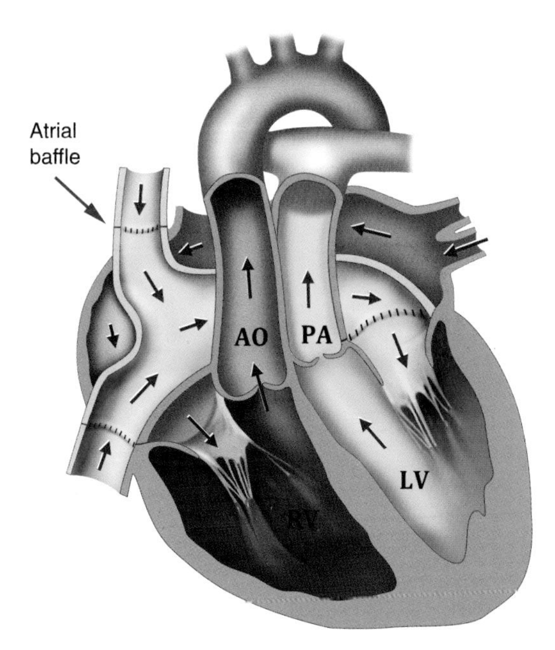

FIGURE 18–28. Atrial switch procedure. (RV, right ventricle; LV, left ventricle; PA, pulmonary artery; AO, aorta.)

return is rerouted through the tricuspid valve into the right ventricle and the aorta. This results in a physiologic correction but not an anatomic correction, as the right ventricle remains the chamber ejecting into the systemic circulation. Long-term complications include tricuspid regurgitation, atrial rhythm disturbances, right ventricular dysfunction, and sudden death.

Echocardiographic Assessment. Typical echocardiographic findings include right ventricular hypertrophy and a convex appearance of the interventricular septum towards the left ventricle as right ventricular pressure exceeds left ventricular pressure. TEE is extremely valuable in patients who have undergone a Mustard or Senning procedure because the systemic venous baffle and pulmonary venous confluence are posterior structures.[24] The combination of the transverse, longitudinal, and modified planes allows for visualization of the caval junctions, the entrance of the pulmonary veins, and the midportion of the baffle. The baffle is typically seen as an oblique, linear echo within the left atrium. Color and spectral Doppler interrogation of venous inflows aids in the detection of turbulence, increased velocity (faster than 1 m/s), and abnormal flow patterns due to baffle obstruction. Baffle leaks are best assessed by using contrast echocardiography and the ME four-chamber view. Baffle obstruction results in the generation of collaterals from the superior to the inferior vena cava. Hence, imaging of the inferior vena cava during injection of agitated saline solution through a peripheral or superior central vein will confirm baffle obstruction by detecting microbubbles in the inferior vena cava. Careful evaluation of RV function, the systemic ventricle, and the tricuspid valve (the systemic atrioventricular valve) for regurgitation completes the examination.

The Rastelli Procedure

The Rastelli procedure is used to correct certain combinations of congenital heart defects. Transposition of the great arteries (d-TGA) with a VSD and right ventricular outflow tract obstruction (RVOTO), or overriding aorta plus VSD and RVOTO, or double-outlet right ventricle with a VSD and RVOTO are all indications for a Rastelli repair. In this repair, a Gore-Tex patch is used as an intraventricular baffle to direct oxygenated blood from the left ventricle to the aorta, while at the same time closing the VSD. The pulmonary valve is surgically closed and an artificial conduit and valve is placed from the right ventricle to the pulmonary artery bifurcation, allowing oxygen-depleted blood to travel to the lungs for reoxygenation.

Echocardiographic Assessment. Satisfactory postoperative hemodynamics are dependent upon free, unobstructed egress of blood from both the left ventricle and the right ventricle. Obstruction to either outflow tract will contribute to ventricular failure. TEE is useful for assessing both the proximal and distal ends of the conduit for stenosis at the anatomosis to the right ventricle or pulmonary artery. Continuous-wave Doppler directed into the conduit promotes detection of high-velocity jets, indicating the presence of an obstruction.

REFERENCES

1. Warnes CA, Liberthson R, Danielson GK, et al. Task force 1: the changing profile of congenital heart disease in adult life. *J Am Coll Cardiol.* 2001;37(5):1170-1175.
2. Webb GD, Harrison DA, Connelly MS. Challenges posed by the adult patient with congenital heart disease. *Adv Intern Med.* 1996;41:437-495.
3. Tynan MJ, Becker AE, Macartney FJ, Jimenez MQ, Shinebourne EA, Anderson RH. Nomenclature and classification of congenital heart disease. *Br Heart J.* 1979;41(5) 544-553.
4. Chassot PG, Bettex DA. Anesthesia and adult congenital heart disease. *J Cardiothorac Vasc Anesth.* 2006;20(3):414-437.
5. Brickner ME, Hillis LD, Lange RA. Congenital heart disease in adults. Second of two parts. *N Engl J Med.* 2000;342(5): 334-342.
6. Haddad F, Couture P, Tousignant C, Denault AY. The right ventricle in cardiac surgery, a perioperative perspective: I. Anatomy, physiology, and assessment. *Anesth Analg.* 2009;108(2) :407-421.
7. Overell JR, Bone I, Lees KR. Interatrial septal abnormalities and stroke: a meta-analysis of case-control studies. *Neurology.* 2000;55(8):1172-1179.
8. Homma S, Di Tullio MR, Sacco RL, Mihalatos D, Li Mandri G, Mohr JP. Characteristics of patent foramen ovale associated with cryptogenic stroke. A biplane transesophageal echocardiographic study. *Stroke.* 1994;25(3):582-586.
9. Meier B, Lock JE. Contemporary management of patent foramen ovale. *Circulation.* 2003;107(1):5-9.
10. Brickner ME, Hillis LD, Lange RA. Congenital heart disease in adults. First of two parts. *N Engl J Med.* 2000;342(4). 256-263.
11. Oh JK, Seward JB, Tajik AJ. *The Echo Manual.* 2nd ed. Philadelphia: Lippincott, Williams & Wilkins; 1999.
12. Sabry AF, Reller MD, Silberbach GM, Rice MJ, Sahn DJ. Comparison of four Doppler echocardiographic methods for calculating pulmonary-to-systemic shunt flow ratios in patients with ventricular septal defect. *Am J Cardiol.* 1995;75(8):611-614.
13. Rastelli G, Kirklin JW, Kincaid OW. Angiocardiography of persistent common atrioventricular canal. *Mayo Clin Proc.* 1967;42(4):200-209.
14. Otto CM. *Textbook of Clinical Echocardiography.* 2nd ed. Philadelphia: W.B. Saunders; 2000.
15. Miller-Hance WC, Silverman NH. Transesophageal echocardiography (TEE) in congenital heart disease with focus on the adult. *Cardiol Clin.* 2000;18(4):861-892.
16. Hayes CJ, Gersony WM, Driscoll DJ, et al. Second natural history study of congenital heart defects. Results of treatment of patients with pulmonary valvar stenosis. *Circulation.* 1993;87(2 Suppl): I28-37.
17. Li W, Henein M, Gatzoulis MA. *Echocardiography in Adult Congenital Heart Disease.* London: Springer; 2007.

18. Dabizzi RP, Caprioli G, Aiazzi L, et al. Distribution and anomalies of coronary arteries in tetralogy of fallot. *Circulation.* 1980;61(1):95-102.
19. Hobbs RE, Millit HD, Raghavan PV, Moodie DS, Sheldon WC. Coronary artery fistulae: a 10-year review. *Cleve Clin Q.* 1982;49(4):191-197.
20. Sakakibara S, Konno S. Congenital aneurysm of the sinus of Valsalva. Anatomy and classification. *Am Heart J.* 1962;63:405-424.
21. Sanders SP, MacPherson D, Yeager SB. Temporal flow velocity profile in the descending aorta in coarctation. *J Am Coll Cardiol.* 1986;7(3):603-609.
22. Khairy P, Poirier N, Mercier LA. Univentricular heart. *Circulation.* 2007;115(6):800-812.
23. Calder L, Van Praagh R, Van Praagh S, et al. Truncus arteriosus communis. Clinical, angiocardiographic, and pathologic findings in 100 patients. *Am Heart J.* 1976;92(1):23-38.
24. Russell IA, Rouine-Rapp K, Stratmann G, Miller-Hance WC. Congenital heart disease in the adult: a review with internet-accessible transesophageal echocardiographic images. *Anesth Analg.* 2006;102(3):694-723.

REVIEW QUESTIONS

Select the best answer for the following questions (single response).

1. A rare finding in an adult with pulmonary stenosis is:
   a. Pulmonary insufficiency
   b. Poststenotic dilatation of the main pulmonary artery
   c. Calcification of the pulmonary valve
   d. Thickened valve with commissural fusion

2. In moderate pulmonary stenosis (peak gradient of 30 to 50 mm Hg), the likelihood of requiring intervention is:
   a. 20%
   b. 30%
   c. 40%
   d. 50%

3. Which of the following is not a classic echocardiographic finding in pulmonary stenosis?
   a. Systolic doming of the pulmonary valve leaflets
   b. Thickened pulmonary valve leaflets
   c. Poststenotic dilatation of the main pulmonary artery
   d. Calcification of the pulmonary valve

4. Which of the following statements regarding balloon valvuloplasty of pulmonary stenosis is false?
   a. A small pulmonary annulus predicts a poor response.
   b. Pulmonary stenosis with a gradient less than 35 mm Hg requires balloon valvuloplasty.
   c. Patients with significant infundibular hypertrophy may demonstrate a high postprocedural gradient.
   d. Markedly thickened cartilaginous leaflets predict a poor response.

5. Which of the following statements regarding pulmonary stenosis is true?
   a. It has a higher prevalence in men.
   b. It is usually detected in childhood.
   c. It generally follows a benign course with advancing age.
   d. Pulmonary stenosis usually is not an isolated finding.

6. Which of the following statements regarding mitral valve cleft is false?
   a. It usually presents with clinical findings of mitral insufficiency.
   b. A mitral valve cleft is usually seen in the anterior leaflet.
   c. It always presents as a part of the complex involving defects in the atrioventricular septum.
   d. Mitral valve repair may be possible.

7. Which of the following is true regarding double-orifice mitral valve?
   a. It usually presents with two equal orifices.
   b. It results from an abnormal fusion of the embryonic endocardial cushions.
   c. It usually presents as a stenotic lesion.
   d. There is always an associated ASD.

8. The most common sinus of Valsalva aneurysm is:
   a. Noncoronary sinus
   b. Left coronary sinus
   c. Right coronary sinus
   d. Between the right and noncoronary sinuses

9. The common termination site for the sinus of Valsalva aneurysm is:
   a. Right ventricle
   b. Left atrium
   c. Right atrium
   d. Left ventricle

10. Regarding sinus of Valsalva aneurysms, which of the following statements is true?
    a. Aneurysms of the noncoronary sinus usually terminate in the right ventricle.
    b. They can present with features of coronary artery compression.
    c. They usually burrow into the interventricular septum.
    d. Acute rupture of a small aneurysm always presents with chest pain.

11. In a patient with sinus of Valsalva aneurysm, a recent finding of severe aortic insufficiency should raise the suspicion of aneurysm rupture into the:
    a. Left atrium
    b. RV outflow tract
    c. LV outflow tract
    d. Right atrium

12. To differentiate the sinus of Valsalva aneurysm from the membranous interventricular septal aneurysm, which of the following is most helpful?
    a. Lack of extended aneurysmal channel
    b. Origin of the aneurysm above the plane of the aortic valve
    c. Aortic insufficiency
    d. LV outflow tract obstruction

13. Which of the following statements is true about sinus of Valsalva aneurysms?
    a. The most common sinus of Valsalva aneurysm involves the left coronary sinus.
    b. Mild aortic insufficiency is seen due to root enlargement and aortic cusp distortion.
    c. In adults, it almost always presents as congestive heart failure.
    d. It is always complicated by infective endocarditis.

14. With regard to sinus of Valsalva aneurysms, which of the following statements is true?
    a. They are thought to result from a weakness in the aortic media.
    b. They are thought to result from a weakness in the aortic intima.
    c. They are thought to result from an abnormal fusion of the annulus fibrosus.
    d. They are thought to result from a weakness in the aortic adventitia.

15. Which of the following echocardiographic findings is not found in sinus of Valsalva aneurysms?
    a. Turbulent flow within the aneurysm and into the receiving chamber
    b. Finger-like "windsock" extending from the base of the sinus
    c. Enlarged sinus from which the aneurysm is originating
    d. Aneurysm originating from below the plane of the aortic valve

16. The most common associated defect seen with the coarctation of the aorta is:
    a. VSD
    b. Patent ductus arteriosus
    c. Bicuspid aortic valve
    d. Subaortic stenosis

17. Which one of the following is not a finding in aortic coarctation?
    a. Hypertension
    b. Elevated systolic blood pressure in upper extremities
    c. Diastolic murmur at the right upper sternal border
    d. Radial to femoral pulse delay

18. Which one of the following is not a Doppler flow profile in aortic coarctation?
    a. Delay in systolic upstroke
    b. Varying degrees of diastolic antegrade flow
    c. Rapid diastolic downstroke
    d. Turbulence in systole

19. Which one of the following is not an echocardiographic finding in coarctation of the aorta?
    a. Systolic flow acceleration
    b. Narrowed flow stream at the point of coarctation
    c. Decreased systolic flow velocity with continuous-wave Doppler
    d. Thoracic aorta dilatation distal to the coarctation

20. Which one of the following is not an indication for intervention in coarctation of the aorta?
    a. Significant pressure gradient between upper and lower extremities
    b. Reduction in luminal diameter greater than 50%
    c. Reduction in luminal diameter greater than 30%
    d. Reduction in luminal diameter greater than 70%

21. Which one of the following is the most common congenital anomaly recognized at birth?
    a. ASD
    b. VSD
    c. Bicuspid aortic valve
    d. Patent ductus arteriosus

22. The most common type of VSD is:
    a. Perimembranous
    b. Supracristal
    c. Muscular
    d. Atrioventricular canal

23. Gerbode defect is one in which there is a communication from the:
    a. LV outflow tract into the right ventricle
    b. Left atrium to the right ventricle
    c. LV outflow tract to the right atrium
    d. RV outflow tract to the left atrium

24. Gasul phenomenon is seen in which type of VSD?
    a. Perimembranous
    b. Muscular

c. Supracristal
d. Atrioventricular canal

25. In Gasul phenomenon:
 a. Pulmonary hypertension is avoided by the development of muscular hypertrophy of the RV outflow tract.
 b. Pulmonary hypertension is avoided by supravalvular dilation of the pulmonic artery.
 c. Right-to-left shunting is limited by a moderator band.
 d. There is spontaneous closure of the VSD.

26. The supracristal VSD is seen more commonly in patients of:
 a. Asian origin
 b. African origin
 c. European origin
 d. Polynesian origin

27. Which type of VSD is associated with a higher incidence of aortic insufficiency?
 a. Perimembranous
 b. Muscular
 c. Supracristal
 d. Atrioventricular canal

28. Atrioventricular canal type VSD is commonly associated with:
 a. Secundum ASD
 b. Primum ASD
 c. Sinus venosus
 d. Unroofed coronary sinus

29. Which of the following statements is not true with regard to management of VSDs?
 a. Surgical intervention is not necessary for an adult with a small VSD and normal pulmonary artery pressures.
 b. Patients with a large VSD and irreversible pulmonary hypertension should have corrective surgery as soon as possible.
 c. Endocarditis prophylaxis is important in patients with VSD.
 d. Periodic follow-up is necessary to assess pulmonary artery pressures.

30. Membranous VSD is visualized with TEE as:
 a. An echo dropout area beneath the aortic valve
 b. An echo dropout area beneath the mitral area
 c. A distortion in the septum just adjacent to the apex of the left ventricle
 d. A bombed-out appearance of the middle part of the septum

31. Membranous VSD is best seen in which of the following TEE imaging plane combinations?
 a. ME four-chamber and two-chamber views
 b. ME RV inflow-outflow view
 c. ME long-axis and deep transgastric views
 d. Aortic arch long-axis view

32. Which of the following statement is not true regarding muscular VSDs?
 a. It can be located anywhere within the trabecular septum.
 b. It is the most common VSD in adults.
 c. It is associated with pulmonary vascular obstructive disease.
 d. Smaller defects often close spontaneously.

33. The following statements about atrioventricular canal type VSDs are true except:
 a. They are commonly associated with primum ASD.
 b. They are usually due to a defect in the formation of the atrioventricular septum.
 c. They are associated with clefts in the pulmonary valve.
 d. They are associated with clefts in the mitral valve.

34. Regarding patent ductus arteriosus, which of the following statements is not true?
 a. It is found in 2% of adults with congenital heart disease.
 b. It spontaneously closes within 24 to 48 hours of life.
 c. It usually is not an isolated anomaly.
 d. Aneurysm of the ductus can occur.

35. In an adult with patent ductus arteriosus, all of the following statements are true except:
 a. Clinical presentation depends on the size of the shunt.
 b. Patients with large shunts develop atrial arrhythmias.
 c. With onset of pulmonary hypertension, differential cyanosis of upper extremities is noted.
 d. Small ductal shunts can produce a continuous murmur at the left upper sternal border.

36. All of the following statements regarding patent ductus arteriosus are true except:
 a. Clinical presentation depends on the size of the shunt.
 b. Right-to-left shunting commonly occurs with normal pulmonary artery pressures.
 c. Flow may be bidirectional.

d. Knowing the peak systolic velocity of the patent ductus arteriosus jet will help in calculating the systolic gradient between the aorta and the pulmonary artery.

37. With regard to management of the patent ductus arteriosus, which of the following statements is not true?
   a. Surgical mortality with repair is low.
   b. Percutaneous closure of the ductus may be preferred in some adults.
   c. Endocarditis prophylaxis is important.
   d. In adults, indomethacin helps in spontaneous closure.

38. Regarding coronary fistula, which one of the following statements is not true?
   a. Most are congenital.
   b. 90% of the fistulas terminate in the left side of heart.
   c. "Coronary steal" can occur, which rarely causes myocardial infarction.
   d. Location of the fistula, termination site, and degree of shunting determine the clinical presentation.

39. All of the following are true regarding coronary artery fistulas except:
   a. There is proximal enlargement of the involved coronary artery.
   b. There is continuous flow within the involved coronary artery.
   c. The affected coronary artery often can be traced to the site of termination.
   d. The termination site is mostly to the left side of the heart.

40. With regard to coronary artery fistula, which of the following statements is false?
   a. Small, clinically silent fistulas do not require closure.
   b. Severe pulmonary hypertension is rare even with large shunts.
   c. Coronary angiography is generally necessary for full evaluation of the fistula.
   d. When the fistula communicates with the left ventricle, the murmur is audible only in systole.

41. All of the following are true in tetralogy of Fallot except:
   a. There is a large VSD
   b. There is an overriding pulmonary artery.
   c. There is RV hypertrophy.
   d. There is pulmonic stenosis.

42. Regarding associated lesions seen with tetralogy of Fallot, which of the following is not true?
   a. There is atrial septal communication in 10% to 15% of patients.
   b. There is a right aortic arch in 25% of patients.
   c. There is anomalous origin of the right coronary artery in 10% of patients.
   d. There is absence of a pulmonary valve in some patients.

43. The common TEE findings of tetralogy of Fallot include all of the following except:
   a. A large malaligned VSD
   b. Anterior deviation of the conal septum
   c. Small pulmonary annulus
   d. Narrowed LV outflow tract

44. All the following statements are true regarding truncus arteriosus except:
   a. A large VSD is usually present.
   b. It is commonly due to improper septation of the primitive arterial trunk.
   c. Survival beyond 1 year of age is common without surgical intervention.
   d. Several types are described, depending on the origin of the pulmonary arteries from the main trunk.

45. The following are true regarding the semilunar valve in truncus arteriosus except:
   a. It has thickened valve leaflets.
   b. It may be stenotic or regurgitant.
   c. It is a bicuspid valve in 50% of patients.
   d. It can have more than three cusps.

46. With TEE, the differentiating findings of truncus arteriosus from tetralogy of Fallot include all of the following except:
   a. Commonly, the aortic valve in truncus is normal.
   b. There is no semblance of an RV outflow tract in truncus.
   c. In truncus, the main pulmonary artery or its branches arise from the ascending trunk.
   d. There is a right aortic arch in 30% of cases.

47. The following statements regarding tricuspid atresia are true except:
   a. It constitutes 1% to 3% of all cases of congenital heart disease.
   b. Fewer than 30% of patients survive beyond childhood even after palliative surgery.
   c. The right ventricle is variably underdeveloped.
   d. A VSD is often present.

48. TEE findings in tricuspid atresia include all of the following except:
    a. A thick band of fibromuscular tissue in place of tricuspid valve
    b. No evidence of flow across the valve
    c. Enlarged left ventricle
    d. Normal right atrium

49. Which of the following statements is not true regarding tricuspid atresia?
    a. LV systolic function may be impaired from volume overload.
    b. A large ASD is present.
    c. Progressive restriction of the VSD may occur.
    d. Adults with uncorrected tricuspid atresia are not susceptible to brain abscess.

50. Regarding management of Fontan procedure, which of the following statements is false?
    a. The Fontan procedure directs systemic venous return to the pulmonary artery.
    b. Patients with pulmonary vascular disease are amenable to surgical intervention.
    c. Ideal candidates for the Fontan procedure should have good LV function.
    d. Significant mitral insufficiency is a contraindication to the Fontan procedure.

51. In patients with a bicuspid aortic valve, which of the following is true?
    a. Coarctation of the aorta is present in 50%.
    b. The aortic root may be inherently abnormal.
    c. Poststenotic dilatation may be present.
    d. Options b and c.

52. Which of the following statements is true for patients with bicuspid aortic valves?
    a. LV hypertrophy or dilatation may be present.
    b. Stenosis of the abnormal valve commonly develops early in life.
    c. Infective endocarditis is not a common complication.
    d. The short-axis view of the aortic valve allows for a true estimate of the area of the valve.

53. Ebstein's anomaly is:
    a. An anomaly of the tricuspid and mitral valve
    b. A common congenital heart defect
    c. An anomaly of all three of the tricuspid leaflets
    d. An anomaly of the septal and posterior tricuspid leaflets only

54. In Ebstein's anomaly, the size of the atrialized right ventricle is best imaged:
    a. In a ME four-chamber view
    b. In an RV inflow-outflow view
    c. In a short-axis transgastric view, with manipulation of the probe toward the right
    d. In a bicaval view

55. An atrialized-to-functional right ventricle ratio greater than x is associated with poor RV systolic function when x equals:
    a. 0.3
    b. 0.8
    c. 0.5
    d. 0.6

56. Which of the following statements about subaortic stenosis is false?
    a. It is commonly associated with an ASD.
    b. It is caused most commonly by a discrete membranous type of obstruction.
    c. Aortic regurgitation may occur secondary to structural damage to the aortic valve.
    d. Options a and c.

57. The evaluation of supravalvular aortic stenosis includes:
    a. Defining the diameter of the ascending aorta
    b. Detection of associated pulmonary artery stenosis
    c. Doppler echocardiography to evaluate for aortic regurgitation
    d. Options a, b, and c
    e. Options a and b

58. Supravalvular aortic stenosis does not lead to:
    a. Dilated and tortuous coronary arteries
    b. LV hypertrophy
    c. Sudden death
    d. Poststenotic dilatation of the ascending aorta

59. Which of the following statements is false regarding ASDs?
    a. ASD accounts for about one-third of all cases of congenital heart disease.
    b. They occur in women two to three times as often as in men.
    c. They may go undetected until adulthood.
    d. Ostium secundum type ASD is associated with a cleft mitral valve leaflet.

60. Which of the following statements regarding PFO is true?
    a. Detection of a PFO in an elderly patient at the time of surgery is an indication for PFO closure.
    b. Paradoxical embolism in the presence of a PFO associated with an atrial septal aneurysm is an indication for PFO closure.

c. PFO occurs in about 10% of the general population.
d. Transthoracic echocardiography as compared with TEE allows for better definition of a PFO.

61. The best view for defining sinus venosus defects is:
    a. RV inflow-outflow view
    b. ME four-chamber view
    c. Bicaval view
    d. Upper esophageal five-chamber view

62. The eustachian valve is found in the:
    a. Right atrium
    b. Right ventricle
    c. Left atrium
    d. Superior vena cava

63. Saline contrast injection allows:
    a. Confirmation of right-to-left shunting
    b. Estimation of the size of the defect
    c. Detection of a negative contrast effect in the right atrium
    d. Options a and c

64. The recommended maneuver to use when performing a transesophageal contrast examination in a patient with a possible PFO is:
    a. Squatting
    b. Supine to standing
    c. Valsalva maneuver
    d. Intravenous phenylephrine

65. The congenital heart defect most often associated with Down syndrome is:
    a. Coarctation of the aorta
    b. Tricuspid atresia
    c. Tetralogy of Fallot
    d. Endocardial cushion defect

66. Cardiac chambers that are commonly enlarged in ASD include all of the following except:
    a. Left atrium
    b. Right atrium
    c. Right ventricle
    d. Main pulmonary artery

67. A complete atrioventricular canal defect is an ostium primum ASD with:
    a. Coarctation
    b. Cleft mitral valve, patent ductus arteriosus
    c. Canal-type VSD, tricuspid atresia
    d. Canal-type VSD, common atrioventricular valve

68. All of the following statements are true for patients with complete transposition of the great arteries except:
    a. Surgical management includes the Jatene procedure.
    b. Some communication at the level of the atria, ventricles, or great arteries is essential for survival.
    c. The right ventricle acts as the systemic ventricle.
    d. There is discordance at an atrioventricular level.

69. Which of the following statements is true regarding patients with DORV?
    a. The most common type of VSD found in DORV is a subaortic type.
    b. Coarctation of the aorta is not associated with this lesion.
    c. A Glenn shunt is used as a palliative procedure in these patients.
    d. A common feature of these lesions is complete mixing of the systemic and pulmonary venous blood at the atrial level.

70. Which of the following findings may alert the echocardiographer to the presence of anomalous pulmonary venous drainage?
    a. The presence of a sinus venosus ASD
    b. An enlarged right atrium
    c. An enlarged right ventricle
    d. An enlarged left atrium
    e. Options a, b, and c
    f. All of the above

Cardiac Masses

19

Jose Coddens

Echocardiography is a powerful tool in the differential diagnosis of cardiac masses. Although echocardiography cannot replace pathologic examination in obtaining an exact diagnosis, characteristic features of the ultrasound images can help to differentiate these masses. Combining clinical data such as sex, age, signs of an extracardiac primary tumor, and response to therapy (anticoagulation or antibiotics) with morphologic properties, such as location, attachment site, size, mobility, texture, and number of tumors, often produces an accurate diagnosis. A correct diagnosis is crucial in therapeutic decision making, but because pathology specimens usually are obtained only during surgical resection, it is important to recognize the typical indirect and direct echocardiographic features of the various tumors. Echocardiography is the technique of choice; further, because of its close proximity to the heart, transesophageal echocardiography (TEE) in general is superior to transthoracic echocardiography (TTE).

Some normal structures may mimic cardiac masses: the eustachian (inferior caval vein) valve, the thebesian (coronary sinus) valve, a Chiari network, crista terminalis, pectinate muscles, atrial chords, a moderator band, trabeculations, ventricular noncompaction, the apical form of hypertrophic cardiomyopathy, and the ridge between the left upper pulmonary vein and left atrial appendage may all be misinterpreted as cardiac masses (see Chapter 3).[1] With the development of three-dimensional real-time TEE, multislice imaging of cardiac masses is possible, allowing for better visualization of tumor morphology and location, which in turn may help to improve decision making during surgical resection.[2] Real-time three-dimensional TEE may become the technique of choice for noninvasive evaluation of tumor size.[3]

Cardiac tumors may be primary or secondary and malignant or benign. Of all primary cardiac tumors 75% are benign and 25% are malignant. Of the *benign tumors* in McAllister and Fenoglio's observations of 533 primary tumors,[4] 24.4% were myxomas, 8.4% were lipomas, 7.9% were papillary fibroelastomas, and 6.8% were rhabdomyomas. Fibromas, hemangiomas, teratomas, atrioventricular nodal mesotheliomas, granular cell tumors, pericardial cysts, and bronchogenic cysts accounted for fewer than 5% each. In the *malignant group*, angiosarcoma (7.3%) and rhabdomyosarcoma (4.9%) were the most frequent, whereas mesothelioma, fibrosarcoma, malignant lymphoma, extraskeletal osteosarcoma, neurogenic sarcoma, malignant teratoma, thymoma, leiomyosarcoma, liposarcoma, and synovial sarcoma were rare conditions. Secondary tumors are more frequently carcinomas than sarcomas, but all types of tumors may be found.

BENIGN PRIMARY CARDIAC TUMORS

Myxoma is the most frequent of the benign cardiac tumors, accounting for 30% to 50% and presenting with a female preponderance (Figure 19–1).[5] They occur most often in the third through sixth decades, and more than 90% are sporadic. Left atrial localization is most frequent (75%),[4,6,7] although 18% are found in the right atrium, 4% in the right ventricle, and another 4% in the left ventricle. Myxomas can present as multiple lesions in the left atrium and may be bilateral, whereas a ventricular location occurs more frequently in children. Myxomas typically are pedunculated, polypoid, friable tumors, sometimes possessing a smooth and rounded surface (Figure 19–2). They are commonly lobulated but can have a villous surface and typically are attached by a narrow stalk to the endocardial surface on the limbus of the left atrial side of the fossa ovalis. However, any other site of attachment is possible.[4] Myxomas contain a mucopolysaccharide myxoid matrix and have a nonhomogeneous appearance on TEE because of the presence of channels, cystic areas, hemorrhage, or calcifications (Figure 19–3). A familial form of myxoma has been described with an autosomal dominant transmission.[4] It occurs at a younger age, is seen more frequently in atypical locations, and is characterized by a higher recurrence rate after surgical resection.[8,9] In contrast, the familial form has a male preponderance and is more frequently bilateral. Routine screening of first-degree relatives of patients with myxoma is therefore indicated, especially in young patients or if multiple tumors are found. Patients with a familial history of myxoma also should be screened carefully for multiple or atypically located myxomas, and repeated postoperative echocardiographic examinations are necessary to detect recurrence.[10] This familial

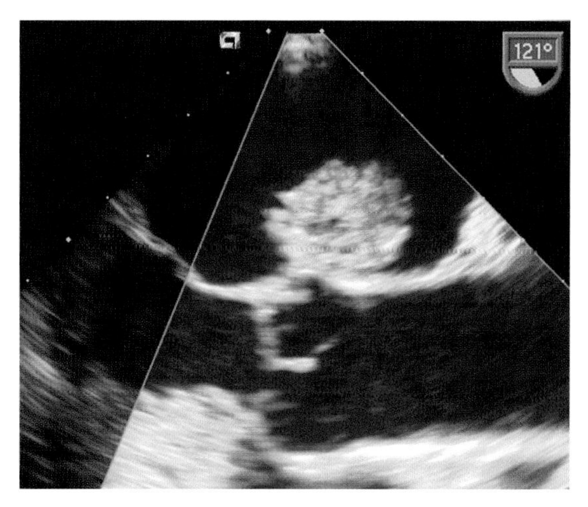

FIGURE 19–1. Long-axis view of the left ventricular outflow tract. Tissue Doppler energy mode is activated. A well-delineated spherical left atrial myxoma is attached to the anterior wall of the left atrium dorsal of the ascending aorta.

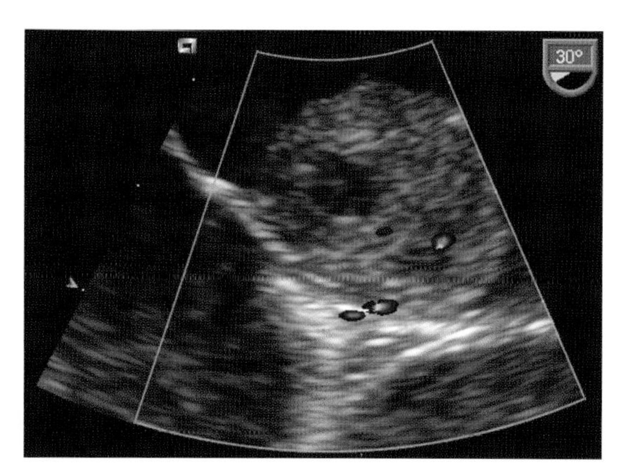

FIGURE 19–3. High-resolution picture of the same myxoma shown in Figure 19–1. Color-flow mapping is activated. The heterogeneous appearance with translucent zones is clearly visible. Tiny blood vessels are detected with color Doppler echocardiography.

variety may be part of a syndrome (Carney's complex, NAME syndrome, or LAMB syndrome).[11]

A typical triad of symptoms includes embolization, obstruction, and constitutional symptoms such as dyspnea, position-related palpitations, syncope, congestive heart failure, and even sudden death. Emboli may cause neurologic deficit or coronary events, but any systemic vessel may be involved. Obstructive symptoms, detected as turbulence on color-flow Doppler, can present with any intracavitary tumor and may involve the mitral or tricuspid valve (atrial myxomas), pulmonic or aortic valve (ventricular myxoma), or venous inflow to the atria.[12,13] If the mitral or tricuspid valve is obstructed, a typical tumor "plop" can be heard after the second heart sound on auscultation.

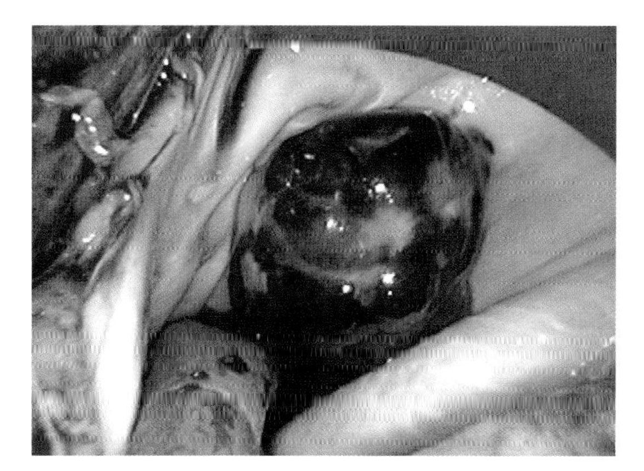

FIGURE 19–2. Intraoperative view of the same left atrial myxoma shown in Figure 19–1. The smooth surface and spherical shape are nicely demonstrated.

Except for detecting ventricular locations, TEE is superior to TTE. It allows for detailed description of tumor morphology and attachment, and for detection of multiple tumors. A bilateral dumbbell shape myxoma may pass through the foramen ovale and may be fixed to the margin of this foramen.[14] Right atrial myxomas tend to be more solid, have wider attachments, and may be fixed to the inferior rim of the fossa ovalis, the tricuspid valve, or the eustachian valve. Obstruction of the tricuspid valve or caval veins is possible.[15,16] Left ventricular myxomas are rare, occur at younger age, and are three times more frequent in women than in men. In these cases, cerebral embolism is frequent and subaortic or aortic obstruction is possible. Right ventricular myxomas also are infrequent and may cause pulmonary embolism and outflow obstruction.

Rhabdomyoma is the most frequent cardiac tumor in infants and children and is associated with tuberous sclerosis.[17,18] Of these, three fourths occur before the age of 1 year. It is usually multiple and frequently involves the right ventricular myocardium. Occasionally, it may project into the ventricular cavity and even move freely as a pedunculated tumor.[19] It can cause obstruction of the right ventricular outflow tract, and diagnosis by fetal echocardiography before birth is possible. Rhabdomyomas may regress spontaneously after birth.

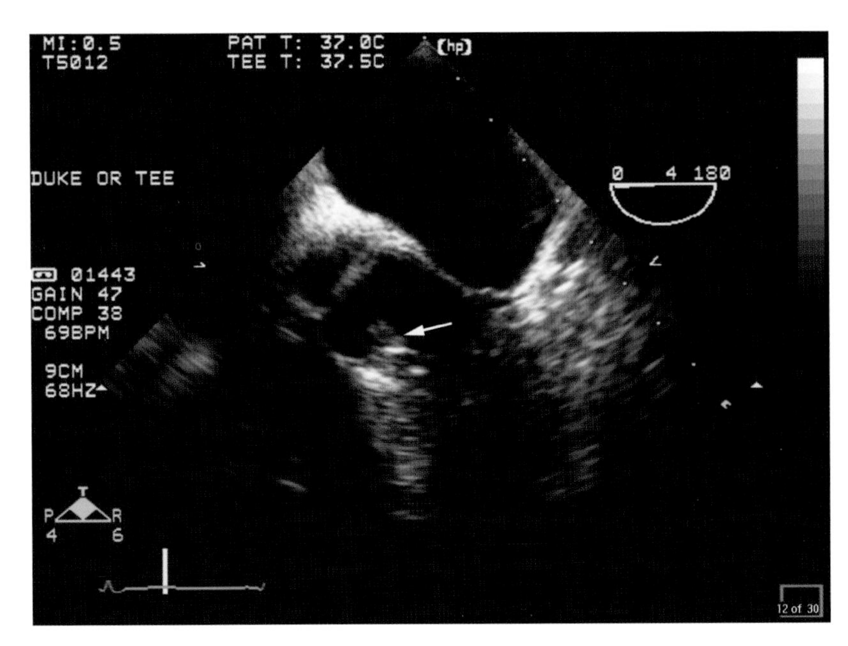

FIGURE 19–4. A highly mobile papillary fibroelastoma *(arrow)* with a short pedicle and multiple fronds is seen in the left ventricular outflow tract.

Fibromas are ventricular intramural tumors that are frequently calcified. They occur more frequently in infants and children.[20]

Papillary fibroelastomas are small (usually <1 cm), homogeneous, mobile tumors, often with a stalk, originating from the cardiac valves or, less frequently, from the ventricular endocardium. Papillary fibroelastomas originate from the atrial side of the atrioventricular valves or from either side of the semilunar valves and frequently are a coincidental finding. The most common locations are on the aortic valve cusps (44.5%) and mitral valve leaflets (36.4%). Attachment to the ventricular septum or close to the left ventricular outflow tract or to the subvalvular mitral apparatus has been described (Figure 19–4). They can cause angina and infarction by coronary ostial occlusion or embolism,[21,22] but systemic embolism is also possible so surgical resection is advocated. They occur most commonly in patients older than 50 years but rarely occur on the right side of the heart.[17,23,24] Multiple fibroelastomas occur in 6.8% to 7.5% of cases.[25] Fibroelastomas have a short pedicle with multiple papillary fronds, and have to be differentiated from Lambl excrescences, which are degenerative in origin and arise from the ventricular side of the semilunar valves along the coaptation line (Figure 19–5).[17] The exact histogenesis of papillary fibroelastoma is uncertain, and although most investigators classify it as a neoplasm, it may represent exuberant organization of thrombi, similar to Lambl excrescences.[25] Colocalization of Lambl excrescences and fibroelastomas suggest a common origin. A virus-induced tumor hypothesis also has been proposed. Differential diagnosis from endocarditis and vegetations may be difficult and depends on the clinical presentation of the patient. However, in contrast to endocarditis, valvular dysfunction (insufficiency) is uncommon.

Lipomas affect the entire heart and pericardium and can be massive.[26] They may produce a pericardial effusion. Intramyocardial lipomas are well encapsulated and small.[17] Occasionally, a lipoma may arise from the mitral or tricuspid valve, and differential diagnosis with a myxoma becomes necessary.[27]

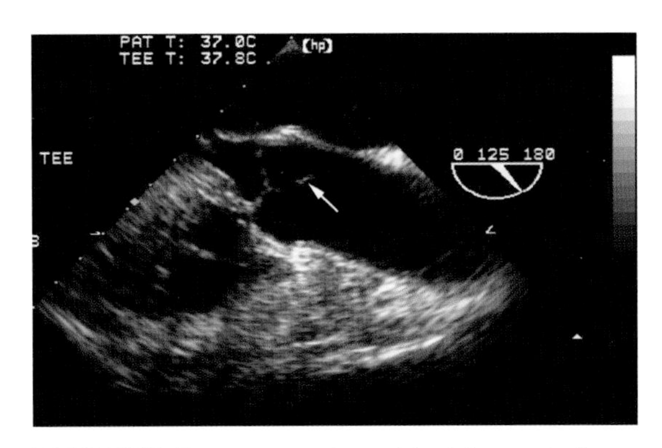

FIGURE 19–5. Long-axis view of the left ventricular outflow tract and ascending aorta showing Lambl excrescences *(arrow)*.

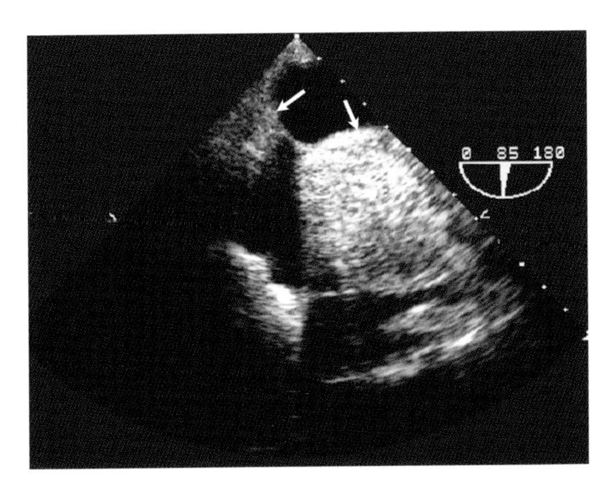

FIGURE 19–6. Lipomatous infiltration of the interatrial septum is visible on the bicaval view as a septum with a "dumbbell" shape.

Lipomatous hypertrophy of the interatrial septum is a form of hyperplasia of adipose tissue (Figure 19–6). It presents as atrial septal thickening with a bilobed or "dumbbell" appearance due to sparing of the fossa ovalis.

MALIGNANT PRIMARY CARDIAC TUMORS

Most malignant primary cardiac tumors are sarcomas, most frequently *angiosarcomas* originating in the right atrium or pericardium.[28,29] They demonstrate a male preponderance. Angiosarcomas often (25%) grow partially intracavitary and may cause caval or valvular obstruction.[30] Cardiac rupture,[6] right heart failure, and pericardial tamponade have been described.

Rhabdomyosarcoma is the second most frequent primary cardiac sarcoma. It is also more frequent in males, has no predilection for any cardiac chamber, is often multiple, and frequently causes obstruction of at least one valve.[31]

Liposarcoma, fibrosarcoma, primary malignant lymphoma, and sarcomas of other cell lines are rare. Any of these also can cause obstruction or result in peripheral embolism.

TUMORS OF THE PERICARDIUM

Pericardial cysts are the most frequent tumors of the pericardium. They are benign, occur most often in the third and fourth decades of life, and are as frequent in men as in women. They appear as fluid-filled, well-delineated, more or less rounded structures. A frequent location is the right costophrenic angle,[32] and rare cases of cardiac-chamber compression have been described.[33]

Echinococcus cysts, caused by a parasite endemic to Greece and Turkey, can involve the left ventricular free wall, the interventricular septum, the right ventricle, and the pericardium. They are usually septated and can calcify.

Blood cysts are found on the closure lines of the valvular endocardium. They are well-circumscribed masses with thin walls and echolucent core. They are presumed to be of congenital origin.[1] *Teratomas* occur most frequently in infants and children, with a female preponderance.[17] They are benign tumors with an extracardiac but intrapericardial location in most cases, and are noted for containing hair, teeth, or other epidermal structures. Blood supply for these tumors arises from the aortic root or pulmonary artery via vasa vasorum. Recurrent, nonbloody pericardial effusion in a child is highly suggestive of pericardial teratoma.

Mesotheliomas are the third most frequent malignant primary tumors of the heart and pericardium.[4] The highest incidence occurs in the third to fifth decades of life, with men being affected twice as often as women. Their symptomatology is similar to those of pericarditis, constrictive pericardial disease, and caval obstruction.

PRIMARY TUMORS OF THE AORTA

Aortic tumors are rare and most frequently are malignant sarcomas. These may involve any segment of the aorta and cause symptoms similar to those of aortic dissection and atherosclerotic occlusive disease. Peripheral metastases are common.

SECONDARY TUMORS OF THE HEART

Metastases may involve the heart, the pericardium, myocardium, endocardium, valves, and coronary arteries. Direct invasion through caval or pulmonary veins is also possible. They occur more frequently in people older than 50 years and affect men and women with similar frequency. Metastatic carcinomas are more frequent than sarcomas, but all types of primary tumors may metastasize to the heart, and metastases are, most often, multiple. Malignant melanoma has a tendency to spread to the heart in more than 50% of cases,[33] but cardiac metastases most frequently originate from the more common bronchogenic and breast carcinomas (lung > breast).[6] If the pericardium is involved, they can cause pericardial fluid accumulation and symptoms of pericarditis or tamponade with typical diastolic collapse of the right atrium and ventricle, inferior caval vein distention, and blunting of the normal inspiratory response. Direct myocardial involvement can result in

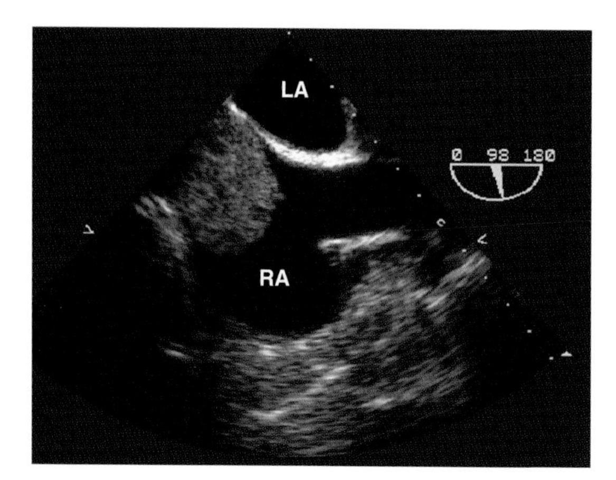

FIGURE 19–7. Bicaval view demonstrating a renal cell carcinoma extending through the inferior vena cava into the right atrium. (LA, left atrium; RA, right atrium.)

extrasystolic beats, conduction disturbances, and arrhythmias resistant to therapy.[34] If coronary arteries are affected, myocardial ischemia or infarction may result. There also may be external compression, tumor embolization, concomitant coronary atherosclerosis, or fibrosis due to radiation therapy.[35] Renal cell carcinoma, hepatocellular carcinoma, and uterine leiomyomatosis may extend along the inferior caval vein toward the right atrium and cause venous inflow and even valvular obstruction (Figure 19–7).

Leukemic myocardial infiltration may cause congestive heart failure, mitral valve dysfunction, myocardial rupture, or pericardial effusion and tamponade.[6,35]

Malignant lymphomas frequently involve the heart but this is rarely discovered before death. Hodgkin's and non-Hodgkin's lymphomas can metastasize to the heart through the blood or lymph, or they can invade the heart directly from another intrathoracic location. In most cases, the epicardium and pericardium are affected.

Carcinoid tumors are never primary cardiac tumors and only rarely metastasize to the heart. Most frequently, the tumor resides in the gastrointestinal tract (ileum) and causes carcinoid disease of the heart by the release of products such as serotonin, 5-hydroxytryptamine, and bradykinin into the venous blood.[36-39] Only patients with liver metastases develop cardiac lesions. The right heart is affected more commonly than the left heart, but bronchial carcinoid tumors are more likely to result in carcinoid disease of the left heart. The presence of an interatrial connection or massive right heart involvement also may cause left heart contamination. Carcinoid disease produces deposits on pulmonary and tricuspid valves and on right atrial and ventricular endocardia. Regurgitation and stenosis of pulmonary and tricuspid valves may arise, and the endocardial involvement causes a restrictive myopathy. Echocardiography typically shows right ventricular volume overload and pulmonary and tricuspid abnormalities. The tricuspid valve appears thickened, retracted, and fixed in a semi-open position with diastolic doming if stenosis is predominant, but most often tricuspid regurgitation is present. Pulmonary valve abnormalities occur in more than 50% of patients with predominant stenosis. Mitral involvement is rare, but, if the mitral valve is affected, insufficiency and stenosis are also possible.

CARDIAC THROMBI

Intracardiac thrombi may mimic cardiac tumors. Left atrial thrombi most often appear in the left atrial appendage in patients with atrial fibrillation, rheumatic mitral stenosis, left atrial enlargement, prosthetic mitral valve disease, and low cardiac output. Right atrial thrombi can obstruct the tricuspid valve or cause pulmonary embolism or paradoxical embolism via a patent foramen ovale (PFO). Pacemaker wires, central venous catheters, or pulmonary artery catheters increase the risk for thrombus formation. TEE is superior to TTE to describe thrombus size, mobility, attachment site, and involvement of superior or inferior caval veins; to detect entrapment by eustachian valve (Figure 19–8) or Chiari network; to search for extension to the left atrium via a patent

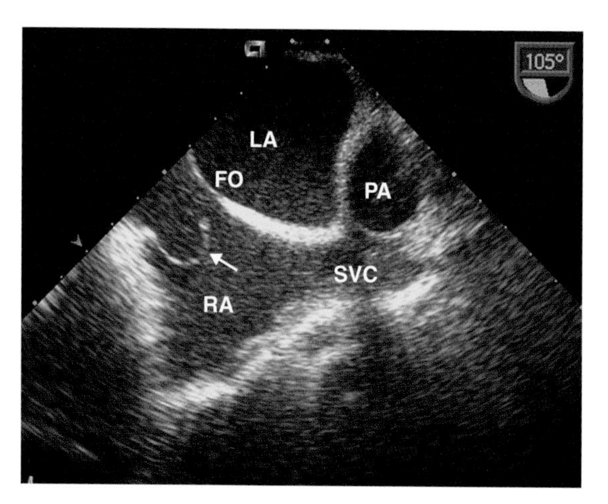

FIGURE 19–8. Longitudinal view through the right atrium, left atrium, and interatrial septum. (*Arrow*, eustachian valve with free edge and attached to the atrial opening of the inferior vena cava; FO, fossa ovalis of interatrial septum; LA, left atrium; PA, transverse section through right main pulmonary artery; RA, right atrium; SVC, superior vena cava.)

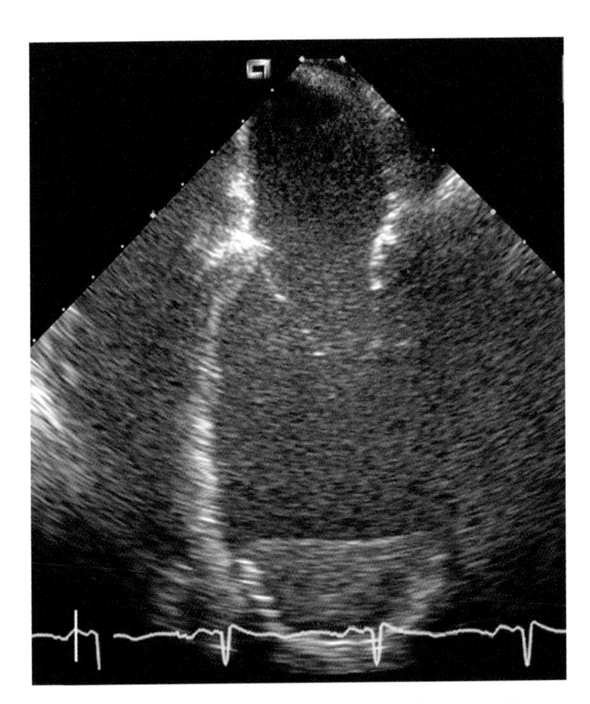

FIGURE 19–9. Four-chamber view. In the apex of the left ventricle, a large, homogeneous, mural thrombus with smooth surface is shown. Note left ventricular dilatation.

foramen ovale, extension to the right ventricle, or the pulmonary artery; and to differentiate them from atrial myxoma.[40-44] Thrombi typically appear as coiled, mobile, serpiginous masses with no clear point of attachment, but sometimes present as a more sessile mass. They can be fixed to the lateral atrial wall, inferior or superior vena cava, interatrial septum, eustachian valve, or Chiari network. Thrombolytic or anticoagulant therapy is indicated when intracardiac thrombi are detected. Disappearance of these masses with therapy confirms the diagnosis and illustrates the need for repeated echocardiographic examination. TEE examination before cardioversion for atrial fibrillation is essential to prevent thromboembolic complications.

Ventricular thrombi occur in patients with large myocardial infarction, ventricular aneurysm, and dilated cardiomyopathy, or in patients with the hypereosinophilic syndrome. Most thrombi reside in the apex of the left ventricle and may be isolated, multiple, laminar, spherical, pedunculated and mobile, or filamentous with a fixed base (Figures 19–9 and 19–10). They are often homogeneous and smooth but may be cavitary and heterogeneous (Figure 19–11). Mobile thrombi with shaggy, irregular borders in patients with ventricular aneurysm or dilated cardiomyopathy have been

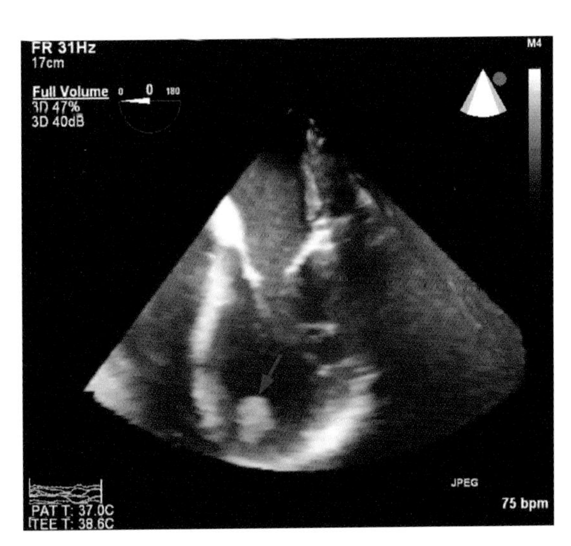

FIGURE 19–10. Three-dimensional image of a thrombus *(arrow)* in the apex of the left ventricle.

associated with an increased risk for embolization. The use of contrast echocardiography has been advocated recently as a technique for successful differentiation between a thrombus and a cardiac mass. In contradistinction to the filling defect seen with a thrombus, significant uptake of contrast agent into the mass confirms the diagnosis of a cardiac tumor. TTE or epicardial echocardiography may be superior to TEE for identification of left ventricular apical thrombi.[45] Some authors describe an entity called "calcified amorphous

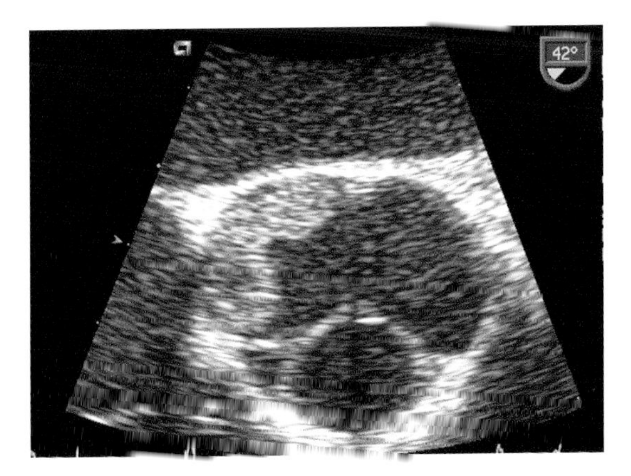

FIGURE 19–11. Short axis view through the aortic valve showing a bilobulated mural thrombus attached to the wall of the noncoronary sinus of Valsalva. The thrombus has a heterogeneous texture.

tumor of the heart" (CAT). CATs are poorly characterized nonneoplastic, endocardially based intracavitary cardiac masses.[46]

ATRIAL SEPTAL ANEURYSMS

An atrial septal aneurysm is a rare condition (0.22% to 1% of adults) defined as an aneurysmal bulging of the interatrial septum, most often at the level of the fossa ovalis. The septum is described as aneurysmal if it has a base wider than 15 mm and the phasic left-to-right excursion during the cardiac cycle is longer than 15 mm (Figure 19–12). Aneurysmal excursion can be best recorded on an M-mode echocardiogram on the bicaval view with TEE. This lesion is associated with atrial septal defects (often multiple) and commonly a patent foramen ovale, and with mitral valve prolapse.[47-50] TEE is most sensitive to detect, describe, and differentiate this abnormality. Atrial septal aneurysm is not a neoplastic disease but causes its morbidity and mortality by thromboembolic mechanisms. Spontaneous contrast and thrombus entrapment have been described in the aneurysmal pocket and may necessitate differentiation from a cardiac tumor. The presence of atrial septal aneurysm has been associated with a PFO and higher incidences of cryptogenic[51] and recurrent[52] strokes.

ENDOCARDITIS

Endocarditis also may result in cardiac masses. Vegetations differ from thrombi and tumors in several morphologic characteristics. Vegetations occur often in patients with normal ventricular function; they move in phase with valve motion because they are attached to valvular structures; and they are associated with valvular regurgitation, flail leaflets, ring abscesses, sinus of Valsalva aneurysms, paravalvular leaks, and clinical sepsis. Vegetations most frequently originate from the atrial side of the atrioventricular valves (Figure 19–13) and from the ventricular side of the aortic or pulmonic valve. They can be mobile, irregularly shaped, and heterogeneous, and are prone to embolization. For the diagnosis and fine description of endocarditis, TEE is superior to TTE. TEE is also very accurate in detecting complications of endocarditis and for monitoring therapy. Vegetations can change in size or, ideally, disappear after weeks to months of antibiotic therapy; thus, repeated echocardiography is essential.

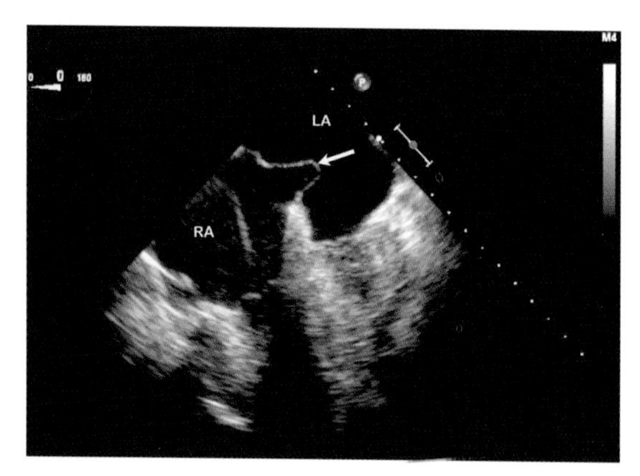

FIGURE 19–12. Atrial septal aneurysm bulging into the left atrium.

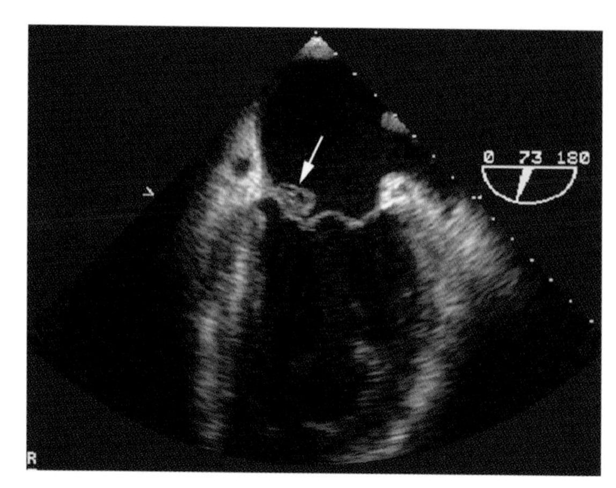

FIGURE 19–13. Vegetation on the atrial side of the mitral valve.

REFERENCES

1. Peters PJ, Reinhardt S. The echocardiographic evaluation of intracardiac masses: a review. *J Am Soc Echocardiogr.* 2006;19(2):230-240.
2. Muller S, Feuchtner G, Bonatti J, et al. Value of transesophageal 3D echocardiography as an adjunct to conventional 2D imaging in preoperative evaluation of cardiac masses. *Echocardiography.* 2008;25(6):624-631.
3. Asch FM, Bieganski SP, Panza JA, Weissman NJ. Real-time 3-dimensional echocardiography evaluation of intracardiac masses. *Echocardiography.* 2006;23(3):218-224.
4. McAllister HA, Fenoglio JJ. Tumors of the cardiovascular system. In: Firminger HI, ed. *Atlas of Tumor Pathology.* 2nd Series, fascicle 15. Washington, DC: Armed Forces Institute of Pathology; 1978:46-52.
5. Colucci WS, Braunwald E. Primary tumors of the heart. In: Braunwald E, ed. *Heart Disease: A Textbook of Cardiovascular Medicine.* 4th ed. Philadelphia: W.B. Saunders Co; 1992:1451.
6. McAllister HA Jr, Hall RJ, Cooley DA. Tumors of the heart and pericardium. *Curr Probl Cardiol.* 1999;24(2):57-116.
7. Burke A, Virmani R. Tumors of the heart and great vessels. In: Rosai J, Sobin LH, eds. *Atlas of Tumor Pathology.* 3rd Series, fascicle 16. Washington, DC: Armed Forces Institute of Pathology; 1996:231.

8. Reynen K. Cardiac myxomas. *N Engl J Med.* 1995;333(24):1610-1617.
9. Singh SD, Lansing AM. Familial cardiac myxoma—a comprehensive review of reported cases. *J Ky Med Assoc.* 1996;94(3):96-104.
10. McCarthy PM, Piehler JM, Schaff HV, et al. The significance of multiple, recurrent, and "complex" cardiac myxomas. *J Thorac Cardiovasc Surg.* 1986;91(3):389-396.
11. Mahilmaran A, Seshadri M, Nayar PG, Sudarsana G, Abraham KA. Familial cardiac myxoma: Carney's complex. *Tex Heart Inst J.* 2003;30(1):80-82.
12. Peters MN, Hall RJ, Cooley DA, Leachman RD, Garcia E. The clinical syndrome of atrial myxoma. *JAMA.* 1974;230(5):695-701.
13. Obeid AI, Marvasti M, Parker F, Rosenberg J. Comparison of transthoracic and transesophageal echocardiography in diagnosis of left atrial myxoma. *Am J Cardiol.* 1989;63(13):1006-1008.
14. Peachell JL, Mullen JC, Bentley MJ, Taylor DA. Biatrial myxoma: a rare cardiac tumor. *Ann Thorac Surg.* 1998;65(6):1768-1769.
15. Kuroda H, Nitta K, Ashida Y, Hara Y, Ishiguro S, Mori T. Right atrial myxoma originating from the tricuspid valve. *J Thorac Cardiovasc Surg.* 1995;109(6):1249-1250.
16. Teoh KH, Mulji A, Tomlinson CW, Lobo FV. Right atrial myxoma originating from the eustachian valve. *Can J Cardiol.* 1993;9(5):441-443.
17. McAllister HA Jr. Primary tumors and cysts of the heart and pericardium. *Curr Probl Cardiol.* 1979;4(2):1-51.
18. Braunwald E, Zipes DP, Libby P. *Heart Disease: A Textbook of Cardiovascular Medicine.* 6th ed. Philadelphia: WB Saunders Co; 2001.
19. Howanitz EP, Teske DW, Qualman SJ, Finck S, Kilman JW. Pedunculated left ventricular rhabdomyoma. *Ann Thorac Surg.* 1986;41(4):443-445.
20. Busch U, Kampmann C, Meyer R, Sandring KH, Hausdorf G, Konertz W. Removal of a giant cardiac fibroma from a 4-year-old child. *Tex Heart Inst J.* 1995;22(3):261-264.
21. Lee CC, Celik C, Lajos TZ. Excision of papillary fibroelastoma arising from the septal leaflet of the tricuspid valve. *J Card Surg.* 1995;10(5):589-591.
22. Paelinck B, Vermeersch P, Kockx M. Calcified papillary fibroelastoma of the tricuspid valve. *Acta Cardiol.* 1998;53(3):165-167.
23. Eckstein FS, Schafers HJ, Grote J, Mugge A, Borst HG. Papillary fibroelastoma of the aortic valve presenting with myocardial infarction. *Ann Thorac Surg.* 1995;60(1):206-208.
24. Prahlow JA, Barnard JJ. Sudden death due to obstruction of coronary artery ostium by aortic valve papillary fibroelastoma. *Am J Forensic Med Pathol.* 1998;19(2):162-165.
25. Neuman Y, Luthringer DJ, Kobal S, Miyamoto T, Trento A, Siegel RJ. Multiple aortic valve papillary fibroelastoma: an unusual presentation of a rare tumor. *J Am Soc Echocardiogr.* 2003;16(5):494-496.
26. Sankar NM, Thiruchelvam T, Thirunavukkarasu K, Pang K, Hanna WM. Symptomatic lipoma in the right atrial free wall. A case report. *Tex Heart Inst J.* 1998;25(2):152-154.
27. Barberger-Gateau P, Paquet M, Desaulniers D, Chenard J. Fibrolipoma of the mitral valve in a child. Clinical and echocardiographic features. *Circulation.* 1978;58(5):955-958.
28. Raaf HN, Raaf JH. Sarcomas related to the heart and vasculature. *Semin Surg Oncol.* 1994;10(5):374-382.
29. Adachi K, Tanaka H, Toshima H, Morimatsu M. Right atrial angiosarcoma diagnosed by cardiac biopsy. *Am Heart J.* 1988;115(2):482-485.
30. Uchita S, Hata T, Tsushima Y, Matsumoto M, Hina K, Moritani T. Primary cardiac angiosarcoma with superior vena caval syndrome: review of surgical resection and interventional management of venous inflow obstruction. *Can J Cardiol.* 1998;14(10):1283-1285.
31. Schmaltz AA, Apitz J. Primary rhabdomyosarcoma of the heart. *Pediatr Cardiol.* 1982;2(1):73-75.
32. Stoller JK, Shaw C, Matthay RA. Enlarging, atypically located pericardial cyst. Recent experience and literature review. *Chest.* 1986;89(3):402-406.
33. Ng AF, Olak J. Pericardial cyst causing right ventricular outflow tract obstruction. *Ann Thorac Surg.* 1997;63(4):1147-1148.
34. Sheldon R, Isaac D. Metastatic melanoma to the heart presenting with ventricular tachycardia. *Chest.* 1991;99(5):1296-1298.
35. Terry LN Jr, Kligerman MM. Pericardial and myocardial involvement by lymphomas and leukemias. The role of radiotherapy. *Cancer.* 1970;25(5):1003-1008.
36. Schiller VL, Fishbein MC, Siegel RJ. Unusual cardiac involvement in carcinoid syndrome. *Am Heart J.* 1986;112(6):1322-1323.
37. Le Metayer P, Constans J, Bernard N, et al. Carcinoid heart disease: two cases of left heart involvement diagnosed by transthoracic and transoesophageal echocardiography. *Eur Heart J.* 1993;14(12):1721-1723.
38. Pellikka PA, Tajik AJ, Khandheria BK, et al. Carcinoid heart disease. Clinical and echocardiographic spectrum in 74 patients. *Circulation.* 1993;87(4):1188-1196.
39. Strickman NE, Hall RJ. Carcinoid heart disease. In: Kapoor AS, Reynolds RD, eds. *Cancer and the Heart.* New York: Springer-Verlag; 1986:135.
40. Martens PR, Driessen JJ, Vandekerckhove Y, Muyldermans L. Transesophageal echocardiographic detection of a right atrial thrombus around a pulmonary artery catheter. *Anesth Analg.* 1992;75(5):847-849.
41. Mugge A, Daniel WG, Haverich A, Lichtlen PR. Diagnosis of noninfective cardiac mass lesions by two-dimensional echocardiography. Comparison of the transthoracic and transesophageal approaches. *Circulation.* 1991;83(1):70-78.
42. Holman WL, Coghlan CH, Dodson MR, Balal R, Nanda NC. Removal of massive right atrial thrombus guided by transesophageal echocardiography. *Ann Thorac Surg.* 1991;52(2):313-315.
43. Pasierski TJ, Alton ME, Van Fossen DB, Pearson AC. Right atrial mobile thrombus: improved visualization by transesophageal echocardiography. *Am Heart J.* 1992;123(3):802-803.
44. Farah MG, Cater GN. Tranesophageal echocardiographic diagnosis and management of right atrial thrombi. [illegible]
45. Otto CM. Echocardiographic evaluation of cardiac masses and potential cardiac "source of embolus". In: Otto CM, ed. *Textbook of Clinical Echocardiography.* Philadelphia: WB Saunders Co; 2000:351-371.

46. Reynolds C, Tazelaar HD, Edwards WD. Calcified amorphous tumor of the heart (cardiac CAT). *Hum Pathol.* 1997;28(5):601-606.
47. Hanley PC, Tajik AJ, Hynes JK, et al. Diagnosis and classification of atrial septal aneurysm by two-dimensional echocardiography: report of 80 consecutive cases. *J Am Coll Cardiol.* 1985;6(6):1370-1382.
48. Roberts WC. Aneurysm (redundancy) of the atrial septum (fossa ovale membrane) and prolapse (redundancy) of the mitral valve. *Am J Cardiol.* 1984;54(8):1153-1154.
49. Iliceto S, Papa A, Sorino M, Rizzon P. Combined atrial septal aneurysm and mitral valve prolapse: detection by two-dimensional echocardiography. *Am J Cardiol.* 1984;54(8):1151-1153.
50. Rahko PS, Xu QB. Increased prevalence of atrial septal aneurysm in mitral valve prolapse. *Am J Cardiol.* 1990;66(2):235-237.
51. Cabanes L, Mas JL, Cohen A, et al. Atrial septal aneurysm and patent foramen ovale as risk factors for cryptogenic stroke in patients less than 55 years of age. A study using transesophageal echocardiography. *Stroke.* 1993;24(12):1865-1873.
52. Mas JL, Arquizan C, Lamy C, et al. Recurrent cerebrovascular events associated with patent foramen ovale, atrial septal aneurysm, or both. *N Engl J Med.* 2001;345(24):1740-1746.

REVIEW QUESTIONS

Select the *one* best answer for each of the following questions.

1. Which of the following statements is correct regarding the use of TEE for the diagnosis of cardiac tumors?
   a. It is unnecessary for prognostic reasons.
   b. It can be obtained with a high grade of certainty with TEE.
   c. It has an accuracy similar to that of pathologic examination.
   d. It is a necessary part of the follow-up after starting the proper therapy.

2. Which of the following may help in identifying the type of tumor with TEE?
   a. Age and sex
   b. A history of nicotine abuse
   c. A history of alcohol abuse
   d. Hemoptysis
   e. All of the above

3. Morphologic properties that may be helpful in the TEE diagnosis of cardiac tumors include:
   a. Tumor location
   b. Attachment site
   c. Tumor size
   d. Mobility
   e. All of the above

4. Other morphologic properties that may be helpful in TEE diagnosis of cardiac tumors include:
   a. Tumor disappearance with anticoagulant or antibiotic therapy
   b. The texture of the tumor
   c. The number of tumors
   d. Familial occurrence
   e. All of the above

5. Which of the following statements is correct regarding primary benign cardiac tumors?
   a. Myxomas are most frequent, accounting for more than 60%.
   b. Lipomas make up some 30% of benign cardiac tumors.
   c. Rhabdomyomas are the third most frequent.
   d. Eight percent are papillary fibroelastomas.

6. Which of the following statements is correct regarding primary benign cardiac tumors?
   a. Lipomas are more frequent than myxomas.
   b. Papillary fibroelastomas are more frequent than lipomas.
   c. Rhabdomyomas are more frequent than fibroelastomas.
   d. Other tumors such as fibromas, hemangiomas, and teratomas each account for less than 5%.

7. Which of the following statements is correct regarding primary malignant cardiac tumors?
   a. Angiosarcoma is the most frequent.
   b. Malignant lymphoma accounts for 7%.
   c. Rhabdomyosarcoma accounts for 20%.
   d. Atrioventricular nodal mesotheliomas account for less than 5%.

8. Which of the following statements best describes secondary or metastatic tumors?
   a. Most often they are sarcomas.
   b. Most often they are lymphomas.
   c. They never affect the pericardium.
   d. They may be of any type of tumor.

9. Which of the following best describes cardiac myxoma?
   a. It accounts for more than 60% of primary benign cardiac tumors.
   b. It has a male preponderance.
   c. It occurs most often in the third through sixth decades of life.
   d. It occurs sporadically half the time.

10. Which of the following statements is correct regarding familial cardiac myxoma?
    a. It occurs at older ages.
    b. It is never multiple.

c. It occurs more frequently in atypical locations.
d. It is linked to multiple endocrine neoplasia syndrome.

11. Which of the following statements best describes the location of classical myxoma?
 a. It is most often in the left atrium.
 b. It is in the right atrium in 30% of cases.
 c. It is right ventricular in 10%.
 d. It is left ventricular in 10% of cases.
 e. All of the above statements are correct.

12. Correct statements regarding the typical morphologic characteristics of cardiac myxomas include:
 a. The absence of calcifications
 b. A homogeneous texture
 c. A broad attachment to the interatrial septum
 d. A polypoid form

13. All the following statements concerning the morphologic properties of cardiac myxomas are correct EXCEPT:
 a. They are pedunculated.
 b. They are friable.
 c. They are lobulated.
 d. They have a ragged, irregular surface.

14. Which of the following statements regarding patients with familial myxoma is correct?
 a. They may have a variety of features called syndrome myxoma or Carney syndrome.
 b. They may have spotty pigmentation, pigmented nevi, or both.
 c. They may have endocrine hyperactivity such as Cushing syndrome.
 d. They may have multiple cerebral fusiform aneurysms.
 e. All of the above statements are correct.

15. Syndromes associated with atrial myxomas include:
 a. NAME syndrome
 b. Noonan syndrome
 c. Wermer syndrome (MEN type 1)
 d. Osler-Weber-Rendu syndrome
 e. All of the above

16. Correct statements regarding cardiac myxomas include:
 a. They are never found in the left atrial appendage.
 b. They never contain channels.
 c. They do not show areas of hemorrhage.
 d. They can have a heterogeneous appearance caused by cystic areas

17. Which of the following statements is correct regarding multiple myxomas?
 a. They do not occur in the left atrium.
 b. They are never bilateral.
 c. They are never found simultaneously in the atrium and ventricle.
 d. They occur more frequently in children.

18. Which of the following statements is correct regarding familial myxomas?
 a. They may have an autosomal dominant transmission.
 b. They have a female preponderance.
 c. They are seldom bilateral.
 d. They occur at older age.

19. Which of the following statements is correct regarding familial myxomas?
 a. They are characterized by a low recurrence rate.
 b. A careful search for multiple locations is not important.
 c. If multiple myxomas are found in a patient, screening of first-degree relatives is indicated.
 d. Myxomas found in young patients are more often of familial origin.

20. Typical clinical symptoms of myxoma include:
 a. Embolization
 b. Signs of pulmonary hypertension
 c. Fever
 d. Signs of pericarditis

21. Embolic symptoms of myxoma may cause:
 a. Upper limb ischemia
 b. Acute coronary events
 c. Neurologic deficit
 d. Lower limb ischemia
 e. All of the above

22. Correct features of LAMB syndrome include:
 a. Lentigines, atrial myxoma, and blue nevi
 b. Lung AVMs, muscle dystrophy, and blue nevi
 c. Lentigines, atrial myxoma, blurred vision
 d. None of the above

23. All the following statement regarding obstruction by cardiac tumors are correct EXCEPT:
 a. It can involve the mitral or tricuspid valve.
 b. It can involve the aortic or pulmonic valve.
 c. It can involve the caval or pulmonary veins.
 d. It can cause a typical tumor "plop" after the first heart sound on auscultation if the atrioventricular valves are involved.

24. Constitutional symptoms related to cardiac myxomas include:
    a. Arterial desaturation in the upright position
    b. Dyspnea
    c. Angina pectoris
    d. Position-related palpitations
    e. All of the above

25. Which of the following conditions is associated with cardiac myxomas?
    a. Ischemic cardiomyopathy
    b. Dressler syndrome
    c. Sudden death
    d. Pleurodynia

26. Which of the following statements is true regarding the utility of intravenous ultrasound contrast agents in the evaluation of cardiac masses?
    a. Contrast agents should be administered intravenously at a declining rate.
    b. Malignancies appear hypoenhanced.
    c. Myxomas appear hyperenhanced.
    d. The use of contrast agents can potentially avoid unnecessary diagnostic surgery or inappropriate anticoagulation.

27. Compared with left atrial myxomas, right atrial myxomas:
    a. Have a narrow attachment
    b. Are the most common site of attachment is the posterior atrial wall
    c. Tend to be less solid
    d. Can be attached to the tricuspid or eustachian valve

28. Which of the following statements is correct regarding cardiac myxomas?
    a. They may pass through the foramen ovale.
    b. They occur at older age if they are located in the left ventricle.
    c. They have a male preponderance if they are located in the left ventricle.
    d. They may cause pulmonary embolism if they have a left ventricular location.

29. Which of the following statements is correct regarding cardiac rhabdomyoma?
    a. It is the most frequent tumor in infants and children.
    b. It is always solitary.
    c. It most often involves the left ventricular myocardium.
    d. It may involve mitral or tricuspid valve leaflets.

30. Which of the following statements is correct regarding cardiac rhabdomyoma?
    a. It may project into the ventricular cavity.
    b. It may obstruct right ventricular outflow.
    c. It can be diagnosed before birth with fetal echocardiography.
    d. It may regress spontaneously after birth.
    e. All of above statements are correct.

31. Which of the following characteristics of fibromas is correct?
    a. Originate from epicardial connective tissue
    b. Always calcified
    c. Typical tumors of the fifth to sixth decades of life
    d. Ventricular intramural tumors

32. Which of the following statements is correct concerning papillary fibroelastomas?
    a. They commonly arise from the cardiac valves.
    b. They arise more frequently from the ventricular endocardium.
    c. They occur most often in patients younger than 50 years.
    d. They are frequently associated with thromboembolism.

33. Which of the following statements is correct concerning papillary fibroelastomas?
    a. They originate from the ventricular side of the atrioventricular valves.
    b. They originate from either side of the semilunar valves.
    c. They occur on the aortic valve cusps in 67.5% of cases.
    d. They occur on the mitral leaflets in 67.5% of cases.

34. All of the following are locations for papillary fibroelastomas EXCEPT:
    a. The ventricular septum
    b. Close to the left ventricular outflow tract
    c. The junction between inferior vena cava and right atrium
    d. The right side of the heart

35. Papillary fibroelastomas:
    a. May cause angina and infarction by coronary ostial occlusion.
    b. May cause angina and infarction by embolism.
    c. May cause systemic embolism.
    d. May have to be surgically resected because of the embolic risk.
    e. All of the above statements are correct.

36. Papillary fibroelastomas:
    a. May be multiple in 70% of cases
    b. Have a long pedicle with single papillary fronds
    c. Must be differentiated from Lambl excrescences
    d. Must be differentiated from cardiac rhabdomyoma

37. The histogenesis of papillary fibroelastoma:
    a. Is neoplastic according to most investigators
    b. May be similar to that of cardiac rhabdomyoma
    c. May be bacteria induced
    d. May be induced by mycoplasma

38. In contrast to papillary fibroelastoma, Lambl's excrescences:
    a. Are rheumatic in origin
    b. Arise from the aortic or pulmonary arterial side of the semilunar valves along the coaptation line
    c. May be caused by exuberant organization of thrombi
    d. Are less mobile

39. Lipomas:
    a. Are localized tumors limited to the heart
    b. May cause pericardial effusion
    c. Are large, diffuse, and not well delineated if they are intramyocardial
    d. May arise from the pulmonary and aortic valves

40. Malignant primary cardiac tumors:
    a. Most frequently are rhabdomyosarcomas
    b. Include liposarcomas, fibrosarcomas, or malignant lymphomas
    c. Are almost never sarcomas
    d. Never cause obstruction and peripheral embolism

41. Angiosarcomas:
    a. Are the most frequent cardiac sarcomas
    b. Most often affect the right ventricle
    c. Show a female preponderance
    d. Grow partially intracavitary but never cause valvular obstruction

42. Rhabdomyosarcomas:
    a. Have no predilection for one or another cardiac chamber
    b. Show female preponderance
    c. Are frequently single
    d. Almost never cause valvular obstruction

43. Primary pericardial tumors:
    a. Most often are fibrosarcomas
    b. Most often are pericardial cysts
    c. Most often are mesotheliomas
    d. In children are most frequently lymphomas

44. Pericardial cysts:
    a. Are benign
    b. Occur most often in infants and children
    c. Are more frequent in men
    d. Are the second most frequent pericardial tumors

45. Pericardial cysts:
    a. Are frequently located in the left costophrenic angle
    b. Appear as solid structures on TEE
    c. Can cause valvular obstruction
    d. May compress a cardiac chamber

46. Which of following statements is correct regarding teratomas?
    a. They show a male preponderance.
    b. They are frequent in old age.
    c. They receive their blood supply from coronary arteries.
    d. They have an extracardiac but intrapericardial location.

47. Which of following statements is correct regarding teratomas?
    a. They have been diagnosed by fetal echocardiography.
    b. They manifest most often as recurrent nonbloody pericardial effusions.
    c. They may contain hair or teeth.
    d. They may compromise cardiac function by compression due to considerable expansion.
    e. All of the above statements are correct.

48. Which of the following statements regarding mesotheliomas is correct?
    a. They are benign pericardial tumors.
    b. They may cause constrictive pericardial disease
    c. They affect males and females with the same frequency.
    d. They occur with the highest incidence in the fifth to seventh decades of life.

49. The following statement regarding secondary tumors of the heart is true:
    a. Sarcomas are more frequent than carcinomas.
    b. They more often affect people older than 50 years.
    c. They do not cause arrhythmias if the myocardium is involved.
    d. They occur in more than 70% of patients with malignant melanoma.

50. Which of the following statements is correct regarding cardiac metastases?
    a. They may involve the pericardium, myocardium, endocardium, valves, and coronary arteries.
    b. They may cause aortic dissection.
    c. They may cause restrictive cardiomyopathy.
    d. They are found in more than 30% of patients with primary tumors.

51. Angina or myocardial infarction in patients with cardiac metastases:
    a. Can be due to coronary artery spasm
    b. Can result from concomitant atherosclerosis or fibrosis aggravated by radiation therapy
    c. Can be caused by secretion of active products such as serotonin and bradykinin
    d. Is the most frequent first clinical sign of these metastases

52. Direct tumor extension into the heart:
    a. May occur along the superior vena cava.
    b. Presents as an endocardial mass.
    c. Is frequent with renal cell carcinoma, hepatocellular carcinoma, and primary leiomyosarcoma of the uterus.
    d. May cause mitral valve obstruction.
    e. All of the above statements are correct.

53. Which of the following statements is correct concerning pericardial constrictive signs in patients with cardiac metastases?
    a. They have to be differentiated from right atrial or tricuspid valve obstruction.
    b. They are never caused by previous radiotherapy.
    c. They are characterized by systolic collapse of right atrium and ventricle, inferior caval vein collapse, and blunted expiratory response.
    d. They cannot be differentiated from obstructive mechanisms on TEE.

54. Which of the following statements is correct regarding carcinoid tumors?
    a. They belong to the group of primary cardiac tumors.
    b. They are never secondary cardiac tumors.
    c. They are typically located in the left ventricular wall.
    d. They secrete active products such as serotonin and bradykinin.

55. Typical echocardiographic signs of carcinoid heart disease include:
    a. Signs of constrictive cardiomyopathy caused by endocardial involvement
    b. Frequent involvement of the left heart
    c. Billowing tricuspid valve leaflets
    d. Right ventricular volume overload

56. Which of the following statements is correct regarding carcinoid heart disease?
    a. Bronchial tumors are prone to carcinoid disease of the right heart.
    b. Gastrointestinal tumors cause carcinoid disease of the right heart.
    c. The left heart is affected more frequently than the right heart.
    d. It causes deposits on mitral and aortic valves and on the left atrial and ventricular endocardium.

57. Typical echocardiographic features of carcinoid heart disease include:
    a. A flail tricuspid valve
    b. Systolic doming of the tricuspid valve
    c. Tricuspid insufficiency on color-flow mapping in most patients
    d. Pulmonary valve abnormalities, predominantly stenosis, in most patients

58. The differential diagnosis of intracardiac masses includes:
    a. Primary and secondary cardiac tumors
    b. Intracardiac thrombi
    c. Endocarditis with vegetations
    d. Normal cardiac structures
    e. All of the above

59. All the following are predisposing factors for left atrial thrombi except:
    a. Atrial fibrillation
    b. Right atrial enlargement
    c. Rheumatic mitral stenosis
    d. Prosthetic valve endocarditis

60. Predisposing factors for right atrial thrombi include:
    a. The presence of an LVAD
    b. The presence of a central venous catheter
    c. The presence of an ASD
    d. Female sex

61. Which of the following characteristics is correct regarding cardiac vegetations?
    a. Homogeneous
    b. Regularly shaped

c. Almost always calcified
d. Mobile and prone to embolization

62. Morphologic aspects of atrial thrombi that may help to differentiate them from other cardiac tumors include:
 a. Attachment to the posterior atrial wall
 b. Appearance as mobile, serpiginous, and coiled masses
 c. Attachment to inferior or lateral ventricular wall
 d. No increase in size with anticoagulant therapy

63. TEE examination prior to cardioversion:
 a. Is optional
 b. Is always indicated immediately after cardioversion
 c. Does not help to prevent thromboembolic complications
 d. Is indicated in patients with chronic atrial fibrillation with recently initiated anticoagulant therapy

64. Which of the following statements is correct regarding ventricular thrombi?
 a. They occur in patients with large myocardial infarction.
 b. They occur in patients with restrictive cardiomyopathy.
 c. They occur most often in the base of the heart.
 d. They always appear as laminar structures adhering to the ventricular wall.

65. Which of the following statements is correct regarding ventricular thrombi ?
 a. They are most often multiple.
 b. They are never pedunculated with a narrow stalk.
 c. They are always laminar.
 d. They are often homogeneous but also may be cavitary and heterogeneous.

66. Which of the following TEE findings may increase the risk for embolization of ventricular thrombi?
 a. Shaggy, irregular borders
 b. Mobility
 c. Coexistence of dilated cardiomyopathy or ventricular aneurysm
 d. Apical location
 e. All of the above findings

67. Which of the following statements is correct regarding an atrial septal aneurysm?
 a. It is a normal cardiac structure.
 b. It may have to be differentiated from a cardiac tumor.
 c. It occurs in 5% of adults.
 d. It is frequently associated with ventricular septal defects.
 e. All of the above statements are correct.

68. Correct statements regarding an atrial septal aneurysm include:
 a. Frequent association with multiple atrial septal defects or mitral valve prolapse.
 b. Phasic right-to-left excursions during the cardiac cycle of less than 1.5 cm.
 c. Undetectable flow in the aneurysmal pocket.
 d. Aneurysmal bulging of the interatrial septum protruding greater than 1.5 cm beyond the level of the interatrial septum.
 e. All of the above statements are correct.

69. Which of the following statements is correct regarding an atrial septal aneurysm?
 a. It causes morbidity and mortality via thromboembolic mechanisms.
 b. It can be detected and differentiated on TEE with high sensitivity.
 c. It can be nicely documented on an M-mode echocardiogram.
 d. It can be filled with thrombus.
 e. All of the above statements are correct.

70. Which of the following morphologic characteristics is typical for vegetations and helps differentiating vegetations from thrombi?
 a. Coexistence of a decreased ventricular function
 b. Movement independent of valvular structures in the cardiac phase
 c. Association with valvular regurgitation
 d. Attachment to the downstream side of atrioventricular or semilunar valves
 e. All of the above

71. Which of the following statements is correct regarding the diagnosis of endocarditis?
 a. TEE and TTE are equally valuable.
 b. TEE is not accurate in describing late complications.
 c. TEE is very accurate in monitoring therapy with antibiotics.
 d. Repeat TEE has no proven benefit.

Epicardial Echocardiography and Epiaortic Ultrasonography

20

Stanton K. Shernan and Kathryn E. Glas

Despite its overwhelming popularity and favorable influence on perioperative clinical decision making and outcome, the transesophageal echocardiographic (TEE) approach to a comprehensive echocardiographic examination may be limited by impaired imaging of the distal ascending aorta and aortic arch, difficulty in advancing the probe within the esophagus in some patients, and contraindications for probe placement in those with gastroesophageal pathology. Furthermore, TEE may be rarely associated with perioperative morbidity from oropharyngeal and gastroesophageal injury.[1,2] In recognition of these potential limitations, the Society of Cardiovascular Anesthesiologists (SCA), American Society of Anesthesiologists (ASA), and American Society of Echocardiography (ASE) currently recommend that advanced intraoperative ultrasonographers also become familiar with epicardial echocardiography and epiaortic ultrasound in addition to TEE.[3,4] The ASE and SCA have subsequently published guidelines specifically focused on acquisition techniques and indications for both epicardial echocardiography and epiaortic ultrasonography.[5,6] Thus, while TEE remains the most frequently used intraoperative tool for imaging cardiac and intrathoracic vascular structures, it is imperative for an experienced intraoperative ultrasonogapher to also be familiar with other imaging modalities including epicardial echocardiographic and epiaortic ultrasound techniques in order to conduct a comprehensive perioperative echocardiographic examination.

EPICARDIAL AND EPIAORTIC PROBE PREPARATION

Epicardial and epiaortic imaging are performed by placing the ultrasound transducer on the surface of the heart or aorta, respectively, to acquire two-dimensional (2D), and color-flow and spectral Doppler images in multiple planes. Due to the proximity of the probe to the heart, these techniques typically use higher frequency probes (5 to 12 MHz). Epicardial and epiaortic imaging require adherence to strict sterile technique while manipulating the probe within the operative field. Consequently, these images may only be obtained by an operator who is wearing a sterile gown and gloves. The probe is placed in a sterile sheath along with sterile acoustic gel or saline in order to optimize acoustic transmission. Warm sterile saline can be poured into the mediastinal cavity to further enhance acoustic transmission from the probe to the cardiac or aortic surface. Additional manipulation of depth, transmit focus, gain, and transducer frequency may be required to optimize the image.

EPICARDIAL ECHOCARDIOGRAPHY IMAGING PLANES

The ASE/SCA guidelines currently recommend that the following seven epicardial echocardiographic imaging planes be obtained to perform a comprehensive 2D and Doppler echocardiographic evaluation.[5] However, the guidelines also recognize that individual patient characteristics, anatomic variations, or time constraints may limit the ability to obtain every component of the recommended comprehensive epicardial echocardiographic examination. Furthermore, modification of the recommended views may be required to obtain a more detailed interrogation of specific anatomy or pathology.

Epicardial Aortic Valve Short-Axis View

The ultrasound transducer is placed on the aortic root above the aortic valve (AV) annulus, with the ultrasound beam directed towards the AV in a short-axis (SAX) orientation to obtain the epicardial AV SAX view (Figure 20–1). Appropriate transducer alignment requires up to 30° of clockwise rotation with the orientation marker (indentation) on the transducer directed toward the patient's left.

Epicardial Aortic Valve Long-Axis View

The epicardial aortic valve long-axis (LAX) view is obtained from the epicardial AV SAX view by positioning the probe

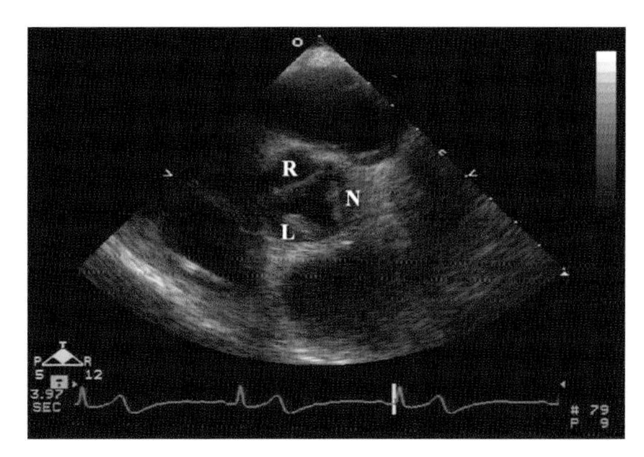

FIGURE 20–1. Epicardial aortic valve short-axis view. When the orientation marker (indentation) on the transducer is pointed towards the patient's left, the right coronary cusp (R) will be at the top of the monitor screen, the left coronary cusp (L) is on the bottom left, and the noncoronary cusp (N) is on the right side of the screen adjacent to the interatrial septum.

upward along the right-side surface of the aortic root with the orientation marker slightly rotated clockwise and directed toward the patient's left. The ultrasound beam is directed posteriorly to visualize the left ventricular outflow tract (LVOT) and AV (Figure 20–2).

Epicardial Left Ventricle Basal SAX View

The epicardial left ventricular (LV) basal SAX view is obtained from the epicardial AV SAX position by moving the probe towards the apex along the right ventricle (RV) with the transducer orientation marker again directed towards the patient's left (Figure 20–3). In this view, the RV is on top in the near field, while the LV is below in the far field of the ultrasound beam sector. The mitral valve (MV) is visualized including both leaflets forming the classic "fish mouth" appearance, with the anterior leaflet on the top of the screen and the posterior leaflet underneath. The anterolateral commissure lies on the right, and the posteromedial commissure on the left of the screen.

Epicardial Left Ventricle Mid SAX View

Angulating the probe inferiorly and to the left from the epicardial LV basal SAX view in an apical direction along the RV myocardial surface allows visualization of the RV and LV in SAX at the level of the papillary muscles (Figure 20–4). When the transducer orientation marker faces the patient's left, the anterolateral papillary muscle will be on the right side of the display and the posteriomedial papillary muscle will be on the left side. The septal wall of the LV is displayed on the left followed by the anterior, lateral, and inferior walls, respectively, in a clockwise rotation. The RV can be evaluated

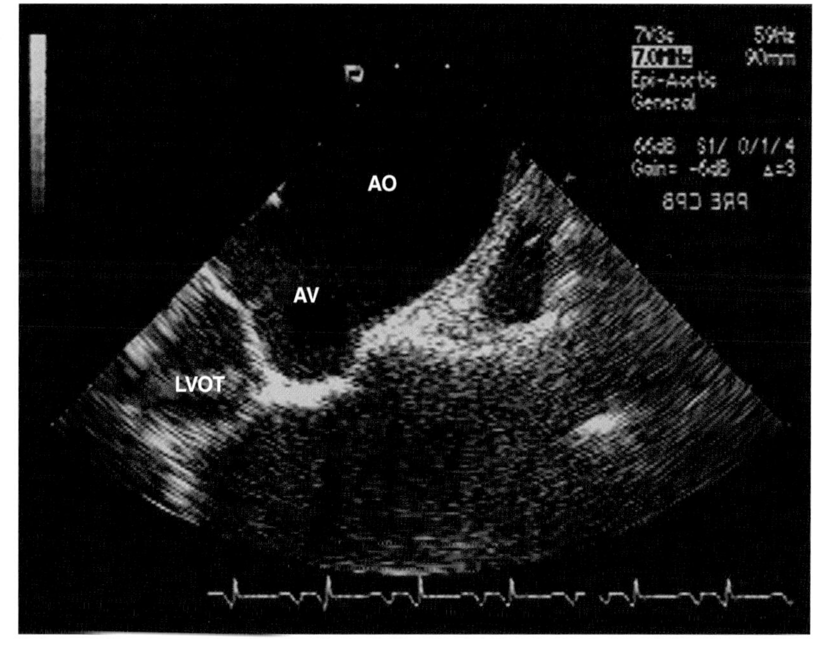

FIGURE 20–2. Epicardial aortic valve long-axis view. This view is optimal for measuring left ventricular outflow tract (LVOT), aortic annulus, and sinotubular junction diameters. Long-axis orientation permits continuous-wave and pulsed-wave Doppler ultrasound beam assessment of pressure gradients across the aortic valve (AV) and LVOT. Similarly, color-flow Doppler interrogation of the AV can be utilized to grade the degree of aortic insufficiency. (AO, proximal ascending aorta.)

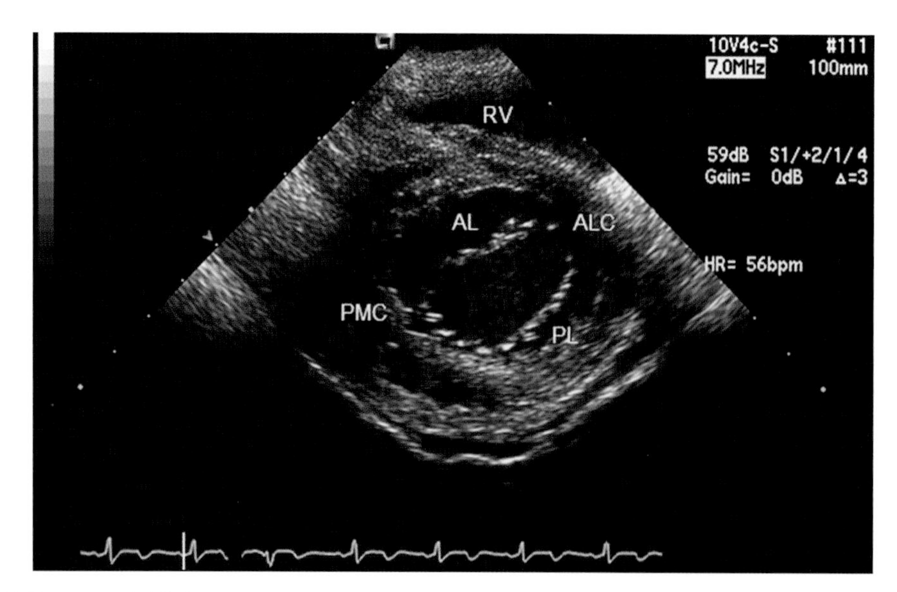

FIGURE 20–3. Epicardial left ventricle basal short-axis view. The epicardial left ventricle (LV) basal short-axis (SAX) view can be used to evaluate the mitral valve annulus and both anterior (AL) and posterior (PL) leaflets. Color-flow Doppler can also be used to determine the origin of mitral regurgitation jets and obtain an estimate of the regurgitant orifice area. Finally, basal LV regional wall motion can be assessed utilizing the same LV wall orientation as seen in the epicardial left ventricle mid SAX. (ALC, anterolateral commissure; PMC, posteromedial commissure; RV, right ventricle.)

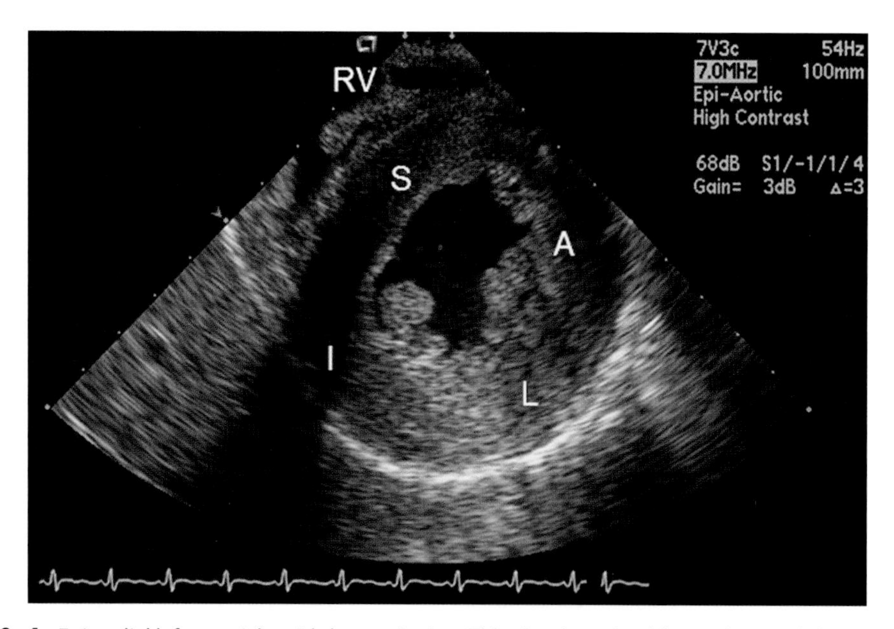

FIGURE 20–4. Epicardial left ventricle mid short-axis view. This view is optimal for evaluating left ventricle (LV) and right ventricle (RV) global and regional function. (S, interventricular septum; A, LV anterior wall; L, LV lateral wall; I, LV inferior wall.)

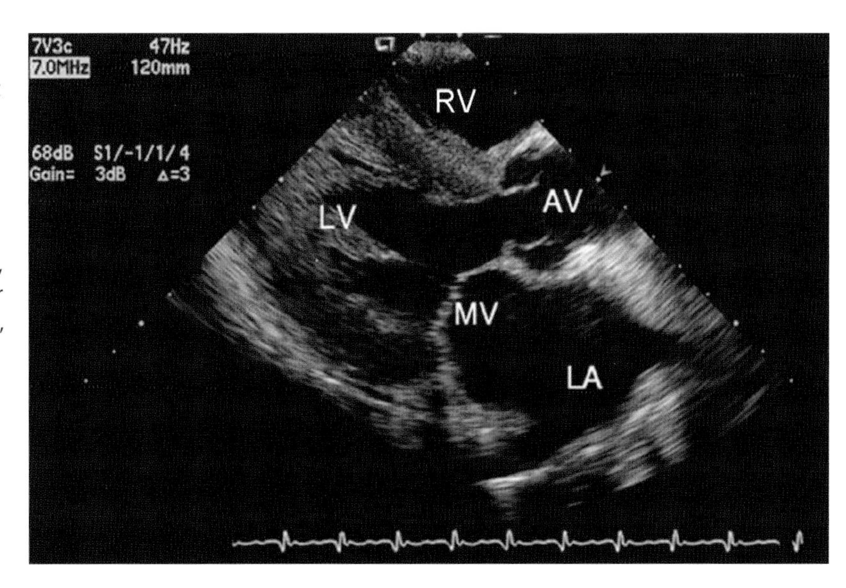

FIGURE 20–5. Epicardial left ventricle long-axis view. This view allows visualization of the inferolateral (far field) and anteroseptal (near field) walls of the left ventricle (LV) as well as the right ventricle (RV), left atrium (LA), left ventricular outflow tract, aortic valve (AV), and mitral valve (MV). Rightward orientation of the beam allows evaluation of the right atrium and tricuspid valve. This view is also useful for diagnosing and quantifying aortic, mitral, and tricuspid regurgitation.

similarly by moving the transducer further towards the patient's right.

Epicardial Left Ventricle Long-Axis view

From the epicardial LV mid SAX view, the ultrasound beam can be angled superiorly and rotated towards the patient's right shoulder to generate the epicardial LV LAX view (Figure 20–5).

Epicardial Two-Chamber View

From the epicardial LV LAX view, movement of the probe toward the anterior surface of the LV and further clockwise rotation will develop the epicardial two-chamber view, permitting evaluation of the LA, left atrial appendage, MV, and LV (Figure 20–6). Basilar and mid segments of the anterior and inferior walls of the LV can be assessed in this view.

Epicardial Right Ventricular Outflow Tract View

The epicardial right ventricular outflow tract (RVOT) view is developed by moving the transducer over the RVOT and directing the ultrasound beam towards the patient's left shoulder (Figure 20–7). The RVOT,

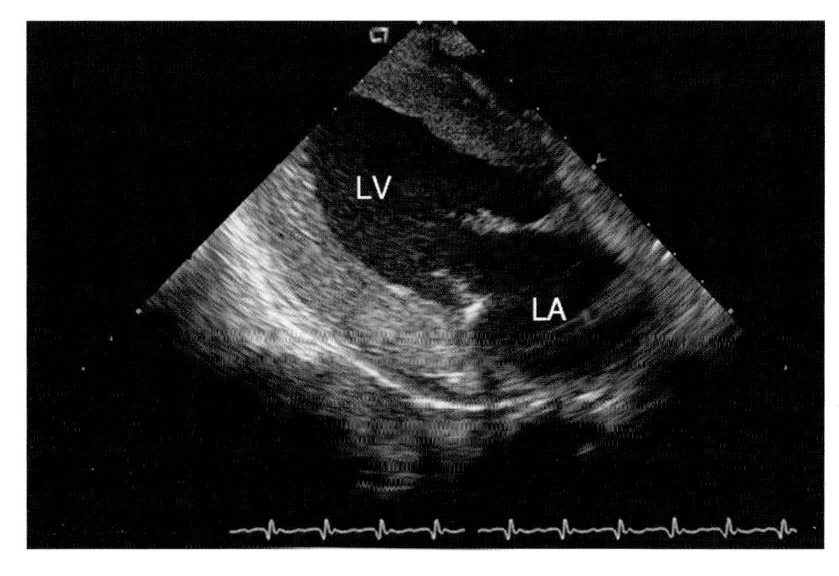

FIGURE 20–6. Epicardial two-chamber view. This view can be used to evaluate left atrial (LA) size and pathology, as well as mitral valve (MV) anatomy and leaflet motion. Regional wall motion of the basal and mid segments of the anterior (near field) and inferior (far field) left ventricular (LV) walls can also be obtained.

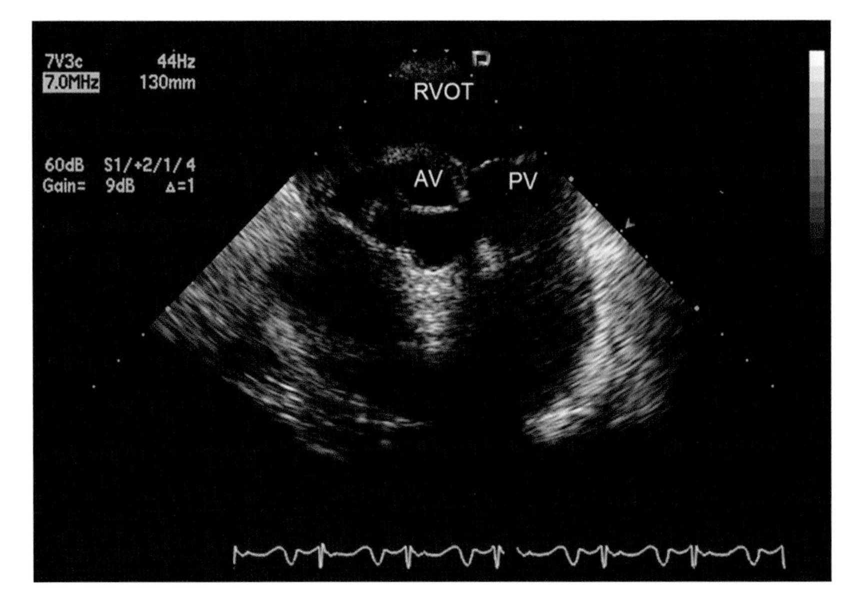

FIGURE 20–7. Epicardial right ventricular outflow tract view. This view permits visualization of the right ventricular outflow tract (RVOT), pulmonic valve (PV), proximal main pulmonary artery, and aortic valve (AV). Orienting a spectral and color-flow Doppler beam parallel to blood flow permits the evaluation of chamber pressures, and quantification of pulmonic regurgitation or stenosis. This view is also useful for diagnosing a proximal pulmonary embolism or assisting with positioning a pulmonary artery catheter.

pulmonic valve (PV), and proximal main pulmonary artery (PA) can be visualized.

EPIAORTIC ULTRASOUND IMAGING PLANES

The ASE/SCA recommended comprehensive epiaortic ultrasound examination includes a minimum of five views for the evaluation of the ascending aorta from the sinotubular junction to the origin of the innominate artery, and the aortic arch.[6] The ascending aorta should be assessed in SAX in each of the proximal, mid, and distal segments. A LAX view of the ascending aorta including visualization of the proximal, mid, and distal segments should also be acquired. A LAX epiaortic ultrasound examination of the arch includes visualization of the proximal arch, and ideally all three arch vessel origins.

The ASE/SCA guidelines recommend that the ascending aorta be divided into 12 areas including the anterior, posterior, and left and right lateral walls within the proximal, mid, and distal ascending aorta segments.[6] The proximal ascending aorta is defined as the region from the sinotubular junction to the proximal intersection of the right pulmonary artery (RPA). The mid ascending aorta includes that portion of the aorta that is adjacent to the RPA. The distal ascending aorta extends from the distal intersection of the RPA to the origin of the innominate artery. The diameter of each aortic segment should be measured as the maximum diameter in the SAX orientation, from the near-field inner edge to the far-field inner edge (internal diameter).[6]

While epiaortic scanning may be used to evaluate ascending aortic aneurysms and dissection, this technique is most commonly utilized to evaluate the extent of aortic atherosclerotic burden to guide the surgical approach towards cannulation for cardiopulmonary bypass with the intention of avoiding the generation of emboli and excessive aortic trauma. While several grading systems have been recommended,[7-10] a comprehensive epiaortic ultrasonographic examination should include an evaluation of each of the following measurements for each of the three ascending aortic short-axis segments and for the aortic arch: (1) maximal plaque height/thickness, (2) location of the maximal plaque within the ascending aorta, and (3) presence of mobile components. Additional measurements indicating the extent of atheroma burden, such as circumferential area of maximal plaque obtained by planimetry, may also be acquired. When plaque area is measured, aortic diameter should also be noted to quantify atheroma burden as a ratio of plaque area to aortic area.[11] Measurements may be repeated as necessary for multiple plaques. Due to the preponderance of data demonstrating an increased risk of adverse neurological outcomes associated with plaques that are greater than 5 mm in thickness, or those that possess a mobile component,[7-10] the presence and location of these plaques should be discussed with the surgeon prior to aortic manipulation.

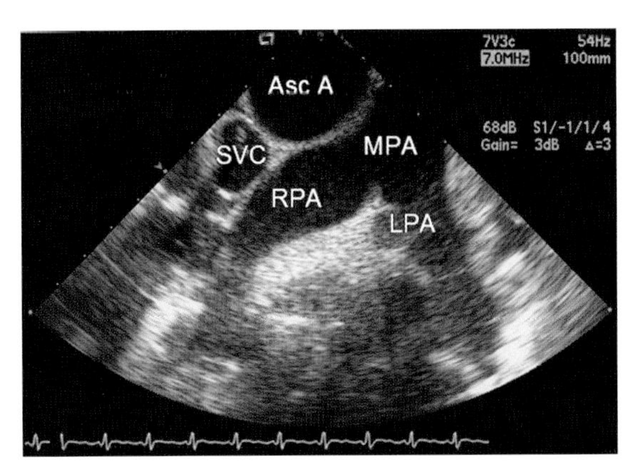

FIGURE 20–8. Short-axis epiaortic ultrasonographic image of the ascending aorta (Asc A). (MPA, main pulmonary artery; LPA, left pulmonary artery; RPA, right pulmonary artery; SVC, superior vena cava.)

SAX Examination

The ultrasound probe is positioned on the ascending aorta as proximal to the aortic valve as possible, with the orientation marker directed toward the patient's left shoulder to obtain an imaging window that is perpendicular to the LAX of the aorta (Figures 20–8 and 20–9). After identifying the proximal ascending aorta and AV, slowly advancing the probe distally in a cephalad direction along the aorta permits visualization of the mid ascending aorta, and the distal ascending aorta towards the aortic arch at the origin of the innominate artery. Advancing the probe slightly further permits examination of the proximal aortic arch.

LAX Examination

The LAX orientation is achieved by rotating the probe 90° from the SAX orientation (Figure 20–10). Proximally, the sinus of Valsalva, sinotubular junction, and aortic valve can be visualized. The probe is then advanced distally in a cephalad direction along the aorta, changing the rotation and angulation accordingly to keep the aorta in a longitudinal LAX view (Figure 20–11). Imaging of the ascending aorta should extend towards the aortic arch with visualization of the innominate, left common carotid, and left subclavian artery origins (Figure 20–12).

EPICARDIAL ECHOCARDIOGRAPHY AND EPIAORTIC ULTRASONOGRAPHY TRAINING GUIDELINES

Compared to TEE, epicardial echocardiography and epiaortic ultrasonography are unique in requiring a collaborative effort with the cardiac surgeon to either allow the echocardiographer to guide them in obtaining images, or alternatively permit the echocardiographer to have direct access to the epicardial or epiaortic surface within the operative field. In addition, experience in epicardial echocardiography is considered an important component of advanced, rather than basic, perioperative echocardiographic training. Current guidelines published by the ASE and SCA recommend that epicardial echocardiographic and epiaortic ultrasonographic training should include the study of 25 examinations, of which five are personally directed under the supervision of an advanced echocardiographer, before a trainee should pursue independent interpretation and

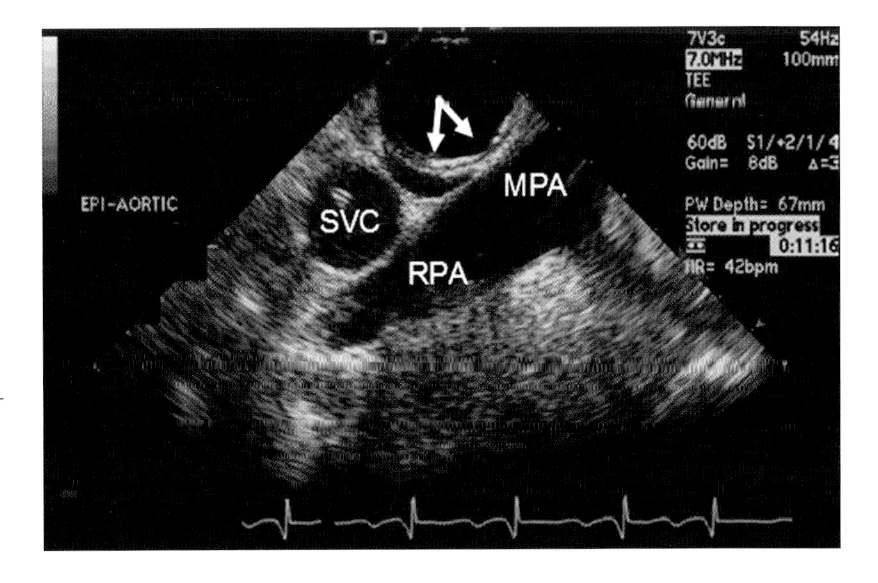

FIGURE 20–9. Short-axis epiaortic ultrasonographic image of echo-dense atherosclerotic plaque *(arrows)* in the ascending aorta. (MPA, main pulmonary artery; RPA, right pulmonary artery; SVC, superior vena cava.)

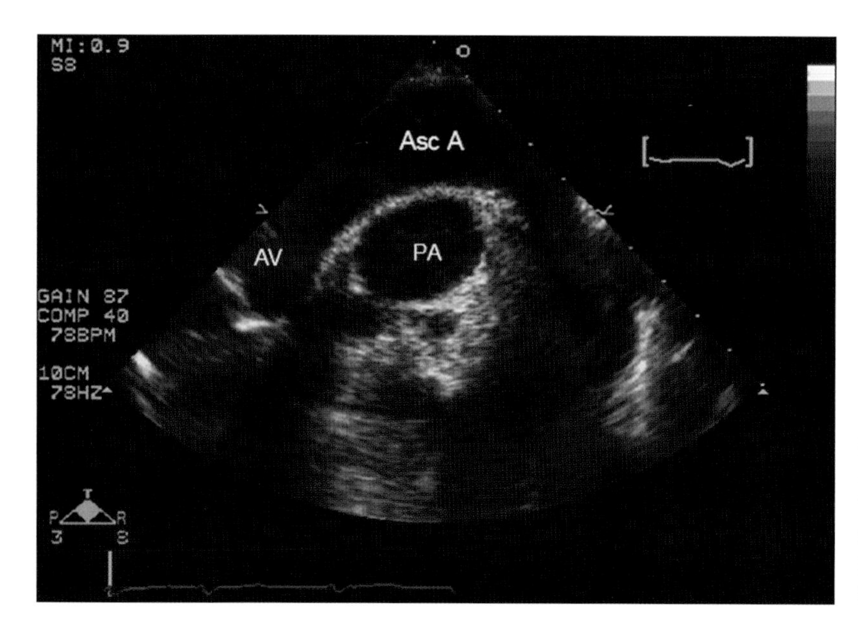

FIGURE 20–10. Long-axis epiaortic ultrasonographic image of the proximal and mid ascending aorta (Asc A). (AV, aortic valve; PA, pulmonary artery.)

application of the information to perioperative clinical decision making.[5,6]

CONCLUSION

A comprehensive epicardial echocardiographic and epiaortic ultrasonographic examination can be performed efficiently and safely,[12] and may be the most practical intraoperative imaging technique when a TEE probe cannot be inserted or when probe placement is contraindicated. In addition, these techniques may offer better windows for imaging anterior cardiac structures including the aorta, AV, pulmonic valve, and pulmonary arteries, and therefore they may have a favorable influence on perioperative surgical decision making.[13-15] Rosenberger et al analyzed the medical records of 6051 consecutive cardiac surgical patients who underwent epiaortic ultrasonography to determine a potential impact on intraoperative surgical decision making.[16] The overall impact of epiaortic ultrasonography on surgical decision

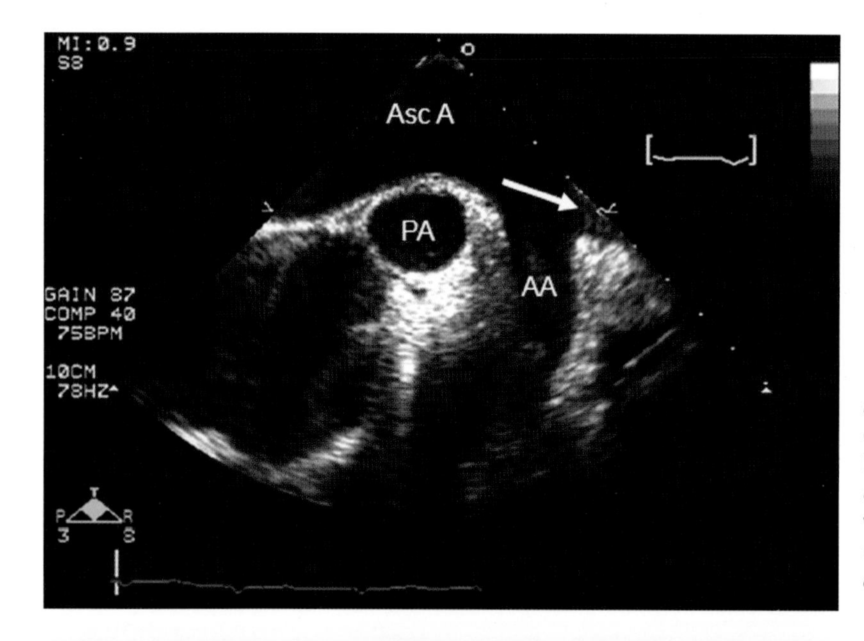

FIGURE 20–11. Long-axis epiaortic ultrasonographic image of the mid and distal ascending aorta (Asc A), as well as proximal aortic arch (AA). (PA, pulmonary artery; *arrow*, innominate artery.)

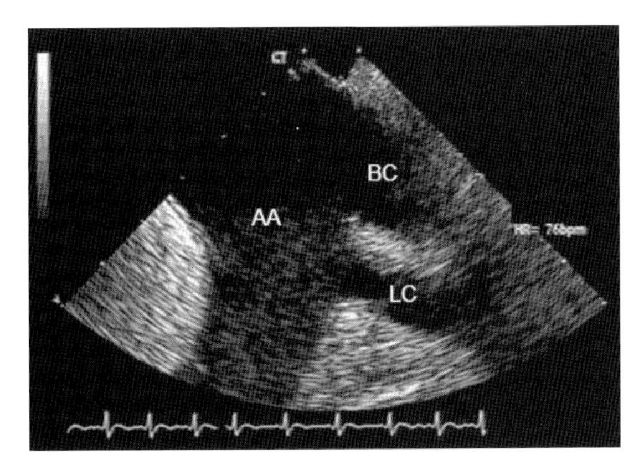

FIGURE 20–12. Long-axis epiaortic ultrasonographic image of the aortic arch (AA) including the origins of the brachiocephalic (BC) and left common carotid (LC) arteries.

making was 4.1%, and included a change in the technique for inducing cardiac arrest during cardiopulmonary bypass in 1.8%, aortic atherectomy or replacement surgery in 0.8%, requirement for off-pump coronary artery bypass grafting in 0.6%, avoidance of aortic cross-clamping and use of ventricular fibrillatory arrest in 0.5%, change in arterial cannulation site in 0.2%, or avoidance of aortic cannulation in 0.2%. In addition, the authors noted that the overall stroke rate was lower in patients in whom intraoperative epiaortic ultrasonography was performed, compared with all patients undergoing cardiac surgical procedures. Nonetheless, epicardial and epiaortic imaging do have certain limitations, including a requirement for a sternotomy to permit direct access to the anterior surface of the heart and aorta, the inability to perform continuous monitoring, and the requirement for at least a brief interruption of the surgical procedure. Despite these limitations, a fundamental understanding of the skills required to obtain and interpret epicardial echocardiographic and epiaortic ultrasound images is an advantageous adjunct to intraoperative TEE in performing a comprehensive intraoperative echocardiographic examination.

REFERENCES

1. Kallmeyer IJ, Collard CD, Fox JA, Body SC, Shernan SK. The safety of intraoperative transesophageal echocardiography: a case series of 7200 cardiac surgical patients. *Anesth Analg.* 2001;92(5):1126-1130.
2. Lennon MJ, Gibbs NM, Weightman WM, Leber J, Ee HC, Yusoff IF. Transesophageal echocardiography-related gastrointestinal complications in cardiac surgical patients. *J Cardiothorac Vasc Anesth.* 2005;19(2):141-145.
3. Practice guidelines for perioperative transesophageal echocardiography. A report by the American Society of Anesthesiologists and the Society of Cardiovascular Anesthesiologists Task Force on Transesophageal Echocardiography. *Anesthesiology.* 1996;84(4):986-1006.
4. Cahalan MK, Abel M, Goldman M, et al. American Society of Echocardiography and Society of Cardiovascular Anesthesiologists task force guidelines for training in perioperative echocardiography. *Anesth Analg.* 2002;94(6):1384-1388.
5. Reeves ST, Glas KE, Eltzschig H, et al. Guidelines for performing a comprehensive epicardial echocardiography examination: recommendations of the American Society of Echocardiography and the Society of Cardiovascular Anesthesiologists. *J Am Soc Echocardiogr.* 2007;20(4):427-437.
6. Glas KE, Swaminathan M, Reeves ST, et al. Guidelines for the performance of a comprehensive intraoperative epiaortic ultrasonographic examination: recommendations of the American Society of Echocardiography and the Society of Cardiovascular Anesthesiologists; endorsed by the Society of Thoracic Surgeons. *J Am Soc Echocardiogr.* 2007;20(11):1227-1235.
7. Katz ES, Tunick PA, Rusinek H, Ribakove G, Spencer FC, Kronzon I. Protruding aortic atheromas predict stroke in elderly patients undergoing cardiopulmonary bypass: experience with intraoperative transesophageal echocardiography. *J Am Coll Cardiol.* 1992;20(1):70-77.
8. Ferrari E, Vidal R, Chevallier T, Baudouy M. Atherosclerosis of the thoracic aorta and aortic debris as a marker of poor prognosis: benefit of oral anticoagulants. *J Am Coll Cardiol.* 1999;33(5):1317-1322.
9. Trehan N, Mishra M, Kasliwal RR, Mishra A. Reduced neurological injury during CABG in patients with mobile aortic atheromas: a five-year follow-up study. *Ann Thorac Surg.* 2000;70(5):1558-1564.
10. van der Linden J, Hadjinikolaou L, Bergman P, Lindblom D. Postoperative stroke in cardiac surgery is related to the location and extent of atherosclerotic disease in the ascending aorta. *J Am Coll Cardiol.* 2001;38(1):131-135.
11. Mackensen GB, Swaminathan M, Ti LK, et al. Preliminary report on the interaction of apolipoprotein E polymorphism with aortic atherosclerosis and acute nephropathy after CABG. *Ann Thorac Surg.* 2004;78(2):520-526.
12. Eltzschig HK, Kallmeyer IJ, Mihaljevic T, Alapati S, Shernan SK. A practical approach to a comprehensive epicardial and epiaortic echocardiographic examination. *J Cardiothorac Vasc Anesth.* 2003;17(4):422-429.
13. Frenk VE, Shernan SK, Eltzschig HK. Epicardial echocardiography: diagnostic utility for evaluating aortic valve disease during coronary surgery. *J Clin Anesth.* 2003;15(4):271-274.
14. Edrich T, Shernan SK, Smith B, Eltzschig HK. Usefulness of intraoperative epiaortic echocardiography to resolve discrepancy between transthoracic and transesophageal measurements of aortic valve gradient—a case report. *Can J Anaesth.* 2003;50(3):293-296.
15. Hilberath JN, Shernan SK, Segal S, Smith B, Eltzschig HK. The feasibility of epicardial echocardiography for measuring aortic valve area by the continuity equation. *Anesth Analg.* 2009;108(1):17-22.
16. Rosenberger P, Shernan SK, Loffler M, et al. The influence of epiaortic ultrasonography on intraoperative surgical management in 6051 cardiac surgical patients. *Ann Thorac Surg.* 2008;85(2):548-553.

TEE for Noncardiac Surgery

21

Angus Christie and Frederick W. Lombard

INTRODUCTION

Transesophageal echocardiography (TEE) is remarkably efficient and effective in revealing a wide spectrum of new findings and information during periods of hemodynamic instability. Since TEE technology is now readily accessible in most settings, TEE is increasingly used during noncardiac surgical procedures. However, in contrast to the cardiac surgery setting, little evidence supports the routine use of TEE in noncardiac surgery. This is largely due to the fact that the validated indications for intraoperative TEE are for use as a diagnostic tool, and not a monitor (Table 21–1). The majority of established indications in cardiac surgery directly pertain to the planned surgical procedure, or the assessment of relevant anatomical structures. To date, no large randomized trials have assessed the impact of intraoperative TEE on outcome in noncardiac surgery. Several reviews, however, have debated the use of TEE in noncardiac surgery.[1-8]

ACUTE HEMODYNAMIC DECOMPENSATION

Life-threatening intraoperative hemodynamic collapse is an indication for the use of TEE (ASA/SCA guidelines).[9] TEE in this setting could rapidly identify abnormalities and help in establishing a diagnosis, monitor the response to treatment, and may have some prognostic value.

The etiology of precipitating events may be difficult to diagnose, since these are often only transiently manifested. Nevertheless, TEE can be useful in diagnosing the majority of specific cardiovascular abnormalities associated with cardiovascular collapse. These include pulmonary embolism, myocardial ischemia, hypovolemia and pericardial tamponade. Specific conditions that have to be ruled out systematically are listed in Table 21–2. The transgastric midpapillary short-axis view is a useful starting point in the evaluation of acute hemodynamic disturbances. From this view contractility and preload can be readily assessed.

Acute Hypovolemia

Hypovolemia is a common finding in perioperative hemodynamic decompensation. Several techniques have been validated to objectively quantify left ventricular (LV) chamber dimensions. However, these usually require measurement of LV dimensions in short- and long-axis views to incorporate into a volume formula, which can be time consuming. In the setting where several potential precipitating causes of hemodynamic collapse have to be rapidly ruled out, more accurate volume calculations probably add little additional value over instant qualitative assessment or simple area measurements. Obliteration of the LV cavity is said to provide an instant diagnosis of inadequate LV preload. However, 20% of cases with systolic cavity obliteration may occur in the setting of reduced afterload and/or increased ejection fraction, and not hypovolemia.[10] Furthermore, patients with chronic dilated cardiomyopathy may require more filling than patients with normal cardiac function, and hypovolemia is more difficult to recognize in this situation. Taking multiple measurements and evaluating filling in multiple imaging planes can improve the accuracy of TEE estimates of LV volumes. When compared with more traditional hemodynamic parameters of LV volume, such as central venous pressure (CVP) and pulmonary artery wedge pressure (PAWP), which are dependent on compliance, TEE provides a more sensitive and reliable method for detecting hypovolemia.[11] Even though it provides a good starting point in rapidly assessing volume status, the transgastric midpapillary short-axis view does not provide a good estimate of right ventricular (RV) volume, and relying on this imaging plane alone in guiding volume replacement can lead to RV distention.

Pulmonary Embolism

In suspected pulmonary embolism, TEE allows direct visualization of the venae cavae, the right atrium (RA), the RV, the right ventricular outflow tract, and the right pulmonary artery (PA). The two key features of acute pulmonary embolism are thrombus in the right heart (Figure 21–1) and acute right ventricular dysfunction (Figure 21–2 and Table 21–3). Since the right PA is in greater flow continuity with the pulmonary trunk, emboli are consistently found on the right, but in severe cases, the distribution of emboli is most commonly bilateral. Pulmonary embolism cannot be excluded

Table 21–1. Recommendations for the Use of TEE in the Perioperative Period.

I. Cardiac and Thoracic Aortic Procedures

- ***Cardiac and Thoracic Aortic Surgery***
  - For adult patients without contraindications, TEE should be used in all open heart (eg, valvular procedures) and thoracic aortic surgical procedures, and should be considered in CABG surgeries as well to:
    - Confirm and refine the preoperative diagnosis
    - Detect new or unsuspected pathology
    - Adjust the anesthetic and surgical plan accordingly
    - Assess results of the surgical intervention
    - In small children, the use of TEE should be considered on a case-by-case basis because of risks unique to these patients (eg, bronchial obstruction)
- ***Catheter-Based Intracardiac Procedures***
  - For patients undergoing transcatheter intracardiac procedures, TEE may be used

II. Noncardiac Surgery

- TEE may be used when the nature of the planned surgery or the patient's known or suspected cardiovascular pathology might result in severe hemodynamic, pulmonary, or neurologic compromise
- If equipment and expertise are available, TEE should be used when unexplained life-threatening circulatory instability persists despite corrective therapy

III. Critical Care

- For critical care patients, TEE should be used when diagnostic information that is expected to alter management cannot be obtained by TTE or other modalities in a timely manner

TEE, transesophageal echocardiography; TTE, transthoracic echocardiography; CABG, coronary artery bypass graft.
Reproduced with permission from Practice Guidelines for Perioperative Transesophageal Echocardiography. An Updated Report by the American Society of Anesthesiologists and the Society of Cardiovascular Anesthesiologists Task Force on Transesophageal Echocardiography. Anesthesiology 2010;112:1084-1096.

based on absence of thrombus alone. Conversely, pulmonary embolism should always be suspected in the presence of acute right ventricular pressure overload, and hemodynamically significant pulmonary embolism can essentially be ruled out in the absence of right ventricular dysfunction. RV dysfunction has been recognized in the International Cooperative Pulmonary Embolism Registry as an independent predictor of death.[12] In prolonged cardiac arrest, about 20 minutes following the initiation of cardiopulmonary resuscitation, intracardiac thrombus could develop as a result of the low flow state.[13] This is associated with a very poor prognosis, but should not be confused with thromboembolism.

Table 21–2. Potential Causes of Hemodynamic Disturbances.

1. Right or left ventricular dysfunction (global or regional; systolic or diastolic)
2. Significant valvular disease
3. Hypovolemia
4. Dynamic left ventricular outflow tract obstruction
5. Pulmonary embolism
6. Pericardial tamponade
7. Aortic dissection
8. Intracardiac shunts

MONITORING

An ideal monitor should have a high sensitivity and specificity, should be easy to learn and use, and should provide real-time continuous and reproducible information. The unique versatility of TEE in rapidly assessing left and right ventricular function, fluid status, and the effect of therapeutic interventions with great precision is unrivaled, and associated risks are minimal. Therefore, it is increasingly utilized as a monitoring device in high-risk patients undergoing all types of surgery. TEE as a complement to invasive monitoring, or as a stand-alone physiologic monitor has not been shown to improve patient outcome. Nevertheless, when it comes to the assessment of myocardial contractility,

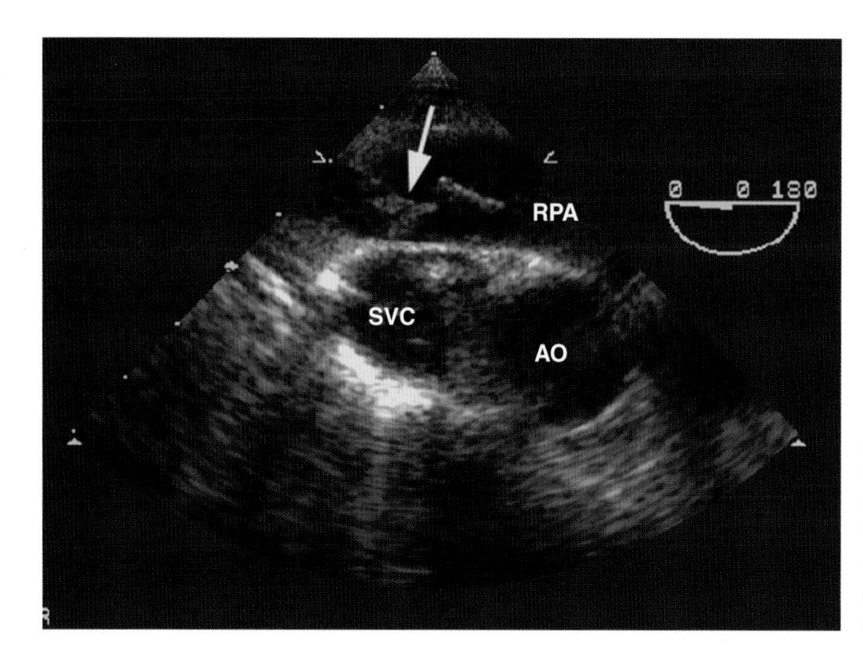

FIGURE 21–1. Thrombus in the right pulmonary artery in a patient with pulmonary embolism. (AO, ascending aorta; RPA, right pulmonary artery; SVC, superior vena cava.)

preload, and ischemia, TEE may offer valuable additional information.

Myocardial Ischemia Monitoring

TEE-based ischemia monitoring in patients at increased risk of myocardial ischemia or infarction remains a common indication.[9] In addition to appreciating the additional benefit TEE could provide over standard electrocardiographic (ECG) monitoring, the clinician should also have a detailed understanding of the shortcomings of TEE as an ischemia monitor.

The movement of the heart during a cardiac cycle is a complex three-dimensional motion captured in real time by TEE as a two-dimensional or M-mode image. There are two distinct events during normal systole: thickening

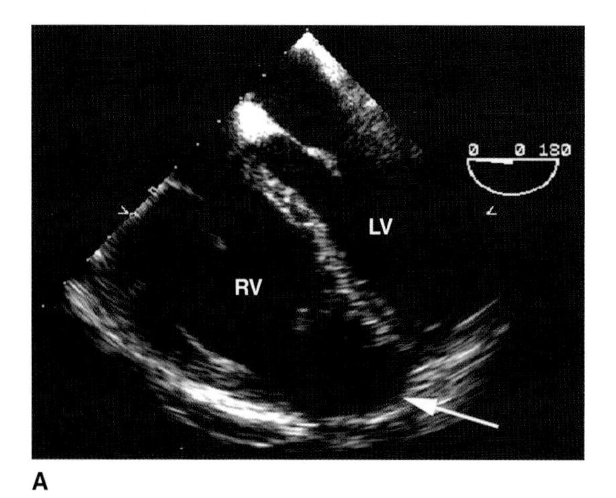

A

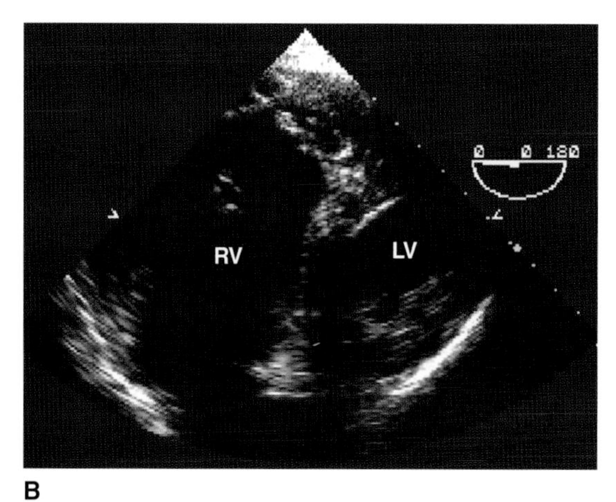

B

FIGURE 21–2. Acute right ventricular failure. **A:** In the long-axis view, the right ventricle is dilated and appears to be greater than two-thirds the size of the left ventricle, and the apex of the heart includes the right ventricle *(arrow)*. **B:** In the short-axis view, a small, hyperdynamic left ventricle is seen with a dilated right ventricle. (LV, left ventricle; RV, right ventricle.)

Table 21–3. TEE Characteristics of Pulmonary Embolism.

Thrombus	Acute Right Ventricular Dysfunction
1. Distinct edges	1. Elevated RA/RV pressure gradient (>30 mm Hg)
2. Protrudes into vascular lumen	2. Dilation of RV, RA, and IVC
3. Visible in multiple planes	3. Leftward bulging of interatrial septum
4. Moves distinct from vascular wall or blood	4. Flattening of interventricular septum

RA, right atrium; RV, right ventricle; IVC, inferior vena cava.

of the myocardial wall and endocardial excursion (inward movement of the endocardial surface during systole). Normal LV wall motion is defined as 30% to 50% thickening of the myocardium during systole at the midpapillary level. Greater degrees of thickening occur at the apex as opposed to the base. Wall thickening is an important component of evaluation, because it may help distinguish between ischemic and nonischemic (variable loading conditions, rhythm disturbances, etc) wall motion abnormalities.

TEE has been demonstrated to be more sensitive than ECG in detecting ischemia. Wall motion abnormalities have been reported to occur within 15 seconds of coronary occlusion, whereas ST segment elevations are seen after only 30 to 60 seconds. While this time difference may not have much clinical relevance, echocardiography is able to detect reductions (as opposed to total occlusion) in coronary blood flow more readily than surface electrocardiography. ECG changes do not occur until coronary flow is decreased by 75%, whereas segmental contraction abnormalities are evident with a 50% decrease in flow.[14] The occurrence of new regional wall motion abnormalities (RWMAs) after cardiopulmonary bypass (CPB) has been correlated with adverse clinical outcomes in patients undergoing cardiac surgery.[15-17] In contrast, RWMA in patients undergoing noncardiac surgery correlates poorly with postoperative cardiac complications.[18]

Although the sensitivity for ischemia detection by TEE is established, the specificity and implications of a transient RWMA are less clear. The normal ventricle displays a wide range of contraction patterns under normal circumstances.[19] This is thought to occur in part because different segments of the ventricle reach their peak contraction at different points within the cardiac cycle. Identification of abnormal contraction patterns based solely on a comparison with adjacent ventricular segments may therefore be an inadequate indicator of myocardial ischemia. Further, although dyskinesia and akinesia are rarely found in the normal heart, mild hypokinesia is frequently observed and may represent normal regional heterogeneity. The normal myocardium also displays transmural heterogeneity of contraction, decreasing from endocardium to epicardium.

Apart from normal heterogeneity, other factors that could cause RWMAs should also be considered. Acute alterations in LV loading conditions (decreased preload or increased afterload) may depress LV function without directly affecting coronary flow. Similarly, myocardial "stunning" may result in the persistence of an RWMA well after the restoration of normal coronary blood flow. Moreover, tethering of normal cardiac tissue to an ischemic area of muscle may result in an area of dysfunctional myocardium that appears larger than the actual ischemic zone. Nonischemic causes of RWMAs are listed in Table 21–4.

Additional limitations to the use of TEE as a method for diagnosing myocardial ischemia arise because of variations in coronary artery distribution. Approximately 70% of patients have a right-dominant coronary circulation in which the posterior descending artery arises from the right coronary circulation to supply the inferior and inferoseptal walls. In 10% of patients, the coronary circulation is left dominant, in that the posterior descending artery arises from the circumflex artery, and the remaining 20% are co-dominant. There is also marked individual variability in the blood supply to the LV apex. Although the midpapillary short-axis view is ideal for monitoring ischemia in areas supplied by the major epicardial vessels, it may

Table 21–4. Nonischemic Causes of Regional Wall Motion Abnormalities.

Coronary artery disease related:
Infarcted myocardium
Stunned myocardium
Altered loading:
Severe increases in afterload
Marked reduction in preload
Tethering
Normal regional heterogeneity:
Range of segmental radial shortening: 0% to 100%
Range of segmental wall thickening: 0% to 150%
Abnormal conduction:
Left bundle branch block
Paced rhythm

not reflect ischemia involving more peripheral and smaller coronary arterioles. As a result, basilar, apical, or RV ischemia may go undiagnosed. In fact, the sensitivity and specificity of recognizing intraoperative ischemic episodes echocardiographically in real time are only moderate (76% for both), with substantial variability in evaluating the severity of regional dysfunction.[20] This could partly explain the discordance between TEE and ECG changes reported in surgical populations. In studies comparing ECG and TEE, only about 25% of patients had temporal overlap between TEE and ECG ischemic changes,[18] and only 15% of patients who developed postoperative myocardial infarction were identified by both modalities.[15] Another potential explanation for the observed discordance is that ECG does not readily detect repolarization abnormalities in the inferior wall, an area where RWMAs are commonly observed. Monitoring the long-axis of the left ventricle in addition to the standard short-axis view may increase the detection of ischemia by approximately 40%. Advancements in technology that permit simultaneous multiplane imaging of a coronary distribution (eg, real-time three-dimensional echocardiography) may improve the ischemia detection capacity of TEE (see Chapter 24).

Hemodynamic Monitoring

The introduction of the pulmonary artery catheter (PAC) in the 1970s dramatically changed the perioperative management of critically ill patients. The use of the PAC significantly increased diagnostic ability, allowing clinicians to optimize cardiac output (CO) and oxygen delivery, while reducing the risk of pulmonary edema by avoiding excessive increases in PAWP. Although previously established that PAC-guided hemodynamic optimization of high-risk patients, prior to the onset of organ failure, significantly reduces mortality, more recent data have implicated the use of the PAC in increasing mortality.[21]

The information derived from a PAC is based on pressure and flow measurements. In comparison, TEE allows the anesthesiologist to visualize the heart and measure filling volumes more accurately, while offering a less invasive alternative for measuring CO. TEE provides real-time evaluation of both cardiac anatomy and function that complements invasive hemodynamic monitoring. Its use in patients undergoing major noncardiac surgery may benefit the clinician in making decisions regarding fluid management, initiation of vasoactive infusions, and evaluation of myocardial ischemia. However, whether a TEE-guided treatment algorithm could be used to guide hemodynamic optimization has yet to be determined. It may be difficult to establish an outcome benefit, given the nature of associated complications and the improvement in both intraoperative and postoperative management of high-risk surgical patients in recent years.

Measurement of Cardiac Output

The ability to steer a pulsed-wave or continuous-wave Doppler beam parallel to the direction of blood flow makes TEE CO measurement possible in more than 95% of patients.[22] The flow volume passing through a vessel or an orifice can be calculated as the product of the velocity-time integral (VTI) and the cross-sectional area (CSA). The preferred sites for determining stroke volume (SV) and CO are the left ventricular outflow tract (LVOT), the aortic annulus, the mitral annulus, and the pulmonic annulus. Of these sites, the LVOT is used most often, since the entire systemic SV traverses the LVOT, flow is usually laminar, and the LVOT is a circular structure with a relatively constant diameter throughout systole. SV is derived as:

$$SV = CSA \times VTI$$

Since the area of a circle = πr^2, CSA can be derived from diameter (D) as:

$$CSA = D^2 \times \frac{\pi}{4} = D^2 \times 0.785$$

To determine CO through the LVOT, diameter is measured during mid-systole in the midesophageal long-axis view. Care has to be taken to avoid foreshortening of the LVOT, and the measurement is made immediately proximal to the aortic valve annulus (see Chapter 4). Since the LVOT diameter is squared, this is the most important measurement in determining CO. Depending on which view allows parallel alignment to the flow of blood, the LVOT VTI is measured from the transgastric or deep transgastric long-axis view. Pulsed-wave Doppler is used, although in the absence of aortic stenosis, a continuous-wave Doppler beam across the aortic valve is also acceptable.

Studies have demonstrated good correlation between TEE and thermodilution CO measurements ($r = 0.90$ to 0.98) with good accuracy (bias 0.01 to 0.17 L/min).[22] It therefore appears that TEE-guided CO measurement could offer an acceptable alternative to the PAC thermodilution method.

Measurement of LV Preload

The ventricular pressure-volume relationship is variable between patients, and may even change during a surgical procedure. Unlike the PAC, TEE does not rely on pressure-derived volume estimates that are subject to the confounding influences of ventricular compliance, positive pressure ventilation, or valvular disease. It is therefore not surprising that TEE is more sensitive in detecting changes in preload than PAWP.[11,23]

Various techniques are available for measuring LV volumes, each offering distinct advantages and limitations. Instant qualitative estimation of LVEDA in the midpapillary transgastric view might provide valuable information in the hemodynamically unstable patient, where cavity obliteration or marked ventricular dilation could provide sufficient information to guide immediate therapy. However, more objective measurements of LV volumes are often required to maintain euvolemia and guide interventions, especially in the patient with compromised ventricular function. The ideal assessment of LV preload would be a three-dimensional assessment of end-diastolic volume, using geometric models to estimate LV end-diastolic volume. Among the various models that have been described, three methods have been validated by TEE: the length-diameter (or prolate-ellipsoid) method, the modified Simpson rule (Figure 21–3), and the cylinder–hemi-ellipsoid method. An acceptable compromise for monitoring purposes, quantitative LVEDA measurement takes advantage of the fact that 90% of the stroke volume is derived from shortening of the ventricular short axis. Several investigators have shown that compared to radionuclide angiography, quantitative LVEDA measurement can provide adequate estimates of LV end-diastolic volume.[24,25] Furthermore, correlations between LVEDA and stroke volume are acceptable ($r = 0.90$; $P < .001$), while PAWP correlates poorly with stroke volume, especially in the presence of impaired LV systolic and diastolic function.[26-28]

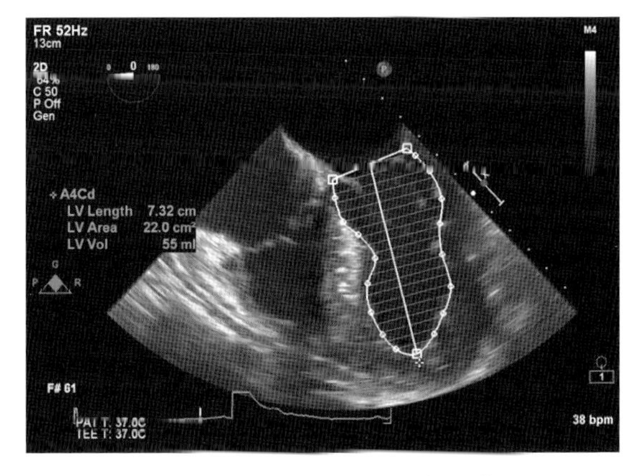

FIGURE 21–3. Left ventricular end-diastolic or end-systolic volumes can be estimated more accurately, in particular in irregularly shaped ventricles, using the modified Simpson rule where the left ventricle is modeled as a series of stacked cylindrical disks.

Newer techniques, such as harmonic imaging, that are aimed at more clearly delineating the endocardial border may further improve the TEE assessment of intravascular volume. Three-dimensional echocardiography has demonstrated superior accuracy and reproducibility for measurement of LV volume (see Chapter 24). Calculating volume in three dimensions overcomes the most basic shortcoming of two-dimensional echocardiography, namely that it does not require any geometric model assumptions. In addition, this technique adapts well to asymmetric ventricles, provides the ability to delineate the entire endocardial contour, and eliminates the need to assume the appropriate short-axis plane relative to the long-axis plane.

PRELOAD RECRUITABLE STROKE VOLUME

Occult hypovolemia is thought to be a key factor in the etiology of postoperative morbidity, and may not be detected by routine heart rate and arterial pressure measurements.[29] Intraoperative gut hypoperfusion, which may occur in about 60% of patients during major surgery, is associated with increased morbidity and postoperative hospital stay.[29] "Goal-directed fluid therapy," wherein preload-recruitable stroke volume and the associated increase in CVP or PAWP are measured in response to an intravenous bolus of fluid, has recently been shown to improve gut perfusion and postoperative outcome. Thus, the current consensus on protocolized intraoperative fluid management is that judicious perioperative fluid management should be practiced, avoiding tissue hypoperfusion, while at the same time avoiding fluid overload and its associated complications.[30]

During hypervolemic hemodilution, volume administration has been demonstrated to significantly increase stroke volume and LVEDA up to a threshold, beyond which no further increases were observed,[31] despite continued increases in PAWP. LVEDA is therefore able to detect the upper threshold or end point, beyond which additional fluid is not warranted. However, it was not possible to identify an overall optimal LVEDA below which most patients demonstrate volume-recruitable increases in stroke volume.[28] It appears also that patients who do not increase their stroke volume by more than 20% in response to a bolus of fluid are more likely to have diastolic dysfunction, which can be measured by TEE. In fact, mitral Doppler indices of diastolic dysfunction might be superior to two dimensional echocardiographic and hemodynamic variables in predicting responsiveness of cardiac output to fluid therapy.[32] The impact of diastolic dysfunction on occult hypovolemia and outcomes in goal-directed fluid therapy has not yet been investigated.

Table 21–5. Estimation of Intracardiac Pressures.

Pressure	Equation
RVSP or PASP	4 (peak TR velocity^2) + RAP
MPAP	4 (peak PI velocity^2) + RAP
PADP	4 (end-diastolic PI velocity^2)
LAP	Systolic BP – 4 (peak MR velocity^2)
LVEDP	Diastolic BP – 4 (end-diastolic AI velocity^2)

RVSP, right ventricular systolic pressure; PASP, pulmonary artery systolic pressure; TR, tricuspid regurgitation; RAP, right atrial pressure; MPAP, mean pulmonary artery pressure; PI, pulmonary insufficiency; PADP, pulmonary artery diastolic pressure; LAP, left atrial pressure; MR, mitral regurgitation; LVEDP, left ventricular end-diastolic pressure; AI, aortic insufficiency

MEASUREMENT OF INTRACARDIAC PRESSURES

Pressure gradients between chambers of the heart can be calculated at various locations by using the modified Bernoulli equation (pressure gradient = $4V^2$). If the absolute pressure in one of the chambers is known, the pressure in the other chamber can be calculated. If right atrial pressure (RAP) or CVP is known, peak RV systolic pressure can be estimated by adding CVP to the peak systolic pressure gradient across the tricuspid valve, which can be determined by measuring the peak velocity of a tricuspid regurgitant jet using continuous-wave Doppler. In the absence of pulmonic stenosis, peak RV systolic pressure equals PA systolic pressure. Other pressures that can be estimated similarly include LA, PA diastolic, and LV end-diastolic pressure by measuring the velocities of mitral regurgitation, pulmonic regurgitation, and aortic regurgitation jets (Table 21–5; see Chapter 4).

TRANSPLANT SURGERY

Solid organ transplantation continues to be the definitive treatment for end-stage disease of the heart, lung, liver, and kidneys. The disease processes that result in end-organ failure are complex and multifactorial, and all have a deleterious effect on cardiac function. Regardless of the failing organ system, a thorough preoperative cardiac evaluation is essential to the care of these patients; both transthoracic echocardiography (TTE) and TEE are utilized extensively in the initial evaluation of this patient population.

Lung Transplantation

Intraoperative management of patients undergoing lung transplantation (LTX) provides the clinician with a unique set of challenges. Patients have limited pulmonary reserve, require one-lung ventilation, and undergo rapid, significant hemodynamic disturbances throughout the procedure. Anesthetic monitoring often includes TEE as it allows the clinician to track changes in preload and to diagnose and manage hypotension, hypoxemia, and graft dysfunction.

INDUCTION OF ANESTHESIA

Induction of general anesthesia in patients undergoing LTX is associated with a significant risk of cardiovascular collapse. Dynamic hyperinflation or auto–positive end-expiratory pressure (PEEP) may occur following initiation of positive-pressure ventilation in patients with chronic obstructive pulmonary disease (COPD), which could result in cardiovascular collapse due to decreased venous return, similar to tamponade.[33] The TEE findings are similar to cardiac tamponade without evidence of pericardial fluid. Right atrial and right ventricular compression can be seen, and compression of the left atrium (LA) and ventricle (LV) is also common. Rapid diagnosis is essential because the treatment is simply to disconnect the patient from the ventilator. Hypotension should gradually resolve as the lungs passively deflate and normal chamber size returns on TEE imaging.

Significant hypoxemia may also be encountered following induction and intubation. The causes of hypoxemia are multifactorial and require rapid assessment and diagnosis. The most likely causes should be ruled out first—fiberoptic bronchoscopy should confirm proper tube placement and position as well as evaluate for secretions and plugs. TEE can be used to further eliminate other causes of hypoxemia such as intracardiac shunts (eg, atrial septal defect [ASD], patent foramen ovale [PFO]) and RV failure. If inadequate oxygenation persists, CPB may be required to successfully complete the operation.

Patients presenting for LTX often have significant pulmonary hypertension. Estimation of PA systolic pressure is accomplished by measuring the maximum velocity jet of tricuspid regurgitation and using the simplified Bernouli equation. However, Doppler-derived pressure gradients of pulmonary artery pressures may be inaccurate in patients with advanced lung disease.[34] The right ventricle compensates for pulmonary hypertension via hypertrophy and dilation. Right ventricular reserves are therefore limited, and failure may be precipitated by inadequate oxygenation and ventilation or clamping of the pulmonary artery. TEE provides an excellent diagnostic tool for evaluation of right ventricular failure.

PULMONARY ARTERY CLAMPING

The initial response to ipsilateral PA clamping is an increase in PA pressure, which could precipitate RV failure.

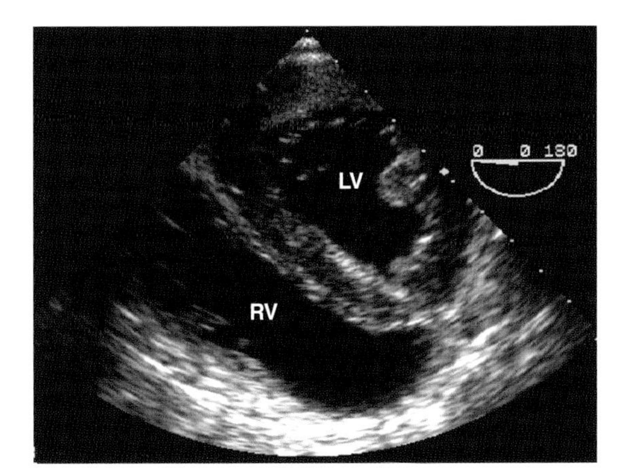

FIGURE 21–4. Flattening of the interventricular septum leading to a D-shaped left ventricle as a consequence of increased right ventricular volume or pressure. (LV, left ventricle; RV, right ventricle.)

If the RV does not tolerate PA clamping, CPB might be required. The echocardiographic signs of impending RV failure include (1) RV dilation with resultant tricuspid regurgitation; (2) RV hypokinesis, especially of the free wall; (3) systolic and diastolic flattening of the interventricular septum, leading to a D-shaped LV (Figure 21–4); (4) paradoxical septal motion—the RV becomes more concentric and the LV more crescent shaped; and (5) dilation of the RA, inferior vena cava (IVC), and PA.

Assessment of Vascular Anastomoses

Elevated PA pressures following reperfusion of lung allografts are concerning for elevated pulmonary vascular resistance, pulmonary edema, and ultimately graft failure. There are multiple causes of elevated PA pressures, which include strictures of the pulmonary artery or venous anastomoses, intrapulmonary thrombi, or acute graft rejection. TEE rapidly provides accurate information that complements invasive hemodynamic monitoring.

The right and left pulmonary arteries are imaged using the midesophageal ascending aortic short-axis view (Figure 21–5). Careful evaluation of the anastomoses, particularly with respect to the location of the PAC, is important since PA pressures may not accurately reflect lung perfusion pressures if the catheter is placed proximal to an anastomotic stricture. Pressure gradients up to 20 mm Hg across an anastomosis are acceptable.

Pulmonary vein flow should also be evaluated using both color-flow Doppler and pulsed-wave Doppler. Additionally, the anastomotic diameter should be measured. Anastomoses greater than 0.5 cm and peak systolic velocities less than 100 cm/s are considered acceptable.[35,36] Causes of increased pulmonary vein flow velocities to consider include pulmonary venous stricture, external compression by either thrombus or pericardial wrap, and intracardiac thrombus.

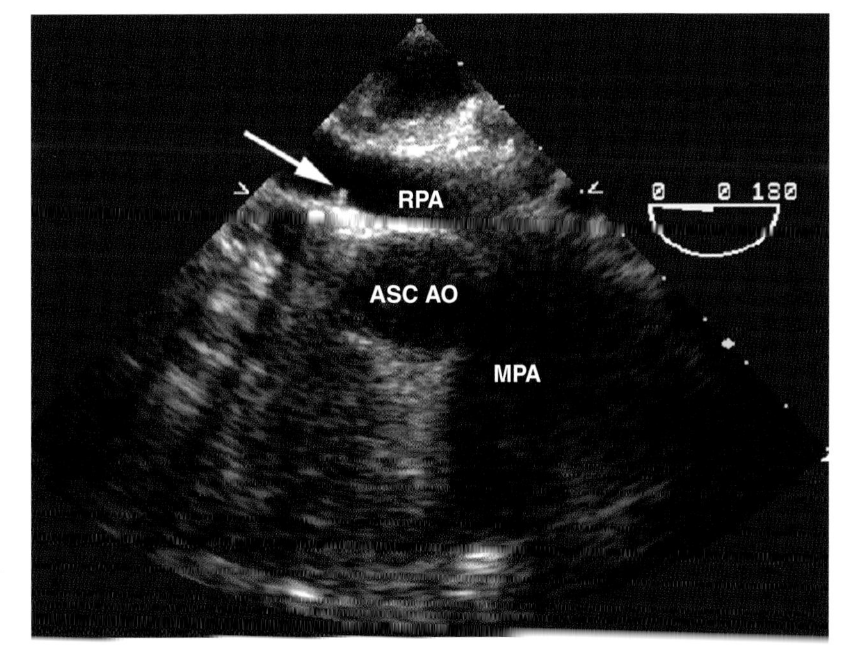

FIGURE 21–5. Right pulmonary artery anastomosis *(arrow)* imaged with transesophageal echocardiography. (ASC AO, ascending aorta; MPA, main pulmonary artery; RPA, right pulmonary artery.)

Vascular complications following LTX have a high mortality. Furthermore, reoperation to repair anastomotic stenosis often requires CPB, inflicting further ischemic injury to lung allografts. Before committing to reoperation, accurate assessment must be performed. Because TEE is often able to visualize anastomoses, it provides information that is not available through traditional hemodynamic monitoring.

POSTOPERATIVE CARE

Postoperative care of the lung transplant patient is as critical to success as intraoperative management. Declining pulmonary function is often subtle and requires a high degree of suspicion and early evaluation. Focused examination of right ventricular function, pulmonary arterial and venous anastomoses, and cardiac structure should help guide therapy. Identification of pulmonary venous thrombosis is critical. While resolution of small thrombi has been reported in the literature, large thrombi are associated with increased risk of morbidity and mortality.[36]

Liver Transplant

Patients presenting for liver transplantation often suffer from multiorgan system failure and limited reserve to respond to the significant physiological stress imposed by liver transplant surgery. End-stage liver disease may affect the cardiovascular, pulmonary, renal, and central nervous systems as well as the coagulation system. The cardiovascular system is noted to be hyperdynamic with markedly increased cardiac output and decreased systemic vascular resistance. The use of TEE as an adjunct to traditional hemodynamic monitoring, which includes PAC monitoring, continues to increase, and has been shown to be helpful in managing fluid therapy, monitoring myocardial function, the management of pulmonary hypertension, and identifying intraoperative complications such as air embolism or thromboembolism.[37,38]

The risk of bleeding from variceal injury remains a concern. In spite of the widespread use of TEE during liver transplantation, there are no reports in the literature of variceal bleeding associated with TEE.[39] Nevertheless, it seems prudent to restrict the use of TEE in patients with known varices to those with strong clinical indications and to account for additional risk factors such as the grade of varices and presence of coagulopathy.[40] Even though a history of variceal bleeding is not viewed as a contraindication, the use of TEE should probably be discouraged in patients with a history of recent or recurrent variceal bleeding.

Intraoperative TEE is particularly useful in assessing and managing patients with portopulmonary hypertension (POPH). The presence of POPH increases the risk for perioperative and long-term morbidity and mortality associated with liver transplantation. POPH is defined as a mean pulmonary arterial pressure (MPAP) of greater than 25 mm Hg with a PAWP of less than 15 mm Hg. While mild POPH (MPAP 25 to 35 mm Hg) does not appear to adversely impact liver transplantation, patients with preoperative mean pulmonary artery pressures of or exceeding 50 mm Hg have mortality rates of 60% to 100%, and are not suitable candidates for surgery.[41] For patients with mean pressures between 35 and 50 mm Hg, mortality rates are 35% to 40%, and this group of patients requires meticulous assessment of right ventricular function prior to surgery. In the absence of RV dysfunction, surgery is not contraindicated, and intraoperative TEE-guided management of RV filling and function could be particularly useful.

Liver transplantation can be divided into three distinct phases, each with its own set of management challenges: dissection, anhepatic, and reperfusion.

DISSECTION PHASE

Hemodynamic instability during dissection is most often caused by hypovolemia from drainage of ascites, compression of major vessels, clinically significant acute blood loss, or "third-space" fluid loss. TEE is an excellent monitor to guide fluid management during this phase, but requires a complete examination at baseline for comparison. There are several case reports in the literature demonstrating the utility of intraoperative TEE in patients with dynamic LVOT obstruction, wherein maintenance of preload and afterload is critical to reduce the gradient across the LVOT.[42]

ANHEPATIC PHASE

Hemodynamic disturbances during the anhepatic phase are most likely caused by inadequate preload due to a reduction in venous return. However, there is some evidence that both RV and LV dysfunction could occur during the anhepatic stage, which may be attributable to endotoxemia.[43] Hemodynamic support during this phase is best achieved with inotropic support and cautious fluid therapy, in anticipation of the restoration of normal venous return and a potential hypertensive pulmonary response following reperfusion.

REPERFUSION PHASE

Reperfusion of the transplanted liver can be associated with significant hemodynamic fluctuation as a consequence of hypovolemia, metabolic derangements, pulmonary embolism, pulmonary hypertension, and right or left ventricular dysfunction. TEE can be used to accurately diagnose the underlying abnormality and guide treatment.

Pulmonary hypertension is a common response to reperfusion, progressing to right ventricular dysfunction and tricuspid regurgitation. The etiology is probably

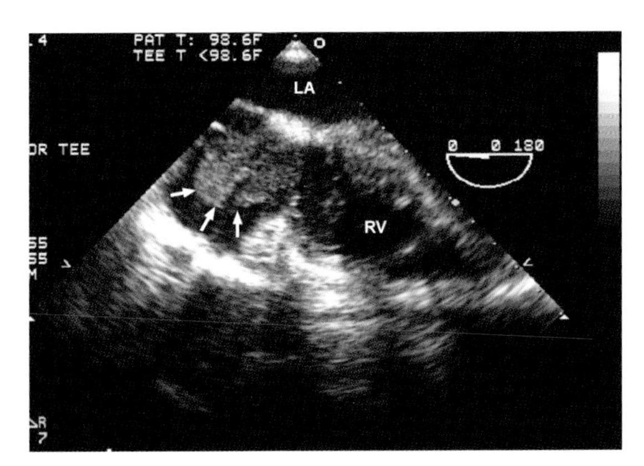

FIGURE 21–6. Large thrombus *(arrows)* seen in the right atrium during the reperfusion phase of liver transplantation. (LA, left atrium; RV, right ventricle.)

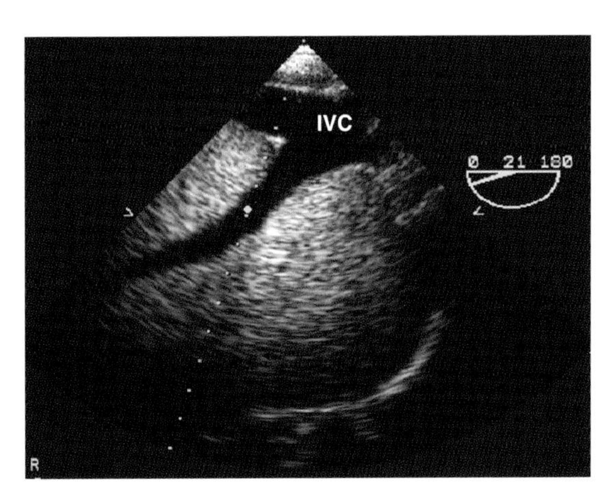

FIGURE 21–7. Assessment of the inferior vena cava and hepatic vein using transesophageal echocardiography. A pulsed-wave Doppler cursor is positioned on the hepatic vein, which usually enters the inferior vena cava tangentially as shown. (IVC, inferior vena cava.)

related to metabolic changes and embolic phenomena. Virtually all patients experience venous microemboli at the time of reperfusion, while macroemboli (Figure 21–6) ranging from 1 to 5 cm have been observed in almost 25% of patients.[44] Right ventricular dysfunction, and in particular tricuspid regurgitation, can result in venous congestion of the liver allograft, which is particularly poorly tolerated and should be avoided and aggressively treated. Venous congestion in the absence of an elevated CVP should raise the suspicion of outflow obstruction at the level of the suprahepatic cava or hepatic vein. To visualize the IVC and hepatic veins the IVC is followed down from where it enters the right atrium in the bicaval view. The liver and hepatic veins can then be brought into view by turning the probe to the right (Figure 21–7; see Chapter 12).

PREGNANCY

Peripartum Cardiomyopathy

Peripartum cardiomyopathy (PPCM) is a rare, life-threatening disease of unknown etiology. The diagnostic criteria for PPCM include (1) development of congestive heart failure (CHF) due to decreased left ventricular systolic function, (2) no pre-existing cardiac dysfunction, (3) no other cause of cardiomyopathy, and (4) ejection fraction less than 40% by echocardiography.[45] Variable numbers are reported worldwide, but the incidence in the United States is about 1 per 3000 to 4000 pregnancies.[45,46] Even though 50% of women will recover ventricular function within 6 months, women with continued ventricular dysfunction have a reported mortality rate of 85%.[47,48]

Obstetrical management requires communication and careful planning between obstetrics, cardiology, and anesthesiology. Elective induction of labor at term is preferred in medically stable patients. Early neuroaxial analgesia is suggested to limit the hemodynamic changes associated with labor. Invasive monitoring with an arterial and central venous catheter is recommended. Emergent cesarean section may be necessary due to acute maternal decompensation. TEE is an excellent complement to invasive hemodynamic monitoring in patients requiring general anesthesia.

Amniotic Fluid Embolism

Amniotic fluid embolism (AFE) is a rare obstetrical emergency with estimated incidence of 1 in 8000 to 1 in 50,000. The pathophysiology of AFE is poorly understood with several hypothesized triggers. Signs and symptoms of AFE occur in a two stage process. In the first stage, pulmonary hypertension leads to RV failure, hypotension, and hypoxia. Hypoxia further exacerbates myocardial damage, ultimately leading to LV failure, while alveolar damage progresses to acute respiratory distress syndrome. Echocardiographic findings are consistent with pulmonary hypertension and RV failure. There is a leftward shift of the interatrial septum and a bowing of the interventricular septum. In the acute setting, LV function is preserved; however, as the disease evolves there is subsequent LV failure. The mortality during the first stage is estimated to be 37% to 80%.[49] TEE provides a rapid, accurate diagnostic tool as well as a subsequent monitor to guide medical management in patients with amniotic fluid embolism.

REFERENCES

1. Maslow A, Bert A, Schwartz C, Mackinnon S. Transesophageal echocardiography in the noncardiac surgical patient. *Int Anesthesiol Clin.* 2002;40(1):73-132.
2. Mahmood F, Christie A, Matyal R. Transesophageal echocardiography and noncardiac surgery. *Semin Cardiothorac Vasc Anesth.* 2008;12(4):265-289.
3. Bilotta F, Tempe DK, Giovannini F, Rosa G. Perioperative transoesophageal echocardiography in noncardiac surgery. *Ann Card Anaesth.* 2006;9(2):108-113.
4. Catena E, Mele D. Role of intraoperative transesophageal echocardiography in patients undergoing noncardiac surgery. *J Cardiovasc Med (Hagerstown).* 2008;9(10):993-1003.
5. Hofer CK, Zollinger A, Rak M, et al. Therapeutic impact of intraoperative transoesophageal echocardiography during noncardiac surgery. *Anaesthesia.* 2004;59(1):3-9.
6. Kneeshaw JD. Transoesophageal echocardiography (TOE) in the operating room. *Br J Anaesth.* 2006;97(1):77-84.
7. Schulmeyer MC, Santelices E, Vega R, Schmied S. Impact of intraoperative transesophageal echocardiography during noncardiac surgery. *J Cardiothorac Vasc Anesth.* 2006;20(6):768-771.
8. Subramaniam B, Park KW. Impact of TEE in noncardiac surgery. *Int Anesthesiol Clin.* 2008;46(2):121-136.
9. Practice Guidelines for Perioperative Transesophageal Echocardiography. An Updated Report by the American Society of Anesthesiologists and the Society of Cardiovascular Anesthesiologists Task Force on Transesophageal Echocardiography. Anesthesiology 2010;112:1084-1096.
10. Leung JM, Levine EH. Left ventricular end-systolic cavity obliteration as an estimate of intraoperative hypovolemia. *Anesthesiology.* 1994;81(5):1102-1109.
11. Swenson JD, Bull D, Stringham J. Subjective assessment of left ventricular preload using transesophageal echocardiography: corresponding pulmonary artery occlusion pressures. *J Cardiothorac Vasc Anesth.* 2001;15(5):580-583.
12. Torbicki A, Galie N, Covezzoli A, Rossi E, De Rosa M, Goldhaber SZ. Right heart thrombi in pulmonary embolism: results from the International Cooperative Pulmonary Embolism Registry. *J Am Coll Cardiol.* 2003;41(12):2245-2251.
13. Varriale P, Maldonado JM. Echocardiographic observations during in hospital cardiopulmonary resuscitation. *Crit Care Med.* 1997;25(10):1717-1720.
14. Waters DD, Da Luz P, Wyatt HL, Swan HJ, Forrester JS. Early changes in regional and global left ventricular function induced by graded reductions in regional coronary perfusion. *Am J Cardiol.* 1977;39(4):537-543.
15. Comunale ME, Body SC, Ley C, et al. The concordance of intraoperative left ventricular wall-motion abnormalities and electrocardiographic S-T segment changes: association with outcome after coronary revascularization. Multicenter Study of Perioperative Ischemia (McSPI) Research Group. *Anesthesiology.* 1998;88(4):945-954.
16. Leung JM, O'Kelly B, Browner WS, Tubau J, Hollenberg M, Mangano DT. Prognostic importance of postbypass regional wall-motion abnormalities in patients undergoing coronary artery bypass graft surgery. SPI Research Group. *Anesthesiology.* 1989;71(1):16-25.
17. Swaminathan M, Morris RW, De Meyts DD, et al. Deterioration of regional wall motion immediately after coronary artery bypass graft surgery is associated with long-term major adverse cardiac events. *Anesthesiology.* 2007;107(5):739-745.
18. London MJ, Tubau JF, Wong MG, et al. The "natural history" of segmental wall motion abnormalities in patients undergoing noncardiac surgery. S.P.I. Research Group. *Anesthesiology.* 1990; 73(4):644-655.
19. Pandian NG, Skorton DJ, Collins SM, Falsetti HL, Burke ER, Kerber RE. Heterogeneity of left ventricular segmental wall thickening and excursion in 2-dimensional echocardiograms of normal human subjects. *Am J Cardiol.* 1983;51(10):1667-1673.
20. Bergquist BD, Leung JM, Bellows WH. Transesophageal echocardiography in myocardial revascularization: I. Accuracy of intraoperative real-time interpretation. *Anesth Analg.* 1996;82(6): 1132-1138.
21. Kern JW, Shoemaker WC. Meta-analysis of hemodynamic optimization in high-risk patients. *Crit Care Med.* 2002;30(8): 1686-1692.
22. Perrino AC Jr, Harris SN, Luther MA. Intraoperative determination of cardiac output using multiplane transesophageal echocardiography: a comparison to thermodilution. *Anesthesiology.* 1998;89(2):350-357.
23. Costachescu T, Denault A, Guimond JG, et al. The hemodynamically unstable patient in the intensive care unit: hemodynamic vs. transesophageal echocardiographic monitoring. *Crit Care Med.* 2002;30(6):1214-1223.
24. Ryan T, Burwash I, Lu J, et al. The agreement between ventricular volumes and ejection fraction by transesophageal echocardiography or a combined radionuclear and thermodilution technique in patients after coronary artery surgery. *J Cardiothorac Vasc Anesth.* 1996;10(3):323-328.
25. Clements FM, Harpole DH, Quill T, Jones RH, McCann RL. Estimation of left ventricular volume and ejection fraction by two-dimensional transoesophageal echocardiography: comparison of short axis imaging and simultaneous radionuclide angiography. *Br J Anaesth.* 1990;64(3):331-336.
26. Cheung AT, Savino JS, Weiss SJ, Aukburg SJ, Berlin JA. Echocardiographic and hemodynamic indexes of left ventricular preload in patients with normal and abnormal ventricular function. *Anesthesiology.* 1994;81(2):376-387.
27. Thys DM, Hillel Z, Goldman ME, Mindich BP, Kaplan JA. A comparison of hemodynamic indices derived by invasive monitoring and two-dimensional echocardiography. *Anesthesiology.* 1987;67(5):630-634.
28. Tousignant CP, Walsh F, Mazer CD. The use of transesophageal echocardiography for preload assessment in critically ill patients. *Anesth Analg.* 2000;90(2):351-355.
29. Mythen MG, Webb AR. Intra-operative gut mucosal hypoperfusion is associated with increased post-operative complications and cost. *Intensive Care Med.* 1994;20(2):99-104.
30. Joshi GP. Intraoperative fluid restriction improves outcome after major elective gastrointestinal surgery. *Anesth Analg.* 2005;101(2): 601-605.
31. van Daele ME, Trouwborst A, van Woerkens LC, Tenbrinck R, Fraser AG, Roelandt JR. Transesophageal echocardiographic monitoring of preoperative acute hypervolemic hemodilution. *Anesthesiology.* 1994;81(3):602-609.
32. Lattik R, Couture P, Denault AY, et al. Mitral Doppler indices are superior to two-dimensional echocardiographic and hemodynamic variables in predicting responsiveness of cardiac output to a rapid intravenous infusion of colloid. *Anesth Analg.* 2002;94(5):1092-1099, table of contents.

33. O'Donnell DE, Laveneziana P. The clinical importance of dynamic lung hyperinflation in COPD. *COPD.* 2006;3(4): 219-232.
34. Arcasoy SM, Christie JD, Ferrari VA, et al. Echocardiographic assessment of pulmonary hypertension in patients with advanced lung disease. *Am J Respir Crit Care Med.* 2003;167(5): 735-740.
35. Michel-Cherqui M, Brusset A, Liu N, et al. Intraoperative transesophageal echocardiographic assessment of vascular anastomoses in lung transplantation. A report on 18 cases. *Chest.* 1997;111(5):1229-1235.
36. Schulman LL, Anandarangam T, Leibowitz DW, et al. Four-year prospective study of pulmonary venous thrombosis after lung transplantation. *J Am Soc Echocardiogr.* 2001;14(8):806-812.
37. Wax DB, Torres A, Scher C, Leibowitz AB. Transesophageal echocardiography utilization in high-volume liver transplantation centers in the United States. *J Cardiothorac Vasc Anesth.* 2008;22(6):811-813.
38. De Wolf AM, Aggarwal S. Monitoring preload during liver transplantation. *Liver Transpl.* 2008;14(3):268-269.
39. Spier BJ, Larue SJ, Teelin TC, et al. Review of complications in a series of patients with known gastro-esophageal varices undergoing transesophageal echocardiography. *J Am Soc Echocardiogr.* 2009;22(4):396-400.
40. Spencer KT. Transesophageal echocardiography in patients with esophageal varices. *J Am Soc Echocardiogr.* 2009;22(4):401-403.
41. Rodriguez-Roisin R, Krowka MJ, Herve P, Fallon MB. Pulmonary-hepatic vascular disorders (PHD). *Eur Respir J.* 2004;24(5): 861-880.
42. Cywinski JB, Argalious M, Marks TN, Parker BM. Dynamic left ventricular outflow tract obstruction in an orthotopic liver transplant recipient. *Liver Transpl.* 2005;11(6):692-695.
43. Guimond JG, Pinsky MR, Matuschak GM. Effect of synchronous increase in intrathoracic pressure on cardiac performance during acute endotoxemia. *J Appl Physiol.* 1990;69(4):1502-1508.
44. Suriani RJ, Cutrone A, Feierman D, Konstadt S. Intraoperative transesophageal echocardiography during liver transplantation. *J Cardiothorac Vasc Anesth.* 1996;10(6):699-707.
45. Pearson GD, Veille JC, Rahimtoola S, et al. Peripartum cardiomyopathy: National Heart, Lung, and Blood Institute and Office of Rare Diseases (National Institutes of Health) workshop recommendations and review. *JAMA.* 2000;283(9):1183-1188.
46. Abboud J, Murad Y, Chen-Scarabelli C, Saravolatz L, Scarabelli TM. Peripartum cardiomyopathy: a comprehensive review. *Int J Cardiol.* 2007;118(3):295-303.
47. Demakis JG, Rahimtoola SH, Sutton GC, et al. Natural course of peripartum cardiomyopathy. *Circulation.* 1971;44(6):1053-1061.
48. Sutton MS, Cole P, Plappert M, Saltzman D, Goldhaber S. Effects of subsequent pregnancy on left ventricular function in peripartum cardiomyopathy. *Am Heart J.* 1991;121(6 Pt 1):1776-1778.
49. Tuffnell DJ. United Kingdom Amniotic Fluid Embolism Register. *BJOG.* 2005;112(12):1625-1629.

REVIEW QUESTIONS

Select the *one* best answer for each of the following questions.

1. Indications for intraoperative TEE during cardiac surgery include:
   a. Confirm and refine the preoperative diagnosis
   b. Detect new or unsuspected pathology
   c. Adjust the anesthetic and surgical plan
   d. Assess results of the surgical intervention
   e. All of the above

2. Of the following options, which provides the best intraoperative estimation of inadequate preload?
   a. Reduced RV volume
   b. Low LVEDA
   c. Systolic cavity obliteration
   d. Paradoxical septal motion
   e. Turbulence in the LVOT

3. Which of the following would be the most useful echocardiographic finding in assessing a patient with intraoperative hypotension not responding to inotropic support?
   a. Interatrial septal excursion of more than 1 cm
   b. Systolic flow reversal in the descending aorta
   c. Dilated RV with rightward bulging of the interatrial septum
   d. Systolic anterior motion of the mitral valve
   e. Inferior LV hypokinesis

4. Which of the following is **NOT** seen in a pericardial tamponade?
   a. Systolic collapse of the right ventricle
   b. Diastolic collapse of the right atrium
   c. Abnormal ventricular septal motion
   d. Respiratory variation in ventricle chamber size
   e. Plethora of the inferior vena cava

5. Which of the following is not a potential cause of RWMA?
   a. Left bundle branch block
   b. Right bundle branch block
   c. Increased afterload
   d. Stunned myocardium
   e. AV pacing

6. Which of the following views is used in determining stroke volume?
   a. ME LAX
   b. TG mid SAX
   c. Four-chamber view
   d. Bicaval view
   e. Mitral commissural view

7. TEE is superior to the PA catheter in the determination of:
   a. Cardiac output
   b. Mixed venous saturation
   c. Pulmonary arterial pressure

d. Preload
e. Afterload

Use the following information to answer questions 8 through 10:

Central venous pressure = 10 mm Hg

Heart rate = 80 beats per minute

Peak blood velocity across the aortic valve = 300 cm/s

Peak blood velocity across the pulmonary valve = 200 cm/s

Peak velocity of the tricuspid regurgitant jet = 300 cm/s

Time velocity interval of blood flow through the left ventricular outflow tract = 15 cm

Left ventricular outflow tract diameter = 20 mm

8. Which is the peak instantaneous pressure gradient across the aortic valve?
   a. Cannot be calculated
   b. 26 mm Hg
   c. 36 mm Hg
   d. 46 mmHg
   e. 56 mm Hg

9. What is the best estimate of the cardiac output?
   a. 4.5 L/min
   b. 3.8 L/min
   c. 4.8 L/min
   d. 2.8 L/min
   e. 5.8 L/min

10. What is the best estimate of the pulmonary artery systolic pressure?
    a. 46 mm Hg
    b. 36 mm Hg
    c. 30 mm Hg
    d. 40 mm Hg
    e. 20 mm Hg

11. Dynamic hyperinflation:
    a. May occur in patients with obstructive lung disease
    b. Leads to right ventricular dilation and tricuspid regurgitation
    c. Causes flattening of the interventricular septum
    d. Could be treated by pleural aspiration
    e. All of the above

12. The following finding in patients with elevated PA pressures following reperfusion during lung transplant surgery may indicate surgical revision:
    a. A 23 mm Hg gradient across a PA anastomosis
    b. A pulmonary vein anastomotic diameter of 3 mm
    c. Peak systolic pulmonary vein flow velocity of 120 cm/s
    d. All of the above

13. During liver transplant surgery, TEE is used to:
    a. Detect possible obstruction to venous drainage of the allograft
    b. Assess right ventricular function in patients with pulmonary hypertension
    c. Diagnose possible causes of hypotension in reperfusion syndrome
    d. Diagnose embolism
    e. All of the above

14. In patients with documented esophageal varices undergoing liver transplant surgery:
    a. TEE should not be performed if a history of recent variceal bleeding is present.
    b. The potential benefit of intraoperative TEE always outweighs the risk for bleeding.
    c. TEE has not been documented to cause variceal bleeding, and can be performed safely in all patients undergoing liver transplant surgery.
    d. TEE can be performed safely even in coagulopathic patients.
    e. TEE is absolutely contraindicated.

15. The diagnostic criteria for peripartum cardiomyopathy include:
    a. Severe diastolic dysfunction
    b. A history of rheumatic fever
    c. No history of pre-existing cardiac dysfunction
    d. EF of less than 25%
    e. All of the above

16. In amniotic fluid embolism:
    a. TEE could provide a rapid and accurate diagnosis.
    b. Initial pulmonary hypertension leads to RV failure.
    c. ARDS is a prominent feature of the syndrome.
    d. LV function is preserved initially, but could fail as a result of myocardial injury.
    e. All of the above.

TEE in the Critical Care Unit

22

Jordan Hudson and Andrew Shaw

INTRODUCTION

In addition to its role as an intraoperative diagnostic tool, transesophageal echocardiography (TEE) has been shown to be increasingly useful in the critical care setting. Patients in the critical care unit may have impaired cardiac function due to comorbidities or as a result of their critical illness. Indeed, cardiac dysfunction is one of the most common causes of hemodynamic instability and death in critically ill patients.[1] Unlike many other diagnostic modalities available to the intensivist, TEE is minimally invasive and can be rapidly performed at the bedside. It can be used to provide valuable information on cardiac function, guide resuscitation and management, and diagnose a wide range of pathologies that may have a negative impact on the critically ill patient (Table 22–1). TEE was initially applied in the intensive care unit (ICU) for the postoperative evaluation of unstable cardiac surgery patients. However, TEE has also been shown to be beneficial in the general ICU setting, changing management in up to two-thirds of cases.[2,3] In addition to the fact that the use of echocardiography has a positive impact on the management of patients in the general ICU,[4] there is also evidence to support its therapeutic impact and its value in predicting mortality.[5] Surprisingly, despite all these advantages, echocardiography is still not yet available in most ICUs, being largely limited by the availability of trained providers.[5]

INDICATIONS

The indications for TEE, as previously discussed in this manual, also apply to critically ill patients. The ACC/AHA/ASE guidelines define hemodynamic instability and suspected aortic dissection as class I indications for echocardiography in the ICU (ACC/AHA/ASE 2003 guidelines) (Table 22–2). Acutely ill trauma patients should also undergo an echocardiographic evaluation if they are suspected to have cardiac tamponade or aortic injury. The most common indication for which TEE is performed in the ICU is hemodynamic instability, followed by endocarditis, assessment of ventricular function, aortic pathology, and miscellaneous others.[2]

TTE VERSUS TEE

In the general population, transthoracic echocardiography (TTE) is typically the first modality used, as it is noninvasive and more widely available. In the ICU population, however, up to one-half of mechanically ventilated patients cannot be imaged adequately via TTE.[6] Barriers to adequate TTE imaging include mechanical ventilation with positive end-expiratory pressure, wounds and dressings, and body habitus. In addition, many ICU and trauma patients may be too unstable to be positioned in the left lateral decubitus position for TTE imaging. In a study comparing TTE to TEE in patients with unexplained hypotension in the ICU, TTE images were inadequate in over 60% of cases, while TEE provided new, clinically significant diagnoses in 28% that were not seen by TTE.[7] The American College of Cardiology deems TEE a reasonable first test (versus TTE) in patients who are intubated, recently postoperative, or who have chronic obstructive pulmonary disease (COPD) or chest wall abnormalities, which may impair TTE examinations.[8]

In addition, there are certain structures and pathologies that are best visualized using TEE. These include the mitral valve, prosthetic valves, great vessels, and atria, as well as endocarditis and intracardiac thrombi (Table 22–3).[8,9] This is particularly important in trauma patients who may be at risk of cardiac tamponade, aortic injuries, and traumatic valvular disruption or septal defects. Finally, TEE is indicated in critically ill patients requiring echocardiographic evaluation in whom TTE images are inadequate.

COMPLICATIONS

As with TEE in the general population, transesophageal echocardiography has a very low incidence of complications in critical care patients.[2,10] Excluding feeding tube dislodgement, TEE had a complication rate of 2.6% in a review comprising 2508 examinations in the ICU.[2] The most common complications included oropharyngeal mucosal lesions (0.7%), hypotension (0.6%), and coughing (0.3%). TEE should not be performed in any patient with esophageal perforation or in whom

Table 22–1. TEE Diagnoses in the Hemodynamically Unstable Patient.

Acute myocardial infarction
Cardiac tamponade
Aortic dissection
Valvular dysfunction
Endocarditis
Source of embolism
Pulmonary embolus (central)
Pleural effusion

From Cheitlin MD, Armstrong WF, Aurigemma GP, et al. ACC/AHA/ASE 2003 guideline update for the clinical application of echocardiography—summary article: a report of the American College of Cardiology/American Heart Association Task Force on Practice Guidelines (ACC/AHA/ASE Committee to Update the 1997 Guidelines for the Clinical Application of Echocardiography). J Am Coll Cardiol. 2003;42(5):954-970.

esophageal pathology or other comorbidities prevent safe and atraumatic insertion of the TEE probe.

TEE EVALUATION OF THE CRITICALLY ILL PATIENT

Patient Preparation

Prior to performing a TEE examination, appropriate equipment for airway management, suctioning, and resuscitation should be available. Standard monitoring should be used including pulse oximetry, invasive or noninvasive blood pressure monitoring, and continuous electrocardiogram. It may be beneficial to have a second physician present to assist with management during the examination of hemodynamically unstable patients.

For elective TEE examinations, the patient should fast for 4 hours prior to the procedure to facilitate gastric emptying. Topical anesthesia with aerosolized or viscous local anesthetic should be performed prior to probe insertion. Judicious sedation may be used at the intensivist's discretion, depending on the patient's clinical presentation. Small titrated doses of benzodiazepines and/or opioids are commonly used, with reversal agents readily available.

For emergent TEE, gastric contents should first be suctioned via orogastric or nasogastric tube if in situ. In a patient with cardiopulmonary instability and an unsecured airway, endotracheal intubation prior to TEE may be clinically indicated. While TEE can be an invaluable tool for diagnosis, its use should not delay appropriate resuscitation and management of the unstable patient.

Imaging

Many TEE studies in the ICU are performed to facilitate diagnosis and management of an unstable patient, or to rule out a specific disease such as tamponade or endocarditis. Thus, while a comprehensive TEE exam as described in the ASE/SCA guidelines should be performed in all cases,[11] the intensivist performing echocardiography should initially focus the exam based upon the patient's clinical status and suspected diagnosis. The following is a brief summary of the intensivist's echocardiographic approach to various clinical presentations and diagnoses—a thorough discussion of each topic can be found in earlier chapters.

HEMODYNAMIC INSTABILITY

Hypovolemia and Preload Assessment

Significant hypovolemia is seen on TEE as decreased left ventricular (LV) filling and commonly demonstrated by obliteration of the LV cavity ("kissing" papillary muscles)

Table 22–2. Recommendations for Echocardiography in the Critical Care Unit.

ACC/AHA/ASE Class I Recommendations for Echocardiography in the Critically Ill
1. The hemodynamically unstable patient
2. Suspected aortic dissection (TEE)
ACC/AHA/ASE Class I Recommendations for Echocardiography in the Critically Injured
1. Serious blunt or penetrating chest trauma (suspected pericardial effusion or tamponade)
2. Mechanically ventilated multiple-trauma or chest trauma patient
3. Suspected pre-existing valvular or myocardial disease in the trauma patient
4. The hemodynamically unstable multiple-injury patient without obvious chest trauma but with a mechanism of injury suggesting potential cardiac or aortic injury (deceleration or crush)
5. Widening of the mediastinum, postinjury suspected aortic injury (TEE)
6. Potential catheter, guidewire, pacer electrode, or pericardiocentesis needle injury with or without signs of tamponade

Table 22–3. Indications for TEE.

TEE should be first choice
1. Endocarditis
2. Prosthetic valve dysfunction
3. Mitral valve anatomy before and after mitral valve repair
4. Aortic dissection
5. Left atrial thrombus
6. Aortic dissection
7. Posterior structures in congenital heart disease
TEE superior to TTE
1. Mechanically ventilated
2. Hemodynamically unstable
3. Chest trauma
4. Postoperative
5. Cardiac tamponade
6. Central pulmonary emboli
7. Suspected intracardiac source of embolus
8. Assist devices (IABP, LVAD, RVAD)

IABP, intra-aortic balloon pump; LVAD, left ventricular assist device; RVAD, right ventricular assist device.

in the transgastric (TG) midpapillary short-axis (SAX) view. However, systolic cavity obliteration may also occur in the setting of reduced afterload and/or increased ejection fraction in 20% of cases, and may not reflect hypovolemia.[12] Furthermore, visual detection of small (< 10%) yet potentially important changes is difficult and more objective measurements of LV volumes are required, especially in patient with compromised ventricular function (see Chapter 21). A left ventricular end-diastolic area (LVEDA) in the TG SAX view less than 6.3 cm^2/m^2 (women) or 7.5 cm^2/m^2 (men) could be consistent with hypovolemia as these values define the lower limits of normal in subjects under general anesthesia.[13] Unfortunately, there is a wide range of normal values and as a consequence, visual estimation of LV volume is limited to the extremes—cavity obliteration or marked ventricular dilation.

Despite the fact that pulmonary artery occlusion pressure (PAOP) does not accurately reflect preload or volume responsiveness, it is still used as supportive criterion for the diagnosis of acute respiratory distress syndrome and heart failure. Noninvasive estimation of PAOP is feasible using TEE-derived simple Doppler variables, but not in every patient. In fact, Vignon and colleagues[14] prospectively assessed the ability of TEE to predict PAOP in mechanically ventilated patients with a pulmonary artery catheter. In the initial group of patients, the correlations between simple Doppler variables and PAOP were better in patients with depressed LV systolic function than in those with normal LV systolic function. PAOP 18 mm Hg or less could be predicted by an E-wave/A-wave ratio greater than 1.4, E-wave deceleration time greater than 100 milliseconds, atrial filling fraction greater than 31%, and systolic fraction of pulmonary venous flow greater than 44%. In a second group, these cutoff values were prospectively validated and the utility of color M-mode Doppler flow propagation velocity (Vp) and the maximal early diastolic velocity of the lateral mitral annulus by tissue Doppler (E′) were assessed. An E/E′ ratio less than 8 and an E/Vp ratio less than 1.7 were predictive for PAOP 18 mm Hg or less, but the predictive value of these variables was not different from the "simpler" pulsed Doppler variables.[14]

Regional Wall Motion Abnormalities

A thorough survey of the left ventricle using the midesophageal (ME) four-chamber, two-chamber, and long-axis (LAX) views, as well as the TG basal, midpapillary, and apical SAX views allows the intensivist to identify regional wall motion abnormalities. It is important to examine each segment for thickening as well as motion, and to observe each segment in multiple views. Comparison with previous echocardiographic exams is helpful to determine whether any abnormalities are new or pre-existing. A new regional wall motion abnormality is consistent with myocardial ischemia. Although the sensitivity for ischemia detection by TEE is established, the specificity and implications of a transient wall motion abnormality are less clear (see Chapter 21).

Left Ventricular Function

Contractility can be inferred from the left ventricular ejection fraction (LVEF). There are several methods by which TEE can estimate the LVEF, including fractional area change, visual assessment, Simpson's rule, area length method, and three-dimensional (3D) modeling. Cardiac output can be calculated using the continuity equation from the LV outflow tract area and velocity-time integral. These techniques are described in earlier chapters. It is also important to note the presence of associated left ventricular hypertrophy or dilatation.

Right Ventricular Function

Although right ventricular function can be more difficult to quantify than left ventricular function, it is possible nonetheless to identify patients with impaired RV performance. Acute right ventricular dysfunction in the critically ill patient may signify pulmonary embolus, acute pulmonary hypertension, or right coronary artery disease. The right ventricle is a thin-walled structure; thus, RV thickening should not be used to quantify function. Tricuspid annular displacement toward the RV apex in the ME four-chamber view, fractional area change in the TG short-axis view, and 3D imaging can all be used to quantify RV function. Other signs of RV dysfunction include flattening of the septum (creating a "D-shaped" left ventricle) and right ventricular enlargement.

Diastolic Function

Impaired cardiac filling can cause cardiac failure in the setting of normal systolic function. Diastolic dysfunction differs from systolic dysfunction in pathophysiology and therapeutic approach; therefore, this diagnosis is important for the intensivist in planning management. A clinical finding of acute cardiogenic pulmonary edema, in the presence of normal systolic function by TEE, is highly suggestive of diastolic dysfunction.[15] Diagnosis of diastolic dysfunction with TEE requires the use of pulsed-wave Doppler of mitral inflow and pulmonary venous flow (see Chapter 12). However, Sadler et al[16] confirmed the load dependence of the pulsed-wave Doppler parameters used to evaluate LV diastolic properties. The abrupt preload reduction induced by ultrafiltration in ICU patients with renal failure significantly decreased E-wave maximal velocities and the E/A ratio because A-wave velocities remained unaffected. Both the isovolumic relaxation time and E-wave deceleration time were significantly prolonged by volume reduction. Also, changes in the pulmonary vein D wave paralleled that of mitral E wave, and the S/D ratio increased after hemodialysis. Therefore, conventional pulsed-wave Doppler parameters to identify transient LV diastolic dysfunction in clinical settings characterized by abrupt changes in loading conditions should be interpreted with caution.[17] On the other hand, E′ velocity from the lateral mitral annulus may be less preload dependent.[17]

Valvular Function

Each valve should be examined for stenosis and regurgitation, as well as abnormalities such as vegetations, thickening, calcification, and prolapse. While valvular lesions may cause hemodynamic instability, their presence may also have implications for management. Severe tricuspid regurgitation, for instance, may result in spurious measurements of cardiac output using thermodilution. Mitral regurgitation may occur as a result of ischemic disease and papillary muscle rupture. Aortic stenosis may be associated with secondary diastolic dysfunction as a result of ventricular remodeling.

Cardiac Tamponade

In the intensive care unit, cardiac tamponade may occur following cardiac surgery, traumatic injury, pericardial effusion, or as a result of myocardial infarction with wall rupture. Rarely, tamponade may occur as a complication of central venous line placement or other procedures. Clinically, cardiac tamponade may present with Beck's triad of hypotension, elevated jugular venous pressure, and muffled heart sounds. However, the absence of these symptoms does not exclude the diagnosis of tamponade, as lesser volumes or chronic accumulation may present with more subtle clinical findings. TEE is highly sensitive and specific in the detection of pericardial tamponade, with accuracy greater than 99%.[9] Pericardial fluid can often be detected in the TG midpapillary SAX, TG LAX, and ME four-chamber views (Figure 22–1). Restriction of cardiac filling and equalization of pressures between the left and right heart may manifest via flattening of the interventricular septum, decreased left ventricular end-diastolic volume, decreased LV size during inspiration, and diastolic posterior motion of the RV.

Miscellaneous

Other causes of unexplained hypotension that may be diagnosed with TEE include pulmonary embolus, hypertrophic obstructive cardiomyopathy, and intracardiac thrombus.

Pulmonary embolus is not normally seen with TEE, with the exception of central emboli involving the pulmonary trunk or main pulmonary arteries. Echocardiographic signs suggestive of pulmonary embolus include new-onset RV dilatation and dysfunction, acute tricuspid regurgitation, and elevated right-side pressures, in the appropriate clinical context.

Hypertrophic cardiomyopathy may result in dynamic obstruction of the left ventricular outflow tract (LVOT) in up to 25% of patients. This obstruction may be intermittent, and is typically exacerbated by hypovolemia, tachycardia, increased contractility, and decreased afterload. In the ME four-chamber and ME aortic valve (AV) LAX views, left ventricular hypertrophy is often seen, particularly septal hypertrophy. Diastolic dysfunction is common in this population. Left ventricular outflow obstruction can cause high flow velocities in the LVOT, increased LV pressures, and a dagger-shaped pattern of flow on pulsed-wave Doppler or continuous-wave Doppler of the outflow tract.

Intracardiac thrombi can be seen in patients with ventricular aneurysm, dilated cardiomyopathy, coagulopathic states, and dysrhythmias. Thrombi appear as echogenic, mobile masses that may be freely floating or attached to a cardiac structure, and may mimic intracardiac tumors.

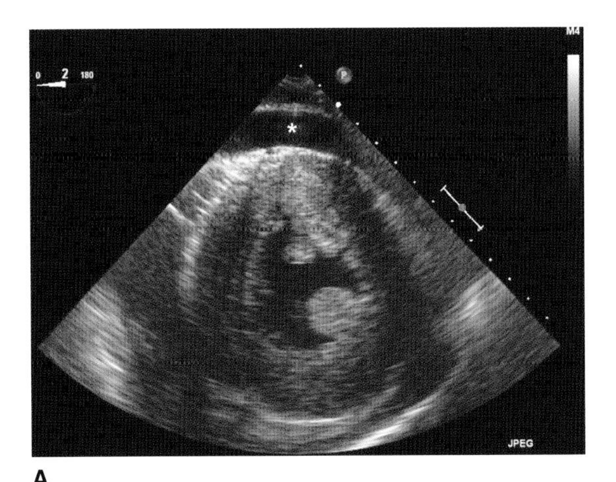

A

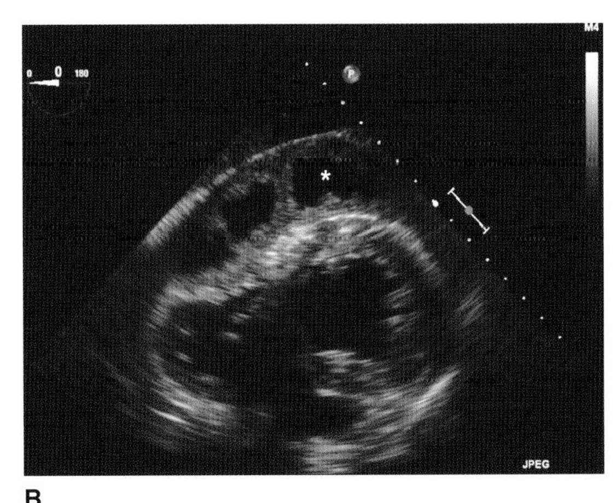

B

FIGURE 22–1. Acute **(A)** and chronic **(B)** pericardial effusions *(asterisk)*.

Clinically, pulmonary or systemic thromboembolic disease may arise as a result.

HYPOXEMIA

TEE can be a useful diagnostic tool in the critically ill patient with unexplained hypoxemia. Causes of hypoxemia that can be detected with TEE include left ventricular failure, valvular pathology, cor pulmonale, pulmonary hypertension, pulmonary vein stenosis, central pulmonary embolus, right to left shunts, and pleural effusions (Figure 22–2).[18]

Echocardiographic findings consistent with pulmonary hypertension include right ventricular dilatation and dysfunction. In the presence of tricuspid regurgitation, the pulmonary artery systolic pressure (PASP) can be estimated by the modified Bernoulli equation ($PASP = 4(V_{TR})^2 + CVP$, where V_{TR} is the maximal flow in m/s of the tricuspid regurgitant jet and CVP is central venous pressure). Pulmonary vein stenosis is an uncommon cause of pulmonary hypertension whose incidence has been increasing as a result of transcatheter radiofrequency pulmonary vein isolation for the treatment of atrial fibrillation.

Right-to-left shunts may also cause unexplained hypoxemia in the ICU in patients with elevated right heart pressures. Shunts may be intracardiac (patent foramen ovale, atrial septal defect, ventricular septal defect) or intrapulmonary. Intracardiac shunting can be detected with color-flow Doppler, or by the venous injection of agitated saline for contrast.

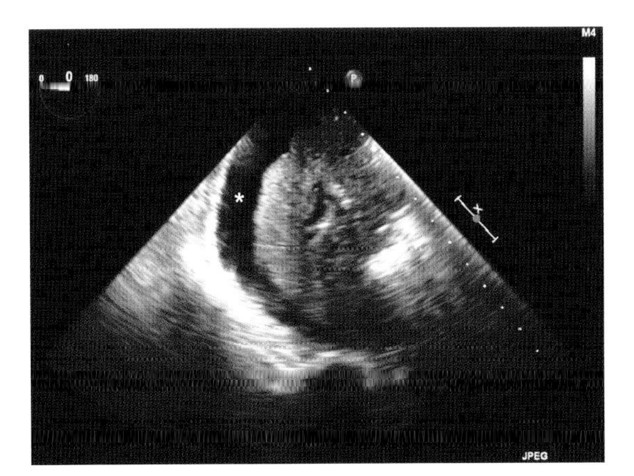

FIGURE 22–2. Right pleural effusion *(asterisk)*.

ENDOCARDITIS

Febrile patients in the ICU may require evaluation for the presence of endocarditis. In these patients, TEE is the gold standard for noninvasive assessment of endocarditis, with a sensitivity of 88% to 98%.[19-21] In contrast, TTE has a sensitivity of 58% to 62%.[19,21] TEE should be performed to rule out endocarditis in patients with a high index of suspicion and a negative TTE, for suspected prosthetic valve endocarditis, in patients with bacteremia of unknown source (or refractory to antibiotic therapy), and to assess complications of known endocarditis.[22]

Echocardiographic signs of infective endocarditis include vegetations on valves, cardiac structures, or devices, dehiscence of prosthetic valves, new onset of valvular regurgitation, and abscesses.[23] Vegetations on native or prosthetic valves occur most commonly on the

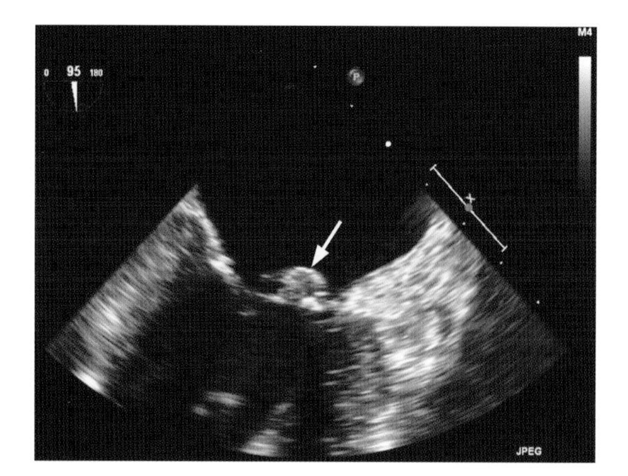

FIGURE 22–3. Mitral valve endocarditis *(arrow)*.

atrial side of the mitral and tricuspid valves and the ventricular side of the aortic and pulmonary valves (Figure 22–3). Vegetations are frequently oscillatory, moving in sync with the cardiac cycle and valvular motion. Repeat TEE examinations are often necessary over the course of treatment to assess for complications of infective endocarditis and the disappearance of vegetations.

EMBOLIC SOURCE

In the patient with unexplained stroke or peripheral embolic disease, TEE may be helpful to identify intracardiac sources of emboli. These include left-side intracardiac thrombi, endocarditis, tumors, aortic atheromatous disease, and right-side masses in the presence of a right-to-left shunt. Patients with indwelling peripherally inserted central catheter (PICC) lines are at increased risk of catheter-associated thrombus (Figure 22–4), occurring in 15% of cases in a recent prospective study.[24] Prior to elective cardioversion of patients with atrial fibrillation or flutter, TEE may be indicated to rule out the presence of thrombi in the left atrium, left atrial appendage, and left ventricle.[20] Patients with a history of atrial dysrhythmia greater than 48 hours who are not therapeutically anticoagulated are at increased risk of thrombus development and stroke following cardioversion.

TRAUMA

TEE is of particular value in the unstable trauma patient, particularly those with blunt or penetrating chest trauma. In such patients, TTE is most often unsatisfactory due to contusions, wounds, subcutaneous emphysema, mechanical ventilation, and/or difficulty with positioning. Patients with traumatic chest injury are at risk for aortic dissection and injury, myocardial contusion and acute dysfunction, traumatic ventricular septal defect, cardiac tamponade, and hemothorax, all of which can be visualized by TEE. TEE should not be performed if esophageal perforation is suspected.

Aortic Dissection

While angiography remains the gold standard for diagnosis of aortic injury in the trauma patient, it is time-consuming and requires transportation of a patient who may be hemodynamically unstable. TEE can be performed safely and rapidly at the bedside or in the

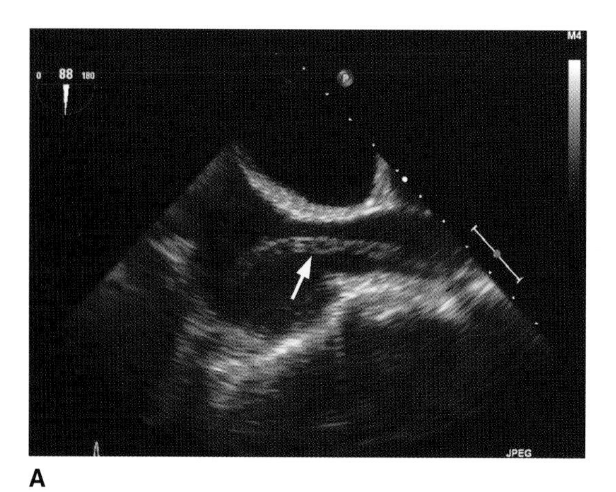

A

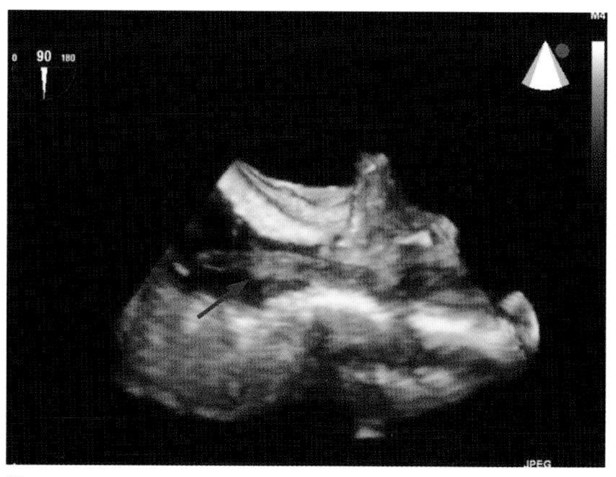

B

FIGURE 22–4. PICC line thrombus *(arrow)* with 2D **(A)** and 3D **(B)** imaging.

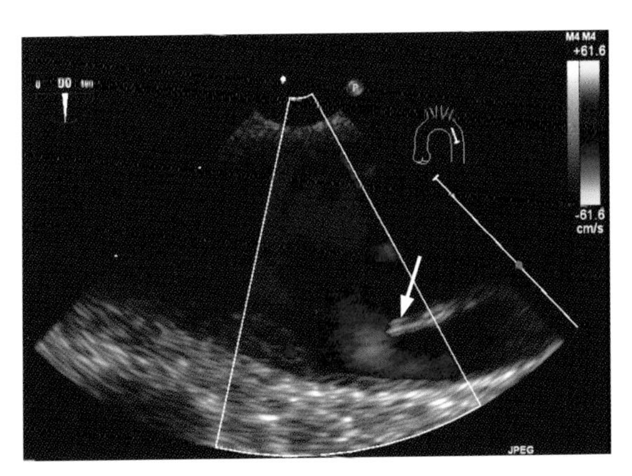

FIGURE 22–5. Aortic dissection flap *(arrow)* with color-flow Doppler imaging.

operating room.[25] The diagnostic accuracy of TEE in patients with suspected acute traumatic aortic injury is comparable to helical computed tomography (CT) but TEE was more sensitive for injuries involving the intimal or medial layers of the thoracic aorta.[26] TEE may miss lesions in the distal ascending aorta and proximal aortic arch due to the interposition of the air-filled trachea between the aorta and the TEE probe.

In a patient with suspected aortic injury, careful inspection of the ascending aorta, aortic arch, and thoracic aorta should be performed. Echocardiographic signs of aortic dissection or disruption include presence of an intimal flap (Figure 22–5), turbulent blood flow in the aorta, evidence of low flow in the aorta visible as spontaneous echo contrast or "smoke," aortic aneurysm, and thrombus.[25]

SUMMARY

TEE is a minimally invasive diagnostic tool that can provide valuable information rapidly and can be performed at the patient's bedside. TEE is increasingly being used by critical care physicians, particularly in hemodynamically unstable and trauma patients. The information obtained from a TEE examination by a skilled operator will often lead to important management changes, as well as alert the intensivist to new diagnoses. Lastly, it is likely that the advent of real-time 3D imaging will only extend the usability of TEE for intensive care physicians

REFERENCES

1. Tuchschmidt JA, Mecher CE. Predictors of outcome from critical illness. Shock and cardiopulmonary resuscitation. *Crit Care Clin.* 1994;10(1):179-195.
2. Huttemann E, Schelenz C, Kara F, Chatzinikolaou K, Reinhart K. The use and safety of transoesophageal echocardiography in the general ICU –a minireview. *Acta Anaesthesiol Scand.* 2004;48(7): 827-836.
3. Porembka DT. Importance of transesophageal echocardiography in the critically ill and injured patient. *Crit Care Med.* 2007;35(8 Suppl):S414-430.
4. Orme RM, Oram MP, McKinstry CE. Impact of echocardiography on patient management in the intensive care unit: an audit of district general hospital practice. *Br J Anaesth.* 2009;102(3): 340-344.
5. Vieillard-Baron A, Slama M, Cholley B, Janvier G, Vignon P. Echocardiography in the intensive care unit: from evolution to revolution? *Intensive Care Med.* 2008;34(2):243-249.
6. Parker MM, Cunnion RE, Parrillo JE. Echocardiography and nuclear cardiac imaging in the critical care unit. *JAMA.* 1985;254(20): 2935-2939.
7. Heidenreich PA, Stainback RF, Redberg RF, Schiller NB, Cohen NH, Foster E. Transesophageal echocardiography predicts mortality in critically ill patients with unexplained hypotension. *J Am Coll Cardiol.* 1995;26(1):152-158.
8. Douglas PS, Khandheria B, Stainback RF, et al. ACCF/ASE/ACEP/ASNC/SCAI/SCCT/SCMR 2007 appropriateness criteria for transthoracic and transesophageal echocardiography: a report of the American College of Cardiology Foundation Quality Strategic Directions Committee Appropriateness Criteria Working Group, American Society of Echocardiography, American College of Emergency Physicians, American Society of Nuclear Cardiology, Society for Cardiovascular Angiography and Interventions, Society of Cardiovascular Computed Tomography, and the Society for Cardiovascular Magnetic Resonance endorsed by the American College of Chest Physicians and the Society of Critical Care Medicine. *J Am Coll Cardiol.* 2007;50(2): 187-204.
9. Cheitlin MD, Armstrong WF, Aurigemma GP, et al. ACC/AHA/ASE 2003 guideline update for the clinical application of echocardiography—summary article: a report of the American College of Cardiology/American Heart Association Task Force on Practice Guidelines (ACC/AHA/ASE Committee to Update the 1997 Guidelines for the Clinical Application of Echocardiography). *J Am Coll Cardiol.* 2003;42(5):954-970.
10. Min JK, Spencer KT, Furlong KT, et al. Clinical features of complications from transesophageal echocardiography: a single-center case series of 10,000 consecutive examinations. *J Am Soc Echocardiogr.* 2005;18(9):925-929.
11. Shanewise JS, Cheung AT, Aronson S, et al. ASE/SCA guidelines for performing a comprehensive intraoperative multiplane transesophageal echocardiography examination: recommendations of the American Society of Echocardiography Council for Intraoperative Echocardiography and the Society of Cardiovascular Anesthesiologists Task Force for Certification in Perioperative Transesophageal Echocardiography. *Anesth Analg.* 1999;89(4):870-884.
12. Leung JM, Levine EH. Left ventricular end-systolic cavity obliteration as an estimate of intraoperative hypovolemia. *Anesthesiology.* 1994;81(5):1102-1109.
13. Skarvan K, Lambert A, Filipovic M, Seeberger M. Reference values for left ventricular function in subjects under general anaesthesia and controlled ventilation assessed by two-dimensional transoesophageal echocardiography. *Eur J Anaesthesiol.* 2001;18(11):713-722.

14. Vignon P, AitHssain A, Francois B, et al. Echocardiographic assessment of pulmonary artery occlusion pressure in ventilated patients: a transoesophageal study. *Crit Care.* 2008;12(1): R18.
15. Pirracchio R, Cholley B, De Hert S, Solal AC, Mebazaa A. Diastolic heart failure in anaesthesia and critical care. *Br J Anaesth.* 2007;98(6):707-721.
16. Sadler DB, Brown J, Nurse H, Roberts J. Impact of hemodialysis on left and right ventricular Doppler diastolic filling indices. *Am J Med Sci.* 1992;304(2):83-90.
17. Munt B, Jue J, Gin K, Fenwick J, Tweeddale M. Diastolic filling in human severe sepsis: an echocardiographic study. *Crit Care Med.* 1998;26(11):1829-1833.
18. Hoole SP, Falter F. Evaluation of hypoxemic patients with transesophageal echocardiography. *Crit Care Med.* 2007;35(8 Suppl): S408-413.
19. Shively BK, Gurule FT, Roldan CA, Leggett JH, Schiller NB. Diagnostic value of transesophageal compared with transthoracic echocardiography in infective endocarditis. *J Am Coll Cardiol.* 1991;18(2):391-397.
20. Beaulieu Y. Bedside echocardiography in the assessment of the critically ill. *Crit Care Med.* 2007;35(5 Suppl):S235-249.
21. Karalis DG, Chandrasekaran K, Ross JJ Jr, et al. Single-plane transesophageal echocardiography for assessing function of mechanical or bioprosthetic valves in the aortic valve position. *Am J Cardiol.* 1992;69(16):1310-1315.
22. Colreavy FB, Donovan K, Lee KY, Weekes J. Transesophageal echocardiography in critically ill patients. *Crit Care Med.* 2002;30(5):989-996.
23. ACC/AHA guidelines for the management of patients with valvular heart disease. A report of the American College of Cardiology/American Heart Association. Task Force on Practice Guidelines (Committee on Management of Patients with Valvular Heart Disease). *J Am Coll Cardiol.* 1998;32(5):1486-1588.
24. Worth LJ, Seymour JF, Slavin MA. Infective and thrombotic complications of central venous catheters in patients with hematological malignancy: prospective evaluation of nontunneled devices. *Support Care Cancer.* 2009;17(7):811-818.
25. Tousignant C. Transesophageal echocardiographic assessment in trauma and critical care. *Can J Surg.* 1999;42(3):171-175.
26. Vignon P, Boncoeur MP, Francois B, Rambaud G, Maubon A, Gastinne H. Comparison of multiplane transesophageal echocardiography and contrast-enhanced helical CT in the diagnosis of blunt traumatic cardiovascular injuries. *Anesthesiology.* 2001; 94(4): 615-622.

REVIEW QUESTIONS

Select the *one* best answer for each of the following questions.

1. Indications for echocardiography in the ICU include all of the following EXCEPT:
   a. Hemodynamic instability
   b. Suspected abdominal aortic injury
   c. Unexplained hypoxemia
   d. Suspected cardiac tamponade

2. All of the following are barriers to transthoracic echocardiography (TTE) EXCEPT:
   a. Chest wall contusions
   b. Recent cardiothoracic surgery
   c. Spontaneous ventilation
   d. Subcutaneous emphysema

3. Transthoracic echocardiography (TTE) is inadequate in what percentage of ICU patients with unexplained hypotension?
   a. 10%
   b. 30%
   c. 60%
   d. 90%

4. TEE is superior to TTE in the evaluation of which valve?
   a. Mitral valve
   b. Aortic valve
   c. Pulmonic valve
   d. Tricuspid valve

5. In which condition does TEE represent a reasonable first test (vs TTE)?
   a. Coronary artery disease
   b. Scleroderma
   c. Congestive heart failure
   d. COPD

6. The most common complication of TEE performed in the ICU is:
   a. Hypotension
   b. Coughing
   c. Esophageal perforation
   d. Feeding tube dislodgement

7. Which of the following is an absolute contraindication to TEE in the ICU?
   a. Hypotension
   b. Gastroparesis
   c. Esophageal perforation
   d. Difficult airway

8. TEE evidence of hypovolemia includes all of the following EXCEPT:
   a. "Kissing" papillary muscles
   b. Left ventricular end-diastolic area of 10 cm^2/m^2
   c. Left ventricular end-diastolic area less than 6 cm^2/m^2
   d. Decreased LV filling

9. To estimate cardiac output by continuity equation, which of the following variables are required?
   a. LV outflow tract area and velocity-time integral
   b. LV outflow tract area and fractional area change
   c. Fractional area change and tissue Doppler
   d. Velocity-time integral alone

10. Methods of quantifying RV dysfunction include all of the following EXCEPT:
    a. Tricuspid annular displacement
    b. Fractional area change
    c. 3D imaging
    d. RV thickening

11. A flattened intraventricular septum is consistent with which of the following diagnoses?
    a. Acute MI
    b. Hypovolemia
    c. Aortic stenosis
    d. Pulmonary embolus

12. Which of the following TEE modalities is used across the mitral valve to diagnose diastolic dysfunction?
    a. Continuous-wave Doppler
    b. Pulsed-wave Doppler
    c. Tissue Doppler
    d. M-mode

13. Common TEE views for the diagnosis of pericardial effusion include all of the following EXCEPT:
    a. TG midpapillary SAX
    b. TG LAX
    c. ME bicaval
    d. ME four chamber

14. Which of the following echocardiographic signs indicates cardiac tamponade?
    a. Presence of pericardial fluid
    b. Right atrial enlargement
    c. Diastolic posterior motion of the RV
    d. Diastolic dysfunction

15. All of the following TEE findings are consistent with pulmonary embolus EXCEPT:
    a. RV dilatation
    b. Tricuspid regurgitation
    c. RV dysfunction
    d. RA enlargement

16. Which of the following complications may be seen on TEE following ablation for atrial fibrillation?
    a. Pulmonary vein stenosis
    b. Myocardial infarction
    c. Ventricular septal defect
    d. LV outflow tract obstruction

17. All of the following findings are consistent with infective endocarditis EXCEPT:
    a. Mass in LA appendage
    b. Oscillatory cardiac mass
    c. New aortic regurgitation
    d. Prosthetic valve dehiscence

18. The gold standard for diagnosis of aortic injury in the trauma patient is:
    a. CT scan
    b. TEE
    c. Angiography
    d. MRI

19. Echocardiographic signs of aortic injury include all of the following EXCEPT:
    a. Presence of intimal flap
    b. Turbulent aortic blood flow
    c. Spontaneous aortic echo contrast
    d. Diastolic aortic flow reversal

20. Common sites of intracardiac thrombus include all of the following EXCEPT:
    a. Left atrium
    b. Left atrial appendage
    c. Left ventricular apex
    d. Coronary sinus

TEE in the Emergency Department 23

Svati H. Shah

Echocardiography has been a component of emergency medicine practice for over 20 years, and serves as an integral diagnostic tool in the evaluation of patients with cardiac and noncardiac disorders. Echocardiography represents the only diagnostic modality capable of providing real-time bedside information for acutely ill patients in the emergency department (ED). In addition to cardiac anesthesiologists and cardiologists, trainees in U.S.-based emergency medicine residency and fellowship programs now often acquire specialized training in echocardiography.

Transthoracic echocardiography (TTE) has proven to have several applications in routine clinical practice including the detection of cardiac effusion and tamponade, estimating cardiac ejection fraction, and as an important adjunct during specialized procedures such as pericardiocentesis.[1,2] Under certain circumstances, however, TTE may be impractical (ie, during active chest compressions in the arresting patient), impossible (ie, in the morbidly obese patient), or inadequate (ie, definitive imaging of the ascending aorta). In such cases, transesophageal echocardiography (TEE) may be a suitable alternative, and in some cases can be regarded as the first-line echocardiographic investigation. While TEE is still primarily under the purview of the cardiologist or cardiac anesthesiologist, suitably trained emergency medicine physicians have also begun to incorporate TEE into their practice. Regardless, physicians using TEE as a tool for clinical management need to be adequately trained in performance and interpretation, which has prompted the American Society of Echocardiography to publish a policy statement on echocardiography in the ED.[3]

Guidelines for the clinical application of echocardiography in the ED. The ACC/AHA/ASE guidelines for the clinical application of echocardiography (2003) have established recommendations for the use of echocardiography in the critically ill or injured patient (Table 23–1), including that echocardiography is appropriate to use in patients with suspected aortic injury, hemodynamically unstable patients, patients with serious blunt or penetrating chest trauma, and suspected pre-existing valvular or myocardial disease in the trauma patient. Table 23–2 details the specific clinical conditions and diagnoses for which echocardiography can be a useful diagnostic tool in the ED.

Transthoracic versus transesophageal echocardiography in the ED. The ACC/AHA/ASE guidelines for the clinical application of echocardiography (2003) have also delineated the conditions and settings in which TEE (as opposed to TTE) provides the most definitive diagnosis in critically ill or injured patients, including the hemodynamically unstable patient with suboptimal TTE images or those on ventilators; major trauma or postoperative patients; suspected aortic dissection or other aortic injury; and other conditions in which TEE is superior (ie, endocarditis and cardiac source of emboli).[4]

TEE has several general advantages that make it a reasonable and useful imaging modality in the ED. TEE is relatively noninvasive and, once placed within the esophagus posterior to the heart, is capable of transmitting real-time images even during active cardiopulmonary resuscitation (CPR), thus permitting cardiac functional information to be viewed by all providers within range of the display monitor. It has been demonstrated to be safe, with low complication rates when used by experienced operators,[5] and may result in a management change in up to 80% of cases.[6] However, one must exercise added caution when using TEE in the ED given the acuity of the patient population, and only adequately trained providers should perform and interpret studies. For example, one study examining the complication rate in 142 patients undergoing TEE in the ED found a 12.6% complication rate including respiratory issues (n = 7), hypotension (n = 3), emesis (n = 4), agitation (n = 2), cardiac dysrhythmia (n = 1), and death (n = 1),[7] a higher complication rate than reported in other clinical situations.[8] Other disadvantages of the use of TEE in the ED relate to problems with incomplete (or absent) historical details in ED patients about the last oral intake, which can result in a need for gastric aspiration and decompression; the unexpected encountering of contraindications to TEE probe placement (such as esophageal webs, strictures, or varices); or unstable/unconscious patients incapable of providing consent.

Table 23–1. ACC/AHA/ASE Guidelines for the Clinical Application of Echocardiography in Critically Ill and Injured Patients.

Class I
• Hemodynamically unstable patient   • If suboptimal images or on ventilator, then TEE • Suspected aortic dissection (TEE) • Serious blunt or penetrating chest trauma (suspected pericardial effusion or tamponade) • Mechanically ventilated multiple-trauma or chest trauma patient • Suspected pre-existing valvular or myocardial disease in the trauma patient • Hemodynamically unstable multiple-injury patient without obvious chest trauma but with a mechanism of injury suggesting potential cardiac or aortic injury (deceleration or crush) • Widening of the mediastinum, postinjury suspected aortic injury (TEE) • Potential catheter, guidewire, pacer electrode, or pericardiocentesis needle injury with or without signs of tamponade
Class IIa
• Evaluation of hemodynamics in multiple-trauma or chest trauma patients with pulmonary artery catheter monitoring and data disparate with clinical situation. • Follow-up study on victims of serious blunt or penetrating trauma
Class III
• Suspected myocardial contusion in the hemodynamically stable patient with a normal ECG who has no abnormal cardiac/thoracic physical findings and/or lacks a mechanism of injury suggesting cardiovascular contusion. • Hemodynamically stable patient not expected to have cardiac disease. • Re-evaluation follow-up studies on hemodynamically stable patients

In major trauma or postoperative patients unable to be positioned for adequate TTE, TEE is recommended.

Modified from Cheitlin MD, Armstrong WF, Aurigemma GP, et al. ACC/AHA/ASE 2003 guideline update for the clinical application of echocardiography: summary article: a report of the American College of Cardiology/American Heart Association Task Force on Practice Guidelines (ACC/AHA/ASE Committee to Update the 1997 Guidelines for the Clinical Application of Echocardiography). Circulation. 2003;108(9):1146-1162.

While most studies of echocardiography in the ED have employed TTE as the first-line study, in many clinical situations including obesity, mechanical ventilation, lung disease, and poor echocardiographic windows, TTE limits clinical evaluation. For example, in a study by Varriale and Maldonado,[9] they employed TTE as first-line echocardiographic imaging while studying patients with cardiac arrest, but required subsequent TEE to obtain acceptable images in 20% of their patients. In other studies, the failure rate of the transthoracic approach in the ICU setting has been reported to be 10% to 40%.[10-12] The critically ill patient in the ED is often managed by intubation and mechanical ventilation, and up to one-half of such patients cannot be adequately imaged by TTE.[13] TTE can also be impeded by objects on the chest wall such as lines, catheters, and electrocardiographic (ECG) leads, and even if performed by an experienced technician, TTE requires frequent interruption of CPR for repeated, intermittent acquisition of images during resuscitation. This is particularly relevant given the emphasis on minimizing the interruption of chest compressions in ACLS guidelines. Recently, an algorithm has been proposed for the use of TTE in resuscitation, to be executed simultaneously during CPR cycles to reduce interruptions.[14]

With TEE, on the other hand, once the probe is placed, it serves as a continuous monitor as it can remain in the esophagus even during active chest compressions[15] and is not affected by objects on the chest wall. Continuous monitoring permits images to be viewed by the entire resuscitation team if a display-ready monitor is available, and can allow confirmation of adequate chest compressions by observing appropriate changes in chamber size as the heart alternately fills and empties.

There are several specific situations in the ED for which TEE is an important diagnostic tool for clinical care and may be considered the first-line echocardiographic investigation, including assessment of patients presenting with cardiac arrest to identify reversible causes; evaluation of patients with chest pain to rule out acute aortic dissection; evaluation of the patient with chest trauma; and evaluation of the patient with unexplained hypotension. Examples of such situations are reviewed in a case-based format below.

Table 23–2. Conditions and Diagnoses in the Emergency Department for which Echocardiography can be a Useful Diagnostic Tool.

Unexplained hypotension
Hypovolemia
Pulmonary embolus
Myocardial infarction
Valvular disease (mitral regurgitation due to ischemia or papillary muscle rupture)
Ventricular septal defect
Pericardial effusion with tamponade
Unexplained hypoxia
Pulmonary embolus
Pulmonary hypertension
Right ventricular failure
Intracardiac shunt
Chest pain
Aortic dissection
Acute myocardial infarction
Trauma
Pericardial effusion with tamponade
Aortic pathology
Aortic dissection
Intramural hematoma

CASE 1. APPARENT CARDIAC ARREST

A 52-year-old male with a history of coronary artery disease, hypertension, and Type 2 diabetes mellitus arrives via local emergency medical service transport. Approximately 20 minutes prior, the patient had reportedly become short of breath with associated chest pressure and nausea. Thereafter, he became unresponsive. Upon arrival at the home, EMS personnel found him prone on the floor, pulseless and apneic. Standard advanced cardiac life support (ACLS) protocol was initiated; organized electrical activity was present on the monitor, and hence the patient appeared to be in pulseless electrical activity (PEA) arrest. After transport to the ED, CPR was continued. Transthoracic echocardiography was attempted but the cardiac windows were inadequate due to the large body habitus of the patient and the resuscitation paraphernalia.

After several rounds of ACLS, discussion to end the resuscitation was initiated. Simultaneously, a TEE probe was inserted and a midesophageal four-chamber view revealed coordinated myocardial contraction but with severe left ventricular dysfunction and an estimated ejection fraction of 10% to 15% (Figure 23–1). Inotropic support with dobutamine and dopamine was initiated. Two days later, the patient recovered neurologically intact.

TRANSESOPHAGEAL ECHOCARDIOGRAPHY IN CARDIAC ARREST

Despite resources allocated to such initiatives as 911 emergency services, broad distribution of automated electronic defibrillators (AEDs), national campaigns to promote bystander CPR, and standardized ACLS guidelines and training, the most recent data suggest that less than 5% of patients suffering an out-of-hospital cardiac arrest survive to discharge.[16] The presence of comorbidities contributes to worse outcomes after presenting with cardiac arrest.[17,18] In an effort to improve this dismal survival rate, several studies have detailed theoretical and actual benefits of ultrasound in the setting of cardiac arrest, and some have even lobbied for echocardiography to be incorporated into resuscitation protocols for PEA and asystole.[19] Although currently there are no guidelines or recommendations for the use of echocardiography in cardiac arrest, it is thought that a protocol inclusive of echocardiography could lead to a decrease in time between onset of arrest and administration of appropriate therapies.

Role of TEE in the Arresting Patient in the ED

The definitive role of TEE during resuscitation of the arresting patient in the ED and its impact on mortality and morbidity remains to be established. However, a limited number of studies that may be generalizable to this patient population have been suggestive. For example, one small study of in-hospital cardiopulmonary resuscitation using echocardiography found that asystole was initially observed in 90% of patients during CPR; the return of ventricular contractions in four patients prompted positive inotropic therapy. Ventricular wall motion was detected in two patients with bradyarrhythmia (pseudo-electromechanical disassociation) and the causes of cardiac arrest were identified as massive pulmonary embolism and hypovolemia, respectively.[9] In another study specifically evaluating TEE, van der Wouw[15] performed TEE on 48 patients who arrested in either the in- or out-of-hospital setting. Patients underwent resuscitation and TEE anywhere in the hospital (including the ED but excluding the intensive care unit [ICU]). The underlying pathologic process was elucidated in 31 of 48 (64%) patients with 27 of 31 having the diagnosis confirmed by other studies (angiography or postmortem). Based on these results, TEE had a sensitivity of 93% and specificity of 50% with a positive predictive value (PPV) of 87%. Most importantly, in 31% of all cases (15 of 41), the treatment was changed after the TEE established a diagnosis.[15] Memtsoudis et al[20] reported a case series of

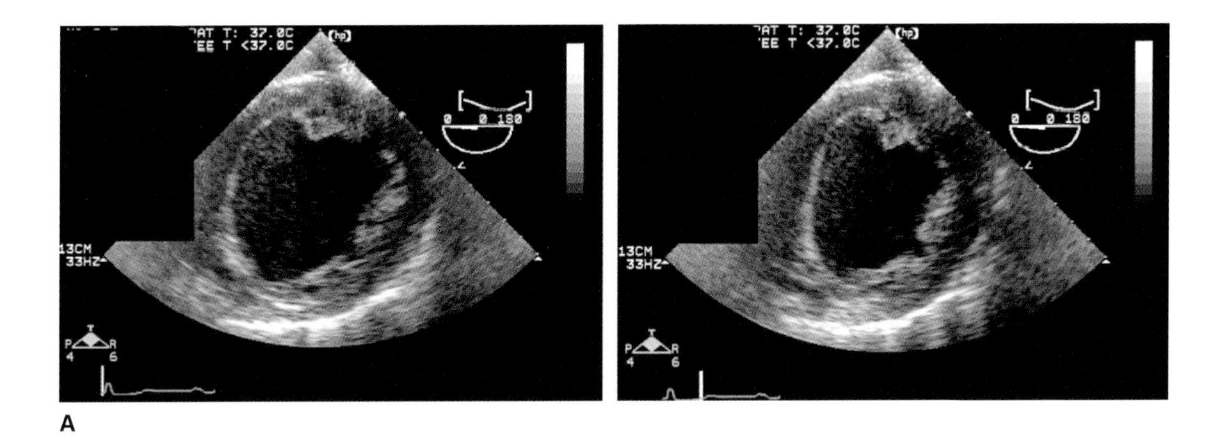

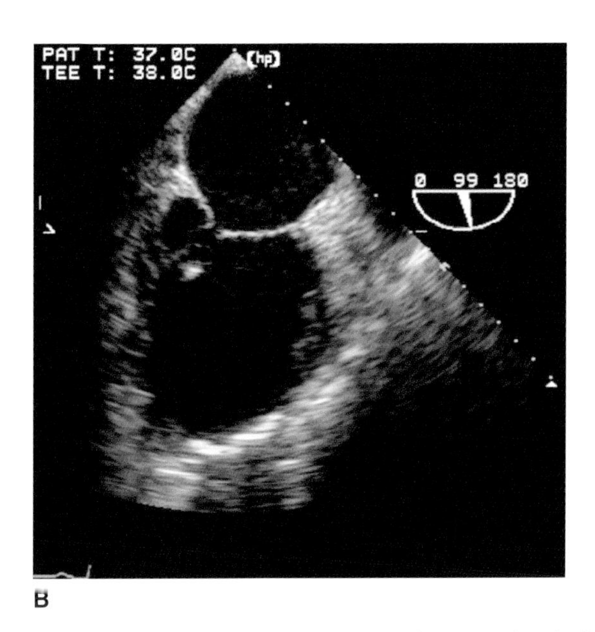

FIGURE 23–1. Transesophageal images of a patient with severe left ventricular dysfunction presenting with cardiac arrest: **(A)** transgastric short-axis view in diastole *(left panel)* and in systole *(right panel)*; **(B)** midesophageal two-chamber view.

TEE performed on 22 patients who had an unexpected arrest during noncardiac operative procedures. A suspected primary diagnosis was established with TEE on 19 of 22 patients, including acute myocardial infarction, thromboembolism, pericardial tamponade, and hypovolemia. The authors state that TEE aided further management in 18 patients.

Although these results suggest the utility of TEE as an adjunctive diagnostic tool for in- or out-of-hospital arrest, they are confounded by the lack of a "gold standard" for comparison and lack of a control comparison group. For example, intracardiac thrombi identified may not represent causal factors in the cardiac arrest, but may just be a side effect of low flow states after cardiac arrest. Further, the diagnostic utility of TEE in myocardial infarction (MI) is limited in differentiation of acute wall motion abnormalities versus old MI, and is contingent upon an organized rhythm, which may be absent during cardiac arrest. Comparative effectiveness analyses are necessary comparing TEE to other diagnostic modalities during cardiac arrest before definitive statements about routine use of echocardiography in cardiac arrest management can be made.

TEE in Patients Presenting With Pulseless Electrical Activity

Often, cardiac arrest is due to pulseless electrical activity (PEA), also known as electromechanical dissociation (EMD). Upon echocardiographic evaluation, many of these cases are actually found to have some degree of cardiac activity, hence representing "pseudo-EMD." Establishment of this condition has important diagnostic and prognostic implications, as patients who do have residual cardiac function (ie, those with severe left ventricular dysfunction like our case example) have a better prognosis than those patients with true EMD.[21] In one study of echocardiography in 169 cardiac arrest victims, cardiac standstill was visualized in 139 patients; of these, none with echocardiographically identified cardiac standstill survived to leave the ED regardless of the initial electrical rhythm.[21] Echocardiography can also be used to confirm asystole and ventricular fibrillation in those patients in whom the rhythm is unclear from the cardiac monitor.

In addition to helping to differentiate the underlying rhythm, echocardiography in cardiac arrest due to PEA or asystole can play an integral and comprehensive role in diagnosing the underlying primary cause (and hence the appropriate treatment), including cardiac effusion with tamponade, pulmonary embolus,[22,23] severe hypovolemia,[24-27] myocardial infarction,[28] myocardial rupture, cardiogenic shock, mitral valve failure or papillary muscle rupture,[29,30] and even tension pneumothorax. Unlike ventricular fibrillation and pulseless ventricular tachycardia, identification of the underlying cause is a key focus of treatment for PEA, and hence echocardiography can play a significant role in patient management.

TEE-Aided Diagnosis of the Underlying Cause in PEA Arrest

Pericardial Effusion

Pericardial effusion is usually easily detected by several routine TEE views, including the transgastric short-axis view and midesophageal four-chamber view (Figure 23–2). One must take care, however, to distinguish pericardial from pleural effusions. In the standard TTE parasternal long-axis view, for example, pericardial effusions normally lie anterior to the aorta, whereas pleural effusions lie posterior to the aorta (Figure 23–3). While visualization of an effusion is relatively straightforward, the diagnosis of pericardial tamponade is more difficult given that traditional echocardiographic evaluations such as mitral inflow respiratory flow variation, absent inferior vena caval inspiratory collapse, and presence of right ventricular diastolic collapse may be very difficult if not impossible in the patient with cardiac arrest. Hence one is reliant upon the physical examination and history to establish a diagnosis of pericardial tamponade. Visualization of a "swinging heart" may also help in diagnosing pericardial tamponade. Pericardial tamponade can be caused by trauma, aortic dissection, infection, neoplasm, congestive heart failure, uremia, autoimmune diseases, and radiation therapy.

Hypovolemia

Hypovolemia can be diagnosed on TTE and TEE by the presence of a small, flattened left ventricle in the four-chamber view. Further interrogation of the left ventricular outflow tract with Doppler echocardiography can help establish whether dynamic outflow obstruction related to the hypovolemia is present. In one study, left ventricular end-diastolic volume was found to correlate well with the presence of blood loss.[31]

Pulmonary Embolism

Pulmonary embolism is typically manifest as right ventricular hypokinesis and/or enlargement, and has been shown to be the cause of almost 5% of cardiac arrests, with PEA being the initial rhythm in 63%.[32] Further details of the echocardiographic evaluation of pulmonary embolism are provided in Case 4.

Primary Cardiac Pathology

Echocardiography can be a very useful adjunct diagnostic tool for primary cardiac pathologies leading to cardiac arrest, including cardiogenic shock, myocardial infarction[28] (diagnosed by findings of wall motion abnormalities in the proper clinical context), and complications of myocardial infarction including myocardial rupture, ventricular septal defect (VSD), mitral valve failure, and/or papillary muscle rupture.[29,30] In an international registry from 19 medical centers of 251 patients after myocardial infarction, the cause of cardiogenic shock was severe left ventricular failure in 85%, mechanical complications in 5%, right ventricular infarct in 2%, and other comorbid conditions in 5%.[33] Cardiac free wall rupture is usually a fatal complication of acute myocardial infarction. Echocardiographic diagnosis requires a careful search for the site of rupture and should be suspected if a region of thin myocardium or a small amount of pericardial effusion is present, particularly if a loculated effusion or clot is detected. Detection of a free wall rupture in such patients can lead to surgical repair with a subsequent

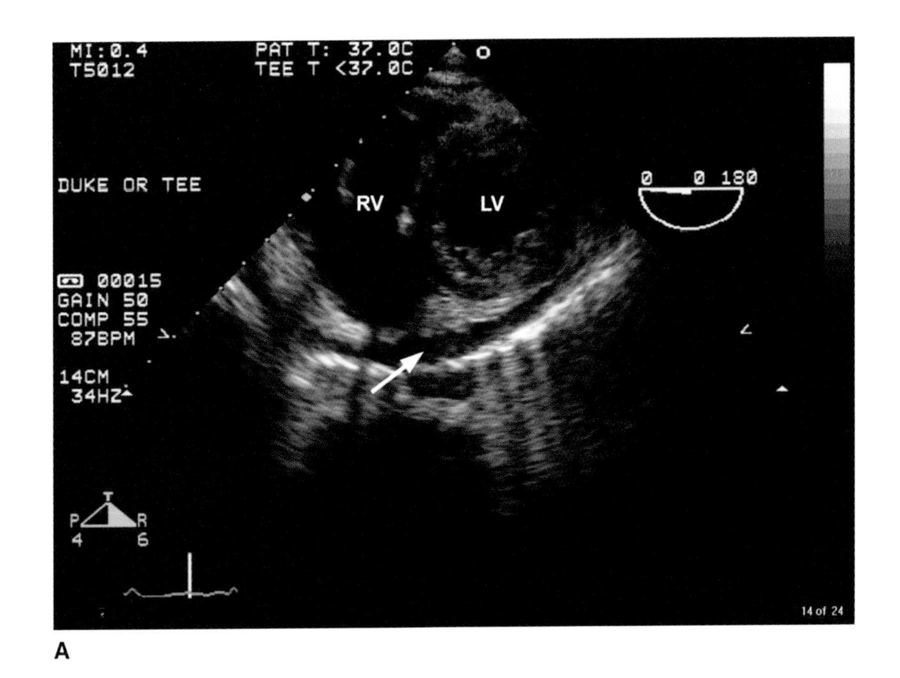

A

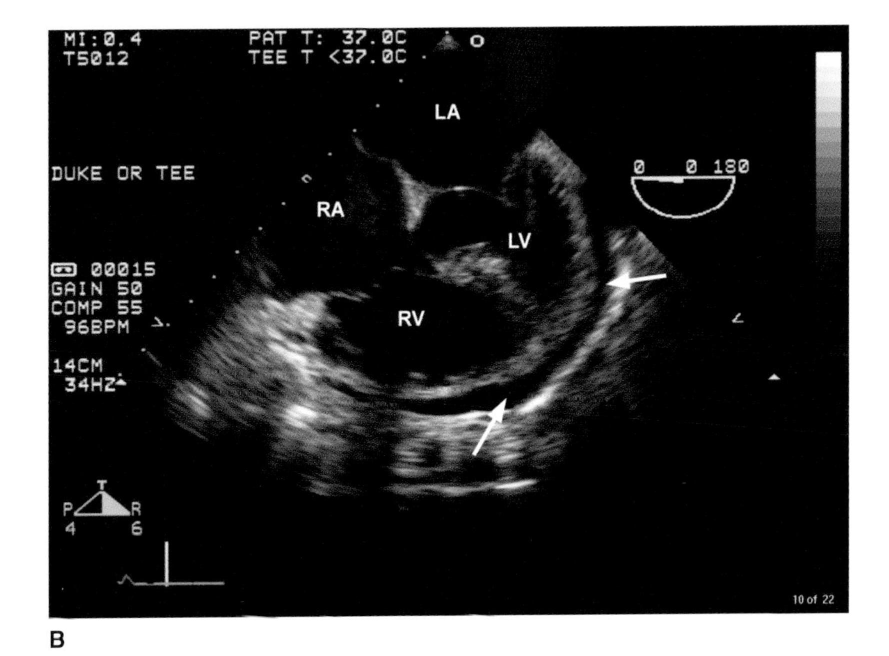

B

FIGURE 23–2. Pericardial effusion visualized on transesophageal echocardiogram: **(A)** transgastric short-axis view and **(B)** midesophageal four-chamber view, demonstrating circumferential pericardial effusion *(arrows)*. (RV, right ventricle; LV, left ventricle; RA, right atrium; LA, left atrium.)

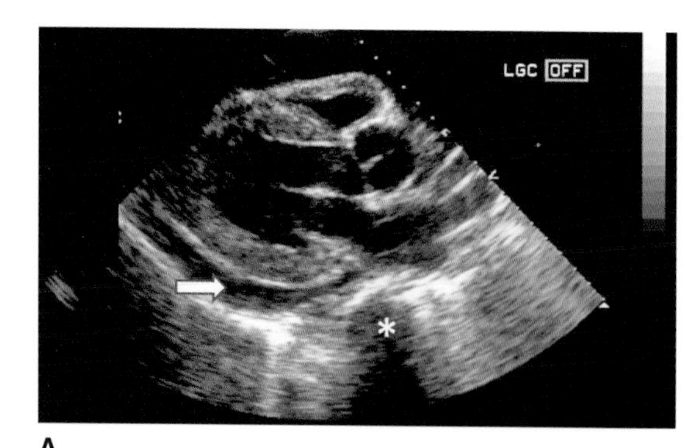

A

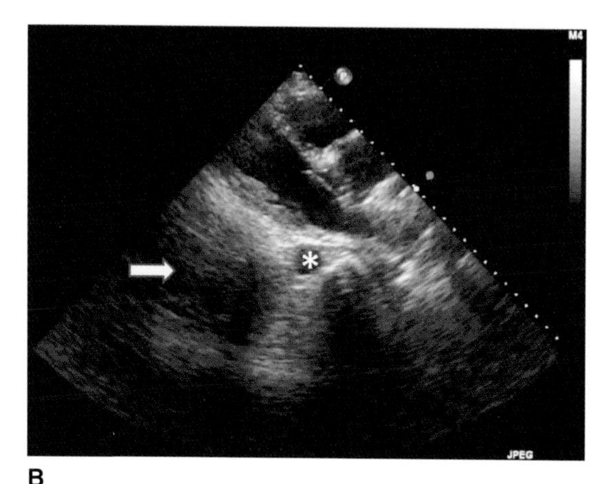

B

FIGURE 23–3. Differentiating pericardial from pleural effusion on transthoracic parasternal long-axis view: **(A)** pericardial effusions *(arrow)* lie anterior to the descending aorta *(asterisk)*, whereas **(B)** pleural effusions *(arrow)* lie posterior to the descending aorta *(asterisk)*.

survival rate of greater than 50%.[34] In some cases, a pseudoaneurysm that forms after a free wall rupture is contained within a limited portion of the pericardial space. This occurs most frequently in the inferolateral wall, and is characterized by a small neck communication between the left ventricle and the aneurysmal cavity, with to-and-fro blood flow through the rupture site seen on Doppler and color-flow imaging.[34] Mitral regurgitation often occurs in the setting of myocardial infarction, can be severe leading to hemodynamic compromise, and can be due to left ventricular dilatation leading to mitral annular dilatation, papillary muscle dysfunction, or papillary muscle rupture (Figure 23–4). Differentiating these causes of mitral regurgitation is important, as papillary muscle rupture is a serious complication that mandates urgent surgical repair.[34]

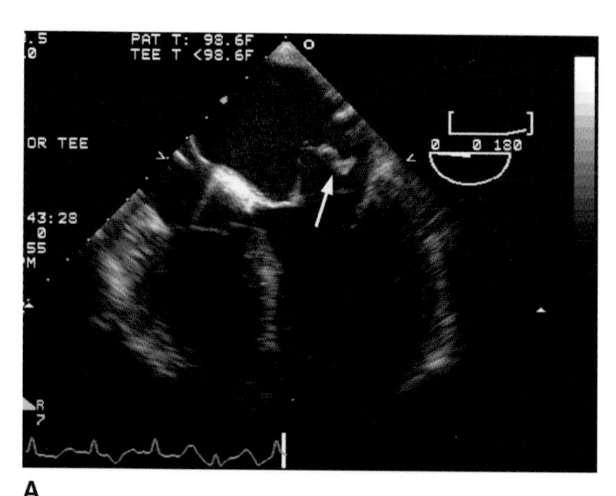

A

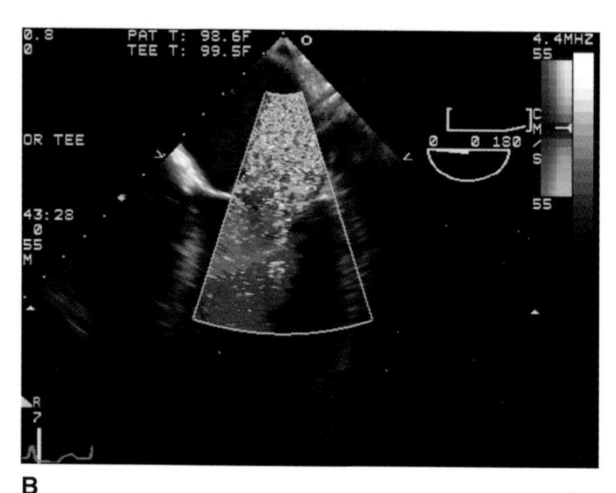

B

FIGURE 23–4. Midesophageal four-chamber TEE view demonstrating **(A)** ruptured papillary muscle *(arrow)* as a mechanical complication of acute myocardial infarction with resultant flail mitral valve leaflet; and **(B)** associated severe mitral regurgitation visualized with color Doppler.

TEE During Cardiopulmonary Resuscitation

In addition to diagnostic utility, TEE can play a role in directing resuscitation efforts and minimizing CPR interruptions by virtue of allowing more rapid assessment of "pulse" following interventions such as defibrillation or epinephrine administration. Survival with shockable rhythms is better with shorter times to defibrillation, and patients who present with a non-shockable rhythm but convert to a shockable one in the ED have better outcomes if the latter is recognized and the appropriate intervention occurs.[35] In this regard, TEE may be the most expedient way to detect such rhythms, particularly during an evolving code where a switch to a different part of the ACLS algorithm may be warranted. Since TEE can differentiate among low ejection fraction, electromechanical dissociation, and asystole, TEE can aid in the decision to cease resuscitative efforts since cardiac standstill (asystole) predicts negative outcome in the ED.[36]

CASE 2. PATIENT WITH ST ELEVATION AND CHEST PAIN

A 68-year-old male presents to a community hospital with severe central substernal chest pain radiating to his neck, jaw, and back. Upon arrival to the ED, he is diaphoretic and complaining of weakness with a blood pressure of 203/99. An ECG performed on arrival reveals anterior ST segment elevation. The nearest cardiac center with catheterization capability is at least 1 hour away, and therefore the decision is made to initiate the thrombolytic protocol established at the hospital.

A portable chest x-ray is completed. The film is difficult to interpret given the patient's body habitus, but a wide mediastinum cannot be excluded. Unequal blood pressures are noted in the arms, being approximately 20 mm Hg less in the left side. Given this physical exam finding and concern for aortic dissection, a TEE probe is placed. The image in Figure 23–5 is obtained, confirming an ascending aortic dissection extending into the left anterior descending artery. Thrombolytic therapy is deferred, and the patient's blood pressure is controlled to 160 mm Hg with esmolol. An emergency consultation with thoracic surgery is obtained, and the patient is taken to the operating room (OR) for primary repair.

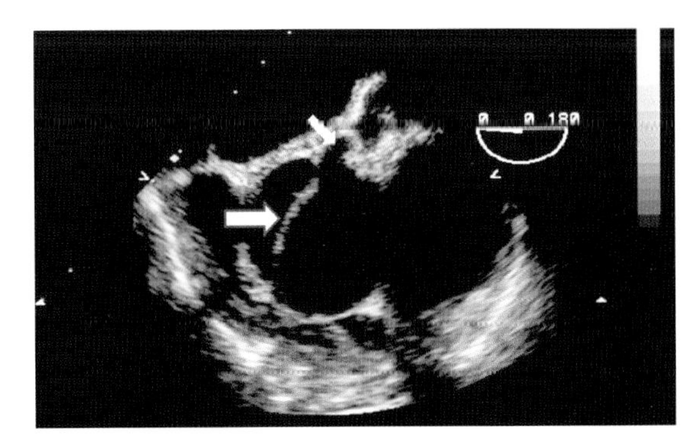

FIGURE 23–5. Upper esophageal short-axis TEE view demonstrating aortic dissection flap *(large arrow)* with dissection into the origin of the left main coronary artery *(smaller arrow)*.

TEE FOR EVALUATION OF AORTIC DISSECTION IN THE ED

Aortic pathology constitutes a subset of cardiovascular disease with high morbidity and mortality; this is compounded by presentation that frequently mimics more common disease processes. ED physicians must maintain a high level of suspicion for aortic disease, as failure to consider it as part of the differential diagnosis can result in delivery of a contraindicated treatment (such as administering thrombolytic therapy in the patient thought to have an ST elevation MI) or a delay in recognition, which could jeopardize outcomes.

Acute aortic dissection occurs with an incidence of 2.9 per 100,000 per year.[37] Any portion of the aorta can dissect. Aortic dissection typically begins with a tear from the lumen of the aorta through the intima into the medial layer. Subsequent propagation extends the intimal dissection away from the media. In addition to the classic aortic dissection instigated by a tear in the lumen of the aorta, spontaneous intramural hematoma is also a cause of aortic dissection. In this case, hemorrhage into the medial layer then dissects without rupture into the lumen. Intramural hematoma is more common in the descending aorta and arch, but can occur at any point along the aorta.

Classification of Aortic Dissections

Aortic dissections are classified by their location, with the most important factor being whether or not involvement of the ascending aorta is present. For example, the Stanford criteria differentiate aortic dissections by whether there is involvement of the ascending aorta, with such involvement classified as Stanford A (regardless of involvement of the descending aorta), and isolated descending aortic dissection classified as Stanford B. In the DeBakey classification, patients with both ascending and descending aortic involvement are classified as DeBakey I; isolated ascending aortic involvement DeBakey II; and isolated descending aortic involvement as DeBakey III. Additionally, isolated aortic arch dissections can occur. Patients with involvement of the ascending aorta have a higher risk of subsequent adverse outcomes, including pericardial effusion/tamponade, rupture, dissection into the coronary arteries, and aortic insufficiency. It should be noted that most dissections will have multiple communication points between the true and false lumens, which may be important for surgical repair.[38]

More recent studies have suggested that intramural hematomas, intramural hemorrhage, and aortic ulcers may represent evolving aortic dissection or dissection subtypes. Therefore, a new classification scheme has been proposed (Table 23–3).[39]

Table 23–3. Alternate Classification Scheme for Aortic Dissection Incorporating Variants of Aortic Pathology.

Class	Description
1	Classical aortic dissection: intimal flap separating true and false lumen
2	Medial disruption with formation of intramural hematoma/hemorrhage
3	Discrete/subtle dissection without hematoma, eccentric bulge at tear site
4	Plaque rupture leading to aortic ulceration, penetrating aortic atherosclerotic ulcer with surrounding hematoma, usually subadventitial
5	Iatrogenic and traumatic dissection

Modified from Erbel R, Alfonso F, Boileau C, et al. Diagnosis and management of aortic dissection. Eur Heart J. 2001;22(18):1642-1681.

TEE in Diagnosis of Aortic Dissection

An ascending aortic dissection is considered a surgical emergency; rapid, accurate diagnostic assessment is associated with improved survival, and hence TEE can play an important role in this assessment. TEE can reliably assess the aorta for atheromatous disease, penetrating ulcers, intramural hematomas, dissection, and rupture, as well as quantification of aortic insufficiency, if present. Although TTE provides a limited view of the ascending aorta, TEE can provide visualization of the entire length of the aorta from the aortic valve to the level of the gastroesophageal junction (although the aortic arch can be difficult to visualize). Other diagnostic modalities include aortic angiography (the traditional gold standard), helical computed tomography (CT), and magnetic resonance imaging (MRI). Each of these modalities plays an important role in the diagnosis of aortic dissection, but the risk-benefit ratio often supports TEE as the first-line imaging technique in suspected aortic injury in the ED.[40]

One study comparing diagnostic modalities for diagnosis of aortic dissection has shown similar sensitivities between single-plane TEE, CT, and MRI with sensitivities of 98% for all three, but with higher specificity for MRI (98%) than TEE (77%).[41] Use of multiplane TEE has been shown to increase the specificity of TEE to greater than 90%.[42] In another study comparing TEE with CT and aortography in the multicenter European Cooperative Study, the sensitivity and specificity of TEE was 99% and 98%, respectively; for CT, 83% and 100%; and for aortography, 88% and 94%.[43] The positive and negative predictive values for TEE were 98% and 99%, respectively; for CT, 100% and 86%; and for aortography, 96% and 84%. Other studies have revealed similar findings for the high accuracy of TEE for diagnosis of aortic dissection, although some do note the lesser sensitivity for dissections in the aortic arch.[44-46] The echocardiographer must also be aware of the not uncommon occurrence of artifactual echos in the assessment of aortic dissection (Figure 23–6).

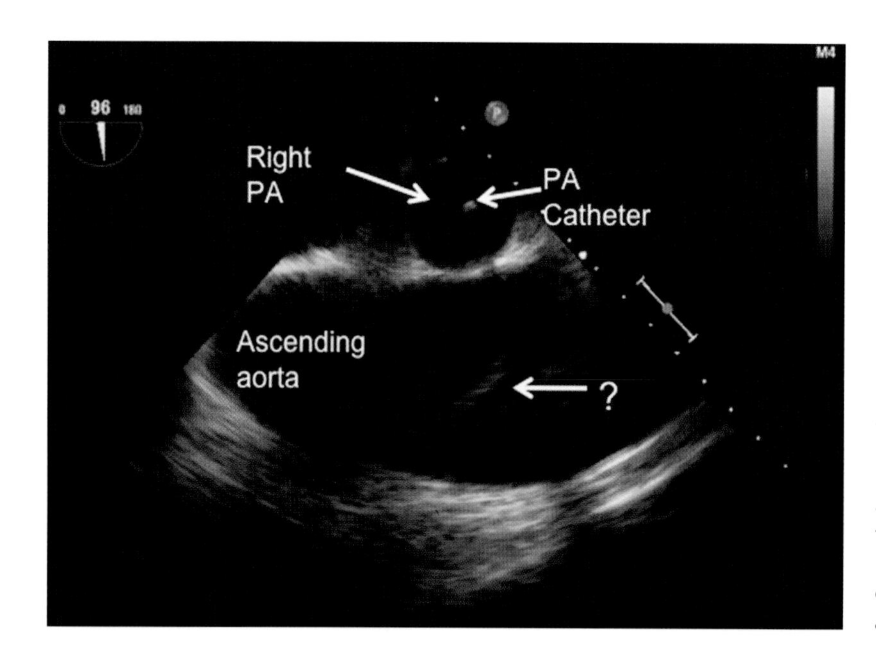

FIGURE 23–6. Midesophageal ascending aortic long-axis view demonstrating a linear artifact *("?" arrow)* in the ascending aorta that could be misinterpreted as an aortic dissection. (PA, pulmonary artery.)

In addition to having a similar sensitivity to other diagnostic modalities, TEE is also the most portable of the available options, which may be the sole determining factor for an unstable patient when transfer to the radiology suite of patient, staff, and equipment is not feasible. TEE has a relatively low cost, does not require contrast, and can provide ongoing, high-resolution image acquisition in real time. It can also provide important information for clinical decision making with regard to surgical candidacy and operative approach by virtue of being able to differentiate dissection from intramural hematoma and penetrating ulcers, localizing primary and secondary entry sites of dissection, differentiating true and false lumens, evaluating the aortic valve for regurgitation, establishing involvement of the coronary arteries, and for ruling out associated conditions such as pericardial effusion and tamponade. In addition, in the setting of trauma when the patient may be expected to have more complex injury patterns, TEE permits assessment of the heart and aortic branches.

TEE Views for Imaging the Aorta

TEE imaging of the aorta usually begins with imaging of the ascending aorta utilizing a 120° imaging plane with the probe in the mid- to upper-esophagus, allowing visualization of the proximal 5 to 10 cm of the ascending aorta. Rotation of the imaging plane to 30° to 60° allows visualization of short-axis views of the proximal ascending aorta and the aortic valve. Next, the probe is moved deeper into the esophagus towards the gastroesophageal junction; rotation of the probe to the left with use of a 0° scanning plane will result in a posterior facing plane and visualization of the descending aorta.[34] The TEE probe is then slowly withdrawn, allowing visualization of the length of the descending aorta through a series of short-axis views, and at several points along the aorta the imaging plane should be rotated to 90°, allowing a longitudinal view of the aorta. As one transitions more proximally in the aorta, the probe position is often less well tolerated by awake patients, making visualization of the aortic arch difficult. The arch is visualized by withdrawing the probe to the level of the left subclavian artery and clockwise rotation with a 0° scanning plane to obtain an elongated view of the arch; rotation to a 90° scanning plane reveals a short-axis view of the arch. Clockwise and counter-clockwise rotation allows full evaluation of the arch with visualization of the takeoff of the great vessels.

Aortic dissections are visualized as an intimal "flap" undulating within the aorta, often demonstrating a "true lumen" and a "false lumen" (Figure 23–7). Intramural hematomas will have the appearance of a smooth, homogeneous thickening of the wall corresponding to thrombus formation between the

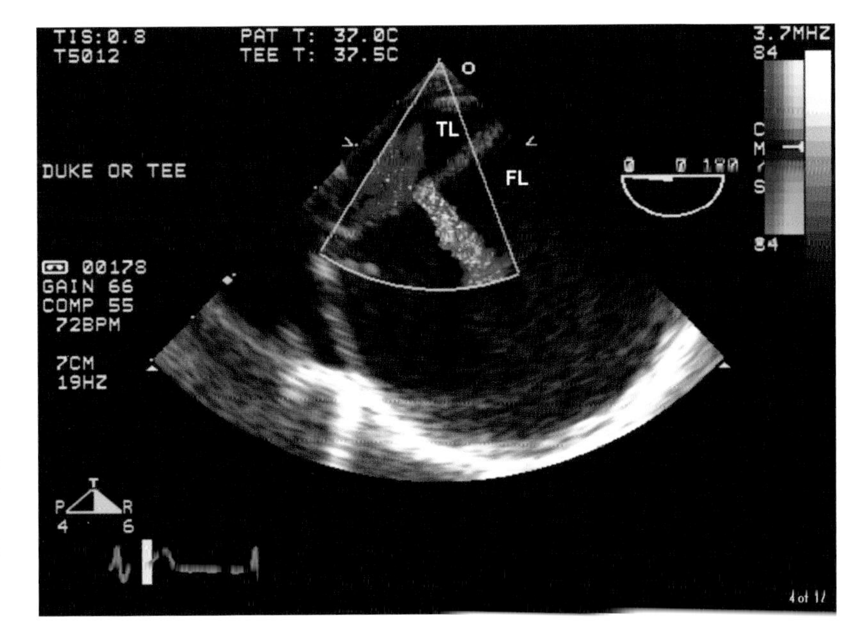

FIGURE 23–7. Transesophageal view of a patient with a descending aortic dissection demonstrating flow entering the false lumen (FL) from the true lumen (TL) through an intimal tear.

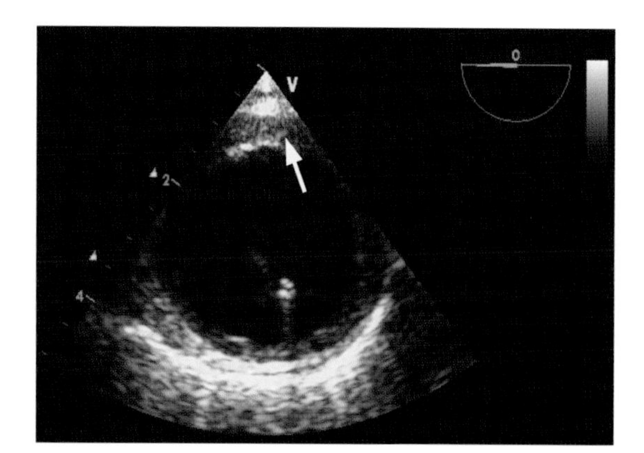

FIGURE 23–8. Descending aorta short-axis view of a patient with an aortic intramural hematoma *(arrow)*. A guidewire for placement of an endovascular stent is also seen in the lumen of the aorta.

intima and adventitia (Figure 23–8), are a precursor for aortic dissection, and should be treated like an aortic dissection. In fact, 15% to 20% of patients with aortic dissection may present with intramural hematoma.[47] The etiology of concurrent aortic insufficiency can also be characterized by TEE, which can occur as a result of dilation of the sinotubular junction and resultant aortic valve malcoaptation, dissection propagation into the sinus of Valsalva, and prolapse of the dissection flap through the aortic valve orifice.

Differentiation of True Aortic Dissection From Artifacts on TEE

Differentiation of true aortic dissection flaps from artifact can be accomplished using several imaging views and using color-flow imaging (a true flap will demonstrate margination of flow, whereas artifact will not disrupt the color Doppler signal). Further, a true flap will show mobility as opposed to artifacts appearing more rigid and fixed in location. Artifacts (see Figure 23–6) are often caused by side lobes of the aortic sinotubular junction, and hence their intensity diminishes in the lumen, whereas a true dissection will not lose its echo density along its course.[38] In addition, venous structures can create an adjacent echo creating the appearance of a linear density suggestive of a dissection flap. Color-flow imaging of this will show that the larger lumen contains pulsatile flow (ie, the true aorta) and that the smaller lumen contains continuous flow typical of a venous pattern.[38] Agitated saline contrast can also be injected to differentiate the venous structure (which is often the brachiocephalic vein). Vignon et al[48] conducted a TEE study of patients with a high risk of aortic dissection (n = 188) or traumatic disruption of the aorta (n = 42; covered later in this chapter), with comparison to final confirmed clinical diagnoses. They found linear artifacts within the ascending and descending aorta in 59 of 230 patients (26%) and 17 of 230 patients (7%), respectively.[48] TEE findings associated with linear artifacts in the ascending aorta (as opposed to true aortic dissection or traumatic disruption of the aorta) included (1) displacement or movement paralleling the aortic walls; (2) similar blood flow velocities on both sides of the "flap"; (3) angle with the aortic wall greater than 85° in short axis; and (4) thickness of "flap" greater than 2.5 mm. Further, none of the patients with linear artifacts within the ascending aorta (as opposed to true aortic pathology) had an associated pericardial effusion or evidence for an entry tear. In a subsequent prospective series of 121 patients, systematic use or these diagnostic criteria resulted in improved TEE specificity for the identification of intra-aortic flaps.[48]

CASE 3. PATIENT IN A MOTOR VEHICLE ACCIDENT

A 29-year-old female was brought in by EMS due to presumed traumatic injuries secondary to a high-speed motor vehicle accident. She was combative and was intubated on-scene. Her initial vital signs showed a blood pressure 80/38, heart rate 122. She had visible facial lacerations, extensive bruising over the precordium, and a slightly distended abdomen with bruising corresponding to the area presumed to be under the location of the lap belt. After completion of the primary survey, the decision was made to take the patient to the OR for explorative laparotomy. Prior to transfer a single portable chest film revealed a widened mediastinum with a mild left pleural effusion. A TEE was able to be rapidly completed and examination of the aorta revealed partial disruption of the aorta (Figure 23–9). Thoracic surgery was immediately consulted, and the patient was taken to the OR for surgical repair.

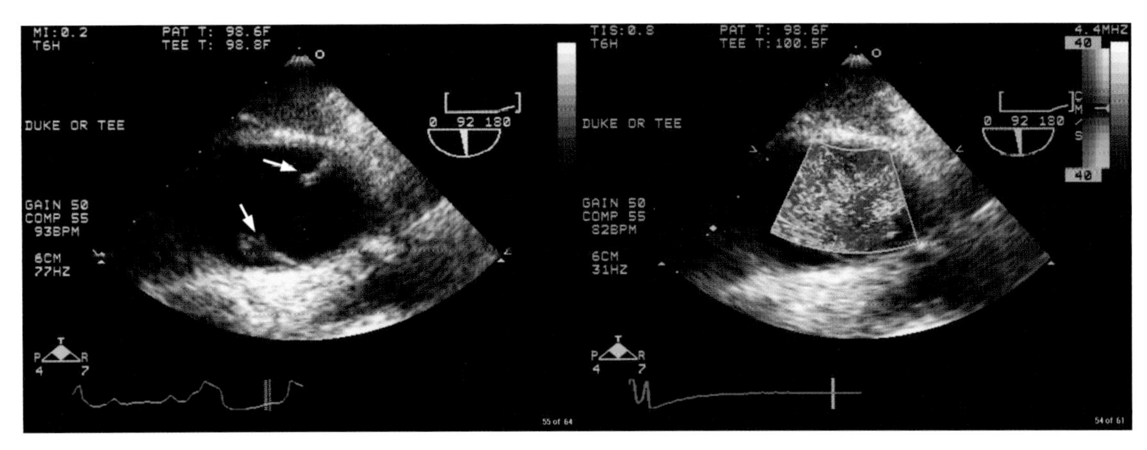

FIGURE 23–9. Transesophageal long-axis view of the descending aorta in a trauma patient demonstrating transection *(arrows)* of the aorta just below the subclavian artery. Note the "thick flap" *(left panel)* and the turbulent flow around the flap *(right panel)*.

TEE IN EVALUATION OF THE PATIENT WITH CHEST TRAUMA

Blunt or penetrating chest trauma can result in myocardial contusion or rupture, pericardial effusion and/or tamponade, hemopericardium, aortic and/or other vascular disruption, septal defects or fistula, and valvular regurgitation.[49] Trauma patients can thus present in cardiogenic shock; in this situation, the most common causes are cardiac tamponade and ventricular akinesia.[50,51]

Both TTE and TEE can be useful diagnostic tools in these situations; however, TEE has been shown to be superior to TTE in the recognition and management of patients with cardiovascular injuries due to blunt chest trauma. For example, in one study of 134 consecutive patients suffering from severe blunt chest trauma, TTE resulted in adequate visualization in only 38% of patients (compared with 98% by TEE).[52] In another study of intubated multiple injury patients not confined to blunt chest trauma, TEE was able to detect unsuspected myocardial contusion, pericardial effusion, and aortic injury.[53] Therefore, although there are no randomized controlled trials, the observational evidence supports that in patients with suspected traumatic aortic injury TEE may be used as a first-line evaluation, especially if hemodynamic instability is present.[54]

Traumatic Aortic Injury in Patients With Chest Trauma

Traumatic aortic injury can range from small intimal tears to catastrophic rupture of the aorta, which usually causes rapid, lethal hemorrhage. Minor arterial wall lesions such as a mural hematoma or a limited intimal flap often have a benign course and regress spontaneously.[55] Pseudoaneurysms can have a more insidious course, and may expand and/or rupture, leading to thromboembolic events, fistualization, or compression of nearby structures.[55,56]

Aortic injury should be particularly suspected when sudden deceleration is present in the history. In fact, up to 18% of deaths in the setting of high-velocity accidents are secondary to rupture of the aorta,[57] and blunt aortic injury is the second most common cause of death in studies of blunt trauma deaths.[4] Unfortunately, 60% to 85% of patients with traumatic aortic injuries die at the site of the accident or within hours of hospital admission.[54,58,59] However, because of improvements in prehospital emergency care, an increasing number of patients with partial aortic rupture arrive at EDs for treatment. Prompt recognition and treatment of traumatic aortic injuries in such patients is vital for survival. Unless suspected early, this partial thickness rupture may not be noticed, especially since 70% to 90% of cases of thoracic trauma are associated with multiple injuries,[60] and clinical attention may be focused (sometimes appropriately) on other even more emergent pathology. However, it is critical to assess possible aortic injuries in a timely fashion, since the goals of ACLS—ie, actively resuscitating someone to a target blood pressure of, perhaps, 90 mm Hg—may be in contrast to optimal management for aortic rupture, where one aims for a reduction in shear forces and hence treats with controlled hypotension.[60]

Furthermore, when secondary to blunt chest trauma, aortic injury frequently coexists with myocardial contusion, which can precipitate myocardial infarction or cardiac tamponade, culminating in overt cardiac failure. Early recognition may allow treatment measures to be instituted quicker. Up to 40% of patients with traumatic injury to the aorta die within 24 hours without surgical intervention.[61]

TEE in the Evaluation of Traumatic Aortic Injury in Patients With Blunt Chest Trauma

TEE plays a key role in the diagnosis of traumatic aortic injury in the patient with blunt chest trauma. In one study, 32 consecutive trauma patients were prospectively evaluated with TEE and the findings compared with aortography, surgery, or necropsy.[62] The authors found two subsets of aortic injury with distinct echocardiographic signs: (1) subadventitial traumatic disruption of the aorta (n = 10), and (2) traumatic intimal tears (n = 3). Eighteen patients had a normal TEE confirmed by aortography. One 2-mm medial tear was missed by TEE (seen on necropsy). They found that the sensitivity of TEE for the diagnosis of subadventitial aortic disruption was 91% and the specificity was 100%.[62] The authors conclude that TEE should be considered as first-line imaging for the evaluation of trauma patients with suspected injuries of the thoracic aorta. Another case series of 101 patients presenting to the ED with a diagnosis of possible traumatic rupture of the aorta who were evaluated simultaneously by TEE and aortography showed that TEE could be successfully performed in 93 patients (others not able to be completed because of lack of cooperation or maxillofacial trauma). No TEE-related complications were noted, and the results showed a sensitivity of 100% and specificity of 98% for the detection of injury to the aorta.[63] A meta-analysis has shown a maximum joint sensitivity and specificity of TEE of 97%, corresponding to a false-positive and false-negative rate of 3%.[54] When only considering studies that compared TEE with the gold standard of aortography, the maximum joint sensitivity and specificity of TEE was slightly lower (93% vs 95% with aortography). However, TEE performed better than aortography in patients with small aortic lesions not requiring surgical repair.[54] Such lesions, though easily missed by aortography, require careful follow-up and can have an unpredictable clinical course.[54] Some have advocated that TEE be routinely performed in patients with violent deceleration collisions even with a normal chest x-ray.[62,64] However, the limitations of TEE should be noted, including limited visualization of branch and proximal arch disruption, which is better visualized with aortography.[65] Of course, TEE should not be attempted in uncooperative, combative patients, or in those with unstable neck injuries.

Diagnosis of Traumatic Aortic Disruption

The most common sites of traumatic aortic injury are the aortic isthmus (at the junction of the relatively mobile aortic arch and the relatively fixed descending aorta) and the ascending aorta just proximal to the origin of the brachiocephalic vessels.[54] Complete aortic transection is a fatal event, but patients with partial aortic disruption may survive and present to the ED. Of the 20% of such patients who survive to reach the ED, 40% die within the first 24 hours.[4] The diagnosis is suggested by history of a deceleration accident and mediastinum greater than 8 cm on chest radiograph. Although CT or angiography has been the primary diagnostic modality, TEE is becoming the first approach in many centers because of the speed and superiority in evaluating aortic disease such as dissection.

The diagnosis of aortic disruption/transection requires the presence of a disrupted aortic wall with blood flow on both sides of the disruption.[62] In the previous case series, TEE findings associated with aortic disruption included the presence of an abnormal intraluminal flap just distal to the aortic isthmus, corresponding to the disrupted wall and consisting of the entire intimal and medial aortic layers, which was thicker than those seen in patients with aortic dissection (4.2 ± 0.8 mm versus 2.2 ± 0.7 mm, respectively), and were usually extremely mobile and oscillating.[62] This "thick flap" was usually accompanied by a regional deformity of the aortic isthmus contour due to formation of an acute localized pseudoaneurysm. In subtotal aortic disruptions (n = 8), this medial flap appeared as a linear structure in a transverse view that corresponded to a spiral tear at surgery. In complete aortic disruption (n = 1), the thick flap appeared as an open circle within the aortic lumen.[62] In partial disruption, the aortic tear was visualized as a discontinuity of the intimal and medial aortic layers, with color flow entering a pseudoaneurysm consisting of the adventitial layer.

With aortic trauma where there has been some partial disruption through the media into the adventitia, often a periadventitial hematoma is encountered. Varying degrees of dissection and intimal tear may be visualized with the TEE probe, or occasionally a focal area of the aorta is visualized where the circular geometry of the aorta is lost and a limited ridge may be seen protruding into the lumen of the aorta.[38] Formation of thrombus within the medial space or in the aortic lumen can also occur, and hence, if such a phenomenon is encountered in a young patient after chest trauma, aortic trauma rather than atheroma should be considered. Other consequences of aortic trauma that can be visualized with TEE include acute rupture of the sinus of Valsalva (typically into the right atrium) and formation of aorta vena caval fistulae, which are visualized as high-volume turbulent flow in the inferior vena cava.[38]

Specific signs of thoracic aortic branch vessel injury are rarely present. For example, pseudocoarctation or decreased blood pressure in the left arm occurs in only 5% of patients with rupture of the aortic isthmus.[66] Clinical signs of injury to an arch artery are more common and include cervical or supraclavicular hematomas, bruits, and diminished peripheral pulses.[67] Patients with rupture or dissection of a common carotid artery can present with coma or hemiparesis, and laceration of the brachial plexus (frequently associated with rupture of the subclavian artery), can present with denervation of the arm.[67]

Table 23–4 details echocardiographic criteria for differentiating between traumatic aortic disruption and acute aortic dissection. Based on their TEE study and previous categorization of nonpenetrating traumatic aortic injuries, Parmley et al[61] suggest a new classification of distinct traumatic aortic injuries: (1) traumatic aortic intimal tears where the integrity of the aortic medial and adventitial layers is preserved—these lesions appear to regress spontaneously; (2) subtotal aortic disruption where more than two-thirds of the aortic wall circumference is involved; (3) complete aortic disruption with involvement of the entire aortic circumference (in both subtotal and complete disruptions, medial flaps are visualized); and (4) partial aortic disruption appearing as a limited discontinuity of both intimal and medial layers.[61]

Echocardiography in the Evaluation of Cardiovascular Injury in Patients With Penetrating Chest Trauma

In patients presenting with penetrating chest trauma (ie, gunshot wound, stabbing, etc), surgical exploration is often required to exclude cardiac injury, but carries a negative exploration rate of 80%. When compared with the usual surgical subxiphoid pericardiotomy, TTE has been found to be 96% accurate, 97% specific, and 90% sensitive in detecting pericardial fluid in juxtacardiac penetrating chest wounds,[68] and hence TTE may prevent unnecessary surgical exploration. In another series of patients with penetrating chest trauma, TTE had an accuracy of 99.2% and positive and negative predictive values of 100% and 98%, respectively.[69] However, others have reported that a normal TTE does not always exclude significant injury; for example, when hemothorax is associated with penetrating injury, TTE is not an adequate replacement for surgical exploration.[70]

Table 23–4. TEE Criteria Differentiating Traumatic Aortic Disruption and Acute Aortic Dissection.

	Traumatic Aortic Disruption	Aortic Dissection
2D TEE	• Thick medial flap • Asymmetric contour of aortic isthmus secondary to aneurysm formation • Mobile, oscillating flap • No entry or reentry tear • Presence of mediastinal hematoma • Absence of thrombus	• Thin medial flap • Symmetric enlargement of aortic isthmus • Less mobile flap • Presence of entry or reentry tear • Absence of mediastinal hematoma • Presence of thrombus in false lumen
Color-flow mapping	• Similar velocities on both sides of flap • Mosaic of colors surrounding disrupted aortic wall	• Different velocities in true and false lumens • Absence of mosaic of colors on both sides of intimal flap
Location	• Limited to the aortic isthmus	• More extensive involvement of the aorta depending on type

Adapted with permission from Vignon P, Gueret P, Vedrinne JM, et al. Role of transesophageal echocardiography in the diagnosis and management of traumatic aortic disruption. Circulation. 1995;92(10):2959-2968.

CASE 4. PATIENT WITH UNEXPLAINED HYPOTENSION

A 47-year-old female with a history of diabetes, hypertension, and breast cancer has an acute onset of chest pain and shortness of breath at rest. Her symptoms progress and she presents to the ED for evaluation. She is initially tachycardic and diaphoretic with a blood pressure of 95/64. Before a 12-lead ECG can be performed, she loses consciousness and is found to have a repeat blood pressure of 63/48. Intravenous fluid boluses are given with no response. Pressors are initiated with some improvement but with sustained hypotension. A 12-lead ECG shows sinus tachycardia with a right bundle branch block. A bedside TEE is performed, which reveals marked right ventricular dysfunction and enlargement (Figure 23–10). A subsequent CT scan confirms a large saddle pulmonary embolus and the patient is successfully treated with thrombolytics.

TEE IN EVALUATION OF UNEXPLAINED HYPOTENSION

Echocardiography can be a valuable tool in evaluation of the patient with unexplained hypotension (see Table 23–2). Both TTE and TEE can help quickly distinguish among a primary cardiac etiology resulting in decreased cardiac output versus a noncardiac etiology such as hemorrhage with hypovolemia. While TTE may provide sufficient imaging in the critically ill patient, visualization of cardiac structures is often impaired and TEE is therefore required. In one series of 2508 TEE studies in critically ill patients over 15 years, hemodynamic instability was the most frequent indication for TEE (39%), followed by suspected endocarditis (19%), assessment of ventricular function (9%), suspected aortic disease (8%), suspected pericardial tamponade (3%), and chest trauma (1%).[71] Similarly, Burns et al[72] demonstrated in acutely ill trauma patients that approximately two-thirds of patients improved because of changes in management resulting from the TEE findings. For example, several patients with what would be deemed as having acceptable filling pressures based on pulmonary arterial catheterization in fact had inadequate filling when visualized on TEE.[72] In another study of 308 critically ill patients, 40% of patients were evaluated by TEE for hypotension; of these, the cause of the hypotension was identified in 67% of the cases, leading to a management change in 31% of patients.[73]

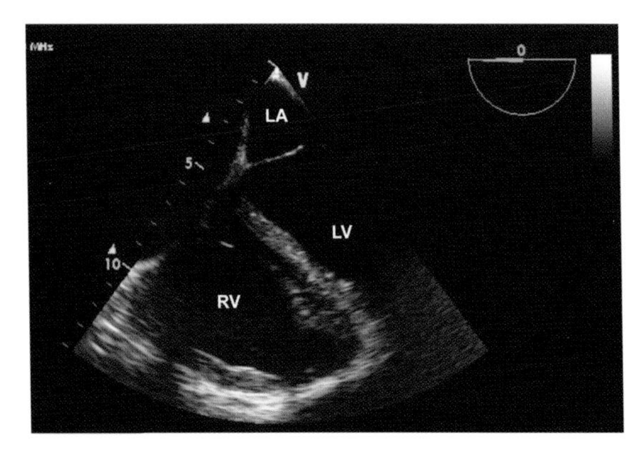

FIGURE 23–10. Midesophageal four-chamber view of a patient with acute pulmonary embolism demonstrating right ventricular dilatation. (LA, left atrium; LV, left ventricle; RV, right ventricle.)

TEE Assessment of Cardiac Etiologies of Hypotension

Echocardiography can delineate the cardiac etiology resulting in hemodynamic instability, ie, cardiogenic shock, acute valvular insufficiency, or concurrent cardiac abnormalities. One of the mainstays of echocardiographic evaluation in patients with unexplained hypotension is left and right ventricular systolic function assessment, which can usually be accomplished by real-time visualization alone through a combination of short-axis and long-axis views of the left and right ventricles. In one study, 115 critically ill patients were evaluated by TEE, with the most common indication being hemodynamic instability (67% of patients).[74] Of these, 26% were found to have left ventricular dysfunction with left ventricular ejection fraction of less than 30%, suggesting that this is not an uncommon cause of hypotension in ill patients. In several series, echocardiography has been found to be more reliable than Swan-Ganz catheter pressure in determining the cause of hypotension.[75-77] Further, left ventricular dysfunction can occur in the setting of septic shock,[78] and hence left ventricular function assessment in such patients can be important to guide subsequent therapy.

In addition to ventricular dysfunction, cardiac hypotension can be caused by pericardial tamponade and/or severe valvular disease. In a study of 61 critically ill patients with unexplained, sustained (>60 minutes) hypotension, a TEE-guided diagnosis of nonventricular limitation to cardiac output (ie, valvular or pericardial) was associated with improved survival to discharge (81%) versus a diagnosis of ventricular disease (41%) or hypovolemia/low systemic vascular resistance (44%).[76] TTE was inadequate in 64% of these patients, and TEE contributed new, clinically significant diagnoses (ie, not seen by TTE) in 28% of patients, leading to surgical interventions in 20%. The authors suggest that TEE makes a clinically important contribution to the diagnosis and management of unexplained hypotension and is prognostic in critically ill patients.[76] TEE can also diagnose myocardial infarction and related mechanical complications as detailed earlier in this chapter.

TEE Assessment of Hypovolemia as a Cause of Hypotension

Echocardiography can represent an important tool for the diagnosis of hypovolemia, documenting a small left ventricular volume and hyperdynamic motion. With TEE, left ventricular volume can be measured by subjective assessment of LV size or by quantitative determination of left ventricular cross-sectional area at end-diastole using the transgastric short-axis view at the level of the midpapillary muscles.[79] In some patients, often those with a history of hypertension, an acquired dynamic left ventricular outflow tract obstruction can occur when volume depletion occurs, with the same hemodynamic consequences as obstructive hypertrophic cardiomyopathy. Elevated left ventricular outflow tract gradients and systolic anterior motion of the mitral valve with secondary mitral regurgitation may be seen, resulting in progressive hypotension and development of a systolic murmur. Gradients exceeding 100 mm Hg have been noted, and hemodynamic assessment with pulmonary artery catheterization may be misleading, showing an elevated pulmonary capillary wedge pressure suggesting an increased left ventricular filling volume.[38] This abnormality resolves with volume repletion and removal of pharmacologic agents aimed at increasing contractility and/or reducing vascular resistance.

TEE Assessment of Pulmonary Embolism as a Cause of Hypotension

Pulmonary embolus (PE) has been shown to be the cause of almost 5% of cardiac arrests, with PEA being the initial rhythm in 63%.[32] In fact, one small study of 25 patients presenting with PEA in whom TEE was routinely performed showed that 14 had evidence of right ventricular enlargement; of these nine were subsequently found to have pulmonary embolism, with the remainder having cardiac contusion, right ventricular infarction, right ventricular hypertrophy, or cor pulmonale.[80] Diagnosis of PE in the setting of cardiac arrest is an important one as prompt treatment with thrombolytics has been shown to result in a significantly higher return of spontaneous circulation than in those patients not receiving thrombolytics (81% vs 43%, respectively).[32]

PE is diagnosed on TEE by findings suggestive of acute right ventricular pressure overload such as right ventricular enlargement and/or hypokinesis in the context of an appropriate clinical scenario. In the absence of myocardial infarction, significant left-side valve or ventricular disease, or known pulmonary disease, this finding indicates a high probability of pulmonary embolus.[4] This can often be accompanied by right atrial enlargement, tricuspid regurgitation, dilation of the inferior vena cava and flattening of the interventricular septum with a "D-shaped" left ventricular geometry in the short-axis views due to pressure overload on the right ventricle, and paradoxical septal motion. Of note, right ventricular dysfunction can also be due to an inferior myocardial infarction, myocardial contusion (ie, in the setting of trauma), sepsis, and acute sickle-cell crisis.[10] Often termed "McConnell sign," a relatively specific sign of right ventricular dysfunction due to pulmonary embolism (as opposed to other causes of right ventricular dysfunction) is characterized by a distinct regional pattern of right ventricular (RV) dysfunction with normal RV apical motion but akinesia of the mid-free RV wall.[81] This regional RV dysfunction was found to have a sensitivity of 77%, specificity of 94%, positive predictive value of 71%, and a negative predictive value of 96% for the diagnosis of PE.

It should be noted that the echocardiographic findings of pulmonary embolus are typically seen after acute obstruction of more than 30% of the pulmonary arterial bed.[82] However, a recent small study has suggested that a decreased acceleration time of pulmonary artery outflow is associated with even small pulmonary emboli obstructing less than 25% of the pulmonary vasculature (acceleration time in pulmonary embolism 85 ± 22 milliseconds vs 117 ± 35 milliseconds in controls without pulmonary embolism).[83] This needs to be further validated before being used clinically, but suggests additional echocardiographic criteria to discriminate smaller pulmonary emboli. In addition, some studies have suggested that the right ventricular to left ventricular end-diastolic diameter ratio (RVEDD/LVEDD) may be an important prognostic factor in patients with pulmonary embolism. In one study of 950 patients hospitalized for acute pulmonary embolism, it was found that the sensitivity and specificity of an RVEDD/LVEDD greater than 0.9 for predicting hospital mortality were 72% and 58%, respectively, with the ratio also being an independent predictor of hospitality mortality (odds ratio 2.66).[84]

Although rarely seen on TTE, TEE may be able to directly visualize pulmonary emboli,[85] usually in the main or right pulmonary arteries (Figure 23–11), with limited sensitivity for more distal or left pulmonary arterial clots. In one study of intraoperative TEE in 46 patients with known PE immediately prior to pulmonary embolectomy, using definitive location of

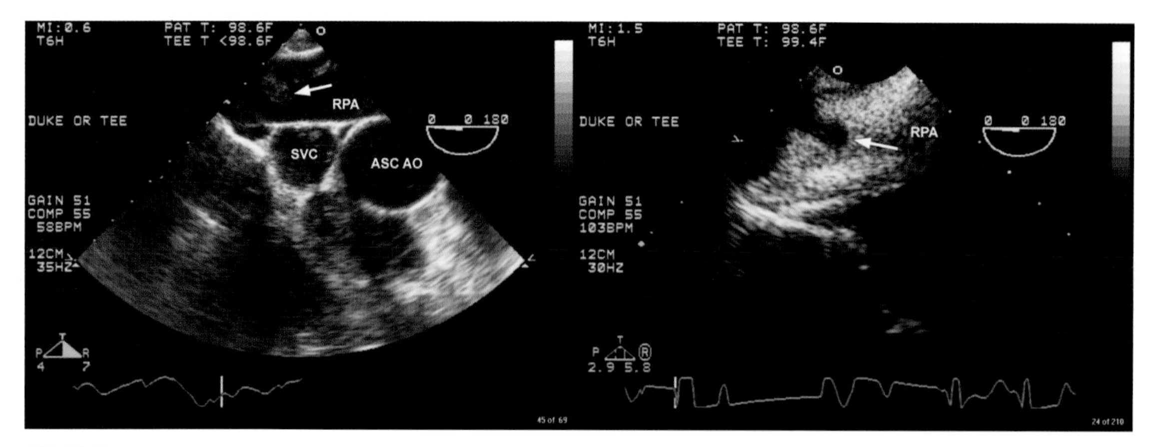

FIGURE 23–11. Upper esophageal ascending aorta (ASC AO) short-axis view demonstrating a pulmonary embolus *(arrow)* in the right pulmonary artery (RPA) *(left panel)*. The embolus is more readily visualized after contrast enhanced ultrasonography *(right panel)*. (SVC, superior vena cava.)

thromboemboli determined from the surgical record as the "gold standard," they found that echocardiographic evidence of right ventricular dysfunction was present in 96% and leftward interatrial septal bowing was present in 98% of examinations. However, the sensitivity of TEE for direct visualization at any specific location was only 26%, with the least sensitivity for the left pulmonary artery.[22] Another study of TEE in patients with known severe PE showed that central pulmonary thromboemboli were directly visualized in 58.3% of patients evaluated, leading the authors to conclude that TEE seems to be a useful method for the diagnosis of severe PE, with the potential ability to clarify the diagnosis within a few minutes without further invasive diagnostic procedures.[85] Regardless, the combination of indirect echocardiographic criteria in combination with potential direct visualization of pulmonary thromboemboli make TEE a valuable tool in the diagnostic workup.

TEE IN EVALUATION OF UNEXPLAINED HYPOXIA

An additional use of echocardiography in the ED and ICU is evaluation of unexplained hypoxia. In such situations, echocardiography can help distinguish causes such as intracardiac shunt, pulmonary embolus, pulmonary hypertension, and right ventricular failure. Often TTE in such critically ill patients is insufficient, and TTE is often insensitive for evaluation of intracardiac shunts, necessitating TEE evaluation. If such an evaluation excludes a primary cardiac abnormality, the ED physician can assume that the cause of the hypoxia is extracardiac.

CONCLUSIONS

Echocardiography remains a mainstay in the diagnosis and management of acutely ill patients presenting to the ED. Given limitations to TTE imaging in this group of patients, TEE can serve as a useful and accurate bedside modality, allowing rapid assessment of a wide range of cardiovascular pathologies observed in patients presenting to the ED.

ACKNOWLEDGMENT

We thank Dr. Robert Preston for his editorial assistance and drafting of the questions associated with this chapter.

REFERENCES

1. Moore CL, Rose GA, Tayal VS, Sullivan DM, Arrowood JA, Kline JA. Determination of left ventricular function by emergency physician echocardiography of hypotensive patients. *Acad Emerg Med.* 2002;9(3):186-193.
2. Jones AE, Craddock PA, Tayal VS, Kline JA. Diagnostic accuracy of left ventricular function for identifying sepsis among emergency department patients with nontraumatic symptomatic undifferentiated hypotension. *Shock.* 2005;24(6):513-517.
3. Stewart WJ, Douglas PS, Sagar K, et al. Echocardiography in emergency medicine: a policy statement by the American Society of Echocardiography and the American College of Cardiology. The Task Force on Echocardiography in Emergency Medicine of the American Society of Echocardiography and the Echocardiography TPEC Committees of the American College of Cardiology. *J Am Soc Echocardiogr.* 1999;12(1):82-84.
4. Cheitlin MD, Armstrong WF, Aurigemma GP, et al. ACC/AHA/ASE 2003 guideline update for the clinical application of echocardiography: summary article: a report of the American

College of Cardiology/American Heart Association Task Force on Practice Guidelines (ACC/AHA/ASE Committee to Update the 1997 Guidelines for the Clinical Application of Echocardiography). *Circulation.* 2003;108(9):1146-1162.

5. Kallmeyer IJ, Collard CD, Fox JA, Body SC, Shernan SK. The safety of intraoperative transesophageal echocardiography: a case series of 7200 cardiac surgical patients. *Anesth Analg.* 2001;92(5):1126-1130.
6. Khoury AF, Afridi I, Quinones MA, Zoghbi WA. Transesophageal echocardiography in critically ill patients: feasibility, safety, and impact on management. *Am Heart J.* 1994;127(5): 1363-1371.
7. Gendreau MA, Triner WR, Bartfield J. Complications of transesophageal echocardiography in the ED. *Am J Emerg Med.* 1999;17(3):248-251.
8. Daniel WG, Erbel R, Kasper W, et al. Safety of transesophageal echocardiography. A multicenter survey of 10,419 examinations. *Circulation.* 1991;83(3):817-821.
9. Varriale P, Maldonado JM. Echocardiographic observations during in hospital cardiopulmonary resuscitation. *Crit Care Med.* 1997;25(10):1717-1720.
10. Beaulieu Y. Bedside echocardiography in the assessment of the critically ill. *Crit Care Med.* 2007;35(5 Suppl):S235-249.
11. Cook CH, Praba AC, Beery PR, Martin LC. Transthoracic echocardiography is not cost-effective in critically ill surgical patients. *J Trauma.* 2002;52(2):280-284.
12. Hwang JJ, Shyu KG, Chen JJ, Tseng YZ, Kuan P, Lien WP. Usefulness of transesophageal echocardiography in the treatment of critically ill patients. *Chest.* 1993;104(3):861-866.
13. Parker MM, Cunnion RE, Parrillo JE. Echocardiography and nuclear cardiac imaging in the critical care unit. *JAMA.* 1985;254(20):2935-2939.
14. Breitkreutz R, Walcher F, Seeger FH. Focused echocardiographic evaluation in resuscitation management: concept of an advanced life support-conformed algorithm. *Crit Care Med.* 2007;35(5 Suppl):S150-161.
15. van der Wouw PA, Koster RW, Delemarre BJ, de Vos R, Lampe-Schoenmaeckers AJ, Lie KI. Diagnostic accuracy of transesophageal echocardiography during cardiopulmonary resuscitation. *J Am Coll Cardiol.* 1997;30(3):780-783.
16. Nichol G, Thomas E, Callaway CW, et al. Regional variation in out-of-hospital cardiac arrest incidence and outcome. *JAMA.* 2008;300(12):1423-1431.
17. Brindley PG, Markland DM, Mayers I, Kutsogiannis DJ. Predictors of survival following in-hospital adult cardiopulmonary resuscitation. *CMAJ.* 2002;167(4):343-348.
18. Taffet GE, Teasdale TA, Luchi RJ. In-hospital cardiopulmonary resuscitation. *JAMA.* 1988;260(14):2069-2072.
19. Hernandez C, Shuler K, Hannan H, Sonyika C, Likourezos A, Marshall J. C.A.U.S.E.: Cardiac arrest ultra-sound exam—a better approach to managing patients in primary non-arrhythmogenic cardiac arrest. *Resuscitation.* 2008;76(2):198-206.
20. Memtsoudis SG, Rosenberger P, Loffler M, et al. The usefulness of transesophageal echocardiography during intraoperative cardiac arrest in noncardiac surgery. *Anesth Analg.* 2006;102(6): 1653-1657.
21. Blaivas M, Fox JC. Outcome in cardiac arrest patients found to have cardiac standstill on the bedside emergency department echocardiogram. *Acad Emerg Med.* 2001;8(6):616-621.
22. Rosenberger P, Shernan SK, Body SC, Eltzschig HK. Utility of intraoperative transesophageal echocardiography for diagnosis of pulmonary embolism. *Anesth Analg.* 2004;99(1):12-16.
23. Vieillard-Baron A, Qanadli SD, Antakly Y, et al. Transesophageal echocardiography for the diagnosis of pulmonary embolism with acute cor pulmonale: a comparison with radiological procedures. *Intensive Care Med.* 1998;24(5):429-433.
24. Fontes ML, Bellows W, Ngo L, Mangano DT. Assessment of ventricular function in critically ill patients: limitations of pulmonary artery catheterization. Institutions of the McSPI Research Group. *J Cardiothorac Vasc Anesth.* 1999;13(5):521-527.
25. Sutton DC, Cahalan MK. Intraoperative assessment of left ventricular function with transesophageal echocardiography. *Cardiol Clin.* 1993;11(3):389-398.
26. Cheung AT, Savino JS, Weiss SJ, Aukburg SJ, Berlin JA. Echocardiographic and hemodynamic indexes of left ventricular preload in patients with normal and abnormal ventricular function. *Anesthesiology.* 1994;81(2):376-387.
27. Cicek S, Demirkilic U, Kuralay E, Arslan M, Tatar H, Ozturk OO. Prediction of intraoperative hypovolemia in patients with left ventricular hypertrophy: comparison of transesophageal echocardiography and Swan-Ganz monitoring. *Echocardiography.* 1997;14(3):257-260.
28. Comunale ME, Body SC, Ley C, et al. The concordance of intraoperative left ventricular wall-motion abnormalities and electrocardiographic S-T segment changes: association with outcome after coronary revascularization. Multicenter Study of Perioperative Ischemia (McSPI) Research Group. *Anesthesiology.* 1998;88(4):945-954.
29. Porter TR, Ornato JP, Guard CS, Roy VG, Burns CA, Nixon JV. Transesophageal echocardiography to assess mitral valve function and flow during cardiopulmonary resuscitation. *Am J Cardiol.* 1992;70(11):1056-1060.
30. Redberg RF, Tucker KJ, Cohen TJ, Dutton JP, Callaham ML, Schiller NB. Physiology of blood flow during cardiopulmonary resuscitation. A transesophageal echocardiographic study. *Circulation.* 1993;88(2):534-542.
31. Brown JM. Use of echocardiography for hemodynamic monitoring. *Crit Care Med.* 2002;30(6):1361-1364.
32. Kurkciyan I, Meron G, Sterz F, et al. Pulmonary embolism as a cause of cardiac arrest: presentation and outcome. *Arch Intern Med.* 2000;160(10):1529-1535.
33. Hochman JS, Boland J, Sleeper LA, et al. Current spectrum of cardiogenic shock and effect of early revascularization on mortality. Results of an international registry. SHOCK Registry Investigators. *Circulation.* 1995;91(3):873-881.
34. Oh JK, Seward JB, Tajik AJ. *The Echo Manual.* Philadelphia: Lippincott Williams and Wilkins; 1999.
35. Olasveengen TM, Samdal M, Steen PA, Wik L, Sunde K. Progressing from initial non-shockable rhythms to a shockable rhythm is associated with improved outcome after out-of-hospital cardiac arrest. *Resuscitation.* 2009;80(1):24-29.
36. Szczygiel M, Wright R, Wagner E, Holcomb MS. Prognostic indicators of ultimate long-term survival following advanced life support. *Ann Emerg Med.* 1981;10(11):566-570.
37. Meszaros I, Morocz J, Szlavi J, et al. Epidemiology and clinicopathology of aortic dissection. *Chest.* 2000;117(5):1271-1278.
38. Feigenbaum H, Armstrong WF, Ryan T. In: Feigenbaum H, Armstrong WF, Ryan T, eds. *Feigenbaum's Echocardiography.* 6th ed. Philadelphia: Lippincott Williams & Wilkins; 2005.

39. Erbel R, Alfonso F, Boileau C, et al. Diagnosis and management of aortic dissection. *Eur Heart J.* 2001;22(18):1642-1681.
40. Willens HJ, Kessler KM. Transesophageal echocardiography in the diagnosis of diseases of the thoracic aorta: part 1. Aortic dissection, aortic intramural hematoma, and penetrating atherosclerotic ulcer of the aorta. *Chest.* 1999;116(6):1772-1779.
41. Nienaber CA, von Kodolitsch Y, Nicolas V, et al. The diagnosis of thoracic aortic dissection by noninvasive imaging procedures. *N Engl J Med.* 1993;328(1):1-9.
42. Keren A, Kim CB, Hu BS, et al. Accuracy of biplane and multiplane transesophageal echocardiography in diagnosis of typical acute aortic dissection and intramural hematoma. *J Am Coll Cardiol.* 1996;28(3):627-636.
43. Erbel R, Engberding R, Daniel W, Roelandt J, Visser C, Rennollet H. Echocardiography in diagnosis of aortic dissection. *Lancet.* 1989;1(8636):457-461.
44. Ballal RS, Nanda NC, Gatewood R, et al. Usefulness of transesophageal echocardiography in assessment of aortic dissection. *Circulation.* 1991;84(5):1903-1914.
45. Barbant SD, Eisenberg MJ, Schiller NB. The diagnostic value of imaging techniques for aortic dissection. *Am Heart J.* 1992;124(2):541-543.
46. Sommer T, Fehske W, Holzknecht N, et al. Aortic dissection: a comparative study of diagnosis with spiral CT, multiplanar transesophageal echocardiography, and MR imaging. *Radiology.* 1996;199(2):347-352.
47. Nienaber CA, von Kodolitsch Y, Petersen B, et al. Intramural hemorrhage of the thoracic aorta. Diagnostic and therapeutic implications. *Circulation.* 1995;92(6):1465-1472.
48. Vignon P, Spencer KT, Rambaud G, et al. Differential transesophageal echocardiographic diagnosis between linear artifacts and intraluminal flap of aortic dissection or disruption. *Chest.* 2001;119(6):1778-1790.
49. Pretre R, Chilcott M. Blunt trauma to the heart and great vessels. *N Engl J Med.* 1997;336(9):626-632.
50. Fulda G, Brathwaite CE, Rodriguez A, Turney SZ, Dunham CM, Cowley RA. Blunt traumatic rupture of the heart and pericardium: a ten-year experience (1979-1989). *J Trauma.* 1991;31(2):167-172; discussion 172-163.
51. Santavirta S, Arajarvi E. Ruptures of the heart in seatbelt wearers. *J Trauma.* 1992;32(3):275-279.
52. Chirillo F, Totis O, Cavarzerani A, et al. Usefulness of transthoracic and transoesophageal echocardiography in recognition and management of cardiovascular injuries after blunt chest trauma. *Heart.* 1996;75(3):301-306.
53. Catoire P, Orliaguet G, Liu N, et al. Systematic transesophageal echocardiography for detection of mediastinal lesions in patients with multiple injuries. *J Trauma.* 1995;38(1):96-102.
54. Cinnella G, Dambrosio M, Brienza N, Tullo L, Fiore T. Transesophageal echocardiography for diagnosis of traumatic aortic injury: an appraisal of the evidence. *J Trauma.* 2004;57(6):1246-1255.
55. Frykberg ER, Crump JM, Dennis JW, Vines FS, Alexander RH. Nonoperative observation of clinically occult arterial injuries: a prospective evaluation. *Surgery.* 1991;109(1):85-96.
56. Pretre R, LaHarpe R, Cheretakis A, et al. Blunt injury to the ascending aorta: three patterns of presentation. *Surgery.* 1996;119(6):603-610.
57. Greendyke RM. Traumatic rupture of aorta; special reference to automobile accidents. *JAMA.* 1966;195(7):527-530.
58. Fabian TC, Richardson JD, Croce MA, et al. Prospective study of blunt aortic injury: Multicenter Trial of the American Association for the Surgery of Trauma. *J Trauma.* 1997;42(3):374-380; discussion 380-373.
59. Minard G, Schurr MJ, Croce MA, et al. A prospective analysis of transesophageal echocardiography in the diagnosis of traumatic disruption of the aorta. *J Trauma.* 1996;40(2):225-230.
60. Balm R, Hoornweg LL. Traumatic aortic ruptures. *J Cardiovasc Surg (Torino).* 2005;46(2):101-105.
61. Parmley LF, Mattingly TW, Manion WC, Jahnke EJ Jr. Nonpenetrating traumatic injury of the aorta. *Circulation.* 1958;17(6):1086-1101.
62. Vignon P, Gueret P, Vedrinne JM, et al. Role of transesophageal echocardiography in the diagnosis and management of traumatic aortic disruption. *Circulation.* 1995;92(10):2959-2968.
63. Smith MD, Cassidy JM, Souther S, et al. Transesophageal echocardiography in the diagnosis of traumatic rupture of the aorta. *N Engl J Med.* 1995;332(6):356-362.
64. Vignon P, Lagrange P, Boncoeur MP, Francois B, Gastinne H, Lang RM. Routine transesophageal echocardiography for the diagnosis of aortic disruption in trauma patients without enlarged mediastinum. *J Trauma.* 1996;40(3):422-427.
65. Ben-Menachem Y. Assessment of blunt aortic-brachiocephalic trauma: should angiography be supplanted by transesophageal echocardiography? *J Trauma.* 1997;42(5):969-972.
66. Cowley RA, Turney SZ, Hankins JR, Rodriguez A, Attar S, Shankar BS. Rupture of thoracic aorta caused by blunt trauma. A fifteen-year experience. *J Thorac Cardiovasc Surg.* 1990;100(5):652-660; discussion 660-651.
67. Rosenberg JM, Bredenberg CE, Marvasti MA, Bucknam C, Conti C, Parker FB Jr. Blunt injuries to the aortic arch vessels. *Ann Thorac Surg.* 1989;48(4):508-513.
68. Jimenez E, Martin M, Krukenkamp I, Barrett J. Subxiphoid pericardiotomy versus echocardiography: a prospective evaluation of the diagnosis of occult penetrating cardiac injury. *Surgery.* 1990;108(4):676-679; discussion 679-680.
69. Nagy KK, Lohmann C, Kim DO, Barrett J. Role of echocardiography in the diagnosis of occult penetrating cardiac injury. *J Trauma.* 1995;38(6):859-862.
70. Meyer DM, Jessen ME, Grayburn PA. Use of echocardiography to detect occult cardiac injury after penetrating thoracic trauma: a prospective study. *J Trauma.* 1995;39(5):902-907; discussion 907-909.
71. Huttemann E, Schelenz C, Kara F, Chatzinikolaou K, Reinhart K. The use and safety of transoesophageal echocardiography in the general ICU—a minireview. *Acta Anaesthesiol Scand.* 2004;48(7):827-836.
72. Burns JM, Sing RF, Mostafa G, et al. The role of transesophageal echocardiography in optimizing resuscitation in acutely injured patients. *J Trauma.* 2005;59(1):36-40; discussion 40-32.
73. Colreavy FB, Donovan K, Lee KY, Weekes J. Transesophageal echocardiography in critically ill patients. *Crit Care Med.* 2002;30(5):989-996.
74. Bruch C, Comber M, Schmermund A, Eggebrecht H, Bartel T, Erbel R. Diagnostic usefulness and impact on management of transesophageal echocardiography in surgical intensive care units. *Am J Cardiol.* 2003;91(4):510-513.
75. Chan KL. Transesophageal echocardiography for assessing cause of hypotension after cardiac surgery. *Am J Cardiol.* 1988;62(16):1142-1143.

76. Heidenreich PA, Stainback RF, Redberg RF, Schiller NB, Cohen NH, Foster E. Transesophageal echocardiography predicts mortality in critically ill patients with unexplained hypotension. *J Am Coll Cardiol.* 1995;26(1):152-158.
77. Jardin F, Valtier B, Beauchet A, Dubourg O, Bourdarias JP. Invasive monitoring combined with two-dimensional echocardiographic study in septic shock. *Intensive Care Med.* 1994;20(8): 550-554.
78. Parker MM, Shelhamer JH, Bacharach SL, et al. Profound but reversible myocardial depression in patients with septic shock. *Ann Intern Med.* 1984;100(4):483-490.
79. Troianos CA, Porembka DT. Assessment of left ventricular function and hemodynamics with transesophageal echocardiography. *Crit Care Clin.* 1996;12(2):253-272.
80. Comess KA, DeRook FA, Russell ML, Tognazzi-Evans TA, Beach KW. The incidence of pulmonary embolism in unexplained sudden cardiac arrest with pulseless electrical activity. *Am J Med.* 2000;109(5):351-356.
81. McConnell MV, Solomon SD, Rayan ME, Come PC, Goldhaber SZ, Lee RT. Regional right ventricular dysfunction detected by echocardiography in acute pulmonary embolism. *Am J Cardiol.* 1996;78(4):469-473.
82. Torbicki A, Pruszczyk P. The role of echocardiography in suspected and established PE. *Semin Vasc Med.* 2001;1(2): 165-174.
83. Kjaergaard J, Schaadt BK, Lund JO, Hassager C. Quantification of right ventricular function in acute pulmonary embolism: relation to extent of pulmonary perfusion defects. *Eur J Echocardiogr.* 2008;9(5):641-645.
84. Fremont B, Pacouret G, Jacobi D, Puglisi R, Charbonnier B, de Labriolle A. Prognostic value of echocardiographic right/left ventricular end-diastolic diameter ratio in patients with acute pulmonary embolism: results from a monocenter registry of 1,416 patients. *Chest.* 2008;133(2):358-362.
85. Wittlich N, Erbel R, Eichler A, et al. Detection of central pulmonary artery thromboemboli by transesophageal echocardiography in patients with severe pulmonary embolism. *J Am Soc Echocardiogr.* 1992;5(5):515-524.

REVIEW QUESTIONS

Select the *one* best answer for each of the following questions.

1. TEE applications for patients in the emergency department include:
   a. Detection of pleural effusions
   b. Diagnosis of hepatic contusion
   c. Adjunct tool for pleurocentesis
   d. Assessing the adequacy of resuscitative efforts

2. TEE (as opposed to TTE) may be particularly useful when:
   a. Patient is thin with good cardiac windows
   b. Active chest compressions are ongoing
   c. Patient has known esophageal strictures
   d. Patient has a low body mass index

3. TEE imaging of the aorta can best be described as:
   a. Inadequate for most elderly patients
   b. Unreliable during ongoing resuscitation efforts
   c. The preferred first line imaging modality in all patients
   d. Limited in visualization of the aortic arch

4. TEE should be the first line imaging modality:
   a. When aortic injury is suspected in a hemodynamically stable trauma patient
   b. When any operator is readily available
   c. In an obese, hypotensive patient with suspected aortic pathology
   d. Only when active chest compressions have been suitably interrupted

5. TEE is preferred over TTE under which of the following circumstances?
   a. When body habitus allows adequate cardiac windows
   b. When the patient is hemodynamically stable
   c. When a posterior pericardial effusion is suspected
   d. When the patient is not receiving active chest compressions

6. Which of the following is a class I guideline for performing TEE as recommended by the ACC/AHA/ASE?
   a. Suspected myocardial contusion in the hemodynamically stable patient
   b. Re-evaluation of hemodynamically stable patient
   c. Suspected aortic dissection
   d. Evaluation of hemodynamics in trauma patients

7. Factors that will likely lead to increased use of TEE in the ED include:
   a. Escalating costs associated with TTE hardware and interpretation
   b. Decreasing trend for miniaturization of ultrasound hardware and esophageal probes
   c. More patients presenting to ED with atypical chest pain
   d. Increasing proportion of critically ill patients "boarding" in the ED

8. Which of the following is an advantage of TEE over TTE?
   a. Issues related to medical consent
   b. More likely to result in a management change
   c. Cost
   d. Unreliable during ongoing resuscitation efforts

9. Which of the following is an absolute contraindication to the use of TEE?
   a. Presence of esophageal varices
   b. Asystole
   c. Esophageal rupture
   d. Hemodynamic instability

10. All the following actions should routinely be performed prior to inserting the esophageal TEE probe *except*:
    a. Application of topical anesthetic to posterior tongue and pharynx
    b. Conform patient has been NPO or if not, evacuate stomach with a nasogastric tube
    c. Consent patient or designee unless under emergency conditions
    d. Perform endoscopy to ensure no esophageal structural abnormalities

11. The following best describes the current state of TEE usage in the ED:
    a. Emergency physicians cannot gain credentialing in TEE performance
    b. TEE has a well-defined list of indications for use in the ED
    c. TEE is now incorporated into the ACLS protocol to confirm cardiac standstill prior to ending a resuscitation
    d. A rapid, focused TEE exam can aid in management decisions, particularly in hemodynamically unstable patients.

12. TEE may be the preferred first-line echocardiographic modality in certain patients. The percentage of patients in whom TTE fails due to inadequate cardiac windows may be as high as:
    a. 5%
    b. 10%
    c. 20%
    d. 60%

13. During the resuscitation of a patient found in cardiac arrest, all of the following are true with regard to the utility of TEE *except*:
    a. Allows rapid assessment of pulse after defibrillation or medication administration
    b. Cannot differentiate between low ejection fraction, electromechanical dissociation and asystole
    c. Minimizes CPR interruptions while permitting constant monitoring
    d. Can change patient management

14. TEE can reliably exclude all of the following causes of hypotension *except*:
    a. PE in the left PA
    b. Pericardial tamponade
    c. Papillary muscle rupture
    d. Hypovolemia.

15. Which of the following statements is correct?
    a. Type A aortic dissections are usually managed medically
    b. Type A aortic dissections are usually managed surgically
    c. TEE cannot reliably detect aortic dissections
    d. Type B aortic dissections are usually managed surgically

16. Which of the following trauma patients most likely stands to benefit from a TEE?
    a. Patient with hypotension, multiple limb fractures and a head injury after a 20 foot fall off a ladder
    b. Hemodynamically stable patient with trauma to chest and abdomen from a rollover MVC
    c. Hypotensive patient with blunt abdominal trauma and a positive DPL
    d. Patient with a stab wound to the chest with a significant pericardial tamponade on chest wall echo (TTE).

17. The main advantage of using TEE in the ED for the detection of aortic injury over MRI or angiography is:
    a. Better sensitivity and specificity
    b. Cost
    c. Lack of need for informed consent
    d. Portability

18. The presence of a dilated right ventricle and right atrium in a patient with tachycardia and shortness of breath suggests the following diagnosis:
    a. Hypovolemia
    b. Cardiac tamponade
    c. Papillary muscle rupture
    d. Pulmonary embolus

19. In patients already on a ventilator with an endotracheal tube, measures to aid successful placement of the esophageal TEE probe include:
    a. Temporary extubation and re-intubation
    b. Placement of a nasogastric tube to provide a guide to location of the esophagus
    c. Placement under direct laryngoscopic view
    d. Additional inflation of the endotracheal tube cuff to avoid entering the trachea

20. The most common reason to obtain a TEE study in the ED is:
    a. Assessment of valve competency
    b. Hemodynamic instability
    c. Persistent fever
    d. Assessing aortic pathology

For questions 21-35, indicate "True" or "False"

21. TEE can differentiate between penetrating aortic ulcers and intramural hematomas.

22. In trauma patients, TEE permits visualization of the heart and the proximal aorta, but will miss injuries to the main aortic branches.

23. The most vulnerable area of the aorta is the ascending aorta.

24. The hemodynamic management for a trauma patient is the same whether traumatic disruption of the aorta is present or not.

25. An aortic injury secondary to blunt trauma frequently co-exists with a cardiac contusion and can be life threatening.

26. TEE examination may reveal an ejection fraction compatible with life in patients without palpable pulses.

27. Use of TEE can result in a significant change in management without the need for further laboratory investigations or imaging.

28. A patient in apparent PEA undergoing active chest compressions is an unsuitable candidate for TEE examination

29. A nasogastric tube is advisable prior to esophageal placement of the TEE probe.

30. There are no major risks to the TEE procedure.

31. Esophageal stricture is a contraindication to esophageal placement of the TEE probe.

32. Topical anesthesia is not needed prior to esophageal placement of the TEE probe in hemodynamically unstable trauma patients.

33. TEE has a sensitivity and sensitivity of approximately 98% for aortic dissection.

34. TEE should never be the initial imaging modality in patients with suspected aortic or cardiac pathology in the ED.

35. Benzocaine spray is an acceptable pharyngeal anesthetic for use prior to esophageal placement of the TEE probe.

For questions 36-45 fill in the blank

36. The most useful TEE window during active resuscitation is typically __________

37. Regional wall motion abnormality assessment with echocardiography can only be performed when there is an __________ rhythm

38. The percentage of patients with aortic rupture who survive to hospital presentation may be as high as __________

39. The most concerning type of dissection, Type A, involves the __________ aorta.

40. A high suspicion of aortic injury must be maintained when patients undergo a __________ injury, such as the case in a motor vehicle accident at high speed or a fall from significant height.

41. Approximately __________ % of cardiac arrests may be due to pulmonary embolus.

42. When assessing for the presence of aortic dissection, a true flap can be differentiated from artifact by __________ of flow of the color Doppler signal.

43. The diagnosis of aortic disruption/transaction requires the presence of a disrupted aortic wall with __________ on both sides of the disruption

44. A small, flattened LV as visualized in the mid-esophageal 4-chamber view suggests __________

45. In a nonfasting patient, __________ is of particular concern in the patient who does not have their airway secured with an endotracheal tube.

For questions 46-50, each diagnosis listed may be best characterized by the following findings on TEE

a. Right ventricular hypokinesis and dilation with sparing of the RV apex
b. Small, flat left ventricle
c. Wall motion abnormality
d. Oscillating flap with severe aortic insufficiency
e. Ruptured chordae tendinae with retrograde, turbulent diastolic blood flow

46. Myocardial infarction

47. PE

48. Aortic Dissection

49. Acute valvular insufficiency

50. Hypovolemia

Emerging Applications of Perioperative Echocardiography

24

Carlo Marcucci, Bettina Jungwirth, G. Burkhard Mackensen, and Aman Mahajan

Advances in echocardiography have been responsible for enhancing our understanding of the mechanisms and progression of cardiovascular diseases. The introduction of new echocardiographic imaging modalities has greatly aided our ability to obtain early and precise disease diagnosis, while simultaneously allowing better means to guide medical or surgical care for patients with heart diseases. In this chapter, we discuss the role of these emerging echocardiographic technologies in the perioperative period.

THREE-DIMENSIONAL ECHOCARDIOGRAPHY

Three-dimensional (3D) echocardiography has a long history with the first 3D-reconstruction of two-dimensional (2D) images described in 1974 and the first human 3D–transesophageal echocardiogram (TEE) performed in 1992.[1,2] Until recently, 3D-TEE was performed using a rotational approach for sequential data acquisition, gated to electrocardiography (ECG) and respiration.[2,3] Volume rendering and cropping of these reconstructed 3D volume data sets allowed display of structures of interest. However, these earlier approaches were limited by time-consuming acquisition and reconstruction processes (15 to 30 minutes), frequent artifacts, and the need for offline processing.[4,5] As a consequence, reconstructive 3D-TEE remained primarily a research tool and did not make it into routine clinical practice. With the recent introduction of a 3D fully sampled matrix array TEE transducer, many of these limitations have been overcome. Based on novel electronic circuitry and a matrix array design of piezoelectric crystals within an otherwise conventional TEE probe, this new technology allows both real-time acquisition as well as live display of 3D images. This real-time 3D-TEE (RT-3D-TEE) system allows for excellent visualization of the mitral valve (MV), the interatrial septum (IAS), the left atrial appendage (LAA), pulmonary veins, and the left ventricle (LV), while imaging of the aortic valve (AV) and tricuspid valve (TV) will require further technological improvements.[6,7] Due to its unique features of real-time acquisition, online rendering and cropping capabilities, accurate identification of the precise pathology and location of cardiac disease, and prompt quantification of 3D structures with built-in software, RT-3D-TEE is expected to soon become a standard of perioperative care and clinical practice. However, this emerging technology requires the echocardiographer to acquire new sets of skills to acquire and manipulate the 3D data sets so that they can reveal valuable information. With an emphasis on RT-3D-TEE, the following sections will combine practical recommendations with some of the key features of the emerging 3D technology.

Imaging Technology

Technologic advances in the 1990s have allowed improved reconstructive 3D echocardiography based on the acquisition of multiple, gated image planes using ECG and respiratory gating that limits the amount of motion artifacts. Post-processing of acquired images results in further optimization of these reconstructive 3D images. One significant drawback of these approaches to 3D echocardiography was that live, real-time (RT) imaging could not be achieved because the different imaging planes are acquired sequentially. Further, sequential and gated acquisition frequently resulted in motion artifacts. In the late 1980s, a sparse array matrix transducer containing 256 elements was designed to develop a new approach to 3D echocardiography and to overcome some of these issues. While this transducer generated different cut-planes from a 3D volume online, it ultimately displayed RT rendered 3D images.[8-10] Further advances in crystal and computer technology allowed for the introduction of matrix-array transducers for use in transthoracic echocardiography (TTE). Matrix-array transducers utilize a greater number of imaging elements (>2500), which are capable of generating RT rendered 3D images.[11,12] More recently, the reduction in the size of the transducer footprint along with improved ultrasound crystal technology led to the introduction of the RT-3D-TEE transducers and real-time capable ultrasound systems.

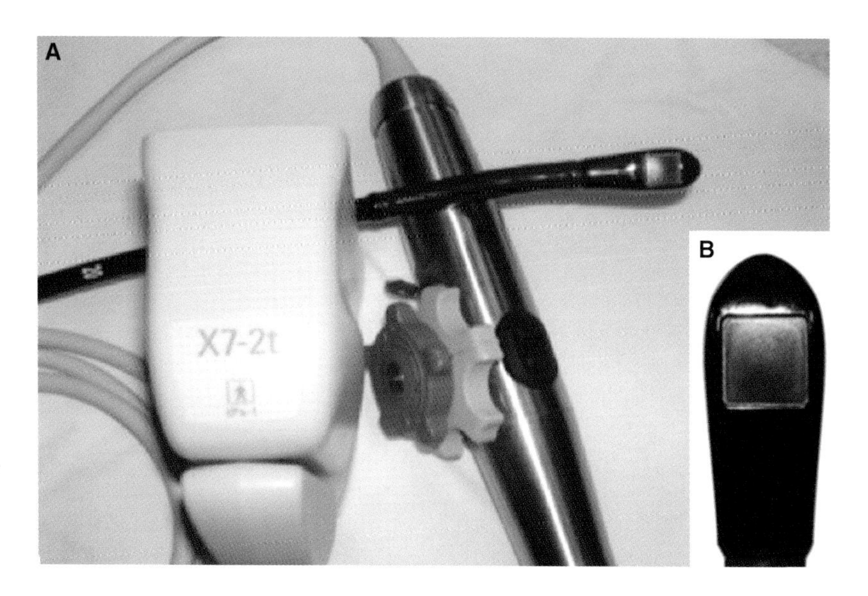

FIGURE 24–1. A real-time 3D transesophageal echocardiographic transducer **(A)**, the X7-2t (see text for details). **(B)** shows an enlarged image of the tip of the transducer.

The first and currently only clinically available RT-3D-TEE transducer is the X7-2t TEE (Philips Medical Systems, Andover, MA, USA) transducer, which combines xMATRIX technology and PureWave crystal technology (Figure 24–1). PureWave crystal technology represents a new class of piezoelectric crystals with remarkably enhanced electromechanical properties. With the power of 150 computer boards, xMATRIX technology utilizes 2500 fully sampled elements for 360° focusing and steering. This cutting-edge technology creates two live full-resolution planes created simultaneously (xPlane imaging) and, therefore, enables the parallel acquisition of diagnostic data without changing the scan angle (Figure 24–2). Further, the system enables live or RT volume imaging over a single heartbeat with unlimited planes in all directions, allowing the acquisition and rendering of true

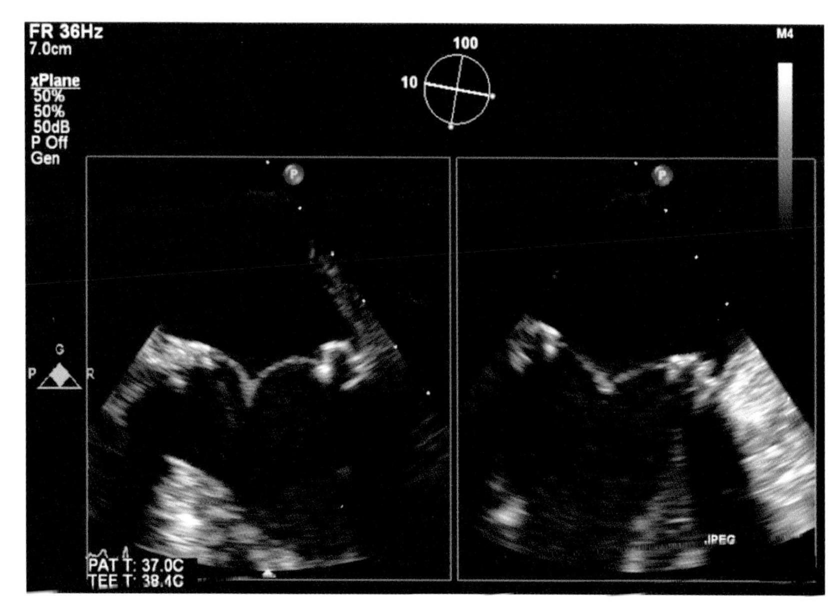

FIGURE 24–2. Bioprosthetic mitral valve as imaged with the xPlane mode (biplane mode). This mode displays two full-resolution planes created simultaneously and therefore enables the parallel acquisition of diagnostic data without changing the scan angle. The scan angle of the left plane (10°) is selected before initiating xPlane imaging; the scan angle of the right plane (100°) can be freely adjusted while imaging.

RT-3D full volume data. Gated images are acquired over multiple heartbeats and are displayed as a loop generated by stitching together subvolumes over consecutive cardiac cycles. Similar to other ultrasound technologies, RT-3D-TEE imaging obeys the laws of physics and is limited by frame rate, image resolution, and sector size.[13] Importantly, RT-3D systems provide all conventional modalities such as 2D multiplane imaging, M-mode, pulsed- and continuous-wave Doppler, as well as color Doppler imaging. In addition, the system offers the following four 3D imaging modes:

- *Live 3D*: This real-time mode displays a fixed pyramidal data set of approximately 50° × 30° by the depth of the initial 2D image that conveniently can be used to visualize any cardiac structure located in the near field (Figure 24–3). Movement of the TEE probe will result in a live (real-time) change of the 3D image. Live 3D allows for quick 3D imaging and immediate return to a 2D mode. Using live 3D, a thick slice (90° × 1°) representing an enhanced 2D image may also be displayed and rotated in space.
- *3D Zoom*: This displays a truncated but magnified pyramidal data set of variable size (pyramidal dimensions vary from 20° × 20° up to 90° × 90°). Upon activation, the 3D-zoom mode displays a biplane preview screen showing the original view and the correspondent orthogonal image. Careful placement and sizing of the zoom sector over the region of interest with minimized sector-width to improve temporal resolution are important to optimize image quality and frame rate (Figure 24–4).

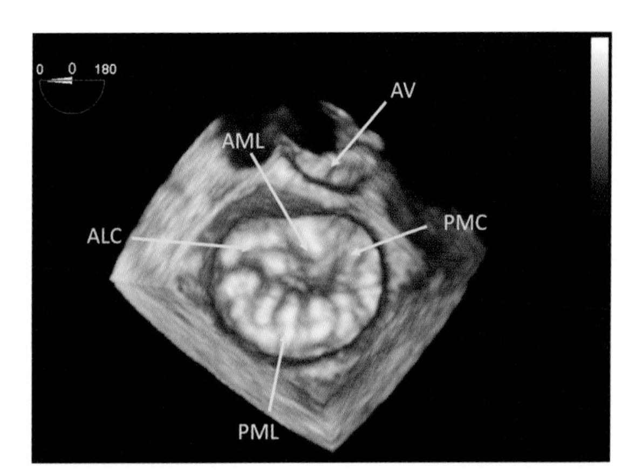

FIGURE 24–4. Three-dimensional TEE zoom *en face* view of a normal mitral valve with the anterior mitral leaflet (AML) on the top and the posterior mitral leaflet (PML) on the bottom. The orientation of the image is similar to the surgeon's view. (AV, aortic valve; ALC, anterolateral commissure; PMC, posteromedial commissure.)

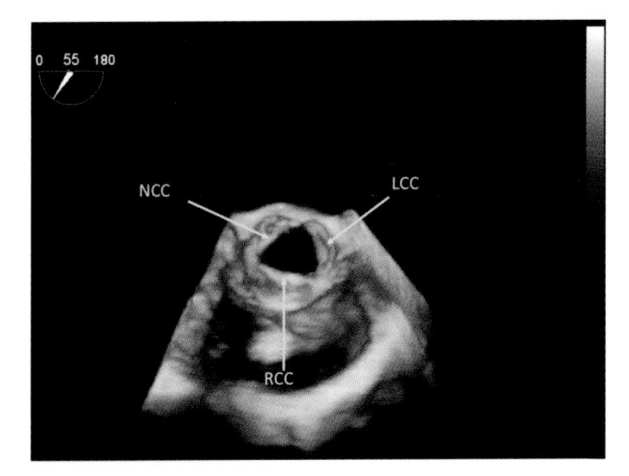

FIGURE 24–3. Live 3D-TEE image of a normal aortic valve. Live 3D obtains a fixed pyramidal data set of approximately 50° × 30°. (NCC, noncoronary cusp; RCC, right coronary cusp; LCC, left coronary cusp).

- *Full Volume*: This mode provides a pyramidal data set (approximately 65° × 60° up to 100° × 100°), which allows the inclusion of a larger cardiac volume at frame rates greater than 30 Hz. The wide-angle data set is compiled by merging four to seven narrower RT-3D pyramidal wedges or subvolumes obtained over four to seven heartbeats. To minimize artifacts in the anesthetized patient, full volume loops should be acquired when ventilation is held and electrocautery is not used. With the goal of minimizing artifacts in the intraoperative setting, it is recommended that full volume loops be acquired at the beginning of the comprehensive TEE exam, before the start of surgery. Artifacts cannot be avoided in patients with arrhythmias, and stitch artifacts delineate subvolumes and may make the interpretation of imaged structures impossible (Figure 24–5). A full volume loop of the LV is acquired based on the 2D midesophageal four-chamber view. Once the full volume mode is activated, a biplane image with the four-chamber view and the correspondent orthogonal plane is displayed on the screen. The first obtained 3D volume is displayed as an automatically cropped image showing 50% of the volume and mirroring the midesophageal four-chamber view (Figure 24–6A). Resetting the crop plane allows display of the entire pyramidal data set (Figure 24–6B). The full volume can be further processed offline by rotating and cropping to visualize specific structures inside the pyramid. Cropping can be performed either by using one of six available cropping planes selected from a 3D cropping box or by

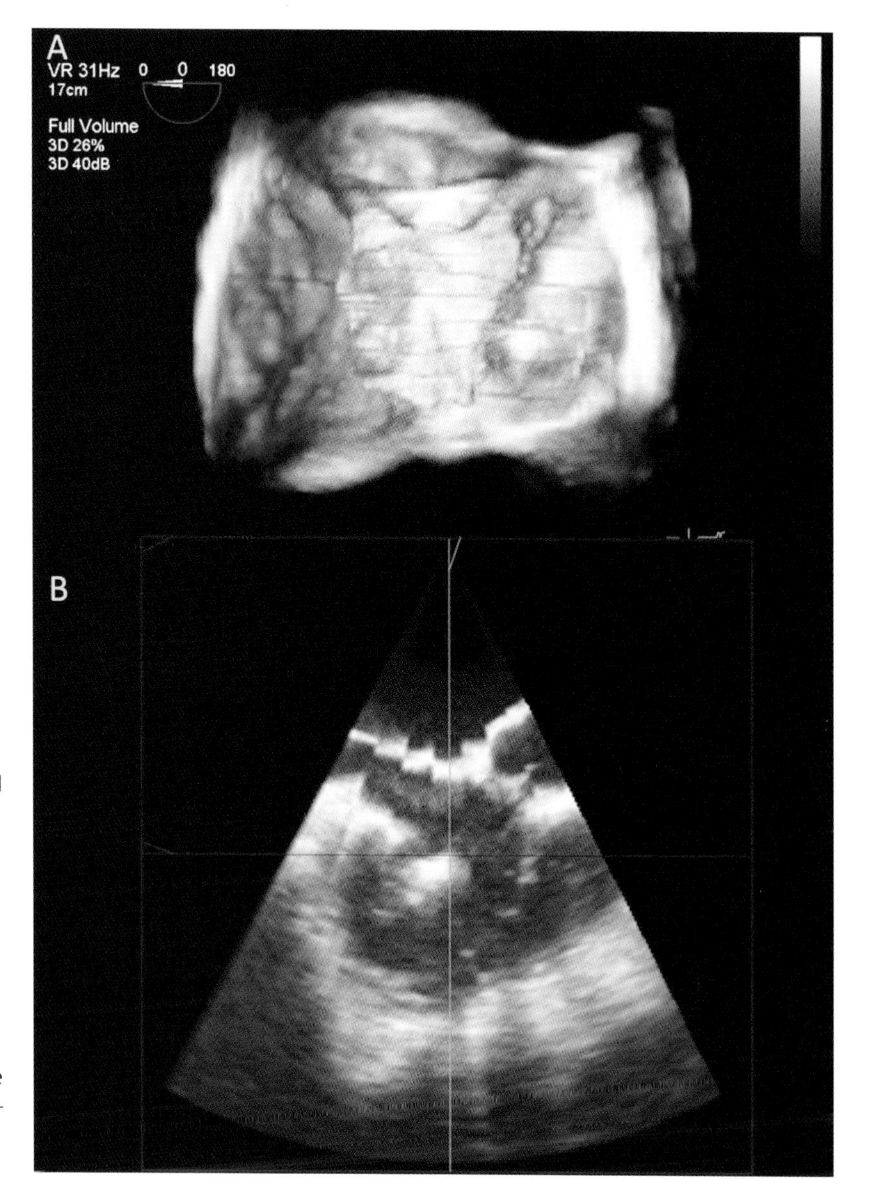

FIGURE 24–5. A 3D-TEE full volume data set is compiled by merging four to seven narrower 3D pyramidal wedges or subvolumes obtained over four to seven undisturbed heartbeats. The enface image in **(A)** demonstrates stitch artifacts (demarcation lines) that delineate subvolumes and may make the interpretation of the imaged structures impossible. **(B)** delineates the subvolumes in a cropped version of the same full volume data set.

using a freely adjustable plane. Acquired full volumes can also be used for volumetric quantification of the LV using available built-in software (QLAB, Philips Medical Systems, Andover, MA, USA, version 6.0).

- *3D Color Full Volume*: Similar to the acquisition of a full volume, the wide-angle color data set is compiled by merging 7 to 14 narrower RT-3D pyramidal wedges and is similarly prone to artifacts introduced by arrhythmias, movement, or electrocautery (Figure 24–7). For this mode, it is important to place the area of interest (eg, the regurgitant jet) in the center of the sector. The remainder of the acquisition is identical to that used for full volume acquisition. Due to the large amount of data incorporated in 3D color Doppler full volume data sets, the resulting pyramidal volumes do not exceed 60° × 60° and have a limited frame rate (<20 Hz).

Approximate measurements on acquired images can be performed easily by using the 3D grid with a specified dot-to-dot distance for estimating dimensions of cardiac structures such as the mitral valve annulus. More

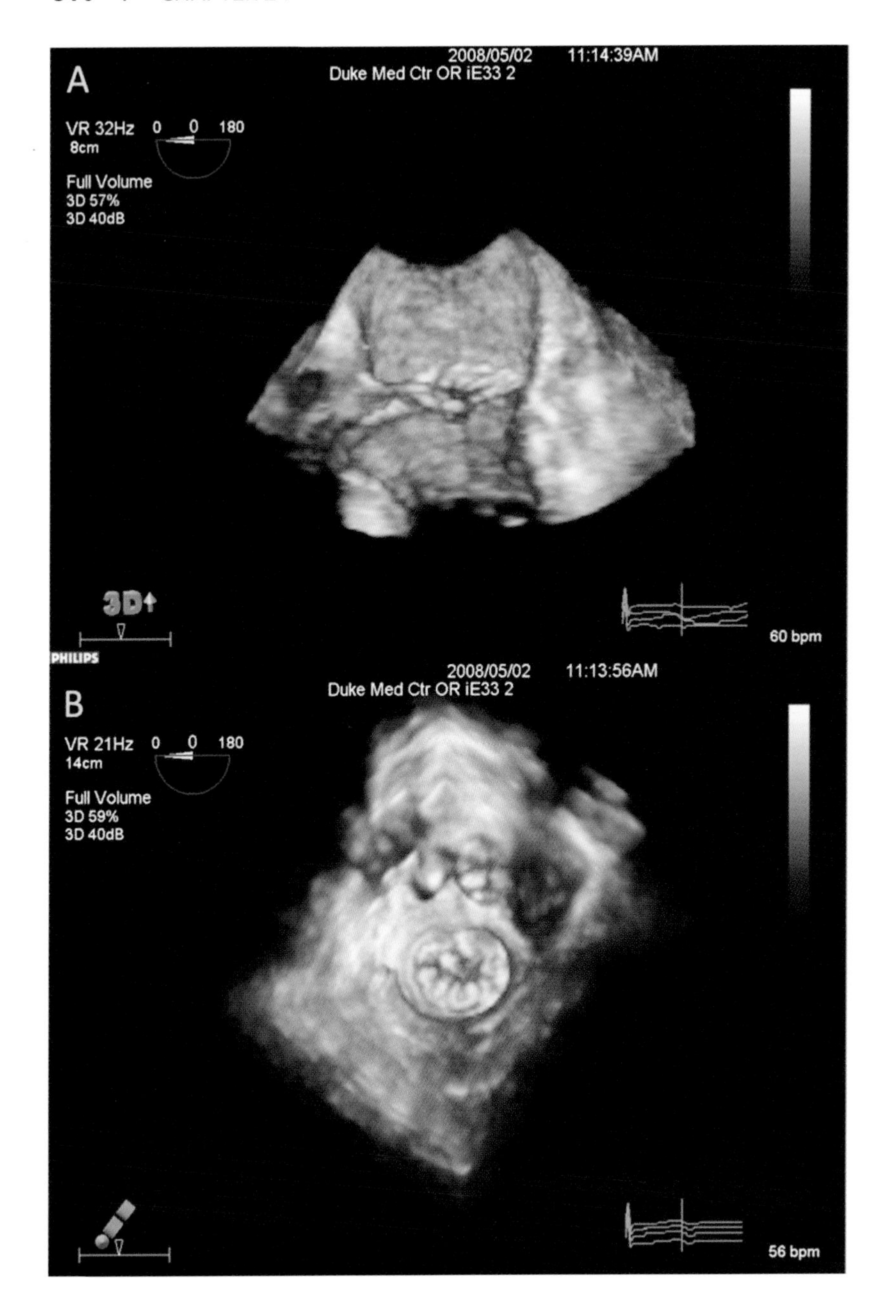

FIGURE 24–6. Following acquisition of a 3D full volume of a mitral valve, **(A)** shows a typical auto-cropped image revealing only 50% of the larger full volume data set. Resetting the crop plane allows the display of a full volume pyramidal data set that can be further rotated and cropped **(B)**.

sophisticated and accurate measurements require the use of built-in software (QLAB). This software contains several programs including the Mitral Valve Quantification (MVQ), the 3D Quantification Advanced (3DQAV), and the simpler 3D Quantification (3DQ). MVQ and 3DQAV are described in detail below. 3DQ allows simple quantitative assessment of any 3D data set (eg, area, distance).

Acquired 3D images should always be rotated and orientated to display a specific anatomic or surgical perspective. Cropping (or slicing) of the 3D image along all three axes (X, Y, and Z) is made possible along six orthogonal planes or based on multiplanar reconstruction planes (Figure 24–8A). In addition, a freely adjustable cropping plane allows more sophisticated cropping in alignment to any cardiac structure of interest (Figure 24–8B).

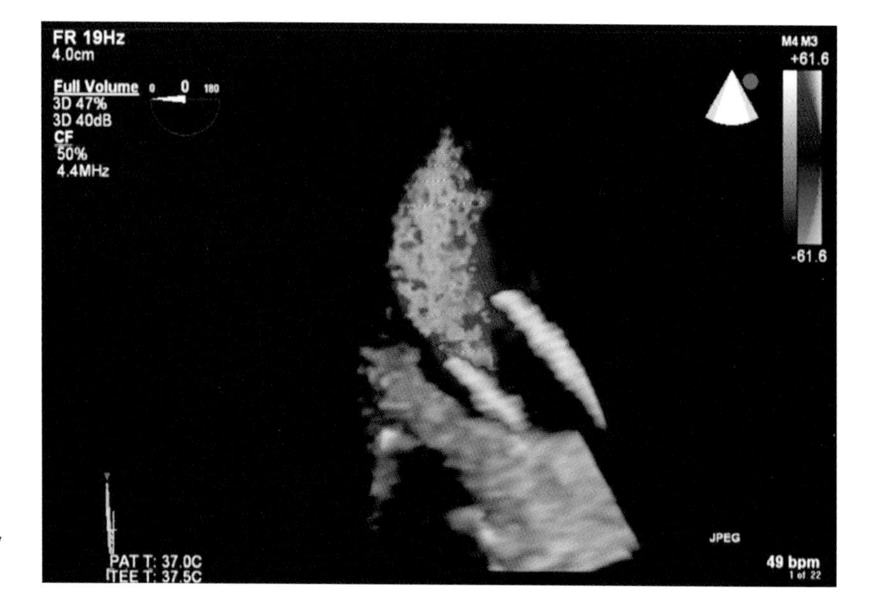

FIGURE 24–7. Three-dimensional TEE color full volume acquisition demonstrating flow from an aortic cannula positioned within the ascending aorta for the conduct of cardiopulmonary bypass.

Simply touching the reset-cropping button can reverse any cropping and will restore the original 3D image.

Clinical Applications

Mitral Valve

The mitral valve (MV), with its complex saddle-shaped configuration, presents one of the most challenging structures to be assessed with 2D-TEE. Two-dimensional TEE imaging of the MV requires a mental integration of several views for accurate assessment and is, therefore, dependent on observer experience and expertise. In addition to its complex anatomic structure, the interrelationship of the MV to chordae, papillary muscles, and myocardial walls makes it particularly suited to 3D assessment. In this context, 3D echocardiography allows a more accurate identification of the etiology and mechanism of MR and is more sensitive than 2D echocardiography in identifying the location of the pathology leading to MR, especially in patients with bileaflet and commissural defects.[4,14-16] In addition, the severity of MR can be more accurately determined using 3D color Doppler echocardiography,[17] and specific geometric shapes for different MR pathologies can be identified.[18-20]

With 3D-TEE, the effective mitral valve area (MVA) may be assessed by carefully cropping through the MV annular plane. In this context, studies have confirmed that 3D echocardiography provides a more accurate measurement of the MVA compared to standard 2D-based measurements and shows the best agreement with invasive methods.[21-23] Importantly, the 3D measurements had the additional advantage of being associated with lower intraobserver and interobserver variability. Further, 3D echocardiography has been used for guidance during percutaneous mitral valvuloplasty and has been shown to be a suitable technique for monitoring its efficacy and complications.[23-25] This technique has become the procedure of choice in patients who are considered at high surgical risk, eg, pregnant women;[26,27] however, the need for surgery after MV valvuloplasty is not uncommon.[28] RT-3D-TEE might become a gold standard in describing the morphology of commissures, which in turn predicts outcome after percutaneous balloon mitral valvuloplasty.[29]

RT-3D-TEE provides superb visualization of prosthetic MVs and annuloplasty rings (Figure 24–9);[6,30] thus, it might help in identifying the location of a paravalvular leak.[31] Three-dimensional TEE has been shown to provide complimentary information in patients with an Alfieri stitch and may aid in long-term follow-up (Figure 24–10).[32] Three-dimensional TEE provides additional information in patients with a postoperative MV dehiscence, and thus may help in planning an optimal surgical intervention.[30] Prosthetic valve endocarditis remains a challenging diagnosis, especially for TEE. However, initial experiences suggest that 3D-TTE might improve the sensitivity of detecting endocarditis.[33]

It is expected that RT-3D-TEE will soon be integrated into routine perioperative practice in patients with MV pathologies. Its unique ability of real-time acquisition, online rendering and cropping capabilities,

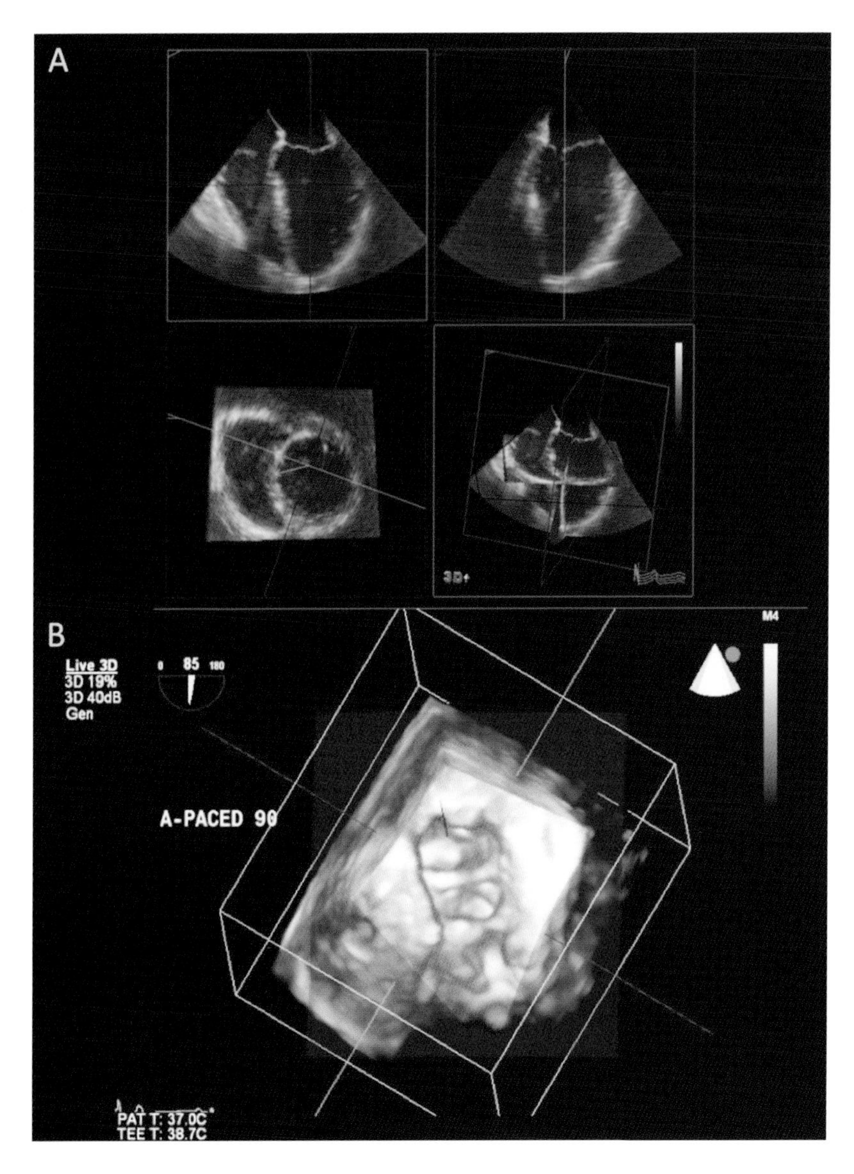

FIGURE 24–8. Full volume data set **(A)** of the left ventricle displayed in three multiplanar reconstruction planes (green, four-chamber view; red, two-chamber view; and blue, short-axis view) along with the 3D image displayed in a slice plane fashion (right lower quadrant). Using a cropping box tool, cropping (or slicing) of the 3D image can be achieved along six orthogonal planes. **(B)** illustrates alternative cropping using a freely adjustable cropping plane that allows more sophisticated cropping in alignment with any cardiac structure of interest. The image shows the purple cropping plane placed over a bilobed left atrial appendage.

and accurate identification of the precise location and pathology leading to MV disease, together with its ability to define the severity of mitral regurgitation/mitral stenosis (MR/MS) by direct assessment of effective regurgitant orifice and volume, even for asymmetrically shaped regurgitant jets, will likely help to transition this modality into standard of care.

Imaging Techniques. With RT-3D-TEE, a comprehensive assessment of the MV involves the acquisition of an *en face* view, a full volume image, and a 3D color full volume image. The *en face* view mirrors the surgical view from the left atrium down to the MV. This view is routinely generated using the 3D-zoom mode based on the midesophageal four-chamber view, and by rotating the obtained image to display the aortic valve at the 12 o'clock position as the midpoint of the anterior annulus. Depending on the frame rate and line density settings, this commonly results in superior-quality volume-rendered images of the anterior leaflet at the top and the posterior leaflet at the bottom of the image (see Figure 24–4). Three-dimensional zoom MV images may then be manipulated such that the MV may be viewed from either atrial or ventricular perspectives,

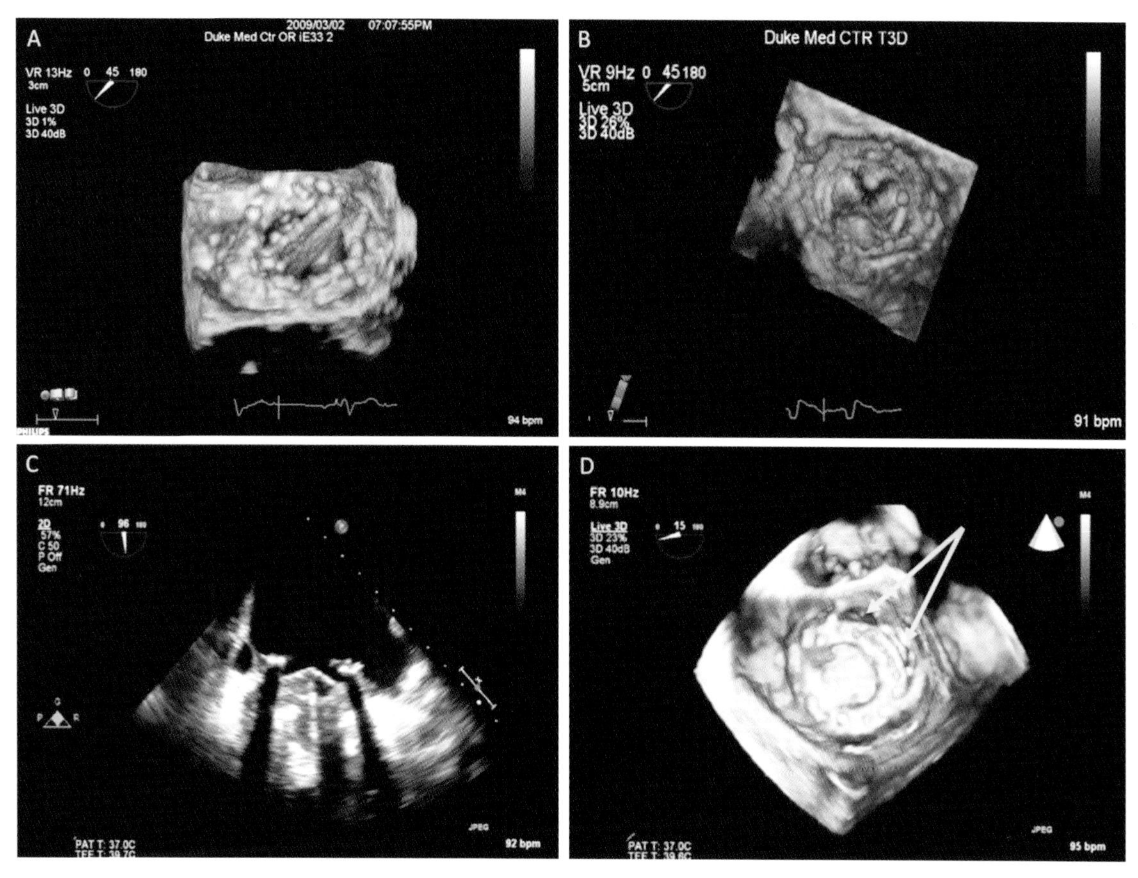

FIGURE 24–9. *En face* view of a mechanical double tilting disc MV prosthesis **(A)**. A stented bioprosthetic MV is displayed in **(B)** as viewed from the left ventricular side. **(C)** represents a 2D-TEE image of a mechanical double tilting disc MV prosthesis. Imaged with the multiplane angle at 90°, this image reveals the significant anterior dehiscence of this MV prosthesis that is easily recognized in the RT-3D-TEE *en face* view displayed in **(D)**.

which is another unique feature of 3D imaging. The full volume data set allows assessment of the interrelationship between the MV, the papillary muscles, the myocardial walls, and the left ventricular outflow tract. Using 3D color, the size and geometry of regurgitant jets can be visualized and the exact quantification of effective regurgitant orifice areas (EROAs) can be obtained (Figure 24–11). These images can be supplemented by 3D quantitative assessment of the MV using built-in software (MVQ, QLAB). The MV Quantification (MVQ) feature offers a semiautomated analysis package for accurate modeling of the mitral annulus, valve commissures, leaflet coaptation, leaflet topography, aortic orifice to mitral valve angle, etc. (Figure 24–12). Reconstructive approaches to assess the MV with 3D-TEE (Siemens, Mountainview, CA, USA) paired with online computer software (TomTec Imaging Systems GmbH, Munich, Germany) allow for similar quantification of the MV.[34]

LEFT VENTRICLE

The evaluation of global and regional left ventricular (LV) function is an essential part of a routine perioperative TEE examination. To date, the assessment of the LV ejection fraction (EF) is mainly performed by "eye-balling," which relies on the echocardiographer's experience and ability to visually integrate spatial information. Further limitations of 2D-TEE assessment of the LV EF are attributed to the use of foreshortened views of the LV and the reliance on geometric assumptions to calculate volumetric parameters. The addition of a third dimension is expected to overcome some of these limitations, especially in patients with cardiomyopathies or wall motion abnormalities where

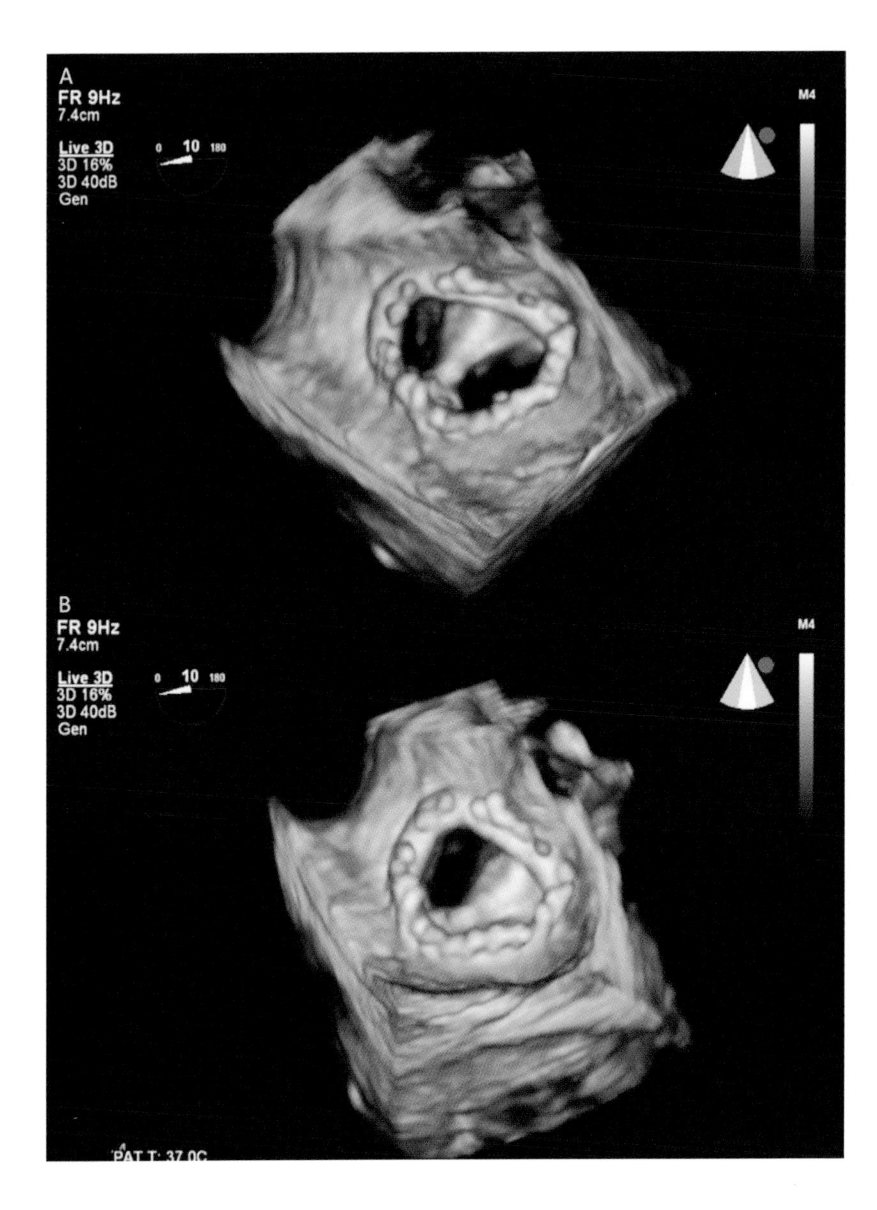

FIGURE 24–10. Postoperative RT-3D-TEE zoom *en face* view of a repaired MV **(A)**. The image clearly reveals the MV ring and an Alfieri stitch between A2 and P2. **(B)** shows the same valve, now tilted to show the anterolateral opening of the MV.

the geometric assumptions may lead to incorrect estimations of LV function. In this context, 3D echocardiography along with built-in quantification software that is based on semiautomated endocardial border detection allows the echocardiographer to obtain fast and accurate measurements of global and regional LV function.[35-37] Studies comparing magnetic resonance imaging (MRI) with 3D echocardiography for the assessment of LV mass and function show very good correlation and agreement that is superior to 2D echocardiography.[38] This also holds true for RT-3D-TTE assessment of patients with cardiomyopathies or regional wall motion abnormalities secondary to myocardial infarction, where LV geometry is frequently abnormal.[39-41] A recent study suggests that LV function assessment based on 3D-TEE data offers more reliable perioperative quantification, especially for less experienced users.[42] However, further research comparing 3D-TEE to a gold standard such as MRI is required to confirm that 3D-TEE is superior to 2D-TEE in assessing LV function.

Imaging Techniques. The best mode to assess global and regional LV function by 3D-TEE is the full volume mode, which is acquired from the midesophageal

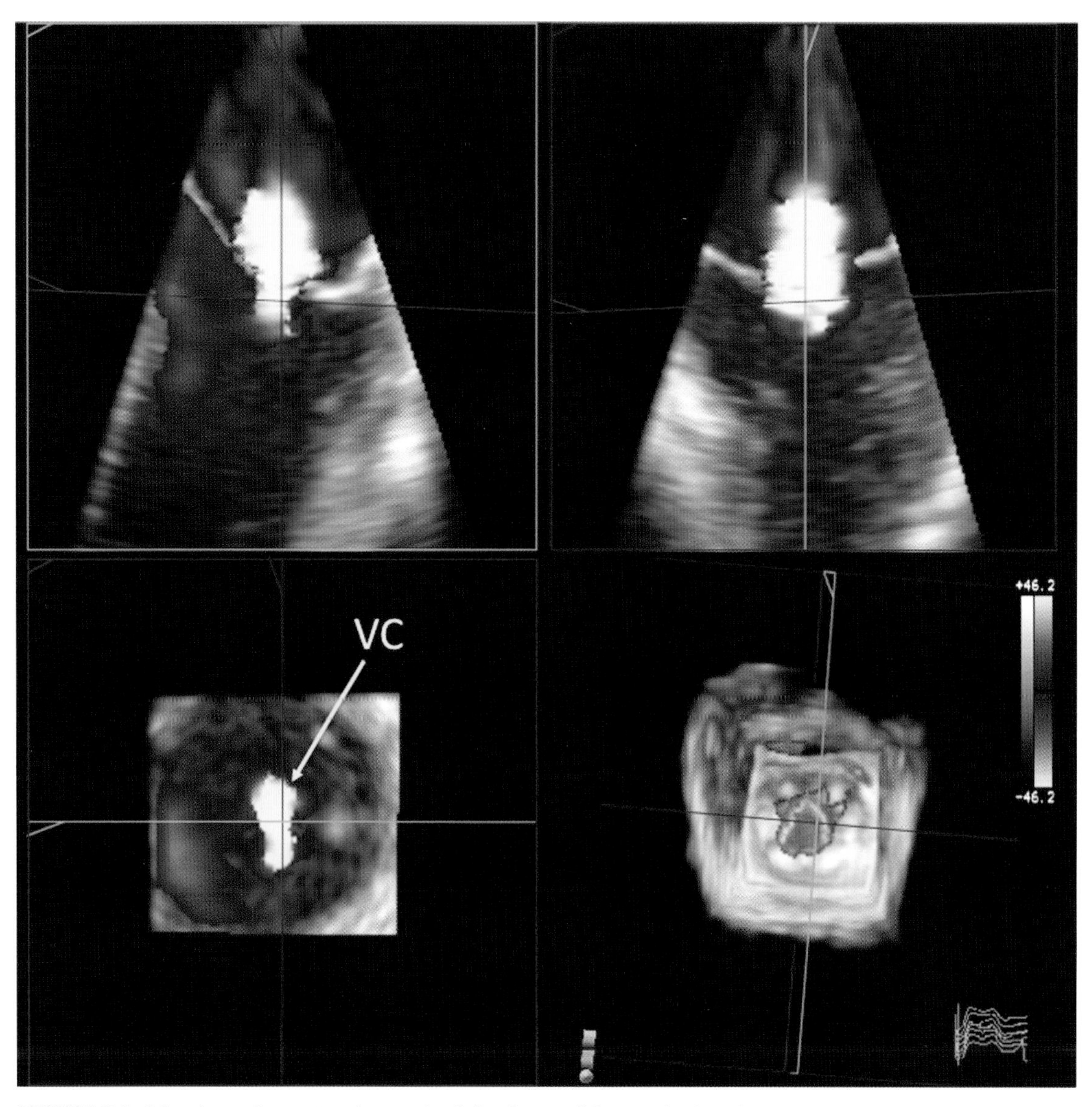

FIGURE 24–11. Three-dimensional TEE color full volume of the MV displayed in three multiplanar reconstruction planes (green, red, and blue MPRs) along with the 3D image displayed as an *en face* view of the MV (right lower quadrant). The left lower quadrant (blue MPR) depicts an elliptical-shaped vena contracta (VC) as often seen in functional mitral regurgitation. This was achieved by carefully cutting the MV at the annular plane.

four-chamber view. Using built-in software, the 3D Quantification Advanced (3DQAV) program, data for both global LV function as well as regional wall motion abnormalities are obtained in a semiautomated fashion. The system relies on automatic endocardial border detection and border tracking algorithms, which can be edited manually. The first step after acquisition is a manual definition of the septal, lateral, anterior, inferior, and apical endocardial border of the LV in the end-systolic and the end-diastolic frames, followed by activation of an automatic border-tracking algorithm (Figure 24–13A). The system will then calculate end-systolic as well as the end-diastolic volumes by summation of the voxels enclosed by the endocardial borders. Thereafter, global stroke volume and EF are derived. The obtained "shell view" is subdivided into 17 regions,

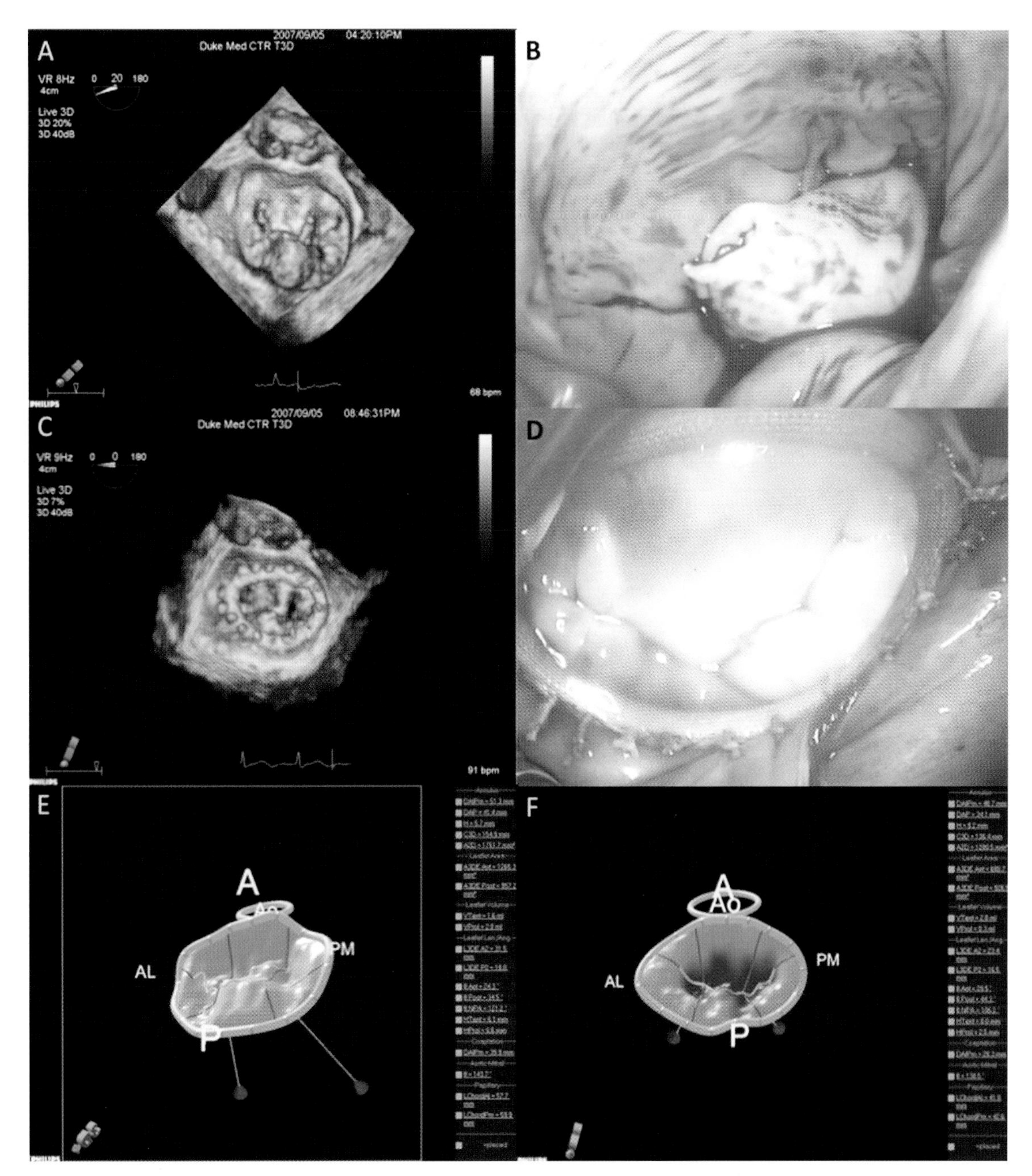

FIGURE 24–12. **(A)** through **(F)** display the RT-3D-TEE views as well as the corresponding digital pictures of the surgical view of a mitral valve (MV) and 3D reconstructions (MV model) in a patient with a large P2 prolapse, ruptured chords, and severe mitral regurgitation. **(A)** shows the 3D zoom *en face* view of this MV, **(B)** the corresponding digital picture taken by the surgeon, **(C)** the 3D zoom *en face* view of the repaired MV (ring annuloplasty, Goretex chords, and Alfieri stitch), and **(D)** shows the digital picture taken by the surgeon following repair. Finally, **(E)** demonstrates the 3D quantitative assessment of the MV using built-in software (MVQ, QLAB) before the repair and following repair **(F)**. The MV quantification software offers a semiautomated analysis package for accurate modeling of the mitral annulus, valve commissures, leaflet coaptation, and leaflet topography. (Al, anterolateral commissure; PM, posteromedial commissure)

which are analyzed separately by performing the "segment analysis," and 17 segmental time-volume waveforms are displayed simultaneously, offering the possibility of more objective wall motion comparisons (Figure 24–13B). Activation of the "show reference mesh" feature within the software displays the end-diastolic surface mesh as a diastolic reference point (Figure 24–13D). Other viewing modes include the "iSlice" view, which displays up to 16 simultaneously moving short-axis views of the LV and allows verification of appropriate endocardial border detection, as well as the "Slice Plane" view, which shows a moving LV surface mesh within three orthogonal axis planes (Figure 24–13C).

Aortic Valve, Tricuspid Valve, and Pulmonic Valve

Three-dimensional assessment of the native AV and TV is more difficult when compared to 3D imaging of the MV. Both valves can be optimally visualized only in 18% (AV) and 11% (TV) when using RT-3D-TEE, largely because these valves are anterior structures with a longer distance from the transducer, are associated with a less favorable angle of insonation, and have thinner leaflets compared to the MV.[6]

Imaging Techniques. The best mode to assess the AV appears to be the Live 3D mode (see Figure 24–3), while the TV is best assessed using the 3D-zoom or full

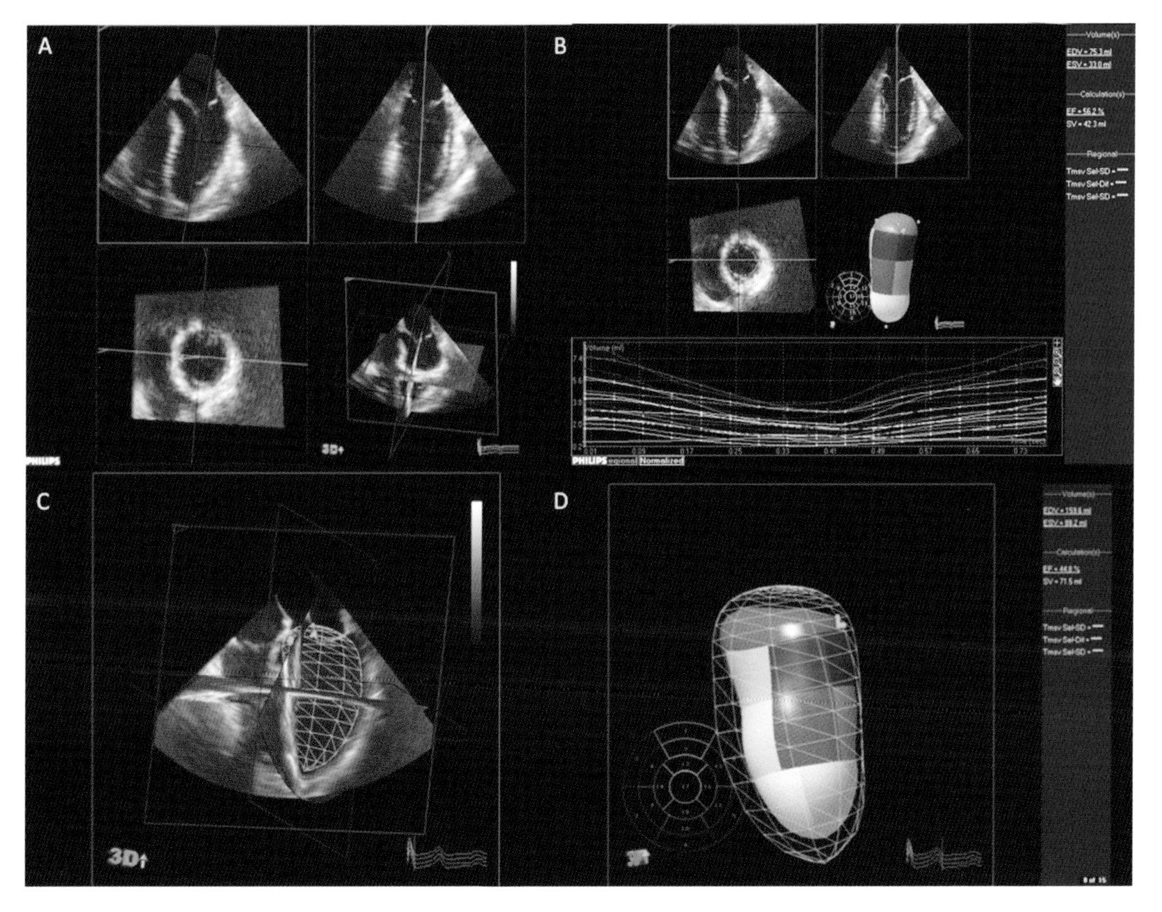

FIGURE 24–13. **(A)** shows a 3D-TEE full volume of the entire heart displayed in three multiplanar reconstruction planes (MPRs) (green, four-chamber view; red, two-chamber view; and blue, midpapillary short-axis view) along with the 3D image displayed as a slice plane view demonstrating the heart within these three MPRs (right lower quadrant). Manual definition of the septal, lateral, anterior, inferior, and apical endocardial border of the LV in end-systole and end-diastole, followed by an automatic border-tracking algorithm and segmental analysis, will display the LV shell in 17 segments **(B)** along with the corresponding segmental time-volume waveforms. The slice plane view **(C)** and the shell view **(D)** with an end-diastolic reference mesh are alternative options for display of the data.

volume mode. Occasionally, the 3D full volume mode might offer more detailed information because of higher frame rates. This mode will also allow assessment of both atrioventricular valves and the AV simultaneously. Thickening and calcification of the AV cusps mostly facilitates RT-3D-TEE imaging of the AV, but significant calcification results in similar drop-out (shadowing) as seen with 2D-TEE. Cropping of a 3D-TEE image assists in the planimetric assessment of the AV area. RT-3D-TEE may also be of benefit in differentiating bicuspid from tricuspid anatomy (Figure 24–14A), assessing involvement of the AV or coronary arteries during acute dissections (Figure 24–14B) of the ascending aorta, or in diagnosing AV endocarditis.

Optimal visualization of the TV using RT-3D-TEE is achieved only in a small percentage of patients (Figure 24–14C).[6] It remains to be seen if RT-3D-TEE will improve the accuracy in the assessment of TV dysfunction similar to what has been described for the MV. Early reports using 3D-TTE suggest that assessment of tricuspid regurgitation is feasible in most patients and that the shape of the vena contracta is more ovoid than that of mitral regurgitant jets.[43]

Three-dimensional echocardiographic imaging of the pulmonic valve is even more difficult. This is due to the fact that the pulmonic valve is located most anteriorly and its cusps are the thinnest of all cardiac valves. The use of RT-3D-TTE suggests that pulmonic

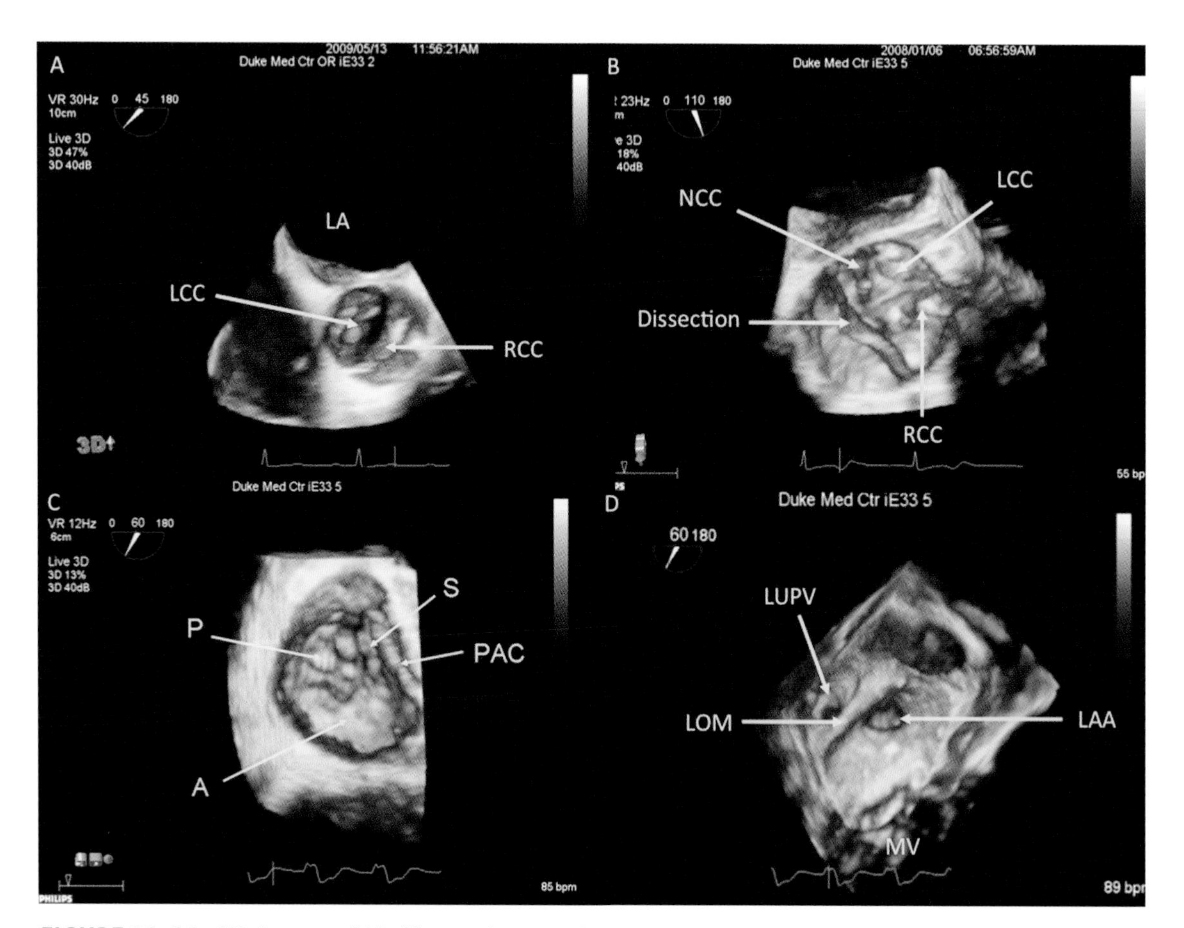

FIGURE 24–14. **(A)** shows a calcified bicuspid aortic valve (AV) imaged with live 3D in an open position. **(B)** displays a dissection of the ascending aorta originating very close to the AV. **(C)** displays the *en face* view of a normal tricuspid valve with a pulmonary artery catheter in place acquired using 3D zoom. **(D)** demonstrates a 3D zoom of the left atrial appendage adjacent to the ligamentum of Marshall, the left upper pulmonary vein, and the mitral valve. (LA, left atrium; NCC, noncoronary cusp; RCC, right coronary cusp; LCC, left coronary cusp; P, posterior leaflet; S, septal leaflet; A, anterior leaflet; PAC, pulmonary artery catheter; LUPV, left upper pulmonary vein; LOM, ligament of Marshall; LAA, left atrial appendage; MV, mitral valve.)

insufficiency may be assessed more accurately and with a lower intra- and interobserver variability when compared with 2D imaging.[44] To date, no studies have assessed the utility of RT-3D-TEE for the assessment of pulmonic stenosis or insufficiency.

LEFT ATRIAL APPENDAGE

TEE is considered the gold standard imaging modality for detection of left atrial appendage (LAA) thrombi. Despite a relatively high specificity, 2D-TEE imaging may overestimate the incidence of thrombi partly due to the complex 3D morphology of multi-lobed appendages.[45] The complex structure of the LAA lends itself well to 3D assessment. Several case reports using RT-3D-TTE or reconstruction 3D-TEE showed that 3D assessment enables excellent visualization of the LAA anatomy and function (see Figure 24–8B).[46,47] Further, RT-3D-TEE provides excellent visualization of the LAA orifice, which may optimize the guidance for the placement of LAA occlusion devices.[48] Successful application of RT-3D-TEE to confirm stable catheter position along the entire length of the ligament of Marshall during left atrial catheter ablation for atrial fibrillation has also been described. RT-3D-TEE could potentially enhance lesion delivery during left atrial catheter ablation for atrial fibrillation to improve efficacy and safety.[49] Further, RT-3D-TEE might become the method of choice to more accurately assess the LAA, especially to distinguish thrombi from anatomical variants, and might alter the course of therapy in patients with atrial fibrillation, particularly during placement of an LAA occlusion device.[50]

Imaging Techniques. The LAA can be best visualized by using the 3D-zoom mode obtaining the *en face* view of the LAA with the adjacent ligament of Marshall (see Figure 24–14D).

Limitations

Although the introduction of RT-3D-TEE to the operating room has truly added a new dimension to perioperative imaging, a number of significant limitations remain. First, while 3D zoom and Live 3D present truly real-time modes, the acquisition of a 3D full volume as well as a 3D color full volume are based on automatic reconstruction from multiple subvolumes, and, therefore, are prone to artifacts resulting from arrhythmias, ventilation, and other movements. Second, as RT-3D-TEE obeys the same physical laws as 2D ultrasound, poor 2D image quality will likely translate into similarly poor 3D image quality that adds little to no value to the overall assessment. Third, image acquisition of 3D full volumes and 3D color full volumes and associated quantification remain time-consuming. Fourth, although built-in software offers a truly novel and promising approach to quantitative assessment of 3D data sets of the MV and LV, this assessment is static, and dynamic changes during the cardiac cycle are not reflected. Finally, as RT-3D-TEE technology represents a brand-new technology, its use will naturally prolong a comprehensive TEE examination. This is especially true when more sophisticated quantification using built-in software is performed.

CONTRAST-ENHANCED ULTRASONOGRAPHY

Ultrasound contrast bubbles were initially used almost 30 years ago when Gramiak and Shah[51] observed that the injection of free gas bubbles produce an enhancement of the ultrasound image. However, it took almost another 20 years of development for the first commercially produced intravenous contrast agent to become available in 1989. The ideal contrast agent should be small and have rheologic properties similar to those of red blood cells. Normal pulmonary capillaries are 5 to 8 μm in diameter; therefore, microbubbles also have to be smaller than this to avoid entrapment in the pulmonary microvasculature.[52] However, since the sound-scattering potential of a microbubble is proportional to the sixth power of its radius, the microbubble may not be adequately visualized if it is too small. Thus, the ideal microbubble diameter should be between 4 and 6 μm. Microbubbles also should be stable on intravenous injection, have good in-vivo persistence to allow imaging from multiple imaging planes, and be neutrally buoyant (do not float out of emulsion). They also should be safe, nontoxic, and readily metabolized.

Contrast agents generally consist of air- or gas-encapsulated microbubbles. The physical behavior of the microbubble is determined by the composition of the outer shell and the gas contained within. The first generation of contrast agents was produced by sonication of 5% human serum albumin, resulting in microbubbles of air covered by a thin shell of denatured albumin. These bubbles cleared the microcirculation after venous injection because of their small size (mean of 4.3 μm) and could opacify the left ventricular (LV) cavity. This bubble held great promise for endocardial border detection during routine echocardiography and dobutamine-stress studies, but high LV pressure during systole resulted in excessive bubble compression and destruction, with rapid loss of the contrast effect. Further, direct intracoronary injection was required to opacify the myocardium. Second-generation contrast agents have demonstrated improvements in their ability to traverse the pulmonary vascular bed (due to encapsulation), stability (decreased solubility of gases), and acoustic properties and backscatter enhancement (particulate or polymer shells). At present two second-generation contrast agents are approved by the U.S. Food and Drug Administration (FDA) for clinical use: Optison® and Definity®. Optison® consists of perfluoropropane-filled albumin microspheres (mean diameter of 3.9 μm, concentration of 5×10^8/mL). It is excreted unchanged by the lungs in minutes, whereas the liver metabolizes the albumin component. Optison® has been shown to be superior to first-generation agents for LV cavity opacification and endocardial border delineation in patients with suboptimal echocardiograms.[53] Definity® is perfluoropropane microbubbles, coated with a phospholipid shell, which shows improved stability and high enhancement at low doses. Mean diameter is only 1.5 μm, with a half-life of only 1.3 minutes. In addition, Definity® microbubbles are neutrally buoyant (do not float out of emulsion) and are effective at very high dilutions, making this agent ideal for continuous infusion and prolonged imaging.

Imaging Technique

Simultaneous with the emergence of novel contrast agents, new ultrasound technologies have been developed to improve microbubble detection. These include nonlinear harmonic imaging, intermittent harmonic power Doppler, power modulation, and pulse inversion imaging. Microbubbles produce their effects by resonating in an ultrasound beam, ie, rapidly contracting and expanding in response to the pressure changes of the sound wave. This results in significant enhancement of the reflected ultrasound signal, thus allowing differentiation from normal body tissues. Unlike tissue, bubble behavior differs according to the intensity of ultrasound exposure. The output intensity of the ultrasound system is expressed in terms of the mechanical index (MI), defined as the peak negative pressure divided by the square root of the ultrasound frequency. In clinical ultrasound systems, the MI lies between 0.1 and 2.0, but it is only an estimate of the pressure to which the tissue is exposed. Classically, microbubbles display three broad patterns of scattering behavior in response to incident intensity[54]:

1. At low transmit intensity, the backscatter enhancement is typically linear, resulting in augmentation of the echo from blood. With conventional gray-scale imaging, endocardial border enhancement is typical. Enhancement of the Doppler spectral display also has been reported, with increases in the technical success rates of Doppler assessment of aortic stenosis, mitral regurgitation, and pulmonary venous flow.
2. As the transmit intensity is increased (but still below the level used in most diagnostic scans), the microbubble backscatter pattern begins to display nonlinear characteristics, such as the emission of harmonics. The harmonic response varies between contrast agents and is dependent on the pressure produced by the ultrasound on the microbubble, the size distribution of the bubbles, and the mechanical properties of the bubble capsule. Typically, in harmonic mode, the ultrasound system transmits at one frequency (eg, 1.5 to 3 MHz) but is tuned to receive at double that frequency (3 to 6 MHz); this is known as the *second harmonic*. Echoes from tissue and tissue-mimicking material are greatly reduced but not completely eliminated.
3. At the highest output power setting of the ultrasound system (approaching an MI of 2.0), the bubbles are disrupted and degraded, producing a strong, transient echo.

Detection of these echoes currently forms the basis of intermittent, or triggered, myocardial perfusion imaging. Controlled destruction of the bubbles also may have a role in emerging therapeutic applications such as targeted drug and gene delivery.

Clinical Applications

In 2007, ultrasound contrast agents were subject to a black box warning by the FDA following reports of 11 deaths associated with the use of these agents. A subsequent review involving 18,671 consecutive patients found no increased mortality risk for patients who received contrast-enhanced echocardiography compared with patients who were imaged without the agent, despite evidence for higher clinical acuity and more comorbid conditions in patients undergoing contrast studies.[55] This led the FDA to ease its restrictions, however, contrast agents are still contraindicated in patients with known or suspected right-to-left or bidirectional cardiac shunts and hypersensitivity to perflutren.[56]

DIAGNOSTIC USE

Diagnostic applications of contrast-enhanced ultrasound techniques include contrast-enhanced color Doppler, endocardial border detection, and organ (myocardial, renal, and hepatic) perfusion imaging.

Improved delineation of the endocardial border has perhaps been the greatest effect of contrast agents. Accurate endocardial definition is important when assessing regional wall motion abnormalities, estimating ejection fraction, and detecting LV thrombi and masses. Assessment of LV function is central to the management of many cardiac conditions. Microbubble contrast agents make the blood-tissue interface much clearer (Figure 24–15), and several studies have validated the effectiveness of contrast-enhanced ultrasound in improving the accuracy of global and regional assessments of LV function.[57,58] In one such study, Daniel and colleagues examined 50 patients with technically difficult echocardiograms in the intensive care unit.[59] The imaging modalities employed included fundamental, harmonic, fundamental plus Optison®, and harmonic plus Optison®. For each set of images, myocardial segments (n = 22) were given an endocardial

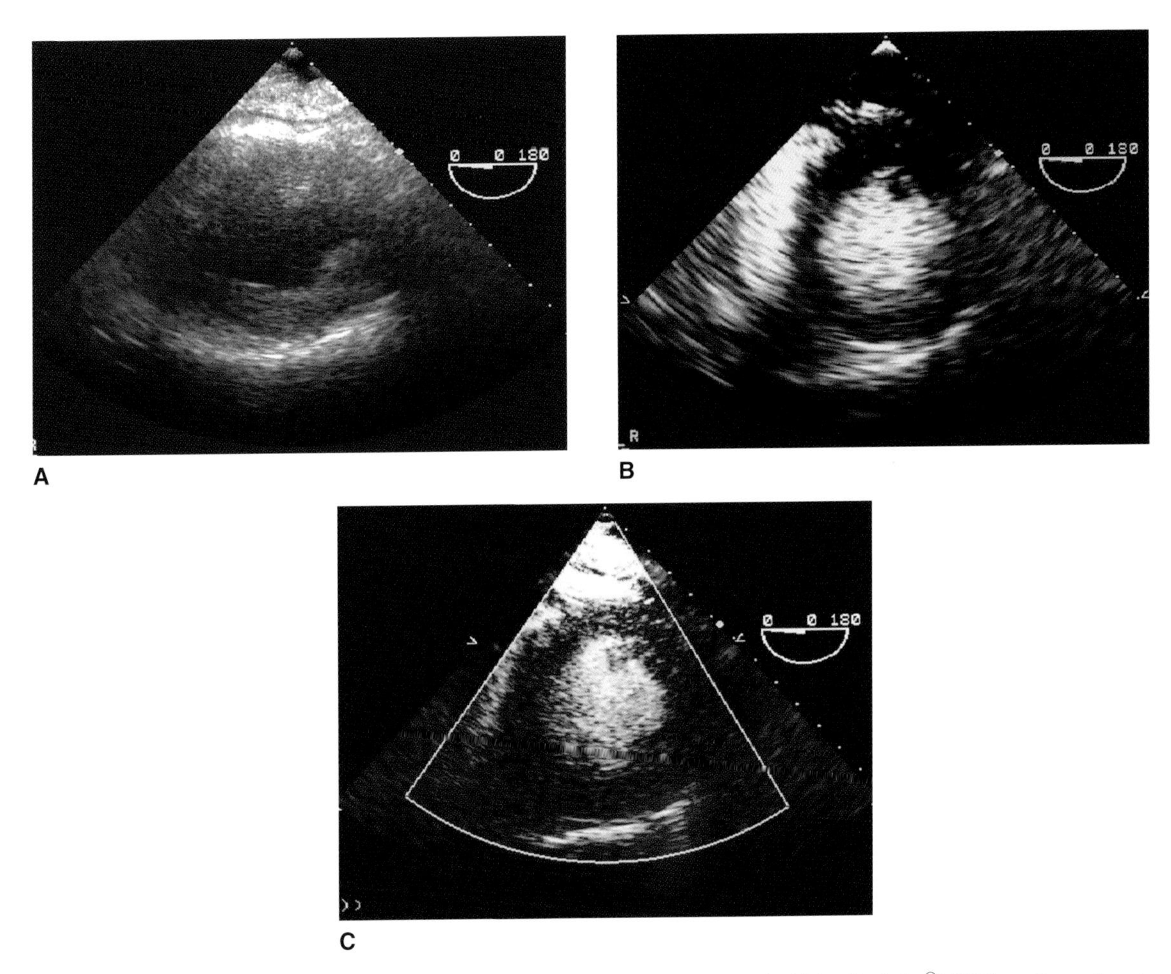

FIGURE 24–15. Enhanced delineation of the endocardial border using microbubbles (Definity®). **(A)** Two-dimensional TEE without harmonics. **(B)** Two-dimensional TEE with harmonics and contrast. **(C)** Two-dimensional TEE with harmonic power Doppler and contrast.

border visualization score of 0 if not visualized, 1 if visualized in systole or diastole, and 2 if visualized in both. There was stepwise improvement in endocardial border visualization, with mean endocardial border visualization scores of 1.09 ± 0.83 (fundamental), 1.33 ± 0.81 (harmonic), 1.64 ± 0.62 (fundamental plus Optison®), and 1.90 ± 0.35 (harmonic plus Optison®; $P < .001$). Endocardial border enhancement can be achieved by using bolus or continuous infusions of contrast agent.

Perfusion imaging, such as myocardial contrast echocardiography (MCE), is based on the seminal work of Wei and Kaul.[60] Quantitative assessment of myocardial blood flow is best obtained by using continuous infusions of contrast (eg, Definity® mixed as 1.5 mL in 50 mL of normal saline delivered at 1.5 mL/min through a syringe infusion pump), although qualitative data can be obtained with bolus injections (eg, 0.2 to 0.3 mL of Definity® followed by a slow saline flush). MCE has the potential to provide the clinician with qualitative and quantitative information on myocardial perfusion that will complement the anatomic, functional, and hemodynamic information derived from a standard 2D echocardiographic examination. The advances and refinements in harmonic imaging and Doppler technology have enabled visualization of tiny amounts of contrast with very high spatial resolution, thus allowing real-time assessment of myocardial perfusion.

In TEE, the use of contrast agents is limited to transgastric views. The interposition of the left atrium between the ultrasound transducer and the ventricle, in all the midesophageal views, causes the contrast-filled atrium to cast an acoustic shadow over the entire left ventricular cavity. MCE in the operating room is performed by obtaining views of the left ventricle at baseline and during constant infusion of contrast agent. Contrast agents should be withdrawn from the vial and delivered to the patient through large-bore needles (eg, 16 gauge) to avoid bubble disruption. Avoiding stopcocks and acute angles in the delivery pathway also enhances bubble preservation. The contrast images can be obtained with triggered harmonic imaging (MI of 1.0 and pulsing intervals of 1, 3, 5, 8, 10, 15, and 20 beats) or with real-time imaging (MI of 0.3 with 10- to 15-beat acquisitions after impulse delivery aimed at destroying the bubbles). Digitally stored images are then analyzed with video densitometry software to determine the amount of contrast with respect to the baseline images. Video intensity is plotted against pulsing interval to give an exponential function: video intensity = $A\,(1 - e^{-\beta t})$ (Figure 24–16). From this exponential function, tissue blood fraction (A), microbubble velocity (β), and myocardial blood flow or perfusion ($A \times \beta$) can be determined.

MCE has been used to assess coronary blood flow reserve, myocardial viability after infarction, and the spatiotemporal discordance between perfusion and function. These advances have provided a means to diagnose acute myocardial infarction, determine the area of myocardium at risk, and evaluate the success of subsequent medical and surgical coronary revascularization interventions (Figure 24–17). Perfusion imaging for the

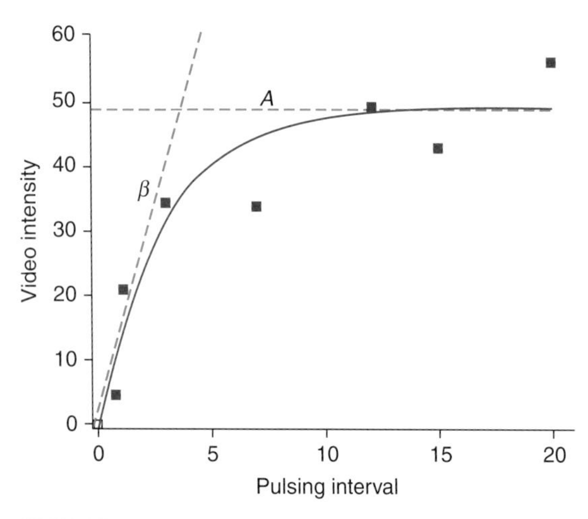

FIGURE 24–16. Plot of pulsing interval versus video intensity fitted to the exponential equation: video intensity, $A\,(1 - e^{-\beta t})$, where A represents the plateau of video intensity, which is equal to the microvascular cross-sectional area; β is rate of rise (slope) of video intensity, which equals microbubble velocity; and $A \times \beta$ equals blood flow.

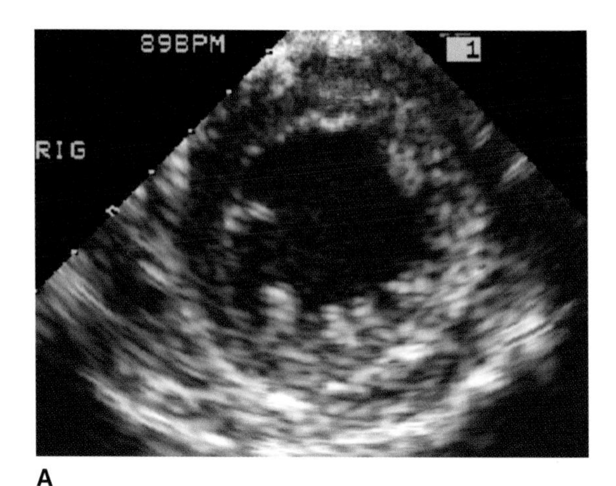

A

85BPM
20
RIG

B

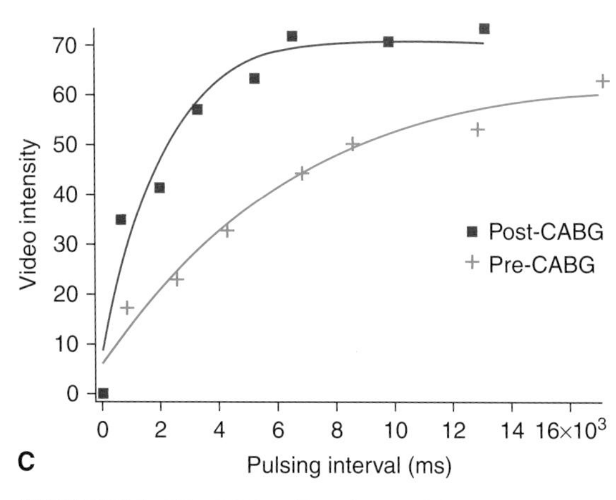

C

FIGURE 24–17. **(A)** Baseline short-axis TEE image. **(B)** Contrast-enhanced ultrasound image at a pulsing interval of 20 beats. **(C)** Pulsing interval versus tissue video intensity showing increased blood flow after revascularization.

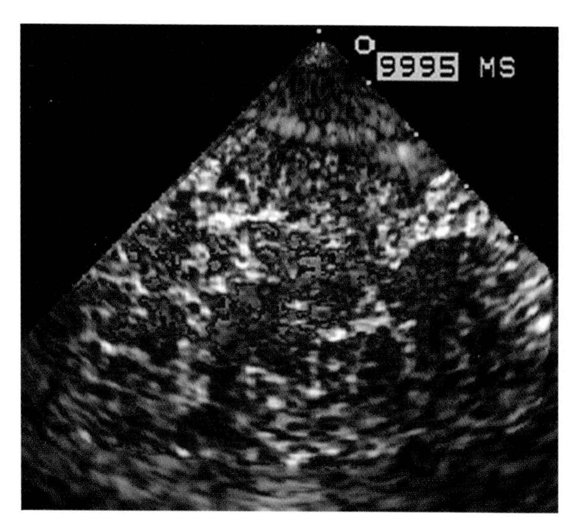

FIGURE 24–18. Renal perfusion imaging using transesophageal echocardiography and Definity®.

liver, kidney, and colon also holds some promise, particularly for the detection and localization of primary and metastatic carcinomas (Figure 24–18).

Therapeutic Use

The role of therapeutic ultrasound is constantly expanding and it is being used currently in a number of medical scenarios such as treatment of glaucoma, cataract, and vitreous hemorrhage; lithotripsy of renal calculi; and the debulking and treatment of certain tumors. Adjunctive administration of microbubbles and contrast agents has opened up new possibilities such as enhanced thrombolysis therapy, modulation of tissue injury, and locally targeted drug and gene delivery.

Many of these emerging applications exploit the bioeffects of ultrasound. Sonothrombolysis is the concept of augmentation of clot lysis by the application of external ultrasound. Microbubbles naturally exist within clots and enhance clot thrombolysis through acoustic cavitation when exposed to ultrasound. Concomitant administration of external microbubbles accelerates this process, probably by lowering the threshold for acoustic cavitation, and may have a role in the treatment of acute and chronic thrombotic coronary occlusions. A thrombus-specific ultrasound contrast agent has been developed that facilitates sonothrombolysis.[61]

Perhaps the most exciting emerging application for microbubbles is targeted drug and gene delivery. Microbubbles can be engineered to carry drugs and genetic material within their core or on their surface. Once injected intravenously, the microbubbles can be followed to the target tissue, at which point a high-energy impulse of ultrasound is delivered, resulting in cavitation, microbubble disruption, and delivery of the drug or genetic material to the target tissue. The accuracy of this system can be increased by incorporating ligands into the outer shell of the microbubbles that specifically target receptors on cell membranes or tissues. The efficacy of this delivery system was validated by Shohet and associates,[62] who successfully delivered an adenoviral transgene to rat myocardium by ultrasound-mediated microbubble destruction. Ultrasound also has been shown to transiently increase the porosity of biological membranes, thereby facilitating delivery of large compounds such as proteins and DNA into cells.[63] Further, disruption of the microbubbles within the capillary bed increases dispersion of the therapeutic payload within the target tissue. As with sonothrombolysis, externally administered microbubbles substantially reduce the power or energy required to produce these effects.

Echo Particle Image Velocimetry

Particle image velocimetry (PIV) is a novel technique used to quantify flow characteristics of fluids and gases by adding particles to the medium. Using a powerful laser flash, the backscatter that reflects off of the particles is recorded by a camera. By cross correlation of two consecutive images, multi-component velocity vectors can be calculated and flow characteristics, such as vortex formation, analyzed. Optical PIV is used extensively in a wide range of fields, but can only be used in transparent media where light propagates freely; it is useless in opaque biological tissues such as blood. Echo PIV is based on the same principles, but uses the backscatter generated by contrast particles when interrogated by ultrasound. When two consecutive B-mode images with high temporal resolution are generated, displacement of the contrast microbubbles in the second image, relative to the first, represents the flow of blood. Because of the high velocity of blood within the cardiac cavities (up to 1.5 m/s), frame rates of more than 200 frames per second are necessary to obtain adequate temporal resolution. The contrast particles must be neutrally buoyant, show a density similar to blood, and not cause any change in flow dynamics. Echo-PIV has been validated in-vitro in an artery model against optical PIV with good results,[64] and in-vivo in a canine model and in patients undergoing electrophysiology studies.[65] Possible applications of this new technique are the quantification of wall and fluid shear stresses in arteries and cardiac cavities, and the measurement of velocity profiles in complex flows such as insufficient or stenotic valves, prosthetic valves, ventricular filling, aortic flow, and congenital cardiac malformations.

Sengupta et al[66] examined intraventricular flow profiles during sinus and paced rhythms. During left ventricular pacing, there was a delay in the redirection of blood flow and in reaching peak longitudinal velocities directed toward the LV base and outflow tract. The pre-ejection blood flow changed from a normal apex-to-base to a base-to-apex direction in the paced ventricle, resulting in turbulence and loss of a well-organized vortex formation across the inflow-outflow region. They found that echo-PIV had several advantages over color Doppler for displaying information on instantaneous intracavitary flow vector fields (Figure 24–19). The exploration of echo-PIV as a potential clinical tool has only just begun, but the fact that the concentration of contrast agent used is much smaller than in conventional contrast echocardiography could allow for its use with TEE.

MYOCARDIAL DEFORMATION IMAGING

Assessment of LV wall motion traditionally has been performed through visual inspection of endocardial thickening and excursion in 2D images. This subjective method has a high degree of inter- and intraobserver variability amongst experienced cardiologists and anesthesiologists.[67,68] Over the past few years, introduction of the concepts of strain and strain rate and development of new technologies have allowed for the objective quantification of myocardial deformation during a cardiac cycle. These techniques are grouped under the name myocardial deformation imaging and comprise tissue Doppler strain (TDS), 2D speckle tracking (2DST), and velocity vector imaging (VVI).

Strain is a measure of the change in length of an object and is calculated as:

$$\varepsilon = \frac{L_1 - L_0}{L_0}$$

where ε is strain, L_0 is the baseline length, and L_1 is the final length of the object. An object that lengthens ($L_1 > L_0$) will have positive strain, and an object that shortens ($L_1 < L_0$) will have negative strain. Strain rate is the rate of change in length over time and is calculated as:

$$SR = \frac{\varepsilon}{\Delta t}$$

where SR is strain rate, ε is strain, and Δt is the time form baseline to final length.

Myocardial strain rates can be measured in the radial (transmural), circumferential, and longitudinal directions, with myocardial fibers shortening in the longitudinal

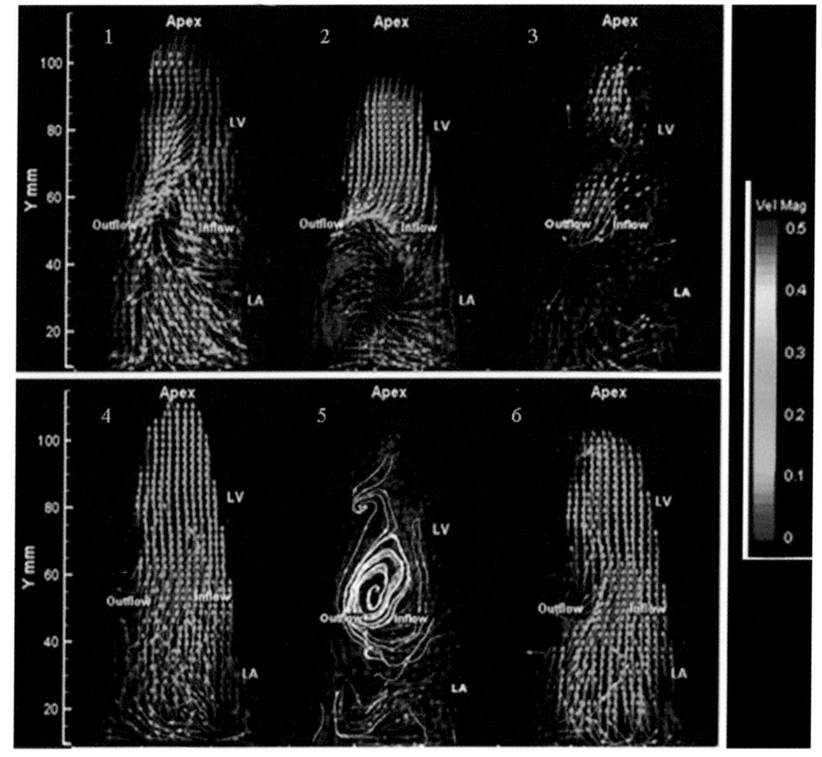

FIGURE 24–19. Echo particle image velocimetry profiles of blood flow in left atrium and ventricle. **(A)** Normal sinus rhythm: pre-ejection phase (1), ejection phase (2), isovolumic relaxation (3), early diastole (4), diastasis (5), late diastole (6).

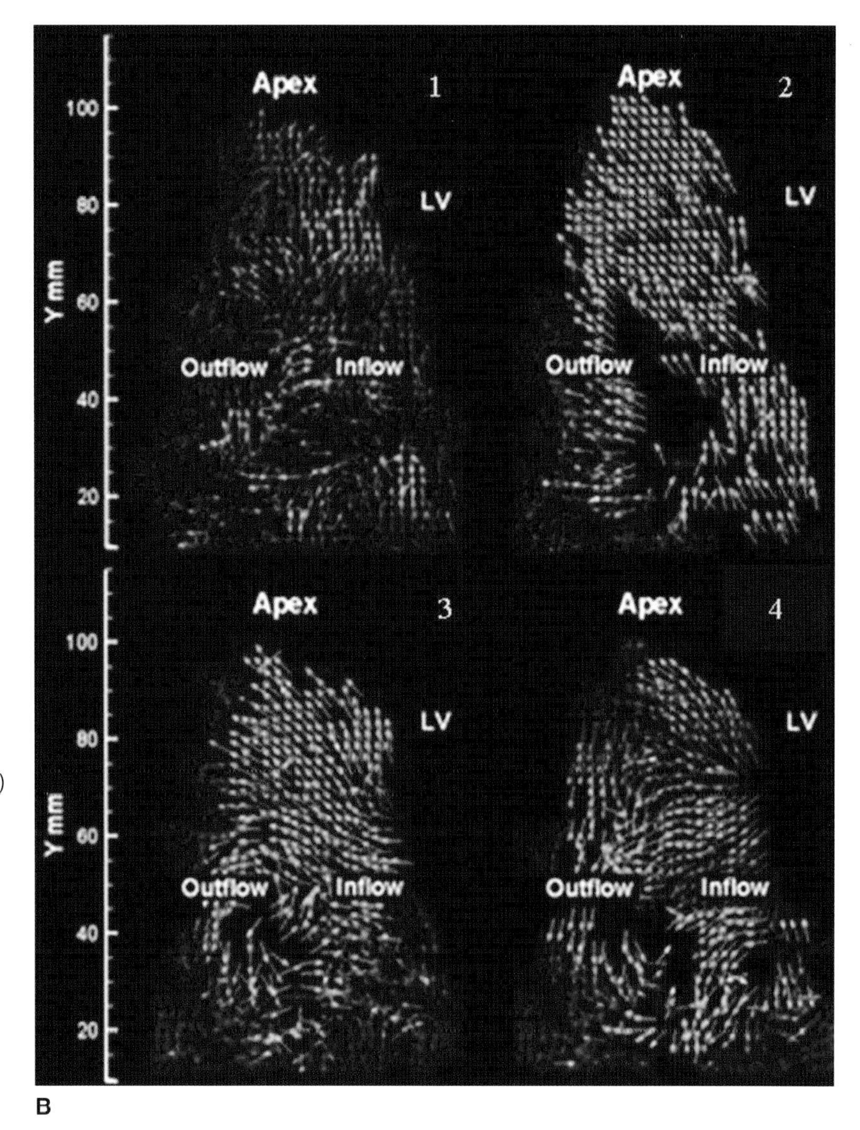

FIGURE 24–19. *(Continued)* **(B)** Epicardial pacing: four consecutive frames are all taken in the pre-ejection phase; the abnormal base-to-apex direction persists for a prolonged time and delays redirection of flow and closure of the mitral valve. (LA, left atrium; LV, left ventricle; Vel Mag, velocity magnitude.)

and circumferential directions, and thickening in the radial direction. Longitudinal strain shows a base-to-apex gradient, with higher strains measured at the level of the apex. Radial strain rates are commonly twice the longitudinal values, and higher strain rates are detected in the subendocardial layers as opposed to the epicardium. Strain rates are distributed more homogeneously from apex to base.[69] The changing length and thickness of myocardial tissue during the cardiac cycle can be graphically displayed in strain and strain rate curves (Figure 24–20). On a strain curve, the length of the myocardial segment is set at baseline (end-diastolic volume) at the onset of systole. During the isovolumic contraction period (IVC), intraventricular pressure rises but no myocardial shortening occurs, thus the strain curve remains at baseline. With the opening of the aortic valve, the ejection phase starts and the myocardium shortens (negative strain) until the aortic valve closes at peak systole. During the following isovolumic relaxation period (IVR), intraventricular pressure drops without a change in myocardial length. When the pressure drops below the aortic pressure, the mitral valve opens and early diastolic filling (E) occurs. The myocardial segments lengthen to a level short of baseline since

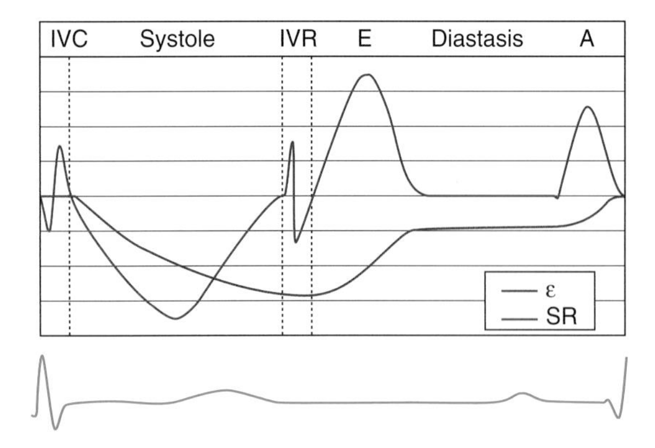

FIGURE 24–20. Normal strain and strain rate curves. (IVC, isovolumic contraction; IVR, isovolumic relaxation; E, early diastole; A, late diastole; ε, strain; SR, strain rate.)

ventricular filling is not complete until atrial contraction (A) brings the ventricular volume back to its maximum. In the period between early diastolic filling and atrial contraction—the diastasis—no volume is added to the ventricle, and thus no change in length of the myocardium will be measured. Strain rate curves are usually noisier than strain curves but have distinct features. The sequential contraction and relaxation of subendo- and subepicardial layers during IVC and IVR is reflected in the biphasic character of the strain rate curve during these phases. After IVC, the rate of shortening of the fibers reaches its maximum in midsystole and drops back to zero by the end of systole. Following IVR, the E and A peaks can be recognized, representing the rate of lengthening of the fibers during early diastolic filling and atrial contraction. During diastasis no change in length of the myocardial fibers occurs, thus strain rate is zero.

Ventricular performance is highly dependent on prevailing loading conditions, according to the Frank-Starling mechanism. Measurements of ventricular performance can thus be strongly influenced by pre- and afterload. Strain measurements are sensitive to both preload and afterload, whereas strain rate seems less influenced by preload, but still shows a strong dependency on afterload. Maximum strain rate acceleration measured in the isovolumic contraction phase is shown to be the most robust, load-independent measurement.[70]

Tissue Doppler Strain

The physical principles of Doppler tissue imaging (DTI) are analogous to those of conventional pulsed-wave Doppler. The main sources of Doppler shift from the pulsed ultrasound waves are blood cells with a normal velocity of up to 150 cm/s and solid tissues with usual velocities rarely faster than 15 cm/s. In conventional pulsed-wave Doppler studies, the low-frequency, high-amplitude, high-energy signals of wall motion are filtered out, leaving only Doppler signals from blood flow. With DTI, the opposite is true, and red blood cell Doppler shifts are filtered, leaving only tissue velocity data. The velocity data can be displayed as a spectral tracing or as color-coded tissue Doppler images. In the latter a color is attributed to every pixel of the 2D image according to its velocity and direction of its motion. DTI allows for the measurement of myocardial wall displacement, velocities, and acceleration. An important limitation of this technique is the influence of tethering on velocity profiles. For example, an infarcted, noncontractile myocardial segment gets pulled along with the adjacent, contracting segment and will appear to have a similar velocity when interrogated with DTI. To overcome this problem, tissue Doppler strain (TDS) has been developed.

During systole, the cardiac structures move in the direction of the apex while the myocardium shortens in the longitudinal axis and thickens in the radial axis. This implies a longitudinal and radial velocity gradient over the entire myocardium. Local strain rate can be calculated parallel to a pulsed-wave Doppler beam as the velocity difference between two points divided by the distance between these two points, and is given by the formula: ($Velocity_2 - Velocity_1$)/Distance (Figure 24–21).[69] Integration of the strain rate value with respect to time yields myocardial strain, which is expressed as a percentage. Since TDS

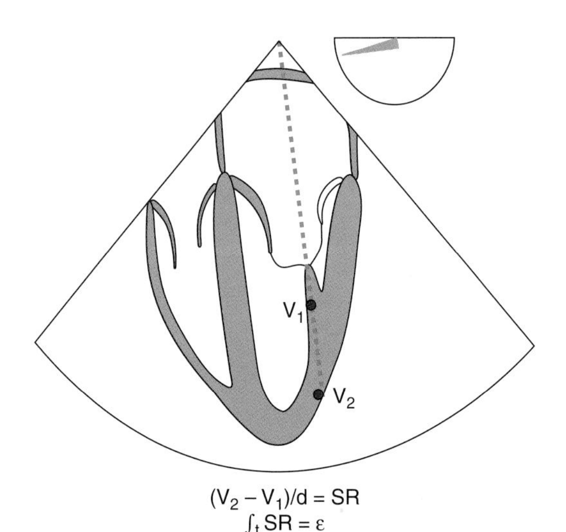

FIGURE 24–21. Doppler-based strain rate and strain calculation. Local strain rate is calculated as the velocity difference between two points divided by their distance. Integration of strain rate in time yields strain. (V_1, velocity 1; V_2, velocity 2; d, distance; ε, strain; SR, strain rate.)

measures local myocardial shortening, and not mere local velocity, the problem of tethering is largely eliminated. TDS measurement is subject to several limitations. First, since it is a Doppler-based technique, only velocities parallel to the insonated ultrasound beam will be accurately measured. Myocardial tissue deforms in several dimensions, and longitudinal shortening occurs simultaneously with radial thickening. When the Doppler beam deviates from the parallel line, components of both velocities will be measured, falsely increasing or reducing the calculated strain and strain rates. Thus, deviations of more than 15° to 20° should be avoided. Second, strain and strain rate calculations are based on velocity gradients from neighboring portions of the myocardium. Stationary artifacts (like reverberations and side lobes) have a velocity close to zero and will cause an overestimation of strain and strain rate in the area below the artifact, a reversal of velocities directly above the artifact, and an underestimation of myocardial velocities in the region above the artifact.[71]

TDI-derived strain and strain rate measurements have been validated using gelatin phantoms, microsonometry crystals, and tagged MRI.[72-74]

Imaging Technique

To obtain reliable results, the image acquisition needs to be optimized and the region of interest (ROI) carefully chosen. A clear ECG signal is mandatory for the timing of events such as the isovolumic phases. The images need to show a clear delineation between the blood pool and endocardial border, and between the myocardium and the extracardiac structures. To increase temporal resolution, the sector width and depth have to be adjusted to contain only slightly more than the interrogated myocardial wall. The optimal frame rate for tissue strain imaging is more than 150 frames per second. The actual strain and strain rate measurements are done offline on digitally stored images. Three consecutive cardiac cycles need to be recorded for the software to be able to filter out noise during post-processing. Assuming myocardial length returns to baseline at the end of the cardiac cycle, calculated strain should return to zero. The integration of strain rate in time can result in drifting of the strain curve. Drift compensation can be applied to the data and is an automatic feature of TDS software, but can introduce an error in strain calculations. The operator places a sampler, of which the length can be chosen, on the ROI, and the software displays velocity, strain, and strain rate curves calculated from the points at the extremities of the sampler. Usually three different portions, corresponding to the basal, midpapillary, and apical segments, of the interrogated myocardial wall are analyzed.

Clinical Applications

Peak systolic strain rates have been shown to correlate with peak contractility by experimental measurements of peak elastance.[75] Similarly, during myocardial ischemia, the homogeneous distribution of systolic strain rates from apical to basal segments is lost and replaced with asynchronous contraction. Strain and strain rates, measured by TDS, are significantly reduced in regional ischemia and can differentiate infarcted and ischemic from normal myocardium.[73,76] TDS can identify the extent of transmural infarction,[77] helps identify viable myocardium,[78] and can predict recovery after revascularization.[79] Thus, changes in strain and strain rate can be used to rapidly diagnose and treat a variety of conditions including myocardial ischemia, systolic or diastolic dysfunction, and ventricular asynchrony. Left atrial strain and strain rate measurement have been proposed as predictors for successful cardioversion.[80] TDS evaluation of regional ischemia with TEE is feasible in the operating room, although incompletely studied.[81,82]

2D Speckle Tracking Echocardiography

Two-dimensional speckle tracking (2DST) is a new echocardiographic technique developed to measure myocardial strain and strain rate independent of the insonation angle. When an ultrasound pulse interacts with tissue, the pulse gets distorted in a way that is highly dependent on the ultrastructure of that tissue. Within the myocardium there are ultrasound reflectors that will distort the sound wave in a relatively constant way throughout the cardiac cycle, so-called natural acoustic markers. These natural acoustic markers have an even distribution throughout the myocardium and produce a consistent gray-scale pattern in consecutive 2D image frames when interrogated by ultrasound. Speckles are groups of 20 to 40 pixels, each with their distinct gray-scale color, representing these natural acoustic markers.[83] Using pattern recognition algorithms, the position of these speckles can be tracked from image to image in a digitally stored cineloop of a cardiac cycle. The displacement of the speckle in both dimensions of the 2D image can thus be measured throughout diastole and systole. By simultaneously tracking multiple speckles, myocardial displacement, velocity, strain, strain rate, and ventricular twist and torsion can be quantified. In the long axis views, longitudinal and radial strain can be calculated. In the short-axis views, circumferential and radial strain, as well as ventricular twist and torsion can be measured.

The major advantage of 2DST over TDS is the angle independence of the technique, but some limitations exist. Two-dimensional speckle tracking is performed on digitized standard 2D gray-scale images and is thus highly dependent on the image quality and resolution. Lateral resolution is lower than longitudinal, which makes the calculations of radial strain less robust. Acoustic shadowing will cause drop-out zones where no tracking is possible, and stationary artifacts like reverberations will erroneously be tracked and cause overestimation of strain distal to the artifact and underestimation proximal to the artifact. Another limitation is that, in some of the commercially available software packages, regional strain and strain rates are the calculated means of all the speckles tracked in one segment. Subsegmental pathology will thus not be detected by speckle tracking. Furthermore, for optimal results, a frame rate of 60 to 90 frames per second is needed, yielding a temporal resolution that is considerably lower than TDS, which may lead to undersampling for high-frequency or short-lived events like the isovolumic phases of ventricular contraction/ relaxation. On the other hand, the lower frame rate allows for the entire left ventricular cavity to be visualized and analyzed in a single cardiac cycle. During ventricular contraction and relaxation, the myocardium twists around its longitudinal axis and moves toward the apex. This will cause speckles to moves out of the 2D scanning plane, leading to a loss of tracking. The software compensates for this by sequentially tracking multiple speckles as they move in and out of the scanning plane. Low frame rates or exaggerated out-of-plane motion will exhaust the software's ability to compensate and lead to loss of tracking.

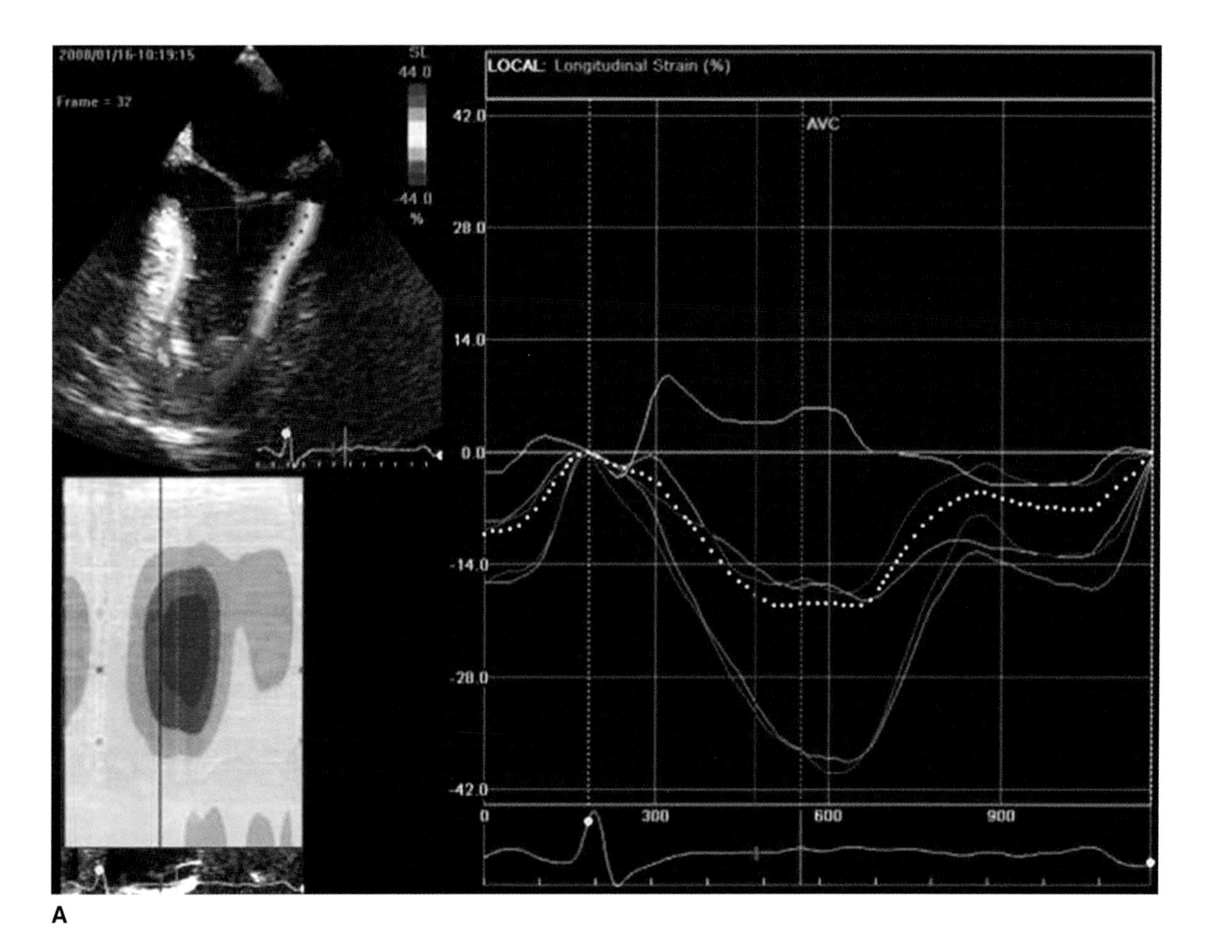

FIGURE 24–22. Two-dimensional speckle tracking on images obtained by transesophageal echocardiography. **(A)** Left ventricular longitudinal strain (midesophageal four-chamber view). **(B)** Left ventricular circumferential strain (transgastric midpapillary short-axis view). **(C)** Left ventricular radial strain rate (transgastric apical short-axis view). **(D)** Left ventricular apical rotation (transgastric apical short-axis view). The white dotted line represents global ventricular deformation; the colored lines correspond to color-coded segments and represent regional deformation. Rotation at the apex occurs counterclockwise (when looking from apex to base) and is by convention positive. (AVC, aortic valve closure.)

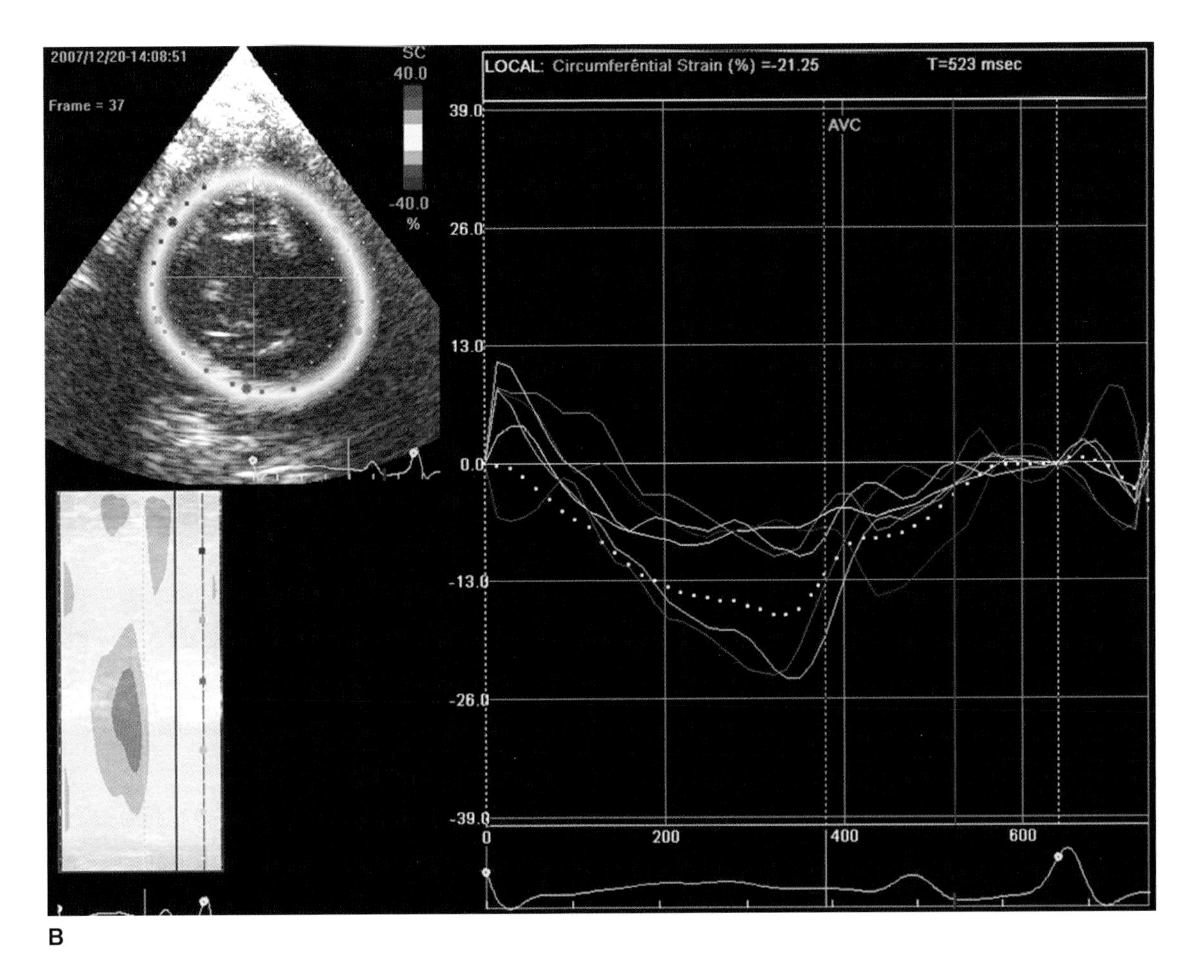

B

FIGURE 24–22. *(Continued)*

The calculation of regional myocardial strain and strain rate by speckle tracking has been validated in vitro using ultrasound phantoms, and in vivo against Doppler tissue imaging, microsonometry, and tagged cardiac MRI.[83-86]

Imaging Technique

For adequate event timing a clear ECG signal has to be displayed on the ultrasound machine, and aortic valve opening and closure must be timed; continuous Doppler through the aortic valve usually does this. A stable heart rate and rhythm are necessary. Two-dimensional speckle tracking is performed on digitally stored 2D gray-scale images. To obtain a frame rate between 60 and 90 frames per second, imaging settings may have to be adjusted (sector width, scanning depth, single focus). Large dilated ventricles may require settings that reduce the frame rate below the lower limit, and limiting the scanning sector to a specific ventricular wall may be necessary to obtain adequate temporal resolution. The focus must be placed at the level of the segment of interest. Usually, three consecutive cardiac cycles are recorded, out of which the cycle with the best image quality is visually chosen for analysis. The software prompts the operator to delineate the endocardial border in one image frame and arbitrarily defines an ROI encompassing the entire ventricular wall, the width of which can be manually adjusted. The ROI is automatically divided into six equally sized, color-coded parts representing the six myocardial segments visualized in the chosen view. After analysis, global and regional myocardial displacement, velocity, strain, and strain rate curves are displayed (Figure 24–22). For the short-axis views, angular rotation and rotation rates can be graphically displayed.

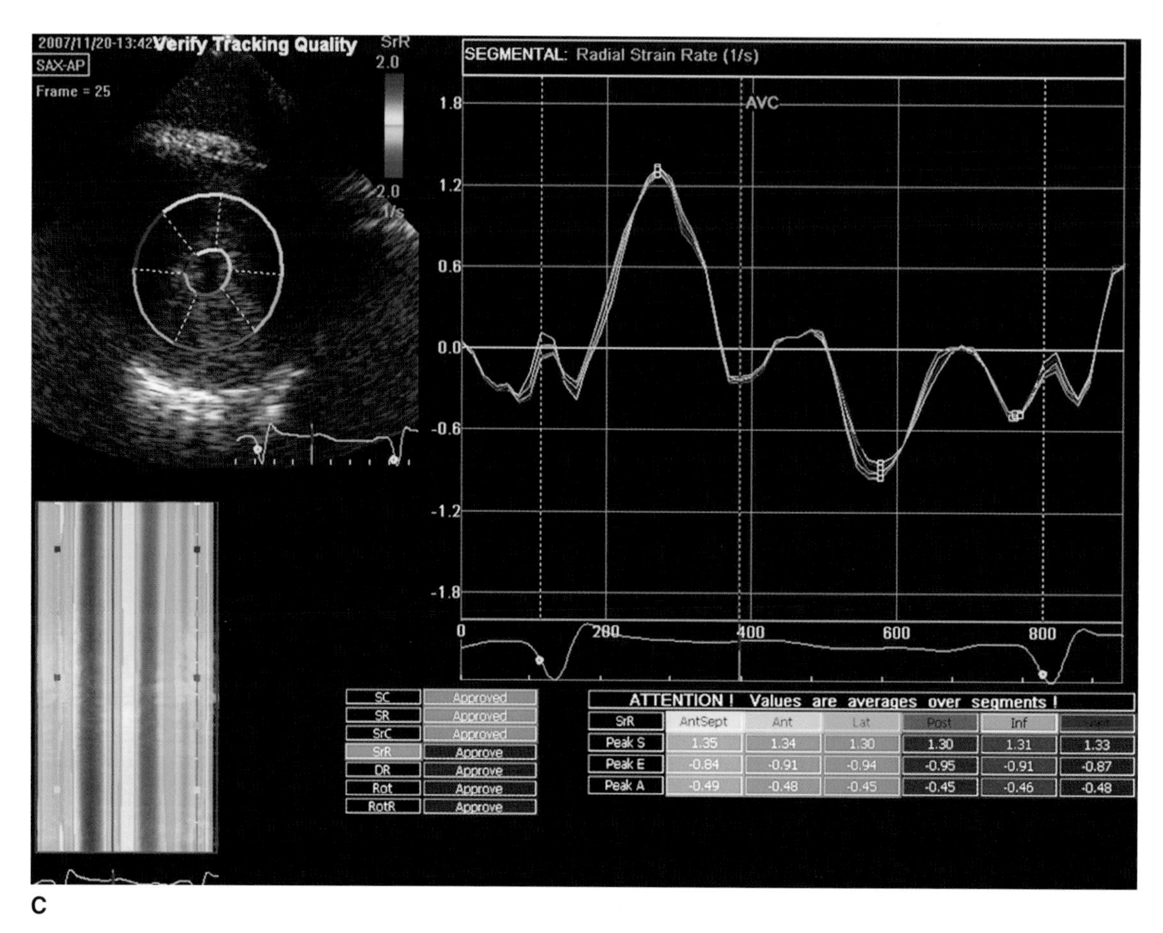

C

FIGURE 24–22. *(Continued)*

Clinical Applications

EF calculated using speckle tracking techniques correlates closely with visual estimation and Simpson's method (r = 0.82).[87] Global longitudinal strain has been proposed as a new index for left ventricular systolic function with a high specificity and sensitivity for the diagnosis of myocardial infarction.[88] Reductions in global longitudinal strain closely correlate to infarct size in chronic ischemic heart disease.[89] Regional reductions in strain correlate well to angiographic findings of coronary artery disease, and speckle tracking can distinguish different states of transmurality of myocardial infarctions.[87,90,91] In patients with subclinical hypertrophic cardiomyopathy, 2DST shows early decreases in global longitudinal, radial, and circumferential strain.[92]

Global diastolic strain rates in the isovolumic relaxation phase correlate to diastolic function.[93] The quantification of left ventricular twist and torsion by 2DST has been used to study changes in ventricular rotation and rotation rate in the elderly,[94] and in patients with essential hypertension,[95] myocardial ischemia,[96] ventricular hypertrophy,[97] dilated cardiomyopathy,[98] and chronic mitral regurgitation.[99] The rate of early diastolic untwist has been correlated to the degree of diastolic dysfunction defined by classic echocardiographic measures.[100]

Cardiac resynchronization therapy (CRT) has been shown to improve heart failure functional class, exercise capacity, quality of life, and survival in patients with heart failure and dyssynchrony.[101] In the perioperative period, biventricular (BiV) pacing with epicardial pacing leads on the RV and LV has been shown to improve ventricular function in patients undergoing cardiac surgery.[102,103] In the majority of patients with reduced LV function, temporary biventricular pacing acutely improved cardiac output and arterial blood pressure after surgery, especially when LV dilatation was present.[102]

Yet, significant proportions (~30%) of patients do not seem to benefit from short- or long-term CRT. Proper

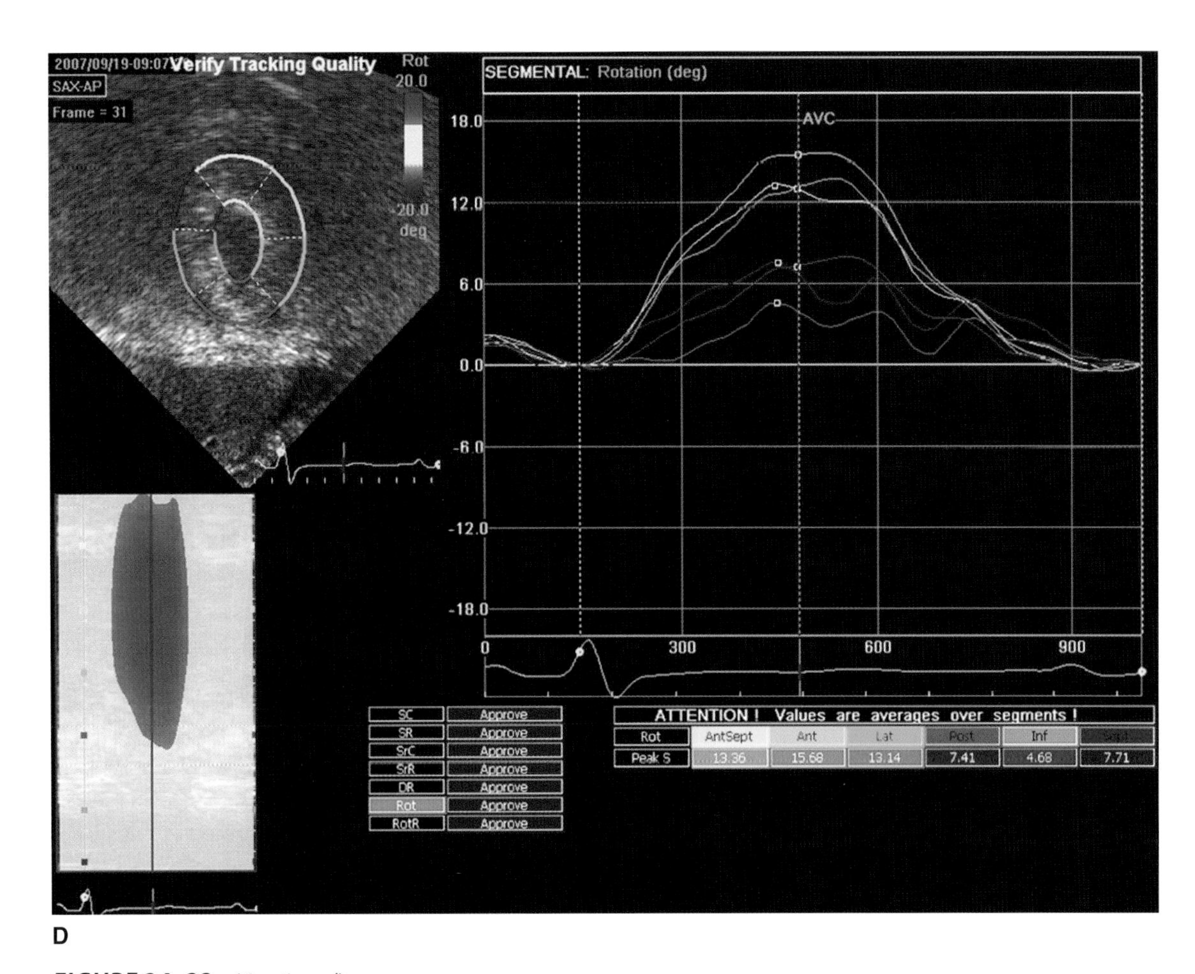

D

FIGURE 24–22. *(Continued)*

diagnosis and quantification of dyssynchrony by echocardiographic techniques is likely to improve patient selection for CRT. However, a recent multicenter trial evaluating conventional echocardiographic parameters including M-mode, pulsed-wave Doppler, and tissue Doppler methods as predictors of clinical or LV remodeling response was unable to recommend any method for improving patient selection despite promising single-center studies using these modalities.[104] Speckle tracking offers the possibility of timing myocardial deformation in six segments simultaneously and is used in numerous trials as a tool to diagnose dyssynchrony and guide CRT (Figure 24–23).[105,106] Nevertheless, because of the much lower temporal resolution compared to tissue Doppler measurements, speckle tracking may be less adapted to distinguish events separated by only a few milliseconds. With further refinements in 2D speckle tracking technology, such limitations can be easily overcome. A consensus statement by the ASE recognizes that many of these parameters are under investigation, and that an ideal approach has not yet been identified.[101] Therefore, the authors currently do not recommend that echocardiographic measures of dyssynchrony be used as a basis to withhold CRT from patients otherwise meeting accepted criteria. Neither can we recommend that CRT be applied to borderline patients without consideration of individual case features.

Two-dimensional speckle tracking can be applied to images obtained by transesophageal echocardiograpy (TEE), but to date, no reports of its use in an intraoperative setting have been published. We compared the results of 2DST performed on images obtained by TEE with equivalent images obtained by transthoracic echocardiography (TTE) in a group of patients undergoing cardiac surgery.[107] We found a moderate correlation between TEE and TTE for global longitudinal strain ($r = 0.5$), with a bias indicating slight overestimation by TEE (-3.4 ± 4.9). The correlation was moderate

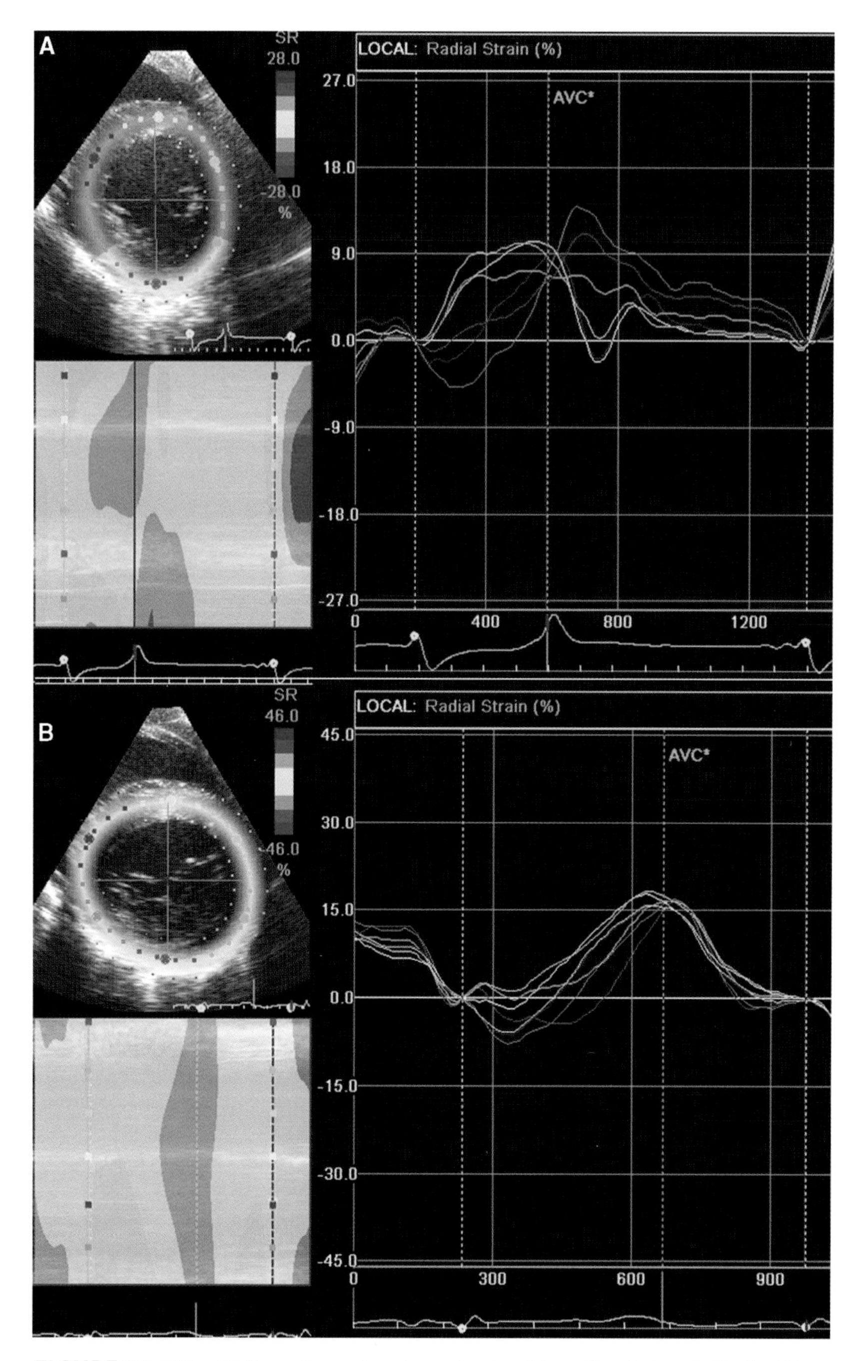

FIGURE 24–23. **(A)** Two-dimensional speckle tracking of radial strain in the LV basal short-axis view demonstrating marked dyssynchrony (time to peak strain) of the regional myocardial segments. **(B)** Improved synchronization of regional radial strain is achieved following simultaneous electrical activation of myocardial segments using CRT. (AVC, aortic valve closure.)

for the four-chamber and two-chamber views (r = 0.6) but poor for the apical long-axis view (r = 0.4). Correlation for global circumferential strain was also moderate between TEE and TTE (r = 0.5) with again a small bias for TEE (−2.1 ± 7.0). Circumferential strain in the transgastric apical short-axis view showed the best correlation of all (r = 0.7) and inter- and intraobserver variability for 2DST on the TEE images was very low (0.4 ± 4.0% and 1.4 ± 4.0% respectively), making it an attractive tool for the quantification of intraoperative changes in myocardial function.

REFERENCES

1. Dekker DL, Piziali RL, Dong E Jr. A system for ultrasonically imaging the human heart in three dimensions. *Comput Biomed Res.* 1974;7(6):544-553.
2. Pandian NG, Nanda NC, Schwartz SL, et al. Three-dimensional and four-dimensional transesophageal echocardiographic imaging of the heart and aorta in humans using a computed tomographic imaging probe. *Echocardiography.* 1992;9(6): 677-687.
3. Roelandt JR, Thomson IR, Vletter WB, Brommersma P, Bom N, Linker DT. Multiplane transesophageal echocardiography: latest evolution in an imaging revolution. *J Am Soc Echocardiogr.* 1992;5(4):361-367.
4. Agricola E, Oppizzi M, Pisani M, Maisano F, Margonato A. Accuracy of real-time 3D echocardiography in the evaluation of functional anatomy of mitral regurgitation. *Int J Cardiol.* 2008;127(3):342-349.
5. Garcia-Orta R, Moreno E, Vidal M, et al. Three-dimensional versus two-dimensional transesophageal echocardiography in mitral valve repair. *J Am Soc Echocardiogr.* 2007;20(1): 4-12.
6. Sugeng L, Shernan SK, Salgo IS, et al. Live 3-dimensional transesophageal echocardiography initial experience using the fully-sampled matrix array probe. *J Am Coll Cardiol.* 2008;52(6): 446-449.
7. Jungwirth B, Mackensen GB. Real-time 3-dimensional echocardiography in the operating room. *Semin Cardiothorac Vasc Anesth.* 2008;12(4):248-264.
8. Sheikh K, Smith SW, von Ramm O, Kisslo J. Real-time, three-dimensional echocardiography: feasibility and initial use. *Echocardiography.* 1991;8(1):119-125.
9. von Ramm OT, Smith SW. Real time volumetric ultrasound imaging system. *J Digit Imaging.* 1990;3(4):261-266.
10. Snyder JE, Kisslo J, von Ramm O. Real-time orthogonal mode scanning of the heart. I. System design. *J Am Coll Cardiol.* 1986;7(6):1279-1285.
11. Ota T, Kisslo J, von Ramm OT, Yoshikawa J. Real-time, volumetric echocardiography: usefulness of volumetric scanning for the assessment of cardiac volume and function. *J Cardiol.* 2001;37 Suppl 1:93-101.
12. Sugeng L, Weinert L, Thiele K, Lang RM. Real-time three-dimensional echocardiography using a novel matrix array transducer. *Echocardiography* 2003;20(7):623-635.
13. Salgo IS. Three-dimensional echocardiographic technology. *Cardiol Clin.* 2007;25(2):231-239.
14. Veronesi F, Corsi C, Sugeng L, et al. Quantification of mitral apparatus dynamics in functional and ischemic mitral regurgitation using real-time 3-dimensional echocardiography. *J Am Soc Echocardiogr.* 2008;21(4):347-354.
15. Jungwirth B, Glower D, Swaminathan M, et al. Is real-time-3D superior to 2D-transesophageal echocardiography to identify segmental involvement of the mitral valve in mitral regurgitation? In: *30th Annual Meeting and Workshops, Society of Cardiovascular Anesthesiologists.* Vol 106. Vancouver, BC, Canada: Anesthesia & Analgesia; 2008:SCA112.
16. Grewal J, Mankad S, Freeman WK, et al. Real-time three-dimensional transesophageal echocardiography in the intra-operative assessment of mitral valve disease. *J Am Soc Echocardiogr.* 2009;22(1):34-41.
17. Little SH, Igo SR, Pirat B, et al. In vitro validation of real-time three-dimensional color Doppler echocardiography for direct measurement of proximal isovelocity surface area in mitral regurgitation. *Am J Cardiol.* 2007;99(10):1440-1447.
18. Matsumura Y, Fukuda S, Tran H, et al. Geometry of the proximal isovelocity surface area in mitral regurgitation by 3-dimensional color Doppler echocardiography: difference between functional mitral regurgitation and prolapse regurgitation. *Am Heart J.* 2008;155(2):231-238.
19. Song JM, Kim MJ, Kim YJ, et al. Three-dimensional characteristics of functional mitral regurgitation in patients with severe left ventricular dysfunction: a real-time three-dimensional colour Doppler echocardiography study. *Heart.* 2008;94(5): 590-596.
20. Kahlert P, Plicht B, Schenk IM, Janosi RA, Erbel R, Buck T. Direct assessment of size and shape of noncircular vena contracta area in functional versus organic mitral regurgitation using real-time three-dimensional echocardiography. *J Am Soc Echocardiogr.* 2008;21(8):912-921.
21. Binder TM, Rosenhek R, Porenta G, Maurer G, Baumgartner H. Improved assessment of mitral valve stenosis by volumetric real-time three-dimensional echocardiography. *J Am Coll Cardiol.* 2000;36(4):1355-1361.
22. Chu JW, Levine RA, Chua S, et al. Assessing mitral valve area and orifice geometry in calcific mitral stenosis: a new solution by real-time three-dimensional echocardiography. *J Am Soc Echocardiogr.* 2008;21(9):1006-1009.
23. Zamorano J, Cordeiro P, Sugeng L, et al. Real-time three-dimensional echocardiography for rheumatic mitral valve stenosis evaluation: an accurate and novel approach. *J Am Coll Cardiol.* 2004;43(11):2091-2096.
24. Langerveld J, Valocik G, Plokker HW, et al. Additional value of three-dimensional transesophageal echocardiography for patients with mitral valve stenosis undergoing balloon valvuloplasty. *J Am Soc Echocardiogr.* 2003;16(8):841-849.
25. Dobarro D, Gomez-Rubin MC, Lopez-Fernandez T, et al. Real time three-dimensional transesophageal echocardiography for guiding percutaneous mitral valvuloplasty. *Echocardiography.* 2009;26(6):746-748.
26. Esteves CA, Munoz JS, Braga S, et al. Immediate and long-term follow-up of percutaneous balloon mitral valvuloplasty in pregnant patients with rheumatic mitral stenosis. *Am J Cardiol.* 2006;98(6):812-816.
27. Notrica M, Wisner J, Villagra L, et al. Life-saving percutaneous mitral valvuloplasty on a pregnant woman with refractory cardiogenic shock. *Heart Lung Circ.* 2009; 18(4): 301-304.

28. Zimmet AD, Almeida AA, Harper RW, et al. Predictors of surgery after percutaneous mitral valvuloplasty. *Ann Thorac Surg.* 2006;82(3):828-833.
29. Fatkin D, Roy P, Morgan JJ, Feneley MP. Percutaneous balloon mitral valvotomy with the Inoue single-balloon catheter: commissural morphology as a determinant of outcome. *J Am Coll Cardiol.* 1993;21(2):390-397.
30. Kronzon I, Sugeng L, Perk G, et al. Real-time 3-dimensional transesophageal echocardiography in the evaluation of post-operative mitral annuloplasty ring and prosthetic valve dehiscence. *J Am Coll Cardiol.* 2009;53(17):1543-1547.
31. Karthik S, Sundar S, Lerner A, Panzica P, Subramaniam B, Mahmood F. Intraoperative assessment of perivalvular mitral regurgitation: utility of three-dimensional echocardiography. *J Cardiothorac Vasc Anesth.* 2008;22(3):431-434.
32. Agrawal R, Rangasetty UC, Kollar A, Tuero E, Ahmad M. Live three-dimensional echocardiography in evaluation of Alfieri mitral valve repair a case report. *Echocardiography.* 2008;25(2):214-216.
33. Kort S. Real-time 3-dimensional echocardiography for prosthetic valve endocarditis: initial experience. *J Am Soc Echocardiogr.* 2006;19(2):130-139.
34. Mahmood F, Karthik S, Subramaniam B, et al. Intraoperative application of geometric three-dimensional mitral valve assessment package: a feasibility study. *J Cardiothorac Vasc Anesth.* 2008;22(2):292-298.
35. Corsi C, Coon P, Goonewardena S, et al. Quantification of regional left ventricular wall motion from real-time 3-dimensional echocardiography in patients with poor acoustic windows: effects of contrast enhancement tested against cardiac magnetic resonance. *J Am Soc Echocardiogr.* 2006;19(7):886-893.
36. Caiani EG, Corsi C, Zamorano J, et al. Improved semiautomated quantification of left ventricular volumes and ejection fraction using 3-dimensional echocardiography with a full matrix-array transducer: comparison with magnetic resonance imaging. *J Am Soc Echocardiogr.* 2005;18(8):779-788.
37. Sugeng L, Mor-Avi V, Weinert L, et al. Quantitative assessment of left ventricular size and function: side-by-side comparison of real-time three-dimensional echocardiography and computed tomography with magnetic resonance reference. *Circulation.* 2006;114(7):654-661.
38. Mor-Avi V, Sugeng L, Weinert L, et al. Fast measurement of left ventricular mass with real-time three-dimensional echocardiography: comparison with magnetic resonance imaging. *Circulation.* 2004;110(13):1814-1818.
39. Soliman OI, Krenning BJ, Geleijnse ML, et al. Quantification of left ventricular volumes and function in patients with cardiomyopathies by real-time three-dimensional echocardiography: a head-to-head comparison between two different semiautomated endocardial border detection algorithms. *J Am Soc Echocardiogr.* 2007;20(9):1042-1049.
40. Arai K, Hozumi T, Matsumura Y, et al. Accuracy of measurement of left ventricular volume and ejection fraction by new real-time three-dimensional echocardiography in patients with wall motion abnormalities secondary to myocardial infarction. *Am J Cardiol.* 2004;94(5):552-558.
41. Chan J, Jenkins C, Khafagi F, Du L, Marwick TH. What is the optimal clinical technique for measurement of left ventricular volume after myocardial infarction? A comparative study of 3-dimensional echocardiography, single photon emission computed tomography, and cardiac magnetic resonance imaging. *J Am Soc Echocardiogr.* 2006;19(2):192-201.
42. De Lange F, Karhausen J, Phillips-Bute B, Swaminathan M, Mackensen GB. Left ventricular ejection fraction assessed by 2D and 3D echocardiography; does experience matter? In: *2009 Annual Meeting, American Society of Anesthesiologists.* Vol 111. New Orleans, LA: Anesthesiology; 2009:A353.
43. Sugeng L, Weinert L, Lang RM. Real-time 3-dimensional color Doppler flow of mitral and tricuspid regurgitation: feasibility and initial quantitative comparison with 2-dimensional methods. *J Am Soc Echocardiogr.* 2007;20(9):1050-1057.
44. Pothineni KR, Wells BJ, Hsiung MC, et al. Live/real time three-dimensional transthoracic echocardiographic assessment of pulmonary regurgitation. *Echocardiography.* 2008;25(8):911-917.
45. Agmon Y, Khandheria BK, Gentile F, Seward JB. Echocardiographic assessment of the left atrial appendage. *J Am Coll Cardiol.* 1999;34(7):1867-1877.
46. Agoston I, Xie T, Tiller FL, Rahman AM, Ahmad M. Assessment of left atrial appendage by live three-dimensional echocardiography: early experience and comparison with transesophageal echocardiography. *Echocardiography.* 2006; 23(2):127-132.
47. Khan GN, Dairywala IT, Liu Z, Li P, Carroll J, Vannan MA. Three-dimensional echocardiography of left atrial appendage thrombus. *Echocardiography.* 2001;18(2):163-166.
48. Perk G, Lang RM, Garcia-Fernandez MA, et al. Use of real time three-dimensional transesophageal echocardiography in intracardiac catheter based interventions. *J Am Soc Echocardiogr.* 2009;22(8):865-882.
49. Mackensen GB, Hegland D, Rivera D, Adams D, Bahnson T. Real-time 3-dimensional transesophageal echocardiography during left atrial radiofrequency catheter ablation for atrial fibrillation. *Circ: Cardiovasc Imag.* 2008;1:85-86.
50. Mizuguchi KA, Burch TM, Bulwer BE, Fox AA, Rizzo RJ, Shernan SK. Thrombus or bilobar left atrial appendage? Diagnosis by real-time three-dimensional transesophageal echocardiography. *Anesth Analg.* 2009;108(1):70-72.
51. Gramiak R, Shah PM. Echocardiography of the aortic root. *Invest Radiol.* 1968;3(5):356-366.
52. Grayburn PA. Current and future contrast agents. *Echocardiography.* 2002;19(3):259-265.
53. Cohen JL, Cheirif J, Segar DS, et al. Improved left ventricular endocardial border delineation and opacification with OPTISON (FS069), a new echocardiographic contrast agent. Results of a phase III multicenter trial. *J Am Coll Cardiol.* 1998;32(3):746-752.
54. Burns PN. Instrumentation for contrast echocardiography. *Echocardiography.* 2002;19(3):241-258.
55. Kusnetzky LL, Khalid A, Khumri TM, Moe TG, Jones PG, Main ML. Acute mortality in hospitalized patients undergoing echocardiography with and without an ultrasound contrast agent: results in 18,671 consecutive studies. *J Am Coll Cardiol.* 2008;51(17):1704-1706.
56. Mulvagh SL, Rakowski H, Vannan MA, et al. American Society of Echocardiography consensus statement on the clinical applications of ultrasonic contrast agents in echocardiography. *J Am Soc Echocardiogr.* 2008;21(11):1179-1201; quiz 1281.

57. Reilly JP, Tunick PA, Timmermans RJ, Stein B, Rosenzweig BP, Kronzon I. Contrast echocardiography clarifies uninterpretable wall motion in intensive care unit patients. *J Am Coll Cardiol.* 2000;35(2):485-490.
58. Yong Y, Wu D, Fernandes V, et al. Diagnostic accuracy and cost effectiveness of contrast echocardiography on evaluation of cardiac function in technically very difficult patients in the intensive care unit. *Am J Cardiol.* 2002; 89(6): 711-718.
59. Daniel GK, Chawla MK, Sawada SG, Gradus-Pizlo I, Feigenbaum H, Segar DS. Echocardiographic imaging of technically difficult patients in the intensive care unit: use of optison in combination with fundamental and harmonic imaging. *J Am Soc Echocardiogr.* 2001;14(9):917-920.
60. Wei K, Jayaweera AR, Firoozan S, Linka A, Skyba DM, Kaul S. Quantification of myocardial blood flow with ultrasound-induced destruction of microbubbles administered as a constant venous infusion. *Circulation.* 1998;97(5):473-483.
61. Wu Y, Unger EC, McCreery TP, et al. Binding and lysing of blood clots using MRX-408. *Invest Radiol.* 1998;33(12): 880-885.
62. Shohet RV, Chen S, Zhou YT, et al. Echocardiographic destruction of albumin microbubbles directs gene delivery to the myocardium. *Circulation.* 2000;101(22):2554-2556.
63. Liu J, Lewis TN, Prausnitz MR. Non-invasive assessment and control of ultrasound-mediated membrane permeabilization. *Pharm Res.* 1998;15(6):918-924.
64. Kim HB, Hertzberg J, Lanning C, Shandas R. Noninvasive measurement of steady and pulsating velocity profiles and shear rates in arteries using echo PIV: in vitro validation studies. *Ann Biomed Eng.* 2004;32(8):1067-1076.
65. Shandas R, Hyoung-Bum K, Hertzberg J, G. DC, Monet E, Valdes-Cruz L. In vivo validation of the echo-PIV technique: animal and clinical studies. Summer Bioengineering Conference. Key Biscane, FL; 2003.
66. Sengupta PP, Khandheria BK, Korinek J, et al. Left ventricular isovolumic flow sequence during sinus and paced rhythms: new insights from use of high-resolution Doppler and ultrasonic digital particle imaging velocimetry. *J Am Coll Cardiol.* 2007;49(8):899-908.
67. Bergquist BD, Leung JM, Bellows WH. Transesophageal echocardiography in myocardial revascularization: I. Accuracy of intraoperative real-time interpretation. *Anesth Analg.* 1996;82(6): 1132-1138.
68. Hoffmann R, von Bardeleben S, ten Cate F, et al. Assessment of systolic left ventricular function: a multi-centre comparison of cineventriculography, cardiac magnetic resonance imaging, unenhanced and contrast-enhanced echocardiography. *Eur Heart J.* 2005;26(6):607-616.
69. Pislaru C, Abraham TP, Belohlavek M. Strain and strain rate echocardiography. *Curr Opin Cardiol.* 2002;17(5):443-454.
70. Missant C, Rex S, Claus P, Mertens L, Wouters PF. Load-sensitivity of regional tissue deformation in the right ventricle: isovolumic versus ejection-phase indices of contractility. *Heart.* 2008;94(4):e15.
71. Teske AJ, De Boeck BW, Melman PG, Sieswerda GT, Doevendans PA, Cramer MJ. Echocardiographic quantification of myocardial function using tissue deformation imaging, a guide to image acquisition and analysis using tissue Doppler and speckle tracking. *Cardiovasc Ultrasound.* 2007;5:27.
72. Belohlavek M, Bartleson VB, Zobitz ME. Real-time strain rate imaging: validation of peak compression and expansion rates by a tissue-mimicking phantom. *Echocardiography.* 2001;18(7):565-571.
73. Edvardsen T, Gerber BL, Garot J, Bluemke DA, Lima JA, Smiseth OA. Quantitative assessment of intrinsic regional myocardial deformation by Doppler strain rate echocardiography in humans: validation against three-dimensional tagged magnetic resonance imaging. *Circulation.* 2002;106(1):50-56.
74. Urheim S, Edvardsen T, Torp H, Angelsen B, Smiseth OA. Myocardial strain by Doppler echocardiography. Validation of a new method to quantify regional myocardial function. *Circulation.* 2000;102(10):1158-1164.
75. Greenberg NL, Firstenberg MS, Castro PL, et al. Doppler-derived myocardial systolic strain rate is a strong index of left ventricular contractility. *Circulation.* 2002;105(1):99-105.
76. Heimdal A, Stoylen A, Torp H, Skjaerpe T. Real-time strain rate imaging of the left ventricle by ultrasound. *J Am Soc Echocardiogr.* 1998;11(11):1013-1019.
77. Weidemann F, Wacker C, Rauch A, et al. Sequential changes of myocardial function during acute myocardial infarction, in the early and chronic phase after coronary intervention described by ultrasonic strain rate imaging. *J Am Soc Echocardiogr.* 2006;19(7):839-847.
78. Hoffmann R, Altiok E, Nowak B, et al. Strain rate measurement by doppler echocardiography allows improved assessment of myocardial viability in patients with depressed left ventricular function. *J Am Coll Cardiol.* 2002;39(3):443-449.
79. Hanekom L, Jenkins C, Jeffries L, et al. Incremental value of strain rate analysis as an adjunct to wall-motion scoring for assessment of myocardial viability by dobutamine echocardiography: a follow-up study after revascularization. *Circulation.* 2005;112(25):3892-3900.
80. Leung DY, Boyd A, Ng AA, Chi C, Thomas L. Echocardiographic evaluation of left atrial size and function: current understanding, pathophysiologic correlates, and prognostic implications. *Am Heart J.* 2008;156(6):1056-1064.
81. Simmons LA, Weidemann F, Sutherland GR, et al. Doppler tissue velocity, strain, and strain rate imaging with transesophageal echocardiography in the operating room: a feasibility study. *J Am Soc Echocardiogr.* 2002;15(8):768-776.
82. Skarvan K, Filipovic M, Wang J, Brett W, Seeberger M. Use of myocardial tissue Doppler imaging for intraoperative monitoring of left ventricular function. *Br J Anaesth.* 2003; 91(4): 473-480.
83. Leitman M, Lysyansky P, Sidenko S, et al. Two-dimensional strain–a novel software for real-time quantitative echocardiographic assessment of myocardial function. *J Am Soc Echocardiogr.* 2004;17(10):1021-1029.
84. Amundsen BH, Helle-Valle T, Edvardsen T, et al. Noninvasive myocardial strain measurement by speckle tracking echocardiography: validation against sonomicrometry and tagged magnetic resonance imaging. *J Am Coll Cardiol.* 2006; 47(4):789-793.
85. Korinek J, Wang J, Sengupta PP, et al. Two-dimensional strain—a Doppler-independent ultrasound method for quantitation of regional deformation: validation in vitro and in vivo. *J Am Soc Echocardiogr.* 2005;18(12):1247-1253.
86. Toyoda T, Baba H, Akasaka T, et al. Assessment of regional myocardial strain by a novel automated tracking system from digital image files. *J Am Soc Echocardiogr.* 2004;17(12):1234-1238.

87. Perk G, Tunick PA, Kronzon I. Non-Doppler two-dimensional strain imaging by echocardiography—from technical considerations to clinical applications. *J Am Soc Echocardiogr.* 2007;20(3): 234-243.
88. Reisner SA, Lysyansky P, Agmon Y, Mutlak D, Lessick J, Friedman Z. Global longitudinal strain: a novel index of left ventricular systolic function. *J Am Soc Echocardiogr.* 2004; 17(6):630-633.
89. Gjesdal O, Hopp E, Vartdal T, et al. Global longitudinal strain measured by two-dimensional speckle tracking echocardiography is closely related to myocardial infarct size in chronic ischaemic heart disease. *Clin Sci (Lond).* 2007; 113(6): 287-296.
90. Becker M, Hoffmann R, Kuhl HP, et al. Analysis of myocardial deformation based on ultrasonic pixel tracking to determine transmurality in chronic myocardial infarction. *Eur Heart J.* 2006;27(21):2560-2566.
91. Hanekom L, Cho GY, Leano R, Jeffriess L, Marwick TH. Comparison of two-dimensional speckle and tissue Doppler strain measurement during dobutamine stress echocardiography: an angiographic correlation. *Eur Heart J.* 2007; 28(14): 1765-1772.
92. Serri K, Reant P, Lafitte M, et al. Global and regional myocardial function quantification by two-dimensional strain: application in hypertrophic cardiomyopathy. *J Am Coll Cardiol.* 2006;47(6):1175-1181.
93. Wang J, Khoury DS, Thohan V, Torre-Amione G, Nagueh SF. Global diastolic strain rate for the assessment of left ventricular relaxation and filling pressures. *Circulation.* 2007;115 (11): 1376-1383.
94. Zhang L, Xie M, Fu M. Assessment of age-related changes in left ventricular twist by two-dimensional ultrasound speckle tracking imaging. *J Huazhong Univ Sci Technolog Med Sci.* 2007;27(6):691-695.
95. Han W, Xie M, Wang X, Lu Q. Assessment of left ventricular global twist in essential hypertensive heart by speckle tracking imaging. *J Huazhong Univ Sci Technolog Med Sci.* 2008;28(1): 114-117.
96. Bansal M, Leano RL, Marwick TH. Clinical assessment of left ventricular systolic torsion: effects of myocardial infarction and ischemia. *J Am Soc Echocardiogr.* 2008; 21(8): 887-894.
97. Takeuchi M, Borden WB, Nakai H, et al. Reduced and delayed untwisting of the left ventricle in patients with hypertension and left ventricular hypertrophy: a study using two-dimensional speckle tracking imaging. *Eur Heart J.* 2007; 28(22):2756-2762.
98. Popovic ZB, Grimm RA, Ahmad A, et al. Longitudinal rotation: an unrecognised motion pattern in patients with dilated cardiomyopathy. *Heart.* 2008;94(3):e11.
99. Borg AN, Harrison JL, Argyle RA, Ray SG. Left ventricular torsion in primary chronic mitral regurgitation. *Heart.* 2008;94(5):597-603.
100. Perry R, De Pasquale CG, Chew DP, Joseph MX. Assessment of early diastolic left ventricular function by two-dimensional echocardiographic speckle tracking. *Eur J Echocardiogr.* 2008; 9(6):791-795.
101. Gorcsan J 3rd, Abraham T, Agler DA, et al. Echocardiography for cardiac resynchronization therapy: recommendations for performance and reporting—a report from the American Society of Echocardiography Dyssynchrony Writing Group endorsed by the Heart Rhythm Society. *J Am Soc Echocardiogr.* 2008;21(3):191-213.
102. Hanke T, Misfeld M, Heringlake M, Schreuder JJ, Wiegand UK, Eberhardt F. The effect of biventricular pacing on cardiac function after weaning from cardiopulmonary bypass in patients with reduced left ventricular function: a pressure-volume loop analysis. *J Thorac Cardiovasc Surg.* 2009;138(1): 148-156.
103. Cannesson M, Farhat F, Scarlata M, Cassar E, Lehot JJ. The impact of atrio-biventricular pacing on hemodynamics and left ventricular dyssynchrony compared with atrio-right ventricular pacing alone in the postoperative period after cardiac surgery. *J Cardiothorac Vasc Anesth.* 2009; 23(3): 306-311.
104. Chung ES, Leon AR, Tavazzi L, et al. Results of the Predictors of Response to CRT (PROSPECT) trial. *Circulation.* 2008;117(20):2608-2616.
105. Gorcsan J 3rd, Tanabe M, Bleeker GB, et al. Combined longitudinal and radial dyssynchrony predicts ventricular response after resynchronization therapy. *J Am Coll Cardiol.* 2007;50 (15): 1476-1483.
106. Suffoletto MS, Dohi K, Cannesson M, Saba S, Gorcsan J 3rd. Novel speckle-tracking radial strain from routine black-and-white echocardiographic images to quantify dyssynchrony and predict response to cardiac resynchronization therapy. *Circulation.* 2006;113(7):960-968.
107. Marcucci M, Keller D, Mackensen GB, et al. Measurement of left ventricular systolic strain: a comparison of transthoracic and transesophageal echocardiographic studies. In: *American Society of Echocardiography.* Vol 21. Toronto, Canada: J Am Soc Echocardiogr; 2008:582.

REVIEW QUESTIONS

Select the *one* best answer for each of the following questions.

1. Real-time 3D-TEE imaging using the 3D zoom mode will allow good visualization of this cardiac structure in more than 50% of all patients:
   a. Aortic valve
   b. Tricuspid valve
   c. Pulmonic valve
   d. Mitral valve
   e. Right superior pulmonary vein

2. Which statement in regard to 3D-TEE image acquisition is correct?
   a. 3D-TEE imaging obeys the same ultrasound physics as 2D-TEE.
   b. 3D-TEE imaging follows unique ultrasound physics that are different from 2D-TEE.
   c. 3D-TEE image quality is independent of frame rate.
   d. 3D-TEE does not allow imaging with color.
   e. 3D-TEE routinely uses higher frame rates compared to 2D-TEE.

3. What statement in regard to ECG-gated 3D image acquisition is *true*?
   a. All currently available 3D-TEE image acquisition systems require ECG-gating.
   b. Real-time 3D-TEE acquisition is independent of ECG and respiratory gating.
   c. ECG-gating is not affected by the patient's underlying heart rhythm.
   d. ECG-gated 3D image acquisition does not require an undisturbed ECG signal.
   e. Real-time 3D-TEE acquisition depends upon ECG-gating.

4. Which of the following statements *best* describes the elements of the mitral valve apparatus that are routinely displayed by a 3D *en face* view of the mitral valve?
   a. Mitral valve commissures and chords
   b. All three posterior leaflet scallops, the anterior leaflet, and anterolateral commissure
   c. Posterior scallops, papillary muscles and chords
   d. Mitral valve annulus, anterior leaflet, and papillary muscle tips
   e. Anterior leaflet, posterior leaflet scallops and chords

5. Which of the statements in regard to 3D-TEE color Doppler imaging of a mitral regurgitant jet is *true*?
   a. The current quality of 3D-TEE color Doppler imaging does not offer any diagnostic value.
   b. 3D-TEE color Doppler imaging allows for easy volumetric assessment of mitral regurgitation.
   c. 3D-TEE color Doppler echocardiography may assist in grading the severity of mitral regurgitation.
   d. 3D-TEE color Doppler imaging is independent of ECG-gating.
   e. 3D-TEE color Doppler acquisition routinely allows capture of the entire mitral regurgitant jet.

6. 3D-TEE imaging of the left atrial appendage (LAA):
   a. Represents the gold standard in ruling out LAA thrombus
   b. Does not add any information to 2D-TEE imaging of the LAA
   c. Allows only poor visualization of the LAA
   d. May assist in the assessment of LAA geometry and pathology
   e. Is impossible in cases of left atrial spontaneous echo contrast

7. Which of the following statements regarding 3D-TEE left ventricular (LV) volumetric assessment is *false*?
   a. 3D-TEE volumetric assessment of the LV relies on semiautomatic endocardial border detection and border tracking algorithms, which can be edited manually.
   b. 3D-TEE volumetric assessment of the LV allows the determination of the LV stroke volume.
   c. 3D-TEE volumetric assessment of the LV is based on the acquisition of a full volume 3D image of the left ventricle.
   d. 3D-TEE volumetric assessment of the LV is fully automated and relies on endocardial border detection.
   e. 3D-TEE volumetric assessment of the LV allows the determination of LV end-diastolic and end-systolic volumes.

8. Which of the following statements is *true* about the mitral valve apparatus?
   a. The posterior leaflet height exceeds that of the anterior leaflet.
   b. The anterior leaflet consists of three scallops.
   c. The anterior leaflet has a crescent shape.
   d. Compared to the anterior leaflet, the posterior leaflet demonstrates a greater attachment to the mitral valve annulus.
   e. In patients with a normal mitral valve, the ratio between anteroposterior (septolateral) and transverse diameter of the mitral annulus is 4:3 during systole.

9. Which of the following statements is true?
   a. Biplane imaging requires the acquisition of two separate views of the same structure.
   b. Biplane imaging can be accomplished with conventional 2D-TEE systems.
   c. Biplane imaging enables the parallel acquisition of diagnostic data without changing the scan angle.
   d. Biplane imaging results in improved image quality with higher frame rates than multiplane imaging.
   e. Biplane scan angles on the two full-resolution planes are preset at 90° and cannot be changed during imaging.

10. Which statement regarding 3D-TEE imaging is true?
   a. Before acquisition of a 3D full volume data set, compression and gain should be kept at the lowest possible setting.
   b. Higher line density settings usually result in improved resolution and lower frame rates.
   c. Live 3D imaging usually results in larger pyramidal data sets than full volume acquisition.
   d. Sparse array transducers usually have a higher number of imaging elements than matrix array transducers.
   e. Live 3D imaging is not affected by artifacts.

11. Decreasing the line density in the imaging sector will result in:
    a. Lower frame rate
    b. Superior temporal resolution
    c. Superior spatial resolution
    d. No change in the frame rate
    e. Longer time per frame

12. Clinical methods used to evaluate left ventricular systolic function include all the following *except*:
    a. Fractional area change
    b. dP/dt
    c. 3D ejection fraction
    d. Systolic pulmonary vein pattern
    e. Fractional shortening

13. While performing contrast-enhanced echocardiography, which of the following statements is true about the use of microbubbles at a transmit intensity of 2 MI?
    a. Microbubbles enhance visualization of the blood/tissue interface, and can thus be used to improve endocardial border delineation.
    b. In the left atrium microbubbles cast strong acoustic shadows over the left ventricle rendering the evaluation of the latter impossible in the midesophageal four-chamber view.
    c. Microbubbles produce a strong transient echo, and are disrupted.
    d. Microbubbles start to behave in a nonlinear way, generating harmonic frequencies of the incident ultrasound pulse.

14. All of the following are imaging modalities developed for improved microbubble detection, *except*:
    a. Intermittent harmonic power Doppler
    b. Pulse inversion imaging
    c. Power modulation
    d. Color Doppler tissue imaging

15. Which statement/s about microbubbles is true?
    a. They lower the threshold for acoustic cavitation.
    b. They are naturally present in blood clots.
    c. They produce linear backscatter at low transmit intensity.
    d. All of the above.

16. Echo particle image velocimetry:
    a. Requires frame rates of at least 150 frames per second
    b. Allows for the calculation of myocardial strain and strain rates
    c. Allows for the calculation of shear stresses and flow profiles
    d. Employs Fournier analysis to correct for the periodicity of cardiac motion

17. The units of measurement for strain and strain rate are, respectively:
    a. m and m/s
    b. % and m/s
    c. % and m/s^2
    d. % and s^{-1}

18. At end-systole (aortic valve closure) normal left ventricular strain is:
    a. Zero
    b. Maximum
    c. Positive
    d. None of the above

19. A true statement about strain rate in a normal left ventricle is:
    a. Strain rate is zero at end-systole and during diastasis.
    b. Strain rate is zero during isovolumic contraction and isovolumic relaxation.
    c. Strain rate is zero during atrial contraction and isovolumic contraction.
    d. Strain rate is zero in late systole and late diastole.

20. What does positive regional strain indicate about cardiac function?
    a. Enhanced myocardial contractility
    b. Dyskinesia
    c. Reduced myocardial compliance
    d. Normal diastolic filling

21. Doppler based myocardial deformation imaging:
    a. Gives reliable results if the insonation angle is less or equal to 30°
    b. Is based on the Doppler shift of low frequency, high amplitude signals from wall motion
    c. Requires frame rates of at least 150 frames per second
    d. Is characterized by an underestimation of strain and strain rate in the area below a stationary artifact

22. In Doppler strain imaging, strain is calculated as which of the following?
    a. It is the velocity gradient between two points divided by the distance.
    b. It is the time integration of the velocity gradient between two points.

c. It is the velocity gradient between two points divided by the frame rate.
d. It is the time integration of the velocity gradient between two points divided by the distance.

23. A true statement about "natural acoustic markers" includes:
 a. They have a homogeneous spread throughout the myocardium.
 b. They show a relative constant backscatter pattern throughout the cardiac cycle.
 c. They can be recognized by feature tracking algorithms.
 d. All of the above.

24. Compared to tissue Doppler strain imaging, 2D speckle tracking:
 a. Has a higher temporal resolution
 b. Is less influenced by stationary artifacts
 c. Is less suited for the evaluation of the isovolumic phases of the cardiac cycle
 d. All of the above

25. Which of the following is *false*?
 a. Low frame rates will lead to loss of tracking due to exaggerated out-of-plane motion of speckles.
 b. Drift compensation is the process that corrects for the out-of-plane motion of speckles due to displacement and rotation of the myocardium.
 c. Drift occurs when strain and strain rate do not return to baseline at the end of the cardiac cycle.
 d. Due to the lower temporal resolution, speckle tracking may be inferior to tissue Doppler for the evaluation of intraventricular dyssynchrony.

The Nuts and Bolts of a Perioperative TEE Service

25

Shahar Bar-Yosef, Rebecca Schroeder, and Jonathan B. Mark

INTRODUCTION

Over the past decade, the practice of perioperative transesophageal echocardiography (TEE) has evolved to the point that many anesthesiology departments own and operate their own ultrasound equipment and offer comprehensive perioperative TEE services, rather than "borrowing" equipment from cardiology colleagues or requesting their professional assistance in the operating room. The successful initiation and delivery of perioperative TEE services requires attention to a number of organizational details. First, practitioners with adequate training should be credentialed by the hospital for performance of perioperative TEE. Additionally, each program requires building a system for report generation and data storage, allocation of capital resources as well as skilled technical personnel to maintain and operate equipment, and implementation of a Continuous Quality Improvement (CQI) process. Finally, an efficient reimbursement infrastructure will ensure the program's fiscal viability. Although specific organizational details will depend on the individual institution and setting, the current chapter provides practical general guidelines that may be implemented to achieve success.

EQUIPMENT AND PROBE MAINTENANCE

The TEE probe in use today has changed little in concept from that originally introduced by Hisanaga in 1977.[1] Most probes are a modified gastroscope with an ultrasound transducer mounted on the tip. They are 80 to 100-cm long with a shaft diameter of 10 mm, a tip width of 12 to 14 mm, and are latex-free. Newer three-dimensional (3D) probes are approximately 1 mm wider at the tip than existing two-dimensional (2D) probes. Rotary dials in the handheld housing control a series of cables sealed within the shaft that allow flexion and extension as well as side-to-side lateral bending of the tip. Range of motion of the tip varies slightly among manufacturers but is approximately 60° up and down as well as 60° to the right and left. Buttons on the side of the housing electronically steer the ultrasound transducer at the tip, providing full 180° rotation.

A grounded shield covers all active circuits distal to the control housing, making electrical injury highly unlikely unless the outer layer of the shaft is cracked. However, the probe should always be disconnected prior to external defibrillation, as any minor defect in the covering could allow secondary arcing, potentially causing severe burns. Generally, the probe should be disconnected if left in place and unused for extended periods of time, such as during cardiopulmonary bypass, to prevent thermal injury or interaction with electrosurgical units. Electrical integrity of the TEE probe should be tested by a qualified technician as part of preventive maintenance, according to the manufacturer's protocol. This includes conducting frequent "bite hole" inspections as well as annual temperature calibration and current-leakage tests.

Current ultrasound machines are equipped with safety features to minimize risks of injury to the patient. Units will "time out" after a designated period, often 10 minutes, of inactivity to avoid probe overheating. In addition, there is an auto-cool feature that will interrupt ultrasound transmission if the transducer becomes excessively hot. Current models will freeze scanning at 41°C, although this can be overridden, usually to a maximum of 42.7°C. At this point, scanning will freeze until a designated cooler threshold is reached. In addition, scanning is frozen at less than 18°C. Although no bioeffects have been demonstrated at acoustic output levels used during echocardiography, it is prudent to maintain ultrasound energy exposure at ALARA (as low as reasonably allowable) levels.[2] As such, the power settings should be set at the lowest level compatible with adequate image acquisition.

Handling of the TEE probe requires care and attention as the fragile elements in the tip must be protected from accidental damage. Prior to connecting the probe to the ultrasound machine, it is important to inspect the entire probe for damage to the probe covering and test the motion of the probe tip. Excessive motion of the tip is indicative of a malfunctioning probe. The contact pins should also be quickly examined to ensure that none are broken or bent. Successful connection is confirmed when the appropriate probe icon appears on the ultrasound machine screen. Multiplane probes autocalibrate each time the probe is connected—a process that is most efficient when the probe shaft is straight.

When used in the operating room, some mechanism should be used to secure the housing in a fixed position, allowing continuous monitoring of a particular view while preventing injury to the patient and keeping the probe from dropping to the floor. A variety of sheaths to cover the probe are available to protect it from contamination, although clear benefit from these has not been demonstrated.

Cleaning procedures for the TEE probe should follow manufacturer's recommendations. The probe is disconnected from the machine and the shaft soaked in mild soapy water to remove all organic matter. Enzymatic cleaners with a moderate pH work well, but iodine-containing solutions should be avoided. Furthermore, use of these enzymatic cleaners helps prevent accumulation of residue from the disinfecting solutions that can turn the patient's lips and tongue black. The shaft and tip should be wiped carefully with gauze pads, and the housing and shaft inspected for cracks, dents, holes, or bumps. Disinfection procedures follow, most often using glutaraldehyde-based solutions or various hydrogen peroxide solutions. Manufacturer's instructions should be carefully followed concerning dilution and soak times. Exceeding these guidelines will weaken the covering of the probe shaft. Disinfectants such as 70% isopropyl alcohol, phenol, benzoyl peroxide, or benzothonium chloride should not be used on the tip or the shaft. Probes should never be autoclaved or disinfected by ultraviolet radiation, steam, gas, or heat sterilization systems. After disinfection, the shaft should be rinsed copiously with sterile water and dried with a soft cloth, while the housing and steering mechanism are wiped down with 70% alcohol. Following cleaning and disinfection, the probe is stored with shaft and tip straight, shielded from direct sunlight and extremes of temperature. The case provided by the manufacturer should only be used for transportation to avoid prolonged storage in a coiled position.

ORGANIZATIONAL LOGISTICS FOR A TEE SERVICE

General organization of a TEE service must be based on the needs and resources of each specific department. Many institutions are able to fulfill their clinical needs with several probes but fewer ultrasound machines. In such cases, two or more patients may have TEE probes in place, and a single ultrasound machine is transported wherever it is needed next. With due diligence and care, this can be done safely and allows maximal flexibility and patient service in a world of limited resources. Furthermore, with currently available equipment that incorporates multiple ultrasound modalities with extremely small footprint units, the ability to share between locations and even between services is greatly enhanced.

If ultrasound equipment is shared with the cardiology department, probes are ideally cleaned, disinfected, and stored in a single location by dedicated technicians familiar with these procedures. In this case, transportation of the probes to and from the operating room may best be done in the carrying case if the distance is far, or by hand with the tip protector in place. Transporting probes that are resting on top of a cart carries a high risk of costly damage to the probe and should not be done.

Competent technical assistance is a key element to a successful perioperative TEE service. For anesthesiology departments, it is often the anesthesia technicians that are responsible for cleaning and maintaining TEE probes, as well as ordering supplies and identifying problems. Also, log books should be kept of probe and machine maintenance activity along with written protocols for equipment cleaning and sterilization. While rarely employed in the operating room setting, a skilled sonographer is invaluable in other critical care settings. Space is often limited, and it is frequently necessary for the machine to be on the opposite side of the bed from the physician performing the exam. A skilled assistant speeds the examination, as the physician can concentrate on manipulating the probe rather than constantly switching hands to operate the ultrasound machine. Regardless of the setting, all TEE exams require the focused attention of the physician performing the procedure. A collaborative relationship with sonographers and cardiologist-echocardiographers often improves the quality of the perioperative TEE service.

PREPARATION FOR THE TEE EXAMINATION

In all clinical settings outside of the operating room, there should always be at least one assistant to monitor the patient's vital signs, administer medications, suction secretions, and otherwise attend to the patient's needs. Sonographers are not typically credentialed to monitor the sedated patient or administer medications, and therefore the presence of a skilled nurse or another physician is usually required. In the operating room, the anesthesiologist-echocardiographer may be responsible for performing the TEE examination and administering the anesthetic. However, owing to the significant workload and attention required of both tasks, a resident anesthesiologist, nurse anesthetist, or other technical assistant is extremely valuable, especially during busy moments.

Written informed consent for TEE outlining the risks and benefits, as well as the indication for the examination, is necessary outside of the operating room. In addition, a thorough discussion of the procedure improves patient cooperation for those studies performed in awake patients. Relative and absolute contraindications must be assessed and discussed with the patient, including a history of gastric or esophageal pathology and abnormalities of the airway and pharynx. In the operative environment, current recommendations are that informed consent be obtained and documented in the patient's chart, either separately or as part of the general anesthetic consent.[3]

In all settings in which TEE is performed, additional required equipment includes suction apparatus, supplemental oxygen, emergency cart with airway equipment and resuscitation drugs, monitors, bite guards, intravenous access supplies, and universal precautions equipment for the staff. Oxygen supplementation is advisable whenever patients are sedated.[4]

Monitoring for all patients should include continuous electrocardiographic and pulse oximetry recording and intermittent blood pressure measurements, in accordance with guidelines for conscious sedation.[4] Patients should have been fasting for at least 6 hours and dentures should be removed. An intravenous catheter should be inserted even if sedation is not anticipated, since it will provide immediate vascular access if needed for resuscitation. When possible, the patient is placed in the left lateral decubitus position to reduce the risk of aspiration.

Topical anesthesia of the mouth and pharynx facilitates all TEE examinations performed in patients who are not heavily sedated or under general anesthesia. Most often viscous lidocaine (2%) gargle or atomized lidocaine (4%) are used as topical agents and carry significantly less risk of methemoglobinemia compared to benzocaine-containing local anesthetics.[5] Superior laryngeal nerve blocks may be performed, or lidocaine-soaked gauzes may be placed in the piriform sinuses with Krause forceps. Adequacy of topical anesthesia can be tested with a tongue blade or suction tip. Successful TEE examination in the awake patient is most likely if adequate time is allowed for the topical anesthesia to become effective.

Intravenous sedation is administered to most patients undergoing elective TEE outside of the operating room, and has been shown to decrease procedure-associated retching as well as post-procedure sore throat.[6] Choice of agents and depth of sedation must be tailored to the patient. Most commonly, fentanyl and midazolam in small doses are administered prior to attempted placement of the probe. Although an unusually cooperative patient may be able to swallow the TEE probe without sedation, a more apprehensive patient may require heavy sedation or even a short-acting hypnotic. Interestingly, additional sedation is rarely required after initial placement of the probe.

Endocarditis temporally related to TEE has been described in only one case report.[7] In contrast, a very low incidence of bacteremia induced by TEE examination was found in several studies (4 out of 500 patients in total).[8-12] A recent editorial noted that most of the organisms isolated in these studies were skin commensals, probably representing contamination rather than true TEE-related bacteremia.[13] Authors of a recent review of 17 databases comprising more than 42,000 adult patients have recommended prophylaxis "in cases of poor oral hygiene, prolonged or traumatic TEE procedures, or in subjects undergoing TEE in the first two months after valve replacement."[14] In contrast, the updated American College of Cardiology/American Heart Association guidelines for management of valvular heart disease do not recommend antibiotic prophylaxis before any gastrointestinal procedure, including TEE.[15]

PROBE INSERTION

Following attention to the preparatory details of informed consent, topical anesthesia, and intravenous sedation described above, the TEE probe is inserted with ease in the majority of adequately prepared awake patients. The probe's control wheels should be tested prior to insertion, to confirm proper function. A bite guard should be used in all patients with teeth to prevent injury to the patient or the probe shaft, even when used in anesthetized patients. Appropriate acoustic coupling gel should be placed on the probe tip prior to insertion to optimize imaging. Although any glycerol or other water-based lubricating medium is acceptable, mineral oil or other oil-based coupling gels will damage the probe's outer covering. After insertion of the bite block, the lubricated probe is introduced into the patient's pharynx, at a depth of approximately 15 to 20 cm from the teeth. Gentle steady pressure to advance the probe is applied, and the patient is asked to swallow. For many patients, this verbal instruction is all that is required—swallowing will close the vocal cords and relax the cricopharyngeus muscle.[14] Flexing the patient's neck or slight flexion of the probe tip may assist its passage past the base of the tongue. Neck flexion also prevents stretching of the esophagus, a condition which might increase the risk of a mucosal tear or perforation.[14] Under no circumstances should the TEE probe be forced into the esophagus. It may also be helpful to hold the small wheel on the housing at a neutral position, to avoid undesirable lateral bending during probe insertion. The large wheel, controlling flexion/extension, should never be locked. If there are feeding or nasogastric tubes in place, the TEE probe can usually be placed alongside these devices, but often they must be removed to allow adequate imaging. Prior to introducing the TEE probe in tracheally intubated patients, many physicians place an orogastric tube to evacuate the stomach contents.

When an endotracheal tube is in place, the TEE probe is placed most easily by manually distracting the patient's mandible by inserting a gloved thumb behind the lower molars and lifting the jaw upward. This maneuver, also known as the Esmarch-Hein maneuver, opens the pharynx and allows the tip of the probe to be guided with ease directly into the mouth, pharynx, and esophagus. On occasion, turning the patient's head to the right or left will be helpful. While the use of direct laryngoscopy is not usually necessary for probe placement, a recent study did show that its use results in successful placement with fewer attempts and reduces complications like odynophagia and minor oropharyngeal injuries.[16]

It should be kept in mind that unsuspected pathology may impede advancement of the probe. Any unusual resistance to probe insertion should prompt abandonment of the procedure. Failure to place the probe is rare. Chee et al found a 1.2% rate of failure among 901 TEE exams.[17] In another review, 98.5% of failures were due to lack of cooperation or lack of operator experience, while only 1.5% were due to anatomic abnormalities.[18] Other authors have identified prominent vertebral spurs associated with cervical spondylosis as a common cause (16 of 40) of failure of probe placement.[19] In intubated patients, briefly deflating the endotracheal tube cuff should be considered as this may ease passage of the probe tip.[14]

When unusual resistance is encountered during attempts to advance or withdraw the probe, the physician should consider that the tip may have "folded" 180° onto itself, so called "buckling" of the probe.[14] This mechanical problem should be suspected when probe movement is difficult, image quality is very poor, and the control wheels are bound and difficult to move. If the physician believes this has occurred, the probe should be advanced gently into the stomach, the tip straightened, and the probe removed and inspected. Under the rare circumstance that the TEE probe cannot be moved without exerting undue force, a radiograph may help determine the probe position and guide the next intervention. In very unusual circumstances, if the deflector mechanism is completely jammed inside the patient and all efforts to release it have failed, the probe should be removed from the unit, and the entire probe shaft should be cut with heavy-duty pliers or other suitable tool. This will release the deflecting mechanism, allow the tip to straighten, and facilitate probe removal.[2]

INDICATIONS FOR TEE IN THE PERIOPERATIVE PERIOD

Indications for performance of a TEE examination are very broad and vary according to practice locations. General indications for perioperative TEE include definition of ventricular and valvular function, identification of intracardiac masses and sources of embolization, evaluation of intracardiac shunt, and assessment of aortic pathology. The most common indication for urgent TEE examination is differential diagnosis of severe hemodynamic instability, including cardiac compression and tamponade following cardiac surgery, suspected pulmonary embolus, acute myocardial ischemia, or aortic dissection. In 2010, the American Society of Anesthesiologists (ASA) and the Society of Cardiovascular Anesthesiologists (SCA) updated the practice guidelines for perioperative TEE (Table 25–1).[20]

The first area in which perioperative TEE achieved routine use was the cardiac surgical operating room. In this setting, TEE is most useful for evaluating ventricular function, detecting wall motion abnormalities indicative of acute myocardial ischemia, and evaluating native or prosthetic valve function immediately following valve replacement or repair (see Table 25–1).[20,21] TEE also has an especially important role in the intraoperative management of surgery for congenital heart disease.[22]

In a large prospective cohort study, Mishra et al found that 36% of 5016 cardiac surgical patients benefited from the pre-cardiopulmonary bypass TEE study and a similar number from the post-bypass study.[23] The TEE examination was most useful for the identification of intracardiac thrombus, aortic atheroma, mitral leaflet configuration, changes in valvular function, and in guiding de-airing procedures prior to separation from bypass. It was also judged essential for transmyocardial laser revascularization and port-access procedures.[23] In some centers, TEE has replaced transthoracic echocardiography (TTE) as the preferred initial imaging study in post-cardiac surgery patients requiring emergent evaluation owing to the superior image quality of TEE compared with chest wall echocardiography. In one report, the average time to reach a diagnosis was 11 minutes, and the etiology of refractory hypotension was clearly identified in 76% of patients.[24]

As more anesthesiologists become skilled in the performance and interpretation of TEE, its use during noncardiac surgery has increased (see Table 25–1). Suriani et al reported the use of TEE in 123 orthotopic liver transplants.[25] In 15% of cases, TEE was critical in altering

Table 25–1. Recommendations for the Use of TEE in the Perioperative Period.

I. Cardiac and Thoracic Aortic Procedures
• ***Cardiac and Thoracic Aortic Surgery*** • For adult patients without contraindications, TEE should be used in all open heart (eg, valvular procedures) and thoracic aortic surgical procedures, and should be considered in CABG surgeries as well to: • Confirm and refine the preoperative diagnosis • Detect new or unsuspected pathology • Adjust the anesthetic and surgical plan accordingly • Assess results of the surgical intervention • In small children, the use of TEE should be considered on a case-by-case basis because of risks unique to these patients (eg, bronchial obstruction) • ***Catheter-Based Intracardiac Procedures*** • For patients undergoing transcatheter intracardiac procedures, TEE may be used
II. Noncardiac Surgery
• TEE may be used when the nature of the planned surgery or the patient's known or suspected cardiovascular pathology might result in severe hemodynamic, pulmonary, or neurologic compromise • If equipment and expertise are available, TEE should be used when unexplained life-threatening circulatory instability persists despite corrective therapy
III. Critical Care
• For critical care patients, TEE should be used when diagnostic information that is expected to alter management cannot be obtained by TTE or other modalities in a timely manner

TEE, transesophageal echocardiography; TTE, transthoracic echocardiography; CABG, coronary artery bypass graft.
Reproduced with permission from Practice Guidelines for Perioperative Transesophageal Echocardiography. An Updated Report by the American Society of Anesthesiologists and the Society of Cardiovascular Anesthesiologists Task Force on Transesophageal Echocardiography. Anesthesiology 2010;112:1084-1096.

surgical or anesthetic technique, treating life-threatening events, or directing further postoperative evaluation. In this population, TEE can also be useful in diagnosing hepatopulmonary syndrome by identification of bubbles in the pulmonary veins after a bubble test.[26] TEE is of immense value in managing intraoperative hemodynamic instability. Feierman reported the use of intraoperative TEE to identify unsuspected dynamic left ventricular outflow tract obstruction, allowing crucial redirection of management strategy.[27] Brandt et al reviewed 66 cases in which intraoperative TEE was emergently requested to diagnose severe left ventricular dysfunction, aortic dissection, new myocardial wall motion abnormalities, patent foramen ovale, localized cardiac tamponade, and right ventricular dilatation consistent with a pulmonary embolism.[28]

TEE use is becoming more and more common in critical care areas, sometimes performed by cardiologists, but more frequently by anesthesiologists and intensivists.[29] Two recent studies examined the indications for and impact of TEE studies in the intensive care unit (ICU). In a total of 379 studies, the most common indications were for evaluation of unexplained hypotension, left ventricular function, pulmonary edema, and suspected endocarditis. The TEE studies had an immediate impact on management in 30% to 50% of the cases.[30,31] Others have reported using TEE in intensive care units to guide central line placement, evaluate patients with unexplained hypoxemia, or to evaluate potential heart donors.[32,33]

In the setting of hemodynamically significant pulmonary embolism, both TEE and transthoracic echocardiography will demonstrate signs of cor pulmonale, including right ventricular dilatation, right ventricular dysfunction, tricuspid regurgitation, and pulmonary hypertension. TEE will be able to demonstrate emboli in the main or right pulmonary artery with a high degree of sensitivity. However, TEE is not sensitive enough for detection of left pulmonary artery or lobar pulmonary artery emboli.[34] Therefore, in a patient with cor pulmonale and suspected pulmonary embolism, TEE can rapidly confirm the diagnosis; however, a negative TEE study should be followed by computed tomography (CT) angiography to rule out left lung or peripheral pulmonary emboli.[29]

The proximity of the esophagus to the aorta allows precise and accurate diagnosis of certain types of aortic pathology using TEE, and this application has found a specific niche in the emergency room. Minard et al compared TEE with aortography to evaluate possible aortic disruption.[35] Diagnosed abnormalities included intimal flaps, pseudoaneurysms, intra- or extraluminal hematomas, and gross dissections with identification of false and true lumens. However, the sensitivity and specificity of TEE were lower than aortography, most likely due to the inability of TEE to image the distal third of the ascending aorta and the aortic arch.[35,36] While some forms of aortic pathology are not completely assessed with TEE, this technique is very valuable in ruling out aortic dissection. Yalcin et al reported TEE to be 98% sensitive and 99% specific for detection of aortic dissection.[37] In addition, of significant importance is the fact that TEE is often safer than other imaging modalities in hemodynamically unstable patients. Overall, despite its known deficiencies, TEE remains the first-line test for evaluation of aortic pathology, owing to its portability, low cost, low level of invasiveness, rapidity, and low complication rate. In the presence of a negative study, however, it is often necessary to proceed to further radiologic imaging if the clinical suspicion of aortic pathology remains high.[36-39]

CONTRAINDICATIONS TO TEE

There are very few absolute contraindications to TEE, and an individualized cost/benefit analysis must influence each decision. Esophageal pathology is probably the most controversial source of risk. Problems such as severe esophageal reflux disease, dysphagia, and odynophagia are considered to be relative contraindications in some centers. However, there are reports of the safe use of TEE even in patients with known esophageal varices. Generally, the presence of esophageal masses, strictures, and large varices are considered strong contraindications to performing TEE. Other conditions such as unstable cervical spine injuries, a history of mediastinal radiation, or upper airway pathology (eg, severe facial trauma or pharyngeal tumors) should be considered relative contraindications. Recent oral intake or an uncooperative patient can make performance of the TEE difficult and may result in a higher rate of complications or an inadequate study. When TEE is being considered as an important diagnostic test and the patient is known to have a history of significant esophageal pathology, it is reasonable to request endoscopic evaluation of the esophagus by a gastroenterologist prior to performing TEE. However, a normal endoscopic evaluation does not eliminate the risk of TEE- induced gastrointestinal injury.[40] In a patient with partial or total gastrectomy, it would be prudent to limit the TEE examination to the upper and midesophageal views and avoiding insertion of the probe to the depth of the surgical site.[14]

COMPLICATIONS AND SAFETY OF TEE

In contrast to the benign nature of TTE, TEE is an invasive procedure, albeit of minimal degree. Furthermore, perioperative TEE is often performed in patients who are either critically ill or are undergoing major surgery and more likely to suffer a variety of adverse events. While a low rate of complications would be expected based upon the similarity of TEE to upper gastrointestinal endoscopy (UGED), there are several pertinent factors that may make TEE fundamentally different from UGED. Many patients undergoing UGED have suspected local pathology, while TEE is avoided in such patients, thereby reducing the risk of probe-induced injury. On the other hand, the TEE probe is inserted blindly rather than under fiberoptic guidance. Furthermore, patients undergoing TEE tend to have more advanced cardiopulmonary disease.[18] Taken together, these factors would indicate that the risk of TEE should probably not be based on generalizations from UGED.

Most descriptions of the complications of TEE are based on published case reports. These can be broadly divided into complications related to upper airway and gastrointestinal injury during probe insertion and manipulation, those related to compression and pressure by the probe on adjacent organs, those related to the sedation used to facilitate the study in non-anesthetized patients, and those complications resulting from the hemodynamic responses to the procedure (Table 25–2).[14] Case reports, however, are deceiving for two main reasons. First, case reports of complications do not identify the prevalence of the complication. Second, some complications ascribed to TEE during cardiac surgery may have another etiology. For example, in one study, the incidence of recurrent laryngeal nerve injury after cardiac surgery was similar with and without TEE.[41] Another study has reported 10 cases of upper gastrointestinal bleeding in 8559 patients undergoing cardiac surgery without the use of TEE (0.1%).[42] Had TEE been used in these cases, the observed gastrointestinal bleeding would likely have been attributed to this procedure.

With the limitations of case reports clearly in mind, several large series have examined complications related to TEE in different settings (Table 25–3). Overall, the risk of major complications in adults was 0.07% to 0.2%, and the risk of all complications was 0.2% to 0.7%. In addition to the studies mentioned in Table 25–3, another large series of 2070 TEE studies performed in a cardiology laboratory described several complications including laryngospasm, hypotension, pulmonary edema, and one death from cardiac arrest possibly related to sedation, for an overall rate of major complications of 0.5%.[43]

Table 25–2. Possible Complications of Transesophageal Echocardiography.

Mechanism	Complication	Possible risk factors
Gastrointestinal effects of probe insertion and manipulation	Hypopharyngeal/esophageal/gastric laceration or perforation	Esophageal pathology (tumor, diverticulum, stricture), aggressive probe manipulation, locked control wheel
	Lip/dental injury	Poor dentition
	Upper GI bleeding	Upper GI pathology, coagulopathy
	Thermal/electrical/chemical burn	Prolonged use, external defibrillation, damaged probe, inadequate rinsing
	Dysphagia/odynophagia	
	Bacteremia/endocarditis	Damaged or prosthetic valves, poor oral hygiene
Compression of adjacent organs	Increased ventilatory pressure/airway obstruction	Small children, aortic aneurysm/dissection
	Endotracheal tube malposition/extubation	Small children
	Arrhythmias (esp. atrial fibrillation)/conduction block	Large left atrium
	Vocal cord injury/paralysis	Asthenia
Over-sedation	Hypotension	Older age, mechanical ventilation, depressed ventricular function, hypovolemia
	Hypoxemia/respiratory arrest	Morbid obesity, lung disease
	Upper airway obstruction	Sleep apnea, morbid obesity
	Methemoglobinemia	Excessive local anesthetic spray (benzocaine)
Hemodynamic stress response and under-sedation	Hypertension and tachycardia	Obesity, baseline hypertension
	Vagotonic responses (bradycardia/conduction block/vasovagal syncope)	
	Myocardial ischemia/infarction	Ischemic heart disease
	Ruptured aortic aneurysm/dissection	Aortic pathology
	Bronchospasm/laryngospasm	Hyper-reactive airways
	Vomiting	Non-fasting
	Aspiration	Non-fasting, unprotected airway

In contrast to these relatively favorable studies, other studies have emphasized a significant risk of TEE-induced major gastrointestinal injury. A 2006 literature review described 12 case reports of major esophageal injury after perioperative TEE.[44] In a series of 860 patients undergoing cardiac surgery, Lennon et al reported a 1.2% incidence of major complications in patients who had TEE compared to 0.3% in those who did not have TEE done.[45] These complications included partial thickness tears or perforations of the esophagus or stomach, as well as upper gastrointestinal (GI) bleeding requiring transfusion and/or endoscopic or surgical interventions. Two-thirds of the complications were not evident until more than 24 hours after surgery. In a recent retrospective database study including more than 16,000 patients undergoing cardiac surgery with TEE, the incidence of esophageal or gastric tears and perforation was small (0.09%) but carried a significant 20% mortality rate.[46]

Other studies have demonstrated an eightfold increase in the risk of transient dysphagia associated with intraoperative use of TEE.[47] Barium studies have confirmed that swallowing abnormalities after cardiac surgery were more common when TEE was used intraoperatively, and these were associated with an increased risk of pneumonia and prolonged mechanical ventilation and ICU stay.[48] Both the incidence of failure to insert the probe and the risk of complications appear to be lower for intraoperative TEE compared to TEE performed in the nonoperative setting. The most likely explanation for these findings is that patients undergoing intraoperative TEE are anesthetized and paralyzed, have their airways protected, and are invasively monitored. However, it should be stressed that an anesthetized patient is not able to assist with probe insertion by swallowing and will not complain of pain as a warning sign of impending injury.

Table 25–3. Complications Related to Transesophageal Echocardiography—Large Case Series.

Study	Daniel et al[18]	Chan et al[71]	Kallmeyer et al[72]	Stevenson[50]
Settings and population	Cardiology lab (mostly)	Cardiology lab—ambulatory patients	Intraoperative TEE, adult cardiac surgery	Intraoperative TEE, pediatric cardiac surgery
N	10,419	1500	7200	1650
Method	Retrospective	Prospective	Retrospective	Prospective
Failure to insert probe	201 (1.9%)	11 (0.7%)	13 (0.18%)	13 (0.79%)
Death	1 (0.01%)	0	0	0
Patient intolerance	65 (0.62%)	0	N/A[a]	N/A
Pulmonary complications (bronchospasm, aspiration, hypoxemia, inadvertent extubation)	8 (0.08%)	1 (0.07%)	2 (0.03%)	9 (0.55%)
Cardiac complications (arrhythmia, ischemia, vascular compression)	8 (0.08%)	2 (0.13%)	0	0
Major GI bleeding	1 (0.01%)	0	2 (0.03%)	0
Esophageal perforation	0	0	1 (0.015%)	0
Any major complication	18 (0.17%)	3 (0.2%)	5 (0.07%)	10 (0.61%)[b]
Tracheal intubation	0	4 (0.27%)	N/A	N/A
Severe nausea/vomiting	5 (0.05%)	3 (0.2%)	N/A	N/A
Dysphagia/odynophagia	0	0	7 (0.1%)	Not assessed
Minor GI bleeding	1 (0.01%)	0	0	0
Dental injury	0	0	2 (0.03%)	0
Other minor	0	0	0	29 (1.76%)[c]
Any minor complication	6 (0.06%)	7 (0.47%)	9 (0.13%)	29 (1.76%)
Any complication	24 (0.23%)	10 (0.67%)	14 (0.19%)	39 (2.36%)

[a]N/A, not applicable.
[b]One patient had gastric laceration during sternotomy.
[c]Complications included an increase in airway pressure (14), advancement of the endotracheal tube into the right main-stem bronchus (3), dampening of arterial waveform (10), obstruction of venous return (1), and laceration of lip (1).

The incidence of minor complications depends to a large extent on the way these are defined and diagnosed. For example, in a case-control series of 664 patients undergoing TEE mostly in the cardiology lab and ICU, changes in blood pressure and hemoglobin oxygen saturation were strictly defined and closely monitored.[49] These authors reported transient hypotension in 5.4% of the examinations, transient hypertension in 8.6%, and desaturation in 3.2%. The overall incidence of minor complications (defined as those not requiring therapy or those reversed by simple interventions) was 16.3%, with only three major complications (0.45%).

Compared to adults, pediatric patients are at a higher risk from TEE, both for failure of probe insertion as well as for complications (see Table 25–3). The child's small oropharynx and the proximity of the relatively large TEE probe to the more pliable great vessels and airway most likely explain the high incidence of hypotension from vascular compression or airway problems like unintentional tracheal extubation and right main-stem bronchial intubation.[50] Fortunately, these problems are easily recognized and resolve with TEE probe removal.

The risk of TEE exams might be higher in other settings and with special patient populations. Critically ill patients may be at a higher risk of complications owing to unstable hemodynamics and coagulopathy. However, in one report of 308 TEE studies performed in critical care units, only two patients developed hypotension requiring pharmacological support, one had a clinically evident aspiration, and one had an oropharyngeal bleeding.[30] In a smaller series of 62 TEE examinations in critical care patients, one patient developed hypotension, one vomited, and one patient with known seizures receiving anticonvulsant therapy had a grand mal seizure soon after start of the TEE study.[51] Generally, it appears that TEE can be performed safely in the intensive care unit.

In contrast, TEE performed in the emergency room (ER) appears to be associated with an increased risk, probably related to the precarious clinical status of the patients and possibly associated with the failure to secure the airway prior to the TEE examination. One study reported 142 TEE examinations performed in the ER with complications occurring in 18 (12.6%).[38] One patient died from rupture of a thoracic aneurysm during the TEE study, seven developed respiratory insufficiency, four required tracheal intubation, and 10 patients suffered other minor complications. When clinically feasible, it may be safer to admit these patients to the ICU and stabilize them prior to performing the TEE study.

Obesity is considered to be a possible risk factor for increased complications after TEE. A case-control study has shown a 2.7-fold increased risk of transient hypoxemia in obese patients.[49] Increased heart size, especially left atrial dilatation, which may compress and distort the esophagus and gastroesophageal junction, has been reported to increase the risk for major gastrointestinal injury during TEE.[44] A recent large study has found significantly increased risk for esophageal and gastric injury in women compared to men, especially those older than 70 years of age.[46]

IMAGE ACQUISITION, STORAGE, RETRIEVAL, AND ARCHIVING

Traditional videotape libraries of echocardiograms are rapidly becoming relegated to the dusty backrooms of medical records departments for a variety of reasons, most importantly because the crucial value of rapid acquisition, retrieval, manipulation, and comparison has been recognized. Despite the obvious technical issues, digital studies do not degrade over time, they can be easily tracked over time to evaluate disease progression, they are available for teaching and research, and they are rapidly searchable in a way not dependent on the memory of the reader or investigator.

Echo signals emerge from the ultrasound transducer in an analog format as continuous voltage signal patterns. These are immediately translated into digital form by a scan converter and undergo a series of transformations. Such signal processing varies between manufacturers but generally improves image quality by screening out superficial structures and improving fine detail, contrast resolution, and spatial focusing. Images are captured at a rate of 25 to 30 frames per second, the minimal rate required for the human eye to perceive smooth motion.[52,53] Historically, the ultrasound machine then converts the image back to analog format for display on the monitor and directs similar analog signals to the video output for recording on videotape. In newer systems, the digital signal is directly stored on a hard drive or optical disc and then transmitted to a distant site for storage on a common server or workstation via network connection.

The advantages of a digital system are immediately obvious and include the ability to record a single image and view it as a continuous loop, review multiple loops on the screen simultaneously, and even compare similar loops from separate studies. Furthermore, the latest systems allow the reviewer to perform off-line spectral Doppler and M-mode analysis at a distant workstation, and some manufacturers allow off-line analysis in nonscanned planes (eg, M-mode scanning in any direction within the 2D scan plane). Studies are immediately available for viewing by the referring physician, and can be transmitted with ease to distant sites for additional opinions or even "tele-cardiology" consults when an expert echocardiographer is not available. The stability of binary code also prevents degradation of data over time. Study archiving and retrieval is tremendously simplified, as patient identifiers included in study information can be stored in databases. Studies are also directly available for educational purposes, as databases can include any quantitative or descriptive information the managers choose to include. Such global digitization of echo studies has been shown to decrease physician interpretation time by greater than 30%.[54] Digital structured reporting, which merges qualitative and quantitative reporting by automatically populating as much data as possible directly from the machine and providing a format for the rest of the report from drop-down menus, showed dramatic improvements in productivity. This advance has been seen for individuals, as well as departments as a whole, even though some variability among physicians remained.[55] All perioperative echocardiographers are therefore urged to move toward this digital standard by incorporating the Digital Imaging and Communications in Medicine (DICOM) format, high-speed networking, and permanent storage with built-in redundancy.[3]

The issue of digital storage capacity deserves special mention in the setting of a digital echo library. Each image requires approximately 1 Mb of memory per frame, or 30 Mb per second for digital storage. For an average 10-minute study, this is 18 gigabytes of memory, exceeding the storage capacity of 28 CD discs or 4 DVDs![56] In addition, transmitting this amount of data over a T1 network line would require approximately 7 hours.[57]

Therefore, data compression strategies have been developed to improve the efficiency of data storage and transfer. One such method preserves the ability to reconstruct the image exactly from the compressed data and is known as "lossless" compression. Only very limited degrees of compression are possible with lossless methods (eg, 3:1 up to possibly 7:1).[56] Alternatively, in "lossy" compression techniques, some information is lost and exact replication of the image is not possible. Joint Photographic Experts Group (JPEG) is an example of a lossy format that can compress in the range of 5:1 and up to 80:1.[58] Further compression is possible with Moving Pictures Expert Group (MPEG) compression. Such lossy techniques take advantage of redundant information both within and between frames and can compress data at rates of up to 200:1 with little degradation in diagnostic content. Such compression decreases the time required for data transmission from hours to minutes. Several studies have compared compressed images and digital video and have shown excellent concordance in visible image quality and diagnostic accuracy.[57,59]

For purposes of standardization, the American College of Radiology and the National Electrical Manufacturers Association formed a joint committee in 1983 to develop the Digital Imaging and Communication in Medicine (DICOM) standard.[58] The latest version (3.0) was released in 1993, and has been endorsed by the American Society of Echocardiography (ASE), the American College of Cardiology (ACC), and the European Society of Cardiology.[54] DICOM specifies how images are to be stored and transmitted over networks, as well as ways to incorporate patient information and image calibration data. The latest systems marketed by TEE manufacturers are able to export images in a variety of formats, including JPEG, Audio Video Interleave (AVI), and MPEG compression.

DATABASE MANAGEMENT

In a world of increasing reliance on electronic data management, it is important to keep several points in mind when choosing a software platform.

1. *Comprehensiveness.* All potentially useful data fields should be included in the original design. Published TEE examination guidelines are a useful starting point to decide upon these fields.[60]
2. *Recording.* Traditionally, a dedicated medical clerk enters test results from hand-written forms completed by the echocardiographer, a system plagued by clerical errors and inefficiencies. Alternatively, the echocardiographer can enter data directly into the database using a Web-enabled application at the time of interpretation or some handheld device at the time of the examination itself. The data input interface can be optimized for efficient data entry and minimal requirement for textual input using check boxes, drop boxes, and shortcuts for repetitive data (eg, "no change" between the pre-operative and post-operative TEE studies). Options can be programmed as mutually exclusive to prevent errors in data entry.[61] The report can even be signed electronically.
3. *Flexibility.* The database should allow insertion of new fields in the future, as methods and study techniques evolve.
4. *Connectivity.* Ideally, the TEE images are digitally archived and a linking field can be used to couple the database record with matching images from the TEE archive.
5. *Security.* Like all medical databases, security measures should conform to current HIPPA regulations.

REPORT GENERATION

When a TEE examination is performed in the operating room, the main findings are always communicated directly to the surgeon and anesthesiologist caring for the patient. Similarly, a TEE performed in the ER or in the ICU is often performed for a specific diagnostic question that needs an urgent answer, and therefore the TEE findings should again be conveyed orally to the appropriate caregivers. However, a signed, written report should always follow any TEE examination for all the standard reasons of officially documenting any medical procedure (Table 25–4).[62] Furthermore, producing a report is one of the requirements for proper training in echocardiography.[63] When a trainee performs a TEE, the supervising echocardiographer should confirm the findings and co-sign the report. A copy of the report should be placed in the patient record, whether in electronic or paper-based format. Ideally, the report should be completed within 24 hours of performing the study.[3]

The SCA and the ASE have published recommendations for the content of a perioperative TEE report, including a sample report template (Table 25–5).[64] The report should reflect the comprehensive adult perioperative TEE examination guidelines published by the SCA and ASE,[60] and include an assessment of the degree of severity of any detected abnormality. Although specific quantitative measurements are not required by this practice guideline, these measurements should be performed and recorded as needed to create a complete description of any cardiac abnormality and its severity.

Table 25–4. Goals of the Perioperative Transesophageal Echocardiography Report.

1. Guide to current therapy
2. Serial study comparisons
3. Research database
4. Billing
5. Risk management
6. Continuous quality improvement
7. Serving to create a case log for training purposes

Table 25–5. Components of the Perioperative Transesophageal Echocardiography Report.

1. Patient demographics:
   a. Name, age, sex
   b. Date of study
   c. Location of, and indication for, the study
   d. Billing information—CPT and ICD-9 codes
2. Echocardiographic 2D and Doppler findings:
   a. Left and right ventricle—structure and function
   b. Regional left ventricle function
   c. Atria/septa/pericardium
   d. Aorta (ascending/arch/descending)
   e. All 4 cardiac valves—structure and function
3. Post-intervention study (if applicable)—note any change in ventricular or valvular function.
4. Complications—directly related to probe insertion and manipulation.
5. Echo impact—How the echo study results affected the surgical plan, if at all.
6. Summary:
   a. List of all pathological findings
   b. Specific answer to the referring physician's question (if any)
   c. Any significant intraoperative change

From Recommendations for a standardized report for adult perioperative echocardiography: from the Society of Cardiovascular Anesthesiologists/American Society of Echocardiography Task Force for a Standardized Perioperative Report. http://www.scahq.org/sca3/peri_op_report4-02.rtf (accessed May 9, 2003).

Left ventricular regional wall motion should be evaluated and described according to standard nomenclature.[62,65] A graphic representation of regional ventricular function facilitates transforming the real-time echocardiographic loops into an easily interpreted picture of left ventricular function.[65]

CONTINUOUS QUALITY IMPROVEMENT (CQI)

Published practice guidelines describe the indications and contraindications,[20] training requirements,[63] study performance procedures,[60] report generation,[64] and clinical competence evaluation[66] for perioperative TEE. Drawing on these documents and on previously published guidelines for CQI in general echocardiography,[67] the ASE and SCA have recently developed and published guidelines for a CQI program in perioperative echocardiography.[3] It is strongly recommended that all practitioners take part in the CQI process to enhance their individual as well as departmental improvement.

The aim of any CQI program is to enable the involved practitioners to identify possible problems early, analyze their causes, develop solutions, and test them. [67] The primary tenets of a CQI program are having an ongoing, continuous process that strives to do the right thing in the right way and results in ongoing practice improvement. Table 25–6 lists the main

Table 25–6. Main Components of a Continuous Quality Improvement Program in Perioperative Transesophageal Echocardiography.

1. Adequate primary training—including theoretical knowledge of ultrasound physics, cardiovascular anatomy and physiology, and surgical techniques, in addition to personally performing and interpreting perioperative TEE studies.
2. Skill maintenance—interpretation of 50 TEE studies per year, at least 25 of them personally performed, and at least 15 CME hours every 3 years.
3. Supervision—a supervising physician should be identified and available at all times for studies performed by a trainee or practitioner with a basic skill level.
4. Periodic review—review of caseload, performance, interpretation, record keeping, and equipment. For each echocardiographer, 5 studies should be reviewed each year by another physician-expert and assessed for study indication, performance, and interpretation.
5. Equipment maintenance—a routine maintenance schedule should be followed, including calibration and current-leakage testing of TEE probes every 3 months.
6. Use review—once a year, a review should be performed to examine the adequacy of the indications for performed studies, the appropriate use of different technologies, the timely completion of a formal study report within 24 hours, and whether the study performed did answer the clinical question.
7. Documentation—an official TEE service policy manual should be available to all service members. All credentialing and training certificates, post-training caseloads, annual case reviews including corrective actions, CME activities, and equipment maintenance activities should be documented. A yearly report should be generated.

CME, continuing medical education.
From Mathew JP, Glas K, Troianos CA, et al. American Society of Echocardiography/Society of Cardiovascular Anesthesiologists recommendations and guidelines for continuous quality improvement in perioperative echocardiography. J Am Soc Echocardiogr. 2006;19(11):1303-1313.

components of a CQI program adapted for the practice of perioperative TEE.[3] It is important that all practitioners who perform echocardiography participate in the CQI process and that these activities be documented. Although the emphasis placed on various numerical requirements that appear in CQI recommendations has been questioned, these numbers, derived from expert opinion, can serve as a reasonable guide to ensure staff proficiency and allow early detection of clinical problems.[68]

BILLING AND REIMBURSEMENT

The cost of establishing and maintaining a perioperative TEE service is significant, and appropriate reimbursement is required to ensure the long-term viability of the service. As stated by the ASA, intraoperative TEE is a new diagnostic tool and service that "extends beyond the scope of standard perioperative anesthesia care." It is "in addition to the anesthesia service being provided," and is not "incorporated within the usual basic or time units of the ASA Relative Value Guide."[69] It comes as no surprise, then, that a study examining Medicare policies for perioperative TEE reimbursement has shown marked variation between local carriers. Only two-thirds had a specific policy for intraoperative TEE performed by an anesthesiologist, and almost half of the carriers denied all payments for this procedure. Reimbursement uncertainties are also shared by anesthesiologists. Almost 30% of those practicing in states where reimbursement does exist have reported that they never bill for TEE. Attesting to the integrity and professionalism of these anesthesiologists, TEE utilization rate was not affected by the availability of reimbursement.[70]

Billing for intraoperative TEE is done using specific Current Procedural Terminology (CPT) codes (Table 25–7). Different codes describe the purpose of the exam (diagnostic vs monitoring), the specific task performed (probe insertion or image acquisition, interpretation, and report, or both), and the modality employed (2D echo vs color-flow Doppler or pulsed-wave/continuous-wave Doppler). For reimbursement of any CPT code, the patient must have a condition corresponding to one or more of 100-plus listed International Classification of Diseases, Ninth Revision, Clinical Modification (ICD9-CM) diagnosis codes (Table 25–8), and these codes should be listed as well on the billing sheet.

Table 25–7. Current Procedural Terminology (CPT) Codes for Transesophageal Echocardiography.

93312—TEE, 2D imaging (w/ or w/o M-mode); including probe placement, image acquisition, interpretation and report, all performed by one person
93313[a]—Probe insertion only
93314[a]—Image acquisition, interpretation, and report only
93315—TEE for congenital cardiac anomalies; including probe placement, image acquisition, interpretation, and report, all performed by one person
93316[a]—Probe insertion only
93317[a]—Image acquisition, interpretation, and report only
93318—TEE for monitoring purposes, including probe placement, real-time 2D image acquisition, and interpretation leading to ongoing (continuous) assessment of (dynamically changing) cardiac pumping function and to therapeutic measures on an immediate time basis. Report is not necessary.
List separately in addition to the above codes for 2D imaging:
93320—PWD and/or CWD; complete study
93321—PWD and/or CWD; a follow-up or limited study
93325—Color-flow Doppler for velocity mapping
Modifiers:
26—Professional/physician component of a service (used when the physician does not own the ultrasound equipment and bills only the professional component of the service).
TC—Technical component: Payment for all the technical and clerical aspects of the exam that are not part of the physician work (providing the equipment and cleaning it, operating the US machine, recovering the patient [non-OR setting], processing the report, dictation, distributing the report, etc). Can only be billed by the owner of the equipment (ie, the hospital).
59—Distinct procedural service: Indicates that a procedure or service was distinct or independent from other services performed on the same day.

[a]Codes 93313 and 93314 (or 93316 and 93317) should not be used together by the same provider (use instead code 93312 or 93315, respectively).

Table 25–8. ICD-9 Diagnostic Codes for Medical Conditions.

Aorta Assessment (Cannulation)	
440.0	Atherosclerosis of aorta
Aorta Assessment (Trauma)	
441.01	Dissection of aorta, thoracic
441.03	Dissection of aorta, thoracoabdominal
441.1	Thoracic aneurysm, ruptured
441.2	Thoracic aneurysm, without mention of rupture
441.6	Thoracoabdominal aneurysm, ruptured
441.7	Thoracoabdominal aneurysm, without mention of rupture
444.1	Embolism or thrombosis of thoracic aortic
Hypotension	
276.5	Volume depletion
429.4	Functional disturbances following cardiac surgery
458.9	Hypotension, unspecified
785.50	Shock, unspecified
785.51	Cardiogenic shock
785.59	Other shock without mention of trauma (incl. septic)
958.4	Traumatic shock
998.0	Postoperative shock, not otherwise specified
Volume Assessment	
276.5	Volume depletion
276.6	Fluid overload
Ventricular Assessment	
414.10	Aneurysm of heart (wall)
414.19	Aneurysm of heart, other
422.91	Idiopathic myocarditis
422.92	Septic myocarditis
425.1	Hypertrophic obstructive cardiomyopathy
429.71	Acquired cardiac septal defect
459.2	Compression of vein
785.51	Cardiogenic shock
999.1	Air embolism—complications of medical care
V15.1	Personal history of surgery to heart and great vessels
Valvular Assessment (Native)	
391.1	Acute rheumatic endocarditis
394.0	Mitral stenosis
394.1	Rheumatic mitral insufficiency
394.2	Mitral stenosis with insufficiency
395.0	Rheumatic aortic stenosis
395.1	Rheumatic aortic insufficiency
395.2	Rheumatic aortic stenosis with insufficiency
396.0	Mitral valve stenosis and aortic valve stenosis
396.1	Mitral valve stenosis and aortic valve insufficiency
396.2	Mitral valve insufficiency and aortic valve stenosis
396.3	Mitral valve insufficiency and aortic valve insufficiency
396.8	Multiple involvements of mitral and aortic valves
397.0	Diseases of tricuspid valve
397.1	Rheumatic diseases of pulmonary valve

(Continued)

Table 25–8. ICD-9 Diagnostic Codes for Medical Conditions. *(Continued)*

421.0	Acute and subacute bacterial endocarditis
421.1	Acute and subacute infective endocarditis in diseases classified elsewhere
424.0	Mitral valve disorders
424.1	Aortic valve disorders
424.2	Nonrheumatic tricuspid valve disorders
424.3	Pulmonary valve disorders
424.91	Endocarditis in diseases classified elsewhere
429.5	Rupture of chordae tendineae
429.6	Rupture of papillary muscle
429.81	Other disorders of papillary muscle
Valvular Assessment (Prosthesis)	
996.02	Mechanical complication of heart valve prosthesis
996.71	Other complication due to heart valve prosthesis
V43.3	Heart valve replacement
Congenital Heart Disease	
745.0	Common truncus
745.7	Cor biloculare
745.10	Complete transposition of great vessels
745.11	Double-outlet right ventricle
745.12	Corrected transposition of great vessels
745.19	Other transposition of great vessels
745.2	Tetralogy of Fallot
745.3	Common ventricle
745.4	Ventricular septal defect
745.5	Ostium secundum type atrial septal defect
745.60	Endocardial cushion defect, unspecified type
745.61	Ostium primum defect
745.69	Other endocardial cushion defects
745.7	Cor biloculare
746.00	Congenital pulmonary valve anomaly, unspecified
746.01	Atresia of pulmonary valve, congenital
746.02	Stenosis of pulmonary valve, congenital
746.09	Other congenital anomalies of pulmonary valve (incl. Fallot's triad)
746.1	Tricuspid atresia and stenosis, congenital
746.2	Ebstein anomaly
746.3	Congenital stenosis of aortic valve
746.4	Congenital insufficiency of aortic valve
746.5	Congenital mitral stenosis
746.6	Congenital mitral insufficiency
746.7	Hypoplastic left heart syndrome
746.81	Subaortic stenosis, congenital
746.82	Cor triatriatum
746.83	Infundibular pulmonic stenosis, congenital
746.84	Congenital obstructive anomalies of heart, not elsewhere classified
746.85	Coronary artery anomaly, congenital
747.0	Patent ductus arteriosus
747.10	Coarctation of aorta (preductal) (postductal)
747.11	Interruption of aortic arch
747.21	Congenital anomalies of aortic arch
747.22	Congenital atresia and stenosis of aorta
747.29	Other congenital anomalies of aorta (incl. aneurysm of sinus of Valsalva)
747.3	Congenital anomalies of pulmonary artery

(Continued)

Table 25–8. ICD-9 Diagnostic Codes for Medical Conditions. *(Continued)*

747.40	Congenital anomaly of great veins, unspecified
747.41	Total anomalous pulmonary venous connection
747.42	Partial anomalous pulmonary venous connection
Heart/Lung Transplant	
V42.1	Heart transplant status
V42.6	Lung transplant status
Tumor	
164.1	Malignant neoplasm of heart
198.89	Secondary malignant neoplasm
212.7	Benign neoplasm of heart
238.8	Neoplasm of uncertain behavior of the heart
239.8	Neoplasms of unspecified nature of the heart
Other Diagnoses	
414.11	Coronary vessel aneurysm
415.0	Acute cor pulmonale
415.11	Iatrogenic pulmonary embolism and infarction
415.19	Other pulmonary embolism and infarction
417.0	Arteriovenous fistula of pulmonary vessels
417.1	Aneurysm of pulmonary artery
427.31	Atrial fibrillation
427.32	Atrial flutter
436	Stroke
996.01	Mechanical complication of cardiac pacemaker (electrode)
996.61	Infection and inflammatory reaction due to cardiac device, implant, and graft
996.72	Other complications due to other cardiac device, implant, and graft (not including prosthetic valve)
998.5	Other postoperative infection

From Recommendations for a standardized report for adult perioperative echocardiography: from the Society of Cardiovascular Anesthesiologists/American Society of Echocardiography Task Force for a Standardized Perioperative Report. http://www.scahq.org/sca3/peri_op_report4-02.rtf (accessed May 9, 2003).

The CPT codes for TEE are commonly bundled into the anesthesia codes. The "59" modifier should therefore be used to override the bundling in cases where intraoperative TEE is performed by the same individual responsible for the rest of the anesthesia care. In such cases, the TEE is a reimbursable service under Medicare guidelines only when it was performed for specific diagnostic purposes and a written report is generated. Use of TEE for monitoring is described by CPT code 93318, which does not require a written report. This code is particularly controversial with regard to Medicare billing. Most carriers view this use of TEE as an integral part of anesthesia care and therefore bundled with the base units of anesthesia and not separately reimbursable. Some carriers, however, will allow billing for probe placement in this situation (CPT codes 93313/93316), and some may even opt to allow full payment for the 93318 code.

Most Medicare carriers will require the provider of TEE services to be specifically credentialed in echocardiography. Since these policies change regularly and depend on the local Medicare carrier, every anesthesiologist should be familiar with the most updated local policies for reimbursement.

REFERENCES

1. Frazin L, Talano JV, Stephanides L, Loeb HS, Kopel L, Gunnar RM. Esophageal echocardiography. *Circulation.* 1976;54(1): 102-108.
2. *User's manual: TEE probes.* Horten: GE Medical Systems; 2007.
3. Mathew JP, Glas K, Troianos CA, et al. American Society of Echocardiography/Society of Cardiovascular Anesthesiologists recommendations and guidelines for continuous quality improvement in perioperative echocardiography. *J Am Soc Echocardiogr.* 2006;19(11):1303-1313.

4. Practice guidelines for sedation and analgesia by non-anesthesiologists. *Anesthesiology.* 2002;96(4):1004-1017.
5. Jacka MJ, Kruger M, Glick N. Methemoglobinemia after transesophageal echocardiography: a life-threatening complication. *J Clin Anesth.* 2006;18(1):52-54.
6. Aeschbacher BC, Portner M, Fluri M, Meier B, Luscher TF. Midazolam premedication improves tolerance of transesophageal echocardiography. *Am J Cardiol.* 1998;81(8):1022-1026.
7. Foster E, Kusumoto FM, Sobol SM, Schiller NB. Streptococcal endocarditis temporally related to transesophageal echocardiography. *J Am Soc Echocardiogr.* 1990;3(5):424-427.
8. Steckelberg JM, Khandheria BK, Anhalt JP, et al. Prospective evaluation of the risk of bacteremia associated with transesophageal echocardiography. *Circulation.* 1991;84(1):177-180.
9. Nikutta P, Mantey-Stiers F, Becht I, et al. Risk of bacteremia induced by transesophageal echocardiography: analysis of 100 consecutive procedures. *J Am Soc Echocardiogr.* 1992;5(2): 168-172.
10. Shyu KG, Hwang JJ, Lin SC, et al. Prospective study of blood culture during transesophageal echocardiography. *Am Heart J.* 1992;124(6):1541-1544.
11. Roudaut R, Lartigue MC, Texier-Maugein J, Dallocchio M. Incidence of bacteraemia or fever during transoesophageal echocardiography: a prospective study of 82 patients. *Eur Heart J.* 1993;14(7):936-940.
12. Mentec H, Vignon P, Terre S, et al. Frequency of bacteremia associated with transesophageal echocardiography in intensive care unit patients: a prospective study of 139 patients. *Crit Care Med.* 1995;23(7):1194-1199.
13. Chambers JB, Klein JL, Bennett SR, Monaghan MJ, Roxburgh JC. Is antibiotic prophylaxis ever necessary before transoesophageal echocardiography? *Heart.* 2006;92(4):435-436.
14. Cote G, Denault A. Transesophageal echocardiography-related complications. *Can J Anaesth.* 2008;55(9):622-647.
15. Bonow RO, Carabello BA, Chatterjee K, et al. 2008 Focused update incorporated into the ACC/AHA 2006 guidelines for the management of patients with valvular heart disease: a report of the American College of Cardiology/American Heart Association Task Force on Practice Guidelines (Writing Committee to Revise the 1998 Guidelines for the Management of Patients With Valvular Heart Disease): endorsed by the Society of Cardiovascular Anesthesiologists, Society for Cardiovascular Angiography and Interventions, and Society of Thoracic Surgeons. *Circulation.* 2008;118(15):e523-661.
16. Na S, Kim CS, Kim JY, Cho JS, Kim KJ. Rigid laryngoscope-assisted insertion of transesophageal echocardiography probe reduces oropharyngeal mucosal injury in anesthetized patients. *Anesthesiology.* 2009;110(1):38-40.
17. Chee TS, Quek SS, Ding ZP, Chua SM. Clinical utility, safety, acceptability and complications of transoesophageal echocardiography (TEE) in 901 patients. *Singapore Med J.* 1995;36(5): 479-483.
18. Daniel WG, Erbel R, Kasper W, et al. Safety of transesophageal echocardiography. A multicenter survey of 10,419 examinations. *Circulation.* 1991;83(3):817-821.
19. Tam JW, Burwash IG, Ascah KJ, Baird MG, Chan KL. Feasibility and complications of single-plane and biplane versus multiplane transesophageal imaging: a review of 2947 consecutive studies. *Can J Cardiol.* 1997;13(1):81-84.
20. Practice Guidelines for Perioperative Transesophageal Echocardiography. An Updated Report by the American Society of Anesthesiologists and the Society of Cardiovascular Anesthesiologists Task Force on Transesophageal Echocardiography. *Anesthesiology.* 2010;112:1084-1096.
21. Lambert AS, Mazer CD, Duke PC. Survey of the members of the cardiovascular section of the Canadian Anesthesiologists' Society on the use of perioperative transesophageal echocardiography—a brief report. *Can J Anaesth.* 2002;49(3):294-296.
22. Ayres NA, Miller-Hance W, Fyfe DA, et al. Indications and guidelines for performance of transesophageal echocardiography in the patient with pediatric acquired or congenital heart disease: report from the task force of the Pediatric Council of the American Society of Echocardiography. *J Am Soc Echocardiogr.* 2005;18(1):91-98.
23. Mishra M, Chauhan R, Sharma KK, et al. Real-time intraoperative transesophageal echocardiography—how useful? Experience of 5,016 cases. *J Cardiothorac Vasc Anesth.* 1998;12(6): 625-632.
24. Cicek S, Demirilic U, Kuralay E, Tatar H, Ozturk O. Transesophageal echocardiography in cardiac surgical emergencies. *J Card Surg.* 1995;10(3):236-244.
25. Suriani RJ, Neustein S, Shore-Lesserson L, Konstadt S. Intraoperative transesophageal echocardiography during noncardiac surgery. *J Cardiothorac Vasc Anesth.* 1998;12(3):274-280.
26. De Wolf A. Transesophageal echocardiography and orthotopic liver transplantation: general concepts. *Liver Transpl Surg.* 1999;5(4):339-340.
27. Feierman D. Case presentation: transesophageal echocardiography during orthotopic liver transplantation—not only a different diagnosis, but different management. *Liver Transpl Surg.* 1999;5(4):340-341.
28. Brandt RR, Oh JK, Abel MD, Click RL, Orszulak TA, Seward JB. Role of emergency intraoperative transesophageal echocardiography. *J Am Soc Echocardiogr.* 1998;11(10):972-977.
29. Beaulieu Y. Bedside echocardiography in the assessment of the critically ill. *Crit Care Med.* 2007;35(5 Suppl):S235-249.
30. Colreavy FB, Donovan K, Lee KY, Weekes J. Transesophageal echocardiography in critically ill patients. *Crit Care Med.* 2002;30(5):989-996.
31. Orme RM, Oram MP, McKinstry CE. Impact of echocardiography on patient management in the intensive care unit: an audit of district general hospital practice. *Br J Anaesth.* 2009;102(3):340-344.
32. Skiles JA, Griffin BP. Transesophageal echocardiographic (TEE) evaluation of ventricular function. *Cardiol Clin.* 2000;18(4):681-697, vii.
33. Heidenreich PA. Transesophageal echocardiography (TEE) in the critical care patient. *Cardiol Clin.* 2000;18(4):789-805, ix.
34. Vieillard-Baron A, Qanadli SD, Antakly Y, et al. Transesophageal echocardiography for the diagnosis of pulmonary embolism with acute cor pulmonale: a comparison with radiological procedures. *Intensive Care Med.* 1998;24(5):429-433.
35. Minard G, Schurr MJ, Croce MA, et al. A prospective analysis of transesophageal echocardiography in the diagnosis of traumatic disruption of the aorta. *J Trauma.* 1996;40(2):225-230.
36. Evangelista A, Avegliano G, Elorz C, Gonzalez-Alujas T, Garcia del Castillo H, Soler-Soler J. Transesophageal echocardiography in the diagnosis of acute aortic syndrome. *J Card Surg.* 2002;17(2):95-106.
37. Yalcin F, Thomas JD, Homa D, Flachskampf FA. Transesophageal echocardiography: first-line imaging for aortic diseases. *Cleve Clin J Med.* 2000;67(6):417-418, 421-418.

38. Gendreau MA, Triner WR, Bartfield J. Complications of transesophageal echocardiography in the ED. *Am J Emerg Med.* 1999;17(3):248-251.
39. Stoddard MF, Longaker RA. The safety of transesophageal echocardiography in the elderly. *Am Heart J.* 1993;125(5 Pt 1): 1358-1362.
40. Ghafoor AU, Schmitz ML, Mayhew JF. Esophageal mucosal tear from a transesophageal echocardiography probe despite preliminary assessment via esophagoscopy in a patient with esophageal disease. *J Cardiothorac Vasc Anesth.* 2004;18(1):78-79.
41. Kawahito S, Kitahata H, Kimura H, Tanaka K, Oshita S. Recurrent laryngeal nerve palsy after cardiovascular surgery: relationship to the placement of a transesophageal echocardiographic probe. *J Cardiothorac Vasc Anesth.* 1999;13(5): 528-531.
42. Egleston CV, Wood AE, Gorey TF, McGovern EM. Gastrointestinal complications after cardiac surgery. *Ann R Coll Surg Engl.* 1993;75(1):52-56.
43. Khandheria B, Seward J, Bailey K. Safety of transesophageal echocardiography: Experience with 2070 patients [abstract]. *J Am Soc Echocardiogr* 1991;17:20.
44. Augoustides JG, Hosalkar HH, Milas BL, Acker M, Savino JS. Upper gastrointestinal injuries related to perioperative transesophageal echocardiography: index case, literature review, classification proposal, and call for a registry. *J Cardiothorac Vasc Anesth.* 2006;20(3):379-384.
45. Lennon MJ, Gibbs NM, Weightman WM, Leber J, Ee HC, Yusoff IF. Transesophageal echocardiography-related gastrointestinal complications in cardiac surgical patients. *J Cardiothorac Vasc Anesth.* 2005;19(2):141-145.
46. Piercy M, McNicol L, Dinh DT, Story DA, Smith JA. Major complications related to the use of transesophageal echocardiography in cardiac surgery. *J Cardiothorac Vasc Anesth.* 2009;23(1):62-65.
47. Rousou JA, Tighe DA, Garb JL, et al. Risk of dysphagia after transesophageal echocardiography during cardiac operations. *Ann Thorac Surg.* 2000;69(2):486-489; discussion 489-490.
48. Hogue CW Jr, Lappas GD, Creswell LL, et al. Swallowing dysfunction after cardiac operations. Associated adverse outcomes and risk factors including intraoperative transesophageal echocardiography. *J Thorac Cardiovasc Surg.* 1995;110(2) :517-522.
49. Garimella S, Longaker RA, Stoddard MF. Safety of transesophageal echocardiography in patients who are obese. *J Am Soc Echocardiogr.* 2002;15(11):1396-1400.
50. Stevenson JG. Incidence of complications in pediatric transesophageal echocardiography: experience in 1650 cases. *J Am Soc Echocardiogr.* 1999;12(6):527-532.
51. Pearson AC, Castello R, Labovitz AJ. Safety and utility of transesophageal echocardiography in the critically ill patient. *Am Heart J.* 1990;119(5):1083-1089.
52. Pincetl PS, Merril JR, Piemme TE. Fundamentals of image processing for personal computers. *MD Comput.* 1993;10(1): 42-49.
53. Feigenbaum H. Digital recording, display, and storage of echocardiograms. *J Am Soc Echocardiogr.* 1988;1(5):378-383.
54. Bansal S, Ehler D, Vacek JL. Digital echocardiography: its role in modern medical practice. *Chest.* 2001;119(1):271-276.
55. Frommelt P, Gorentz J, Deatsman S, Organ D, Frommelt M, Mussatto K. Digital imaging, archiving, and structured reporting in pediatric echocardiography: impact on laboratory efficiency and physician communication. *J Am Soc Echocardiogr.* 2008;21(8): 935-940.
56. Chandra S, Thomas JD. Digital storage and analysis of color Doppler echocardiograms. *Echocardiography.* 1997;14(1):91-102.
57. Spencer K, Weinert L, Mor-Avi V, et al. Electronic transmission of digital echocardiographic studies: effects of MPEG compression. *Int J Cardiol.* 2000;75(2-3):141-145.
58. DICOM Strategic Document, Version 2.1. http://medical.nema.org/dicom.geninfo/dicom_strategy/Strategy_2003-02-07.htm (accessed April 21, 2003).
59. Soble JS, Yurow G, Brar R, et al. Comparison of MPEG digital video with super VHS tape for diagnostic echocardiographic readings. *J Am Soc Echocardiogr.* 1998;11(8):819-825.
60. Shanewise JS, Cheung AT, Aronson S, et al. ASE/SCA guidelines for performing a comprehensive intraoperative multiplane transesophageal echocardiography examination: recommendations of the American Society of Echocardiography Council for Intraoperative Echocardiography and the Society of Cardiovascular Anesthesiologists Task Force for Certification in Perioperative Transesophageal Echocardiography. *Anesth Analg.* 1999;89(4): 870-884.
61. Podgoreanu M, Hansley W, Mathew JP. Intraoperative transesophageal echocardiography data collection using a personal digital assistant. *J Am Soc Echocardiogr.* 2001;14(5):433.
62. Douglas PS, Hendel RC, Cummings JE, et al. ACCF/ACR/AHA/ASE/ASNC/HRS/NASCI/RSNA/SAIP/SCAI/SCCT/SCMR 2008 Health Policy Statement on Structured Reporting in Cardiovascular Imaging. Endorsed by the Society of Nuclear Medicine [added]. *Circulation.* 2009;119(1): 187-200.
63. Cahalan MK, Stewart W, Pearlman A, et al. American Society of Echocardiography and Society of Cardiovascular Anesthesiologists task force guidelines for training in perioperative echocardiography. *J Am Soc Echocardiogr.* 2002;15(6):647-652.
64. Recommendations for a standardized report for adult perioperative echocardiography: from the Society of Cardiovascular Anesthesiologists/American Society of Echocardiography Task Force for a Standardized Perioperative Report. http://www.scahq.org/sca3/peri_op_report4-02.rtf (accessed May 9, 2003).
65. Cerqueira MD, Weissman NJ, Dilsizian V, et al. Standardized myocardial segmentation and nomenclature for tomographic imaging of the heart: a statement for healthcare professionals from the Cardiac Imaging Committee of the Council on Clinical Cardiology of the American Heart Association. *Circulation.* 2002;105(4):539-542.
66. Quinones MA, Douglas PS, Foster E, et al. ACC/AHA clinical competence statement on echocardiography: a report of the American College of Cardiology/American Heart Association/American College of Physicians-American Society of Internal Medicine Task Force on clinical competence. *J Am Soc Echocardiogr.* 2003;16(4):379-402.
67. Recommendations for continuous quality improvement in echocardiography. American Society of Echocardiography. *J Am Soc Echocardiogr.* 1995;8(5 Pt 2):S1-28.
68. Kisslo J. Reconsidering quality. *Heart.* 1998;80 Suppl 1:S27-29.
69. Statement on Transesophageal Echocardiography. www.asahq.org/publicationsAndServices/standards/TEE.htmwww.asahq.org/publicationsAndServices/standards/TEE.htm (accessed May 6, 2003).

70. Morewood GH, Gallagher ME, Gaughan JP. Does the reimbursement of anesthesiologists for intraoperative transesophageal echocardiography promote increased utilization? *J Cardiothorac Vasc Anesth*. 2002;16(3):300-303.
71. Chan KL, Cohen GI, Sochowski RA, Baird MG. Complications of transesophageal echocardiography in ambulatory adult patients: analysis of 1500 consecutive examinations. *J Am Soc Echocardiogr*. 1991;4(6):577-582.
72. Kallmeyer IJ, Collard CD, Fox JA, Body SC, Shernan SK. The safety of intraoperative transesophageal echocardiography: a case series of 7200 cardiac surgical patients. *Anesth Analg*. 2001;92(5):1126-1130.

Training and Certification in Perioperative Transesophageal Echocardiography

26

Jack Shanewise

Over the past 25 years, transesophageal echocardiography (TEE) has become an integral part of the care received by patients undergoing heart surgery. The interest in the perioperative application of TEE (PTE) continues to broaden and now includes, to name just a few, liver transplantation, lung transplantation, major vascular surgery, and persistent hemodynamic instability in the operating room. Anesthesiologists have been actively involved with PTE from its inception, and some degree of training in PTE has become an integral, accepted component of all anesthesiology residencies. The program requirements for anesthesiology training state that residents should have "significant experience with . . . the use of TEE."[1] This chapter reviews the issue of training for anesthesiologists in PTE and discusses the development of certification in this area.

EARLY STEPS IN PTE TRAINING

One of the first publications addressing training in PTE came from the Cleveland Clinic Foundation, the largest center for heart surgery in the United States.[2] The authors described an extensive training program developed for the cardiac anesthesiologists using TEE during heart surgery at their institution. The training took place over a year and started off with 6 months devoted to full-time training, initially in the echocardiography laboratory and then divided between the lab and the cardiac operating room (OR). The second 6 months consisted of closely supervised intraoperative echocardiography experience integrated with anesthesiology responsibilities. The program included extensive training and experience with transthoracic echocardiography (TTE) as well as TEE. The editorial accompanying this publication thoughtfully supported the importance of training in PTE, but pointed out the impracticality of extended, full-time training for many anesthesiologists, and advocated in favor of an "on the job" approach to training through a mentoring program with an experienced expert in PTE to be available at critical times during the procedure.[3] The editorial also put forth the view that training in TTE was not the most efficient way for practitioners exclusively using TEE to be trained. Both approaches have been successfully applied in different ways at various institutions, and many TEE education programs provide a combination of intensive full-time echo lab experience with mentoring in the OR.

Perhaps the most important early document to address training and the use of TEE in the perioperative setting was the seminal *Practice Guidelines for Perioperative Transesophageal Echocardiography*,[4] jointly developed by the American Society of Anesthesiologists (ASA) and the Society of Cardiovascular Anesthesiologists (SCA) and published in 1996. It was written by a task force formed in 1993 that was led by Daniel Thys, MD, and consisted of nine anesthesiologists, two cardiologists, and one methodologist who reviewed over 500 publications relevant to PTE. While this document focused primarily on the various indications for TEE in the perioperative setting, it did discuss training and fairly specifically defined the cognitive and technical skills needed for training in PTE at two levels, basic and advanced (Tables 26–1 and 26–2). Basic training was defined as the use of TEE in the customary practice of anesthesiology and included such applications as monitoring for myocardial ischemia, evaluation of ventricular function, and assessment of hemodynamic instability. Advanced training included using the full diagnostic potential of TEE such as quantification of cardiac valve lesions and evaluation of valve repairs and complex congenital heart defects. Subsequent PTE guidelines and certification processes have continued to refer to these cognitive and technical skills.

DEVELOPMENT OF THE PTEeXAM

The next major step in the development of training and certification was the formation in 1995 of the SCA Task Force for Certification in Perioperative Transesophageal Echocardiography. This group was led by

Table 26–1. Specific Training Objectives for Basic Training in PTE from the Practice Guidelines for Perioperative Transesophageal Echocardiography.

Cognitive Skills
1. Knowledge of the physical principles of echocardiographic image formation and blood velocity measurement
2. Knowledge of the operation of ultrasonographs including all controls that affect the quality of data displayed
3. Knowledge of the equipment handling, infection control, and electrical safety associated with the techniques of perioperative echocardiography
4. Knowledge of the indications, contraindications, and potential complications for perioperative echocardiography
5. Knowledge of the appropriate alternative diagnostic techniques
6. Knowledge of the normal tomographic anatomy as revealed by perioperative echocardiographic techniques
7. Knowledge of commonly encountered blood flow velocity profiles as measured by Doppler echocardiography
8. Knowledge of the echocardiographic manifestations of native valvular lesions and dysfunction
9. Knowledge of the echocardiographic manifestations of cardiac masses, thrombi, cardiomyopathies, pericardial effusions, and lesions of the great vessels
10. Detailed knowledge of the echocardiographic presentations of myocardial ischemia and infarction
11. Detailed knowledge of the echocardiographic presentations of normal and abnormal ventricular function
12. Detailed knowledge of the echocardiographic presentations of air embolization
Technical Skills
1. Ability to operate ultrasonographs including the primary controls affecting the quality of the displayed data
2. Ability to insert a TEE probe safely in the anesthetized, tracheally intubated patient
3. Ability to perform a comprehensive TEE examination and differentiate normal from markedly abnormal cardiac structures and function
4. Ability to recognize marked changes in segmental ventricular contraction indicative of myocardial ischemia or infarction
5. Ability to recognize marked changes in global ventricular filling and ejection
6. Ability to recognize air embolization
7. Ability to recognize gross valvular lesions and dysfunction
8. Ability to recognize large intracardiac masses and thrombi
9. Ability to detect large pericardial effusions
10. Ability to recognize common echocardiographic artifacts
11. Ability to communicate echocardiographic results effectively to health care professionals, the medical record, and patients
12. Ability to recognize complications of perioperative echocardiography

From Practice guidelines for perioperative transesophageal echocardiography. A report by the American Society of Anesthesiologists and the Society of Cardiovascular Anesthesiologists Task Force on Transesophageal Echocardiography. Anesthesiology. 1996;84(4):986-1006.

Solomon Aronson, MD, and consisted of 10 SCA members with considerable experience and expertise in TEE. Over the next 2 years, this group met regularly and developed what is now called the Examination of Special Competence in Perioperative Echocardiography (PTEeXAM). The PTEeXAM covers perioperative applications of TEE at the advanced level, and is intended primarily for anesthesiologists using TEE during cardiac surgery, although other physicians are eligible and have taken it. Early on, the task force considered whether to create certification processes at both the basic and advanced level, and after much discussion the decision was to address only the advanced level, and defer basic level certification to another time and place. Besides the cognitive and technical skills described for the advanced level in the practice guidelines, the test writers had in mind the level of knowledge in PTE that a candidate would have after completing a 1-year fellowship in cardiothoracic anesthesiology. The SCA worked with the National Board of Medical Examiners in developing the PTEeXAM to assure the quality of the examination and the certification process.

The examination was administered in a pilot form to a group of volunteers at the SCA annual meeting in 1997 in order to assess the quality of the questions and to help establish the level of knowledge, or standard, required to pass the test. The PTEeXAM was then offered for certification to interested physicians at the SCA annual meeting in 1998 and has been given every year since that time. Over 4000 physicians, the vast majority anesthesiologists, have taken it. The same level of knowledge (standard) was used to determine the passing score for the PTEeXAM through 2001 and then, because of a steadily increasing passing rate of well over 80%, a

Table 26–2. Specific Training Objectives for Advanced Training in PTE from the Practice Guidelines for Perioperative Transesophageal Echocardiography.

Cognitive Skills
1. All the cognitive skills defined under basic training
2. Detailed knowledge of the principles and methodologies of qualitative and quantitative echocardiography
3. Detailed knowledge of native and prosthetic valvular function including valvular lesions and dysfunction
4. Knowledge of congenital heart disease (if congenital practice is planned then this knowledge must be detailed)
5. Detailed knowledge of all other diseases of the heart and great vessels that is relevant in the perioperative period (if pediatric practice is planned then this knowledge may be more general than detailed)
6. Detailed knowledge of the techniques, advantages, disadvantages, and potential complications of commonly used cardiac surgical procedures for treatment of acquired and congenital heart disease
7. Detailed knowledge of other diagnostic methods appropriate for correlation with perioperative echocardiography
Technical Skills
1. All the technical skills defined under basic training
2. Ability to acquire or direct the acquisition of all necessary echocardiographic data including epicardial and epiaortic imaging
3. Ability to recognize subtle changes in segmental ventricular contraction indicative of myocardial ischemia or infarction
4. Ability to quantify systolic and diastolic ventricular function and to estimate other relevant hemodynamic parameters
5. Ability to quantify normal and abnormal native and prosthetic valvular function
6. Ability to assess the appropriateness of cardiac surgical plans
7. Ability to identify inadequacies in cardiac surgical interventions and the underlying reasons for the inadequacies
8. Ability to aid in clinical decision making in the operating room

From Practice guidelines for perioperative transesophageal echocardiography. A report by the American Society of Anesthesiologists and the Society of Cardiovascular Anesthesiologists Task Force on Transesophageal Echocardiography. Anesthesiology. 1996;84(4):986-1006.

somewhat higher standard was set, essentially raising the bar, in order to keep the PTEeXAM a credible test of advanced knowledge in PTE. This new standard has been used to determine the passing score since 2002. Over the first 4 years the test was given, overall performance was positively related to having 3 or more months of training in echocardiography or performing at least six TEE examinations per week.[5]

FORMATION OF THE NATIONAL BOARD OF ECHOCARDIOGRAPHY

The National Board of Echocardiography (NBE) currently develops and administers the PTEeXAM and certifies individual practitioners in advanced PTE. The origins of the NBE date from 1992, when the American Society of Echocardiography (ASE) formed the ASEeXAM parent committee, which was chaired by Arthur "Ned" Weyman, MD, and was charged with developing a process by which physicians could demonstrate special competence in adult echocardiography. The result was what is now called the Examination of Special Competence in Adult Echocardiography (ASCeXAM), which has been given at the ASE annual meeting since 1995. The ASCeXAM is a general test of knowledge in adult echocardiography including transthoracic and stress echo, and is intended mainly for cardiologists, although other physicians including anesthesiologists are eligible and have taken it. But it was primarily out of concern that the ASCeXAM was not an appropriate measure of knowledge in PTE for most anesthesiologists that the SCA formed the Task Force for Certification in Perioperative TEE, which developed the PTEeXAM. In 1996, in order to deal with potential conflict of interest issues that arose with the ASE certifying practitioners in echocardiography, the ASEeXAM parent committee became an independent corporation called ASEeXAM, Incorporated. In 1998, as a result of negotiations between ASEeXAM, Inc and the SCA, ASEeXAM, Inc took on writing and administration of the PTEeXAM and changed its name to the NBE.

Anesthesiologists are well represented at the NBE. Three members of the NBE Board of Directors must belong to the SCA. It takes a supermajority to change the NBE bylaws, so that at least one anesthesiologist must support any future bylaws changes. In fact, there have been no significantly contentious issues dividing the cardiologists and anesthesiologists within the NBE. The cardiology members have been very accommodating and supportive of the efforts of the anesthesiologists to develop a credible, fair process by which anesthesiologists can demonstrate their competence in advanced PTE. As a matter of fact, an anesthesiologist, Daniel Thys, has served as president of the NBE.

NBE CERTIFICATION IN ECHOCARDIOGRAPHY

After 1998, the NBE was writing and administering two examinations in echocardiography: the ASCeXAM primarily for cardiologists and the PTEeXAM primarily for anesthesiologists. But the certificates issued could only attest to the fact that someone had passed the test, not that they had demonstrated competence in echocardiography. Board certification in a medical specialty typically requires individuals to demonstrate competency by completing a specific training program and then passing a board examination. In addition, for some period of time newly created specialties usually allow current practitioners to substitute practice experience for training. In 2001, the NBE initiated a certification process based on training guidelines for echocardiography published in the cardiology literature by which physicians could, by passing the ASCeXAM and providing documentation of specified training and experience, become certified as Diplomates of the NBE in adult echocardiography. The NBE began using the term "testamur" (ie, one who has passed a test) to refer to those who had passed an examination but had not become certified by submitting documentation of the required training or experience.

TRAINING GUIDELINES IN PERIOPERATIVE ECHOCARDIOGRAPHY

In order for PTEeXAM certification to remain credible compared to ASCeXAM certification, a similar process of submitting documentation of training or experience had to be developed for the PTEeXAM. However, there were no published training guidelines in PTE for the NBE to refer to in developing advanced PTE certification. Previously published guidelines for training in TEE were intended for cardiologist echocardiographers and recommended at least 6 months of training in transthoracic echocardiography as a prerequisite to TEE.[6] Consequently, in 2000 the ASE and SCA formed the Task Force for Training Guidelines in Perioperative Echocardiography, chaired by Michael Cahalan, MD, to formulate training guidelines and, by the same token, facilitate the development of a certification process in advanced PTE. The task force consisted of the chair, four cardiologists, and four anesthesiologists with experience and expertise in PTE. This group produced several drafts before developing a set of acceptable guidelines that were subsequently adopted by both the SCA and ASE Boards of Directors.

The guidelines for training in perioperative echocardiography made recommendations for training in both basic and advanced PTE as described in the 1996 ASA/SCA Practice Guidelines in PTE. For basic training, the task force recommended study of 150 complete TEE examinations under appropriate supervision, including the full spectrum of commonly encountered perioperative diagnoses and at least 50 comprehensive intraoperative TEE examinations personally performed, interpreted, and reported by the trainee. For advanced-level training the recommendation was the study of 300 complete examinations under appropriate supervision, including a wide spectrum of cardiac diagnoses and at least 150 comprehensive intraoperative TEE examinations personally performed, interpreted, and reported by the trainee. The guidelines recognize that physicians in practice may be able to acquire the requisite knowledge and skills without enrolling in a formal, supervised training program, as long as they can document their experience in detail and be able to demonstrate its equivalence to the supervised training guidelines.

The guidelines were published in 2002[7,8] and adopted by the NBE as requirements for training and experience for advanced PTE certification. It is important to note that the training requirements for certification were not arbitrarily developed by the NBE, but came from a document that was developed and adopted by the SCA and ASE through an insightful and extensive process involving several iterations of feedback and modification. The NBE issued applications for certification in advanced PTE in late 2003 and began certifying individual practitioners in February 2004. As of February 2009 over 1200 physicians have been certified as Diplomates of the NBE in PTE; all but a few are anesthesiologists. Because NBE certification is a requirement, the advanced PTE certification process has made it possible for many anesthesiologists to become Fellows of the American Society of Echocardiography (FASE).

REQUIREMENTS FOR ADVANCED PTE CERTIFICATION

There are five requirements for certification by the NBE in advanced PTE. The applicant must have:

1. Passed the advanced PTEeXAM within 10 years
2. A current, unrestricted license to practice medicine
3. Board certification in a medical specialty recognized by the American Board of Medical Specialties (ABMS)
4. Training or experience in the perioperative care of patients with cardiovascular disease
5. Training or experience in advanced perioperative TEE

Requirement 4—training or experience in the perioperative care of patients with cardiovascular disease—may be accomplished through one of two pathways: the supervised training pathway or the practice experience pathway. The supervised training pathway requires completion of at least 1 year of fellowship training in cardiovascular disease after core residency. This most commonly is a cardiothoracic anesthesiology fellowship, but could be fellowship training in cardiology, critical care medicine, or thoracic surgery as long as there is extensive perioperative experience. The practice experience pathway specifies that the applicant must have at least 24 months of experience in perioperative care of patients with cardiovascular disease, including at least 150 patients in each of the 2 years prior to application for certification. These patients do not necessarily have to be undergoing heart surgery, but must have significant cardiovascular disease.

Similarly, requirement 5, training or experience in PTE, may be fulfilled through a supervised training or a practice experience pathway. For supervised PTE training, applicants must study 300 complete perioperative TEE examinations under appropriate supervision. These examinations must include a wide spectrum of cardiac diagnoses and at least 150 comprehensive intraoperative TEE examinations personally performed, interpreted, and reported by the applicant. With the practice experience pathway applicants must perform and interpret at least 300 perioperative transesophageal echocardiograms within 4 consecutive years immediately preceding application with no less than 50 in any year in which any of the 300 echocardiograms were performed. At least 150 of the 300 TEE examinations must be intraoperative. The practice experience pathway also requires at least 50 hours of American Medical Association (AMA) category 1 level continuing medical education devoted to echocardiography be obtained within 4 years of application. For applicants completing their core residency training (usually in anesthesiology) after June 30, 2009, requirement 5 must be fulfilled through the supervised training pathway; the practice experience pathway will remain open indefinitely for those who have finished their core residency on or before that date. Applications from candidates outside of North America are considered based on the equivalency of training compared to the United States and Canada.

RECERTIFICATION IN PTE

All certificates issued by the NBE expire after 10 years, so recertification processes for both the ASCeXAM and PTEeXAM have been developed. The first advanced PTEeXAM certificates were issued in 1998, and the recertification exam for advanced PTE (RePTE) was given for the first time in 2007. Candidates for recertification may take the RePTE the year their certificate expires, the year before, or the year after. Those who fail to recertify by the year after expiration of their certificate will have to retake and pass the PTEeXAM and fulfill the requirements for initial certification again in order to regain advanced PTE certification. The RePTE exam has been a subset of questions from the PTEeXAM that are focused on clinical issues. There are four requirements for recertification by the NBE in advanced PTE. The applicant must have:

1. Passed the RePTE exam before the 1-year anniversary of the expiration of their PTEeXam certificate
2. A current, unrestricted license to practice medicine
3. Performed and interpreted at least 50 perioperative TEEs per year in 2 of the 3 years immediately preceding application
4. At least 15 hours of AMA category 1 continuing medical education devoted to echocardiography obtained during the 3 years immediately preceding application

Another important advance made by the NBE for all of its examinations is the move from paper testing forms to computer-based testing. As of 2009, candidates will take an NBE examination by going to a local testing center on a specified date.

ACGME ACCREDITATION OF ADULT CARDIOTHORACIC ANESTHESIOLOGY FELLOWSHIPS

In 2007, the Accreditation Council for Graduate Medical Education (ACGME) began accrediting adult cardiothoracic anesthesiology (ACTA) fellowships, culminating an almost 10-year process of application and reapplication pursued persistently by the SCA. These fellowships last 1 year and require successful completion of an accredited anesthesiology residency as a prerequisite. In developing the ACTA fellowship program requirements, the anesthesiology Residency Review Committee of the ACGME essentially adopted the ASE/SCA Guidelines for Training in Perioperative Echocardiography recommendations for advanced PTE.[9] As a result, trainees completing an accredited ACTA fellowship are eligible for NBE certification in advanced PTE, provided they pass the PTEeXAM. This has afforded an objective measure and accomplishment by which those completing ACTA fellowships can validate their subspecialty training, in lieu of subspecialty certification in adult cardiothoracic anesthesiology. Now that there is accredited subspecialty training in ACTA, the issue of whether or not to provide subspecialty board certification in this area is due to be addressed by the American Board of Anesthesiology around 2012. It seems certain that any such certification process would have to include an assessment of knowledge of advanced PTE.

BASIC PTE CERTIFICATION

In 2006, the ASA House of Delegates passed a resolution directing the ASA to create a certification process for PTE at the basic level. A primary motivation for this was the belief that many anesthesiologists regularly use TEE in their practice at a frequency insufficient to obtain advanced PTE certification. The ASA approached the NBE regarding this issue, and the two organizations have developed a basic PTE certification process that was launched in 2009. The scope of practice for basic PTE is defined by the ASA and NBE as follows:

> *The application of a basic perioperative TEE examination is limited to non-diagnostic monitoring within the customary practice of anesthesiology. Because the goal of training in basic PTE is focused on intraoperative monitoring rather than specific diagnosis, except in emergent situations, diagnoses requiring intraoperative cardiac surgical intervention or post-operative medical/surgical management must be confirmed by an individual with advanced skills in TEE or by an independent diagnostic technique.*

Besides the cognitive and technical skills described for basic PTE in the practice guidelines, the level of knowledge intended for practitioners of basic PTE would enable them to use TEE as a hemodynamic and cardiac monitor during general anesthesia, but not direct surgical decisions during heart surgery. The basic TEE exam consists of the midesophageal four-chamber, two-chamber, long-axis, and right ventricular (RV) inflow-outflow views; the transgastric mid short-axis view; and views of the thoracic aorta from the diaphragm to the arch, with views of the valves repeated using color-flow Doppler. There is at least one study suggesting that a limited, basic TEE examination can acquire most of the information obtained in a comprehensive exam.[10]

The NBE is developing an examination assessing knowledge in basic PTE, which is scheduled to be given in the fall of 2010 (www.echoboards.org). Until the basic PTEeXAM is available, candidates may fulfill the examination requirement for basic PTE certification by passing the advanced PTEeXAM. There are four requirements for certification by the NBE in basic PTE. The applicant must have:

1. Passed the basic or advanced PTEeXAM within 10 years
2. A current, unrestricted license to practice medicine
3. Board certification in anesthesiology
4. Training or experience in basic perioperative TEE

There are three pathways offered by the NBE to fulfill the echocardiography training requirement for basic PTE certification that are based on the ASE/SCA Guidelines for Training in Perioperative Echocardiography: the supervised training pathway, the practice experience pathway, and the extended continuing medical education (CME) pathway. For the supervised pathway, applicants must study at least 150 basic perioperative TEE examinations under appropriate supervision. Of these, the applicant must personally perform and interpret at least 50 basic intraoperative TEE examinations. Supervised training in basic perioperative TEE is limited to accredited anesthesiology residency programs, and must be accomplished within a 4-year period of time or less. For the practice experience pathway, applicants must perform and interpret at least 150 basic intraoperative TEE examinations within 4 consecutive years with no less than 25 in any year. In addition, applicants must obtain at least 40 hours of AMA category 1 continuing medical education devoted to perioperative TEE obtained within 4 years. The practice experience pathway will not be available to those completing tier anesthesiology residency training after June 30, 2016. For the extended CME pathway, applicants must have personally performed and interpreted at least 50 basic intraoperative TEE examinations within 2 years of the application with at least 25 within 1 year of the application. Applicants must also study, personally interpret, and subsequently review, either under direct supervision or in an electronic format acceptable to the NBE and ASA, at least 100 basic perioperative TEEs from a banked source. This education program must be accredited for at least 30 AMA category 1 CME hours. Applicants must also have at least 10 additional hours of AMA category 1 CME devoted to perioperative TEE within 2 years.

TEE ACCREDITATION IN EUROPE

Accreditation in adult TEE is a joint initiative of the European Association of Echocardiography and the European Association of Cardiothoracic Anesthesiologists (http://www.escardio.org/communities/EAE/accreditation/TEE/Pages/aims.aspx) that was launched in 2005. Currently, specific certification in PTE is not offered. The accreditation process consists of two parts: (a) written exam of multiple-choice questions (single best answer) with 50 questions related to cases displayed on a screen and 100 questions related to theory, and (b) practical assessment accomplished by submitting a case log of 125 exams performed within a 12-month period from which 15 cases are chosen randomly and reviewed by graders. Accreditation will last only for 5 years and a re-accreditation process is currently under development.

PTE ACCREDITATION IN AUSTRALIA AND NEW ZEALAND

There is no formal process for accreditation in Australia, but the Australian and New Zealand College of Anaesthetists (ANZCA) has issued guidelines for the training and practice of perioperative TEE (http://www.anzca.edu.au/resources/professional-documents/professional-standards/pdfs/PS46.pdf/). The period of training is defined as the equivalent of 50 days full-time over a minimum period of 10 weeks to a maximum of 2 years. During the period of training, the trainee is expected to perform and report 50 complete TEE examinations under supervision, 50 unsupervised examinations, and at least 100 additional supervised reviews. Ongoing competence requires performance of at least 30 examinations and reviews of at least 50 recorded exams every year. Completion of the PTEeXAM or the Postgraduate Diploma in Perioperative and Critical Care Echocardiography from the University of Melbourne is also strongly recommended. Practitioners of TEE should additionally satisfy the requirements of the Australian Society of Ultrasound in Medicine (Intercollegiate Consensus Statement 1995) and the Cardiac Society of Australia and New Zealand for training in echocardiography. The latter society recommends intraoperative training to consist of 150 studies in basic monitoring, of which 50 have been personally performed, and 150 advanced (valve) studies, of which 50 have been personally performed.

CONCLUSIONS

Now that training and certification requirements are clearly defined, it seems likely that some anesthesiology residencies will begin to offer basic PTE training to at least some of their residents. If this trend does in fact develop, it seems possible that more and more residencies would provide basic PTE training in order to remain competitive and attract the best residents. And it's not entirely impossible to envision a day—probably many years from now, despite the current lack of sufficient equipment, clinical material, and expertise at many if not most training programs—when all anesthesiology residents are trained in basic PTE and every certified anesthesiologist is competent to use TEE as a hemodynamic and cardiac monitor during general anesthesia.

REFERENCES

1. ACGME Program Requirements for Graduate Medical Education in Anesthesiology. http://www.acgme.org/acWebsite/downloads/RRC_progReq/040_anesthesiology_07012008_u03102008.pdf.
2. Savage RM, Licina MG, Koch CG, et al. Educational program for intraoperative transesophageal echocardiography. *Anesth Analg.* 1995;81(2):399-403.
3. Cahalan MK, Foster E. Training in transesophageal echocardiography: in the lab or on the job? *Anesth Analg.* 1995;81(2):217-218.
4. Practice guidelines for perioperative transesophageal echocardiography. A report by the American Society of Anesthesiologists and the Society of Cardiovascular Anesthesiologists Task Force on Transesophageal Echocardiography. *Anesthesiology.* 1996;84(4):986-1006.
5. Aronson S, Butler A, Subhiyah R, et al. Development and analysis of a new certifying examination in perioperative transesophageal echocardiography. *Anesth Analg.* 2002;95(6):1476-1482, table of contents.
6. Pearlman AS, Gardin JM, Martin RP, et al. Guidelines for physician training in transesophageal echocardiography: recommendations of the American Society of Echocardiography Committee for Physician Training in Echocardiography. *J Am Soc Echocardiogr.* 1992;5(2):187-194.
7. Cahalan MK, Abel M, Goldman M, et al. American Society of Echocardiography and Society of Cardiovascular Anesthesiologists task force guidelines for training in perioperative echocardiography. *Anesth Analg.* 2002;94(6):1384-1388.
8. Cahalan MK, Stewart W, Pearlman A, et al. American Society of Echocardiography and Society of Cardiovascular Anesthesiologists task force guidelines for training in perioperative echocardiography. *J Am Soc Echocardiogr.* 2002;15(6):647-652.
9. Program Requirements for Fellowship Education in Adult Cardiothoracic Anesthesiology. http://www.acgme.org/acWebsite/downloads/RRC_progReq/041pr206.pdf.
10. Miller JP, Lambert AS, Shapiro WA, Russell IA, Schiller NB, Cahalan MK. The adequacy of basic intraoperative transesophageal echocardiography performed by experienced anesthesiologists. *Anesth Analg.* 2001;92(5):1103-1110.

The TEE Board Exam

27

Matthew Wood and Katherine Grichnik

EXAM NEED

The American Society of Echocardiography (ASE) developed the initial formal exam in echocardiography over the years of 1993 to 1995. Following the pilot exam in 1995, the first exam was administered in 1996 and has been administered yearly since by ASEcXAM, Inc, an independent corporation designed to reduce any potential conflicts of interest between the professional society and the certifying entity. The ASEeXAM exam was designed to test all aspects of echocardiography and was intended primarily for cardiologists with additional training in echocardiography. Many in anesthesiology felt that this exam might result in their exclusion from using transesophageal echocardiography (TEE) perioperatively. Thus, in 1996 the Society of Cardiovascular Anesthesiologists (SCA) convened a task force for certification in perioperative transesophageal echocardiography.[1] This committee was responsible for defining the appropriate fund of knowledge, for outlining the exam content based on this fund of knowledge, and for the development of fair multiple-choice questions.

EXAM DEVELOPMENT

The initial step in exam development was to define the content outline. The task force, with input from cardiology colleagues, set forth 23 initial knowledge categories that emphasized basic echocardiography and ultrasound principles, assessment and interpretation of echocardiographic images, Doppler calculations, and intraoperative applications. The next step for the committee was to write the questions with each member being given a category from the content outline on which to base their questions. All questions were then reviewed by both the committee and a medical editor for the National Board of Medical Examiners (NBME) for content, accuracy, clinical significance, and relevance.[2] The pilot examination was given to 95 representative participants in 1997; this exam contained two parts. Part 1 was allotted 60 minutes and consisted of 15 videotaped echocardiography cases with two to four questions per case for a total of 43 questions. Part 2 consisted of both A-type (single best answer) and K-type (complex multiple choice) multiple-choice questions from one of two exam booklets.[2] The initial responses to a survey about the initial exam were positive. Following question analysis and recommendations of the NBME, the K-type questions were removed for future exams. The first formal perioperative transesophageal exam (PTEeXAM) was administered by the SCA the following year. In 1998 the SCA and ASCeXAM, Inc, formed the National Board of Echocardiography (NBE). Within its charter, three of the 10 NBE members are anesthesiologists, and eight members are required to change any bylaws. Thus, anesthesiologists are appropriately represented within the NBE. Yearly since 1998, the NBE has developed and administered both the ASCeXAM and the PTEeXAM.

EXAM APPLICATION, CONTENT, AND PREPARATION: NUTS AND BOLTS

The PTEeXAM is now administered as a computer-based exam. The exam is currently administered once per calendar year at Prometric Testing Centers within the United States, U.S. territories, and Canada, but may increase in administration frequency in the future. The test is given in a standardized fashion; all personal belongings are to be left in a locker outside the testing room. A laminated note board, dry erase markers, and an eraser are provided by the testing center. Calculators are not allowed in the exam, but a simple calculator will be available on the computer. The application fee for the 2009 PTEeXAM was 995 USD.[3] Though the certification requirements are significant and at times confusing (see Chapter 26), the application process is fairly straightforward. The application for the exam can be found at the NBE website (www.echoboards.org), and includes instructions and a checklist required for completion. After the applicant has applied for the exam, the NBE will confirm receipt of the application. The NBE will then provide a scheduling permit for the exam no later than 2 months prior to the test date. The applicant may also seek advanced perioperative transesophageal (PTE) board certification at the same time as applying to take the PTEeXAM. The requirements for board certification are also discussed in Chapter 26. It should be noted that the practice experience pathway is not available to those finishing their core residency after June 30th, 2009, and the fellowship pathway will be the sole pathway to advanced PTE board certification. The application for certification is located at the same NBE website and also contains an extensive checklist of required documentation. After the PTEeXAM is passed, the Committee for Certification reviews the certification application and, if appropriate, grants Board certification. The effective date of Board certification is actually retroactive and is the date the PTEeXAM was passed. The Board certification is valid for 10 years, after which a recertification process must be undertaken. This includes taking the RePTE exam and documenting continued competence and experience in echocardiography (50 TEEs per year in 2 of the 3 prior years and 15 hours of continuing medical education [CME] in the 3 prior years). The RePTE exam consists of a subset of questions from the PTEeXAM. Further details can be found at www.echoboards.org.

EXAM FORMAT

The exam consists of four blocks with 50 multiple-choice questions in each block. The first part consists of three blocks of 150 single answer-type questions with 60 minutes allotted for completion. The fourth block of 50 single answer-type questions is allotted 90 minutes and is video and case-based. Typically, there is a clinical vignette accompanied by a series of related videos and/or images followed by 2-4 questions based on the presented case. All questions are presented in digital format, including images and video loops that are imbedded within the questions. Thus, there is no longer a need to project the clips on a screen for all examinees to view at the same time, allowing examinees to advance at their own pace. Image quality may be variable as a consequence of the varying sources of the video loops and the need to use older loops, which are associated with questions that have previously met the rigorous validation and verification processes. While the questions are both challenging and fair, they are also designed to judge whether examinees have the requisite knowledge. There are appropriate distracters among the possible response options, which are of similar length and grammar and are unlikely to contain opposites. There is only one correct option given and there is no ambiguity. Further, in general, negative or exclusion-type ("except") questions are discouraged.

COURSE OF STUDY

The NBE does not recommend any particular course of study for any of its examinations. However, the NBE does publish the content outline each year for the PTEeXAM; see Table 27–1 for the complete 2009 content outline.[4] The outline is extensive and all components of the outline are tested. However, not all of the components are equally weighted throughout the exam. As determined by the PTEeXAM writing committee, more important components are more extensively tested, and questions may require the knowledge of multiple topics to reach the correct answer. Many questions are designed to ensure that the practitioner is performing a complete echocardiographic exam and is focusing on all structures seen in the ultrasound images, not just the primary one. Examinees must be able to identify well-known structures in lesser-known views and lesser-known structures in well-known views. Of note, it is important to study all topics including those not directly related to a specific pathological condition, such as the physics of ultrasound and diastolic heart function.

EXAM RESULTS

The results of the PTEeXAM are posted 10 weeks after the exam. Certificates are then mailed 8 weeks after this date to those who pass. Even though the test is administered on computer, the delay between the test date and the posting of the results is a consequence of the need to review each question for validity and performance by the testing committee. If statistical evaluation of a question reveals that a large number of examinees consistently answer with the same incorrect response, then the question is closely evaluated for accuracy. If there are any inaccuracies noted, the question may be discarded or re-scored to ensure valid scores and a fair test. The passing score is determined by the NBE with regard to a minimum amount of knowledge required to pass. Candidates are not measured against each other and the test is not scored on a curve. The passing rate for the 2008 PTEeXAM was 76%,[5] but varies from year to year. Test performance data are available from the pilot exam and the first four PTEeXAMs administered over 1998 to 2001. The variables evaluated in the *pilot* exam were length and type of dedicated echocardiography training, primary setting, primary clinical area, time spent in echocardiography practice, and number of echocardiograms interpreted weekly. The examinees who performed or interpreted more than six exams per week, had formal echocardiography training, were postgraduate year (PGY) 5 or greater, or had taken time off from practice for training attained higher scores.[2] The results of the comparison of examinee subgroups from 1998 to 2001 are shown in Table 27–2. Again, the examinees at the PGY 5 or greater level of training and those performing more than three to five exams per week had higher passing rates.[2]

Table 27–1. 2009 PTeXAM Content Outline.

1. Principles of Ultrasound
   a. Nature of ultrasound: compression and rarefaction
   b. Frequency, wavelength, tissue propagation velocity
   c. Properties of ultrasound waves
   d. Ultrasound/tissue interactions
   e. Tissue characterization
2. Transducers
   a. Piezoelectric effect
   b. Crystal thickness and resonance
   c. Damping
3. Sound Beam Formation
   a. Focusing
   b. Axial and lateral resolution
   c. Arrays
4. Equipment, Infection Control, and Safety
   a. Clinical dosimetry
   b. Biological effects of ultrasound
   c. Electrical and mechanical safety
   d. Infection control
   e. TEE probe insertion and manipulation
   f. Contraindications to transesophageal echocardiography
   g. Complications of transesophageal echocardiography
5. Imaging
   a. Instrumentation
   b. Displays
   c. B-mode, M-mode, and two-dimensional echocardiography
   d. Signal processing and related factors
6. Principles of Doppler Ultrasound
   a. Doppler effect
   b. Doppler equation
   c. Doppler shift frequencies and influencing factors
   d. Nyquist limit
   e. Spectral analysis and display characteristics
   f. Pulsed-wave Doppler
   g. High pulse repetition frequency pulsed-wave Doppler
   h. Continuous-wave Doppler
   i. Color-flow Doppler
   j. Color M-mode
7. Quantitative M-Mode and Two-Dimensional Echocardiography
   a. Edge recognition
   b. Edge components
   c. Temporal resolution
   d. Referencing centroids, fixed and floating axes
   e. Center-line method
   f. Global function; measurements and calculations
   g. Geometric, spectral, and other methods
8. Quantitative Doppler
   a. Types of velocity measurements
   b. Volumetric measurements and calculations
   c. Valve gradients, areas, and other measurements
   d. Cardiac chamber and great vessel pressures
   e. Tissue Doppler
9. Doppler Profiles and Assessment of Diastolic Function
   a. Tricuspid valve and right ventricular inflow
   b. Pulmonary valve and right ventricular outflow
   c. Mitral valve and left ventricular inflow
   d. Aortic valve and left ventricular outflow
   e. Non-valvular flow profiles
10. Cardiac Anatomy
    a. Imaging planes
    b. Cardiac chambers and walls
    c. Cardiac valves
    d. Cardiac cycle and relation of events relative to ECG
11. Pericardium and Extracardiac Structures—Anatomy and Pathology
    a. Pericardium and pericardial space
    b. Pulmonary arteries
    c. Pulmonary veins
    d. Vena cavae and hepatic veins
    e. Coronary arteries
    f. Aorta and great vessels
       i. Anatomy
       ii. Atherosclerosis
       iii. Aneurysm
       iv. Dissection and traumatic injury of the aorta
    g. Pleural space
12. Pathology of the Cardiac Valves
    a. Acquired valve diseases
       i. Endocarditis
       ii. Rheumatic
       iii. Myxomatous
       iv. Calcific/degenerative
       v. Traumatic
    b. Tricuspid
    c. Pulmonary
    d. Mitral
       i. Mitral regurgitation
       ii. Ischemic mitral valve dysfunction
       iii. Mitral stenosis
       iv. Systolic anterior motion of mitral valve (SAM)
    e. Aortic
       i. Aortic regurgitation
       ii. Aortic stenosis
13. Intracardiac Masses and Devices
    a. Tumors
    b. Thrombi
    c. Devices and foreign bodies
14. Global Ventricular Systolic Function
    a. Normal left ventricular systolic function
    b. Abnormal left ventricular systolic function
       i. Etiologies including ischemia
       ii. Assessment/ejection fraction
       iii. Confounding factors
    c. Right ventricular systolic function

(Continued)

Table 27–1. 2009 PTeXAM Content Outline. (*Continued*)

d. Cardiomyopathies
   i. Hypertrophic
   ii. Restrictive
   iii. Dilated

15. Segmental Left Ventricular Systolic Function
   a. Myocardial segment identification
   b. Coronary artery distribution and flow
   c. Normal and abnormal segmental function
      i. Assessment and methods
      ii. Differential diagnosis
      iii. Confounding factors
   d. Left ventricular aneurysm
   e. Left ventricular rupture
16. Assessment of Perioperative Events and Problems
   a. Hypotension and causes of cardiovascular instability
   b. Cardiac surgery: techniques and problems
      i. Assessment of bypass and cardioplegia
      ii. Cannulae and devices commonly used during cardiac surgery
      iii. Circulatory assist devices
      iv. Intracavity air
      v. Minimally invasive cardiopulmonary bypass
      vi. Off pump cardiac surgery
   c. Coronary surgery: techniques and assessment
   d. Valve surgery: techniques and assessment
      i. Valve replacement: mechanical, bioprosthetic, and other
      ii. Valve repair
   e. Transplantation surgery
      i. Heart
      ii. Lung
      iii. Liver
17. Congenital Heart Disease
   a. Identification and sites of morphologically left and right structures
   b. Atrial septal defects
   c. Ventricular septal defects
   d. Pulmonary valve and infundibular stenosis
   e. Left atrial and mitral valve conditions
   f. Aortic valve and left ventricular outflow tract abnormalities
   g. Coronary artery anomalies
   h. Patent ductus arteriosus
   i. Coarctation of the aorta
   j. Ebstein anomaly
   k. Persistent left superior vena cava
   l. Tetralogy of Fallot
   m. Transposition of great arteries
   n. Atrioventricular septal defect—"AV canal"
   o. Conditions with single ventricle physiology
18. Artifacts and Pitfalls
   a. Imaging artifacts
   b. Doppler artifacts and pitfalls
   c. Structures mimicking pathology
19. Related Diagnostic Modalities
   a. Stress echocardiography
   b. Myocardial perfusion imaging
   c. Epicardial scanning
   d. Contrast echocardiography
   e. Utility of TEE relative to other diagnostic modalities

From National Board of Echocardiography: 2009 PTeXAM Content Outline. http://www.echoboards.org/faq.html (accessed January 29, 2009).

LEARNING PERIOPERATIVE TEE

Though much of this chapter is dedicated to the actual PTEeXAM, the primary goals of the examination and board certification are, as stated by the NBE, to establish practice domains, to assess the level of knowledge of the practitioner, to enhance the quality of perioperative transesophageal echocardiography, to provide formal recognition to those having met the requirements, and to serve the public by outlining quality patient care.[3] In accordance with these principles, the goals of teaching perioperative echocardiography should be quality patient care first and passing the exam second. There are basic skills required to obtain competence in echocardiography. As listed in Table 27–3, training physicians must have a basic knowledge of ultrasound physics, be proficient with technical aspects of the examination, know the cardiovascular anatomy and physiology, and be able to recognize both simple and complex pathology.[6] This education process usually begins with basic two-dimensional (2D) image acquisition and ultrasound physics. The ASE has published guidelines for performing a multiplane TEE exam; these are available at www.asecho.com and are adapted from the original intraoperative guidelines put forth by Shanewise et al[7] for the ASE and SCA in 1999. The natural progression in learning usually follows with 2D image assessment, Doppler assessment, and three-dimensional (3D) image acquisition and assessment. Mastery of these skills requires practice and repetition. The ASE, SCA, and NBE all recognize the importance of repetition in the learning process and have placed minimum requirements for echocardiograms performed and/or interpreted for board certification.

Additionally, the need for extensive reading in all aspects of echocardiography cannot be overemphasized. Though the practitioner may be familiar with most concepts and disease states, the interactions with ultrasound,

Table 27–2. Results of an Analysis of Variance Comparison of Subgroups of Examinees from 1998 to 2001.

Variable	n	% Pass	Significance Level
PGY level training			<0.00001
None	379	72	
PGY 1, 2, or 3	95	74	
PGY 4	152	79	
PGY 5 or more	314	86	
Time off from practice	262	80	
Number of exams per week			<0.00001
None	54	56	
Fewer than 3	412	71	
3 to 5	481	83	
6 to 10	20	87	
More than 10	56	86	

PGY, postgraduate year.
Adapted from Aronson S, et al. Development and analysis of a new certifying examination in perioperative transesophageal echocardiography. Anesth Analg. 2002;95:1481.

the interpretation of images and Doppler, and the anticipation of probable therapeutic interventions with their likely resultant effects must be known in order to appropriately guide complex medical decisions. An example is the use of ultrasound to diagnose and categorize diastolic dysfunction with the goal of guiding therapeutic decisions.

NOVEL EDUCATION TECHNIQUES

Traditional supplements to the actual performance of transesophageal echocardiograms in the learning process have included seminars, books, and video/DVDs. More recently, interactive computer programs and simulation have initiated a transformation in the educational environment. In 2009, most of the simulators were in the early phases of use and had yet to be formally evaluated. The Heartworks simulator and the EchocomTEE simulator are both examples of this technology. The Heartworks simulator uses an accurate 3D virtual heart and the 3D data set then generates a simulated ultrasound image.[8] This allows the user to develop the appropriate spatial anatomical knowledge required to accurately interpret the 2D ultrasound image. Similarly, the EchocomTEE simulator generates the 2D ultrasound images from a 3D data set.[9] Both of these systems have available a mannequin and a dummy TEE probe to practice probe steering and image acquisition with the added 3D guidance. One simulator was evaluated with respect to both realism and usefulness for TEE training as judged by experienced echocardiographers.[9] This group also evaluated novice echocardiographers as to the ease of use and the usefulness of the 3D image for 2D ultrasound image adjustment; 82% of the experts rated the mannequin as realistic and 68% rated the probe handling realistic. All of the experts thought that the simulator successfully established the relationship of the heart, probe, and multiplane ultrasound slice, and the resultant image. Thus, all of the experts would recommend the simulator as an additional aid in echocardiography training. For the novice group, 87% thought that the probe was easy to use and 90% found the virtual heart to be helpful in fine-tuning the image.

Table 27–3. Basic Cognitive Skills Required for Competence in Echocardiography.

Knowledge of physical principles of ultrasound image formation and blood flow velocity measurements
Knowledge of instrument settings required for image optimization
Knowledge of normal anatomy
Knowledge of fluid dynamics of normal blood flow
Knowledge of pathological changes in anatomy and blood flow due to acquired and congenital heart diseases

Adapted from Thys DM. Clinical competence in echocardiography. Anesth Analg. 2003;97:315.

THE FOCUSED BASIC EXAM WITH TEE EDUCATION

In 2006, the American Society for Anesthesiologists (ASA) formally requested a path for anesthesiologists who do not focus in cardiac anesthesia, to obtain experience and privileges in echocardiography as a basic perioperative monitor. Thus, the ASA and the SCA developed a plan for introductory CME courses to be made available four times a year. These are considered an introduction to perioperative echocardiography and teach practitioners the fundamental principles and applications necessary to perform a focused basic exam by transesophageal echocardiography (FBE-TEE). The course is designed for those who want to gain sufficient knowledge and experience to start to integrate basic TEE into clinical practice outside of cardiac surgery. Of note, the course includes a focus on determining which pathologies are appropriate to diagnose with just an introductory level of education and which require consultative assistance. For example, the diagnosis and treatment of hypovolemia would be appropriate with this basic level of training, but the interrogation of a prosthetic valve would require expert consultation. The ASA is also currently developing a Basic Perioperative

TEE examination with the NBE that will be administered for the first time in the fall of 2010. Relevant practice and certification requirements are also being developed with the goal of creating a pathway to attain a Diplomate status in Basic Perioperative Echocardiography (www.echoboards.org).

SUMMARY

The American Society of Echocardiography and the Society of Cardiovascular Anesthesiologists administer the PTEeXAM as a means to promote education, certify basic competence, and promote quality patient care. The exam process is designed to achieve the education necessary to make important clinical decisions based on echocardiographic imaging. In contrast, a new (not yet named) exam is being formulated that will serve to certify individuals in basic echocardiography competence utilizing the FBE-TEE educational process.

REFERENCES

1. Aronson S, Thys DM. Training and certification in perioperative transesophageal echocardiography: a historical perspective. *Anesth Analg.* 2001;93(6):1422-1427, table of contents.
2. Aronson S, Butler A, Subhiyah R, et al. Development and analysis of a new certifying examination in perioperative transesophageal echocardiography. *Anesth Analg.* 2002;95(6):1476-1482, table of contents.
3. National Board of Echocardiography: 2009 PTeXAM Application. http://www.echoboards.org (accessed January 29, 2009).
4. National Board of Echocardiography: 2009 PTeXAM Content Outline. http://www.echoboards.org/faq.html (accessed January 29, 2009).
5. National Board of Echocardiography. http://www.echoboards.org/faq.html (accessed January 29, 2009).
6. Thys DM. Clinical competence in echocardiography. *Anesth Analg.* 2003;97(2):313-322.
7. Shanewise JS, Cheung AT, Aronson S, et al. ASE/SCA guidelines for performing a comprehensive intraoperative multiplane transesophageal echocardiography examination: recommendations of the American Society of Echocardiography Council for Intraoperative Echocardiography and the Society of Cardiovascular Anesthesiologists Task Force for Certification in Perioperative Transesophageal Echocardiography. *J Am Soc Echocardiogr.* 1999;12(10):884-900.
8. Heartworks TEE Simulator. http://www.heartworks.me.uk (accessed February 8, 2009).
9. Weidenbach M, Drachsler H, Wild F, et al. EchoComTEE—a simulator for transoesophageal echocardiography. *Anaesthesia.* 2007;62(4):347-353.

Appendix A: Normal Chamber Dimensions

Structure		Measurement	View	Dimension[a] (cm)
Chambers	Left atrium[b]	Diameter (A)	ME4C or ME2C	2.7-4.0
	Right atrium[c]	Minor axis (B)	ME4C	2.9-4.5
	Left ventricle[d]	Wall thickness (septal) (C)	TGmidSAX	0.6-1.0
		Wall thickness inferolateral (D)	TGmidSAX	0.6-1.0
		Diameter (E)	ME2C or TG2C	3.9-5.9
	Right ventricle	Basal diameter (F)	ME4C	2.0-2.8
		Mid diameter (G)	ME4C	2.7-3.3
		Length (H)	ME4C	7.1-7.9
		Wall thickness (I)	ME4C or RV inflow-outflow	< 0.5
Tracts/Vessels	Right ventricular outflow	RVOT diameter (below PV) (J)	ME AV SAX or RV inflow-outflow	2.5-2.9
		RVOT diameter (above PV) (K)	ME AV SAX or RV inflow-outflow	1.7-2.3
	Aortic root[e]	Sinus of Valsalva (L)	ME AV LAX	2.6-4.0
	Pulmonary artery[f]	Diameter (M)	RV inflow-outflow	1.5-2.1
	Inferior vena cava[g]	Diameter	ME4C (modified)	1.2-1.7

[a]All dimensions are adapted from the ASE guidelines[1] and include the normal ranges for adult men and women.
[b]Left atrium (LA): The LA diameter cannot be reliably measured with TEE. Multiple views are recommended to obtain the diameter.
[c]Right atrium (RA): The RA should be measured from its lateral border to the interatrial septum. The TEE probe should be rotated slightly towards the right from the ME4C view to obtain optimal views of the RA.
[d]Left ventricle (LV): The diameter of the LV should be measured at end-diastole in the two chamber views to avoid foreshortening.
[e]Aortic root: Normal dimensions of the aortic root, LV outflow tract, and aortic annulus are highly variable and dependent on body size. Standardized nomograms have been published elsewhere.[2] These values represent ranges in aortic root diameter measured at the level of the sinus of Valsalva in individuals above 40 years.
[f]Pulmonary artery (PA): There are no standardized TEE views for measuring the PA diameter. These values are adapted from the transthoracic parasternal short-axis view.
[g]Inferior vena cava (IVC): There are no standardized TEE views for measuring the IVC diameter. The IVC may be measured 1 to 2 cm from its junction from the RA by rotating the TEE probe towards the right and withdrawing slightly from the ME4C view and following the IVC into the hepatic parenchyma.

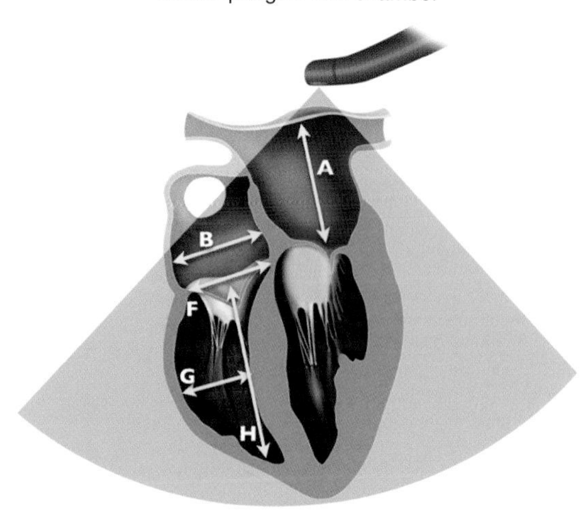

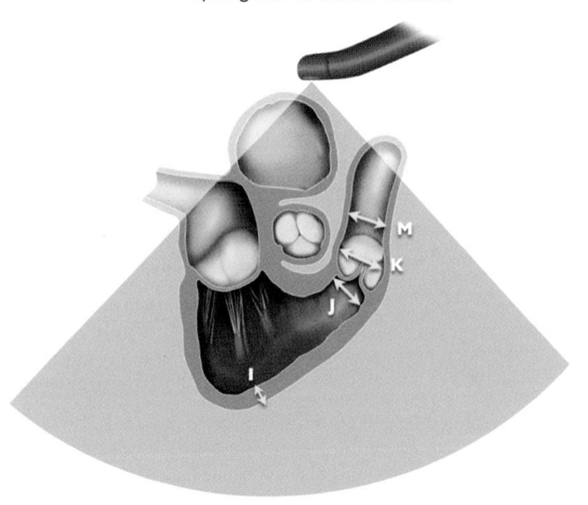

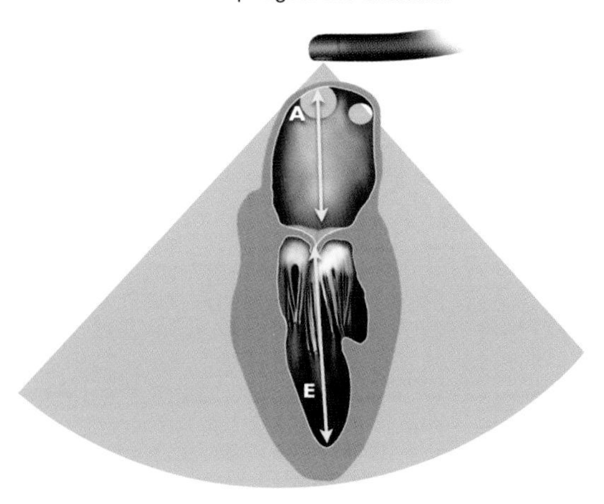

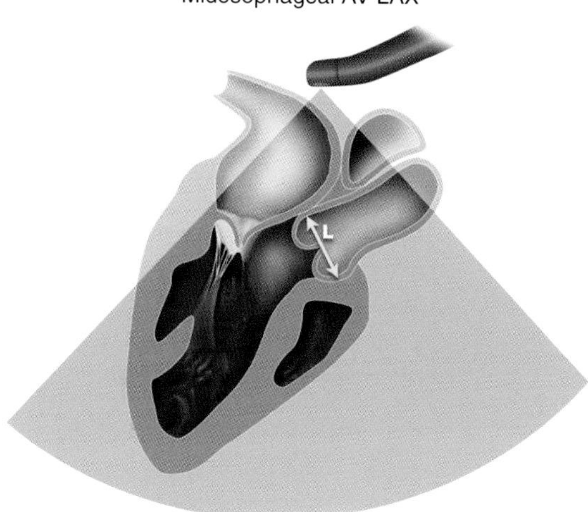

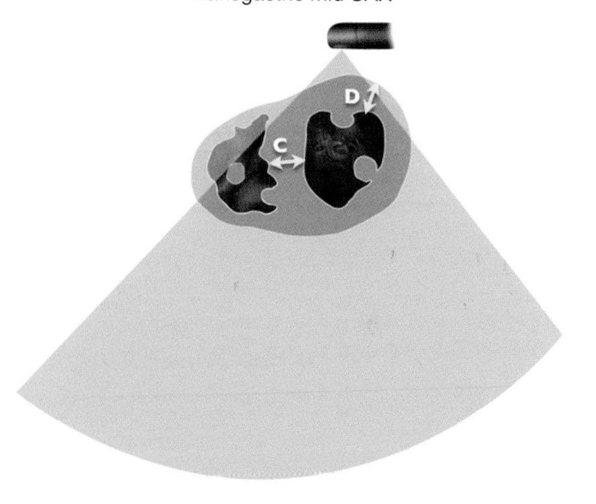

REFERENCES

1. Lang RM, Bierig M, Devereux RB, et al. Recommendations for chamber quantification: a report from the American Society of Echocardiography's Guidelines and Standards Committee and the Chamber Quantification Writing Group, developed in conjunction with the European Association of Echocardiography, a branch of the European Society of Cardiology. *J Am Soc Echocardiogr.* 2005;18:1440-1463.
2. Roman MJ, Devereux RB, Kramer-Fox R, O'Loughlin J. Two-dimensional echocardiographic aortic root dimensions in normal children and adults. *Am J Cardiol.* 1989;64:507-512.

Appendix B: Wall Motion and Coronary Perfusion

SEVENTEEN-SEGMENT MODEL OF THE LEFT VENTRICLE

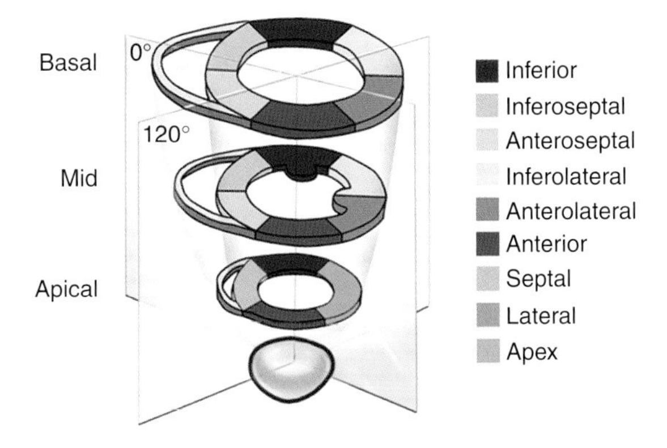

CORONARY PERFUSION IN THE LONG-AXIS VIEWS

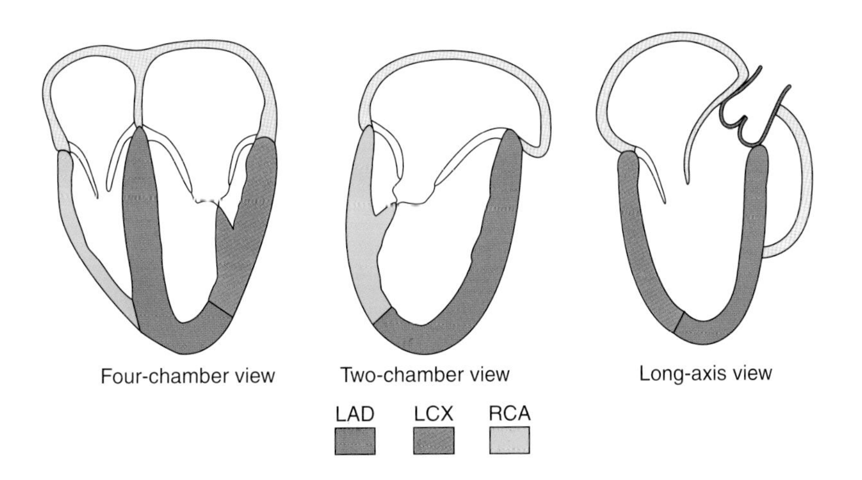

CORONARY PERFUSION IN THE SHORT-AXIS VIEWS

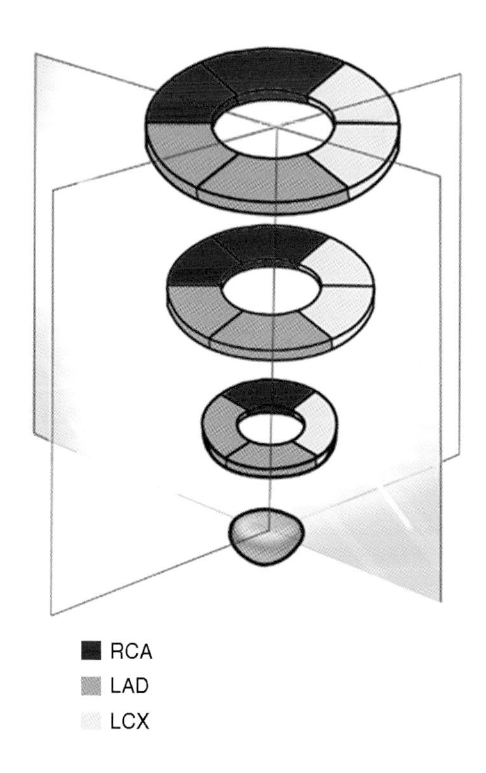

SCORING OF WALL MOTION ABNORMALITIES

Grade	Wall Thickening (%)	Radial Shortening[a] (%)
1 = Normal	>30	>30
2 = Mild hypokinesis	10-30	10-30
3 = Severe hypokinesis	<10	<10
4 = Akinesis	None	None
5 = Dyskinesis	Systolic thinning	Systolic increase in radius

[a]Radial shortening is defined as the percent shortening of an imaginary radius from the endocardial border to the center of the left ventricle

Appendix C: Diastolic Function

CLASSIFICATION OF DIFFERENT STAGES OF DIASTOLIC DYSFUNCTION

	Normal	Impaired Relaxation	Pseudonormal	Restrictive Filling
TMF				
E/A	0.8-1.5	<0.8	0.8-1.5	≥2
DT (ms)	150-220	>200	150-220	<160
IVRT (ms)	60-100	>100	>100	<60
PVF				
PV-S/PV-D	>1	>1	<1	<1
PV-AR (cm/s)	<35	<35	>35	>35
ARdur–Adur (ms)	<30	<30	>30	>30
Vp (cm/s)	>55	<45	<45	<45
E′ (cm/s)	>8 (septal)	>8 (septal)	<8 (septal)	<8 (septal)
	>10 (lateral)	>10 (lateral)	<10 (lateral)	<10 (lateral)
E/E′	<8	<8	9-12	>13
(see footnote a)				

[a] Average of septal and lateral velocities. TMF, transmitral flow; E, early filling peak velocity; A, late-filling peak velocity; DT, deceleration time of E wave; IVRT, isovolumic relaxation time; PV-S, peak velocity of systolic component; PV-D, peak velocity of diastolic component; PV-AR, peak velocity of atrial reversal flow; PV-ARdur, duration of atrial reversal flow; Adur, duration of A wave; PVF, pulmonary venous flow; E′, peak tissue velocity in early diastole; Vp, velocity of propagation.

ALGORITHM FOR GRADING DIASTOLIC DYSFUNCTION[1]

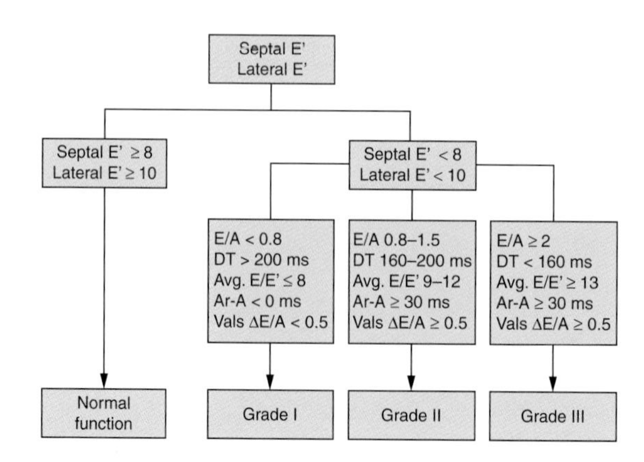

EFFECT OF AGE ON DOPPLER-DERIVED DIASTOLIC MEASUREMENTS

		Age Group (years)		
Doppler Parameter	**Measurement**	**<20**	**21-60[a]**	**>60**
Transmitral low	IVRT (ms)	50 ± 9	67-74	87 ± 7
	E/A ratio	1.9 ± 0.5	1.5-1.3	1.0 ± 0.2
	DT (ms)	142 ± 19	166-181	200 ± 29
	A dur (ms)	113 ± 17	127-133	138 ± 19
Pulmonary vein flow	S/D ratio	0.8 ± 0.18	1.0-1.2	1.4 ± 0.5
	Ar (cm/s)	16 ± 10	21-23	25 ± 9
	Ar dur (ms)	66 ± 39	96-112	113 ± 30
Lateral annulus tissue velocity	E′ (cm/s)	21 ± 3.8	20-16	13 ± 3.5
	E′/A′ ratio	3.1	1.9-1.5	0.9 ± 0.4

Values are expressed as mean ± standard deviation.
[a]For the age group 21-60, values are expressed as range of means.
A′, late lateral annulus tissue velocity; A, late transmitral velocity; Ar, pulmonary venous atrial reversal velocity; D, pulmonary venous diastolic velocity; DT, deceleration time; dur, duration; E′, early lateral annulus tissue velocity; E, early transmitral velocity; IVRT, isovolumic relaxation time; ms, milliseconds; S, pulmonary venous systolic velocity.

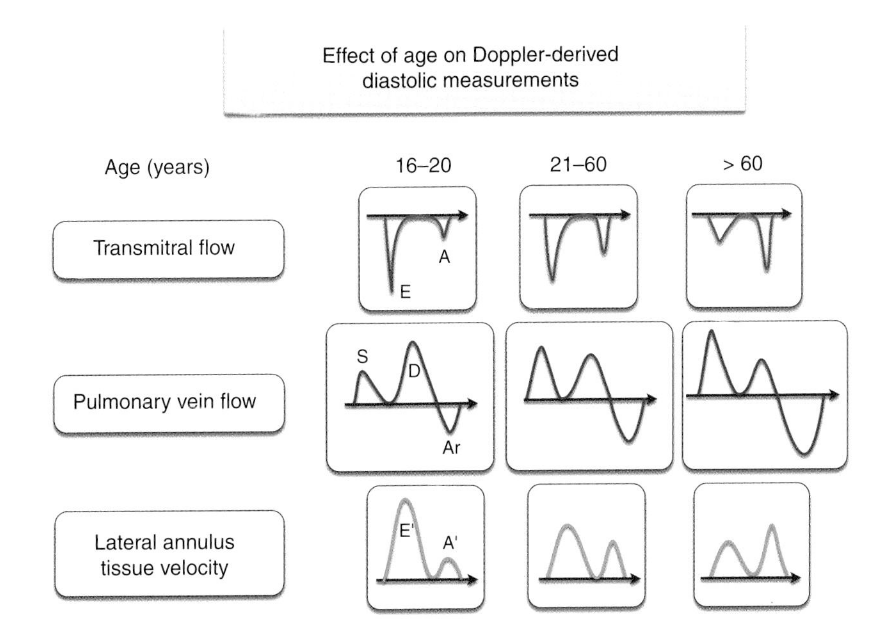

REFERENCE

1. Nagueh SF, Appleton CP, Gillebert TC, et al. Recommendations for the evaluation of left ventricular diastolic function by echocardiography. *J Am Soc Echocardiogr.* 2009;22:107-133.

Appendix D: Native Valve Areas, Velocities, and Gradients

NORMAL VALVE AREAS

Mitral valve	4-5 cm^2
Aortic valve	3-4 cm^2
Pulmonic valve	3.5-4.5 cm^2
Tricuspid valve	5-8 cm^2

MITRAL VALVE

Parameters for the Determination of the Severity of Mitral Regurgitation[1]

	Mild	**Moderate**	**Severe**
Structural Parameters			
LA size	Normal[a]	Normal or dilated	Usually dilated[b]
LV size	Normal[a]	Normal or dilated	Usually dilated[b]
Mitral leaflets or support apparatus	Normal or abnormal	Normal or abnormal	Abnormal, flail leaflet, or ruptured papillary muscle
Doppler Parameters			
Color flow jet area[c]	Small, central jet (usually <4 cm^2 or <20% of LA area)	Variable	Large central jet (usually >10 cm^2 or >40% of LA area) or variable size wall-impinging jet swirling in LA
Mitral inflow–PW	A-wave dominant[d]	Variable	E-wave dominant[d] (E usually 1.2 m/s)
Jet density–CW	Incomplete or faint	Dense	Dense
Jet contour–CW	Parabolic	Usually parabolic	Early peaking–triangular
Pulmonary vein flow	Systolic dominance[e]	Systolic blunting[e]	Systolic flow reversal[f]
Quantitative Parameters[g]			
VC width (cm)	<0.3	0.3-0.69	≥0.7
R Vol (mL/beat)	<30	30-44, 45-59	≥60
RF (%)	<30	30-39, 40-49	≥50
EROA (cm^2)	<0.20	0.20-0.29, 0.30-0.39	≥0.40

CW, continuous-wave Doppler; LA, left atrium; EROA, effective regurgitant orifice area; LV, left ventricle; PW, pulsed-wave Doppler; RF, regurgitant fraction; R Vol, regurgitant volume; VC, vena contracta.
[a]Unless there were other reasons for LA or LV dilation. Normal 2D measurements: LV minor axis ≤2.8 cm/m^2, LV end-diastolic volume ≤82 mL/m^2, maximal LA anteroposterior diameter ≤2 cm/m^2, maximal LA volume ≤36 mL/m^2.
[b]Exception: acute mitral regurgitation.
[c]At a Nyquist limit of 50-60 cm/s.
[d]Usually above 50 years of age or in conditions of impaired relaxation, in the absence of mitral stenosis or other causes of elevated LA pressure.
[e]Unless other reasons for systolic blunting (eg, atrial fibrillation, elevated left atrial pressure).
[f]Pulmonary venous systolic flow reversal is specific but not sensitive for severe MR.
[g]Quantitative parameters can help sub-classify the moderate regurgitation group into mild-to-moderate and moderate-to severe.

Calculation of the Quantitative Parameters of Mitral Regurgitation

1. ***Vena Contracta***

   Narrowest width of the mitral regurgitation jet as it *emerges* from the coaptation site of the leaflets

2. ***Regurgitant Volume***

   $$\text{Regurgitant Volume } (\text{RVol}_{\text{Mitral}}) = \text{SV}_{\text{MV}} - \text{SV}_{\text{LVOT}}$$
   $$\text{SV}_{\text{MV}} = \text{MV Annulus}_{\text{Area}} \times \text{Mitral Valve}_{\text{TVI}} \text{ (at the level of MV annulus)}$$
   $$\text{MV Annulus}_{\text{Area}} = (\text{Mitral Annulus Diameter})^2 \times 0.785$$
   $$\text{SV}_{\text{LVOT}} = \text{LVOT}_{\text{Area}} \times \text{LVOT}_{\text{TVI}}$$

3. ***Regurgitant Fraction***

   $$\text{Regurgitant Fraction (RFMitral)} = \left(\frac{\text{RVol}_{\text{Mitral}}}{\text{SV}_{\text{MV}}}\right) \times 100$$

4. ***Effective Regurgitant Orifice Area (EROA)***

   $$\text{EROA}_{\text{Mitral}} = \frac{\text{RVol}_{\text{Mitral}}}{\text{TVI of the Mitral Regurgitant Jet}}$$

5. ***Proximal Isovelocity Surface Area***

   $\text{Flow Rate} = 2\pi r^2 v$

   r = Radius of the proximal isovelocity contour, in cm

   v = Aliasing velocity, in cm/s

   EROA = Flow Rate/V

   V = Maximal velocity of the mitral regurgitant jet by CW, in cm/s

   $\text{RVol}_{\text{Mitral}} = \text{EROA} \times \text{CW TVI of the Mitral Regurgitation Jet}$

Parameters for the Determination of the Severity of Mitral Stenosis[2]

Indicator	Mild	Moderate	Severe
Mean pressure gradient (mm Hg)	<5	5-10	>10
Pressure half-time (ms)	90-150	150-219	>220
Mitral valve area (cm^2)	>1.5	1.0-1.5	<1.0
Pulmonary artery pressure (mm Hg)	<30	30-50	>50
Mitral valve resistance ($dyne.s.cm^{-5}$)			>85

Methods for Determining Mitral Valve Area (MVA)

1. ***Planimetry***

   Tracing the mitral orifice obtained from the TG basal SAX view

2. ***Pressure Gradient***

   Tracing the entire envelope of the CWD spectrum of mitral inflow, from the beginning of early diastolic flow (E wave) to the end of flow due to atrial contraction (A wave)

3. ***Pressure Half-time ($P_{1/2T}$)***

$$\text{MVA (cm}^2\text{)} = \frac{220}{P_{1/2T}}$$

4. ***Deceleration Time***

$$\text{MVA (cm}^2\text{)} = \frac{759}{\text{Deceleration Time (ms)}}$$

5. ***Continuity Equation***

   1—Determine the diameter (D) of the LVOT in the ME LAX view: Cross-Sectional Area (CSA_{LVOT}) = 0.785* D^2

   2—Utilizing the PW Doppler in the transgastric view, determine the VTI in the LVOT: VTI_{LVOT}

   3—In the midesophageal four-chamber view, determine the VTI of the mitral valve: VTI_{MV}

$$\text{MVA (cm}^2\text{)} = \frac{CSA_{LVOT}\ (\text{cm}^2)^*\ VTI_{LVOT}\ (\text{cm})}{VTI_{MV}\ (\text{cm})}$$

6. ***Proximal Isovelocity Surface Area (PISA)***

$$\text{MVA} = \frac{(\text{PISA} * \text{Velocity}_{\text{Aliasing}})}{\text{Peak Velocity}_{\text{Transmitral}}}$$

   where PISA (surface area of the hemisphere) = 2π * (radius of the shell)^2 * $\alpha/180$,

   where α = Angle subtended by the mitral leaflets

Echo Score Index for Rheumatic Mitral Stenosis[3]

Grades	Mobility	Leaflet Thickening	Subvalvular Thickening	Calcification
1	Highly mobile valve, only leaflet tips are restricted	Normal thickness (4-5 mm)	Minimal thickening just below leaflets	Single area of increased echo brightness
2	Leaflet mid and base portions have normal mobility	Mid leaflets are normal, marked thickening of margins (5-8 mm)	Thickening of chordal structures extending up to one-third chordal length	Scattered areas of brightness confined to margins
3	Valve continues to move forward in diastole	Entire leaflet is thickened (5-8 mm)	Thickening of chordal structures to the distal one-third	Brightness to midportions of leaflets and leaflet margins
4	No or minimal movement forward	All leaflet tissue has marked thickening (>8-10 mm)	Extensive thickening and shortening of all chordal structures down to papillary muscles	Extensive brightness through much of leaflet tissue

AORTIC VALVE

Parameters for the Determination of the Severity of Aortic Regurgitation[1]

	Mild	Moderate	Severe
Structural Parameters			
LA size	Normal[a]	Normal or dilated	Usually dilated[b]
Aortic leaflets	Normal or abnormal	Normal or abnormal	Abnormal, flail, or wide coaptation defect
Doppler Parameters			
Jet width in LVOT–color flow[c]	Small in central jets	Intermediate	Large in central jets; variable in eccentric jets
Jet density–CW	Incomplete or faint	Dense	Dense
Jet deceleration rate–CW (PHT, ms)[d]	Slow >500	Medium 500-200	Steep <200
Diastolic flow reversal in descending aorta–PW	Brief, early diastolic reversal	Intermediate	Prominent holodiastolic reversal
Quantitative Parameters[e]			
VC width (cm)[c]	<0.3	0.3-0.60	>0.6
Jet width/LVOT width (%)[c]	<25	25-45, 46-64	≥65
Jet CSA/LVOT CSA (%)[c]	<5	5-20, 21-59	≥60
R Vol (mL/beat)	<30	30-44, 45-59	≥60
RF (%)	<30	30-39, 40-49	≥50
EROA (cm^2)	<0.10	0.10-0.19, 0.20-0.29	≥0.30

AR, aortic regurgitation; CSA, cross-sectional area; CW, continuous-wave Doppler; EROA, effective regurgitant orifice area; LV, left ventricle; LVOT, left ventricular outflow tract; PHT, pressure half-time; PW, pulsed-wave Doppler; R Vol, regurgitant volume; RF, regurgitant fraction; VC, vena contracta.

[a]Unless there were other reasons for LV dilation. Normal 2D measurements: LV minor axis ≤2.8 cm/m^2.

[b]Exception would be acute AR, in which chambers have not had time to dilate.

[c]At a Nyquist limit of 50-60 cm/s.

[d]PHT is shortened with increasing LV diastolic pressure and vasodilator therapy, and may be lengthened in chronic adaptation to severe AR.

[e]Quantitative parameters can sub-classify the moderate regurgitation group into mild-to-moderate and moderate-to-severe regurgitation as shown.

Calculation of the Quantitative Parameters of Aortic Regurgitation

1. ***Vena Contracta***

   Narrowest width of the aortic regurgitation jet at or just distal to the orifice

2. ***Regurgitant Volume***

   $$\text{Regurgitant Volume } (RVol_{Aortic}) = SV_{LVOT} - SV_{MV}$$

   $$SV_{MV} = \text{MV Annulus}_{Area} \times \text{Mitral Valve}_{TVI} \text{ (at the level of MV annulus)}$$

   $$\text{MV Annulus}_{Area} = (\text{Mitral Annulus Diameter})^2 \times 0.785$$

   $$SV_{LVOT} = LVOT_{Area} \times LVOT_{TVI}$$

3. ***Regurgitant Fraction***

   $$\text{Regurgitant Fraction } (RF_{Aortic}) = \left(\frac{RVol_{Aortic}}{SV_{LVOT}}\right) \times 100$$

4. ***Effective Regurgitant Orifice Area (EROA)***

   $$EROA_{Aortic} = \frac{RVol_{Aortic}}{\text{TVI of the Aortic Regurgitant Jet}}$$

Parameters for the Determination of the Severity of Aortic Stenosis[2]

Indicator	Mild	Moderate	Severe
Peak jet velocity (m/s)	<3.0	3.0-4.0	>4.0
Mean gradient (mm Hg)	<20	20-40	>40
Aortic valve area (cm^2)	>1.5	1.0-1.5	<1.0
Dimensionless index	>0.50	0.25-0.50	<0.25
Indexed valve area (cm^2/m^2)	>0.85	0.60-0.85	<0.6

Methods for Determining Aortic Valve Area (AVA)

1. ***Planimetry***

   Tracing the aortic orifice obtained from the ME AV SAX view

2. ***Pressure Gradient***

   Tracing the CWD spectral envelope of the of the flow across the aortic valve obtained in the TG LAX or deep TG LAX views and applying the Bernoulli equation

   Modified Bernoulli: $\Delta P = 4 (V_2^2 - V_1^2)$ where

   V_2 = Transvalvular velocity

   V_1 = Subvalvular (LVOT) velocity

   Simplified Bernoulli: $\Delta P = 4 V_2^2$ if $V_1 < 1.5$ m/s

3. ***Aortic Valve Area (AVA) Using the Continuity Equation***

   1—Determine the diameter (D) of the LVOT in the ME LAX view.
   Cross-sectional area $(CSA_{LVOT}) = 0.785 * D^2$

   2—Utilizing the CW Doppler in the transgastric view, determine the VTI in the ascending aorta: VTI_{Aorta}

   3—Utilizing the PW Doppler in the transgastric view, determine the VTI in the LVOT: VTI_{LVOT}

   $$AVA\ (cm^2) = \frac{(CSA_{LVOT})\ (cm^2) * VTI_{LVOT}\ (cm)}{VTI_{Aorta}\ (cm)}$$

PULMONIC VALVE

Parameters for the Determination of the Severity of Pulmonary Regurgitation[1]

Parameter	Mild	Moderate	Severe
Pulmonic valve	Normal	Normal or abnormal	Abnormal
RV size	Normal[a]	Normal or dilated	Dilated[b]
Jet size by color Doppler[c]	Thin (usually <10 mm in length) with a narrow origin	Intermediate	Usually large, with a wide origin; may be brief in duration
Jet density and deceleration rate–CW[d]	Soft; slow deceleration	Dense; variable deceleration	Dense; steep deceleration, early termination of diastolic flow
Pulmonic systolic flow compared to systemic flow–PW[e]	Slightly increased	Intermediate	Greatly increased

CW, continuous-wave Doppler; PR, pulmonic regurgitation; PW, pulsed-wave Doppler; RA, right atrium; RF, regurgitant fraction; RV, right ventricle.

[a]Unless there are other reasons for RV enlargement. Normal 2D measurements from the apical four-chamber view: RV mediolateral end-diastolic dimension ≤4.3 cm, RV end-diastolic area ≤35.5cm^2.

[b]Exception: acute PR.

[c]At a Nyquist limit of 50-60 cm/s.

[d]Steep deceleration is not specific for severe PR.

[e]Cutoff values for regurgitant volume and fraction are not well validated.

Method for Determining Pulmonic Valve Area

Pressure Gradient
Tracing the CWD spectral envelope of the flow across the pulmonic valve obtained in the UE aortic arch SAX view and applying the Bernoulli equation.

Parameters for the Determination of the Severity of Pulmonary Stenosis[2]

	Stenosis Severity		
	Mild	Moderate	Severe
Two-dimensional findings			
Leaflet morphology	Usually normal	Thickening	Thickening +/– calcifications
Leaflet mobility	Normal	Moderately restricted	Severely restricted; doming
RV hypertrophy	Usually absent		Usually present
Doppler findings			
Color Doppler			Turbulent outflow
Peak velocity (m/s)	<3	3-4	>4
Peak gradient (mm Hg)	<36	36-64	>64

TRICUSPID VALVE

Parameters for the Determination of the Severity of Tricuspid Regurgitation[1]

Parameter	Mild	Moderate	Severe
Tricuspid valve	Usually normal	Normal or abnormal	Abnormal, flail leaflet, poor coaptation
RV/RA/IVC size	Normal[a]	Normal or dilated	Usually dilated[b]
Jet area–central jets (cm^2)[c]	<5	5-10	>10
VC width (cm)[d]	Not defined	Not defined, but <0.7	>0.7
PISA radius (cm)[e]	≤0.5	0.6-0.9	>0.9
Jet density and contour–CW	Soft and parabolic	Dense, variable contour	Dense, triangular with early peaking
Hepatic vein flow[f]	Systolic dominance	Systolic blunting	Systolic reversal

CW, continuous-wave Doppler; IVC, inferior vena cava; RA, right atrium; RV, right ventricle; VC, vena contracta.
[a]Unless there are other reasons for RA or RV dilation. Normal 2D measurements from the apical four-chamber view: RV mediolateral end-diastolic dimension ≤4.3 cm; RV end-diastolic area ≤35.5cm^2; maximal RA mediolateral and superoinferior dimensions ≤4.6 cm and 4.9 cm, respectively; maximal RA volume ≤33 mL/m^2.
[b]Exception: acute TR.
[c]At a Nyquist limit of 50-60 cm/s. Not valid in eccentric jets. Jet area is not recommended as the sole parameter of TR severity due to its dependence on hemodynamic and technical factors.
[d]At a Nyquist limit of 50-60 cm/s.
[e]Baseline shift with Nyquist limit of 28 cm/s.
[f]Other conditions may cause systolic bunting (eg, atrial fibrillation, elevated RA pressure).

Method for Determining Tricuspid Valve Area (TVA)

Pressure Gradient
Tracing the entire envelope of the CWD spectrum of tricuspid inflow, from the beginning of early diastolic flow (E wave) to the end of flow due to atrial contraction (A wave).

Parameters for the Determination of the Severity of Tricuspid Stenosis[2]

	Stenosis Severity		
	Mild	**Moderate**	**Severe**
Two-dimensional findings			
Leaflet morphology	Usually normal	Thickening	Thickening +/– calcifications
Leaflet mobility	Normal	Moderately restricted	Severely restricted; doming
Right-side chambers	Can be normal	Dilated	Significantly dilated
Doppler findings			
Color Doppler			Turbulent inflow
Inflow velocity (m/s)	<0.7	>0.7	>>0.7
Mean diastolic gradient	≤2		≥5
Pressure half-time			≥190 ms
Area by continuity equation			≤1 cm^2

REFERENCES

1. Zoghbi WA, Enriquez-Sarano M, Foster E, et al. Recommendations for evaluation of the severity of native valvular regurgitation with two-dimensional and Doppler echocardiography. *J Am Soc Echocardiogr.* 2003;16:777-802.
2. Baumgartner H, Hung J, Bermejo J, et al. Echocardiographic assessment of valve stenosis: EAE/ASE recommendations for clinical practice. *J Am Soc Echocardiogr.* 2009;22:1-23; quiz 101-102.
3. Wilkins GT, Weyman AE, Abascal VM, Block PC, Palacios IF. Percutaneous balloon dilatation of the mitral valve: an analysis of echocardiographic variables related to outcome and the mechanism of dilatation. *Br Heart J.* 1988;60:299-308.

Appendix E: Measurements and Calculations

LEFT VENTRICLE:

1. Fractional shortening (%) =

$$\frac{\text{(end-diastolic diameter)} - \text{(end-systolic diameter)}}{\text{(end-diastolic diameter)}} \times 100$$

2. Velocity of circumferential fiber shortening (circ/sec) =

$$\text{fractional shortening} \times \text{ejection time}$$

3. Fractional area change (%) =

$$\frac{\text{(end-diastolic area)} - \text{(end-systolic area)}}{\text{(end-diastolic area)}} \times 100$$

4. Ejection fraction (%) =

$$\frac{\text{(end-diastolic volume)} - \text{(end-systolic volume)}}{\text{(end-diastolic volume)}} \times 100$$

5. Volume by Simpson's method of disks where the LV is modeled as a series of stacked cylindrical disks capped by an elliptical disk apex

$$\text{Volume}_{\text{cylindrical disks}} = (\pi \times D_1/2) \times D_2/2) \times H$$

where D_1 and D_2 are orthogonal diameters of the cylinder, and H is the height of the cylinder

and

$$\text{Volume}_{\text{elliptical disk}} = Ah/2 + a^2/b^2 \times \pi \times h^3/6$$

where A is the area of the ellipsoid segment, h is the height of the ellipsoid segment, and a and b are radii of the total ellipsoid.

6. Volume by the area-length method where the LV is modeled as a cylinder–hemi-ellipsoid

$$\text{Volume} = (5 \times \text{area} \times \text{major-axis length})/6$$

where the area is planimetered by using a short-axis view at the level of the mitral valve

7. Volume by the diameter-length method where the LV is modeled as a prolate-ellipsoid

$$\text{Volume} = (\pi \times D1 \times D2 \times \text{major-axis length})/6$$

where $D1$ and $D2$ are orthogonal short-axis diameters

8. Stroke volume (ml) =

$$\text{(end-diastolic volume} - \text{end-systolic volume)}$$

9. Cardiac output (liters/min) = (stroke volume × heart rate)

10. Cardiac index (liters/min/m^2) =

$$\frac{\text{(stroke volume} \times \text{heart rate)}}{\text{body surface area}}$$

11. Meriodinal wall stress

$$\sigma_m = 1.33 \times P\,(A_c/A_m) \times 10^3 \text{ dyne/cm}^2$$

where P represents LV peak pressure, A_c is LV cavity area, and A_m represents LV myocardial area (area of the muscle in the short-axis view)

12. Circumferential wall stress

$$\sigma_c = \left[\frac{(1.33P\sqrt{A_c})}{(\sqrt{A_m + A_c} - \sqrt{A_c})}\right] \times \left[1 - \frac{(4A_c\sqrt{A_c}/\pi L^2)}{(\sqrt{A_m + A_c} + \sqrt{A_c})}\right] \text{dyne/cm}^2$$

where L represents the LV long-axis length

13. Strain (%) =

$$\frac{\text{length} - \text{length}_0}{\text{length}_0}$$

where length_0 is the initial length

14. Strain rate (s^{-1}) =

$$\frac{\text{strain}}{\text{time}}$$

15. LV mass (g) =

$$(1.04 \times [(LVID + PWT + IVST)^3 - LVID^3]) \times 0.8 + 0.6$$

16. dP/dt (mm Hg/s) =

$$32 \times 1000/dt$$

where dt (in msec) is the time for velocity to rise from 1 m/s to 3 m/s on a continuous wave Doppler tracing of mitral regurgitation

17. Myocardial performance index =

$$\frac{\text{(isovolumic contraction time + isovolumic relaxation time)}}{\text{(ejection time)}}$$

RIGHT VENTRICLE

1. Fractional area change (%) =

$$\left[\frac{\text{(end-diastolic area)} - \text{(end-systolic area)}}{\text{end-diastolic area}}\right] \times 100$$

2. Ejection fraction (%) =

$$\frac{\text{(end-diastolic volume)} - \text{(end-systolic volume)}}{\text{(end-diastolic volume)}} \times 100$$

using Simpson's method of disks

3. Tricuspid annular plane systolic excursion (mm)
From the transgastric RV inflow view and using M-mode, the movement of the leading edge of the lateral tricuspid annulus attachment is tracked during systole, and its excursion measured

4. Myocardial performance index =

$$\frac{\text{(isovolumic contraction time + isovolumic relaxation time)}}{\text{(ejection time)}}$$

5. dP/dt (mm Hg/s) =

$$12 \times 1000/dt$$

where dt (in msec) is the time for velocity to rise from 1 m/s to 2 m/s on a continuous wave Doppler tracing of tricuspid regurgitation

DOPPLER-BASED CALCULATIONS:

1. Doppler shift

$$\Delta f = \frac{2f_t \times (v \times \cos\theta)}{c}$$

Δf = Difference between the transmitted frequency (f_t) and received frequency
v = Velocity of red blood cells
θ = Angle between the Doppler beam and the direction of blood flow
c = Speed of ultrasound in blood (1540m/sec)

2. Stroke volume (ml) =

Stroke Distance × Cross Sectional Area (CSA)

where

Stroke Distance = LVOT or RVOT Velocity Time Integral (VTI)

$$CSA = 0.785 \times (\text{LVOT or RVOT Diameter})^2$$

3. Shunt ratios

$Qp/Qs = SV_{RVOT} / SV_{LVOT}$ (for atrial or ventricular septal defects)

$Qp/Qs = SV_{LVOT} / SV_{RVOT}$ (for patent ductus arteriosus)

4. Valve area by conservation of flow

$$\text{Aortic valve area} = \frac{(CSA_{LVOT} \times VTI_{LVOT})}{VTI_{\text{Aortic Valve}}}$$

$$\text{Mitral valve area} = \frac{(CSA_{LVOT} \times VTI_{LVOT})}{VTI_{\text{Mitral Valve}}}$$

5. Mitral valve area by pressure half-time

$$\text{Mitral valve area} = \frac{220}{\text{Pressure half-time}}$$

where

Pressure half-time is measured or calculated as 0.29 × Deceleration time

6. Valve area by flow acceleration

$$CSA_{stenotic\ orifice} = \frac{PISA \times velocity_{aliasing}}{peak\ velocity_{orifice}}$$

$$\text{Mitral valve area} = \frac{2\pi r^2 \times velocity_{aliasing}}{peak\ velocity_{transmitral}}$$

where

r = PISA radius

7. Regurgitant volume (ml)

$$\text{Regurgitant Volume}_{Mitral\ Valve} = SV_{Mitral\ Valve} - SV_{LVOT}$$
$$= (CSA_{Mitral} \times VTI_{Mitral}) - (CSA_{LVOT} \times VTI_{LVOT})$$

$$\text{Regurgitant Volume}_{Aortic\ Valve} = SV_{LVOT} - SV_{Mitral\ Valve}$$
$$= (CSA_{LVOT} \times VTI_{LVOT}) - (CSA_{Mitral} \times VTI_{Mitral})$$

8. Regurgitant fraction (%) =

$$\frac{\text{Regurgitant Volume}_{Valve}}{\text{Stroke Volume}_{Valve}} \times 100$$

9. Effective Regurgitant Orifice Area (EROA) =

$$\frac{\text{Regurgitant Volume}_{Mitral\ Valve}}{VTI_{Mitral\ regurgitant\ jet}}$$

OR

$$\frac{2\pi r^2 \times velocity_{aliasing}}{peak\ velocity_{mitral\ regurgitant\ jet}}$$

where

r = PISA radius

10. Bernoulli Equation

Pressure Difference = Convective Acceleration + Flow Acceleration + Viscous Friction

or

$$P_1 - P_2 = \Delta P = 1/2\rho\,(V_2^2 - V_1^2) + \rho\int_1^2 \frac{dv}{dt}\,ds + R(\mu, v)$$

$P_1 - P_2$ = Pressure difference between the two locations
ρ = Mass density of blood (gm/cm^3)
V_1 = Velocity proximal to stenosis (m/sec)
V_2 = Velocity at vena contracta (m/sec)
$\frac{dv}{dt}$ = Acceleration
s = Distance over which flow accelerates
R = Viscous resistance
μ = Viscosity
v = Velocity of blood flow (m/sec)

11. Modified Bernoulli equation

$$\Delta P = 4(V_2^2 - V_1^2)$$

12. Simplified Bernoulli equation

$$\Delta P = 4V_2^2$$

13. Peak instantaneous gradient =

$$4 \times (V_{Peak})^2$$

14. Intracardiac pressure measurements

$$P_{OC} = 4v^2 + P_{RC}$$

$$P_{RC} = P_{OC} - 4v^2$$

where

P_{OC} = pressure in the origination chamber
P_{RC} = pressure in the receiving chamber

15. Right ventricular systolic pressure (RVSP) using tricuspid regurgitant (TR) jet

$$RVSP = 4\,(V_{Peak\ TR})^2 + \text{right atrial pressure (CVP)}$$

In the absence of pulmonic stenosis or right ventricular outflow tract obstruction, RVSP is equal to pulmonary artery systolic pressure.

16. Right ventricular systolic pressure in the presence of a ventricular septal defect (VSD)

$$RVSP = \text{Left ventricular systolic pressure} - 4\,(V_{Peak\ VSD})^2$$

17. Pulmonary artery mean pressures (PAMP) using pulmonary regurgitant (PR) jet

$$PAMP = 4\,(V_{Peak\ PR})^2 + \text{right atrial pressure (CVP)}$$

18. Pulmonary artery diastolic pressures (PADP) using pulmonary regurgitant (PR) jet

$$PADP = 4\,(V_{End\text{-}diastolic\ PR})^2 + \text{right atrial pressure (CVP)}$$

19. Pulmonary artery systolic pressure (PASP) in the presence of a patent ductus arteriosus (PDA)

$$PASP = \text{Systolic blood pressure} - 4\,(V_{Peak\ PDA})^2$$

20. Left atrial pressure (LAP) from a mitral regurgitant (MR) jet

$$LAP = \text{Left ventricular systolic pressure} - 4\,(V_{Peak\ MR})^2$$

In the absence of aortic stenosis or left ventricular outflow tract obstruction, systolic blood pressure can be substituted for left ventricular systolic pressure.

21. Left atrial pressure in the presence of a patent foramen ovale (PFO).

$$LAP = 4\,(V_{Peak\ PFO})^2 + \text{right atrial pressure (CVP)}$$

22. Left ventricular end-diastolic pressure (LVEDP) from an aortic regurgitatant (AR) jet.

$$LVEDP = \text{Diastolic blood pressure} - 4\,(V_{End\text{-}diastolic\ AR})^2$$

Appendix F: Normal Doppler Echocardiographic Values for Prosthetic Aortic Valves

Valve	Size	Peak Gradient (mm Hg)	Mean Gradient (mm Hg)	Effective Orifice Area (cm²)
ATS *Bileaflet*	19	47.0 ± 12.6	25.3 ± 8.0	1.1 ± 0.3
	21	23.7 ± 6.8	15.9 ± 5.0	1.4 ± 0.5
	23		14.4 ± 4.9	1.7 ± 0.5
	25		11.3 ± 3.7	2.1 ± 0.7
	27		8.4 ± 3.7	2.5 ± 0.1
	29		8.0 ± 3.0	3.1 ± 0.8
ATS AP *Bileaflet*	18		21.0 ± 1.8	1.2 ± 0.3
	20	21.4 ± 4.2	11.1 ± 3.5	1.3 ± 0.3
	22	18.7 ± 8.3	10.5 ± 4.5	1.7 ± 0.4
	24	15.1 ± 5.6	7.5 ± 3.1	2.0 ± 0.6
	26		6.0 ± 2.0	2.1 ± 0.4
Baxter Perimount *Stented bovine pericardial*	19	32.5 ± 8.5	19.5 ± 5.5	1.3 ± 0.2
	21	24.9 ± 7.7	13.8 ± 4.0	1.3 ± 0.3
	23	19.9 ± 7.4	11.5 ± 3.9	1.6 ± 0.3
	25	16.5 ± 7.8	10.7 ± 3.8	1.6 ± 0.4
	27	12.8 ± 5.4	4.8 ± 2.2	2.0 ± 0.4
Biocor *Stented porcine*	23	30.0 ± 10.7	20 ± 6.6	1.3 ± 0.3
	25	23.0 ± 7.9	16 ± 5.1	1.7 ± 0.4
	27	22.0 ± 6.5	15.0 ± 3.7	2.2 ± 0.4
Extended Biocor *Stentless*	19-21	17.5 ± 6.5	9.6 ± 3.6	1.4 ± 0.4
	23	14.7 ± 7.3	7.7 ± 3.8	1.7 ± 0.4
	25	14.0 ± 4.3	7.4 ± 2.5	1.8 ± 0.4
Bioflo *Stented bovine pericardial*	19	37.2 ± 8.8	26.4 ± 5.5	0.7 ± 0.1
	21	28.7 ± 6.2	18.7 ± 5.5	1.1 ± 0.1
Bjork-Shiley *Single tilting disc*	21	38.9 ± 11.9	21.8 ± 3.4	1.1 ± 0.3
	23	28.8 ± 11.2	15.7 ± 5.3	1.3 ± 0.3
	25	23.7 ± 8.2	13.0 ± 5.0	1.5 ± 0.4
	27		10.0 ± 2.0	1.6 ± 0.3
Carbomedics Reduced *Bileaflet*	19	43.4 ± 1.2	24.4 ± 1.2	1.2 ± 0.1

(Continued)

Valve	Size	Peak Gradient (mm Hg)	Mean Gradient (mm Hg)	Effective Orifice Area (cm²)
Carbomedics Standard	19	38.0 ± 12.8	18.9 ± 8.3	1.0 ± 0.3
Bileaflet	21	26.8 ± 10.1	12.9 ± 5.4	1.5 ± 0.4
	23	22.5 ± 7.4	11.0 ± 4.6	1.4 ± 0.3
	25	19.6 ± 7.8	9.1 ± 3.5	1.8 ± 0.4
	27	17.5 ± 7.1	7.9 ± 3.2	2.2 ± 0.2
	29	9.1 ± 4.7	5.6 ± 3.0	3.2 ± 1.6
Carbomedics Tophat	21	30.2 ± 10.9	14.9 ± 5.4	1.2 ± 0.3
Bileaflet	23	24.2 ± 7.6	12.5 ± 4.4	1.4 ± 0.4
	25		9.5 ± 2.9	1.6 ± 0.32
Carpentier Edwards	19	32.1 ± 3.4	24.2 ± 8.6	1.2 ± 0.3
Pericardial	21	25.7 ± 9.9	20.3 ± 9.1	1.5 ± 0.4
Stented bovine pericardial	23	21.7 ± 8.6	13.0 ± 5.3	1.8 ± 0.3
	25	16.5 ± 5.4	9.0 ± 2.3	
Carpentier Edwards	19	43.5 ± 12.7	25.6 ± 8.0	0.9 ± 0.2
Standard	21	27.7 ± 7.6	17.3 ± 6.2	1.5 ± 0.3
Stented porcine	23	28.9 ± 7.5	16.1 ± 6.2	1.7 ± 0.5
	25	24.0 ± 7.1	12.9 ± 4.6	1.9 ± 0.5
	27	22.1 ± 8.2	12.1 ± 5.5	2.3 ± 0.6
	29		9.9 ± 2.9	2.8 ± 0.5
Carpentier Supra-Annular	19	34.1 ± 2.7		1.1 ± 0.1
Stented porcine	21	28.0 ± 10.5	17.5 ± 3.8	1.4 ± 0.9
	23	25.3 ± 10.5	13.4 ± 4.5	1.6 ± 0.6
	25	24.4 ± 7.6	13.2 ± 4.8	1.8 ± 0.4
	27	16.7 ± 4.7	8.8 ± 2.8	1.9 ± 0.7
Cryolife	19		9.0 ± 2.0	1.5 ± 0.3
Stentless	21		6.6 ± 2.9	1.7 ± 0.4
	23		6.0 ± 2.3	2.3 ± 0.2
	25		6.1 ± 2.6	2.6 ± 0.2
	27		4.0 ± 2.4	2.8 ± 0.3
Edwards Duromedics	21	39.0 ± 13		
Bileaflet	23	32.0 ± 8.0		
	25	26.0 ± 10.0		
	27	24.0 ± 10.0		
Edwards Mira	19		18.2 ± 5.3	1.2 ± 0.4
Bileaflet	21		13.3 ± 4.3	1.6 ± 0.4
	23		14.7 ± 2.8	1.6 ± 0.6
	25		13.1 ± 3.8	1.9
Hancock	21	18.0 ± 6.0	12.0 ± 2.0	
Stented porcine	23	16.0 ± 2.0	11.0 ± 2.0	
	25	15.0 ± 3.0	10.0 ± 3.0	
Hancock II	21		14.8 ± 4.1	1.3 ± 0.4
Stented porcine	23	34.0 ± 13.0	16.6 ± 8.5	1.3 ± 0.4
	25	22.0 ± 5.3	10.8 ± 2.8	1.6 ± 0.4
	29	16.2 ± 1.5	8.2 ± 1.7	1.6 ± 0.2

(Continued)

Valve	Size	Peak Gradient (mm Hg)	Mean Gradient (mm Hg)	Effective Orifice Area (cm^2)
Homograft	17-19		9.7 ± 4.2	4.2 ± 1.8
Homograft valves	19-21			5.4 ± 0.9
	20-21		7.9 ± 4.0	3.6 ± 2.0
	20-22		7.2 ± 3.0	3.5 ± 1.5
	22	1.7 ± 0.3		5.8 ± 3.2
	22-23		5.6 ± 3.1	2.6 ± 1.4
	22-24			5.6 ± 1.7
	24-27		6.2 ± 2.6	2.8 ± 1.1
	26	1.4 ± 0.6		6.8 ± 2.9
	25-28			6.2 ± 2.5
Intact	19	40.4 ± 15.4	24.5 ± 9.3	
Stented porcine	21	40.9 ± 15.6	19.6 ± 8.1	1.6 ± 0.4
	23	32.7 ± 9.6	19.0 ± 6.1	1.6 ± 0.4
	25	29.7 ± 15.0	17.7 ± 7.9	1.7 ± 0.3
	27	25.0 ± 7.6	15.0 ± 4.5	
Ionescu-Shiley	17	23.8 ± 3.4		0.9 ± 0.1
Stented bovine pericardial	19	19.7 ± 5.9	13.3 ± 3.9	1.1 ± 0.1
	21	26.6 ± 9.0		
	23		15.6 ± 4.4	
Labcor Santiago	19	18.6 ± 5.0	11.8 ± 3.3	1.2 ± 0.1
Stented bovine pericardial	21	17.5 ± 6.6	8.2 ± 4.5	1.3 ± 0.1
	23	14.8 ± 5.2	7.8 ± 2.9	1.8 ± 0.2
	25	12.3 ± 3.4	6.8 ± 2.0	2.1 ± 0.3
Labcor Synergy	21	24.3 ± 8.1	13.3 ± 4.2	1.1 ± 0.3
Stented porcine	23	27.3 ± 13.7	15.3 ± 6.9	1.4 ± 0.4
	25	22.5 ± 11.9	13.2 ± 6.4	1.5 ± 0.4
	27	17.8 ± 7.0	10.6 ± 4.6	1.8 ± 0.5
MCRI On-X	19	21.3 ± 10.8	11.8 ± 3.4	1.5 ± 0.2
Bileaflet	21	16.4 ± 5.9	9.9 ± 3.6	1.7 ± 0.4
	23	15.9 ± 6.4	8.6 ± 3.4	1.9 ± 0.6
	25	16.5 ± 10.2	6.9 ± 4.3	2.4 ± 0.6
Medtronic Advantage	23		10.4 ± 3.1	2.2 ± 0.3
Bileaflet	25		9.0 ± 3.7	2.8 ± 0.6
	27		7.6 ± 3.6	3.3 ± 0.7
	29		6.1 ± 3.8	3.9 ± 0.7
Medtronic Freestyle	19		13.0 ± 3.9	
Stentless	21		9.1 ± 5.1	1.4 ± 0.3
	23	11.0 ± 4.0	8.1 ± 4.6	1.7 ± 0.5
	25		5.3 ± 3.1	2.1 ± 0.5
	27		4.6 ± 3.1	2.5 ± 0.1
Medtronic Hall	20	34.4 ± 13.1	17.1 ± 5.3	1.2 ± 0.5
Single tilting disc	21	26.9 ± 10.5	14.1 ± 5.9	1.1 ± 0.2
	23	26.9 ± 8.9	13.5 ± 4.8	1.4 ± 0.4
	25	17.1 ± 7.0	9.5 ± 4.3	1.5 ± 0.5
	27	18.9 ± 9.7	8.7 ± 5.6	1.9 ± 0.2

(Continued)

Valve	Size	Peak Gradient (mm Hg)	Mean Gradient (mm Hg)	Effective Orifice Area (cm²)
Medtronic Mosaic	21		14.2 ± 5.0	1.4 ± 0.4
Stented porcine	23	23.8 ± 11.0	13.7 ± 4.8	1.5 ± 0.4
	25	22.5 ± 10.0	11.7 ± 5.1	1.8 ± 0.5
	27		10.4 ± 4.3	1.9 ± 0.1
	29		11.1 ± 4.3	2.1 ± 0.2
Mitroflow *Stented bovine pericardial*	19	18.6 ± 5.3	13.1 ± 3.3	1.1 ± 0.2
Monostrut Bjork-Shiley	19		27.4 ± 8.8	
Single tilting disc	21	27.5 ± 3.1	20.5 ± 6.2	
	23	20.3 ± 0.7	17.4 ± 6.4	
	25		16.1 ± 4.9	
	27		11.4 ± 3.8	
Prima	21	28.8 ± 6.0	13.7 ± 1.9	1.4 ± 0.7
Stentless	23	21.5 ± 7.5	11.5 ± 4.9	1.5 ± 0.3
	25	22.1 ± 12.5	11.6 ± 7.2	1.8 ± 0.5
Omnicarbon	21	37.4 ± 12.8	20.4 ± 5.4	1.3 ± 0.5
Single tilting disc	23	28.8 ± 9.1	17.4 ± 4.9	1.5 ± 0.3
	25	23.7 ± 8.1	13.2 ± 4.6	1.9 ± 0.5
	27	20.1 ± 4.2	12.4 ± 2.9	2.1 ± 0.4
Omniscience	21	50.8 ± 2.8	28.2 ± 2.2	0.9 ± 0.1
Single tilting disc	23	39.8 ± 8.7	20.1 ± 5.1	1.0 ± 0.1
Starr Edwards	23	32.6 ± 12.8	22.0 ± 9.0	1.1 ± 0.2
Caged ball	24	34.1 ± 10.3	22.1 ± 7.5	1.1 ± 0.3
	26	31.8 ± 9.0	19.7 ± 6.1	
	27	30.8 ± 6.3	18.5 ± 3.7	
	29	29.0 ± 9.3	16.3 ± 5.5	
Sorin Bicarbon	19	30.1 ± 4.5	16.7 ± 2.0	1.4 ± 0.1
Bileaflet	21	22.0 ± 7.1	10.0 ± 3.3	1.2 ± 0.4
	23	16.8 ± 6.1	7.7 ± 3.3	1.5 ± 0.2
	25	11.2 ± 3.1	5.6 ± 1.6	2.4 ± 0.3
Sorin Pericarbon	19	36.5 ± 9.0	28.9 ± 7.3	1.2 ± 0.5
Stentless	21	28.0 ± 13.3	23.8 ± 11.1	1.3 ± 0.6
	23	27.5 ± 11.5	23.2 ± 7.6	1.5 ± 0.5
St. Jude Medical	19	28.5 ± 10.7	17.0 ± 7.8	1.9 ± 0.1
Haem Plus	21	16.3 ± 17.0	10.6 ± 5.1	1.8 ± 0.5
Bileaflet	23	16.8 ± 7.3	12.1 ± 4.2	1.7 ± 0.5
St Jude Medical Regent	19	20.6 ± 12	11.0 ± 4.9	1.6 ± 0.4
Bileaflet	21	15.6 ± 9.4	8.0 ± 4.8	2.0 ± 0.7
	23	12.8 ± 6.8	6.9 ± 3.5	2.3 ± 0.9
	25	11.7 ± 6.8	5.6 ± 3.2	2.5 ± 0.8
	27	7.9 ± 5.5	3.5 ± 1.7	3.6 ± 0.5

(Continued)

Valve	Size	Peak Gradient (mm Hg)	Mean Gradient (mm Hg)	Effective Orifice Area (cm^2)
St Jude Medical Standard *Bileaflet*	19	42.0 ± 10.0	24.5 ± 5.8	1.5 ± 0.1
	21	25.7 ± 9.5	15.2 ± 5.0	1.4 ± 0.4
	23	21.8 ± 7.5	13.4 ± 5.6	1.6 ± 0.4
	25	18.9 ± 7.3	11.0 ± 5.3	1.9 ± 0.5
	27	13.7 ± 4.2	8.4 ± 3.4	2.5 ± 0.4
	29	13.5 ± 5.8	7.0 ± 1.7	2.8 ± 0.5
St Jude Medical *Stentless*	21	22.6 ± 14.5	10.7 ± 7.2	1.3 ± 0.6
	23	16.2 ± 9.0	8.2 ± 4.7	1.6 ± 0.6
	25	12.7 ± 8.2	6.3 ± 4.1	1.8 ± 0.5
	27	10.1 ± 5.8	5.0 ± 2.9	2.0 ± 0.3
	29	7.7 ± 4.4	4.1 ± 2.4	2.4 ± 0.6

From Zoghbi WA, Chambers JB, Dumesnil JG, et al. Recommendations for evaluation of prosthetic valves with echocardiography and doppler ultrasound: a report From the American Society of Echocardiography's Guidelines and Standards Committee and the Task Force on Prosthetic Valves, developed in conjunction with the American College of Cardiology Cardiovascular Imaging Committee, Cardiac Imaging Committee of the American Heart Association, the European Association of Echocardiography, a registered branch of the European Society of Cardiology, the Japanese Society of Echocardiography and the Canadian Society of Echocardiography, endorsed by the American College of Cardiology Foundation, American Heart Association, European Association of Echocardiography, a registered branch of the European Society of Cardiology, the Japanese Society of Echocardiography, and Canadian Society of Echocardiography. J Am Soc Echocardiogr. 2009;22:975-1014.

Appendix G: Normal Doppler Echocardiography Values for Prosthetic Mitral Valves

Valve	Size	Peak Gradient (mm Hg)	Mean Gradient (mm Hg)	Peak Velocity (m/s)	Pressure Half-Time (ms)	Effective Orifice Area (cm^2)
Biocor	27	13 ± 1				
Stentless bioprosthesis	29	14 ± 2.5				
	31	11.5 ± 0.5				
	33	12 ± 0.5				
Bioflo pericardial	25	10 ± 2	6.3 ± 1.5			2 ± 0.1
Stented bioprosthesis	27	9.5 ± 2.6	5.4 ± 1.2			2 ± 0.3
	29	5 ± 2.8	3.6 ± 1			2.4 ± 0.2
	31	4.0	2.0			2.3
Bjork-Shiley	23			1.7	115	
Tilting disc	25	12 ± 4	6 ±2	1.75 ± 0.38	99 ± 27	1.72 ± 0.6
	27	10 ± 4	5 ±2	1.6 ± 0.49	89 ± 28	1.81 ± 0.54
	29	7.83 ± 2.93	2.83 ± 1.27	1.37 ± 0.25	79 ± 17	2.1 ± 0.43
	31	6 ± 3	2 ± 1.9	1.41 ± 0.26	70 ± 14	2.2 ± 0.3
Bjork-Shiley monostrut	23		5.0	1.9		
Tilting disc	25	13 ± 2.5	5.57 ± 2.3	1.8 ± 0.3		
	27	12 ± 2.5	4.53 ± 2.2	1.7 ± 0.4		
	29	13 ± 3	4.26 ± 1.6	1.6 ± 0.3		
	31	14 ± 4.5	4.9 ± 1.6	1.7 ± 0.3		
Carbomedics	23			1.9 ± 0.1	126 ± 7	
Bileaflet	25	10.3 ± 2.3	3.6 ± 0.6	1.3 ± 0.1	93 ± 8	2.9 ± 0.8
	27	8.79 ± 3.46	3.46 ± 1.03	1.61 ± 0.3	89 ± 20	2.9 ± 0.75
	29	8.78 ± 2.9	3.39 ± 0.97	1.52 ± 0.3	88 ± 17	2.3 ± 0.4
	31	8.87 ± 2.34	3.32 ± 0.87	1.61 ± 0.29	92 ± 24	2.8 ± 1.14
	33	8.8 ± 2.2	4.8 ± 2.5	1.5 ± 0.2	93 ± 12	
Carpentier- Edwards	27		6 ± 2	1.7 ± 0.3	98 ± 28	
Stented bioprosthesis	29		4.7 ± 2	1.76 ± 0.27	92 ±14	
	31		4.4 ± 2	1.54 ± 0.15	92 ± 19	
	33		6 ± 3		93 ± 12	
Carpentier- Edwards	27		3.6	1.6	100	
pericardial	29		5.25 ± 2.36	1.67 ± 0.3	110 ± 15	
Stented Bioprosthesis	31		4.05 ± 0.83	1.53 ± 0.1	90 ± 11	
	33		1.0	0.8	80	
Duromedics	27	13 ± 6	5 ± 3	1.61 ± 0.4	75 ± 12	
Bileaflet	29	10 ± 4	3 ± 1	1.40 ± 0.25	85 ± 22	
	31	10.5 ± 4.33	3.3 ± 1.36	1.38 ± 0.27	81 ± 12	
	33	11.2	2.5		85	

(Continued)

Valve	Size	Peak Gradient (mm Hg)	Mean Gradient (mm Hg)	Peak Velocity (ms)	Pressure Half-Time (m/s)	Effective Orifice Area (cm^2)
Hancock I or not specified	27	10 ± 4	5 ± 2			1.3 ± 0.8
Stented bioprosthesis	29	7 ± 3	2.46 ± 0.79		115 ± 20	1.5 ± 0.2
	31	4 ± 0.86	4.86 ± 1.69		95 ± 17	1.6 ± 0.2
	33	3 ± 2	3.87 ± 2		90 ± 12	1.9 ± 0.2
Hancock II	27					2.21 ± 0.14
Stented bioprosthesis	29					2.77 ± 0.11
	31					2.84 ± 0.1
	33					3.15 ± 0.22
Hancock pericardial	29		2.61 ± 1.39	1.42 ± 0.14	105 ± 36	
Stented bioprosthesis	31		3.57 ± 1.02	1.51 ± 0.27	81 ± 23	
Ionescu-Shiley	25		4.87 ± 1.08	1.43 ± 0.15	93 ± 11	
Stented bioprosthesis	27		3.21 ± 0.82	1.31 ± 0.24	100 ± 28	
	29		3.22 ± 0.57	1.38 ± 0.2	85 ± 8	
	31		3.63 ± 0.9	1.45 ± 0.06	100 ± 36	
Ionescu-Shiley low profile	29		3.31 ± 0.96	1.36 ± 0.25	80 ± 30	
Stented bioprosthesis	31		2.74 ± 0.37	1.33 ± 0.14	79 ± 15	
Labcor-Santiago pericardial	25	8.7	4.5		97	2.2
	27	5.6 ± 2.3	2.8 ± 1.5		85 ± 18	2.12 ± 0.48
Stented bioprosthesis	29	6.2 ± 2.1	3 ± 1.3		80 ± 34	2.11 ± 0.73
Lillehei- Kaster	18			1.7	140	
Tilting disc	20			1.7	67	
	22			1.56 ± 0.09	94 ± 22	
	25			1.38 ± 0.27	124 ± 46	
Medtronic- Hall	27			1.4	78	
Tilting disc	29			1.57 ± 0.1	69 ± 15	
	31			1.45 ± 0.12	77 ± 17	
Medtronic Intact Porcine	29		3.5 ± 0.51	1.6 ± 0.22		
Stented bioprosthesis	31		4.2 ± 1.44	1.6 ± 0.26		
	33		4 ± 1.3	1.4 ± 0.24		
	35		3.2 ± 1.77	1.3 ± 0.5		
Mitroflow	25		6.9	2.0	90	
Stented bioprosthesis	27		3.07 ± 0.91	1.5	90 ± 20	
	29		3.5 ± 1.65	1.43 ± 0.29	102 ± 21	
	31		3.85 ± 0.81	1.32 ± 0.26	91 ± 22	
Omnicarbon	23		8.0			
Tilting disc	25		6.05 ± 1.81	1.77 ± 0.24	102 ± 16	
	27		4.89 ± 2.05	1.63 ± 0.36	105 ± 33	
	29		4.93 ± 2.16	1.56 ± 0.27	120 ± 40	
	31		4.18 ± 1.4	1.3 ± 0.23	134 ± 31	
	33		4 ± 2			

(Continued)

Valve	Size	Peak Gradient (mm Hg)	Mean Gradient (mm Hg)	Peak Velocity (ms)	Pressure Half-Time (m/s)	Effective Orifice Area (cm^2)
On-X	25	11.5 ± 3.2	5.3 ± 2.1			1.9 ± 1.1
Bileaflet	27-29	10.3 ± 4.5	4.5 ± 1.6			2.2 ± 0.5
	31-33	9.8 ± 3.8	4.8 ± 2.4			2.5 ± 1.1
Sorin Allcarbon	25	15 ± 3	5 ± 1	2 ± 0.2	105 ± 29	2.2 ± 0.6
Tilting disc	27	13 ± 2	4 ± 1	1.8 ± 0.1	89 ± 14	2.5 ± 0.5
	29	10 ± 2	4 ± 1	1.6 ± 0.2	85 ± 23	2.8 ± 0.7
	31	9 ±1	4 ±1	1.6 ± 0.1	88 ± 27	2.8 ± 0.9
Sorin Bicarbon	25	15 ± 0.25	4 ± 0.5	1.95 ± 0.02	70 ± 1	
Bileaflet	27	11 ± 2.75	4 ± 0.5	1.65 ± 0.21	82 ± 20	
	29	12 ± 3	4 ± 1.25	1.73 ± 0.22	80 ± 14	
	31	10 ± 1.5	4 ± 1	1.66 ± 0.11	83 ± 14	
St Jude Medical	23		4.0	1.5	160	1.0
Bileaflet	25		2.5 ± 1	1.34 ± 1.12	75 ± 4	1.35 ± 0.17
	27	11 ± 4	5 ± 1.82	1.61 ± 0.29	75 ± 10	1.67 ± 0.17
	29	10 ± 3	4.15 ± 1.8	1.57 ± 0.29	85 ± 10	1.75 ± 0.24
	31	12 ± 6	4.46 ± 2.22	1.59 ± 0.33	74 ± 13	2.03 ± 0.32
Starr- Edwards	26		10.0			1.4
Caged ball	28		7 ± 2.75			1.9 ± 0.57
	30	12.2 ± 4.6	6.99 ± 2.5	1.7 ± 0.3	125 ± 25	1.65 ± 0.4
	32	11.5 ± 4.2	5.08 ± 2.5	1.7 ± 0.3	110 ± 25	1.98 ± 0.4
	34		5.0			2.6
Stentless quadrileaflet	26		2.2 ± 1.7	1.6	103 ± 31	1.7
bovine pericardial	28			1.58 ± 0.25		1.7 ± 0.6
Stentless bioprosthesis	30			1.42 ± 0.32		2.3 ± 0.4
Wessex	29		3.69 ± 0.61	1.66 ± 0.17	83 ± 19	
Stented bioprosthesis	31		3.31 ± 0.83	1.41 ± 0.25	80 ± 21	

Zoghbi WA, Chambers JB, Dumesnil JG, et al. Recommendations for evaluation of prosthetic valves with echocardiography and doppler ultrasound: a report From the American Society of Echocardiography's Guidelines and Standards Committee and the Task Force on Prosthetic Valves, developed in conjunction with the American College of Cardiology Cardiovascular Imaging Committee, Cardiac Imaging Committee of the American Heart Association, the European Association of Echocardiography, a registered branch of the European Society of Cardiology, the Japanese Society of Echocardiography and the Canadian Society of Echocardiography, endorsed by the American College of Cardiology Foundation, American Heart Association, European Association of Echocardiography, a registered branch of the European Society of Cardiology, the Japanese Society of Echocardiography, and Canadian Society of Echocardiography. J Am Soc Echocardiogr. 2009;22:975-1014.

Appendix H: Miscellaneous

GRADING OF ATRIAL SEPTAL ANEURYSMS (1.5 cm of the Atrial Septum and Extending 1.5 cm into Either Atrial Chamber)[1]

IA	Aneurysm bulges continually to the right atrium
IB	Aneurysm predominantly bulges to the right atrium but has a phasic oscillation into the left atrium during the cardiorespiratory cycle
IC	Aneurysm that oscillates between the right and left atrial chambers with each cardiac cycle
II	Aneurysm protruding exclusively into the left atrium

CLASSIFICATION OF THE SEVERITY OF ATHEROSCLEROSIS[2]

Class 1	No or minimal intimal thickening <3 mm
Class 2	Intimal layer thickness >3 mm
Class 3	Protruding atheroma <5 mm
Class 4	Protuding atheroma >5 mm
Class 5	Protuding atheroma >5 mm with a mobile fragment

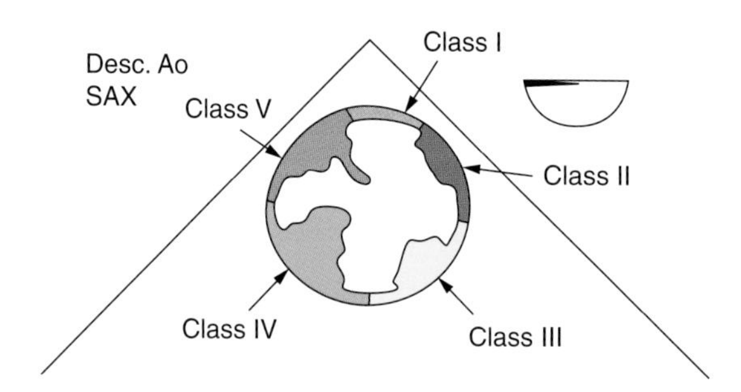

ASSESSMENT OF THE SEVERITY OF PERICARDIAL EFFUSION

Small	<0.5 cm
Moderate	0.5-2 cm
Large	>2 cm

Normal pericardial thickness:1 to 2 mm.

REFERENCES

1. Hanley PC, Tajik AJ, Hynes JK, et al. Diagnosis and classification of atrial septal aneurysm by two-dimensional echocardiography: report of 80 consecutive cases. *J Am Coll Cardiol.* 1985;6:1370-1382.
2. Katz ES, Tunick PA, Rusinek H, Ribakove G, Spencer FC, Kronzon I. Protruding aortic atheromas predict stroke in elderly patients undergoing cardiopulmonary bypass: experience with intraoperative transesophageal echocardiography. *J Am Coll Cardiol.* 1992;20:70-77.

ANSWERS

Chapter 1

Basics of Ultrasound

1. d. The four acoustic variables are pressure, density, distance, and temperature. Intensity is a parameter used to describe a sound wave. It is the concentration of power in a beam.

2. b. US is a wave with a frequency greater than 20 kHz, or 20,000 Hz. Clinical US imaging typically occurs between 2 and 15 MHz.

3. b. Intensity is related to the strength of the sound beam and is equal to the power (watts) divided by the beam area. Frequency is the number of cycles that occur in 1 s. Pulse duration is the time from the beginning to the end of a US pulse (usually made up of three to five cycles). Pulse repetition frequency is the time from the beginning of one US pulse to the beginning of the next pulse.

4. c. Pulse repetition frequency is the number of pulses that occur in 1 s. When a US system images shallower depths, the receive time decreases, thus increasing the pulse repetition frequency.

5. a. Rayleigh scattering is a special type of scattering that occurs when the reflector is much smaller than the wavelength. Scattering increases with higher frequencies. In clinical US, the best example of Rayleigh scattering is the interaction between US and red blood cells.

6. b. Period is the time from the start of one cycle to the start of the next cycle. Period and frequency are reciprocally related, so doubling the frequency halves the period.

7. d.

$$\text{Wavelength} = \text{Propagation Speed in Soft Tissue / Frequency}$$

$$= \frac{1.54 \frac{\text{mm}}{\mu\text{s}}}{2 \text{ MHz}}$$

8. a. The speed of sound is slowest in air (300 m/s), followed by fat (1450 m/s), soft tissue (1540 m/s), and bone (3000 m/s).

9. b. Period, frequency, amplitude, power, and intensity are determined by the sound source. Propagation speed is determined only by the medium. Wavelength is the only parameter that is determined by the sound source and the medium through which sound travels.

10. b. Reflection of a US wave requires a difference in the acoustic impedance at the boundary between two media. Impedance is calculated as the density of the medium multiplied by the propagation speed through the medium.

11. d. Refraction is a change in direction of wave propagation when traveling from one medium to another. It occurs only when there are different propagation speeds *and* oblique incidence. Therefore, it cannot occur with normal incidence or identical propagation speeds. Snell's law describes refraction.

12. a. The angle of reflection is equal to the angle of incidence. The rest of the data provided in the question are not required to obtain the answer.

13. c. Refraction is described by Snell's law, which states:

$$\frac{\text{Sine Transmission Angle}}{\text{Sine Incident Angle}} = \frac{\text{Propagation Speed in Second Medium}}{\text{Propagation Speed in First Medium}}$$

Thus, if the propagation speed in the second medium is slower than the propagation speed in the first medium, then the transmission angle is less than the incident angle. Similarly, if the propagation speed in the second medium is faster than the propagation speed in the first medium, then the transmission angle is greater than the incident angle. If the propagation speed in the second medium is the same as the propagation speed in the first medium, then the transmission angle is the same as the incident angle.

14. d. If it takes 1 s to travel to and from the reflector at a speed of 600 m/s, then the reflector is situated 300 m from the source.

15. a. Amplitude is determined by the sound source, cannot be changed by the sonographer, and is half of the peak-to-peak amplitude.

16. a. Intensity is power divided by beam area. Intensity is proportional to amplitude squared.

17. d. The speed of sound through a medium is determined only by the characteristics of the medium. Speed increases when density decreases and stiffness increases. Elasticity is the opposite of stiffness.

18. b. Increasing the frequency improves axial resolution by decreasing wavelength, spatial pulse length,

period, and pulse duration. Lateral resolution is improved by decreasing beam width and the angle of beam divergence. However, an improved resolution with higher frequencies must be balanced by the decrease in the depth of penetration.

19. c. Propagation speed is the speed at which sound moves through a medium. This speed is determined only by the characteristics of the medium (density and stiffness) and averages 1540 m/s in soft tissue. As a general rule, the speed of sound in a gas is slower than in a liquid, which in turn is slower than in a solid.

20. d. Attenuation is the decrease in intensity, power, and amplitude of a sound wave as it travels and is a consequence of absorption, reflection, and scattering. Absorption results when energy imparted to biologic tissues is converted to another form of energy such as heat. Reflection results in some of the acoustic energy being directed back to the transducer, thus weakening the propagating sound beam. Scattering occurs when the US beam is reflected in a number of different directions.

21. c. Backscatter (diffuse scattering) is scatter returning in the general direction of the transducer. All forms of scatter produce much weaker echoes when compared with specular reflections. Specular reflections occur when the wavelength is much smaller than the irregularities in the boundary and are well seen only when sound strikes the reflector at 90°.

22. d. All of the above along with the pulse duration and repetition period are used to describe pulsed US. Pulse duration is the time from the start to the end of a pulse. Pulse repetition period is the time from the start of one pulse to the start of the next pulse. Pulse repetition frequency is the number of pulses that occur in 1 s. Spatial pulse length is the length or distance that a pulse occupies in space. Duty factor is the fraction of time that a US system is transmitting a pulse.

23. b. Pulse repetition frequency is determined by the sound source but not the medium. Pulse repetition frequency decreases as the imaging depth increases. Because the sonographer can set imaging depth, he or she can change the pulse repetition frequency. Pulse repetition period and pulse repetition frequency are reciprocals.

24. c. Normal incidence is also referred to as *perpendicular, orthogonal, right angle*, and *90°*.

25. c. Sound is a mechanical, longitudinal wave. The particles in a longitudinal wave are displaced in the direction of sound. The particles in a transverse wave are displaced perpendicular to the direction of sound.

Transducers

1. b. The piezoelectric effect is the conversion of sound energy into electrical energy and is seen in the reception phase of clinical imaging. The reverse piezoelectric effect represents the transmission phase in which sound energy is produced by the application of electric energy to a piezoelectric material.

2. d. Naturally occurring piezoelectric materials include quartz, Rochelle salts, and tourmaline. The most common synthetic material contains lead, zirconate, and titanate. Other synthetic materials include barium titanate, lead metaniobate, lithium sulfate, and polyvinyl diflouride.

3. b. The matching layer is the material placed on the surface of the piezoelectric elements to reduce the acoustic impedance mismatch between the elements and soft tissue. Typically, the matching layer has impedance between that of the skin and the piezoelectric elements to increase the percentage of transmitted sound between the skin and the elements. The optimal thickness of the matching layer is one-fourth the wavelength.

4. d. Linear switched or sequential transducers are comparatively large transducers, with multiple elements arranged in a line. The image produced is no wider than the transducer and produces a rectangular image. Multiple piezoelectric crystals are fired at exactly the same time, focusing is fixed, and there is no steering.

5. c. In a phased array transducer, the delivery of electrical pulses to the piezoelectric elements in various patterns (timing) results in focusing and steering of the US beam.

6. b. M-Mode is a continuous B-mode display versus time, allowing comparison of object motion. Time is on the x-axis and reflector depth on the y-axis.

7. d. Damping material is the substance (eg, tungsten powder plus araldite) placed behind the piezoelectric elements to reduce the "ringing" produced by the elements and to absorb the energy directed toward the US system itself. Use of damping material reduces pulse duration, spatial pulse length, duty factor, transducer output intensity, transducer sensitivity, and quality factor, but increases bandwidth. Bandwidth is the difference between the highest and lowest frequencies emitted from the transducer.

8. b. The near zone is also referred to as the *Fresnel zone*, and the far zone (area of the sound beam beyond the focal point) is called the *Fraunhofer zone*. The near zone length is directly proportional to the diameter of the piezoelectric crystal and frequency. The near zone length is increased by larger crystal diameters and higher emitted frequencies.

9. b. For a continuous wave transducer that is not electronically focused, the beam diameter at the end of the near zone (focus) is one-half the transducer diameter.

10. c. A linear phased array produces a sector shape image without blunting. Steering and focusing are accomplished electronically, and crystal defects result in poor steering and focusing.

Instrumentation

1. d. M mode uses a single beam of ultrasound and thus provides a high sampling (frame) rate. Temporal resolution, the ability to accurately locate moving structures at a particular instant in time, is best with M mode.

2. a. Increasing the overall gain results in amplification (making the signals larger), thus affecting the brightness of the entire image. Transducer output is also known as *energy output,* can be controlled by the sonographer, is determined by the excitation voltage from the pulser, and produces an increase in the brightness of the entire image when increased.

3. b. Time gain compensation makes all echoes appear similar regardless of the depth from which they return. Compression decreases the dynamic range of the signals. Demodulation changes the signal into a more suitable form for display. Increasing the overall gain increases the brightness of the entire image but does not create an image with uniform brightness.

4. a. Axial resolution is the ability to distinguish two structures that are close to each other, front to back. It is also called *longitudinal, range, radial,* or *depth resolution* and can be remembered by the acronym LARRD.

5. c. If the system is not displaying weaker echoes, it is likely because the reject (threshold) level is set so that weaker echoes are ignored. Therefore, the most appropriate action is to decrease the reject level.

6. d. The principal display modes are A and B. A mode is also called *amplitude mode* and displays returning energy as spikes. B mode is also called *brightness mode* because returning echoes are displayed as bright dots. M mode is a form of B mode, also called *time motion mode,* and is used to display reflector motion over time.

7. c. Single-focus systems, narrow sectors, and low line density use fewer US pulses and therefore yield a higher frame rate and thus better temporal resolution. A shallower image provides better temporal resolution.

8. d. The six components of a US system are the transducer, pulser, receiver, display, storage, and master synchronizer. The transducer turns electrical energy into acoustic energy during transmission and vice versa during reception. The pulser controls the electrical signals sent to the transducer for pulse generation. The receiver consists of the electronics associated with taking the electronic signal produced by the transducer from the returning echoes and producing a picture. The display is the device associated with the presentation of processed data. Storage is the medium used to store data. The master synchronizer communicates with all of the components and organizes and integrates their functions.

9. c. Lateral resolution is the ability to resolve two closely spaced structures lying perpendicular to the US beam. Lateral resolution is also referred to as *angular, transverse,* or *azimuth resolution* and can be remembered by the acronym LATA. Lateral resolution is improved by increasing transducer diameter, which extends the near zone length and thus reduces beam diameter; by increasing transducer frequency, which reduces beam diameter and extends the near zone length; and by focusing, which decreases the beam diameter in the near zone.

Doppler

1. c. A change in the frequency of sound relative to the motions of the sound source and the receiver is known as the *Doppler principle.* The amount of change in the frequency is known as the *Doppler shift.* A positive shift occurs when the sound source and receiver are approaching each other, and a negative change occurs when the sound source and receiver are moving apart.

2. d. Velocity is defined by a magnitude and a direction, whereas speed is defined by magnitude only.

3. b. The magnitude of the Doppler shift depends on the cosine of the angle between the sound beam and the direction of motion. At 0° or 180°, the measured velocity is equal to true velocity because cosine of 0 and 180 is 1. At 90°, the measured velocity is 0 because the cosine of 90 is 0. At angles between 0° and 90°, only a portion of the true velocity is measured.

4. a. Spectral analysis in conventional Doppler currently is accomplished by a mathematical technique that converts analog signals into digital signals by using fast Fourier transform.

5. b. The modal frequency or velocity represents the greatest amplitude Doppler shift signal. Mean velocity represents the average Doppler velocity, and peak velocity represents the maximum velocity.

6. a. Doppler shift information can be obtained due to wall or blood vessel motion. Wall motion frequency shifts are high-amplitude, low-velocity, and low-frequency signals.

7. b. Doppler wall filters are used to eliminate low Doppler frequency shifts (caused by wall or blood vessel motion) and are therefore considered high-pass filters.

8. c. The maximal detectable frequency shift is equal to one-half the PRF and is known as the Nyquist limit.

9. b. When the Doppler shift exceeds the Nyquist limit, velocities are perceived as going in the opposite direction, or *aliasing.* Aliasing is the most commonly observed artifact in pulsed Doppler imaging. The higher the emitted frequency from the transducer, the more likely aliasing is to occur.

10. b. Color-flow Doppler reports mean velocities.

11. d. Packet size refers to the number of US pulses per scan line. Color-flow Doppler requires a minimum of three US pulses for each scan line. If packet size is increased, the estimate of Doppler shift is enhanced but frame rate decreases.

12. b. This is a velocity map. All of the measured velocities from each packet are averaged to produce a mean velocity. The colors provide information on flow direction. Blue reflects flow away from the transducer, with lighter blue representing higher velocities. Similarly, red represents flow toward the transducer, with yellow representing higher velocities.

13. c. This is a variance map. All of the measured velocities from each packet are averaged to produce a mean velocity. However, if a broad range of velocities is present, then another color signifying variability in velocities is added to the image. The colors provide information on flow direction and turbulence. Blue and green reflect flow away from the transducer, with blue representing laminar flow and green representing turbulent flow. Similarly, red and yellow represent flow toward the transducer, with red representing laminar flow and yellow reflecting turbulent flow.

14. b. Blackness on the color map indicates that no Doppler shift was measured.

15. c. Because the angle between the direction of flow and the direction of the sound beam is 90°, no Doppler shift will be detected (cosine 90 = 0). Thus, no color will appear on the image.

16. b. Laminar flow appears on the left side of a variance map. Since color Doppler aliases, flow above the aliasing velocity will appear on the opposite side of the spectrum.

17. c. By convention, red blood cells moving toward the transducer result in a positive Doppler shift and are displayed above the zero baseline. With a positive Doppler shift, the sound source and reflector are approaching each other and the reflected (received) frequency is greater than the transmitted frequency.

18. b. Continuous-wave Doppler consists of two crystals in one transducer. One crystal is constantly sending out energy and the other is constantly listening. It is able to measure very high velocities and therefore does not have aliasing artifact. Because the velocities can come from anywhere along the length of the beam, it has range ambiguity, or the inability to determine the exact point of increased velocities. Use of continuous-wave Doppler means no damping, narrow bandwidth, and high quality factor.

19. d. The velocity (magnitude and direction) of blood flow is demonstrated in the spectral display. Duration of blood flow is displayed on the x-axis by measuring time. The turbulent or laminar nature of blood flow is demonstrated by the degree of spectral broadening and window fill-in.

20. c. The Nyquist limit is equal to the pulse repetition frequency divided by 2.

21. c. Pulsed-wave Doppler uses longer pulse lengths. It also uses higher pulse repetition frequencies (resulting in shorter pulse repetition periods), and the output power is greater. The combination of longer pulse lengths, greater output power, and higher pulse repetition frequencies means that the patient has greater acoustic exposure when pulsed-wave Doppler is used.

22. a. Color Doppler is a pulsed US technique that reports mean velocities. Therefore, it provides range resolution but is subject to aliasing.

23. d. Color-flow Doppler has poor temporal resolution because of a reduction in frame rate. Flow toward and away from the transducer depends upon the color map being used.

24. c. Sliding one's finger from the color at the top of the map to the bottom of the map is a quick way of determining direction of flow. In this case, starting with a "red" color and moving to a "blue" color indicates that flow is moving from left to right.

Bioeffects

1. a. Spatial peak, temporal average (SPTA) intensities are the most important for thermal bioeffects. SPTP intensities have the highest value.

2. c. M-mode/B-mode (two-dimensional) US has the lowest intensities (0.60 to 200 mW/cm^2 SPTA) in comparison with pulsed-wave Doppler (50 to 290 mW/cm^2 SPTA) or continuous-wave Doppler (110 to 2500 mW/cm^2 SPTA).

3. b. Stable cavitation is the contraction and expansion of gas bubbles. It can be seen with high-intensity-level pulsed-wave US. Transient cavitation is the implosion of a gas bubble.

4. c. Scan conversion make gray-scale images possible and have no relation to US bioeffects.

5. b. Mechanical index is a number developed to predict the likelihood of cavitation-induced bioeffects. Mechanical index settings have been used in the field of contrast echocardiography to preserve (low mechanical index) and burst (high mechanical index) contrast agents.

6. d. Increase in acoustic exposure occurs by increasing examination time, transmit gain (power), and pulse repetition frequency.

Chapter 2

1. b.

2. d.

3. b.

4. c.

5. c.

6. b.

7. a.

8. c.

9. d.

10. a.

11. d.

12. c.

13. d.

14. c.

15. b.

16. b.

17. c.

18. d.

19. a.

20. a.

21. d.

22. b.

23. a.

24. b.

25. b.

Chapter 3

1. a. Chiari network. This is a sinus venosus derived structure that is characterized by a fenestrated undulating appearance.

2. b. Mirror image. This is a mirror image of an aorta with an intra-aortic balloon pump in it. Note that the false image of the balloon pump *(arrow)* is distant to the real image.

3. b. This is a myxoma. The patient also has lipomatous hypertrophy of the interatrial septum but the arrow is pointing to the myxoma.

4. a. This is an atrial septal defect, not a normal anatomic variant.

5. c. This is a large acoustic shadow from the strut of a mechanical valve in the mitral position, which makes evaluation of distal structures difficult.

6. d. This is a left ventricular (LV) thrombus. It is not in the correct location for a papillary muscle or a moderator band. LV bands usually cross the LV but do not appear as an isolated mass at the apex of the LV.

7. c. This is flow away from the probe from the left atrium to the right atrium through a patent foramen ovale. There is color-flow Doppler aliasing seen in the flow as well.

8. c. This is a strong reverberation from air left in the left atrium after an aortic valve replacement.

9. d. This is the brachiocephalic vein in the upper esophageal aortic valve short-axis view.

10. c. This is classic lipomatous hypertrophy of the interatrial septum.

11. b. This is a normal coronary sinus at less than 1 cm wide. Note the tricuspid valve with blue flow indicating blood flowing away from the transducer from the right atrium to the right ventricle.

12. c. This is the transverse sinus, a pericardial space between the ascending aorta, the left atrium, and the pulmonary artery.

13. a. This is a side lobe generated from a pulmonary artery catheter in the right ventricle.

14. b. These are pectinate muscles in the periphery of the right atrium.

15. b. This is a eustachian valve, an embryological remnant that directs blood flow in utero from the inferior vena cava towards the interatrial septum.

16. d. This is endocarditis. The aortic valve leaflets are intact (excluding a flail valve) and the masses are not attached to the aortic valve leaflets (excluding fibroelastoma or Lambl's excrescence).

17. d. This is the ligament of Marshall or the "coumadin ridge." The mitral valve can be seen on the left side of the image.

18. d. This is color-flow Doppler aliasing in the left ventricular outflow tract as the color flow changes from red to blue. One can also see severe mitral regurgitation in this image.

19. c. This is a view of the tricuspid valve in the modified bicaval view.

20. c. Chiari networks are associated with interatrial septal aneurysms.

21. d. This is the coronary sinus as seen in the modified bicaval view.

22. b. This is a left atrial appendage thrombus. The thrombus is different in texture and density from the rest of the surrounding tissue, which differentiates it from anatomic variants.

23. b. This is a classic side lobe from a St. Jude prosthetic valve.

24. c. This is a moderator band, which appears in the apical third of the right ventricle.

25. b. This is an enhancement artifact. The region pointed to by the arrow is brighter because the ultrasound beam has traveled through a region with abnormally low attenuation (amniotic fluid).

26. c. This is a displaced tricuspid valve due to the right atrial tumor.

27. d. This is a dilated coronary sinus cava seen in cross section.

28. a. This is thrombus in the periphery of the right atrium to be distinguished from pectinate muscles that occur in the same location. The density and texture of the thrombus is different from the surrounding heart tissue.

29. b. This is an off-angle view of the ligament of Marshall. The left atrial appendage is readily identified, but the left upper pulmonary vein is barely visible in this view.

30. c. This is a thrombus in the SVC.

31. a. This is a pericardial effusion seen anterior to the right atrium.

32. c. This is the location of the right atrial appendage in the bicaval view.

33. b.
34. d.
35. c.
36. a.
37. c.
38. b.
39. b.
40. b.
41. b.
42. b.
43. c.
44. d.
45. a.
46. c.
47. a.
48. b.
49. c.
50. a.

Chapter 4

1. a.
2. e.
3. a.
4. c.
5. c.
6. d.
7. a.
8. c.
9. d.
10. b.
11. a.
12. c.
13. d.
14. c.
15. a.
16. c.
17. c.
18. d.
19. a.
20. c.
21. e.
22. b.
23. c.
24. a.
25. c.
26. a.
27. a.
28. d.
29. a.
30. e.
31. b.
32. d.
33. c.
34. b.
35. a.
36. a.

37. b.

38. a.

39. a.

40. a.

41. b.

42. d.

43. b.

44. c.

45. a.

46. b.

47. b.

48. d.

$$\Delta P = 4(V_2)^2$$
$$= 4(6.3)^2$$
$$= 158.8 \text{ mm Hg}$$

49. b.

$$\Delta P = 4(V_2)^2$$
$$(V_2)^2 = \Delta P/4$$
$$V_2 = \sqrt{39.6/4}$$
$$= \sqrt{9.9}$$
$$= 3.15 \text{ m/s}$$

50. d.

$$\text{CSA of the PA} = \pi \times r^2 = 0.785 \times D^2$$
$$= 0.785 \times (2.5)^2$$
$$= 4.9 \text{ cm}^2$$

Stroke Volume (SV) = Stroke Distance (VTI) × Cross-Sectional Area (CSA)

$$= 11 \text{ cm} \times 4.9 \text{ cm}^2 = 53.9 \text{ mL}$$

51. c.

$$\text{Cardiac Output} = \text{Stroke Volume} \times \text{Heart Rate}$$
$$= 53.9 \text{ mL} \times 100 = 5.39 \text{ L/min}$$

52. d.

$$\text{Aortic Valve Area} = CSA_{LVOT} \times \left(\frac{V_{LVOT}}{V_{Aortic\ Valve}}\right)$$
$$= 0.785 \times D^2 \times (1/4.5)$$
$$= 0.785 \times (2)^2 \times (1/4.5)$$
$$= 0.69 \text{ cm}^2$$

53. d.

$$\text{RVSP} = 4\,(V_{Peak\ TR})^2 + \text{Right Atrial Pressure (CVP)}$$
$$= 4(4)^2 + 15$$
$$= 64 + 15$$
$$= 79 \text{ mm Hg}$$

54. c.

$$\text{Peak Instantaneous Gradient} = 4 \times (V_{Peak})^2$$
$$= 4\,(4.4)^2$$
$$= 77 \text{ mm Hg}$$

55. c.

$$\text{CSA of the LVOT} = \pi \times r^2 = 0.785 \times D^2$$
$$= 0.785 \times (2.15)^2$$
$$= 3.6 \text{ cm}^2$$

Stroke Volume (SV) = Stroke Distance (VTI) × Cross-Sectional Area (CSA)

$$= 12 \times 3.6 = 43.5 \text{ mL}$$

56. b.

$$\text{Cardiac Output} = \text{Stroke Volume} \times \text{Heart Rate}$$
$$= 43.5 \times 64 = 2.78 \text{ L/min}$$

57. a.

$$\text{Aortic Valve Area} = CSA_{LVOT} \times \left(\frac{VTI_{LVOT}}{VTI_{Aortic\ Valve}}\right)$$

$$= 0.785 \times D^2 \times (12/22)$$

$$= 0.785 \times (2.15)^2 \times (12/22)$$

$$= 1.9\ cm^2$$

58. a.

$$EROA = 2\pi r^2 \times \frac{Velocity_{Aliasing}}{Peak\ Velocity_{Mitral\ Regurgitant\ Jet}}$$

$$= 2 \times 3.14 \times (1)^2 \times 50/500$$

$$= 0.62\ cm^2$$

59. c.

$$LAP = \text{Left Ventricular Systolic Pressure} - 4\,(V_{Peak\ MR})^2$$

$$= 110 - 4(5)^2$$

$$= 110 - 100 = 10$$

60. a.

Stroke Volume (SV) = Stroke Distance (VTI) × Cross-Sectional Area (CSA)

$$\text{CSA of the LVOT} = \pi \times r^2 = 0.785 \times D^2$$

$$= 0.785 \times (2.5)^2$$

$$= 4.9\ cm^2$$

Stroke Volume (SV) = Stroke Distance (VTI) × Cross-Sectional Area (CSA)

$$= 15 \times 4.9 = 73.6\ cm^3\ (mL)$$

61. d.

Stroke Volume (SV) = Stroke Distance (VTI) × Cross-Sectional Area (CSA)

$$\text{CSA of the Mitral} = \pi \times r^2 = 0.785 \times D^2$$

$$= 0.785 \times (3.7)^2$$

$$= 10.7\ cm^2$$

Stroke Volume (SV) MV = Stroke Distance (VTI) MV × Cross-Sectional Area (CSA) MV

$$= 12 \times 10.7 = 129\ cm^3\ (mL)$$

62. b.

$$\text{Regurgitant Volume}_{Mitral\ Valve} = SV_{Mitral\ Valve} - SV_{Aortic\ Valve}$$

$$= 129 - 73.6\ mL$$

$$= 55.4\ mL$$

63. c.

$$\text{Regurgitant Fraction}_{Mitral\ Valve}\ (\%) = \frac{\text{Regurgitant Volume}_{Mitral\ Valve}}{\text{Stroke Volume}_{Mitral\ Valve}} \times 100$$

$$= (55.4/129) \times 100$$

$$= 42.9\%$$

64. b.

$$EROA = \frac{2\pi r^2 \times Velocity_{Aliasing}}{Peak\ Velocity_{Mitral\ Regurgitant\ Jet}}$$

$$= 2 \times 3.14 \times (0.7)^2 \times (45/445)$$

$$= 0.31$$

65. b.

$$PASP = \text{Systolic Blood Pressure} - 4\,(V_{Peak\ PDA})^2$$

$$= 90 - 4(4)^2$$

$$= 26\ mm\ Hg$$

66. e.

$$PAMP = 4\,(V_{Peak\ PR})^2 + \text{Right Atrial Pressure (CVP)}$$

$$= 4\,(1.69)^2 + 10$$

$$= 21.4\ mm\ Hg$$

67. d.

$$PADP = 4\,(V_{End\text{-}Diastolic\ PR})^2 + \text{Right Atrial Pressure (CVP)}$$

$$= 4(1.43)^2 + 10$$

$$= 18.2\ mm\ Hg$$

68. c.

$$LVEDP = \text{Diastolic Blood Pressure} - 4\,(V_{\text{End-Diastolic AR}})^2$$
$$= 60 - 4(2.2)^2$$
$$= 60 - 19.4$$
$$= 40.6 \text{ mm Hg}$$

69. c.

$$\text{Left Ventricular } \frac{dP}{dt} = 32 \times 1000/dt \text{ in Milliseconds}$$
$$LV \frac{dP}{dt} = 32{,}000/42$$
$$= 761 \text{ mm Hg/s}$$

Chapter 5

1. b.
2. c.
3. b.
4. b.
5. a.
6. b.
7. c.
8. c.
9. d.
10. a.
11. c.
12. b.
13. c.
14. a.
15. b.
16. d.
17. c.
18. a.
19. a.
20. d.
21. c.
22. b.
23. b.
24. d.
25. a.
26. c.
27. a.
28. b.
29. c.
30. d.
31. c.
32. d.
33. a.
34. b.
35. b.
36. c.

Chapter 6

1. e.
2. b.
3. d.
4. a. A; b. A; c. A; d. C; e. B.
5. a. B; b. B; c. A; d. A.
6. d.
7. c.
8. d.

9. b.
10. c.
11. d.
12. a.
13. e.
14. c.
15. d.
16. d.
17. a.
18. c.
19. b.
20. b.
21. c.
22. d.
23. c.
24. d.
25. a.

Chapter 7

1. b.
2. b.
3. c.
4. c.
5. c.
6. d.
7. a.
8. c.
9. a.
10. b.
11. c.
12. a.
13. c.
14. a.
15. d.
16. c.
17. b.
18. c.
19. c.
20. d.
21. c.
22. a.
23. d.
24. c.
25. c.
26. d.
27. b.
28. b.
29. c.
30. d.
31. b.
32. d.
33. c.
34. a.
35. d.
36. b.
37. b.

38. c.

39. a.

40A. b.

$$SV = [0.785 \times (LVOT_{Diameter})^2] \times LVOT_{VTI}$$

$LVOT_{Diameter} = 20\ mm = 2\ cm$

40B. b.

40C. c.

$$MVA = SV/Transmitral_{VTI} = 75\ cm^3/80\ cm = 0.94\ cm^2$$

40D. c.

41A. b.

41B. c.

$$\text{Maximum Transmitral Gradient} = 4(V_{max})^2$$

$$V_{max} = \sqrt{16/4} = 2\ m/s$$

$$= 200\ cm/s$$

$$MVA = 2\pi r^2 \times \frac{V_a}{V_{max}}$$

$$= \frac{[2\pi\ (1 cm)^2 \times 21\ cm/s]}{200\ cm}$$

41C. a.

$$SV = MVA \times Transmitral_{VTI}$$

41D. d.

42. a.

43. b.

44A. c.

$$EROA = \frac{(2\pi r^2 \times V_a)}{V_{max}}$$

$$= \frac{[2\pi\ (0.9\ cm)^2 \times 69\ cm/s]}{500\ cm/s}$$

44B. c.

$$R_{Vol} = EROA \times VTI_{Mitral\ Regurgitant\ Jet}$$

$$= 0.70\ cm^2 \times 130\ cm$$

Chapter 8

1. b.

2. c.

3. b.

4. d.

5. d.

6. c.

7. d.

8. b.

9. e.

10. e.

11. b.

12. c.

13. e.

14. e.

15. b.

16. e.

17. d

18. b.

19. b.

20. e.

21. e.

22. b.

23. b.

24. e.

25. d.

Chapter 9

1. e.
2. d.
3. d.
4. b.
5. a.
6. d.
7. d.
8. b.
9. b.
10. c.
11. a.
12. b.
13. a.
14. c.
15. c.
16. a.
17. b.
18. d.
19. d.
20. b.
21. d.
22. c.
23. b.
24. b.
25. a.
26. d.
27. b.
28. a.
29. d.
30. b.
31. a.
32. d.
33. a.
34. c.
35. d.
36. a.
37. b.
38. b.
39. d.
40. b.
41. d.
42. c.
43. a.
44. e.
45. d.

Chapter 10

1. e.
2. d.
3. d.
4. d.
5. b.
6. d.
7. a.

8. d.

9. b.

10. b.

11. c.

12. a.

13. c.

14. d.

15. e.

Chapter 11

1. a. Rocking of the support ring of a mechanical prosthesis suggests suture failure, improper implantation, or ring abscess.

2. c. The maximal opening angle depends on the anatomic position of the valve. When placed in the aortic position, the maximal angle is 75°; in the mitral position, it is designed to open to 70°.

3. a. The constant of 220 milliseconds was derived from native stenotic mitral valves. Use of this constant can overestimate the effective orifice area of a prosthetic valve.

4. b. Regurgitation occurs more frequently than stenosis. Both pathologies occur secondary to calcific degeneration of the valve leaflets, leading to restricted motion, holes, or tears.

5. c. Proper leaflet coaptation in a stentless valve requires the prosthesis to maintain its engineered shape. A dilated STJ can cause the cylindrical shape of the valve to be distorted at the distal end, resulting in failure of apposition of the leaflets during diastole. It is the ascending aorta rather than the STJ that is assessed for post-stenotic dilation.

6. d. The major advantage of tissue valves is that they usually do not require long-term anticoagulation. If the patient is already on anticoagulants for some other reason, such as a history of thrombosis or embolism, persistent atrial fibrillation, or a significantly increased left atrial size, surgeons and cardiologists often recommend the use of a mechanical valve because the major advantage of the tissue valve is nullified.

7. b. Approximately 1.6% per patient-year.

8. a. After passing through the narrowest orifice of a stenotic valve, the jet expands in area and recovers pressure energy. Catheter-derived "peak" pressures are often measured distal to the area of pressure recovery, yielding pressures lower than the actual peak.

9. b. Structural elements such as struts, stents, and occluders are positioned within the sewing ring of these valves and limit the EOA of the prosthesis.

10. a. Calcific degeneration is stiffening of tissue leaflets, usually at the base, caused by calcium deposition that can also lead to perforations, tears, and eventual failure of the prosthesis. This process occurs more slowly in stentless valves because of decreased mechanical stress and differences in leaflet preparation methods.

11. a. The rate of thrombosis of right-side valves can be as high as 20% because of a relatively low flow state.

12. b. The rate for both is approximately 0.5% per year.

13. b. No, but vegetations commonly lead to regurgitation of the valve, whereas thrombosis often leads to obstruction.

14. c. The normal mean gradient is approximately 15 mm Hg, assuming normal LV function.

15. b. In the mitral position, the normal mean gradient is approximately 4.0 mm Hg.

16. d. The gradient across an aortic homograft in an average individual is approximately 7 mm Hg.

17. e. "Washing jets" that extend farther than 2.5 cm into the left atrium are considered abnormal. An exception to this rule is the Medtronic-Hall single tilting disk valve in which the central regurgitant jet can be as long as 5 to 6 cm.

18. d. Starr-Edwards valves normally do not have any washing jets because of the tight fit between the occluder ball and the support ring.

19. e. Aortic pressure is greater than LV pressure throughout diastole; therefore, the washing jets are holodiastolic in nature.

20. d. Trace to mild regurgitant jets are seen in approximately 10% of properly functioning mitral bioprostheses. Moderate regurgitation is pathologic.

21. c. These valves are oriented such that the position of pivots is approximately where the anterolateral and posteromedial commissures were located.

22. d. Many surgeons attempt to orient the major orifice so that it directs the flow toward the greater curvature of the aortic arch.

23. e. Ring or myocardial abscesses are the most common presentations for mechanical prostheses.

24. a. Anterior portions of the valve structure are often poorly visualized because of the greater distance from the probe and artifact from the more posterior aspects of the ring.

25. d. Resistance to infection, no need for long-term anticoagulation, and a favorable hemodynamic profile (especially in smaller sizes) are the major advantages of homografts.

26. d. Pressure gradients, the continuity equation, DVI, and pressure half-time analyses are methods that can be used to grade stenosis in prosthetic valves. It should be remembered that in the assessment of mitral valves using the pressure half-time method, the constant of 220 milliseconds was derived from native stenotic mitral valves. Use of this constant with prosthetic valves can overestimate the effective orifice area.

27. a. The TEE probe is directly posterior to the left atrium and thus has an unobstructed view of the valve and any regurgitant jets without artifact interference. TEE probes are also higher in frequency (3 to 8 MHz), providing a higher-resolution image.

28. a. St. Jude valves commonly have two central convergent jets originating from the hinge points in addition to several peripheral jets from the edge of the disk occluder and the support ring. Ball-in-cage valves normally do not have "washing jets" because the occluder ball seats snugly into the support ring. All single tilting disk valves have two to three peripheral jets from the edge of the occluding disk, whereas the Medtronic-Hall valve has a narrow central jet that emanates from a hole in the occluder disk through which the hinge strut passes. Bioprosthetic valves do not have "washing jets." Approximately 10% of tissue valves will have trace to mild central regurgitation, which is considered normal.

29. c. The major orifice is generally directed toward the lateral LV wall.

30. d. Annular diameters of the aortic and pulmonic valves and diameters of the sinotubular junction and proximal ascending aorta are of interest.

31. b. The deep transgastric long-axis view provides the best alignment with transaortic flow and permits adequate imaging even in the presence of a mitral prosthesis. The transgastric long-axis view (at approximately 110°) also allows for an artifact-free view of the LVOT side of the aortic valve, but can be limited by the presence of a mitral prosthesis.

32. d. For stented prostheses, the aortic annulus diameter is measured. If a stentless valve is to be placed, the diameter of the STJ and proximal ascending aorta are also determined.

33. c. The opening angle of a St. Jude bileaflet prosthetic valve is 85°.

34. e. Pannus, thrombus, inflammatory material, and subvalvular tissue can obstruct a mechanical valve.

35. c. Calcific degeneration and a limited lifespan requiring reoperation if the patient outlives the functionality of the prosthesis are the major disadvantages. Stentless bioprostheses appear to have a slower rate of degeneration than the others.

36. b. Improved hemodynamics, increased EOA, and slower degeneration are all advantages. Neither type requires long-term anticoagulation.

37. d. Doppler-derived data provide the maximal instantaneous gradient calculated by using velocities and the modified Bernoulli equation, whereas catheter techniques measure the peak-to-peak gradient, which is not a true physiologic variable. Maximal instantaneous gradients are always greater than or equal to peak-to-peak gradients.

38. b. Homografts are harvested from human cadavers and are treated with antibiotics and decalcifying agents, and cryogenically treated or preserved before implantation. An autograft is one of the patient's own native valves that is transposed to a new location (eg, pulmonic to aortic) without treatment or preservation. The treatment and preservation processes alter the leaflet tissue resulting in calcific degeneration over time in the homograft, whereas autografts last indefinitely.

39. b. The posterior position of the TEE probe frequently allows visualization of pathology that would be missed with chest wall imaging. Higher-frequency probes allow for better resolution and penetration is dependent upon transducer frequency. Clinical correlation is required for both types of examination.

40. d. Inconsistent occluder opening and closing occurs because of low flows and leads to unacceptably high rates of thrombosis (even with adequate anticoagulation).

41. a. Prosthetic valves are more likely to have ring abscesses, conduction abnormalities, and worse prognosis because of resistance to antibiotics and more complicated and higher-risk surgery, if it is required.

42. c. Endocarditis destroys bioprosthetic valve leaflets with resulting regurgitation, whereas mechanical valves are prone to vegetations leading to obstruction and/or regurgitation. Both can have ring abscesses.

43. d. Perivalvular abscesses should be suspected with rocking motion of the valve (not heart), aortic root thickening, perivalvular lucency, or visualization of a fistula tract.

44. d. Persistent sepsis despite antibiotic treatment, new or worsening heart failure, and development of a new bundle branch block support the diagnosis of a perivalvular abscess.

45. c. Spontaneous contrast in the left atrium, progressive enlargement or thrombus in the *left* atrium or on the valve proper, decreased occluder excursion or decreased leaflet opening, thickened cusps in bioprostheses, and a "low-volume" LV are suggestive of prosthetic mitral valve occlusion.

46. d. The root inclusion technique results in a two-layer proximal ascending aorta, one from the prosthesis and one from the patient's native aorta. It is not uncommon to see a small amount of fluid between the layers.

47. e. Attenuation, reverberation, side lobes, and mirror image are some of the more common imaging artifacts with prostheses containing synthetic materials; however, almost any type of artifact is possible.

48. a. The small (23-mm) Sapien valve is preferred for annular diameters of 18 to 21 mm.

49. b. The use of RT3DTEE has been studied for its effectiveness for the evaluation of prosthetic valves. Three-dimensional matrix array TEE provides excellent visualization of all components of prosthetic mitral valves. However, due to current technological difficulties, optimal visualization of the aortic and tricuspid valves is inconsistent.

50. c. Epicardial echocardiography (EE) has been demonstrated to show high agreement and correlation with established techniques of aortic valve area assessment using the already familiar continuity equation (without correction factors). Even in patients where TEE is not contraindicated, intraoperative EE can be utilized to calculate the aortic valve area when standard TEE views are unable to provide all the information required for the calculation. Epicardial echocardiography has become an important component of advanced echocardiographic training and should be utilized when required.

Chapter 12

1. c. In patients with left ventricle systolic dysfunction an E-wave DT less than 150 milliseconds correlates with grade III diastolic dysfunction (restrictive filling pattern) characterized by elevated filling pressures and PCWP. A DT value between 150 and 220 milliseconds (choices a and e) may represent grade II diastolic dysfunction (pseudonormal pattern) with elevated filling pressures; however, this cannot be confirmed solely on the base of DT—other echocardiographic indicators are necessary.

2. b. IVRT is the interval during which LV relaxation occurs and consequently LV pressure declines until LV pressure is less than the left atrial pressure, leading to the opening of the mitral valve and to the beginning of the rapid diastolic filling.

3. b. Isolated relaxation abnormality with normal filling pressures represents grade I diastolic dysfunction (impaired relaxation) characterized by increased IVRT, decreased E-wave velocity, increased DT of the E wave, and decreased E/A ratio.

4. d. Transmitral E-wave velocity depends on left atrial pressure, left ventricular compliance, and rate of relaxation and heart rate. Left atrial contraction influences the peak velocity of the transmitral A wave.

5. d. Hypovolemia can mimic a relaxation abnormality with an increased DT even in young patients with normal cardiac function, mostly because it decreases the atrioventricular pressure gradient at the beginning of diastole. Hypertension delays the onset of relaxation by prolonging the duration of systole, resulting in impaired relaxation and increased DT. Decreased LV compliance, however, leads to rapid equalization of the pressure gradient between the left atrium and left ventricle during early filling and a reduced DT.

6. b. Mitral stenosis leads to an increase in E-wave deceleration time. Because the LV fills through the stenotic mitral valve during diastole, it takes a long time to equalize the pressures in the left atrium and the left ventricle. The other statements are true (see text for explanation).

7. e. Grade II diastolic dysfunction (pseudonormal pattern) is characterized by a lower than normal systolic filling fraction on the pulmonary venous flow Doppler profile (<50%) reflecting the high filling pressures. Impaired relaxation is also present as shown in a lower than normal LV filling propagation velocity (Vp <50 cm/s) and a lower than normal E′ velocity (E′ velocity <8 cm/s).

8. d. Severely increased LV stiffness results in a restrictive filling pattern characterized by decreased IVRT, increased E-wave velocity, decreased A-wave velocity, increased E/A ratio, and decreased E-wave DT.

9. b. The normal transmitral flow Doppler parameters in conjunction with a lower than normal E′ velocity indicated that this situation, in fact, corresponds with grade II diastolic dysfunction (pseudonormal pattern). A healthy adult would have a normal E′ velocity (>8 cm/s). Hypertrophic cardiomyopathy with normal filling pressures indicate grade I diastolic dysfunction (impaired relaxation pattern) with decreased E-wave velocity, decreased E/A ratio, and increased E-wave DT.

10. d. Septal wall ischemia and paradoxical septal wall motion result in impaired relaxation of the left ventricle. Direct compression of the left ventricle because of right ventricular dilation in an intact pericardium leads to changes in the LV compliance. Tricuspid regurgitation has no impact on LV diastolic function. However, in the long term tricuspid regurgitation can contribute to the volume overload and further dilation of the right ventricle.

11. d. Active atrial relaxation and LV systolic function are the main determinants of the systolic component of the pulmonary venous flow. Elevated LA pressure and atrial fibrillation impair atrial relaxation. LV hypertrophy does not influence the pulmonary venous flow, unless in its most severe form it leads to decreased LV compliance and increased filling pressures.

12. b. Because of the very vigorous elastic recoil of the left ventricle during relaxation, most of the filling of the left ventricle (approximately 80%) occurs in early filling with very little contribution of the atrial systole to the final end-diastolic LV volume. However, with aging there is a gradual decrease in the myocardial elastic recoil, early filling is reduced, and the contribution of atrial systole becomes more important. Atrial systole also contributes more to LV filling in grade I diastolic dysfunction when early filling is reduced as a consequence of impaired relaxation. In grade III diastolic dysfunction, atrial contraction contributes very little to the filling of the noncompliant LV.

13. a. LV end-diastolic pressure correlates well with a pulmonary venous flow AR velocity greater than 35 cm/s, AR duration greater than the transmitral A duration by 30 milliseconds, an E/E′ ratio greater than 15, and an E/Vp ratio greater than 1.5. An E/A ratio less than 0.8 is most likely to be found in grade I diastolic dysfunction with an impaired relaxation pattern and normal filling pressures.

14. d. The transmitral flow Doppler pattern in a young, healthy subject can mimic a restrictive filling pattern with an E/A ratio more than 1.5. Because of the vigorous elastic recoil, most of the ventricular filling occurs in early diastole resulting in a high E-wave velocity and a high E/A ratio. In these subjects, the rest of the parameters are normal (normal IVRT, E′ velocity greater than 8 cm/s, and propagation velocity Vp >55 cm/s).

15. e. A normal E/A ratio in a 70-year-old patient with uncontrolled hypertension most likely represents a pseudonormal pattern. Therefore, the pulmonary venous flow shows diastolic predominance reflecting the high filling pressures. IVRT is decreased due to the high LA pressure, which leads to an earlier opening of the mitral valve. E′ velocity is less than 8 cm/s due to impaired relaxation and the E/E′ ratio is greater than 10.

16. c. A young, healthy subject (as in choice c) can have a transmitral flow Doppler with an E/A ratio more than 1.5 mimicking a restrictive filling pattern in the absence of disease. Severe acute aortic insufficiency, severe mitral regurgitation, and restrictive cardiomyopathy can result in a restrictive filling pattern with an E/A ratio more than 1.5. Chronic aortic regurgitation, however, due to increased LV compliance over time has less impact on the transmitral flow, and a restrictive pattern is less likely in the absence of other concurrent cardiac pathology.

17. e. Mitral annulus tissue Doppler imaging measures high-amplitude, low-velocity signals from the myocardium with velocities less than 15 cm/s. Generally, septal velocities are lower than the lateral velocities.

18. d. Both constrictive pericarditis and restrictive cardiomyopathy show increased E-wave velocity, increased E/A ratio, and reduced E-wave DT. Patients with constrictive pericarditis have a normal Vp, while patients with restrictive cardiomyopathy will have a decreased Vp due to abnormal relaxation. Patients with constrictive pericarditis and normal systolic function have a normal E′ velocity, while patients with restrictive pericarditis have a low E′ velocity.

19. d. The ability of an E/E′ ratio greater than 15 to estimate elevated filling pressure has been validated in patients with atrial fibrillation. The same is true for an E/Vp ratio more than 1.5 and an E0wave deceleration time less than 130 milliseconds.

20. e. Atrial fibrillation can result in late systolic reversal of flow in the absence of significant mitral regurgitation. Severe mitral regurgitation can also result in reversal of the systolic component of the pulmonary venous flow. Impaired LV relaxation, tachycardia, and mitral stenosis do not result in reverse systolic flow.

21. b. Constrictive pericarditis is characterized by a restrictive filling pattern on the transmitral Doppler flow (increased E velocity, high E/A ratio, decreased DT) with normal E′ velocity and normal Vp.

22. e. Strain rate measured by TDI is less susceptible to myocardial tethering but is dependent on the angle of the Doppler beam. Lengthening of the myocardium corresponds with positive strain and shortening with negative strain. Speckle tracking is independent of the angle of the Doppler beam. Both strain rate and speckle tracking measure myocardial deformation.

23. e. Because the Valsalva maneuver decreases the preload and consequently the left atrial pressure, the pseudonormal pattern will change into a pattern of impaired relaxation (E/A ratio will decrease). In reversible restrictive filling (grade IIIa diastolic dysfunction), the Valsalva maneuver may change the pattern to a pseudonormal or even impaired relaxation pattern (E/A ratio will decrease). In a healthy subject, the Valsalva maneuver will decrease both E and A velocities and the E/A ratio will remain unchanged.

24. d. Mitral stenosis results in increased transmitral flow velocities, increased E-wave DT, and fusion of the E and A waves. Increased LA pressure and increased LA stiffness result in systolic blunting on the pulmonary vein flow Doppler profile. E′ may not be accurate in mitral stenosis due to increased stiffness of the mitral annulus. E/E′ ratio does not reflect left ventricular end-diastolic pressure.

25. c. TDI usually interrogates longitudinal fibers, their motion being aligned with the Doppler beam. Fibrotic myocardium may have a normal velocity due to tethering to adjacent segments with normal motion. TDI is not dependent on a high-quality 2D image, but is dependent on the angle of the Doppler beam with respect to the tissue motion.

26. a. The administration of diuretics as well as hypovolemia may mimic a relaxation abnormality in healthy subjects.

27. c. S_1 wave depends on LA relaxation. S_2 wave depends on RV function, LV contraction, LA compliance, and presence of mitral regurgitation. D wave depends on the rate of LV relaxation. AR wave depends on the contractility of the LA as well as compliance of the LA, LV, and pulmonary venous bed.

28. a. The transmitral flow Doppler profile can mimic a restrictive pattern in healthy young individuals with strong elastic recoil. With aging there is a gradual decrease in the myocardial rate of relaxation resulting in an increase in IVRT, decline in the E-wave velocity, decrease in the E/A ratio, and increase in the E-wave DT.

29. e. The initial abnormality of diastolic dysfunction is impaired ventricular relaxation. As the disease progresses, a decrease in LV compliance will follow. LV compliance is dependent on many factors including ventricular interdependence and ventricular stiffness.

30. b. In this young patient with grade II diastolic dysfunction (normal E/A ratio, normal DT, S/D<1), hypovolemia will mimic an impaired relaxation pattern (decreased E/A ratio, prolonged DT).

31. d. This patient most likely has grade II diastolic dysfunction (pseudonormal pattern) with normal values of the transmitral flow parameters and low E′ velocity. A decrease in preload with nitroglycerin infusion will unmask the relaxation abnormality and change the pattern to an impaired relaxation pattern.

32. b. IVRT is decreased in grade III diastolic dysfunction (restrictive filling pattern) due to increased left atrial pressure, which leads to earlier opening of the mitral valve.

33. a. Severe aortic regurgitation results in a restrictive transmitral flow pattern (increased E-wave velocity, decreased A-wave velocity, and decreased E-wave DT) due to rapid increase in the LV pressure. E-wave DT is increased in mitral stenosis, elderly individuals, and in an impaired relaxation pattern.

34. c. Tissue Doppler imaging measures intramyocardial velocities using a pulsed-wave Doppler technique. TDI has a high temporal resolution and it mostly evaluates the axial motion of the LV.

35. c. In atrial fibrillation the systolic component of the pulmonary venous flow will be decreased despite normal filling pressures because atrial relaxation is absent. E-wave velocity by itself does not correlate with filling pressures, and because of the absence of organized atrial contraction the E/A ratio cannot be calculated. Less beat-to-beat variability in mitral inflow parameters has been associated with increased filling pressures.

36. b. The "normal" transmitral flow in this patient with aortic stenosis undergoing aortic valve replacement is most likely grade II diastolic dysfunction with a "pseudonormal" transmitral flow. A decrease in preload (blood loss, nitroglycerin infusion, Valsalva maneuver) will decrease only the E-wave velocity (which is dependent on the pressure gradient between the left atrium and the left ventricle at the beginning of diastole) resulting in a decreased E/A ratio similar to an impaired relaxation pattern.

37. e. In young, healthy subjects, due to the strong elastic recoil in early diastole and because the LA behaves more as a "passive" conduit during early diastole, predominant forward flow occurs in diastole resulting in a blunted systolic component, while in older age adults, forward flow occurs largely in systole. In healthy individuals AR duration is equal or less than the transmitral A duration. In grade I diastolic dysfunction, the pulmonary vein flow D wave correlates well with the mitral E wave; therefore, it will be diminished when compared with the systolic component.

38. e. Increased left atrial pressures in patients with impaired relaxation will restore the normal pressure gradient between the left atrium and left ventricle and will lead to a "pseudonormalization" of the dynamics of left ventricular filling during diastole.

39. e. Both E and E′ velocity are increased in patients with severe mitral regurgitation and normal left ventricular ejection fraction and the E/E′ ratio does not accurately estimate filling pressures in these patients.

40. b. An E/E′ ratio more than 15 is highly sensitive for increased LV filling pressures. An E/A ratio less than 0.8 corresponds to an impaired relaxation pattern (grade I diastolic dysfunction), which is characterized by normal LV filling pressures. E/E′ ratio cannot be used to estimate filling pressures in constrictive pericarditis and mitral stenosis.

41. c. Impaired relaxation leads to a reduction in peak –dP/dt and prolongation of the isovolumic relaxation time and of the time constant of relaxation. Isovolumic relaxation time depends on the timing of aortic valve closure and mitral valve opening.

42. d. Compliance is the ratio of change in volume to unit change in pressure. Stiffness is the ratio of change in pressure to unit change in volume. Compliance affects mostly late diastole while relaxation predominates in early diastole. Active relaxation begins in the second half of the systolic ejection. An increase in afterload will delay myocardial relaxation especially when combined with elevated preload.

43. b. In healthy subjects, E′ occurs before transmitral E wave, reflecting myocardial relaxation before the beginning of flow across the mitral valve. In diastolic dysfunction, TE-E′ is prolonged (see text for details). In constrictive pericarditis, septal E′ may be greater than lateral E′, reflecting the preserved longitudinal expansion of the LV while the lateral and anteroposterior excursions are limited by the pericardial disease. In healthy subjects, E′ velocity is preload dependent.

44. b. Retrograde flow occurs in the hepatic veins at the end of systole (V wave) and at the end of diastole (AR wave). S wave represents antegrade flow at the beginning of systole and it is dependent on right atrium relaxation. Decreased RV compliance is associated with diastolic predominance of the hepatic venous flow.

45. d. Although administration of diuretics may mimic impaired relaxation in young, healthy subjects, it does not lead to diastolic dysfunction. In patients with restrictive filling the administration of diuretics can have a beneficial effect by reducing the intravascular volume and moving the left ventricle to a more favorable position on its end-diastolic pressure-volume curve.

46. e. The modulus of chamber stiffness reflects the relation between ventricular chamber stiffness and pressure. It is proportional to ventricular stiffness and independent of ventricular chamber geometry. Chamber stiffness is not constant, but increases throughout ventricular filling.

47. e. During spontaneous inspiration the intrathoracic pressure will decrease, resulting in increased venous return and increased right ventricular filing. The increased right ventricular filling will lead to increased transtricuspid E-wave velocity.

48. d. Tachycardia does not influence E′ velocity. The rest of the changes could occur with tachycardia (see text for details).

49. d. In the elderly, in the absence of cardiac disease, predominant flow from the pulmonary veins into the left atrium occurs in systole; therefore, the pulmonary venous S wave is greater than the pulmonary venous D wave.

50. e. Placing the patient in steep Trendelenburg will cause an increase in preload, which will most likely increase the pressure gradient between the left atrium and the left ventricle at the beginning of diastole, resulting in a decreased IVRT, increased E wave velocity and decreased E wave DT ("pseudonormalization" of the transmitral flow Doppler pattern).

Chapter 13

1. c.

2. d.

3. d.

4. c.

5. d.

6. c.

7. d.

8. d.

9. d.

10. c.

11. d.

12. b.

13. a.

14. a.

15. d.

16. a.

17. b.

Chapter 14

1. a.

2. a.

3. c.

4. b.

5. b.

6. a.

7. d.

8. c.

9. a.

10. b.

11. c.

12. b.

13. c.

14. c.

15. a.

16. a.

17. d.

18. d.

19. c.

20. c.

21. a.

22. d.

23. b.

24. a.

25. e.

26. b.
27. c.
28. e.
29. d.
30. d.
31. b.
32. a.
33. c.
34. a.
35. d.
36. c.
37. d.
38. c.
39. c.
40. a.
41. e.
42. d.
43. d.
44. a.
45. b.
46. c.
47. b.
48. b.
49. d.
50. b.
51. a.
52. d.
53. c.
54. c.
55. d.
56. a.
57. d.
58. e.

Chapter 15

1. a.
2. b.
3. b.
4. a.
5. e.
6. b.
7. b.
8. a.
9. b.
10. a.
11. a.
12. b.
13. e.
14. a.
15. c.
16. b.
17. c.
18. e.
19. b.
20. a.
21. b.
22. d.

23. b.
24. b.
25. c.
26. b.
27. e.
28. d.
29. a.
30. e.
31. d.
32. b.
33. a.
34. e.
35. b.
36. a.
37. d.
38. a.
39. a.
40. e.
41. b.
42. a.
43. b.
44. b.
45. e.
46. d.
47. b.
48. a.
49. b.

Chapter 16

1. c.
2. b.
3. b.
4. d.
5. d.
6. c.
7. a.
8. c.
9. a.
10. d.
11. a.
12. c.
13. b.
14. d.
15. a.
16. c.
17. a.
18. c.
19. d.
20. a.
21. a.
22. a.
23. c.
24. a.
25. d.
26. b.
27. b.

28. d.
29. d.
30. c.
31. a.
32. c.
33. c.
34. d.
35. c.
36. c.
37. b.
38. c.
39. d.
40. a.

Chapter 17

1. c.
2. d.
3. c.
4. c.
5. d.
6. a.
7. c.
8. d.
9. c.
10. d.
11. d.
12. b.
13. d.
14. a.
15. a.
16. d.
17. b.
18. c.
19. b.
20. c.
21. d.
22. b.
23. c.
24. a.
25. a.
26. c.
27. a.
28. c.
29. c.
30. d.
31. d.
32. a.
33. c.
34. c.
35. a.

Chapter 18

1. c.
2. a.
3. d.
4. b.
5. c.
6. c.

7. b.
8. c.
9. c.
10. b.
11. c.
12. b.
13. b.
14. a.
15. d.
16. c.
17. c.
18. c.
19. c.
20. c.
21. b.
22. a.
23. c.
24. b.
25. a.
26. a.
27. c.
28. b.
29. b.
30. a.
31. c.
32. b.
33. c.
34. c.
35. c.
36. b.
37. d.
38. b.
39. d.
40. d.
41. b.
42. c.
43. d.
44. c.
45. c.
46. a.
47. b.
48. d.
49. d.
50. b.
51. d.
52. a.
53. c.
54. a.
55. c.
56. a.
57. d.
58. d.
59. d.
60. b.
61. c.
62. a.

63. d.

64. c.

65. d.

66. a.

67. d.

68. d.

69. a.

70. e.

Chapter 19

1. b.

2. a.

3. e.

4. e.

5. d.

6. d.

7. a.

8. d.

9. c.

10. c.

11. a.

12. d.

13. d.

14. e.

15. a.

16. d.

17. d.

18. a.

19. c.

20. a.

21. e.

22. a.

23. d.

24. e.

25. c.

26. d.

27. d.

28. a.

29. a.

30. e.

31. d.

32. a.

33. b.

34. c.

35. e.

36. c.

37. a.

38. c.

39. b.

40. b.

41. a.

42. a.

43. b.

44. a.

45. d.

46. d.

47. e.

48. b.
49. b.
50. a.
51. b.
52. c.
53. a.
54. d.
55. d.
56. b.
57. c.
58. e.
59. d.
60. b.
61. d.
62. b.
63. d.
64. a.
65. d.
66. e.
67. b.
68. d.
69. e.
70. c.
71. c.

Chapter 21

1. e.
2. b.
3. d.
4. a.
5. b.
6. a.
7. d.
8. c.
9. b.
10. a.
11. a.
12. d.
13. e.
14. a.
15. c.
16. e.

Chapter 22

1. b.
2. c.
3. c.
4. a.
5. d.
6. d.
7. c.
8. b.
9. a.
10. d.
11. d.
12. b.
13. c.
14. c.

15. d.

16. a.

17. a.

18. c.

19. d.

20. d.

Chapter 23

1. d.

2. b.

3. d.

4. c.

5. c.

6. c.

7. d.

8. b.

9. c.

10. d.

11. d. Currently, the American Society of Echocardiography does not exclude any specific medical specialty's physicians from attempting the credentialing exam provided the training curriculum has been completed. No well-defined indications for TEE currently exist in the ED; rather, the list of indications is continually being expanded. Though it has been proposed, TEE is not yet incorporated into ACLS or ATLS protocols.

12. c. The study by Varriale and Maldonado suggested that, on average, adequate windows could not be obtained in up to 20% of patients.

13. b. It is precisely the ability to differentiate among these three pathologies that illustrates the ability to impact patient care decisions including ceasing resuscitative efforts when cardiac standstill is evident after a prolonged period.

14. a. It is difficult to obtain adequate views of the left pulmonary artery owing to interference from the left main bronchus

15. b. The Stanford classification classifies ascending aortic aneurysms as type A and descending as type B which are typically managed surgically and medically respectively.

16. a. A failure to consider an aortic injury due to deceleration forces in a patient with multiple limb fractures and a head injury could prove catastrophic.

17. d. TEE is relatively low cost, but it is unclear if it is less expensive than other modalities when training and acquisition costs are considered. TEE does require informed consent, except in extreme emergency situations where consent is not readily available. Although the sensitivity and specificity of other modalities may be better than TEE, TEE is the most portable of the available options which may be the sole determining factor for an unstable patient when transfer to the radiology suite is not prudent.

18. d.

19. c. For patients on the ventilator, a number of maneuvers can help with successful probe placement including temporary deflation of the endotracheal tube cuff, removal of the nasogastric tube after aspiration of stomach contents, employing a jaw thrust, application of paralytics, and by attempting placement under direct laryngoscopy.

20. b. The vast number of patients in the ED experiencing hemodynamic instability of unknown etiology suggests a burgeoning area of growth for TEE use in the ED.

21. True.

22. False. The main aortic branches may be assessed, too. TEE may miss aortic pathology in the aortic arch.

23. False. The most vulnerable part is the isthmus.

24. False. If aortic disruption is present, it is critical to identify expediently since active resuscitation consistent with ACLS protocols may result in a "goal" blood pressure (e.g. 90-100mmHg) much higher than that which would be considered optimal for aortic ruptures when one aims for a reduction shear forces and a systolic blood pressure of ~ 80 mmHg (i.e. "controlled hypotension").

25. True.

26. True. Pulses may not be palpable for a number of reasons including low stroke volume, peripheral vascular disease, distorted anatomy and operator (assessor) error.

27. True. A patient seemingly in PEA could be found to be in another rhythm (such as fine ventricular fibrillation) mandating a change to another ACLS/ATLS algorithm.

28. False. This is precisely the patient in whom TEE may provide benefit in the form of a management change, but could be performed simultaneously to, and without the need for interruption of, active chest compressions.

29. True. Inpatients are typically kept NPO for at least 8 hours prior to elective TEE performance, thus evacuation of gastric contents should be performed whenever possible prior to performance in the ED where details of last meal may be unknown or may suggest an inadequate fasting interval.

30. False. Although relatively low-risk, the TEE procedure has several potential complications including esophageal injury and/or rupture, respiratory compromise, and oropharyngeal trauma.

31. True. Likewise, other esophageal pathology such as rings, webs, and suspected perforation should also be viewed as, at minimum, relative contraindications.

32. False. Even in unconscious trauma patients, topical anesthesia should be employed in an effort to blunt reflex activity thus minimizing the degree or incidence of emesis, forceful gag like movements, and bradycardia.

33. True. False positives and negatives do occur, however, most notably due to operator (interpretative) error and occasionally when the dissection is located in the extreme aspect of the ascending aorta, the putative "TEE blind spot".

34. False. While TTE is often the first line echocardiographic technique employed in the ED, TEE can be considered to be the first line echocardiographic imaging technique in patients undergoing active chest compressions or for those in whom cardiac windows may be inadequate owing to high BMI, other body habitus characteristic or deformity, or the presence of various medical devices and resuscitation paraphernalia on the chest wall.

35. False. Historically, benzocaine spray was used in the ED for topical anesthesia. However, aerosolized lidocaine is now preferred owing to the theoretical possibility of developing methemoglobinemia.

36. mid-esophageal four chamber view

37. organized

38. 20 %

39. ascending

40. deceleration

41. 5 %

42. margination

43. blood flow

44. hypovolemia.

45. aspiration

46. c.

47. a.

48. d.

49. e.

50. b.

Chapter 24

1. d.

2. a.

3. b.

4. b.

5. c.

6. d.

7. d.

8. d.

9. c.

10. b.
11. b.
12. d.
13. c.
14. d.
15. d.
16. c.
17. d.
18. b.
19. a.
20. b.
21. b.
22. d.
23. d.
24. c.
25. a.

Index

Page numbers followed by *f* or *t* indicate figures or tables, respectively.

M